1 MONTH OF
FREE
READING

at

www.ForgottenBooks.com

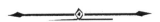

By purchasing this book you are eligible for one month membership to ForgottenBooks.com, giving you unlimited access to our entire collection of over 1,000,000 titles via our web site and mobile apps.

To claim your free month visit:

www.forgottenbooks.com/free889133

ISBN 978-0-266-78612-2
PIBN 10889133

This book is a reproduction of an important historical work. Forgotten Books uses
state-of-the-art technology to digitally reconstruct the work, preserving the original format
whilst repairing imperfections present in the aged copy. In rare cases, an imperfection in
the original, such as a blemish or missing page, may be replicated in our edition. We do,
however, repair the vast majority of imperfections successfully; any imperfections that
remain are intentionally left to preserve the state of such historical works.

THE

LONDON MEDICAL GAZETTE,

BEING A

WEEKLY JOURNAL

OF

Medicine and the Collateral Sciences.

FRIDAY, MARCH 31, 1843.

LECTURES

ON THE

THEORY AND PRACTICE OF MIDWIFERY,

Delivered in the Theatre of St. George's Hospital,

BY ROBERT LEE, M.D. F.R.S.

LECTURE XXI.

On the Symptoms and Treatment of Natural Labours.

WHEN the foetus has completed the period of its existence in the uterus, it can live no longer in the same condition, and the great nervous and muscular structures of the organ, which have lain dormant during pregnancy, are suddenly roused into action in consequence of the stimulus imparted to them by the mature foetus, and the whole contents of the uterus are expelled. This process, which is always attended with pain and danger, is called *labour*, *delivery*, or *parturition;* all the varieties and complications of which have been arranged by Smellie and Denman in a regular systematic manner, under the four following heads:—

1. *Natural labour*, in which the head of the foetus presents or comes first; and the delivery is accomplished in twenty-four hours, by the natural contractions of the uterus and the assistance commonly given.

2. *Lingering, tedious, protracted*, and *difficult labour*, in which the head of the foetus likewise presents, but the labour continues upwards of twenty-four hours, and some unusual assistance is required. Irregular uterine action, nervous exhaustion, rigidity of the parts, cicatrices of the vagina, tumors of various kinds within the pelvis, and distortion of the pelvis, and unfavourable position, or unusual size of the foetal head, are the most common causes of the difficulty experienced in the cases referred to in this class, and which terminate either without manual or instrumental assistance after unusual suffering, or by the employment of the forceps or perforator.

3. *Preternatural labour*, where the nates, the inferior or superior extremities, present; or the umbilical cord is prolapsed; or there is a plurality of children.

4. *Complicated labour*, in which some dangerous accident occurs, unconnected with the presentation of the foetus: as uterine hæmorrhage, retention of the placenta, inversion or rupture of the uterus, puerperal convulsions.

This classification of labours is both natural and artificial; and for all practical purposes it is the best which has yet been proposed.

1. *Of the Symptoms and Treatment of Natural Labour.*

In natural labour the head of the foetus presents, and the delivery is generally completed in twenty-four hours, and no artificial assistance is required. In every case the os uteri, vagina and external parts, are dilated, the membranes ruptured, the child expelled, and the placenta and membranes separated and forced from the uterus. The dilatation of the os uteri, rupture of the membranes, and escape of the liquor amnii, take place in the first stage of labour. When the os uteri is fully dilated, and the head has passed through the os uteri, the first stage of labour is completed. The entire expulsion of the head, trunk, and extremities of the child, is effected in the second stage of labour; and in the third stage the placenta and membranes are detached from the inner surface of the uterus, and completely expelled both from the uterus and vagina. In the greater number of cases, before the first stage of labour has been fully completed, the second has commenced and made some progress; and it is not unusual for the head

B

THE

London

MEDICAL GAZETTE;

BEING A

Weekly Journal

OF

MEDICINE AND THE COLLATERAL SCIENCES.

NEW SERIES.

VOL. II.

FOR THE SESSION 1842—43.

LONDON:

PRINTED FOR LONGMAN, BROWN, GREEN, & LONGMANS,
PATERNOSTER-ROW.

1843.

THE

LONDON MEDICAL GAZETTE,

BEING A

WEEKLY JOURNAL

OF

Medicine and the Collateral Sciences.

FRIDAY, MARCH 31, 1843.

LECTURES

ON THE

THEORY AND PRACTICE OF MIDWIFERY,

Delivered in the Theatre of St. George's Hospital,

BY ROBERT LEE, M.D. F.R.S.

LECTURE XXI.

On the Symptoms and Treatment of Natural Labours.

WHEN the foetus has completed the period of its existence in the uterus, it can live no longer in the same condition, and the great nervous and muscular structures of the organ, which have lain dormant during pregnancy, are suddenly roused into action in consequence of the stimulus imparted to them by the mature foetus, and the whole contents of the uterus are expelled. This process, which is always attended with pain and danger, is called *labour*, *delivery*, or *parturition;* all the varieties and complications of which have been arranged by Smellie and Denman in a regular systematic manner, under the four following heads:—

1. *Natural labour*, in which the head of the foetus presents or comes first; and the delivery is accomplished in twenty-four hours, by the natural contractions of the uterus and the assistance commonly given.

2. *Lingering, tedious, protracted,* and *difficult labour*, in which the head of the foetus likewise presents, but the labour continues upwards of twenty-four hours, and some unusual assistance is required. Irregular uterine action, nervous exhaustion, rigidity of the parts, cicatrices of the vagina, tumors of various kinds within the pelvis, and distortion of the pelvis, and unfavourable position, or unusual size of the foetal head, are the most common causes of

the difficulty experienced in the cases referred to this class, and which terminate either without manual or instrumental assistance after unusual suffering, or by the employment of the forceps or perforator.

3. *Preternatural labour*, where the nates, the inferior or superior extremities, present; or the umbilical cord is prolapsed; or there is a plurality of children.

4. *Complicated labour*, in which some dangerous accident occurs, unconnected with the presentation of the foetus: as uterine hæmorrhage, retention of the placenta, inversion or rupture of the uterus, puerperal convulsions.

This classification of labours is both natural and artificial; and for all practical purposes it is the best which has yet been proposed.

1. *Of the Symptoms and Treatment of Natural Labour.*

In natural labour the head of the foetus presents, and the delivery is generally completed in twenty-four hours, and no artificial assistance is required. In every case the os uteri, vagina, and external parts, are dilated, the membranes ruptured, the child expelled, and the placenta and membranes separated and forced from the uterus. The dilatation of the os uteri, rupture of the membranes, and escape of the liquor amnii, take place in the first stage of labour. When the os uteri is fully dilated, and the head has passed through the os uteri, the first stage of labour is completed. The entire expulsion of the head, trunk, and extremities of the child, is effected in the second stage of labour; and in the third stage the placenta and membranes are detached from the inner surface of the uterus, and completely expelled both from the uterus and vagina. In the greater number of cases, before the first stage of labour has been fully completed the second has commenced and made some progress; and it is not unusual for the head

B

to descend through the brim and cavity to the outlet of the pelvis, and begin to press upon the external parts, before the complete dilatation of the os uteri has been effected.

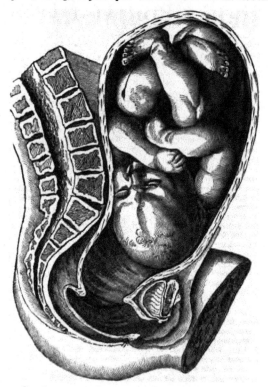

Fig. 1 represents the progress of the first stage of labour.

For several days before labour supervenes there are often certain symptoms observed which have been called the precursory or premonitory symptoms of labour. The first and most striking of these is a subsidence or sinking down of the uterus. The epigastric region, in consequence of this, becomes less distended, respiration is performed with greater ease, and the patient feels herself more comfortable, and more disposed and able to exert herself than she had been for some time before. This sinking down of the uterus is not from a mechanical cause, but from relaxation of the parts, and is often observed in the lower animals before parturition.

A sensation of weight in the inferior part of the pelvis and in the region of the uterus, and irritation of the bladder and rectum, often accompany this subsidence of the uterus. Not only do the parts become soft ... d, but in some women, before any pains of labour are experienced, there is a mucous discharge from the vagina tinged with blood, arising from the dilatation of the orifice of the uterus, and the separation of the membranes. Some women suffer for a week or more before labour begins from sleeplessness at night, irregular pains about the uterus, and a peculiar nervous irritability. Some have at the first a sharp pain or uterine contraction, in a few hours another, and a few more after long intervals ; whilst in others without pains the membranes are ruptured, and the liquor amnii escapes. These pains are sometimes experienced fifteen or twenty hours before the commencement of regular uterine action. They are then slight, produce little effect upon the constitution, and come at intervals of a quarter or half an hour, the intervals gradually becoming shorter, and the uterine contractions stronger. During these periodical pains the os uteri is opened, and its margin becomes tense and stretched, and a slight degree of pressure is felt on the extremity of the finger, if an examination be made. As soon as the pain or uterine contraction subsides, this state of tension or stretching of the lips of the orifice of the uterus ceases, and the orifice itself again closes. The membranes are put upon the stretch also during the pains; but at first they do not protrude through the orifice. Gradually these pains, which are often called cutting or grinding, become more and more severe, continue longer, recur at shorter intervals, and leave a certain degree of uneasiness when they are absent; and each pain is sometimes preceded by a slight tremor or shivering; and sickness, vomiting, restlessness, impatience, and despondency, are often present during the whole of the first stage of labour. The action of the heart and arteries becomes increased, the skin hot, and the countenance flushed. The tone of the voice is peculiar in the first stage of labour. As the dilatation of the os uteri advances, the membranes enter into it during each pain, and its margin becomes softer and thinner, and the head of the child at the same time usually passes down through the brim, and occupies a considerable portion of the cavity of the pelvis. The os uteri becomes at last wholly effaced, and the head of the infant passes through it into the vagina. In most cases the membranes are now ruptured, if they have not previously given way, and the liquor amnii escapes. At other times the membranes are not only pressed into the vagina, but through its orifice upon the external parts, which they assist in dilating. After the rupture of the membranes a short interval of freedom from pain often ensues, and then they become much more acute and severe, and are accompanied with a strong desire to bear down. But there is often great irregularity in the strength, duration, and intervals of the pains. In some women, without any apparent cause, they disappear altogether for a considerable time, and several hours of sleep will follow. Even between the strong expelling pains in the second stage of labour some go to sleep, and the pains are absent for a considerable period. The duration of the first stage of labour varies very much in different cases. In some it is completed by a few pains; in others many hours of severe suffering is required to effect the expulsion of the head through the os uteri. The dilatation usually goes on much more slowly in first than in subsequent labours, and in persons advanced in life than in those who are under thirty years of age. This difference depends fully as much on the condition of the os uteri as on the strength of the uterine contractions. In some it is thin, soft, and dilatable at the commencement of labour; in others thick, rigid, high up, and inclined backward or laterally.

In the second stage of labour the same phenomena are observed as in the first, but in a much more striking degree. The uterine contractions are much more violent, the patient fills the chest with air, closes the glottis to prevent its escape, involuntarily grasps any object near her, and forcibly bears down. The greater part of the head of the child is now in the cavity of the pelvis, and it is forced upon the perineum during each pain. The head most frequently lies obliquely or diagonally in the pelvis, with the occiput directed to the left acetabulum, and the forehead to the right sacro-iliac symphysis, the vertex being the most dependent part. When the membranes are ruptured, the pressure upon the head, during the pain, causes the integuments to become wrinkled, the parietal bones overlap one another, and, if the external parts are rigid and the labour is protracted, a tumor is formed under the scalp from blood being effused into the loose cellular membrane between the bones and integuments. At each succeeding pain the head presses against the parts at the outlet of the pelvis, and pushes them before it. The parts are gradually dilated, and, the head turning slightly round, the occiput is forced out between the labia. The perineum is carried forward by the pressure of the head, and becomes thin and distended. When the pain subsides the head recedes, and, the distension of the perineum being removed, the external parts resume their natural appearances. On the return of pain the head is forced still lower down, the perineum is again put upon the stretch, and to a still greater degree. The anus projects, dilates, and the contents of the rectum escape. The sufferings endured at this period are usually most intense, and the patient expresses the acuteness of her pangs by loud cries, sufficient, sometimes, to make the ears ring, or by deep, stifled, or suppressed groans. If we may judge from appearances, the suffering endured in some cases of labour is equal to what is experienced by those individuals who undergo severe surgical operations, or have the most violent cramps in muscular parts. In other cases the pain endured is trifling, and of such short duration that it is soon forgotten. At last, the head of the child, greatly compressed and swollen if it is a first labour, and there is much resistance at the outlet of the pelvis, is partially forced through the external parts, and does not recede when the pains go off. There is then usually in no long time a succession of strong expelling pain experienced, accompanied with involuntary efforts to bear down, by which the perineum is stretched to the greatest degree; at last it slides back o----

THE

LONDON MEDICAL GAZETTE,

BEING A

WEEKLY JOURNAL

OF

Medicine and the Collateral Sciences.

FRIDAY, MARCH 31, 1843.

LECTURES

ON THE

THEORY AND PRACTICE OF MIDWIFERY,

Delivered in the Theatre of St. George's Hospital,

By ROBERT LEE, M.D. F.R.S.

LECTURE XXI.

On the Symptoms and Treatment of Natural Labours.

WHEN the fœtus has completed the period of its existence in the uterus, it can live no longer in the same condition, and the great nervous and muscular structures of the organ, which have lain dormant during pregnancy, are suddenly roused into action in consequence of the stimulus imparted to them by the mature fœtus, and the whole contents of the uterus are expelled. This process, which is always attended with pain and danger, is called *labour, delivery,* or *parturition;* all the varieties and complications of which have been arranged by Smellie and Denman in a regular systematic manner, under the four following heads:—

1. *Natural labour,* in which the head of the fœtus presents or comes first; and the delivery is accomplished in twenty-four hours, by the natural contractions of the uterus and the assistance commonly given.

2. *Lingering, tedious, protracted,* and *difficult labour,* in which the head of the fœtus likewise presents, but the labour continues upwards of twenty-four hours, and some unusual assistance is required. Irregular uterine action, nervous exhaustion, rigidity of the parts, cicatrices of the vagina, tumors of various kinds within the pelvis, and distortion of the pelvis, and unfavourable position, or unusual size of the fœtal head, are the most common causes of the difficulty experienced in the cases referred to this class, and which terminate either without manual or instrumental assistance after unusual suffering, or by the employment of the forceps or perforator.

3. *Preternatural labour,* where the nates, the inferior or superior extremities, present; or the umbilical cord is prolapsed; or there is a plurality of children.

4. *Complicated labour,* in which some dangerous accident occurs, unconnected with the presentation of the fœtus: as uterine hæmorrhage, retention of the placenta, inversion or rupture of the uterus, puerperal convulsions.

This classification of labours is both natural and artificial; and for all practical purposes it is the best which has yet been proposed.

1. Of the Symptoms and Treatment of Natural Labour.

In natural labour the head of the fœtus presents, and the delivery is generally completed in twenty-four hours, and no artificial assistance is required. In every case the os uteri, vagina, and external parts, are dilated, the membranes ruptured, the child expelled, and the placenta and membranes separated and forced from the uterus. The dilatation of the os uteri, rupture of the membranes, and escape of the liquor amnii, take place in the first stage of labour. When the os uteri is fully dilated, and the head has passed through the os uteri, the first stage of labour is completed. The entire expulsion of the head, trunk, and extremities of the child, is effected in the second stage of labour; and in the third stage the placenta and membranes are detached from the inner surface of the uterus, and completely expelled both from the uterus and vagina. In the greater number of cases, before the first stage of labour has been fully completed the second has commenced and made some progress; and it is not unusual for the head

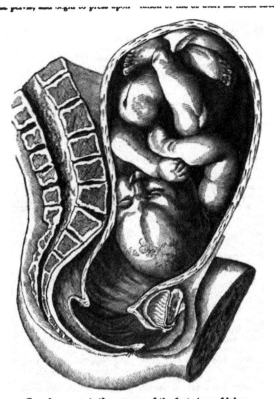

Fig. 1 *represents the progress of the first stage of labour.*

For several days before labour supervenes there are often certain symptoms observed which have been called the precursory or premonitory symptoms of labour.
The first and most striking of these is a
subsidence or sinking down of the uterus.
The epigastric region, in consequence of
this, becomes less distended, respiration is
performed with greater ease, and the patient
feels herself more comfortable, and more
disposed and able to exert herself than she
had been for some time before. This sinking down of the uterus is not from a mechanical cause, but from relaxation of the parts,
and is often observed in the lower animals
before parturition.

A sensation of weight in the inferior part
of the pelvis and in the region of the uterus, and irritation of the bladder and rectum, often accompany this subsidence of the
uterus. Not only do the parts become soft
and relaxed, but in some women, before any

pains of labour are experienced, there is a
mucous discharge from the vagina tinged
with blood, arising from the dilatation of
the orifice of the uterus, and the separation
of the membranes. Some women suffer for
a week or more before labour begins from
sleeplessness at night, irregular pains about
the uterus, and a peculiar nervous irritability. Some have at the first a sharp pain or
uterine contraction, in a few hours another,
and a few more after long intervals; whilst
in others without pains the membranes are
ruptured, and the liquor amnii escapes.
These pains are sometimes experienced fifteen or twenty hours before the commencement of regular uterine action. They are
then slight, produce little effect upon the
constitution, and come at intervals of a
quarter or half an hour, the intervals gradually becoming shorter, and the uterine contractions stronger. During these periodical
pains the os uteri is opened, and its margin

becomes tense and stretched, and a slight degree of pressure is felt on the extremity of the finger, if an examination be made. As soon as the pain or uterine contraction subsides, this state of tension or stretching of the lips of the orifice of the uterus ceases, and the orifice itself again closes. The membranes are put upon the stretch also during the pains; but at first they do not protrude through the orifice. Gradually these pains, which are often called cutting or grinding, become more and more severe, continue longer, recur at shorter intervals, and leave a certain degree of uneasiness when they are absent; and each pain is sometimes preceded by a slight tremor or shivering; and sickness, vomiting, restlessness, impatience, and despondency, are often present during the whole of the first stage of labour. The action of the heart and arteries becomes increased, the skin hot, and the countenance flushed. The tone of the voice is peculiar in the first stage of labour. As the dilatation of the os uteri advances, the membranes enter into it during each pain, and its margin becomes softer and thinner, and the head of the child at the same time usually passes down through the brim, and occupies a considerable portion of the cavity of the pelvis. The os uteri becomes at last wholly effaced, and the head of the infant passes through it into the vagina. In most cases the membranes are now ruptured, if they have not previously given way, and the liquor amnii escapes. At other times the membranes are not only pressed into the vagina, but through its orifice upon the external parts, which they assist in dilating. After the rupture of the membranes a short interval of freedom from pain often ensues, and then they become much more acute and severe, and are accompanied with a strong desire to bear down. But there is often great irregularity in the strength, duration, and intervals of the pains. In some women, without any apparent cause, they disappear altogether for a considerable time, and several hours of sleep will follow. Even between the strong expelling pains in the second stage of labour some go to sleep, and the pains are absent for a considerable period. The duration of the first stage of labour varies very much in different cases. In some it is completed by a few pains; in others many hours of severe suffering is required to effect the expulsion of the head through the os uteri. The dilatation usually goes on much more slowly in first than in subsequent labours, and in persons advanced in life than in those who are under thirty years of age. This difference depends fully as much on the condition of the os uteri as on the strength of the uterine contractions. In some it is thin, so't, and dilatable at the commence-

ment of labour; in others thick, rigid, high up, and inclined backward or laterally.

In the second stage of labour the same phenomena are observed as in the first, but in a much more striking degree. The uterine contractions are much more violent, the patient fills the chest with air, closes the glottis to prevent its escape, involuntarily grasps any object near her, and forcibly bears down. The greater part of the head of the child is now in the cavity of the pelvis, and it is forced upon the perineum during each pain. The head most frequently lies obliquely or diagonally in the pelvis, with the occiput directed to the left acetabulum, and the forehead to the right sacro-iliac symphysis, the vertex being the most dependent part. When the membranes are ruptured, the pressure upon the head, during the pain, causes the integuments to become wrinkled, the parietal bones overlap one another, and, if the external parts are rigid and the labour is protracted, a tumor is formed under the scalp from blood being effused into the loose cellular membrane between the bones and integuments. At each succeeding pain the head presses against the parts at the outlet of the pelvis, and pushes them before it. The parts are gradually dilated, and, the head turning slightly round, the occiput is forced out between the labia. The perineum is carried forward by the pressure of the head, and becomes thin and distended. When the pain subsides the head recedes, and, the distension of the perineum being removed, the external parts resume their natural appearances. On the return of pain the head is forced still lower down, the perineum is again put upon the stretch, and to a still greater degree. The anus projects, dilates, and the contents of the rectum escape. The sufferings endured at this period are usually most intense, and the patient expresses the acuteness of her pangs by loud cries, sufficient, sometimes, to make the ears ring, or by deep, stifled, or suppressed groans. If we may judge from appearances, the suffering endured in some cases of labour is equal to what is experienced by those individuals who undergo severe surgical operations, or have the most violent cramps in muscular parts. In other cases the pain endured is trifling, and of such short duration that it is soon forgotten. At last, the head of the child, greatly compressed and swollen if it is a first labour, and there is much resistance at the outlet of the pelvis, is partially forced through the external parts, and does not recede when the pains go off. There is then usually in no long time a succession of strong expelling pain experienced, accompanied with involuntary efforts to bear down, by which the perineum is stretched to the greatest degree; at last it slides back over the forehead and face of the child, and allows the whole head to escape. The time required for the dilatation of the perineum varies extremely in different cases : in first labours the head often presses upon it for several hours before this is effected, while in other cases only a few pains are required.

After the expulsion of the head, if the mucus in the mouth be cleared away, respiration soon commences. and the child goes on b eathing regularly until another pain is exı er'enced which expels the shoulders and body of the child through the outlet of the pelvis. At other times, and more generally, there is an interval of a minute or two, or still longer, between the pains, and when the uterine contractions are renewed, the occiput usually becomes inclined to the left thigh of the mother, while the chin is turned to the opposite side. The shoulders then pass out of the pelvis, one under the arch of the pubes, and the other along the hollow of the sacrum, during which time the perineum is often again so much stretched as to be in danger of laceration. The transition is sudden from a state of the most intense suffering and anxiety to one of freedom from almost all pain, and the patient is left in a state of great excitement or exhaustion, with a rapid pulse, flushed countenance, and profuse perspiration over the whole body.

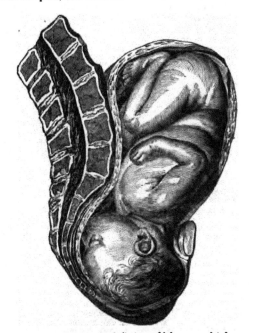

Fig. 2 *represents the first stage of labour completed.*

After a longer or shorter interval the uterus again contracts and expels the placenta, fœtal membranes, and the coagula of blood formed within its cavity. In general the placenta is only partially or not at all detached from the uterus before the birth of the child. The same pain which expelled the child sometimes expels the placenta, but more frequently several minutes elapse, and sometimes half an hour or longer, before the contractions of the uterus are renewed, and the placenta descends through the orifice into the vagina. If slight traction be made upon the cord downward and backward, a few pains are usually sufficient for the entire exclusion of the placenta and membranes.

If no assistance is given the uterus usually moulds the after-birth into a cylindrical form, and gradually forces it through the orifice into the dilated vagina, where it may remain a considerable period, until its presence excites the action of the diaphragm and abdominal muscles. Blood in greater or smaller quantity, fluid and coagulated, continues for some hours to flow from the parts. The uterus, after it has been emptied of its contents, and has properly contracted, forms a round hard tumor like a cricket-ball in the hypogastrium. It often, however, for several hours, or even longer in women who have had many children, alternately contracts and relaxes, and, if the labour is protracted, it is painful on pressure, and prone to inflammation. In the course of a few days the sanguineous fluid which flowed from the exposed vessels of the uterus where the placenta had adhered assumes a greenish hue, and, at a later period, it has sometimes a milky or purulent appearance, and has a peculiar odour. This discharge from the uterus after delivery, called the lochial discharge, does not usually cease altogether until the uterus has contracted greatly and become much reduced in volume by the absorption of its coats, bloodvessels, and nerves. The uterus is much more rapidly absorbed in some women than in others, and this chiefly depends on the previous state of the patient's health, and the nature of the labour. In some women the pulse returns to the natural standard, and the exhaustion disappears quickly; in others, without any disease, the pulse continues rapid for several days, with considerable general febrile excitement. The secretion of milk occasionally commences immediately after delivery, but generally not till the second or third day. Such is a very general description of the phenomena most frequently observed in the progress of natural labours, and I now proceed to consider the treatment required in their different stages.

Treatment of Natural Labour.

The first circumstance to be attended to, when we have been engaged to take charge of a patient in her confinement, is that when sent for we are to proceed as expeditiously as possible to her assistance. We are frequently summoned at the very commencement of labour, or when the pains experienced are false or spurious, but this affords no ground for unnecessary delay in any case, for the whole process of delivery is not unfrequently completed in a short space of time, and with a few pains, and if we are not present fatal accidents may occur. Where the superior extremities present, or the umbilical cord surrounds the neck of the infant, or uterine hæmorrhage occurs, the favourable opportunity for operating may be lost, and the mother and child both sacrificed by unnecessary delay on the part of the medical attendant. Independent of the actual good we may do by immediately proceeding to the assistance of patients when summoned, their confidence in us is deservedly increased by a proper display of activity on our part, and by shewing that we sympathise with them in their sufferings, and

are resolved to do whatever lies in our power to avert the danger to which they are exposed. It is far from my wish to recommend you to practise any unworthy art, to affect an interest in their welfare which you do not feel, to gain the confidence and esteem of your patients; but I would urge you to employ all proper means to acquire their confidence, for without it you will find that it is impossible to conduct any case of midwifery to a satisfactory termination.

Though we should proceed without loss of time to the assistance of our patients in labour, yet we shall do harm if we propose immediately, in an abrupt manner, to ascertain the progress of the labour by an internal examination. No impatience ought to be manifested, or any inquiries made respecting the state of the different functions which could possibly offend their delicacy. No woman's feelings can be hurt by inquiring when the pains commenced—if they came on spontaneously—how often they return—how long they continue—if they begin in the back and come round to the front of the abdomen—and if they are accompanied with shivering and sickness, or a sensation of bearing down. By the answers given to these inquiries, and by the appearance of the countenance during the pains, we are sometimes able to form a tolerably correct judgment of the state of the case, though we cannot be absolutely certain that labour has actually commenced, and can give no positive opinion on the subject until we have been permitted to ascertain the state of the os uteri, or to take a pain, as nurses express it. However strong the pains may be, however regular in their recurrence, they may be false or spurious pains, and we cannot determine their true character if the patient does not allow us to make the proper investigation. Where it is a first child, and the patient feels an unusual dread of an internal examination, the hand may be applied to the abdomen to feel if the uterus becomes hard during a pain, and if so there is the greatest probability that labour has commenced. But, under such circumstances, until the pains have continued so long, and have occurred so frequently and with such force as to lead us to believe that the os uteri is considerably dilated, it is better, perhaps, to wait for a few hours to observe the progress of the symptoms than to urge the patient to submit to an immediate examination. Indeed, the proposal to ascertain the state of the case must not be made directly to the patient, but to the nurse, who, if experienced, will only require a hint, and will find no difficulty in obtaining the requisite consent; every woman being naturally anxious at the commencement of labour to know if she is safe, and if the infant is coming in the usual way. When the con-

orehead and face of the child, and allows
rhole head to escape. The time required
be dilatation of the perineum varies ex-
ely in different cases : in first labours
head often presses upon it for several
s before this is effected, while in other
only a few pains are required.

ter the expulsion of the head, if the
as in the mouth be cleared away, respi-
n soon commences. and the child goes
eathing regularly until another pain is
r'enced which expels the shoulders and
of the child through the outlet of the
s. At other times, and more generally,
is an interval of a minute or two, or still
r, between the pains, and when the

uterine contractions are renewed, the occiput
usually becomes inclined to the left thigh of
the mother, while the chin is turned to the
opposite side. The shoulders then pass out
of the pelvis, one under the arch of the pubes,
and the other along the hollow of the sacrum,
during which time the perineum is often again
so much stretched as to be in danger of
laceration. The transition is sudden from
a state of the most intense suffering and
anxiety to one of freedom from almost all
pain, and the patient is left in a state of
great excitement or exhaustion, with a rapid
pulse, flushed countenance, and profuse
perspiration over the whole body.

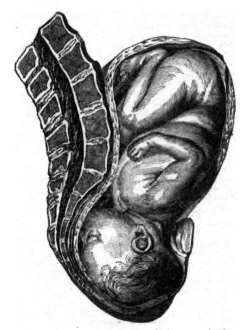

FIG. 2 *represents the first stage of labour completed.*

er a longer or shorter interval the
s again contracts and expels the pla-
, foetal membranes, and the coagula of
formed within its cavity. In general
acenta is only partially or not at all
ned from the uterus before the birth of
aild. The same pain which expelled
ahild sometimes expels the placenta,
ore frequently several minutes elapse,
ometimes half an hour or longer, before
ntractions of the uterus are renewed,
ne placenta descends through the orifice

into the vagina. If slight traction be made
upon the cord downward and backward, a
few pains are usually sufficient for the entire
exclusion of the placenta and membranes.

If no assistance is given the uterus usually
moulds the after-birth into a cylindrical
form, and gradually forces it through the
orifice into the dilated vagina, where it may
remain a considerable period, until its presence excites the action of the diaphragm
and abdominal muscles. Blood in greater
or smaller quantity, fluid and coagulated,

continues for some hours to flow from the parts. The uterus, after it has been emptied of its contents, and has properly contracted, forms a round hard tumor like a cricket-ball in the hypogastrium. It often, however, for several hours, or even longer in women who have had many children, alternately contracts and relaxes, and, if the labour is protracted, it is painful on pressure, and prone to inflammation. In the course of a few days the sanguineous fluid which flowed from the exposed vessels of the uterus where the placenta had adhered assumes a greenish hue, and, at a later period, it has sometimes a milky or purulent appearance, and has a peculiar odour. This discharge from the uterus after delivery, called the lochial discharge, does not usually cease altogether until the uterus has contracted greatly and become much reduced in volume by the absorption of its coats, bloodvessels, and nerves. The uterus is much more rapidly absorbed in some women than in others, and this chiefly depends on the previous state of the patient's health, and the nature of the labour. In some women the pulse returns to the natural standard, and the exhaustion disappears quickly; in others, without any disease, the pulse continues rapid for several days, with considerable general febrile excitement. The secretion of milk occasionally commences immediately after delivery, but generally not till the second or third day. Such is a very general description of the phenomena most frequently observed in the progress of natural labours, and I now proceed to consider the treatment required in their different stages.

Treatment of Natural Labour.

The first circumstance to be attended to, when we have been engaged to take charge of a patient in her confinement, is that when sent for we are to proceed as expeditiously as possible to her assistance. We are frequently summoned at the very commencement of labour, or when the pains experienced are false or spurious, but this affords no ground for unnecessary delay in any case, for the whole process of delivery is not unfrequently completed in a short space of time, and with a few pains, and if we are not present fatal accidents may occur. Where the superior extremities present, or the umbilical cord surrounds the neck of the infant, or uterine hæmorrhage occurs, the favourable opportunity for operating may be lost, and the mother and child both sacrificed by unnecessary delay on the part of the medical attendant. Independent of the actual good we may do by immediately proceeding to the assistance of patients when summoned, their confidence in us is deservedly increased by a proper display of activity on our part, and by shewing that we sympathise with them in their sufferings, and

are resolved to do whatever lies in our power to avert the danger to which they are exposed. It is far from my wish to recommend you to practise any unworthy art, to affect an interest in their welfare which you do not feel, to gain the confidence and esteem of your patients; but I would urge you to employ all proper means to acquire their confidence, for without it you will find that it is impossible to conduct any case of midwifery to a satisfactory termination.

Though we should proceed without loss of time to the assistance of our patients in labour, yet we shall do harm if we propose immediately, in an abrupt manner, to ascertain the progress of the labour by an internal examination. No impatience ought to be manifested, or any inquiries made respecting the state of the different functions which could possibly offend their delicacy. No woman's feelings can be hurt by inquiring when the pains commenced—if they came on spontaneously—how often they return—how long they continue—if they begin in the back and come round to the front of the abdomen—and if they are accompanied with shivering and sickness, or a sensation of bearing down. By the answers given to these inquiries, and by the appearance of the countenance during the pains, we are sometimes able to form a tolerably correct judgment of the state of the case, though we cannot be absolutely certain that labour has actually commenced, and can give no positive opinion on the subject until we have been permitted to ascertain the state of the os uteri, or to take a pain, as nurses express it. However strong the pains may be, however regular in their recurrence, they may be false or spurious pains, and we cannot determine their true character if the patient does not allow us to make the proper investigation. Where it is a first child, and the patient feels an unusual dread of an internal examination, the hand may be applied to the abdomen to feel if the uterus becomes hard during a pain, and if so there is the greatest probability that labour has commenced. But, under such circumstances, until the pains have continued so long, and have occurred so frequently and with such force as to lead us to believe that the os uteri is considerably dilated, it is better, perhaps, to wait for a few hours to observe the progress of the symptoms than to urge the patient to submit to an immediate examination. Indeed, the proposal to ascertain the state of the case must not be made directly to the patient, but to the nurse, who, if experienced, will only require a hint, and will find no difficulty in obtaining the requisite consent; every woman being naturally anxious at the commencement of labour to know if she is safe, and if the infant is coming in the usual way. When the consent of the patient has been obtained, let her lie down near the edge or foot of the bed, on her left side, under the sheet or coverlet, with the knees drawn up to the abdomen, and when a pain comes on, let the fore finger of the right hand, covered with cold cream, lard, soap, or some other unctuous matter, be gently passed from the anus along the perinæum into the vagina, and forward along its posterior surface, as far as the finger can reach. The point should then be drawn forward to the centre of the brim of the pelvis, where the os uteri is most frequently situated, or a little behind this, at the commencement of labour. You cannot fail to reach the os uteri if the finger be passed up along the posterior wall of the vagina, and the point of it be brought forward towards the symphysis pubis. While the pain continues, the most careful examination should be made to ascertain the degree to which the orifice is dilated, the effect produced upon it by the pain, and whether it is thin, soft, and yielding, and low in the pelvis, or high up, thick, rigid, and unyielding. During the pain, we have to ascertain whether the labour has commenced, and if so, the extent to which the os uteri is dilated, and from its condition endeavour to determine the probable duration of the labour. When the pain has subsided, and the os uteri and membranes have collapsed, and not before, the finger is to be passed very cautiously within the orifice, to discover whether the head of the child presents. The head is usually recognised without difficulty by its globular shape, the peculiar hardness of the parietal bones, and by the sutures. If the finger touches the sagittal suture, midway between the fontanelles, the edges of the parietal bones will be distinctly felt through the membranes. If you feel the hard edges of the parietal bones, you can have no doubt about the presentation, although neither fontanelle be touched. In no case is it necessary or proper at the commencement of the labour, before the membranes are ruptured, and the first stage completed, to endeavour to discover in what position the head of the child is placed relatively to the pelvis of the mother; it is enough to know with absolute certainty that the head presents; and this information should be possessed in every case; no doubt should be left on the subject, before the finger be withdrawn. Having ascertained that the pains are those of labour, and that the head presents, we have obtained all the knowledge that can ever be of use in practice. Any attempt to determine in which of the numerous positions described by some authors the head is placed at the brim of the pelvis, would only endanger the rupture of the membranes, and disturb the regular order observed by nature in the process. I am

greatly at a loss to discover what benefit could result from knowing during the first stage of labour, provided you can touch the vertex with the point of the finger, in which of the six or eight positions of Baudelocque, and other foreign authors, the head is placed. The importance attached by some writers to a knowledge of these positions, some of which are wholly imaginary, has probably arisen from the dangerous practice of employing the long forceps before the os uteri is fully dilated, and before the head has passed into the cavity of the pelvis. At this early stage of labour no instrument of this description can be safely used, and if the operation of turning the child were required, the position of the head would have no influence upon the method we would adopt in turning the child. Be sure that the head presents before you state this to the nurse or patient, for they will not soon forget your mistake if it should turn out to be a case of nates presentation.

In some cases where the head presents, it remains so high up, even when the first stage of labour is considerably advanced, that the finger cannot reach it without endangering the rupture of the membranes. Here the patient should be kept in the horizontal position, till the first stage of labour is nearly completed, and the presentation ascertained.

When it is the first labour, and the os uteri is high up in the pelvis, rigid, and little dilated, and the pains are irregular and produce little effect upon it, we infer that many hours will elapse before the labour is completed. As sudden and unexpected changes, however, often occur in the progress of labour, it is necessary to be extremely cautious, both in forming and delivering an opinion respecting its duration in every case. Even when the os uteri is widely dilated, its margin thin and soft, and the pains strong and regular, circumstances which could not have been foreseen may occur to retard delivery many hours beyond the time we expected. The assurance that the labour is natural, that the child is coming as it ought to do, that it is not a cross birth, which all women dread so much, and that there is every reason to expect in due time a successful termination of the labour by the natural efforts, is sufficient to satisfy the mind of every woman possessed of ordinary fortitude and intelligence. But there are some resolute enough in ordinary circumstances whose courage leaves them entirely during labour, and who require not only to be assured again and again that there is no danger, but to be convinced, by our cheerful and composed demeanour, that such is the fact.

I ought to have stated before, that if, on making an internal examination, we find no change produced on the os uteri during the pains, we conclude that the labour has not commenced, and endeavour to discover and remove the cause of the irritation. False or spurious pains are usually vague and irregular, and never cease entirely. They often follow strong exercise, or fatigue from walking, and irregularities of diet, and occur before the full period. There is sometimes tenderness of the uterine region, and febrile excitement. They are to be relieved by opiates, warm fomentations, cathartics, and bleeding, according to the cause on which they depend.

During the first stage of labour the proper arrangements in the dress of the patient, the bed, and apartment, should be made for delivery. The stays, and every thing that can compress the body during the strong muscular efforts, should be removed, and a night-wrapper or loose dressing-gown put on. The mattress should be laid over the feather-bed; and over the dressed sheep's skin or water-proof cloth a blanket should be laid, and this covered by a folded sheet. According to the temperature of the atmosphere at the time, a blanket or coverlet should be placed over the patient when she lies down. The feet are usually pressed against one of the bed-posts during the pains, as she lies on the left side, and a long towel fixed to the other or foot of the bed, on which she can pull when the uterine action is strong. The apartment should be kept moderately warm, and well ventilated during the whole period of labour; and the food and drink should consist of tea, gruel, coffee, barley-water, toast and water, and other diluents. It is only when labour is protracted, and exhaustion takes place, that broth or beef-tea is required, and that a little wine and water, or brandy and water, should be given. If the bowels are confined when labour begins, give a sufficient dose of castor oil, or let a stimulating enema be exhibited. Until the first stage of labour is nearly completed, the patient should be allowed to sit up, to lie down, or walk about and change her position, as she may feel inclined. Even in the second stage of labour, if it is a first child, and the parts at the outlet of the pelvis are rigid, it is often useful to keep the patient for a time out of the recumbent position. Nurses often request them to bear down in the first stage; but this exhausts the strength, and voluntary exertions should never be made at any period of labour. The circumstances of each case will enable us to judge whether it is requisite for us to remain in constant attendance, or if we may with safety absent ourselves altogether for a few hours, and attend to other professional business. Our constant presence in the apartment is rather injurious than beneficial in most cases until

the first stage of labour is nearly completed, and the pains are strong and frequent. If the labour is protracted, it is necessary from time to time, at intervals probably of two or three hours or longer, to repeat the internal examination, that its progress may be ascertained. Women are anxious to know that the labour is advancing, and they are aware that this can only be ascertained by an internal examination, which if properly conducted can neither excite inflammation of the vagina nor produce any other injurious effect; at least I have never seen inflammation of the vagina nor laceration of the perineum where I could fairly attribute them to this cause. It is scarcely necessary for me to point out to you the necessity of examining the hypogastrium from time to time, to be sure that there is no accumulation of urine taking place in the bladder. In all protracted cases there is no circumstance which requires greater attention than this, and the immediate employment of the catheter when the necessity for it arises.

It is always requisite to make a careful internal examination when the membranes burst and the liquor amnii begins to escape, as a loop of the navel-string may descend before the head, or an upper extremity accompany it. The membranes should not be ruptured artificially, and no attempt should be made to dilate the orifice of the uterus or the external parts, in ordinary circumstances. When the head of the child comes to press forcibly against the perineum, and it is greatly distended and in danger of being lacerated, the patient should then be placed upon the left side in bed, and should not quit that position for an instant. The left side is by far the most convenient position both for the patient and her medical attendant, and it is so not only in natural labour but in all cases where the forceps or perforator are to be employed, or the operation of turning performed. The palm of the right hand, with a soft napkin interposed, should be firmly applied over the centre of the perineum, and proper support given during the pains. In first labours, where the head is large and the perineum rigid, and the uterine contractions violent, the parts at the outlet of the pelvis are often extensively torn where this artificial support is not given effectually. Extensive laceration of the perineum very rarely occurs where the necessary assistance is afforded with the palm of the right hand placed over it, and strong counter pressure made during the pains. By counter pressure is meant, pressing the head forward to the symphysis pubis, and preventing the whole force of the uterine action being directed against the perineum. It is sometimes requisite to guard the perineum thus for several hours, and, where it is exposed to great danger, it is useful occasionally to cover it with some unctuous matter, or still better, between the pains, to apply over it a large sponge soaked in hot water. Nothing should be interposed between the hand and perineum when it is in great danger of being torn. The right knee should be supported when the head is thus pressing upon the parts at the head of the pelvis, and the patient strongly urged to abstain from all voluntary efforts to bear down.

When the head has passed, clear away all the mucus in the mouth, that the child may breathe, and feel whether the umbilical cord surrounds the neck. If it does, and is not tight, the best practice is to leave it alone, or slide it up a little over the shoulders when a pain comes on, that they and the body may pass readily through the loop. I prefer doing this, or merely slackening it a little, to pulling the loop entirely over the head, which is sometimes done. If there is no pain to expel the trunk soon after the head is born, make firm pressure over the fundus uteri, and excite it to contract. The child should never be dragged into the world, but the uterus should always be made to expel it: even if several minutes should elapse without any pain occurring, I would not pull the child forward, but wait until it was forced into the world by the action of the uterus. It is of the greatest consequence that the uterus should not be suddenly emptied of its contents. When the shoulders are passing, the perineum should again be supported: then draw the child into the light, and if it has breathed freely and vigorously, apply a good strong ligature very firmly around the cord, about two fingers breadth from the navel. This ligature should be applied with as much care as around a large divided artery, and to make it perfectly secure pass it twice round the cord, and tie it firmly. Apply another ligature an inch or two nearer the placenta, and divide the funis between the ligatures with a pair of scissors, put the child in the flannel receiver, and give it to the nurse. If the respiration is not readily established, recourse must be had in the first instance, before applying the ligatures, to the dashing or sprinkling of cold water over the face and chest, rubbing the chest with brandy, and the application of stimulants to the nostrils. Immersion of the child in warm water, and inflating the lungs, should be employed, and our efforts to excite respiration should not cease until the pulsations in the heart and funis have entirely ceased for some minutes. When this is the case all our efforts to restore animation will be useless.

Next ascertain, by applying the hand over the abdomen, if there be another child within the uterus. If there be a second child the fundus of the uterus will still be in the epigastrium; it will be large and hard, and some part of the child distinctly felt. If there is a doubt about the presence of a second child within the uterus, examine internally, and the second bag of membranes and presenting part, if there are twins, will be distinctly felt. If this could not be ascertained by passing two fingers of the right hand along the cord of the first child, it would be justifiable to introduce the whole hand into the vagina.

I have several times been sent for to deliver a second child when there was nothing within the uterus but an unusually large placenta. When there is not a second child, the fundus uteri is usually felt nearly as low as the umbilicus, and it is greatly reduced in size, and has none of the irregular hardness which is always felt in cases of twins.

The temporary binder, to which I attach the greatest importance, should now be applied firmly around the abdomen. In all cases of labour, immediately after the birth of the child, a broad bandage should be applied around the body. A broad towel or napkin is often employed for this purpose, and, without raising the patient, it may be passed under her. and spread out so as to surround the whole pelvis and abdomen, and firmly fixed with tapes or strong pins. It should be so tightly applied around the lower part of the abdomen as to occasion a slight degree of uneasiness. The firm equal pressure of the binder or bandage over the uterus causes it to contract in a regular manner, and diminishes greatly the risk of syncope, retained placenta, and hæmorrhage. Some have attributed inflammation of the uterus after delivery, and prolapsus, and a great many other evil consequences, to the temporary binder, but, as you may suppose, without the slightest proof or foundation. Some practitioners apply a binder exterior to the clothes at the commencement of labour, and tighten it as the process advances. Even in the eighth month of pregnancy, where there is great relaxation of the abdominal parietes, it might sometimes be proper to give gentle support to the pendulous abdomen with a bandage.

Our great object now is to make the uterus permanently contract, to detach and expel the placenta, and prevent hæmorrhage. For this purpose, if the labour has been tedious, and there is much exhaustion, some stimulant, as a little wine and water, or brandy and water, should be administered; and over the binder, if the uterus is relaxed, and indisposed to contract, the hand should be placed, and firm pressure made. When a pain is felt, slight traction in the direction of the axis of the pelvis, downward and backward, should be made upon the cord, to promote the separation of the placenta from the uterus. By compressing and squeezing the fundus uteri, and gently pulling from time to time upon the cord, the placenta usually descends, and passes through the os uteri into the vagina, in the course of a quarter of an hour, or twenty minutes, or half an hour, after the birth of the child. More anxiety is often felt by us during this period than during the whole of the previous stages of the labour, and not without good reason. In removing the placenta from the vagina, it is necessary to be very careful that the membranes are not torn away from its margin, and left behind. The best method of obviating this accident is slowly to turn the placenta round twice or thrice as we extract it, and if the membranes seem disposed to tear, as we gently draw them out, to seize them with a dry napkin, and very gradually remove them. The placenta may be retained beyond the usual period, by want of uterine action, by morbid adhesion to the uterus, and by premature contraction of the cervix. On whatever cause it depends there are no cases in which the placenta ought to be permitted to remain within the uterus beyond an hour after the birth of the child, and not so long if hæmorrhage takes place. That there may be no misunderstanding on this important practical point, I repeat, that I have never seen a case of retention of the placenta where any thing but mischief resulted from leaving it within the uterus beyond an hour after the expulsion of the child. If the binder has been applied, and pressure made over the fundus uteri, and traction upon the cord properly employed, and the placenta does not descend at the end of an hour, I would not advise you to give the ergot of rye, or to wait longer for its detachment and expulsion, but to put the cord upon the stretch with your left hand, and to introduce your right hand, in a conical form, through the vagina into the uterus, to spread out the fingers to the circumference of the placenta, and to press the mass slowly from the uterus if it still adheres, and to extract it. In the greater number of cases the placenta has been completely or partially detached from the uterus when this requires to be done.

When the placenta has come away, or been removed, make the patient dry and comfortable, by removing all the wet clothes, and applying warm napkins to the external parts, and around the pelvis, and giving her warm gruel, with a little wine or brandy, or some warm tea. As hæmorrhage may occur an hour or more after delivery, you should from time to time feel the pulse, enquire if the patient is faint, ascertain if the uterus is contracted, and if the discharge is not too great. It is a good rule to remain with every patient at least an hour after the expulsion of the placenta, and if there is faintness, and

a disposition to flooding, it is necessary to devote a much longer time to the case.

If severe after-pains soon commence, or if they have occasioned much suffering in former labours, it is useful to administer a draught, with 30 or 40 minims of the Liquor Opii Sedativus. I am an advocate for an opiate after delivery, to soothe the nervous system, if much excited by severe and protracted suffering. If opium be useful in tranquillising the system, and preserving it from febrile excitement and irritation after extensive wounds of the large cavities, surely it cannot but be beneficial after delivery, and it can do no harm, particularly if combined with a saline diaphoretic draught. Where a labour has been severe, and inflammation of the uterus is to be dreaded, it is not only useful to administer a sufficient quantity of an anodyne to quiet the system, but for a day or two to give small doses of Dover's powder to subdue irritation, and promote perspiration. It is beneficial, also, under such circumstances, to cover the hypogastrium with a warm poultice, or occasionally to apply warm fomentations.

Three or four hours ought in all cases to be allowed to pass, after the labour is concluded, before the patient is moved up in the bed, and has her clothes changed, and when this is being done by the nurse, she ought to make no exertion, or to quit the horizontal position. The apartment should be kept moderately warm, and free from all noise and excitement of every kind, and nothing should be given but gruel, tea, or barley water, for 48 or 60 hours, in the majority of cases.

With respect to the infant, it is necessary to see before quitting the house that it is not malformed, that the cord is properly secured, that it is not unnecessarily exposed to cold air, while being washed by the nurse, and that no improper food or medicine is administered. A small tea-spoonful of castor oil may be given to expel the meconium. A little warm milk and water or thin gruel is the only food that is required before applying the child to the breast, which should not be done for at least twelve hours after delivery. Every patient should be seen by her medical attendant within twenty-four hours after delivery, and if possible daily, at least for a week after. The danger of childbearing may now almost be said to commence, for there are very many women who pass through the different stages of labour with impunity, who perish in the puerperal state. Inflammation of the uterus and its appendages is the cause of all the danger, and in the daily visits which you make this is the great point to which your attention should be directed. Pain, increased by pressure over the hypogastrium, suppression of the lochia and milk, rigors, headache, and quick pulse, are the principal diagnostic symptoms. It most frequently commences on the second and third day after delivery, but sometimes within twenty-four hours.

At each daily visit pass the hand over the region of the uterus, press upon the fundus and over the situation of the uterine appendages, and you will sometimes detect uterine inflammation where the complaints of the patient and the statements of the nurse would have given you no reason to suspect its existence. Examine the state of the bladder, the pulse, tongue, lochial discharge, and mark the expression of the countenance, and never fail to inquire if there is milk in the breasts, and if the patient has had any coldness or shivering, or is suffering from headache. If the pulse continues several days after delivery 100 or 110 in the minute, and one or more of these symptoms are present, the patient is not safe.

It is of the utmost importance to form a correct diagnosis between after pains and uterine inflammation. Many women are lost in consequence of this mistake. Generally there are intervals of complete freedom from suffering in the irregular contractions of the uterus which follow delivery, without inflammation, and constitute after pains; they are relieved by pressure over the uterus—they gradually diminish in severity on the second and third days, and they are unaccompanied with rigors, fever, and headache, and the lochial discharge is not suppressed. But if you cannot satisfactorily establish the diagnosis between after-pains and inflammation of the uterus, I would take the least favourable view of the symptoms, and give the patient the benefit of a small general bleeding, or the application of leeches to the region of the uterus. I have seen many puerperal women lost for want of timely depletion; I never saw one suffer in consequence of a moderate quantity of blood being taken from the arm, or from the hypogastrium by leeches.

On the third morning after delivery it is necessary in most cases to administer a mild cathartic, castor-oil, or an aperient draught of senna, sulphate of magnesia and manna, should be given, and where the bowels have not been attended to before the labour, this should be done on the second morning. The diet of puerperal women during the first week should be the same as that allowed to persons who are convalescent from fever, or from severe acute diseases. Until the secretion of milk is established, nothing but gruel, tea, a little thin arrow-root, or panado, should be allowed. On the fourth day, if there is no pyrexia, and the child has taken the breast, and the milk flows freely, a little beef-tea or chicken broth may be given. This should be continued in all cases till the end of the first week, and even at the end of that period, if the tongue is not clean, the pulse quiet, and the abdomen wholly free from tenderness on pressure, the patient should still be kept on low diet. After the ninth day in ordinary cases, some chicken or solid animal food may be allowed with a little wine and water, and after this the patient may gradually return to her accustomed diet.

These are all the observations which I consider it necessary to offer on the phenomena and treatment of natural labours. When I have described all the varieties of difficult, preternatural, and complicated labours, I shall endeavour to give you a full account of the pathology and treatment of the acute, inflammatory, and febrile diseases of puerperal women, and the other diseases which follow delivery.

LECTURES
ON THE
PHYSICAL AND PATHOLOGICAL
CHARACTERS OF URINARY
DEPOSITS,

Delivered at Guy's Hospital, London,

BY DR. GOLDING BIRD.

LECTURE V.

Carbonate of lime. Cause of ammoniacal urine. Presence of phosphates in urine. Solubility of phosphates in ammoniacal salts—in carbonic acid—deposited by boiling—mistaken for mucus—crystalline forms of. Phosphate of lime. Phosphatic urine—varieties of. Sources of phosphates—traced to vegetable ingesta—and destructive assimilation of nervous tissue.

GENTLEMEN — The next constituent of urinary deposit to which I have to direct your attention is one by no means of frequent occurrence, viz:

Carbonate of lime.

This salt, although a constant ingredient in the alkaline urine of graminivorous animals, never occurs in the urine of carnivora or of man; unless as the result of certain secondary changes, of which the most essential is the resolution of urea into carbonate of ammonia, and the consequent formation of carbonate of lime. You have not, I trust, forgotten the explanation I have given you of the probable formation of carbonate of ammonia from urea; the addition of water being sufficient to afford all the elements necessary for the production of the salt under consideration. So that urea may be regarded as carbonate of ammonia *minus* water, or a *carbonamide*. We know that the conversion into the carbonate takes place but slowly in healthy urine out of the body, and with still less rapidity when this substance is dissolved in pure water. Still less frequently does this change take place whilst the urine is retained in the bladder. Under certain circumstances, however, especially where an excess of mucous matter is secreted, this substance acts the part of a ferment, induces a new arrangement of the elements of urea and water, and thus the urine is voided in an ammoniacal condition. Excepting, however, under certain circumstances of by no means constant occurrence, the vital endowments of the bladder are sufficient to preserve the urine from undergoing this change, even if a very considerable quantity of mucus be present. It is only, indeed, when the conservative powers of the nervous influence supplying the bladder become exhausted, that its contents become subject to the ordinary laws of chemistry. Thus, as has been long shewn by Dr. Prout and Sir Benjamin Brodie, blows on the back have a tendency to produce alkaline urine; a fact admitting of ready explanation, by the necessarily depressed condition of the nervous power of the bladder, resulting from the injury to the spine. Even in these cases, however, I doubt considerably whether the urine is by any means generally *secreted alkaline.* From the result of many cases which have occurred in this hospital I am induced to believe that the urine is secreted by the kidneys in the usual subacid condition, and that it becomes alkaline by the subsequent change which it undergoes in the bladder, when the vital endowments of the latter have become depressed, and the mucus acting as a ferment converts the urea into carbonate of ammonia. In confirmation of this view I have repeatedly observed that, in cases where the urine appeared alkaline, on emptying the bladder with a catheter it was found that the partly secreted urine was acid or neutral, and it was only after being retained for some time in the bladder that it presented alkaline properties.

Again, in cases of paraplegia, where the urine is often found to be alkaline, this state may be almost constantly traced to the inability of the patient to empty the bladder; and thus it is the *retained urine* which undergoes change; the freshly secreted portions being nearly natural. In the case of a woman labouring under complete paraplegia, whose urine was seldom voided, and was ropy, alkaline, and offensive, I washed out the bladder with warm water, and left an elastic catheter in the urethra, so that the urine might escape almost as soon as it reached the bladder. Under these circumstances the urine appeared clear, pale, and slightly acid, whilst that voided 24 hours before was dark, offensive, alkaline, and turbid not only from mucus, but from sediment, consisting of carbonate of lime and the earthy phosphates. The best and most satisfactory cases in which

the urine was secreted alkaline are those recorded by Dr. Graves, of Dublin; one of them was a case of adynamic typhus fever, in which an abundance of carbonate of ammonia existed in the urine, and a corresponding deficiency of urea and uric acid existed. *Pari passu* with the convalescence of the patient the carbonate of ammonia vanished, being replaced by an equivalent proportion of urea and uric acid. The second case was one of fatal general anasarca, following exposure to cold; here the urine was loaded with carbonate of ammonia, but neither urea nor albumen existed. After death the bladder appeared perfectly healthy.

Whilst I have thus endeavoured to explain to you the reasons which have induced me to regard the development of carbonate of lime as almost invariably secondary to changes which the urine undergoes in the bladder, I must confess that more information is required on this subject. I have never seen a deposit consisting entirely of carbonate of lime, but have not unfrequently met with it in small quantities in phosphatic deposits. We have, in our hospital museum, but a single specimen in which carbonate of lime occurs in any considerable quantity. It is, however, very remarkable, that an excellent and highly respected provincial surgeon, Mr. Smith, of Bristol, has met with many instances of calculi composed chiefly of this calcareous salt. Should such calculi be again met with, it will be extremely important to carefully examine the urine passed by the patients from whom they were removed. We may thus resolve the curious questions whether in certain states of health the urine is secreted alkaline, like that of herbivora, or whether such an alkaline condition is really secondary.

The next series of deposits that will engage our attention includes those which are composed of ingredients chiefly of inorganic origin. This class contains four varieties of deposits, viz. those composed of phosphate of lime, of triple phosphate, of a mixture of these salts, and of silicic acid. Although this division to a certain extent is practically necessary, yet in our consideration of them I shall explain to you the peculiarities of deposits consisting of phosphates generally, as they are accompanied by analogous phenomena.

Phosphatic Deposits.

You are aware that on an average 6.5 grains of phosphoric acid leave the system in the urine in the course of 24 hours. Although the particular state of combination in which this acid exists may admit of doubt, yet it is evident that a considerable portion of it exists in urine with lime, magnesia, and ammonia. The two latter bases very probably exist in the same combination, forming a double salt; the ammonio-phosphate of magnesia, or triple phosphate, as it is termed.

If you add a very small quantity of ammonia to a large quantity of healthy urine the mixture becomes turbid from a deposit of the triple phosphates, mixed in all probability with phosphate of lime. On placing a drop of this turbid urine under the microscope, myriads of minute prisms of the triple salt, mixed with amorphous granules of the phosphates of lime, will be seen floating in the fluid. These readily disappear on the addition of a drop of almost any acid. As these earthy salts are insoluble in water, it is evident that they must be held in solution in the urine by the free acid which generally exists; this acid is either the phosphoric or lactic, or both. If from any cause the quantity of solvent acid falls below the necessary proportion, the earthy phosphates appear in the urine, forming a deposit. Hence, when the urine is alkaline, phosphatic deposits are necessary consequences. If urine be secreted with so small a proportion of acid as barely to redden litmus paper, a deposit of triple phosphates often occurs a few hours after emission; a phenomenon depending on the influence of the mucous matter present, which exciting a catalytic action like a ferment, induces the decomposition of urea, and the formation of carbonate of ammonia, which by neutralising the solvent acid, throws down the phosphates. The precipitation of the phosphates thus takes place in a manner analogous to that in which carbonate of lime is thrown down, the action being here limited to a neutralisation of a free acid: indeed, where phosphates of lime form the great bulk of a deposit, a certain portion of carbonate is generally present.

It is, however, by no means necessary for urine to be alkaline for a deposit of phosphates to exist; indeed, in the great majority of cases, urine which deposits the triple phosphate is acid at the time of emission, and often for long after. This may appear rather paradoxical, when we recollect the ready solubility of triple phosphate in a very weak acid; but admits of a ready explanation when the fact that a fluid may redden litmus, and still contain no uncombined acid, is borne in mind. Thus, a solution of hydrochlorate of ammonia will redden litmus paper, and yet it contains no free acid; and as this salt exists in the urine, it is quite possible that it may be one of the causes on which its acid reaction depends, where deposits of phosphates exist. It has been rendered very probable, by the interesting experiments of Dr. Rees, that this very salt may in some instances be really the solvent of the earthy phosphates, as they are to a certain extent soluble in solutions of sal-ammonia. These solutions

possess the very remarkable property, first pointed out by the excellent chemist to whom I have just referred, of becoming opaque by ebullition, from a deposition of a portion of the earthy salt. The very same phenomenon often occurs in urine which contains an excess of phosphates. Indeed, it is not unfrequent to meet with urine which does not contain any visible deposit, and yet on the application of heat appears to coagulate, not from the presence of albumen, but from the deposition of earthy phosphates. The addition of a drop of nitric acid immediately dissolves this deposit, and distinguishes it from albumen. A different explanation to this phenomenon has been offered by Dr. Hargrave Brett, and which undoubtedly is perfectly true in many cases, although the hypothesis of Dr. Rees is applicable to the greater number. Dr. Brett's explanation is founded on the solubility of phosphates in water impregnated with carbonic acid. It has been long known that carbonic acid frequently exists in a free state in the urine, and in a large number of specimens examined by Dr. Brett and myself we succeeded in readily isolating it. These experiments were made several years ago, in consequence of our having noticed some curious phenomena presented by the urine of a student of this hospital (since dead), a pupil of the late Mr. Bryant, of Kennington. This gentleman, in endeavouring to raise a heavy sack of Epsom salts, strained his back, and soon after fell into a state of marasmus, with occasional hectic, which ultimately exhausted him. During the last six months of his life he passed a very large quantity of pale acid urine, which by keeping soon became alkaline. This urine was limpid when first passed, but became opaque as soon as it had cooled, still, however, retaining its acidity, so that the deposition of the phosphates did not necessarily depend upon the development of an alkali. On warming the fresh urine an evolution of carbonic acid gas took place, accompanied by a deposition of phosphates. When the two portions of the fresh urine were placed as soon as passed in separate bottles, and left open, and the other closely corked, the urine contained in the latter remained transparent, and that in the former became opaque.

Whenever the triple phosphate occurs in the urine as a deposit, it is always found to be composed of crystals which are generally sharply defined, and extremely regular. You must, however, bear in mind that these crystals may exist in large quantities, and yet escape detection in consequence of their extreme transparency. In cases of this kind the deposit which forms by repose generally presents the appearance of a mere mucous cloud, and it is only distinguished from it by the addition of an acid, which immediatley dissolves it. On decanting such urine and placing the lower turbid portion in a watch-glass, the crystals may be detected by moving the latter near a lighted candle, when a series of glittering points will become visible from the reflection of the light from the facets of the minute prisms of triple salt. On placing the watch-glass under a microscope the crystals may be readily recognised. The depositions of the phosphates may become accelerated by warming the urine in the manner I explained to you when speaking of the oxalate of lime. The exact resemblance presented by the deposits of phosphates to mucous clouds is so very close that the most practised eye can scarcely distinguish between them; indeed, scarcely a week passes but I find myself completely at fault on attempting to distinguish between them by bare inspection. When phosphate of lime exists mixed with the triple salt, the deposit often remains for a long time diffused through the urine, so as to resemble ropelike masses of purulent mucus. Not only do deposits of phosphates resemble mucus and pus in physical appearances, but they frequently co-exist. Indeed, it is very frequent to find fine prisms of triple phosphate entangled in the meshes of the mucous cloud which forms by repose in all urine. When the triple phosphate co-exists with mucus or pus, the microscope will readily detect its presence.

Occasionally, where a small excess of the triple phosphate is present, it is found on the surface of the urine, forming a delicate iridescent scum or pellicle, reflecting coloured bands of light, like a thin layer of oil, or the surface of a soap-bubble.

When a considerable quantity of ammonia is added to urine, a deposit occurs from setting free a triple phosphate of magnesia, which differs from that to which I have just been alluding, in containing half an equivalent more of ammonia; it is in fact a *sesqui-basic*, or, as it is commonly termed, a bibasic triple phosphate of magnesia and ammonia. This is evidently formed by the ammonia playing a double part; it not only neutralises the solvent acid, but combines with the normal phosphate to form a basic salt. This can be readily distinguished from the neutral salt by its crystalline form, as it always presents the form of stellæ, generally six-rayed, often elegantly pinnated, in some cases presenting the appearance of foliaceous crystals resembling fern leaves; this variety, however, being almost always the result of decomposition, when the urine has been kept a long time.

This basic phosphate invariably, and I believe necessarily, exists with alkaline urine; it very rarely occurs in recent urine, and so far as I have had occasion to observe, is always a secondary product.

Before proceeding to explain the genera properties of urine depositing phosphates, I would call your attention to these diagrams, exhibiting the crystalline forms of the phosphatic magnesian salts, as it is important you should be sufficiently familiar with them to enable you to recognise them.

A. *Prisms of neutral triple phosphates.*—These are always exceedingly well defined, the angles and edges of the crystals being remarkably sharp and perfect. The triangular prism is the form most frequently met with, but it presents every variety in its termination. These are sometimes merely truncated, often bevelled off, and not unfrequently the terminal edges are replaced by facets.

FIG. 16.

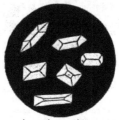

I scarcely know a more beautiful microscopic object than is afforded by a well-marked deposit of this salt. You will frequently be struck with the very different degrees of transparency presented by these crystals; sometimes they are so transparent as to resemble pri ms of glass or crystal; at others presenting an enamel-like opacity, so that they can only be viewed as opaque objects. When preserved in balsam, they depolarise light very beautifully where the axes of the tourmalines or calc-spars are crossed in the polarising microscope.

B. *Simple stellæ of the neutral salt.*—These are in fact minute calculous concretions, and are generally composed of minute prisms cohering at one end, so as to represent simple stellæ. Not unfrequently they adhere so closely and so crowded as to resemble rosettes. I have repeatedly seen small prisms crystallized as one of the fine transparent hairs which are of frequent occurrence in urine. Indeed, if for the word *rhomboids* you substitute *prisms*, the account I have given you in a former lecture of the varieties of the compound crystals of uric acid will apply to the phosphatic magnesian salt, bearing in mind that the latter is invariably colourless, never presenting the yellow or orange hue of uric acid.

C. *Penniform crystals of neutral salt.*—This very elegant variety of the neutral magnesia phosphate has only lately fallen under my notice, and has not hitherto been described. It presents the appearance of striated feather-like crystals,

FIG. 17.

two being generally connected so as to cause them to resemble a pair of wings. I cannot give any satisfactory explanation of the causes of this curious and elegant variety, or whether they differ in any way chemically from the prismatic form. The few specimens I have met with occurred in acid urine.

D. *Stella and foliaceous crystals of basic salt.*—This variety, as I have already told you, cannot generally be regarded in any other light than as a secondary product taking place out of the body. When rapidly

FIG. 18.

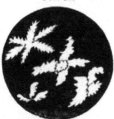

formed, we generally find this salt in the form of six-rayed stars, each ray being serrated, or irregularly crenate, often renunciated, like the leaf of the taraxacum. This, however, presents several subordinate varieties, depending, in all probability, upon accidental circumstances. When this salt is more slowly formed, as on the surface of the urine of pregnancy, it presents large and broad foliaceous laminæ, often so thin and transparent as to escape notice altogether, especially if viewed in too strong a light. I have, indeed, often overlooked them until I illuminated the specimen under the microscope with pulverized light, when they started into view elegantly tinted with colours in which pink and green are the most prominent.

There are no definite microscopic characters by which phosphate of lime can be recognised in deposits; it always appears as a

mere amorphous cloud, made up of extremely minute particles, sometimes presenting a globular arrangement. In this form they are frequently found adhering to prisms of the triple salt, and their nature can be readily made out by the addition of a drop of very dilute hydrochloric acid, in which both phosphates readily dissolve, and by this property are at once distinguished from all organic globules, which are insoluble in that menstruum. These deposits are so readily recognisable with the assistance of the microscope, that it can scarcely be deemed necessary to have recourse to their chemical characters, which are often made out with extreme difficulty, from the small quantity of deposit we have in most cases to operate on. If any doubt should, however, remain regarding the nature of any deposit of this class, it may be sufficient to recollect that of all the deposits possessing a true crystalline form which have yet been examined, the triple phosphate is the only one which is soluble in acetic acid, and of all amorphous deposits, the phosphate of lime is the only one which does not disappear on the addition of liquor potassæ.

The urine, in cases where an excess of phosphates of either kind exists, differs in its physical character very materially. Certainly no general rule can be assigned for the colour, density, or quantity of the urine secreted in these cases, taking them in a mass ; although I think there are certain facts connected with the presence of the phosphatic deposits which serve to connect the colour and quantity of the urine with the pathological conditions producing, or at least co-existing with them.

As a general rule, where copious phosphatic deposits, whether magnesian, calcareous, or both, exist for a considerable time, the urine is pale, often whey-like, and of low specific gravity. This is especially the case where organic lesion of the kidneys exists. On the other hand, when the deposits are of occasional occurrence, often disappearing and recurring in the course of a few days, the urine generally presents a deep amber colour, and is not only of high specific gravity, but often contains an excess of urea, and presents an iridescent pellicle on its surface by repose. This is especially the character of the phosphatic urine secreted under the influence of some forms of irritative dyspepsia, and where the phosphates themselves may be traced to mal-assimilation. Again, phosphatic urine may be met with varying from a pale whey-like hue to deep brown or greenish brown, exceedingly fœtid, generally but not constantly alkaline, and loaded with dense ropy mucus, often tinged with blood, and in which large crystals of the triple phosphate and amorphous masses of phosphate of lime are entangled. This variety is almost always met with either under the irritation of a calculus, or where disease of the mucous membrane of the bladder exists.

It was long ago remarked by Berzelius, that phosphatic deposits were often present in the urine passed in one part of the day, and absent in other specimens. I carefully watched a series of cases where the triple phosphate existed in the urine, with a view to determine the accuracy of this statement, and am convinced that the following may be assumed as a safe induction from these observations. *That where the presence of deposits of phosphates is independent of the irritation of a calculus, or of organic disease, it is most abundant in the urine passed in the evening (urine of digestion), and absent* or replaced by uric acid, or urates, in the morning urine (urine of the blood), the urine being always of tolerably natural colour, never below, and often above the mean density. *Where the presence of phosphatic salt depends on the irritation of a calculus, or of organic mischief in the urinary passages, the urine is pale and whey-like, of a density below the average, often considerably so, and the earthy deposit is nearly equally abundant in the night and morning urine.*

I have arranged, in the table before you, the results of some of my observations on several specimens of urine yielding some copious deposits of triple phosphate, and unconnected with calculus or organic disease.

Urine depositing phosphates without organic disease.

Evening urine.				Morning urine.				
Colour.	Density.	Action on litmus.	Deposit.	Colour.	Density.	Action on litmus.	Deposit	Case.
Pale amber	1.029	Neutral.	Prisms of triple phosphates.	Dark amber.	1.031	Neutral.	Red urates.	Gouty dyspepsia.
Normal	1.028	Alkaline.	Ditto.	Normal.	1.025	Acid.	Ditto.	Ditto.
Pale	1.020	Neutral.	Ditto with phosphate of lime.	Pale.	1.025	Ditto.	Uric acid.	Ditto.
Pale	1.022	Neutral.	Nearly all phosphate of lime.	Normal.	1025	Ditto.	Ditto.	Ditto.
Normal	1.028	Barely alkaline.	Prisms and stellæ of phosphate.	Ditto.	1.031	Neutral.	Ditto and scanty prisms of phosphate.	Dyspepsia of intemperance.
Amber	1.025	Acid.	Prisms of phosphate.	Ditto.	1.020	Acid.	None.	Dyspepsia following fatigue.
Amber	1.025	Acid.	Fine stellæ of triple salt.	Ditto.	1.020	Ditto.	Ditto.	Dysmenorrhœa.

In these examples you have an excellent illustration of the fact announced by Berzelius, that phosphates may be abundantly present in some specimens of urine and deficient in others passed within a few hours of the former. We must next investigate the

Cause of the excess of phosphate in the urine.

I shall not here direct your attention to the immediate cause as connected with the particular function involved, as this has been so well and so accurately explained by Dr. Prout in his elegant and valuable work on "Stomach and Urinary Diseases," that I should feel it quite unjustifiable to occupy your time further than to press you to peruse this excellent volume, unless I had far more information to add to what is there laid down on this important subject, than I really possess. The question for me to take up in this place is the one which, as in the case of uric acid and urates, has been of late much neglected, especially by the disciples of Liebig—on the nature of *the ultimate origin of phosphates in the urine.* When we recollect that combinations of magnesia, lime, potass, and ammonia, exist in great abundance in the articles of food yielded by the vegetable kingdom, we at once discover a probable source of much of the phosphates in the urine, and, indeed, in other fluids and solids of the body. It is easy to prove that much more of the phosphatic salts are thus taken into the system than can possibly be got rid of by the urine, which as we have seen contains as a mean 6.5 grains of phosphoric acid in the secretion of 24 hours. We know also that a large amount of phosphatic earthy salts is laid up in the body in the osseous and cartilaginous textures, and in mucous tissues and secretions, as well as in smaller quantity in all the solids and fluids of the animal frame. In addition to this, part of the phosphoric acid of the ingesta exists, combined with oleine as oleo-phosphoric acid, and is an important ingredient of nervous matter of the brain and its extensions; whilst another portion is deoxidised, and exists in this nervous tissue combined with carbon, nitrogen, hydrogen, and oxygen, under the form of a phosphorised fat or cere-

bric acid. The excess of phosphates which escape the assimilative powers of the stomach may be traced in the fæces. Berzelius found in three ounces of human excrement six grains of earthy phosphates (Swedish weights.)

To shew you how amply any excess of phosphates in the secretions may be accounted for by their presence in the ingesta, I have calculated the quantity of these earthy salts which exist in an ounce of ten articles of food from the vegetable, and two from the animal kingdom, taking care to choose for the basis of my calculation those analyses which appear to be most trustworthy.

Proportion of Phosphates in articles of Diet.

Article of Food,	Grains of phosphates in an ounce.	Authority.
Potato (Solanum Tuberosum) . . .	23.56	Liebig.
Pease (Pisum Sativum)	9.26	Braconnot.
Maize (Zea Mays)	7.2	Gorham.
French Bean (Phaseolus Vulgaris) . .	4.7	Braconnot.
Wheat (Triticum Hybernum). . . .	4.77	Liebig.
Beans (Vicia Faba)	4.7	Einhoff.
Lentil (Ervum Lens)	2.736	Ditto.
Rice (Oryza Sativa)	1.92	Braconnot.
Milk	1.2	Liebig.
Artichoke (Helianthus Tuberosus) . .	0.96	Payen & Braconnot.
Tuberous Vetchling (Lathyrus Tuberosus	0.5760	Ditto.
Beef	0.38	Liebig.

From this table you cannot fail to be struck with the enormous quantity of the earthy phosphates which daily enters the stomach with our food; although you must bear in mind that the numbers I have inserted in the tables cannot be taken as absolutely correct; for in most of the analyses I have consulted, the quantities of earthy salts (phosphates, carbonates, sulphates) are placed together, followed by the remark that the salts were "chiefly composed of phosphates," or "nearly all phosphates."

If, for the sake of illustration, we suppose a person makes a hearty meal of bread, meat, and potatoes, we shall find that he is eating a far greater quantity of earthy phosphates than we should have, *à priori*, supposed: thus, if we suppose a meal to consist of

Four ounces of beef	1·52
Do. of wheaten flour made into bread or pudding	19.08
Three ounces of potatoes . .	94·24
	114·84

it is evident that upwards of 114 grains of earthy salts, consisting chiefly of phosphates, would enter the stomach.

It is obvious that another source of the excretion of phosphate in the urine is to be

found in the destructive or secondary assimilation of nervous matter in which phosphorus enters as a component. This view was propounded and illustrated by Dr. Prout long before Professor Liebig's work appeared, although, in common with the prevailing fashion of the day, and forgetful of the merits of our own illustrious countryman, the disciples and followers of Liebig have given the merit of this idea to him. Most, indeed, of this number appear to have been ignorant that a similar view had been announced by Dr. Prout. As the nervous mass must, in common with other tissues of the body, be daily and hourly undergoing a change, fresh matter being deposited and the old absorbed, during which process its particles undergo a secondary assimilation (Prout), or metamorphosis (Liebig), phosphoric acid is generated, and, combining with bases, escapes in the urine.

The discovery of phosphorus as an element of the mass of the brain is due to Vauquelin; and, according to his analysis, it contains 1·5 per cent. of phosphorus. This statement has been verified by many subsequent observers, especially by M. Couerbe, and more recently by Fremy. According to the latter, the nervous matter consists of

Albumen . . . 7
Fat 5
Water 88
————
100

This cerebral fat is a mixture of olein, margarin, oleic, and margaric acids, with cholesterine, oleo-phosphoric, and cerebric acids; the latter being wholly or partly combined with soda (Annalen der Chimie und Physik. Band, 40). The oleo-phosphoric acid is, by boiling, resolved into olcine and phosphoric acid; the cerebric acid is composed of

Carbon . . . 66·7
Hydrogen . . 10·6
Nitrogen . . 2·3
Oxygen . . . 19·5
Phosphorus . . 0·9
————
100·

In addition to this source of phosphoric acid, we must not overlook the fact of the albuminous tissues containing phosphorus, and hence of their affording, by the process of obstructive assimilation, another supply of this element.

Thus far I have endeavoured to point out

to you the probable source of the phosphates of the urine, more especially of the triple salt. But it is evident that phosphates, especially the calcareous combinations, may be discovered in large quantity in the urine, quite independent of any organic or functional lesion of the kidney. In fact, cases not unfrequently occur in which phosphate of lime in particular, less frequently the magnesian salt, is poured out by the mucous membrane of the bladder, mixed with mucus. All mucous secretions contain the phosphoric acid combined with earthy bases, and hence, if an excess of the latter is secreted with the vesical mucus, it may be washed away by the urine, and form a deposit. This is by no means unfrequent in the irritable bladder depending on the irritation of chronic cystitis, prostatic diseases, &c.: we have a perfect analogy to this in the calculous concretions found in the ducts of glands furnishing mucous secretions. These are all prone to secrete phosphates in too great an excess to be washed away with the secretion; they are, therefore, retained, and form a calculus. These, from whatever part of the body they are obtained, present nearly the same composition.

Composition of phosphatic concretions.

Species	Prostatic	Bronchial	Seminal	Salivary	Pancreatic.
Phosphate of lime .	84·5	80·	90·	75·	80·
Carbonate of lime .	·5	2·3	2·	2·	3·
Animal matter . .	15·0	7·7	10·	23·	7·
Authority . . .	Lassaigne	Brandes	Peschier	G. B.	G. B.

At our next meeting I shall conclude my remarks on this class of sediments, and pass to the consideration of those which present evidence of organization.

ON THE HOMOLOGY OF THE FŒTAL CIRCULATION.

By Thomas Williams, M.B.

Tutor on Healthy and Morbid Microscopic Anatomy, at Guy's Hospital.

(*For the London Medical Gazette.*)

It is now a fundamental principle in the science of embryology that the ovum of the mammiferous animal, during the progress of development, exhibits phases of structure which, although transient in duration, present the most remarkable correspondence with types of structure which belong persistently to animals inferior in the scale. It is therefore admitted to be necessary, in order to the attainment of the greatest perfection in the details of organic structure, that nature should first realise the simplest formative idea, and subsequently make advance along the typical gradations of the extended scale which so remotely separates the most simple from the most complex and perfect of living forms. So that if regarded in the light of a universal and abstract law, language of mathematical exactness and precision might be employed in the enunciation of this developmental principle. If the correctness of this be admitted as a general fact, it may be certainly reduced to the definite proposition that the higher organic form is nothing more than a *multiple* of the lower; the highest only a compound multiple of *all* below it; and conversely, the simplest a remote submultiple of the highest.

When thus contemplated, there is confessedly an imposing air of universality about this principle, which may be apparently received as a trium-present proof that physiological science is susceptible of generalisations more extended and comprehensive than any of which the science of inanimate matter is capable. But there are exceptions in the details of its operation, which arise as real objections against the implicit recognition of this law, at all events against its pretensions to universal applicability. It is at present proposed to consider these exceptions with reference only to a few partial particulars.

The analogy is perhaps admissible which physiologists have generally announced between the character of the circulation, as it primitively appears in the vascular lamina of the mammiferous ovum, and the type of the circulating system which obtains as a permanent formation in many of the inferior orders of invertebrate animals. In the succeeding phase the central vessel assumes the higher characters, which distinguish the propulsive apparatus in the circulation of fishes; a simple auricle, and an equally simple ventricle, now constitute the sum of the cardiac centres. A subdivision, or rather a multiplication of the cardiac cavities, subsequently occurs, which exalts the mechanism of the apparatus to the standard of the reptilian type. It must not be supposed that the bulbus arteriosus of fishes, although it composes a third element in the propulsive system, is a true cardiac cavity; or the analogue of the second auricle of the repitilian heart. It is a collateral or superadded provision, made in obvious accordance with the strictest hydraulic principles. The intervention of the branchial capillaries* between the two segments of the circulating system renders necessary the provision of the auxiliary force realised in the aortic bulb. (This is not the occasion on which to shew the physical principles on which this object is accomplished). The same necessities exist in the case of the fœtus of the higher animal; the existence, namely, of a *branchial* circulation, and it is accordingly proved that the same provisions are temporarily made. This is not true in detail of structure, but only in *type*. Let all these be admitted as correct correspondences, which in great

* Certain remarkable peculiarities in the circulation of fishes, which the author has recently proved, will be disc— future number.

probability is a legitimate admission. The process of evolution proceeds. The aortic dilatation contracts, the rudimentary branchiæ disappear, and a second auricle is developed. It is now that the most interesting part of this subject approaches. It is evident that adapting nature has now advanced the organic standard of the new being into an actual parity with the reptilian model; that is, the ventricular segment of the heart consists only of *one* chamber, while the auricular is subdivided into two.

Like the former correlation, this is not exactly true. If the *right* ventricle in the instance of the fœtus were supposed altogether absent, the three remaining chambers would more completely resemble the cardiac system of the reptile; the single ventricle would assume at once the branchial (placental, or pulmonic) and systemic characters. It is quite capable of demonstration that the septum *ventriculorum* occupies a period of four weeks in its completion; its formation commences at the 4th and is completed by the 8th week. The development of the *auricular* septum, however, does not begin until the 10th or 11th week; and is completed about the 3d month. Before the development of the ventricular septum, it is implied that the propulsive segment of the heart consists only of *one* cavity. In regard to the interposition between the two chambers of the auricular partition, in consequence of the persistence of the oval foramen, it is at once seen that no alteration of *type* is produced by its ordinary and incomplete formation. Let it now then be determined what are the real terms of the alleged analogy between the stage of fœtal evolution, which, indeed, continues throughout the term of utero-gestation, and the form of the circulating system which is proper to and permanent in the reptile. In the crocodilian, the highest, as well as the amphibious, the lowest reptile, the arterial stream which returns from the lungs, and the venous current which reflows from the general system, admingle in the common chamber of the ventricle. In the fœtus this admixture happens in the inferior cava; *here* the confluence occurs between the placental and venous streams. The ductus arteriosus in the mammiferous fœtus cannot be viewed as the analogue of that freer communication which exists between imperfectly divided ventricles of the reptilian heart. In the reptile the blood is exactly the same in every part of the circulating system; with the exception only of that returning from the lungs. In the fœtus, on the contrary, there is an appreciable amount of difference between the cephalic and caudal currents; yet the former, which is the more arterial of the two, possesses only mean qualities, or those precisely intermediate between venous and arterial blood, for the placental and caval streams nearly equal each other in magnitude. In relation, however, to the blood which circulates the posterior extremities, it is at once apparent that in nutrient properties it is inferior to the systemic fluid of the really cold-blooded animal.

From a careful examination of the anatomical character and dependence of the Eustachian valve, notwithstanding the opposing experiments of Dr. John Reid, I have recently convinced myself that it is mechanically inefficient as a means for preserving the individuality of the two caval currents as they traverse the chamber of the right auricle; at the period of its diastole, when the auricle has attained a moderate limit of distension, it may be readily demonstrated that the two streams must freely intermingle. It is not true, therefore, that the difference of quality is so considerable as that generally taught by anatomists between the blood distributed to the anterior segment and that circulating the posterior segment of the body in the fœtus.

It must, then, be admitted that while the detailed mechanism of the cardiac apparatus in the mammalian fœtus is strikingly dissimilar from that which is proper to the reptile, the circulating blood in the two instances is, notwithstanding, assimilated by the most striking affinity of character. But if this similarity of property, and organic character, be fundamentally correct, the reflective inquiries at once suggest themselves—How is it, then, that one is cold-blooded and the other warm-blooded? How is it that the heart of one pulsates with double vigour and frequency, while that of the other struggles out its laborious beats with so much slowness; that the temperature of the one exceeds the limits of the maternal heat, while the other sinks to the standard of the surrounding medium? These inquiries suggest the consideration of several analogous and differential conditions. The temperature in the two instances is certainly determined by that of the surrounding element. The fœtus exhibits exactly the same temperature as the internal surface of the uterine walls, and the liquor amnii. In making other observations upon the pregnant rabbit, I have more than once incidentally proved that the thermometer mounts by several degrees when removed from amid the convolutions of the intestines and planted in the interior of the gravid uterus. The uterine parietes generally are unquestionably the scene of great comparative activity of circulation. The interposed layer of the animal fluid offers a favourable medium for the conveyance of the heat thus rapidly generated towards the exterior of the new being. From recent observations, I am disposed to believe that the temperature of the maternal system is elevated altogether during the period of utero-gestation; but that certainly the temperature of the uterus itself is raised beyond that of the abdominal cavity. So far, then, the correlative conditions in the case of the reptile and the fœtus are closely correspondent. But there are now some discrepant points to be adjusted. Notwithstanding the slowness with which the nutrient process proceeds in the two cases, there are striking differences in the comparative velocities of the two circulations. The fœtal heart performs double the strokes of the maternal organ, and considerably more than double the number of the cardiac pulsations in the reptile. It is evident that the surrounding any more than its own proper heat will not account for this multiple of frequency; for if so, its temperature ought to be double that of the mother, which it is not. There must be some other cause, then, for this remarkably augmented frequency in the cardiac pulsations of the fœtus. It is not apparent that the explanative argument can be derived from the greater excitability of the nervous system. Some physiologists, I believe the idea originated with Dr. Hall, have supposed that this double frequency exactly agrees with the idea that the two ventricles contract at alternate times. The two ventricles are known also, to be supplied by two independent and separate arterial streams, although there is but one coronary vein. But suppose this hypothesis positively to embrace the truth—that the systole of the two ventricles is performed at regularly alternate periods—it must of course follow that the pulsations of the cephalic and brachial system of arteries should be exactly one-half the frequency of the beats in the abdominal and crural : since the out-going current in the ascending aorta and its dependent branches can obey *only* the action of the left ventricle, while confessedly the descending stream would acknowledge the *two-fold* agency of the two ventricles. But let the correctness of this view be momentarily admitted, and let us inquire into the necessary results. It appears almost certain that if the undulations in the two fluid columns—that, namely, urged by the right side through the pulmonary artery and arterial duct, and that driven by the left side through the aortic arch—or, to express the fact in more precise language, if the phases of elevation and depression in these two conjugating currents be not exactly coincident, it obviously follows that the resultant stream would be continuous and *unpulsating* in its course ; and this must be the consequence if it be actually true that the ventricular contractions are alternate, and *not contemporaneous*. So that the eccentric conditions would be realised in the system of the fœtus, of a central organ performing 150 pulsations in a minute, the pulmonary artery and ascending aorta and its branches undulating with a frequency of 75 waves in the same period of time, while positively the descending system does not pulsate at all[*]. This might be readily proved by the obstetrician. But I think it will be admitted that its importance scarcely requires a confutation so grave. It is sufficient to remark in disproof, that the arteries of the funis pulsate synchronously with the fœtal heart.

It now becomes plain that the peculiarities of the fœtal circulation must be explained on some sounder and more philosophic principles : and it was not until a comparatively recent period that these principles could be either recognised or applied. Since the late observations of Dr. M. Barry,

---

[*] I have proved that the abdominal aorta of the fish does not properly *pulsate*.

Gulliver, and Wharton Jones, and the subsequent luminous generalizations of Dr. Carpenter, the conclusion appears well founded that in the blood of the young of all vertebrata the colourless corpuscles preponderate over the red particles, this preponderance being the greater as the fœtus is younger. As regards the diminished proportion of the red particles in the fœtal blood, the fact coincides well with the views of Mr. Wharton Jones in relation to their functions—that, namely, of maintaining the excitability of the nervous and muscular systems. But it does not appear that the number of the red corpuscles in the fœtus is exclusively adequate to the efficient maintenance of its known excitability. Müller has proved by direct observation that the blood of the umbilical vein is scarcely or not at all distinguishable in colour from that of the umbilical arteries, and Dr. Carpenter has instituted a comparison between the contents of the placental vessels and the *chyle*—not the pulmonic blood—of the adult animal. It is believed that in equal volumes of reptilian and fœtal blood, a similar proportion of the *coloured* corpuscles would be found ; while in regard to the *colourless* globules they would be far more numerous in the latter. Since the time of Hunter, two principles have become axiomatic in physiology : first, that the red particles are directly in proportion as the energies and demands of the muscular and nervous systems : and secondly, as the volume of oxygen consumed. The diminished proportion of these corpuscles in fœtal blood conforms with, and confirms, these important principles ; the fact likewise affords clear confirmation to the views of Liebig in reference to the functions of the red particles as vehicles simply for the transmission of oxygen from one part of the system to the other ; while it opposes with almost equal force the hypothesis of Dr. Carpenter, which assigns to these remarkable bodies in part the office of elaborating the liquor sanguinis into some higher organic principle, or of converting albumen into fibrine.

From the concurrent weight of these observations, it may be received as most probable that the blood circulating in the placenta receives only a very small comparative volume of oxygen, and it is in intimate agreement with this circumstance to perceive that positively the fœtal economy requires but a very inconsiderable proportion of this element. According to the recent inductions of Liebig, the most direct agency of oxygen consists in that of oxidising *away* the effete materials of the structure.

In the fœtal organism this process of oxidising disentegration is as obscure as the volume of the consumed oxygen is small. It is unquestionable that the most active organic process in the fœtus is that of growth—the constant superposition of nutrient elements—as in old age it is the process of decay. In the former case, therefore, a small supply only of oxygen is required; while in the latter, the disentegration of the fabric being rapid, the consumption of this element must be great. It becomes consequently apparent, that the most important of all conditions to be realised in the fœtal organism must be that of supplying the materials of growth. Then, since neither a great volume of oxygen, nor a great proportion of red particles, is necessary to the accomplishment of this object, a copious provision of either would be certainly superfluous. In conclusion, then, there are several facts with reference to the character of the fœtal circulation to be accounted for. First, the small amount of red particles, entailing a diminished consumption of oxygen. Secondly, the doubly rapid rate of the circulation. Thirdly, the great preponderance of colourless globules. These are peculiarities which belong exclusively to the uterine fœtus of the mammiferous animal.

It is thus shown that there is a want of proportion between the volume of oxygen consumed, the red particles, the amount of the muscular and nervous expenditure, and the rate of the circulation. The generalisations of Hunter, therefore, encounter a striking exception in the laws of the fœtal economy. I believe the real explanation of these interesting circumstances to be contained in the following reasons. The rate of growth appears to be determined, first, by the proportion of the colourless corpuscules, or of fibrine in the liquor sanguinis; secondly, by the rapidity of the circulating stream. These two conditions are eminently realised in the fœtal system, and the consequence of rapid growth is insured.

As already stated, the quantity of oxygen consumed is small, and the red corpuscules exist only in small proportion, so that neither of these agents can contribute much towards the maintenance of this inordinate rate of circulation. But these conditions would be entirely inoperative in the absence of the proper temperature. In the adult this is immediately dependent upon the mutual agency of atmospheric oxygen and the red particles—the organic process, secondary assimilation; and in the fœtus—not by the analogous process of placental respiration—it is in greatest proportion derived from the heat of the medium which it inhabits. It is the comparatively elevated temperature of the uterine parietes and liquor amnii that occasions and maintains the remarkably rapid rate of its circulation.

When the transition is made from the intra-uterine to the atmospheric mode of living, some of these conditions undergo a most complete reversal. This transition is accomplished by the adoption of the most remarkably foresighted precautions against the injurious operation of the altered circumstances into which the new being is thrown. It was while studying the changes which occur in the lungs, when commencing their functions as agents of atmospheric respiration, that these reflections first presented themselves to my mind. At birth, the physiological dangers which immediately affect the child are twofold. First, if the lungs were to suffer complete and perfect distension by the air at the very first act of inspiration, and the process of atmospheric breathing thus to acquire at once its maximum efficiency, it is unquestionably plain that the few red corpuscules at this period in its blood would be inevitably super-oxidised, and even completely disorganised, just as the voltaic fluid transmitted along a small metallic wire breaks up the arrangement of its component atoms, in consequence of the absence of all relation of equality between the bulk or substance of the wire and the calorific agency of the voltaic current; and so, likewise, in the fœtus, the process of growth would be immediately converted into one of rapidly destructive assimilation. These formidable consequences are, however, wonderfully averted by the creation of a mechanical difficulty against the too abrupt and profuse penetration of the ærating element into the remote parenchyma of the lungs. I have proved, on several occasions, that the few first acts of respiration in puppies, pigs, and also in the child, effect no more than the inflation of a few *vesicles only* in different portions of the organ. In proportion as the process is continued, and as the muscular and nervous systems are developed, the pulmonary structure becomes more uniformly distended, and the area of the breathing surface is correspondingly multiplied. The transition, thus, from a cold-blooded to a warm-blooded character, with respect to the properties of the circulating fluid, is accomplished by steps of the most provident and cautious progression.

By the process of analogical reasoning which I have here attempted to institute and follow out, it certainly appears that a very probable and approximative determination may now be made, in regard to the respiratory value of the placental agency. If it be true that atmospheric breathing commences progressively, the inference must be correctly founded, which argues that the amount of placental æration, as performed for a period of given duration immediately *before* birth, must be very nearly equal to the amount of the process of respiration as accomplished by the lungs within the same period immediately *after* birth; and as it is within the range and power of direct observation to establish that it is mechanically impracticable to introduce any other than a small and gradually increasing volume of oxygen into the blood, through the channel of the collapsed and resisting parenchyma of the unexpanded lungs, at this incipient period of ærial existence, it seems quite legitimate to maintain the associated conclusion that the standard of the placental æration is below the type which is proper even to the inferior reptiles. This inferior measure of oxidation appears likewise satisfactorily to account for the remarkable absence of excreta from the fœtal organism; for continued growth, unfettered by the counterpoising forces of decay; for a wisely regulated addition of materials to, without any appreciable subtraction from, the sum of the increasing organism.

———

INFLUENCE OF THE MOON'S RAYS.

———

To the Editor of the Medical Gazette.

SIR,

IN your valuable periodical of the 24th of February, I noticed with great pleasure an article by Mr. Thompson, on the supposed influence of the moon's rays as a cause of disease in tropical climates, which so closely agrees with the view I had taken of the subject that I feel inclined to offer a few remarks in support of the same.

During an intertropical voyage, I frequently heard from the seamen of all grades long accounts of the dangers of sleeping on deck in the moon's rays; such as being struck moon-blind, palsy of the face, &c. These accidents, I explained, arose, not from the rays of the moon, but from the quantity of moisture in the atmosphere, which is much greater in strong moonlight nights than otherwise; and, of course, a person sleeping in the open air at such a time would be liable to attacks of the kind.

This I constantly maintained was the only cause, and that the rays of the moon had no more to do with it "than the man in the moon:" but I found no converts to my theory; nobody believed a word about it. Again, it was said that meat exposed to the moon's rays during the night would be found putrefied in the morning, and full of maggots. This I also contradicted and proved to be erroneous by the following conclusive experiment. I hung up at night a piece of fresh mutton exposed to the rays of the moon, and, at the same time, another piece in the shade away from its influence; both these pieces, in the morning, presented exactly the same appearances, rather tainted, but no maggots, and not different from what we would expect to find meat in the tropics, where it will not keep sweet more than four-and-twenty hours.

When sailors see a man asleep on deck in a moonlight night, they invariably throw something over his face to screen it from the moon's rays, and prevent the ill consequences supposed to be caused by them. This it certainly might do, but on a different principle: for by covering the person he would not be so likely to take cold from the dampness of the atmosphere, which is the real cause of these pretended moon-strokes. However, it is difficult to overcome a prejudice so deeply rooted, not only amongst seamen, but also amongst very intelligent persons, many of whom I have frequently heard maintain the same erroneous opinion : but "magna est veritas, et prevalebit," The moon's rays have no more to do with it than the moon was supposed by the ancients to influence the catamenial periods ; but as people who have slept exposed to the rays of the moon are frequently found affected in various ways, the conclusion naturally come to by an unscientific observer would be that those diseases were caused by the rays ; and I think, therefore, that the clear and rational explanation of such phenomena, given by Mr. Thompson, cannot be too widely diffused and made known, so as to overthrow a very general popular error, which, I believe, has never before been treated and explained in a manner so able and satisfactory.

I am, sir,

Your obedient servant,

J. BERNCASTLE, M.R.C.S. &c.

London, March 13, 1843.

ON PRIMARY

CANCEROUS DEGENERATION AND ULCERATION OF THE LUNG.

BY D. MACLACHLAN, M.D.

Physician to the Royal Hospital, Chelsea.

(*For the Medical Gazette.*)

PRIMARY cancer of the lung is, I believe, very generally an obscure affection, and even in secondary cases the disease is frequently latent, remaining altogether unsuspected. This obscurity has arisen, in a great measure, from the want of carefully recorded cases, the occasional absence of local symptoms, neglect of the physical signs, or, where these have been noted, their reference to other sources of common occurrence producing similar signs and symptoms, and, by their frequency, exciting little interest in the observer. A post-mortem examination is then, perhaps, omitted, and the case passes away without the true nature of the disease being discovered.

Until the appearance of Laennec's immortal work on Auscultation, very little was known of malignant diseases of the lung. They seem to have been regarded as almost, if not always, secondary affections, and in our own country, so late as 1825, Mr. Wardrop, in his edition of Baillie's Works, vol. 2, p. 67-68, says, "melanoid, hæmathoid, and scirrhus tubercle, when they attack the lungs, appear only as a secondary form of the disease."

There can be no doubt that *primary* cancer of the lung is rare : very few cases are recorded, and whether primarily or secondarily affecting the lungs, the ulceration of cancerous depositions in this situation is still of less frequent occurrence.

Much as we owe Laennec, it is to subsequent writers that we are chiefly indebted for the information we possess on this subject, and to none is the profession under greater obligations than to Dr. Stokes. The work of this eminent physician, on the Diagnosis and Treatment of the Diseases of the Respiratory Organs, published in 1837, contained all the knowledge we had then acquired of the nature of cancer and fungoid disease of the lung. Since then fresh facts have been collected, and a valuable paper published by Dr. Hughes in Guy's Hospital Reports for 1841, details several interesting cases, while the works of Hodgkin, Walshe, and the instructive lecture by Dr. Taylor, in the Lancet for March 1842, give much additional information.

Dr. Stokes has been carefully investigating the subject since his volume issued from the press, and we have the results of his labours in an interesting memoir which is inserted in the Dublin Journal of Medical Science, for May 1842. Those who are desirous of arriving at " the actual state of our knowledge of the history of thoracic cancer" will consult this memoir, and the work of Dr. Walshe, " On the Physical Diagnosis of the Lungs," with great advantage.

These reflections have been suggested by the occurrence of a case of *primary cancerous degeneration, and ulceration* of the *whole* of the right lung, which has recently been under my care in the infirmary of this establishment, the account of which may be considered a contribution to the history and pathology of intra-thoracic cancer; and, as the case presented some peculiarities, it may probably assist the future observer in forming a diagnosis of what may very generally be still regarded as an obscure affection.

J. H., æt. 62, was admitted into the infirmary of this hospital, on the 4th of October 1842, complaining of a very frequent dry cough, difficulty of breathing, especially in the recumbent posture, and general debility. For several weeks before admission he had been attending the dispensary attached to the infirmary, with these symptoms, which had been gradually and progressively increasing from their commencement. He had derived no benefit from the means employed, and passed restless nights, in a sitting posture, with a teazing, tickling dry cough, unaccompanied with pain in the chest, or fever. The face was sallow, and, particularly about the eye-lids, occasionally œdematous. The urine was said to be scanty. He came under my observation on the 9th of the month.

Physical signs.—At this period, the 9th of October, the left side of the chest sounded clear on percussion, and the respiratory murmur was puerile, without râles of any description. The right side was dull all over, but not unequivocally so in the mammary region, and the respiratory murmur, feeble throughout, in some places extinct, was accompanied with an occasional muco-crepitating ronchus along the spine.

No impression was made on the symptoms by medicine. He continued to pass almost sleepless nights with the cough, and the difficulty of breathing forced him to sit half erect in bed, the cough and dyspnœa increasing on his assuming any other position. On the 28th of October, I made a careful examination of the chest, having hitherto found it impossible to satisfy myself as to the precise or even probable nature of the case. This examination, though conducted with great exactitude, and with every attention to the symptoms and collateral circumstances, left me almost equally in doubt and uncertainty.

The dulness on percussion had progressively increased. By this time it was perfect, particularly in the posterior regions of the chest, and the walls resisted the fingers. Respiration had entirely ceased in the lung, and though there continued a slight vocal resonance along the base of the right scapula, it was much less marked than on the opposite side; and no vibration

whatever was communicated on applying the hand. The right side appeared to move *en masse;* the upper intercostal spaces remained natural, neither sunken nor prominent; posteriorly and inferiorly they were less marked. Mensuration detected no difference, but, to the eye, the upper part of the right side was contracted in its anteroposterior diameter, while lower down it was fuller, bulging considerably posteriorly. The right hypochondrium projected, and elicited a dull sound, for two or three inches beyond the ribs, on percussion. No enlarged veins were observed on the chest or abdomen; both jugulars were of natural size, probably a little dilated. The heart's action was normal, and unaccompanied with any murmur. No note was taken of the extent of the sounds, or whether more audible on the right than the left side. The pulse at the wrists was regular but feeble. There was no difficulty in swallowing until two or three days at most before death, and the patient's appetite was but little impaired. He had passed less urine lately. The constant teazing dry cough, and the difficulty of breathing, were the only symptoms of which he complained, and he was still free from any pain in the chest.

From the period of this examination no perceptible change took place in the physical signs: the respiration remained extinct, with diminished vocal resonance; total absence of vibratory sensation on applying the hand to the right side, and universal dulness on percussion; while, on the opposite side, the respiration was puerile, and the resonance natural. The cough, hitherto dry, was at length occasionally accompanied with a scanty brownish mucous expectoration. At no period was there hæmoptysis. On the 7th of November, he, for the first time, complained of uneasiness, scarcely amounting to pain, in the right side of the chest. His face was now generally swollen, especially in the morning, and the conjunctivæ were congested. About this time his wrists and hands became œdematous, and by the 16th the œdema had extended up the arms to the shoulders. The œdema advanced rapidly, extended over the chest, but never affected the lower extremities. He was now wholly confined to bed. On the 18th, his countenance was fearfully altered; the eyes, congested, projected from their sockets; and both arms, enormously swollen, equalled the thighs in circumference. The dyspnœa and cough had increased in proportion. The poor man sat doubled up in bed, his chest resting on his knees, or, turned over on the right side, he sought in vain for relief to his breathing, supporting himself, in this position, with his face on the pillow. His intellects remained clear. At length, exhausted by his suffering, he suddenly expired on the morning of the 22d November, probably about three months from the commencement of the disease.

Anatomical appearances thirty hours after death.

The whole of the right side of the chest was filled with a firm unyielding mass, pushing the liver two or three inches below the margins of the ribs, and adhering so strongly to all the neighbouring structures that it was found impossible to detach it without a tedious dissection, and the attempt to remove the whole lung was abandoned. That portion exposed on raising the sternum presented a rose tint. Cut into at any part, the knife penetrated innumerable excavations, varying in size from a pea to a walnut. These cavities, universally disseminated throughout the lung, were, for the most part, filled with a thick, yellow, fœtid, diffluent pus; others contained thin sanious offensive matters, while a third set, and these were fewest in number, were occupied with a whitish 'pultaceous substance, resembling softened brain. The walls of these various cavities were ragged, broken down, and not lined with any membrane. At the root of the lung, encroaching on the heart, and adhering firmly to the pericardium, there was a large, dense, white, knotty substance, surrounding the vena cava superior, compressing it and the right bronchus, and almost obliterating the right branch of the pulmonary artery. This firm tumor resisted the knife, and the incised surface, of a white colour, presented a fibrous texture resembling true scirrhus. From the cut surfaces there exuded, on pressure, a creamy fluid appearing in drops at various points. Immediately contiguous to this scirrhus mass, the abscesses observed in other portions of 'the lung were here of diminished size;

the nearer the surface, the larger these appeared to be; and where the lugy could be traced it was of a deep green colour. Several enlarged bronchial glands, filled with black carbonaceous matter, adhered firmly to the tumor, and two or three melanotic tubercles were immediately adjacent.

The left side of the chest contained a large quantity of clear serum. The lung itself was perfectly healthy, crepitating, free from adhesions, and the pleura was without any trace of inflammation.

Nothing particular was observed in the heart. The right ventricle was probably a little dilated. As above stated, the right branch of the pulmonary artery was greatly compressed, and nearly flattened.

The liver projected several inches below the ribs, was pale, but, together with the remaining viscera of the abdomen, appeared sound. Excepting in the right lung nothing like cancer existed in any other part of the body; and all the organs but the brain were minutely examined.

REMARKS.—It is not my intention to occupy the reader's time with a lengthened analysis of this important case. The main objects I have had in view are to record the facts relating to the symptoms and physical signs, as far as they were observed, and the morbid alterations exhibited on postmortem examination.

Until far advanced, the case was exceedingly intricate : I had, besides, laboured under the disadvantage of never having seen a case of primary cancer of the lung, where it was settled beyond dispute by subsequent examination. Various opinions were formed, and I never could satisfy myself of their correctness; nor were others able to determine the precise cause of the various phenomena. There were no external tumors, no enlarged or varicose veins on the chest or abdomen; there was no hæmoptysis, and several signs and symptoms of malignant degeneration of the lung were absent. The disease had evidently made considerable progress before the man came under hospital treatment; and on admission it was obvious that the greater portion of the lung was condensed. Extinct here and there, and feeble throughout, the respiratory murmur was accompanied, at the root of the lung, with a muco-crepitating ronchus; and the almost universal dulness on percussion, with the incessant dry cough, led to the opinion that this consolidation proceeded either from tubercles or chronic pneumonia. The rarity of the latter, and the frequency of the former, inclined me to the belief that the case was one of a class sometimes met with, in which, for a long time, only one lung is the seat of crude tubercles. The physical signs, however, together with the general symptoms and history, were, as regards either of these affections, incomplete, and gave other indications. At a more advanced stage the case was almost equally obscure. The total extinction of the respiratory murmur in the lung, the unequivocal and universal dulness, the absence of vibratory fremitus, the descent of the diaphragm and consequent displacement of the liver, the detrusion of the side, and the increasing œdema, all indicated effusion into the chest. There was, however, no obliteration of the upper intercostal spaces, such as would likely have existed had there been effusion sufficient to push down the diaphragm and dilate the chest. The œdema was limited to the face, chest, and upper extremities, and there was still some vocal resonance along the base of the right scapula—a sign, however, comparatively, of less value. The general symptoms were not more decisive than those afforded by auscultation and percussion. There was little or no pain in the chest; the patient never complained of any until pointedly asked the question, and then not until the lung had acquired increased bulk, and pressed in every direction. The cough, almost dry, throughout the progress of the case, and the difficulty of breathing, might have arisen from many causes: in themselves they were little to be depended upon; but, in connection with other phenomena, they yielded negative information. The difficulty of swallowing did not occur till a few days before dissolution; but, as the œdema was confined to the upper extremities, it appeared more than probable that this symptom proceeded from interrupted circulation, and that the seat of the obstruction was somewhere about the superior vena cava. No stethoscopic signs of disease of the heart existed, and

in what this obstruction consisted was questionable. That it arose from cancerous disease of the lung was not improbable, though this opinion was merely conjectural, and formed negatively on a review of the case, and on excluding other diseases with which it was earlier confounded.

The rapid progress of the case is worthy of observation. Although, on presentation, the lung appeared to be extensively consolidated, in about a fortnight afterwards there was perfect and universal dulness on percussion, and all respiration had ceased to be heard. It is very probable that the original seat of the disease was at the root of the lung, that the main bronchial tubes had very soon become obliterated; and this, together with the compression of the right bronchus, accounts for the absence of blowing and cavernous respiration, cavernous gurgling, as well as the total extinction of the vibratory fremitus. The absence of these phenomena is an important feature of the case.

The effusion into the left cavity of the chest was very recent. A physical examination was not made for some days before the death of the patient. As to the treatment, it is needless to state that all means were quite unavailing. Sleep was sometimes procured by opiates. Ether seemed to aggravate the dyspnœa. A drastic purgative had, on one or two occasions, a surprising effect in diminishing the œdema; but the cough and difficulty of breathing were hardly ever alleviated.

MEDICAL GAZETTE.

Friday, March 31, 1843.

" Licet omnibus, licet etiam mihi, dignitatem
Artis Medicæ tueri ; potestas modo veniendi in
publicum sit, dicendi periculum non recuso."
                    CICERO.

COMBINATION.

WHOEVER pays much attention to passing events, must have noticed the remarkable tendency to combination, for different purposes, which prevails on all sides at the present day, and so extensively as to be a leading and characteristic feature of our time. Our own countrymen, whose mental and bodily vigour has enabled them to recognise the value, and labour for the adoption, of whatever can be applied to good purposes, seem to have bestowed more attention on this new element, and made larger use of it, than any nation in the world.

To those who live in London, the number of associations for the promotion of every thing good, and the suppression of every thing evil, has an appearance rather ludicrous than otherwise. The eye is fatigued, and the heart hardened, by the placarding system so profusely adopted by well-intentioned committees. Our city is like a vast fair, where so many dramas are being acted at the same time, that the *bills* we read lose all attraction.

To see the effects of combination where they are most evident, we should watch them in a village, in the small branches of large associations. If possible, we should have no personal interest or acquaintance with the places or the people. The process is, then, about as instructive and certainly as fanciful as zootomy; or, as the objects are small, though the actions are intense, it is zoomicroscopic, showing an exaggeration like that of a frog's foot under natural and unnatural stimuli. It is not that persons of conflicting interests all hate each other with a more perfect hatred in villages than in cities, but they are brought into more immediate opposition. Mr. A. cannot gain, or lose a patient, without directly affecting the interests of Mr. B. of that ilk. The large vessels of the body lie side by side in great comfort, though working in different directions; if one presses for a time on the other, a good deal of disturbance takes place certainly, but if a chill or a heat, a stagnation, or an *error loci*, take place in the capillaries, the mischief is organic as far as it goes,

and takes longer to repair too; for a dyspepsy or a plethora disperses more quickly than a nævus or even a pimple.

Voluntary combination cannot exist without more or less equality among the members; their need of each other's support, by labour or capital, by patronage or sufferage, must be real and reciprocal; this is a simple fact; the mere act of combining is often held to be a proof of equality—this is a mistake. The combination which seems to shew the least of equality, viz. between the great and small, rich and poor, employer and employed; in fact, one of the strongest of all; for their wants and dependence are mutual; so are their will and power to supply those wants. Equality is often assumed, or taken for granted, for the mere purpose of effecting combination where it does not really exist, and this of course is a fiction; but the fact, the mistake, and the fiction, exist together in nearly all voluntary combinations; the first, which is the real element of strength, will be found to depend on the combination being one of real unity, and not of uniformity—unity of interest and of purpose, and consequently of plan and of method. The plan and method, indeed, may differ almost entirely, if real unity of interest and purpose exist. The cohesive force will be sufficient to sustain severe pressure, and to do much work. But the mere uniformity of plan and method cannot bear severe pressure, nor do any work at all. It may present a fair surface, and a broad one, but not a solid nor a strong one. Combinations for purely charitable purposes, or for mutual assurance, can only be strong, permanent, and effective, in proportion as the unity of design and interest is carried out; and if this be really effected, the methods are comparatively unimportant. A hospital or an assurance-office, so defective in principle, or so ill worked, as not to afford relief to sickness, nor security to property, would fall to pieces though not a harsh word were ever heard among the managers. But hospitals and companies do flourish whose board-rooms sorely try the tempers of their managers and governors, so long as there be no *malapraxis* in the wards, or errors in the calculations. But an inefficient medical officer, or a defect in the interest table, will do more harm than half a score of irritable governors.

When earnest men are seen clinging with bigoted tenacity to a particular method of reform or conservancy, making the adoption of a single term the test of approval and fellowship, it may be suspected, if not asserted, that there is more of uniformity than of unity in the combination for which they strive.

There are two principal causes which induce men to unite into brotherhood, or societies for effecting specific objects. One is, the sense of an evil to be removed, a weight to be lifted from themselves, which is too heavy for their private exertions; the other is a strong impulse originating from vivid impressions on the mind of a single individual, and thence communicated to numbers; but, however humiliating it may appear, most of the great social efforts which have agitated the world are traceable to what may well be termed despair or enthusiasm. To have effected what they did effect, these movements must have been produced, and the resulting systems sustained by materials of the firmest texture, and when decay has overtaken them, their solidity can be inferred from the ruins which they have left. No human fabric, material or social, is proof against time and force; there is grandeur in the fall as in the elevation of what is really gigantic, but mere aggregations of material, however bulky, of parts however numerous, can excite no other feeling than contempt when wanting in grandeur of design and solidity of material.

How very few of the associations which have been lately formed have possessed these essential characters—how many are unknown for any useful purposes beyond the precincts of the committee-room. It really seems as if the soundness and efficiency of the whole were inversely as the bustle and tumult at the centre: a really working association is tranquil and dignified at the seat of government, lively and energetic in its distant parts, every member living, feeling, acting, not by convulsive throbs of the centre organ, audible to the by-standers, but by the steady unnoticed current of vigorous health.

It is curious how much of righteous self-discipline, of sound wisdom, is required before men can act together in large numbers with energy and effect. That many fail is most true and lamentable, but that very many are making praiseworthy efforts is matter of sincere rejoicing. It is no small attainment in self-government for a man to sit out a debate of two hours without yielding to the conviction that what he has to say on the subject is better worth hearing than the discourse of his neighbour; the act of speaking one at a time is not attained without labour, nor practised without difficulty. It is a very great attainment to be silent, to go on patiently storing up facts which others may use more than ourselves — to be establishing premises that others may draw inferences, to hand water from the well of truth, that others may quench the flames of error. There are some very well-meaning persons who honestly advocate the extinction of quackery and medical heresy, and other flagrant evils, by act of parliament, and until the authorized brigade shall arrive with its well-appointed engines each man runs hither and thither to dash his bucket of indignation on the flames he would extinguish; much smoke and hissing are thereby produced, and no little confusion, the well-meaning neighbours getting sadly in each other's way; but what is worse, they forget that

> ———"Water thrown on fire
> By sprinkling does but raise it higher."

So, too, the counter-practice of the druggist, fanned and fed by the prescriptions of the physician, threatens to consume and scorch up the general practitioner. Shall we, then, establish a quarantine to ward off the sick from their abodes, and draw a *cordon sanitaire* round each unqualified blue light? shall we hold meetings, and appoint committees of licensed men who have no practice, to watch and report the proceedings of those who have too much? We think not. We would rather say, convert your day-books into records of symptoms; your ledgers into case-books; and your long bills for draughts and powders into commentaries on the bills of mortality; and the enlightened chymist will be your professional ally; the mere retailer of patent medicines, sweetmeats, and cigars, will no longer be confounded with yourselves—he will have his own gains, but not yours.

VACCINE REPORT.

To the Right Hon. the Secretary of State for the Home Department.

IN making another annual report of the progress of vaccination, we are happy to be able to state that a farther experience of that great resource has confirmed our confidence in it.

Wherever vaccination has been practised carefully, and with those precautions which experience has pointed out as necessary, it has been followed almost universally with success. But we lament it, as one of the proofs of the general reliance of medical practitioners in its efficacy as a preservative, that it has been deferred too frequently until the seeds of small-pox have been received into the system and about to produce their natural consequences.

This Board has manifested the propriety of its establishment and maintenance by having never failed to produce efficacious vaccine lymph when called for. This is universally acknowledged to have been a resource in the most urgent circumstances.

HENRY HALFORD—President of the Board.
ARTHUR WHITE—President of the College of Physicians.
HENRY HOLLAND—Senior Censor.
CLEMENT HUE—Registrar.
March 13, 1843.

NOTE IN REPLY TO

DR. GRIFFITH'S REMARKS ON THE BLOOD AND FIBRE.

BY MARTIN BARRY, M.D. F.R.SS.L. & E.

DR. MARTIN BARRY presents his respects to the Editor of the MEDICAL GAZETTE, and requests that he will have the kindness to insert the inclosed, from the Lancet, in reply to the remarks of Dr. Griffith, reprinted in last week's number of the MEDICAL GAZETTE from the Annals and Magazine of Natural History.

London, 27 iii. mo. (March), 1843.

I have to acknowledge the courtesy shown in the remarks of Dr. Griffith, and regret that his opinions differ so widely from my own; but am compelled to say I find nothing in his communication that alters in any particular my views, or that requires more than *general* notice at my hands.

"The appearances observed by Dr. Barry in the blood," which Dr. Griffith thinks were "misinterpreted," I cannot suppose that Dr. Griffith ever *saw*; if I may judge from the description he has given, that they are, however, visible, is proved by the following description given by another, who did see the appearances in question. Whether they have been "misinterpreted" the future may determine.

"Bristol, Aug. 19, 1842.

"Dr. Barry has pointed out to me, among the corpuscles of newt's blood preserved in their own serum, without any re-agent having been applied to them, many which had the form of a flask with a projecting neck, or which might be still better compared to the body of a pair of bellows, with its projecting nozzle. The projecting portion appeared to be a filament, having a much higher refracting power than the general substance of the corpuscle. He also showed me, in a portion of blood to which corrosive sublimate had been added, a corpuscle which was evidently destitute of the ordinary nucleus, and which contained what appeared to be a filament, which presented transverse markings that resembled those of muscular fibrillæ, the interspaces being oblique. The appearance resembled that of Dr. Barry's Fig. 9 β (Phil. Trans., 1842, plate v.), except that there was no trace of nucleus.

(Signed) " W. B. CARPENTER."

My preparations of muscle have been seen by many, to whom I could refer for their opinions regarding them. Among our own countrymen may be mentioned Robert Brown, D.C.L., and Professors Owen and Sharpey, besides the gentlemen from whom I have received the testimonials at foot. To the kindness of Professor Sharpey I am indebted for the beautiful preparation of muscle from the tail of the tadpole mentioned by Dr. Griffith. The following note was sent me by one who had closely examined that preparation :—

" 6, Holles Street, Cavendish Sq.
            "Oct. 12, 1842.

" My dear sir,—On returning home to-day, after seeing your exquisite preparations of muscular tissue, I was anxious to express my thanks for your kindness and patience in exhibiting the series to me. I went to your house by no means prepared to admit the existence of the spiral fibre; on the contrary, somewhat prepossessed against such a theory ; for while I had already made up my mind as to the non-existence of the discs advocated in Mr. Bowman's very ingenious paper in the Philosophical Transactions, I had not been able to bring my belief to the idea of substituting a spiral thread or fibre to account for the peculiar markings on the muscular fasciculi. You have, however, convinced me, for in several instances I was enabled to follow the spiral thread round its axis, and to see the continuity of both sides of the chain. In one or two instances I observed it drawn out or separated so far as not to leave a doubt of its reality. In the same way I distinctly recognised the double spiral (especially in one preparation, where the two spirals had not an equal oblique), and I can conceive that the longitudinal lines or fibrillated appearance of the larger fasciculi depends upon the even juxta-position of many minute spirals.

" The reason, probably, I had failed in previously making out this structure resulted from my expectation of seeing this appearance throughout the whole length of a filament ; but I now observe how minute is the care necessary to separate parts, and how small often is the portion favourably situated or sufficiently isolated to admit of a distinct view of this curious structure. There are,

also, many circumstances connected with the different refrangibility of objects, of great importance in explaining why a spiral fibre should be so much more easily seen in one tissue than another ; and thus it is that reagents are often most usefully applied where different parts of the same object refract the light nearly equally. I think, through your help, I have at last settled my belief as to the true character of the markings of muscle, and for which I beg you to accept the thanks of your's faithfully,

(Signed) " JOHN DALRYMPLE."

" To Martin Barry, M.D."

The following, connected with the same subject, was received from Dr. Carpenter, bearing the same date as his testimonial above given :—

" I have this day had the opportunity, through Dr. Barry's kindness, of examining several of his preparations of muscular fibre, especially those from the heart of the turtle and from the shrimp. I have distinctly seen single spiral threads continuous with fasciculi ; in one or two instances so little elongated as to resemble a corkscrew, in others drawn out more or less straightly. In several fibrillæ, which had been isolated without disturbance of their structure, I have seen appearances closely corresponding with those represented by Dr. Barry in figs. 52 and 56 of his last paper (Phil. Trans., 1842). I may add, that I have seen these appearances even more distinctly under my own microscope, which is furnished with one of Powell's latest 1-16th objectives, than under Dr. Barry's instrument, in which lower powers were used.

(Signed) " WILLIAM B. CARPENTER."

The microscope I use is one of Schick's achromatics, similar to those employed by Professors Ehrenberg, Schwann, and R. Wagner. On this subject I cannot refer to a higher authority than that of Joseph Jackson Lister, who, after a close examination, describes my deeper object-glasses as " very finely corrected every way."

MEDICAL MEETING IN SURREY.

ON Friday the 24th instant, March, 1843, the General Practitioners of the County of Surrey assembled at the Coffee House at Epsom, to consider whether any steps should be taken, relative to measures in contemplation, to regulate the general medical profession.

There were present, practitioners of Epsom, Ewell, Chertsey, Weybridge, Guildford, Godalming, Dorking, Leatherhead, Reigate, Croydon, Carshalton, and other places : Mr. Martin, of Reigate, in the chair.

Whereupon, after mature deliberation, it was proposed by Wallace, of Carshalton, and seconded by Mr. Fletcher, of Croydon, and resolved unanimously,

That under present circumstances it is advisable, *without delay*, to petition both Houses of Parliament on the contemplated legislation respecting the medical profession, and that the following petition to the House of Commons be adopted :—

To the Honourable the Commons of the United Kingdom of Great Britain and Ireland, in Parliament assembled.

The humble Petition of the undersigned, Practitioners of Medicine, Surgery, and Midwifery, or, as they are usually denominated, " General Practitioners of Medicine," residing in the County of Surrey,

Sheweth,

That your Petitioners, assuming that the great body of the General Practitioners are the advisers, in ordinary, of by far the largest portion of the population of the country, it is of essential importance that they should be thoroughly qualified as skilful and able advisers.

And, understanding that measures are in contemplation for reforming and regulating the profession generally, are well assured that no reform can be effectual, or permanent, unless, while it provides for the qualifications, efficiency, and respectability of the profession, it shall also be adapted to the wants of the public, as demonstrated by the universal practice of appealing in all ordinary cases to the skill and care of the General Practitioner.

That the supply of an adequately qualified class of General Practitioners is of national importance, must be felt by every observing and reflecting person ; and that a legislative re-organization of the profession, your humble Petitioners conceive to be of indispensable necessity, from several causes ; and among others, from the various and incongruous modes by which Medical Practitioners procure admission into the profession; there being no less than sixteen different sources, from which certificates may be obtained.

Your Petitioners therefore pray, that on this as well as on other grounds of incongruity and inconsistency in the polity of the Profession, your Honourable House would cause inquiry to be made into the present state of the Medical Profession, and more especially in reference to that of the General Practitioners, in number *ten or twelve thousand*, or perhaps more ; delaying any legislative measure, which might lead to the granting of new Charters to the Colleges of Physicians and Surgeons, until the whole subject of medical regulation and reform has been well and thoroughly investigated by a Committee of your Honourable House, and has undergone adequate discussion in Parliament.

Proposed by Mr. Fletcher, seconded by Mr. J. Wallace, and resolved unanimously,

That one of the Surrey Members be respectfully requested to present the Petition to the House of Commons ; and that the other Members for Eastern and Western Surrey be also requested to favour the Petitioners with their support on the occasion.

Proposed by Mr. Bottomley, seconded by Mr. Nash, and resolved unanimously,

That his Grace the Duke of Richmond be respectfully requested to present the Petition to the House of Peers.

Proposed by Mr. Chaldecott, seconded by Mr. Harcourt, and resolved unanimously,

That a Committee be appointed to observe the proceedings of Parliament and the Government on the subject of medical legislation, to consist of nine Practitioners, with power to add to their number, and to call other General Meetings if they should deem it expedient so to do.

Proposed by Mr. Eager of Ripley, seconded by Mr. Hart, and resolved unanimously,

That members of the Medical Profession be recommended to endeavour to call the attention of Members of both Houses of Parliament to the subject of the legislative regulation of the profession—on the importance of the general practitioners to the health and welfare of the community—and on their present position.

Proposed by Mr. Shelley, seconded by Mr. Bottomley, and resolved unanimously,

That the best thanks of the present meeting are due to Sir James Clark, Bart., for his judicious and able Tracts on the education of Medical Men, and on Medical Polity, in the form of two letters, addressed to the Right Hon. Sir James Graham, Bart., her Majesty's Secretary of State for the Home Department ; and this meeting recommends those letters to the careful perusal of every Medical Man in the kingdom. Also, that a copy of this resolution be sent to Sir James Clark. Adjourned.

ALBERT NAPPER, of Guildford, *Sec.*

REDUCTION OF A PROLAPSUS UTERI

AFTER SIXTEEN YEARS' CONTINUANCE.

M. DURANT records an interesting case of this in the Transactions of the Medical Society of Ghent. The wound protruding beyond the external parts, and covered by the inverted vagina, presented a globular tumor, round and contracted at its origin into the form of a circular appendix. The *os uteri* was clear at its inferior part. The tumor at its middle part was fifteen and a half inches in circumference. Its external surface was brownish red, and covered with crusts and ulcerations. The long continuance of the affection had seriously injured the general health of the patient—she was pale and emaciated, and subject to sleeplessness, and cramps of the stomach.

M. Durant, before attempting reduction, kept the patient on light diet, and at rest in bed in a proper position ; at the same time dressing the tumor with opiated emollient fomentations. Its surface speedily softened, and the crusts fell off, leaving superficial sores. After six days of this treatment, the operation was performed. It having been ascertained that the rectum and bladder were empty, the patient was placed in the position most advantageous for the entrance of the womb. M. D. then introduced the right forefinger into the os uteri, and burying it, pushed upwards in the axis of the tumor, which itself was placed in the axis of the true pelvis—then retaining the uterus in its place with the left hand, withdrew the finger, and, repeating this manipulation with gentleness, just as one turns the finger of a glove outside in, accomplished the reduction in less than half an hour. He then inserted into the vagina a sponge, cut into the form of a cylinder, and saturated with an emollient decoction, the thick end being highest up, and a cord attached to the other, for the purpose of removing it at pleasure. This sponge-pessary was retained in its place by means of compresses, and the T bandage. The patient did well, speedily gaining flesh and strength. During the after-treatment, which continued for about six weeks, emollient and astringent lotions were employed, and an ordinary-sized caoutchouc ring-shaped pessary was used, the saturated sponge and the injections being passed through its centre.— *Journ. de Méd. et de Chirurg. Prat.*

MEDICAL & CHIRURGICAL SOCIETY.

To the Editor of the Medical Gazette.

SIR,

IN the history of almost all societies, whether formed for the cultivation and extension of science or for other purposes, it may be observed that *pari passu* with the prosperity of such institutions, advances a tendency to jobbing and favoritism in their management.

The Royal Medical and Chirurgical Society, I am afraid, is about to add another example to the already long list of mismanagements. Not to take up your time with other examples, let me notice that, although the Royal Medical and Chirurgical Society purports to admit as fellows, medical men of all classes, whether physicians, surgeons, or Apothecaries, there appears in the list of

council, the name of but one surgeon practising generally.

Now, I am not aware of any cause for such departure from the originally intended tripartite character of the society, except, as I before stated, rank favoritism and jobbing. Again, in the list of vice-presidents is to be found the name of a member elected only in 1840, in whose favour many older and equally worthy members have been passed over and neglected.—I am, sir,

Your obedient servant,
JUSTITIA.

March 4, 1843.

A TABLE OF MORTALITY FOR THE METROPOLIS,

Shewing the number of deaths from all causes registered in the week ending Saturday, March 18, 1843.

Small Pox	10
Measles	15
Scarlatina	21
Hooping Cough	60
Croup	8
Thrush	2
Diarrhœa	2
Dysentery	3
Cholera	0
Influenza	3
Typhus	30
Erysipelas	2
Syphilis	3
Hydrophobia	0
Diseases of the Brain, Nerves, and Senses	151
Diseases of the Lungs and other Organs of Respiration	357
Diseases of the Heart and Blood-vessels	14
Diseases of the Stomach, Liver, and other Organs of Digestion	53
Diseases of the Kidneys, &c.	4
Childbed	7
Ovarian Dropsy	0
Disease of Uterus, &c.	2
Rheumatism	5
Diseases of Joints, &c.	2
Ulcer	0
Fistula	2
Diseases of Skin, &c.	0
Diseases of Uncertain Seat	100
Old Age or Natural Decay	92
Deaths by Violence, Privation, or Intemperance	17
Causes not specified	0
Deaths from all Causes	**995**

METEOROLOGICAL JOURNAL.

Kept at EDMONTON, Latitude 51° 37′ 32″ N. Longitude 0° 3′ 51″ W. of Greenwich.

March 1843.	THERMOMETER.		BAROMETER.	
Wednesday 22	from 45 to 58		29·36 to	29·39
Thursday . 23	46	55	29·40	29·53
Friday . . 24	46	61	29·53	29·68
Saturday . 25	39	54	29·72	29·66
Sunday . . 26	35	49	29·73	29·69
Monday . . 27	34	42	29·66	29·67
Tuesday . 28	34	48	29·67	29·76

Wind, S. by E. on the 22d ; S. by W., S., and N.W. on the 23d ; since N.E.

Since the morning of the 22d, when a little rain fell, generally clear.

CHARLES HENRY ADAMS.

WILSON & OGILVY, 57, Skinner Street, London.

THE

LONDON MEDICAL GAZETTE,

BEING A

WEEKLY JOURNAL

OF

𝔐𝔢𝔡𝔦𝔠𝔦𝔫𝔢 𝔞𝔫𝔡 𝔱𝔥𝔢 𝔠𝔬𝔩𝔩𝔞𝔱𝔢𝔯𝔞𝔩 𝔖𝔠𝔦𝔢𝔫𝔠𝔢𝔰.

FRIDAY, APRIL 7, 1843.

LECTURES

ON THE

THEORY AND PRACTICE OF MIDWIFERY,

Delivered in the Theatre of St. George's Hospital,

BY ROBERT LEE, M.D. F.R.S.

LECTURE XXII.

On protracted and difficult labours.

THE second class of labours includes all those cases in which the head of the child presents, and the delivery is not completed in twenty-four hours. It might be objected to this definition, that there are some cases in which it becomes necessary to deliver artificially before the expiration of twenty-four hours from the commencement of labour; and that there are many others in which the process is protracted ten, fifteen, or even twenty hours beyond this period, without any unfavourable symptom occurring, and where the delivery is at last safely accomplished by the natural efforts. I think, however, with Dr. Denman, that this definition will, on the whole, be found to apply to practice in an advantageous and unexceptionable manner, and that it, in particular, affords a remedy against impatience, and is calculated to guard the practitioner in some measure from premature attempts to give assistance, without incurring the danger of those evils which might be apprehended from too long delay. When regular pains have continued twenty-four hours, the patient and her friends naturally feel anxious to know the cause of the protraction, and whether there are any unfavourable symptoms present to excite alarm. When a labour has continued twenty-four hours, and there is a probability that it will not be completed for some time longer, it is a good rule, whether

801.—XXXII.

you are urged or not by the fears and anxieties of others, carefully to examine the condition of the patient—all the symptoms, local and constitutional—to ascertain, if possible, the cause of the delay—closely and calmly to watch the progress of the case, and promptly to employ the appropriate treatment. Beyond a certain period, it is proved by the experience of all practitioners that a woman cannot continue in labour, whatever the cause of the difficulty may be, without certain hazard, and that the danger is, in most cases, proportioned to the duration of the labour. In the course of 57 years, 78,001 women were delivered in the Dublin Lying-in Hospital, of whom one out of every 92 died, and one child out of every 18 was still-born. In women who were in labour with their first children from 30 to 40 hours, one in 34 died, and one child in five was still-born. When labour was protracted from 40 to 50 hours, one in 13 died. If labour were protracted other ten hours, 1-11th of the women died, and when it went on between 60 and 70 hours, 1-8th died, and nearly one-half of the children. It follows from these statements made by Dr. Burns, from the Tables of the Dublin Lying-in Hospital, calculated by Dr. Breen, that when labour is protracted beyond 30 hours, one woman in 34 dies; in other 10 hours, the danger is more than doubled, for one in 13 dies; then one in 11, and next one in 8. A single case of difficult and tedious labour in private practice, where you are left to your own resources, and where you know not how to proceed, or decide erroneously, will probably, however, have more influence in impressing upon your minds the vital importance of this subject than any general statements which I can make.

Protracted and difficult labours can generally be referred to one or several of the following causes :—

1. Feeble, irregular, or partial uterine action, from passions of the mind, original or accidental debility in the mother, and

D

other constitutional causes which impair the energy of the brain and nervous system of the uterus.

2. A rigid, undilatable condition of the os uteri, vagina, and other soft parts.

3. Rigidity of the fœtal membranes; their premature rupture; imperfect discharge of the liquor amnii; over-distension of the uterus by dropsy of the amnion, and a plurality of children.

4. Shortness of the umbilical cord, from being twisted once or several times around the neck and trunk of the child.

5. Unusual size and ossification of the head of the child; hydrocephalus; the forehead situated under the arch of the pubes; presentation of the face; one of the arms with the head; death of the child, and the distension of its abdomen with air or fluid.

6. Distortion and bony tumors of the pelvis

7. Diseases of the uterine organs: as cancer of the os uteri; cicatrices of the vagina, and cohesion of the labia; ovarian and uterine tumors within the pelvis.

1 Of protracted and difficult labours, from feeble, irregular, or partial uterine action.

The uterine contractions may be of short duration, continuing only for a few seconds, or they may return only after long and irregular intervals, so that many hours may elapse before the first stage of labour is considerably advanced, though the orifice of the uterus be soft and dilatable. This does not usually depend on constitutional debility, for in many women exhausted by tubercles of the lungs and hectic fever, the uterus contracts forcibly and regularly in all the different stages of labour, and I do not recollect being obliged to apply the forceps in a single case of this description. Some women are liable to have one labour protracted from this cause without any assignable reason, and all their succeeding labours are speedily accomplished. Others have this slow imperfect action of the uterus in all their labours, and it appears to depend on a sluggish, dull, torpid, inactive condition both of body and mind; in a word, on a want of proper nervous irritability in the constitution. In some women, from observing the progress of former labours, we can almost predict with certainty that in all succeeding labours the first stage at least will go on very slowly, and occupy a considerable number of hours, though there be no rigidity of the os uteri or membranes, or over distension of the uterus, and the umbilical cord does not surround the neck of the child. "The circumstances attending labours," observes Dr. Denman, "are generally alike, yet in many women they are

marked with some peculiarity, most frequently in the time required for their completion. When there has been an opportunity of observing the progress of labour in two or three instances, we shall be able to tell what will be the probable termination of a future labour in the same person, and when it will take place; and we can no more control the order of labour in one woman, so as to make it correspond with, or exactly resemble, that of another, than we can judge of the quantity of food which one person may require by that which is sufficient for another, or regulate any other function of the body. One woman may require twelve hours for the production of the same effects in the time of labour that another may finish in four hours; and it would be in vain to attempt to make an alteration, because the reason exists in some essential property of the constitution, beyond the power of medicine, or of any other method, to alter." You will readily perceive, from this statement, how unnatural the rule must be which some distinguished accoucheurs have laid down for the treatment of all cases of labour, viz., that the first stage should invariably be completed in twelve hours from the commencement of regular pains, and how impossible it is to act upon this principle without producing the greatest mischief.

Sudden and violent emotions of the mind have a powerful influence over the contractions of the uterus, and may at once completely suspend them, or greatly impair their energy. Dr. Merriman relates the case of a woman who was seized with a fit, from which she never recovered, in consequence of a medical practitioner being abruptly introduced into her room to whom she had previously taken a violent dislike. I saw, in consultation with Mr. Jones, Soho Square, a young married lady in labour with her first child, not long since, in whom the uterine action was almost completely suspended, and an attack of puerperal convulsions threatened, from an excessive fear of dying during delivery, or being subjected to some frightful operation. A female friend had put into the hands of this lady, when seven months pregnant, the London Practice of Midwifery, and she could read no other book during the latter months. The consequence was, when labour commenced, she thought of nothing but flooding, convulsions, arrest and impaction of the head, deformed pelvis, and all the operations so minutely described in that work. The uterine action was so completely destroyed by terror, that she would have sunk in a few hours had the delivery not been effected by artificial means. "Such extreme cases as this rarely occur," says Dr. Merriman; "but various kinds of mental excitements continually prevail, and, without producing the more violent ill consequences, tend, however, to disturb and interrupt the favourable process of child-birth. The influence of mental emotions over the act of parturition was strongly and very extensively exemplified not long since on the occasion of the sudden decease, immediately after delivery, of an illustrious and most amiable personage. Indeed, this calamitous event is still found to operate unfavourably on the minds of patients in a certain rank of life."

In protracted labours, arising solely from feeble and irregular uterine action, if the pulse is not much accelerated, the surface cool, little thirst, tongue moist, no tenderness of the abdomen, no unusual sensibility of the vagina and os uteri, and the dilatation is advancing, however slowly, we ought not to interfere. Many hours often elapse before the first stage of labour is completed, yet no bad effects from the pressure of the head of the child upon the soft parts, or exhaustion or fever, will be produced, if the apartment is preserved cool, if all voluntary efforts to bear down are checked, if the posture is occasionally changed, and if nothing but mild nourishment and diluents be allowed. If there is thirst and slight pyrexia, some purgative, as castor-oil, which operates quickly, should be given, or a stimulating enema exhibited. Purgatives and clysters often have the effect of exciting uterine contractions, and they assist in preventing fever and inflammation from being excited in the progress of a tedious labour.

If opiates are ever administered with success in these cases, it can only be at the commencement of the first stage of labour, before the membranes are ruptured, with the view of entirely suspending for a time the uterine contractions, and procuring rest. When the os uteri is fully dilated, and the membranes ruptured, I have never seen opium given with advantage, and I have repeatedly seen it produce bad effects. If the first stage of labour without rigidity of the os uteri is greatly protracted, it is often of advantage to rupture the membranes before it is fully dilated, to raise the head that the liquor amnii may entirely escape, and to make gentle pressure with the finger around the margin of the os uteri during the pains, or to press up the anterior lip where it remains down between the head or symphysis pubis, and when the posterior lip has disappeared. Even in first labours, before the os uteri has been fully dilated, where there has been danger of exhaustion, I have adopted this practice in some cases with the most decided advantage. You will not, however, infer from this, that I wish you to suppose that it is justifiable, in ordinary cases of labour, artificially to rupture the membranes.

It is chiefly in cases of protracted labour from deficient uterine action, that ergot of

rye has lately been so strongly recommended and so generally employed. From the days of Paré and Guillemeau to the present time, the belief has prevailed that certain substances possess a specific power over the actions of the uterus, and promote labour pains. Oil of cinnamon was used by Chapman, and I believe he had great faith in it. In Brachen's time the same opinion was very generally entertained, but he did not believe it to be true. Ergot appears to have been employed by midwives on the continent from time immemorial. Desgranges published his first researches on its properties in 1777, and they have since been examined by several American and French physicians. The results of all the observations hitherto made upon the secale cornutum prove that it does in some cases of labour excite the contractions of the uterus in a very peculiar manner, but that its action is extremely uncertain, and that it often fails to produce the slightest effect. Some deny that it possesses any influence whatever over the uterine contractions; but there can be no doubt that it occasionally does act upon the uterus, and very violently.

As it is impossible to determine in many cases the precise cause of the difficulty in protracted labour, to be sure that the restrained uterine contractions do not depend on some unusual condition of the contents of the uterus, and that the life of the child may not be destroyed by its use, I have never ventured, either in public or private practice, except in cases of accidental uterine hæmorrhage and retained placenta, to administer the ergot of rye to a woman in labour, and I am satisfied that no individual under my care has suffered from the want of it. But I have been consulted in many cases of protracted and difficult labour, where it had previously been administered, and in some I have not opposed its exhibition, where it has been firmly believed by other practitioners that it might be given with safety and advantage. Twenty grains of the powder have been given in a tablespoonful of warm tea, or warm water and sugar, and repeated three or four times at intervals of twenty minutes or a quarter of an hour. Or ʒij. or ʒiij. of the powder have been added to ʒvi. of boiling water, which has been allowed to stand for twenty minutes and then to be strained, and ʒij. of this infusion have been given for a dose at intervals of a quarter of an hour. In other cases the decoction of ergot has been employed, or ʒj. of this preparation, called the liquor secali cornuti, has been repeatedly given, and one fluid drachm of which is said to be equal in effect to ʒj. of the powder. In the greater number of the cases in which I have seen it given, little or no effect has been produced upon the uterine contractions. But the evidence of many others is so strong in favour of its decided influence upon the uterus during labour, that I believe it does sometimes, and in a striking manner, increase the labour pains. The pains produced by it are represented to be different from those nine-tenths of women experience in labour. The contractions excited by the ergot are unusually violent, they occur in rapid succession, so that there are no intervals between them, like those observed in natural labour.

It is agreed on all hands that ergot ought not to be given in first labours, as the rupture of the perinæum would likely be the result ; that it ought not to be administered in any case till the orifice of the uterus is fully dilated, the membranes ruptured, and the presenting part is ascertained. Nor should it be given in any case where there is a suspicion that deformity of the pelvis exists, or disproportion between the head and pelvis from any cause whatever. A foreign accoucheur has, indeed, recommended it to be given in cases of distortion of the pelvis, for the purpose of fixing or jamming the head of the child in the brim, in order that the long forceps might be applied over the occiput and forehead. But where distortion exists, or disproportion between the head and pelvis from any cause, I have never found that the secale was necessary to fix the head in the brim ; this has generally taken place, more speedily than was desired, by the unassisted uterine action, and fatal contusion or rupture of the soft parts has too often been the result of attempting to deliver in such cases without lessening the volume of the head.

It would only be in such a case as the following that the ergot could be given without certain danger, and even in such a case I would prefer trusting to the efforts of nature, and the influence of other remedies whose operation is attended with less hazard to the mother and child. Suppose a woman has had previous labours—has a capacious pelvis—the os uteri soft and widely dilated, the membranes ruptured, the head presenting and low in the pelvis, no fever or inflammation, but the pains are feeble and irregular, and have little effect in pushing forward the head for several hours, and you fear exhaustion from longer continuance of the labour, and time, which you can ill spare from other professional business, is being consumed apparently to no purpose—under such circumstances you might be tempted to exhibit the ergot, and if you did so the probability is that it would produce no effect. But if it did act, and the child, which had been alive a short time before, was born dead, with or without the umbilical cord round the neck, you would then have good reason to regret that the case had not been left to

nature. If in practice you go about constantly armed with this weapon, as many midwives in London now do to my certain knowledge, you will probably be tempted to administer it in cases of protracted labour from great rigidity of the os uteri, hydrocephalus in the child, preternatural presentation, plurality of children, distortion of the pelvis, hæmorrhage from attachment of the placenta to the neck of the uterus, over distended urinary bladder, and other cases where the difficulty and danger are not removed by exciting the contractions of the uterus. Secale is certainly not a remedy which can be safely entrusted to inexperienced practitioners, or which ought to be prescribed in any case without the utmost caution. I have seen a number of cases of first labour, in which the ergot had been given largely though the os uteri was rigid, not more than half dilated, and the membranes unruptured ; violent peritonitis followed in one of these. It was employed not far from this, in a case of protracted labour, where the difficulty arose from an immense accumulation of urine in the bladder ; the bladder was ruptured, and the urine escaped into the sac of the peritoneum. I saw the perforated bladder soon after the occurrence, at the Middlesex Hospital, in the possession of Dr. Hugh Ley. It would have been employed in another case of difficult labour from retention of urine, which I saw in consultation not long after, had I not prevented it. In this case the head was so completely jammed in the pelvis that the catheter could not possibly be introduced into the bladder, and the urine drawn off, till the volume of the head had been lessened by perforation. I was called to a patient of the St. Marylebone Infirmary in 1832, who had been in labour nearly 60 hours, and was attended by one of the parochial midwives, who had given ergot liberally during the labour. The head was extracted with great difficulty after perforation. In 1833 she was delivered safely by the same means, but in 1834 she was attended by two inexperienced accoucheurs, who gave her the ergot of rye in great doses, without reflecting on the distorted condition of the pelvis. The vagina was afterwards lacerated by the forceps, and she died, soon after being delivered by the perforator and crotchet, with incessant vomiting and complete exhaustion. This is not the only case of distorted pelvis which I have seen where ergot has been employed. In other two the women died, and in a third there is an incurable fistulous communication between the bladder and vagina. In more than one case of placental presentation which I have seen, the ergot had been given before it was distinctly ascertained that the hæmorrhage arose from attachment of the placenta to the neck of the uterus. A gentleman who had unbounded faith in the efficacy of secale, and who had prescribed it in a multitude of cases, met with one of protracted labour from congenital hydrocephalus, and here also his favourite remedy was vigorously applied; but the head could not enter the brim of the pelvis, and when the patient was completely exhausted I was requested to see her. A great quantity of fluid escaped on opening the head, which was afterwards readily extracted; but she died in a short time. Ergot was given in a case of difficult labour, from hydrocephalus in the fœtus, which occurred a number of years ago in the neighbourhood of London, and rupture of the uterus was the consequence. In July 1836, a case of arm presentation occurred where ergot was given before the presenting part was felt. Great difficulty was experienced in turning. The child was dead, and the woman died on the 5th day. Not long ago it was given in a case of twins. The arm of the second child presented, and the utmost difficulty was experienced in the operation of turning.

It was observed in America that the children were often still born after the exhibition of ergot of rye, and this led many practitioners in that country to discontinue its use altogether. The same circumstance has likewise been noticed in this country, and it is not difficult to explain the cause. The contractions of the uterus excited by the ergot of rye are different from those of natural labour; they are of much greater strength and longer duration, like a number of violent labour pains continued into one another without intervals. The long interruption to the circulation of the maternal blood in the uterus and placenta, which must take place during these lengthened contractions, and the want of the necessary changes in the fœtal blood, will explain why children are often born in a state of asphyxia, after the administration of the secale cornutum.

2. *Of protracted and difficult labours, from a rigid and undilatable state of the orifice of the uterus, vagina, and other soft parts.*

It is in first labours, and in women advanced in age, that rigidity of the os uteri, and other soft parts, is most frequently met with. Sometimes it is confined to the orifice of the uterus, so that the second stage of labour is very short, when the first has been extremely protracted. More frequently the rigidity exists both in the orifice of the uterus and in the parts at the outlet of the pelvis, so that the first and second stages are both tedious and painful. In the greater number of cases of this description, if no improper treatment be employed, the dilatation of the os uteri and other parts is at last accomplished with safety to the mother and child. It is necessary, however, to be fully

aware that both are exposed to imminent danger if the labour is protracted from rigidity beyond a certain period; and every practitioner ought thoroughly to know the symptoms which indicate that the labour has been left to nature, or allowed to continue as long as is compatible with their safety.

The parts after a certain period become hot, dry, swollen and puffy, from the long continued pressure and interrupted circulation, and so tender that an examination cannot be made without causing pain. The discharge from the vagina becomes offensive, and retention of urine takes place from the pressure of the child's head on the urethra and neck of the bladder, with a sense of soreness and tension of the abdomen. More or less anxiety should always be felt about a case of protracted labour where any of these local symptoms are observed, and especially where the employment of the catheter becomes necessary, and where some difficulty is experienced in passing it into the bladder, and where the head of the child has remained several hours without making any progress, and the bones are compressed, and there is a large tumor under the scalp. The excitement of great constitutional disturbance, with increased determination of blood to particular organs, especially the brain, and exhaustion of the vital powers, are the most unfavourable general symptoms observed in cases of protracted labour from rigidity. The accession of fever in the second stage of labour, or in the first stage after the membranes have long been ruptured, indicated by rigors, a rapid pulse, furred tongue, and flushed countenance, affords additional evidence that the labour cannot be left much longer to the natural efforts; and still more unfavourable is the case if the labour pains have been gradually diminishing in force, if the head has ceased to advance, and symptoms of exhaustion have appeared. One of the most striking circumstances observed in these cases is the sudden manner in which the unfavourable constitutional symptoms manifest themselves, and the necessity which arises for the immediate interference of art. The pains cease almost entirely, the head begins to wander, the face and trunk become covered with a clammy perspiration, the features and tone of the voice become completely changed—so altered that you might almost doubt whether it was the same individual you had been so long watching with anxiety—with constant restlessness and jactitation.

These local and constitutional symptoms may occur before the first stage of labour has been completed, but they are, perhaps, most frequently observed after the head has passed through the os uteri into the pelvis, and has remained there pressing for some time upon the parts at the outlet. While the dilatation is going on, however slowly, and the head is descending, and none of these symptoms are present, the labour may safely be left to nature; but when the process is arrested, and the parts within the pelvis begin to suffer from the pressure, and symptoms of fever and exhaustion appear, it is your duty to interfere, otherwise the strength of the patient may be so exhausted that she will speedily die after delivery from the mere shock of labour, or from hæmorrhage and retained placenta, or, what is, perhaps, worse than death, she may have sloughing of the uterus, vagina, bladder, and rectum. There are few cases in midwifery which require greater practical skill to conduct to a happy issue than some of these cases of protracted labour from rigidity, and which are sometimes complicated with other causes of difficulty.

The most important remedy in cases of rigidity of the os uteri is, doubtless, venesection, which not only promotes the dilatation of the parts, but checks the disposition to inflammation and fever. If the patient is robust, the pulse full, strong, and frequent, and unfavourable symptoms begin to appear, especially congestion of the brain, the abstraction of a moderate quantity of blood from the arm is often followed by relaxation of the os uteri and external organs, efficient pains, and the speedy termination of the labour. In all these cases it is the most safe and powerful remedy we possess, and, if employed with proper caution, can never be injurious where the strength of the patient has not been previously exhausted by the long-continued efforts. You must distinctly understand, however, that blood-letting should be employed in no case of labour unless it is absolutely necessary, and that it is a remedy inapplicable to cases of disproportion between the child and mother, and where the protraction depends on feeble uterine action. Blood-letting during labour sometimes alarms the patient and her attendants, and is absolutely injurious by inducing debility in the puerperal state. Some practitioners have strongly recommended the exhibition of an enema of starch and laudanum in cases of protracted labour from great rigidity of the os uteri, after the employment of venesection.

Where blood-letting fails to relieve the symptoms, and artificial delivery becomes necessary, it may be safely completed with the forceps, if the os uteri is fully dilated, and the head has descended so far into the pelvis that an ear can be felt. Where the second stage of labour has not commenced, and the greater part of the head remains above the brim, and any circumstance occurs demanding immediate delivery, to save the mother's life the perforator and crotchet must be employed.

PUBLIC HEALTH.

An Oration delivered on the 70th Anniversary of the London Medical Society, on Wednesday, 8th of March.

By LEONARD STEWART, M.D.

(For the Medical Gazette.)

THE most general and the most powerful influence exerted upon the constitution of men and animals is that of climate and locality.

Many familiar examples may be given of the force of the endemic causes of disease; which technical expression must be taken as including the telluric as well as the aerial agents prevalent in any given region, whose combined effect is to modify the living principle, and at times quite overcome the normal power of resistance to what is deleterious.

The production of agues in marshy districts; of goitres and cretinism in mountain passes; of dysenteries and liver complaints in various tropical plains; of fatal pestilential fever in other localities; the more familiar evils of scrofula, phthisis, and rickets, (called proverbially the English malady), all these, too surely, and too repeatedly, prove this assertion.

A comparison of the results of particular endemial influences gives us the means of escaping from danger, or of palliating the virulence of morbific agents, by removal to a locality having an opposite character. This mutual exchange of advantages is one of the most successful and gratifying arrangements in our power, for ensuring health and prolonging life; and one of the most reasonable in theory; because, in so doing, we remove the causes of evil, and prove the maxim that " prevention is better than cure."

The statistical information which is now being obtained from many quarters on the subject of medical topography is of the greatest importance in directing the migration of invalids, the route of all expeditions, and the establishment of colonies and new settlements.

It occasionally gives a reason for abandoning regions, which are either too severely cold for the susceptible natives of more sunny skies, or insupportably hot and pestiferous to the labourer from the north. It appears that any frozen climate developes tubercles in the Malay and in the negro; while we are told that the marshy plains of Demerara, though prolific of other diseases to the Anglo-Saxon race, are both preventive and curative of phthisis. There is some reason for believing that the causes of ague and consumption are antagonist powers, and do not commonly prevail in the same localities.

We have before us the good and the evil,

and can at pleasure use, without abusing, the natural influences around us.

Of course it will be recollected that, in speaking upon the subject of health and recovery from disease, the medical man is understood to consider them as objects of paramount importance.

He is not accountable for any obstacle that may lie in the way, connected with politics, commerce, or finance.

His vocation is to establish the laws of his profession, founded as they are upon nature and observation, and to disregard all other considerations but the discovery and declaration of the truth.

In the British Isles there appear to be no peculiar or indigenous diseases, if we except those already named, that are connected with the strumous constitution or diathesis. And even here there are other circumstances, which influence these maladies, if they do not originate them, that are not necessarily connected with our climate and locality.

On the contrary, it is our boast, in the present day, to be secure in the possession of a soil well subdued, and rendered incapable of generating the more noxious forms of malady; and of a temperature favourable to the development of the greatest energy of mind and body, unusually free from extremes of heat and cold, known as a general place of refuge from other malarious and plague infested climes. But notwithstanding our great natural advantages, and the addition of facilities resulting from enterprise and civilization, there does still exist a great amount of disease.

We have frequently wide-spread epidemics, and generally diffused contagious maladies; and the attention of the learned, of the powerful, of the charitable, has been from time to time aroused by the overshadowing of danger more than usually imminent.

The occasional prevalence of puerperal fever; the rapid march of scarlatina, small-pox, and certain eruptive diseases; the pestilential type of typhus in seasons of scarcity; the unexampled intensity and fatality of cholera; have all, in their day, called aloud for public consideration.

From a variety of causes, the desire for statistical and extended information has of late years been more fixed, and the facts already published and laid before the world, by official statements, as well as by individual declarations, have caused more deliberation than at any former period, on the possibility of affording relief.

When we ascertain that there are fewer malarious and atmospheric causes of malady with us than elsewhere, we at once establish the very important conclusion, that the circumstances which generate and diffuse the evils that do exist, are, in their essential nature, more accidental and artificial.

Our prevalent sufferings are therefore connected, it is probable, with modes of life and social conditions which are not incapable of reform. Such, for instance, as the precocious labour of children, and the sedentary occupations of females.

There is a great deal that can be traced to what is familiar and tangible—as to dirty and insufficient clothing, damaged provisions, over-crowded rooms, excessive toil, intemperance—often to ignorance and prejudice.

We cannot for a moment doubt, that by investigating and correcting these and many other improper habits of a similar character, much unmixed good may be done.

The many advantages which arise from "centralization," and the collection of crowds into large towns and capitals, are not without great drawbacks.

The unnumbered conveniences and amusements, which attract equally the industrious and the frivolous, the cooperation for many common objects of business and pleasure, the multiplied choice of occupation, and the demand for the talents of the ingenious or the gifted, in ways unknown or unappreciated in rural life, the privacy, concealment, and mystery, necessary for many modes of existence (adopted by individuals, or forced upon their necessities), the greater liberty and variety offered to all classes, are too generally counterbalanced by striking disadvantages.

The masses have generally herded together without foresight, or due provision for comfort and safety.

This is especially the case in old and populous cities.

We have the narrow streets, dark and crowded passages, with noisome cellars and comfortless attics. There are the suffocating factories and workshops, the damp grounds and yards, the smoking labyrinths of what are called the "back settlements," all swarming with the toil-worn, the debauched, and the brutalized, strangely huddled together. Their scanty or precarious food, dejection of mind, discomfort, ill-regulated or intemperate habits, and filthy places of residence, are altogether the prolific source of disease and infection.

The dangers arising from this want of arrangement, and the absence of the true conditions proper for health, relaxation, and natural recreation, are not limited to the labouring drudges, nor to the abject dwellers in low pauperized localities, but hang over; and frequently involve, those even who appear to be far removed and carefully secured from contact and contamination.

The intercommunion continually going on (however imperceptibly) between the members of any family, their children, domestics, and day-servants, with all the various dependents, messengers, providers, and attendants, forms a chain of connection unbroken between the most epicurean and fastidious, and the most debased and outcast.

Innumerable examples could be quoted to illustrate this position.

It is quite impossible to live and move in society, and to be insured with anything like precision against the attack of some of the most pernicious and loathsome contagions.

" Pallida mors æquo pulsat pede pauperum
        tabernas,
Regumque turres."

There is a striking exemplification of this irresistible truth on record in the death of Louis XV., who, living in the midst of refinements and luxuries, with everything studied with a view to his health and security, after a long and voluptuous life, found his palaces and his parks no sufficient refuge from the terrible invasion of confluent small-pox.

It is for the good of all, then, to promote an improvement in the condition, both moral and physical, of the poorest and most abandoned :

It is twice blessed :
It blesseth him that gives, and him that takes!

In devising and in superintending all plans of medical police, our profession must cooperate with the legislature, the civil authorities, with the architect and engineer. We must call to our aid all the arts and sciences now rendered popular by civilization and enlightened government ; and join in providing due space for ventilation and draining, when they have been of old neglected ; or for additional comfort, cleanliness, and warmth, wherever these are demanded, in new districts.

Already it has been pointed out to the public, and to the proprietors of various works and handicrafts, that many of the desirable ends of skill and enterprise can be obtained at a diminished rate of suffering from noxious materials and from accidents ; but a great deal more is to be done under the personal superintendence of our profession, both by general precaution and the minute adaptation of ingenious contrivances.

Among crowds of people there are many things which oppose the full enjoyment of health ; but it is to be remembered there are some great advantages.

The very circumstance of their residing and acting together supposes more publicity and protection than when their work is done alone, and without assistants and witnesses. This particularly applies to children and young persons, who are often liable to suffer from neglect or tyranny where there is no one by to share their condition.

The forlorn and helpless situation of individuals or small families, when isolated and at a distance from help and attendance, is to none better known than to medical men. It is well worth the attention of philanthropists, and those who desire the well-working of the social mass, to contrive some plan for the protection of children when their parents are away. The infant-schools, and other places of deposit during the day, are shut out from them when ill. The parents (whose occupation often keeps them abroad) are frequently obliged to employ very inefficient persons to supply their place ; or they have the difficult alternative of giving up their work, and forfeiting their only means of support. Even where there is no neglect, it is well known to those who are in the habit of attending the poor at their own homes, that there is too frequently great ignorance and prejudice, and that these helpless objects suffer from all kinds of mismanagement, injudicious meddling, and caprice. Add to all this, the danger continually arising from the number of persons huddled together in one room, frequently in one bed.

Under proper direction, it is probable that some plan of placing sick children under skilful and responsible persons when the parents are compelled to be away, or are incompetent to manage them, would diminish the intensity of the materials of infection, and prevent a great deal of mischief now arising from accident, ignorance, and at times from brutal inattention.

But it is not in cities alone (let it be understood) that our profession has to consider the best arrangements for health and well-being. In rural districts and remote settlements it is more than ever important that the presence of the medical man should witness the fulfilment of his precepts. It is here chiefly that neglect of authority, or blind adherence to custom, is found to prevail without chance of being corrected.

There are bodies of men, too, who are associated, but yet cut off, more or less, from ordinary intercourse with the world, and where the absence of an adviser and protector, with knowledge and influence sufficient to hold over them the shield of the remedial sciences, is felt as the greatest calamity. All rural factories, all mines and collieries, all asylums for the poor, the sick, the superannuated, the helpless, the insane, the captive, the criminal, look to us for fair play.

In an especial manner, as scientific men, we are called upon to be present with all expeditions and emigrations, by land or by water ; always as companions, and not unfrequently as leaders.

Whenever there is a probability of ameliorating the condition of labourers by regulating their work, both with regard to duration and intensity, or by insisting that the stupefying monotony of their toil should have due opportunity of being broken by amusement and heart-easing mirth, we should not be silent.

Whenever we can manage to save them from dangerous accidents, from deleterious materials, unwholesome places of work or of residence, it is the recognized province of our profession to interfere.

Who, so well as we, are entitled to open the door to moral and intellectual sources of improvement?

By no class is the intelligent co-operation of those with whom we have to deal more appreciated or more desired. We have unequalled opportunites for observation and reflection, and, as a consequence, I will boldly ask, where shall we find so little bigotry and prejudice?

I am not ignorant of the great attention which has already been given to many of these matters. I rejoice that much more is likely to be done in this direction; but I think it only right to say, that much more of the control and management of all sanatory regulations should be in the hands of medical men than has hitherto been common.

We have something more to do here than to set other people to work!

Our vocation is administrative as well as legislative: we are not only abstract advisers, but peculiarly and proverbially *practitioners.*

Medical men should be in person ready to superintend the execution of what they may theoretically recommend.

We have the highest *political* authority of the present day declaring that a physician should not prescribe until he is *called* in!

To suppose that there is an inherent virtue in *formulæ*, that enables any one without education or practice to deal with them successfully, is really as absurd as to fancy that the colours and brushes of a portrait-painter constitute the chief part of his skill.

And yet this is common enough! It happened to me, some twenty years since, to be the only passenger in a merchant-ship; and upon the occurrence of some illness in one of the crew, I found the captain about to fire off some article from his medicine chest. I took this opportunity of examining this magazine of *specifics*, which consisted of a box of powders differently sorted—for in those days we had not got to infinitesimals! I was much edified at finding the simplicity and certainty to which the art and mystery of the practice of physic was reduced. There were some of these powders labelled as good for a fever, some for a spitting of blood, for a liver complaint, for rheumatism, and so on through the entire collection, which contained various antidotes for many other nautical maladies, both British and foreign. Upon my venturing to mention the possibility of his giving a wrong direction to

these compositions, (which he was in the habit of inflicting upon his men when slack at their work), and upon hinting that he ought to study diseases, and have some reason for ·his practice, my friend seemed to consider all this a troublesome refinement; as the names were plainly written, and he was not partial to innovations. I found, in short, that it was not easy to move him from the fixed groove in which his ideas ran, or to lessen his conceit of his own infallibility.

The experience of every day teaches us that it is precisely those who know least about anatomy, physiology, and pathology, who talk with the greatest confidence of the efficacy of various specifics, which they seem to consider as if *billeted* to certain maladies, or as so many charms or talismans, capable of producing results without any particular management.

They are deluded by names, and do not understand diseases.

Within my recollection the names and titles of mixtures, powders, and other preparations, were made to indicate the particular diseases and morbid conditions to which they were considered specially adapted. They were named from their supposed effects, and not from their composition and ingredients. This was at regular institutions, hospitals, and under the superintendence of educated practitioners We have, however, made a great stride from this narrow and erroneous view of therapeutics. I do not know that, at present, any formulæ are called after the maladies to which they are considered destined. Their aptitude or affinity is not declared; they are merely named by enumerating their ingredients or qualities. We now do not suppose that because certain drugs (by a peculiar affinity or pre-established harmony) are taken up by the stomach, as ipecacuan; or the intestines, as senna; or the uterus, as ergot of rye, so as to bear a part in modifying the functions of these organs, that therefore these medicines are always to cure the diseases of these regions. In short, we distinguish between the pharmacological and the remedial character of the various substances used for prescriptions.

The familiar titles of emetics, sudorifics, cathartics, diuretics, and so on, are retained more for convenience and classification than as indicating their invariable character. We know that, in the hands of the skilful, they are made to play various and opposite parts.

The past history of medicine shews that many articles of the materia medica, to which at one time great virtue and importance were attributed, have either sunk into total neglect, or are associated with other drugs, and are mere condiments or adjuvants. In this category stand most spices and aromatics. Many spirituous cordials, whose names alone would indicate the possession of the most salutary influence, are now very often strictly forbidden in the very cases where they were once considered sovereign remedies. The names aqua vitæ, usquebaugh, eau de vie, and so on, in all languages were Æsculapian as well as Bacchanalian titles. But physiology is now in the ascendant, and we have discarded most of these old material notions.

In chemical and mechanical operations the action of the substances which meet is mutually balanced, and can be calculated upon. The result is unvaried and certain. There ought to be no irregularities, because these are purely physical experiments; they are of the exact sciences. It is only when the vital energy and organic power is called into play that there is any uncertainty or caprice, or that action and reaction is not reciprocal, and mathematically adjusted. This essential difference, it is very clear, cannot be attributed to the brute substance, the passive inanimate material; but at once marks the peculiar character of organization—the more active *initiative* and independent function of the living fibre.

There seems to be a discriminating power —a force which resists and repels the approach of deleterious matters, and their ingress into the absorbing surfaces. Again, it appears that this power is lost or modified, or possibly inverted, so that what was once excluded by the skin and mucous surfaces is, at these times, attracted and absorbed.

We continually observe the different susceptibility of various constitutions, or of the same persons at different periods, and in the many fluctuating conditions of health. We know that neither food, nor medicines, nor poisons, are acted upon in one invariable mode. Now the moral of all such researches is, that no routine can be established for all emergencies; because the true agents in all remedial transactions are the organs and functions of the living frame, and not the material appliances which are merely the occasions and instruments — the subject matter—of any change.

Too much stress cannot be laid upon this doctrine in our dealings with the public.

The study of the general laws of physiology, as well as a microscopic acquaintance with the most evanescent changes, and the practical application of this knowledge, fully entitle the conscientious practitioner to much weight and influence.

While we have so many fortunes made by hawking about a single recipe; so many laws amended by the development of principles familiar with us; so many characters rescued from aspersion by the display of pathological facts; surely those who stand at the source and fountain-head of all this good ought to be the most considered.

When acting in honourable alliance with all the sciences, keeping up with the march of discovery, and ever ready to suggest useful improvements, they leave behind them single-string practitioners, and the formalists, who adhere to narrow obsolete systems, who follow the *letter* but feel nothing of the *spirit* of their rules.

There is no doubt about the necessity for attending to the skilful preparation and to the dexterous administration of the most ordinary appliances and means, or of the importance of studying the relative and occasional utility of all palliative measures; but it is still more to the interest of the public that the superiority of thought and invention over dull routine should be made clear, and the agency of principles upon details understood.

Were attention generally paid to the natural history of diseases, no one would be satisfied with any single method of treatment; were it a popular conviction that the experienced reflection and vigilance of the practitioner should in every case be applied *before any thing else*, there would be less reliance upon universal nostrums. Even in the boldest empirical or experimental attempts it would be seen that here also there should be a previous knowledge of anatomy, physiology, and pathology.

The plans of unenlightened people are always limited and meagre. They aim at a simplicity which is not borne out by observation and adhesion to truth; they fail, not only in candour, but in variety of resources. It is commonly true, that where they succeed it is by stumbling on a remedy; or still more frequently by claiming as their own what nature was about to do without them. On the other hand, it is certain, that when they are defeated, they are quite bewildered, having no reserve to fall back upon.

I am, for one, little disposed to quarrel with the boldness of any experiment, or the novelty of any theory or any practice; but I like to see the ground cleared, and the conditions well and fairly understood, so that no conclusion may be jumped at, and no victory unworthily trumpeted forth.

The exalted character and multiplied resources of intelligent medicine in its widest signification, would then be sufficient (without any interference from without) to bring into discredit the follies of quacks, and the culpable greediness of the dealers in patent medicines.

Many false promises made by reckless and unfeeling men would be contrasted with the good faith of the considerate adviser and faithful friend of the doomed and hopeless sufferer. Those who *kill* would stand out more distinctly from those who *cure*; and some daylight would be thrown upon the contrivances of those more crafty personages, who, making an even division between the claims of their patients and their own profit, steer a middle course, give placebos only, and take especial care neither to kill nor cure.

But if an acquaintance with the natural history of disease, and the various sciences which are appealed to and put in requisition by the healing art, is necessary to the safe and successful practice of our profession, it follows that the unskilful employment of recipes by the ignorant, by amateurs, or by the followers of *routine*, is dangerous.

It becomes more and more important to supply the personal attendance and assistance of the skilful and experienced as generally and as widely as possible—to spread abroad not only the measures but the men. There can be no discovery, no conquest obtained by the skill or enterprise of our expeditions into various regions, more truly important than the sure victory established on all sides over the mischievous systems and ignorant practices pursued by various less enlightened people. This, although not always the object, is frequently the best result of such undertakings.

It must be consolatory to those who turn with pain from the contemplation of the violence committed when the customs of other countries are interfered with, or when their territory is invaded, to reflect upon the soothing and healing influence of the medical profession. Carried into all parts, and diffusing unnumbered benefits, it seeks, as the only tribute, information and experience —and this is collected and employed for the universal good. It is not always the same with the other professions.

We can well understand the dread and angry feeling which a vanquished and mortified nation may entertain against our naval and military heroes. Experience has shown that the spread of any new religion by persuasion and argument is always a work of time, when opposed by the bigotry of ignorant or interested persons. It is again conceivable that any proposal to fix an entirely new set of legislators and lawyers (with chancery suits and solicitors' bills) upon any people would not be acceded to with great alacrity. And the jealousy and rivalry of traders is always in the way of free and friendly relations with our commercial men. But the medical profession has, on every occasion, been met with confidence and kindness. Its good deeds and benevolent attempts are always hailed with feelings of profound interest, and remembered with gratitude. Syria and China will bear me out in this assertion! It is always something to counterbalance the evils too commonly attendant upon warfare and revolution, and to reconcile the conquered to the presence of strangers and innovators. It is one of the best ways, for all parties, of making compensation. And this debt, which may be considered as due from a powerful and enlightened nation to the barbarians who fall under its sway, it is ever gratifying to contemplate; this is a kind of "national debt" which has indeed some chance of being redeemed.

So great are the resources of the profession, and such the energy and good-will of its members, that we could undertake to scatter on all sides from our "embarras de richesses," and to establish in all quarters the true principles and practice of the healing art.

This would be a twofold advantage; for the glut and stagnation which is so much complained of every where has its parallel in our province also. When we glance at the actual condition of all countries, we shall find that there are strange accumulations of similar conditions; so that distribution seems to be pointed out as the leading duty of the age.

We shall see, on every hand, multitudes existing in the position of the fabled Tantalus —surrounded by the most desirable objects, which they are debarred from using and enjoying. What numbers of persons, of all ages, sexes, and occupations, cramped by sedentary monotonous toil, when half asphyxiated in their close and dusty workshops, would fain escape to the breezes of the hill-side*. Many hunting tribes might safely share the excess of stimulants which the desponding artizan is now tempted to use, and miserably abuse.

We have a sister country exporting substantial food to all parts, yet half starving her own peasantry. In the wild parts of North and South America, the carcases of deer and of cattle are left to rot, while many of our own labourers are limited to vegetable diet, or nearly so. The mountains of Switzerland are carefully cropped and shorn of every blade of grass; the wine countries are tended like gardens; while many of the richest plains, both of the old world and the new, as on the Euphrates and the Mississipi, are either abandoned or unattempted by the hand of the cultivator.

We have, at the present day, the eyes of politicians and of speculators directed to the striking spectacle of the Eastern coast of Asia (with its three hundred millions of Chinese, scantily fed, and often living in boats and on rafts for want of room on shore), as contrasted with the opposite North-west coast of America (or the Oregan territory), whose only civilized inhabitants consist of some few hundred men, the servants of two

---

* " As one who long in populous cities pent, Where houses thick and sewers annoy the air, Forth issuing on a summer's morn to breathe Among the pleasant villages and farms Adjoin'd, from each thing met conceives delight."

or three private companies of merchants. It is no far-fetched improbable theory, to propose the greater equalization of these opposite conditions.

"Nature's full blessings would be well dispens'd
In unsuperfluous even proportion,
And she no whit encumbered with her store."

We may imagine the many powerful elements of knowledge and production, which now jar and fret in opposition and competition, more harmonized and combined in effecting the general advantage.

In cities, in rural districts, in distant settlements, and in home colonies, it is still to be seen whether the peculiar good of each is inseparable from the usual drawback of evil to which each is now subject.

We may fancy such expeditions as have already occasionally taken place made more frequently and systematically, so as to encourage and hasten the progress of unsophisticated nations from barbarism to refinement.

What unnumbered benefits would arise to all, both far and near, from the solution of the great political problem, which proposes so to combine the results of intellectual and associated life, as to bring them to bear upon the rustic and the savage!

Already we have begun to act upon the plan of retaining the strength and creative power of large masses, without permitting the producers and operatives to be oppressed or neglected. We hear already a general desire expressed, that education for the mind, proper exercise for the body, and due repose and recreation for both, should be fully considered in all arrangements for associated life.

The diffusion of all kinds of publications now secures so great an interchange of intelligence as will prevent any isolated members of the human family from becoming torpid and indifferent to the attainments of the rest; and it is not an impossible thing to allow to the peculiarities of individuals much that the necessary order and discipline of the whole body can spare.

Should society, anxious to escape from some of the anomalous difficulties which have been before described, make a general movement on a more comprehensive scale, a speculation of such surpassing interest and importance would find no class of men who would more powerfully contribute to its success than our own.

The members of the medical profession form the truest bond of union between the near and the distant, the savage and the civilized world. We are the only cosmopolites!

There is no occupation which interferes so little with the free agency of others, and when it does command, accomplishes its end by so often appealing to truth, and the laws of nature and necessity.

But in the promotion of any scheme of amelioration, I feel confident that nothing more than a generous emulation would animate our exertions.

I can safely assert, that as a profession we have at no time shown a disposition to claim more than our due. And, as the patriot of old (when not elected to some office, though conscious of deserving it), rejoiced that his country possessed men better than himself, we would gladly say to any people, or sect, or party, or profession, who should engage in this great work, who should take the lead in this glorious mission—

" Master, go on, and I will follow thee,
To the last gasp, with truth and loyalty."

CASE OF

DIABETES MELLITUS,

WITH NUMEROUS OBSERVATIONS,
AND A REVIEW OF THE PATHOLOGY AND
TREATMENT OF THIS DISEASE.

By JOHN PERCY, M.D. (Edin.)

Physician to the Queen's Hospital, and Lecturer on Organic Chemistry at the Royal School of Medicine and Surgery, Birmingham.

(For the London Medical Gazette.)

IT must be admitted that the hospital is the field where disease can be most minutely, most perseveringly, and most extensively studied. Hence arises the responsibility, which devolves upon every hospital practitioner, of exerting himself to the utmost in the promotion of the science of medicine or surgery; and the man who retains his connection with an hospital when he has become incapable, from one cause or another, of promoting this object, does not discharge his duty. The author is deeply impressed with this truth, and is desirous, so far as his humble abilities will permit, of contributing, in some degree at least, to the furtherance of medical science, Extended and correct observations are essential in every science, and, if in one more than another, especially in the science of medicine. Diabetes mellitus is a disease which, notwithstanding all that has yet been accomplished, either by observation or experiment, is involved in great obscurity. This fact is the apology for the publication of the present case. It is possible that multiplied and accurate observations may eventually shed some light upon the pathology of the disease in question. Facts, at first apparently sterile and useless, have not unfrequently been found to admit of valuable and practical application. The case will first be minutely recorded; then will follow a variety of observations, intended to serve as the basis of reasoning; remarks upon the pathology, with the detail of some illustrative experiments; and, lastly, a review of the various methods of treatment which have been recommended. The author can truly declare that he has had but one object in view, and that is the elimination of truth.

Joseph Merchant, æt. 31, admitted in-patient of the Queen's Hospital, August 25th, 1842. Of middle stature, and of moderately robust habit; complexion ruddy; hair and eyes brown. He has always been a remarkably temperate man. For the truth of this statement I did not rely solely upon the testimony of the patient, but upon that of persons who had long been acquainted with him. He was employed in attending to two steam engines connected with coal-pits; one engine was high-pressure, of twelve horse power, the other condensing, of thirty-six horse power. I am particular in relating these circumstances, in order that a proper inference may be drawn in respect to the atmospheric conditions to which he was habitually exposed. His average weight, when in health, was twelve stones and a half. He was married seven years ago, and has three children, of whom the youngest is two years old. Eleven months ago his wife died, and he has since been much distressed at the fact of his children being left motherless. Three months have now elapsed since the commencement of his illness. Before this period he had enjoyed uninterrupted health. He became affected with languor and depression of spirits; his appetite and thirst were inordinately increased; and he observed that he passed urine in much larger quantity, and more frequently, than natural, being obliged to rise several times in the course of the night for the purpose of micturition. From the nature of his employment, he has been exposed to very great and sudden alternations of temperature, to which circumstance he is disposed to attribute his illness. He has also, as might be expected, been accustomed to drink copious draughts of cold water. The preceding symptoms have, in conjunction with gradually increasing debility and loss of flesh, continued to the present time. He has also lost all sexual desire.

Present condition.—His appetite and thirst are inordinate, and he prefers liquids cold. The skin is dry and slightly harsh; the tongue is fissured, red at the edges and tip, and coated in a slight degree in the centre; the gums are spongy and ulcerated round the teeth, and the saliva has an acid reaction. The mouth and fauces are dry, and he complains of a sour taste. The pulse is moderately compressible, and of the natural quickness. The quantity of urine passed will be found registered in the table appended to the case. The bowels are generally irregular and confined, and he is troubled with flatulence. The lower extremities are œdematous. His hair readily falls off, which was not the case previously to his present illness. He has neither pain in the head nor vertigo; both sides of the chest dilate equally; percussion is everywhere natural, respiratory murmur is generally feeble; he is without any cough or dyspnœa; there is nothing unnatural in the appearance of the penis; his sleep is not disturbed, except by calls to pass urine; he has inguinal hernia on the left side. He reports that, so far as his knowledge extends, none of his relatives were ever affected in a manner similar to himself; and this report was confirmed on careful inquiry of his mother. Before admission, he had been bled in the arm without relief.

Habeat Pil. Saponis c. Opio, gr. v. bis quotidie. His body to be sponged every morning with salt and water, and then to be rubbed dry. To have 12oz. of beef or mutton daily, with cabbage, and only a small quantity of bread and potatoes. To have infusion of chamomile for common drink. In other respects, ordinary diet.

August 28th.—Much as before. Pulse 76, soft.

Cont. omnia.

30th.—Complains much of languor and depression, and also of heart-burn. Bowels moved twice yesterday, and once this morning.

Cont. omnia.

31st.—Reports himself improved.

℞ Strychniæ, gr. j.; Sp. Vini Rect. f℥ss.
solve. Dein adde Aquæ, f℥j. M.
ft. mist. Capiat f℥j. ex aquâ ter
indies. Om. Opium.

Sept. 1st.—Reports himself better.
Skin not quite so dry as before; œdema
still continues; tongue red, and saliva
acid.

2d.—He has evidently improved in
appearance. Thirst somewhat diminished.

3d.—Last night he perspired freely
during three hours. Bowels moved
twice this morning. Pulse 84.

4th.—Has had pain in the bowels,
with diarrhœa. Thirst abated; tongue
red and moist; has not perspired; skin
cool, and inclined to be moist. Pulse 80.

6th.—Has suffered from cramp and
pain in the bowels during the night,
and attributes this to the cabbage. It
will, however, be seen in the sequel,
that, for some time after admission, he
was in the habit of swallowing by
stealth even purgative mixture, placed
in the ward for other patients, as he
was ashamed of being observed to drink
so copiously; and, when an opportunity
occurred, he gladly drank water from
the tap.

7th. — Reports himself improved.
The cramp occasionally returns. He
passes the greater part of his urine
during the night.

Om. Mist. Strychniæ.

℞ Infus. Calumbæ, f℥viij.; Ammon.
Carb. ℨiss. solve. ; Capiat f℥j. ter
quotidie.

Omit the cabbage.

10th.—Has not slept so well during
the last two nights. Bowels moved
regularly.

H. s. s. Pulv. Ipecac. co. gr. x.

℞ Tincturæ Capsici, f℥ij. ; Aquæ, f℥viij.
M. Ft. gargarisma, subinde indies
utendum. Cont. alia.

12th.—Thirst not so urgent; appetite
as before; he feels better. Since he has
taken the last mixture, he has discharged a considerable quantity of
flatus; dryness of the mouth somewhat
relieved; has had pain across the
loins; no return of perspiration.

15th.—Thirst less; mouth more moist;
he is drowsy, and much inclined to
sleep.

19th.—Urine discharged involuntarily

during the night; in other respects as
before.

20th.—Passed a restless night.

℞ Calomelanos, gr. iij. ; Pulv. Jacobi
Veri. gr. v. M. Ft. pil. ij. h. s. s.
Cont. alia.

21st.—Œdema of legs and thighs
increased; perspired freely in the
night; he complains of pain extending
down in the direction of the inner side
of the thighs, and in those parts there
is a diffused blush; abdomen enlarged,
with fluctuation; bowels open; the
redness, œdema, and pain described,
continued several days. These symptoms, however, were much relieved by
the application of cloths impregnated
with acetate of lead lotion.

Oct. 4th.—Bowels moved four or five
times daily. It would appear from the
table that the quantity of urine passed
daily is diminished in a remarkable
degree; but, on inquiry, it is found
that he passes some urine at the closet;
still, the diminution is decided.

Mistura Cretæ, Tincture of Catechu, and
Aromatic Confection, had been ordered
during my absence.

7th.—His bowels have been moved
six times during the night; thirst less;
no perspiration; he passed about a
quart of urine at the closet; tenesmus;
tongue clean and moist; œdema of
lower extremities has nearly disappeared; no abdominal fluctuation; no
pain or tenderness of abdomen; pulse
70, feeble and compressible.

H. s. s. Pil. Sap. c. Opio, gr. x. formâ
suppositorii. Cont. Mist. Catechu.

14th.—Feels better; legs less œdematous; bowels moved twice yesterday; wishes to have more meat.

Sumat. "Tannin" gr. ij. f. pil. ter die.
2 ounces of additional meat, and less
bread.

18th.—Purging has returned: much
complaint of languor and debility.
The following mixture was prescribed
in my absence, by the medical officer,
Mr. Swain.

℞ Tinct. "Kino," Tinct. "Catechu," aa.
f℥ij.; Infusi Quassiæ, f℥viij. M.
Capiat. f℥iss. quartis horis.

22d.—Less purging; much as before
in other respects.

℞ Sulphatis Ferri, Ext. Hyoscyami, aa.
gr. ij.; Ft. pilula. Capiat j. ter die.
H. s. s. Pulv. Antimonialis, gr. v.

24th.—Slept pretty well; had a sup-pository of five grains of Pil. Sap. c. Opio. Bowels not moved in the night; complains of looseness of the teeth, of weakness, and of pain across the loins.

Contr. pil. et rep. suppositorium.

Nov. 3d.—Improved; no return of purging; perspired freely in the night; pulse 84; somewhat improved in strength; slight drowsiness; no pain of head, or cough.

4th.—Perspired last night; tongue florid at the tip and edges; mouth dry; fæces dark and offensive, and containing, according to his own re-port, some blood; occasional pain across the loins; pulse 81, regular; counted during one minute while the patient was in a sitting posture; after walking three or four times across the room it rose to 84, counted in a stand-ing posture. Respirations 22 in one minute.

℞ Sulph. Ferri; Camphoræ; Extr. Conii; Extr. Gentianæ; Extr. Rhei aa. gr. xij. M. Fiant. pil. xij.; Capiat. j. ter die.

To have three raw eggs daily, 4 ounces of additional meat, and 6 ounces less bread.

From the beginning of November to the beginning of January, when the patient expired, a register was accurately kept of the food taken, and the urine and fæces evacuated daily. These ob-servations were made by an intelligent patient, who occupied an adjoining bed, and who was in every way quali-fied for the purpose, as he had long officiated as guard of the mail on the London and Holyhead road, and had, therefore, been accustomed to weighing. I am satisfied that this individual took every precaution to ensure accuracy of result. He scarcely ever left the patient Merchant, who could not, if he had been disposed, have deceived his at-tendant, in respect to ingesta or egesta.

9th.—Feels better. He relishes the eggs.

Contr. pil. Habeat ter die Sodæ phos-phatis, ℈ij.

12th.—As before; still some œdema of legs. Wishes to have an onion.

15th.—After exposure, he caught a severe cold, attended with pain of the face and ear on the left side; he has, in consequence, fretted much, and to-day I found him crying.

℞ Sp. Ammon. Aromat. Sp. Lavand. Co. aa. f℥ij.; Mist. Camph. f℥vss. M. Capiat f℥j. p. r. n.

I was sent for in the evening to visit him again. He complained of pain of the left side of the chest below the scapula, increased by pressure, by cough, and by deep inspiration. There was dulness in this situation, and the respiratory murmur was not audible over a limited space. Dyspnœa. In-spirations short and abrupt. I did not detect crepitation.

Lateri Sinistro Applic. Empl. Lyttæ.

℞ Sp. Æth. Nitr. f℥ij.; Tinct. Opii. f℥iss.; Aquæ, f℥iv.; M. Capiat ℥j. p. r. n.

16th.—The blister has not risen; passed a tolerable night; no perspira-tion; pain of side diminished; dyspnœa relieved by the mixture; skin warm and dry; pulse 88, as before; bowels open last evening.

Rep. Pulv. Ipecac. co. gr. x. Cont. Mistura.

17th.—The blister having been left applied has now risen; no return of dyspnœa or of pain of side.

Rep. Pulv. Cont. alia.

23d.—Has been purged five or six times during the night; stools dark and watery; vesicular eruption of lower lip; when hurried or excited, he still has pain in lower part of left side of chest; skin dry, and more harsh.

Cont. Pil. Om. Sodæ Phosphas. Gargar. Boracis.

26th.—Feels much better this morn-ing; perspired freely in the night; mouth less dry; spat freely last even-ing. Says that "when his mouth is dry he is always bad; and when it is moist he is always better." Bowels pretty regular; stools lighter coloured than previously.

Four eggs daily.

Dec. 6th.—I found him in bed cry-ing, in consequence of severe pain referred to left shoulder.

Linim. Camph. Co. Potatoes to be omitted.

8th.—Still complains of aching pain,

referred especially to a small space on the posterior edge of the left scapula, where there is considerable tenderness on pressure; perspires much every night.

Cont. To have carbonate of soda daily.

9th.—Pain is removed from the scapula, and is now referred to left axilla; tenderness on pressure in the situation of the pain; tongue very florid at the tip and edges; mouth still moist; abdomen generally tympanitic.

Epigastrio applic. Hirudines iv.; H. s. s. Pulv. Ipecac. co. gr. x.; cras mane Olei Ricini, f3vj.

10th.—Passed a good night, and perspired copiously; tongue not quite so red at the tip and edges.

21st.—I had been absent for several days from Birmingham. Since I last saw him he appears to have remarkably altered for the worse. Complains much of wandering aching pains, referred to the shoulders, arms, and hips; feels much weaker; face œdematous; pulse feeble; dyspnœa, increased by the recumbent posture; numbness of both arms and legs; he cannot flex the fingers of the left hand; much purged.

Statim Habent. Suppositorium. c. Pil. Sap. c. Opio, gr. x.

R Infusi Calumbæ, Mist. Camph. aa. f3iv.; Tinct. Conii, f3ij.; Ammon. Carb. 3j.; M. Capiat f3j.; ter die. Diet as before. Om. alia.

24th.—Pretty much as before; complains of pain across the loins and shoulders; purging still continues; tongue aphthous; restless night; pale and offensive stools, compared to yeast.

Injic. Enema Amyli c. Tinct. Opii, f3j.

R Opii, Camphoræ, aa. gr. j.; Ext. Hyoscyami, gr. ij. Ft. Pil. Capiat j. bis terve indies.

R Æth. Sulphur. Sp. Lavand. co. Sp. Ammon. Aromat. aa. f3ij.; Mist. Camph. f3vss. M.; Capiat f3j p. r. n. Gargarisma Mellis Boracis. Partibus quâ dolet. Empl. Opii.

28th.—Much complaint of pain and soreness generally, principally referred to shoulders, arms, and loins; no œdema of face; can scarcely bear to be moved; sat up nearly the whole of yesterday; purged five or six times during the night; stools dark; pulse compressible; skin hot and dry; teazing hacking cough; slightest pressure about the shoulders occasions pain.

Cont. Medic. Sumat. Pil. 4tes. indies. H. s. Suppositor. Pil. Sap. c. Opio, gr. x.; Lumbis applic. cucurbit. sine ferro.

R Extracti Conii. 3j.; Aquæ, f3viij.: M. Ft. lotio, partibus dolent. applic.

29th.—Much relief from dry cupping; purging six times in the course of the night.

Contr.

30th.—Passed a quiet night; perspired profusely during the night; he had had forty drops of laudanum. I found him asleep, bathed in perspiration.

Cont. et rep. haustus. Tinct. Opii.

31st.—Passed a tolerably good night; slept well yesterday and during the night; no return of perspiration, which, however, continued the whole of yesterday; pulse 98, compressible; occasional hacking cough; pains much abated; bowels moved last night; stools reported natural in appearance; tongue smooth and red; aphthæ gone; pain across the loins and between the shoulders; thirst much diminished; countenance more cheerful; mouth moist. Has, during the last four days, taken four opium pills daily; numbness of left hand and arm up to the shoulder; can now raise this hand to his mouth, whereas, a few days ago, he had scarcely any power over it.

Capiat Pil. Opii. v. quotidie. Rep. haustus Opii.

Jan. 2d.—In the afternoon of yesterday (Sunday), I visited him. He was much in the same condition as when I last saw him, except that the pulse was considerably weaker, and had evidently begun to fail. He took his opiate draught at about 2 in the morning. He voided urine for the last time at a quarter past 10 in the evening of January 1st, when he went to stool. Between 3 and 4 this morning he attempted to pass fæces, but without effect: at this time he drank copiously of peppermint-water, and was able to hold the bottle to his mouth. He passed fæces in bed at 10 minutes before 6, when it was found that he could not speak. After a few groans, he tranquilly expired at a quarter before 7 this morning. He sat up and was cheerful on the 31st of December. He fully believed that his complaint was removed, and that he should shortly be able to return to his friends, who, however, were apprised of his situation. Mr. Fulford, our intelligent resident-surgeon, informs me that for one or two nights previously to his decease he had obstinate erection, with sexual desire.

By some, perhaps, it may be thought that in recording this case I have entered into superfluous detail. My apology must be, that in the study of a disease like diabetes mellitus, the pathology of which is involved in so much obscurity, minute and persevering observation is essential. My object is truth; and I cherish the hope, that the labour and attention which have been expended in these observations, may tend, in some degree, to promote this object.

Post-mortem examination, Jan. 3, 10 A.M.: present, my colleague Mr. Bolton, Demonstrator of Anatomy; Mr. Fulford, Resident-Surgeon; Mr. Hinds, my industrious clinical clerk, and myself.

The body generally presented the appearance of great emaciation. No œdema. No cadaveric discoloration of depending parts.

Head.—On opening the dura-mater, on each side, a quantity of air-bubbles escaped. Examined the brain *in situ.* A minute quantity of effused liquid in the cavity of the arachnoid. Pia-mater of anterior lobes pale, but vessels of pia-mater of middle, and especially of posterior lobes, contained blood. On the anterior lobes, under the arachnoid, and *between* the convolutions, air, in small bubbles, was accumulated. On the posterior lobe of right hemisphere, on its upper surface, in the centre, and near the falx, there was a small quantity of white flaky deposit beneath the arachnoid in a few points; this matter appeared to be distinct from the membrane itself. On slicing off the hemispheres nothing abnormal was observed. A very small quantity of effusion was found in each lateral ventricle. The choroid plexuses were pale. In the arachnoid, at the base, there was also some serous liquid. The cerebral substance was everywhere firm.

Thorax.—On turning up the sternum, there came into view a superficial abscess, of an irregularly oval form, and about two inches by three, situated on the anterior and inferior part of right lung, and commencing at the cartilage of the third rib and extending to that of the sixth. Immediately beneath this abscess the lung was condensed, and there were several small excavations containing pus; and further in the substance of the lung were found several small collections of softened tubercular matter. Slight pleuritic adhesions on the right as well as the left side, but to a greater extent on the former than on the latter. Right lung weighed 2 lbs. (all the weights avoirdupois); left lung, 1 lb. 1½oz. Both were gorged with red serous liquid, and both contained small collections of tubercular matter, in a crude and also in a softened state, irregularly disseminated throughout their substance. Some of these collections, of the size of a small hazelnut, were immediately beneath the pleura. No pleuritic effusion. *Heart* small, weighing, with the arch of the aorta, 8 oz. 12 drachms. On the surface was a quantity of gelatinous matter, which appeared like translucent fat*. All the valves and all the cavities perfectly natural.

The vagus nerve was very large and firm. The great and lesser splachnic nerves and semilunar ganglion were much larger than natural; and these nerves were so firm as to appear to the touch cartilaginous and chord-like. Thoracic duct of the natural size. The muscles of the chest, and, indeed, the muscles generally, were pale and flabby, and in some parts, for example the recti abdominis, had undergone a kind of gelatinous degeneration.

Abdomen.—No liquid in the peritoneal cavity. The intestines were pale and attenuated; they were generally stained with bile, and where they were not so stained they presented a pale leaden hue. We were remarkably struck with the almost complete absence, in the omentum, mesentery, and the body throughout, of everything that resembled ordinary fat. Except

---

* This matter became opaque by boiling in water. Æther extracted only a trace of fatty matter. By drying, a minute quantity only of residuum was obtained.

E.

in a space of small extent, the omentum had a dark slaty appearance, as though produced by a kind of melanotic deposit. The mesenteric glands were generally enlarged, and, by section, exhibited a somewhat gelatinous aspect. *Liver:* Gall-bladder distended with pale bile. Colour of the liver natural. Some adhesions on upper surface to the diaphragm. Nothing abnormal discovered by section. Liver and gall-bladder weighed 3 lbs. Spleen apparently healthy; weight 6 oz. *Pancreas* also healthy; weight 3 oz. *Stomach* presented nothing abnormal. *Kidneys:* right weighed 6 oz. 5 drs.; *left*, after having been injected with size, weighed 7 oz. 8 drs. Both were more deeply lobulated than usual. They were equal in size. *Right* measured 4½ inches long by 2½ broad. On the surface of the *right* one there were collections of what appeared like caseous matter before section; they were eight in number, varying in size from a pea to a hazel-nut; they were scattered irregularly. By section it was ascertained that they contained true purulent matter. There was no proper fat in the vicinity of the kidneys, but only a substitute of the same gelatinous consistence as that formerly described. The infundibula and calices were all, as might be anticipated, much larger than in ordinary circumstances. The *bladder* was distended with urine of a brown colour. I collected f℥xij.; some, however, escaped on removing the viscus. No morbid appearance. A small collection of pus was found in the vicinity of the prostate.

Table of the quantity of Liquid drunk, and the quantity of Urine evacuated daily, from August 29th, to October 20th.

The first part of this table is doubtless, in some respects, incorrect, from the fact, previously mentioned, that the patient for a short time after admission took liquid by stealth. He confessed this a few days before his death, but affirmed that afterwards he had never deceived us in this respect.

Date.	Pints Liquid drunk.	Pints Urine passed.	Specific gravity.	Date.	Pints Liquid Drunk.	Pints Urine passed.	Specific gravity.
Aug. 29	8	12	037°	Sept. 25	12	18	1036°
30	7	12	40	26	12	18	32
31	6	12	36	27	14	20	34
Sept. 1	5	9	38	28	16	20	32
2	6	12	38	29	18	20	36
3	6	10	39	30	20	20	33
4	6	10	44	Oct. 1	20	20	33
5	6	10	37	2	4	10	38
6	6	12	36	3	6	10	42
7	6	12	35	4	8		
8	6	10		5	8	3	40
9	6	12		6			
10	6	12	36	7	14	4	
11	6	12	34	8	14	8½	31
12	6	12	38	9	14	9½	50
13	6	12	36	10	14	3½	40
14	6	10	38	11	14	3	35
15				12	14	4	35
16	8	12	36	13	14	5	35
17	8	12	36	14	14	8	35
18	10	16	35	15	14	10	35
19	8	14	35	16	14	12	38
20	12	14	36	17	14	14	38
21	12	16	35	18	14	16	36
22	12	20	34	19	14	18	35
23	12	14	35	20	14	18	40
24	12	18	39				

Tables of the quantity of food, liquid and solid, taken by Merchant, from November 2 to January 2 inclusive.

Every single item is introduced, in order to furnish data for any calculations for which these tables may serve as a basis. Dinner means 14 ounces of meat, beef or mutton, cooked; the extra weight is gravy and potatoes. The average amount of gravy may be ascertained by reference to the latter part of the table, when no vegetable matter was taken with the meat. Supper means simply milk. The milk used for tea is included in the supper. The weights are avoirdupois. For gin was occasionally substituted whiskey. 1000·0 grains of beef-tea were found to contain 931·6 of water, 52·8 of animal matter, and 15·6 of saline matter. Peppermint water was common water flavoured with oil of peppermint.

Food taken.	Nov. 2.	Nov. 3.	Nov. 4.	Nov. 5.	Nov. 6.	Nov. 7.	Nov. 8.	Nov. 9.	Nov. 10.	Nov. 11.	Nov. 12.	Nov. 13.	Nov. 14.	Nov. 15.	Nov. 16.	Nov. 17.	Nov. 18.
Bread																	
Dinner																	
Supper																	
Ale																	
Beef-tea																	
Tea																	
Water																	
Peppermint water																	
Eggs																	
Onion																	
Gin																	
Total																	

Food taken.	Nov. 19.	Nov. 20.	Nov. 21.	Nov. 22.	Nov. 23.	Nov. 24.	Nov. 25.	Nov. 26.	Nov. 27.	Nov. 28.	Nov. 29.	Nov. 30.	Dec. 1.	Dec. 2.	Dec. 3.	Dec. 4.	Dec. 5.
Bread																	
Dinner																	
Supper																	
Ale																	
Beef-tea																	
Tea																	
Water																	
Peppermint water																	
Eggs																	
Onion																	
Gin																	
Total																	

Table of the food, &c. taken by Merchant—continued.

Food taken.	Dec. 6.	Dec. 7.	Dec. 8.	Dec. 9.	Dec. 10.	Dec. 11.	Dec. 12.	Dec. 13.	Dec. 14.	Dec. 15.	Dec. 16.	Dec. 17.	Dec. 18.	Dec. 19.
	lbs. oz.	lbs. oz.	lbs. oz.	lbs. oz.	lbs. oz.	lbs. oz.	lbs. oz.	lbs. oz.	lbs. oz.	lbs. oz.	lbs. oz.	lbs. oz.	lbs. oz.	lbs. oz.
Bread	2 6	2 2	2 2	2 2	2 2	2 2	2 2	2 2	2 2	2 2	2 2	2 2	1 13½	1 13
Dinner	1 2¼	0 13½	0 15	0 15¾	1 2	1 0½	1 2	1 2	1 2	1 2	1 2	1 2	1 0	1 0
Supper	2 5¼	2 5¼	2 9	3 3¼	2 7	1 2	2 7	2 6	2 6½	2 7	2 6	2 6	2 6	2 6
Ale	1 13	1 15	1 12	1 10	1 15	1 7½	1 12¾	1 12	1 12	1 12	1 12	1 12	1 12	1 0
Beef-tea	0 14	0 12	0 12	0 11½	0 12	0 13	0 12	0 11½	0 11½	0 11½	0 11½	0 11	0 11	0 10½
Tea	2 7	5 3¼	5 3¼	4 14¼	4 8¾	4 13	5 0¼	4 12¼	4 12½	4 12½	4 12	4 12	4 12	4 12
Water	..	..	2 0	2 0	..	..	..	..	..	..	..	..	..	..
Peppermint Water	2 8	2 8	5 0	2 8½	2 9½	2 9½	..	2 9	2 9	2 9	2 9	2 7	2 9	2 6
Eggs	0 6	0 6½	0 7	0 7	0 7	0 7	0 7	0 7	0 7	0 7	0 7	0 7	0 7	0 6
Onion	0 3	0 3	0 3	0 3	0 3	0 3	0 3	0 3	0 3	0 3	0 3	0 3	0 3	0 3
Gin	0 2	0 2	0 2	0 2	0 2	0 2	0 2	0 2	0 2	0 2	0 2	0 2	0 2	0 2
Total	14 2¾	16 6½	21 1½	18 13¾	16 4	14 11½	14 0	16 3	16 3½	16 4	16 2½	16 0	15 11¼	15 10½

Food taken.	Dec. 20.	Dec. 21.	Dec. 22.	Dec. 23.	Dec. 24.	Dec. 25.	Dec. 26.	Dec. 27.	Dec. 28.	Dec. 29.	Dec. 30.	Dec. 31.	Jan. 1.
	lbs. oz.	lbs. oz.	lbs. oz.	lbs. oz.	lbs. oz.	lbs. oz.	lbs. oz.	lbs. oz.	lbs. oz.	lbs. oz.	lbs. oz.	lbs. oz.	lbs. oz.
Bread	2 12	1 12	1 13	1 12	1 9½	1 9	1 10	1 5	1 7	1 7	1 7	1 7	1 7
Dinner	1 0	1 2	1 2	1 0	1 0	1 0	1 0	0 10	0 12	0 12	0 10	0 10	1 8
Supper	2 0	2 0	2 0	2 0	2 0	2 0	2 0	2 0	2 0	2 0	2 0	2 0	..
Ale	1 8	1 0	1 10	1 8	1 8	1 8	1 8	1 8	1 8	1 8	1 8	1 4	1 8
Beef-tea	0 9	0 5	0 10	0 10	0 10	0 10½	0 10	0 10	0 10	0 10	0 10	0 10	0 10
Tea	4 0	4 0	4 0	4 0	4 0	4 0	4 0	4 0	4 0	4 0	4 0	4 0	4 0
Water	..	..	..	..	..	..	..	..	..	..	..	..	..
Peppermint water	..	2 6	..	..	..	2 6	..	..	..	..	..	2 6	2 6
Eggs	0 6	0 6	0 7	0 6½	0 7	0 7	0 7	0 7	0 7	0 7	0 7	0 7	0 7
Onion	0 3	0 3	0 3	0 3	..	..	..	..	..	..	..	..	..
Gin	0 2	0 2	0 2	0 2	0 3	0 3	0 3	0 3	0 3	0 3	0 3	0 3	0 3
Total	12 8	13 4	11 15	11 9½	11 5½	13 11½	11 6	10 11	10 15	10 15	10 13	12 15	12 1

Tables indicating the daily amount of ingesta and egesta, and the specific gravity of the urine, at different times of the day, from November 2 to January 1. The weights are avoirdupois. The weight of fæces was accurately determined, as the patient always had a chamber-vessel before him during the evacuation of his bowels.

Date.	Food taken.	Urine & fæces passed.	Fæces passed.	Urine passed.	Specific gravity of Urine. Morn.	Noon.	Even.
	lbs. oz.	lbs. oz.	lbs. oz.	lbs. oz.			
Nov. 2.	21 0	23 15½	3 9	20 6½	35	...	...
3.	23 9½	23 0	3 11	19 5	40	...	...
4.	18 10	21 2	7 1	14 1	40	...	...
5.	18 0¾	19 7½	1 7	18 0½	42	...	...
6.	17 7¼	23 15½	3 9	20 6½	35	...	...
7.	19 5¾	17 12	3 2	14 10	33	...	...
8.	18 2½	19 4	4 5	14 15	33	...	...
9.	20 0¾	...	...	15 0¾	35	32½	32
10.	21 12½	21 1	1 6	19 11	31½	33	31½
11.	22 9½	20 14¾	1 15¾	18 15	42½	32	32
12.	20 7¾	20 7	1 9	18 14	42½	41	41
13.	21 5¾	...	...	14 4¼	42½	42	40
14.	19 7½	...	...	...	42½	42	42
15.	20 1¾	15 4¼	1 0½	14 3¾	42½	44	...
16.	16 7¾	17 6½	2 0	15 6½	42½	42½	...
17.	17 15¼	...	...	13 7	42½	...	42
18.	18 11¼	14 9½	4 0½	10 9	42	41	...
19.	18 1	...	...	10 2¾	42	41½	...
20.	16 11½	10 10	5 0	5 10	41	41	...
21.	18 0¼	10 6	4 11½	5 10½	40	41	...

Date.	Food taken.	Urine & fæces passed.	Fæces passed.	Urine passed.	Specific gravity of Urine. Morn.	Noon.	Even.
	lbs. oz.	lbs. oz.	lbs. oz.	lbs. oz.			
Nov. 22	16 3	10 9	3 5	7 4	41	41	...
23	18 8½	17 0¾	2 10½	14 6½	32	38	...
24	16 12¼	10 5½	4 12	5 9½	32	33	...
25	17 4	13 6½	2 11½	10 11	34	33	30
26	18 3½	19 5½	5 10	13 11½	34	...	32
27	16 4¾	...	...	9 2	½35	...	34
28	16 6½	14 9	4 2	10 7	36	...	35½
29	16 13¼	12 6	2 13½	9 8½	31	...	32
30	15 12¾	14 12½	4 2	10 10½	35	...	34
Dec. 1	16 15¼	12 8	1 11½	10 12½	32	...	33
2	16 5¼	13 1	1 8	11 9	30	...	30
3	14 2¼	9 0	3 1½	5 14½	32	...	32½
4	17 3¼	16 3	2 10	13 9	38	...	36
5	17 9½	15 4½	2 7½	12 13	30	...	29
6	14 2¼	...	...	..	30	...	29
7	16 6½	14 3	1 12	12 7	32	...	32
8	21 1¾	...	...	12 14	29	...	29
9	18 13¼	...	...	13 15½	32	...	...
10	16 4	11 15	2 8	9 7	31	...	31
11	14 11½	...	...	6 5	26	...	26

Date.	Food taken.	Urine & fæces passed.	Fæces passed.	Urine passed.	Specific Gravity of Urine. Morn.	Even.
	lbs. oz.	lbs. oz.	lbs. oz.	lbs. oz.		
Dec. 12	14 0	10 7½	2 3	8 4½	29	29
13	16 3	...	...	14 4½	30	30
14	16 3½	9 5¼	4 5	5 0¼	35	35
15	16 4	...	...	9 4½	35	35
16	16 2½	14 14¾	6 1½	8 13¼	35	35
17	16 0	8 3	1 9½	6 9½	32	32
18	15 11¼	7 15¼	3 0	4 15½	29	28
19	15 10½	5 10½	2 8½	3 2¼	32⅛	29
20	12 8	8 12½	5 9½	3 3	32	35
21	13 4	...	...	12 14	29	29
22	11 15	6 4	3 14	2 6	32	35
23	11 9½	11 14½	7 1	4 13	33	34
24	11 5½	9 7	4 10	4 13	34	34
25	13 11½	10 8	5 2	5 6	36	36
26	11 6	10 1	9 3	0 14	30	30
27	10 11	10 9	10 1½	0 7½	22	...
28	10 15	9 0	7 4	1 12	...	...
29	10 15	9 10	7 14	1 12	15	...
30	10 13	...	...	..	...	...
31	12 15	11 12½	8 12	3 0¼	15	17
Jan. 1.	12 1	5 13	4 0	1 13	20	20

Table of Merchant's Weight.

Date.	Morning.			Noon.			Evening.		
	st.	lbs.	oz.	st.	lbs.	oz.	st.	lbs.	oz.
Nov. 5.	...			...			8	9	0
6	8	2	0	8	7	0	...		
7	...			...			8	5	0
8	8	1½	0	8	7	0	8	8	8
9	...			8	6	13	8	9	4
10	8	5	4	8	7	4	8	12	8
11	8	6	8	8	10	4	8	11	0
12	8	5	0½	8	7	0	8	11	0
13	8	2	12	8	6	0	8	6	0
14	8	0	6	8	2	0	8	2	0
15	7	14	0	...			...		
27	...			8	7	0	...		
29	...			8	11	8	...		
Dec. 2.	...			...			8	9	0
5	...			...			8	7	8

[To be continued.]

THE HUMAN SKIN AND ITS PATHOLOGY.

By OTHO WUCHERER, M.D.

Member of the Royal College of Surgeons in
London; Rua de Boa Vista, Lisbon.

(For the London Medical Gazette.)

THE following brief and cursory sketch of the anatomy and physiology of the skin and mucous membrane, is intended merely as a preface to some remarks on cutaneous diseases, and professes to regard only some of the more recent discoveries.

Corium and mucous membrane resemble one another much in structure: in respect of chemical composition, however, they differ; the former giving glue when boiled, the latter not. Both have some resemblance to cellular tissue, consisting of fibres united together to a sort of irregular net-work, but they are easily distinguished from it by a granular appearance, and a more intricate interlacement of their fibres, which have, however, between them an homogeneous structure, bearing a greater resemblance to that tissue. Mucous membrane contains, moreover, as pointed out by Henle, dark bodies equal in diameter to 0·0013 of a Parisian line, of an uncertain shape and unequal distribution, soluble in acetic acid.

The corium presents on its surface slight elevations, the diameter of which is found to be equal to half a Parisian line. They consist of tortuous vessels, and loops of nerves, and seem to be connected with one another at the base: however, they are evidently separated by perceptible grooves; they are pierced by the excretory tubes of the sudorific glands. As in other parts, two and two primitive nervous fibres form loops, but in the elevations now in question these loops do not lie so open to view, being folded together in various ways, so as to form balls, some of which, collected together in the figure of rosettes, may be found on the corium of the ends of the fingers, as shown by Gerber.

Leuwenhoeck long since described, as consistent parts of the skin and epithelium of the mucous membrane in the mouth, pentangular scales, which are constantly cast off from the surface and reproduced underneath: however, Henle was the first to give a proper description of the superficial coverings of the skin and mucous membranes, to which the term of epithelium is applied in common. According to this assiduous anatomist it consists of one or more layers of transparent cells, which cover the corium, in a great part the mucous membranes, the serous membranes, and also the inner tunic of the blood-vessels. These cells have a nucleus, the shape of which is more or less flat and roundish or oval, and in which again are discovered one or two nucleoli. The shape of the nuclei is always the same, but not so that of the cells, which differs in the different kinds of epithelium, as also in the different stages of their development.

The first kind of epithelium described by Henle has in its appearance some resemblance to the pavement of a street; whence the German term, *plaster-epithelium*, for it. It forms a covering for the whole surface of the body, and some parts of the mucous membranes. The cells of which it is composed follow in general the outlines of their nuclei, which they surround as spacious cases. Acetic acid sometimes dissolves only the cells, or only their nuclei, or both, or neither. In all parts, except the excretory ducts of glands and the tympanum, they lie in more than one layer. As they proceed from the surface of the skin propelled by new generations of cells, and so gain at last the outmost position in the whole layer of epithelium, they undergo changes in their structure and shape, arising from their pressure one against the other.

In the layer next to the corium the nuclei are of a yellowish red, and have a slight resemblance to blood-globules; in the beginning they are not surrounded by cells, and when these appear they surround the nuclei very closely. Of this layer acetic acid dissolves both nuclei and cells. In the next more superficial layers the nuclei show a more granular appearance, are of a lighter colour, and appear larger; however, the cells grow still more, and become, in proportion to the nuclei, much larger than in the preceding layer. Still more superficially both cells and nuclei become flatter, till they finally attain the shape of thin scales or disks with their nuclei in the middle. The nuclei become, as the cells proceed to the surface, less and less distinct, particularly when the latter dry up and stick together. The diameter of the nuclei in this kind of epithelium is 0·0012-0·0040 of a Parisian line; that of the cells in the innermost layer 0·0035-0·0072; in the most external or superficial layer 0·010-0·015 of a Parisian line. The thickness of the epithelium never diminishes, and as the most superficial cells are cast off there must be a constant reproduction of cells on the corium. These new cells undergo, then, those changes in structure and shape, as are described above in the different layers of cells. According to Schwann, the nuclei of new cells are formed in a fluid substance, which being the same in which all tissues have their origin, is called by him cytoblastema. This kind of epithelium, as at present described, covers besides the corium some parts of the mucous membranes. The mucous membrane of the eyelids has, according to Henle, cylindrical epithelium, but the lachrymal tube has pavement-like epithelium, which reaches on the septum, as well as on the side-walls of the nose, till to a line which you may imagine extending from the anterior free margin of the nasal bones to the anterior spine of the superior maxillary bone. The tympanum is also laid out with a pavement-like epithelium consisting of very small globular cells. In the neighbourhood of the larynx, the ligaments between the tongue and epiglottis, the upper surface of the latter and the posterior part of its under surface are covered with pavement-like epithelium. On the anterior wall of the larynx it reaches but a short way under the epi-

glottis, on the posterior till about two lines from the aperture of the larynx. Beyond these limits, another, the vibratory epithelium, is found. On the mucous membranes of the digestive tube the pavement-like epithelium is extended over the inside of the mouth, over the pharynx and œsophagus, till to the pylorus, meeting, however, at the cardia with a short interruption. On the uropoetical mucous membrane of the male, pavement-like epithelium is found only in the cells of the prostate, and in the vesiculæ seminales; in the female it covers the inner surface of the labia majora, the nymphæ, clitoris, hymen, vagina, and inferior half of the neck of the uterus.

The second kind of epithelium, as Henle describes it, is the cylindrical epithelium. Its cells are of a conical shape, the point being turned towards the mucous membrane, the base towards the surface, and the nucleus situated about the half of their length on the inner surface of their wall. These cylindrical cells become immediately pale in acetic acid, and after some time they are dissolved by it to the nuclei, which finally also disappear. Ether or alcohol produce no change on them, nor carbonate of ammonia or caustic ammonia, and the strong mineral acids, but they are soluble in carbonate of potash and caustic potassa. Their length is equal to 0·008-0·009 of a Parisian line, the diameter of their thick end to 0·0017-0·0024 of a Parisian line. This epithelium is not constant like the former, but at intervals cast off and reproduced. According to Henle it is found at a point in the stomach just below the cardia, and then from the pylorus till the anus throughout the intestines, covering all the projections. At the anus it stops suddenly, and there is no gradual transition from it to the epithelium of the skin or epidermis. It covers also all the excretory ducts of the glands connected with the digestive tube. In the genital organs of the male it is only wanting in the prostate and vesiculæ seminales. The urinary bladder has an intermediate kind of epithelium, with oblong cells placed perpendicularly.

As a third kind, Henle describes the vibratory epithelium, which consists of cylindrical or conical cells similar to those of the cylindrical epithelium, but they have on this broad end ciliæ 3 to 8 in number. The length of the cells is, according to Henle, equal to 0·008-0·0138; their greatest breadth at the external end 0·0037-0·0025 of a Parisian line. The length of the ciliæ is, according to Treviranus, equal to 0·0018; their thickness 0·0004 of a Parisian line. This epithelium is cast off and reproduced like the former, but at intervals. According to Henle it is found in the respiratory organs beyond the above-defined limits, and in the female genital organs upwards of the middle of the neck of uterus. It is also found on the inner side of the eye-lids, in the lachrymal sac and duct, and finally in the ventricles of the brain. The ciliæ are of an homogeneous structure, and are arranged in a manner similar to that of the lines seen on the palm of the hand. They move during life constantly to and fro, and bend at the same time in which the free ends of the ciliæ describe circles on their ends. A circular motion of the ciliæ, in which the free ends of the ciliæ describe circles, Müller and Rudolph Wagner declare never to have seen.

The nails and hairs may be regarded as a peculiar modification of the epidermis. The nails are received with their posterior part into a fold of the corium, which is, like this, covered with papillæ, differing from those of the corium only in being smaller. The structure of the nails is best seen in the fœtus. If the nail of a full-grown fœtus, or a new-born child, is cut through longitudinally, you perceive it to consist of several layers, the undermost of which are less distinct, particularly in that part concealed in the fold of corium, where they are hardly perceptible at all. This part of the nail is seen to consist of polyhedral cells, many of which show nuclei. Dr. Schwann thinks, that as these cells are pushed forward from their origin in the fold of corium by successive generations of cells, they attain the form of small flat discs, which are found in the front of the nail. But as in this case the nail would be much thinner in its fore-part than behind, Schwann, and also Lauth and Gurlt, are of opinion that the formation of cells takes place also on the under surface of the nail as far as it is adherent. These cells proceed towards the forepart of the nail, in which direction layers increase in number. Before the fifth month of fœtal existence the nail can hardly be distinguished in structure from the epidermis.

The hairs proceed from follicles, which according to Gurlt are nothing but impressions into or bulgings of the epidermis: this is clearly seen if the epidermis is torn off from a piece of skin of a fœtus macerated some time; then these follicles are seen to come off in one continuation with the epidermis. They are widest at their blind end, and narrowest at their neck, or where they open on the surface. At their blind end they have an elevation into their cavity, similar to the bottom of a glass bottle; on this elevation the hairs grow forth. The hairs are, according to Weber and Müller, not round, but rather flat, and the surface they present when cut through is oval or reniform. Gurlt, Heusinger, Eble, Krause, and Valentia, declare them to consist of an external or cortical, and an internal cellular substance. The former is thin, transparent, and evidently of a fibrous structure; the latter is composed of cells arranged in a single row of a diameter equal to 0·0006-0·0015. In a hair are generally distinguished the point, the shaft, and the root. Gurlt says that in the point the cellular substance is wanting, but it is found in the shaft. In the root or bulb both cortical and cellular substance are soft and tender. The elevation on the bottom of the follicle is received into a conical cavity in the bulb of the hair, and Gurlt says that there intervene fine threads or roots between both.

Between corium and epidermis of individuals possessing a dark complexion is found the black pigment. It is contained in cells similar to those of the epidermis, which contain, besides a transparent nucleus, fine particles of pigment. Sometimes these cells are prolonged in three or more directions, and those prolongations that radiate from the central cell are also filled with pigment. Whether these cells of pigment proceed to the surface of the epidermis, like those of the latter, and undergo the same changes till they are cast off, is not yet ascertained.

Albinus* says, there are no sebaceous glands of the skin where there are no hairs, and rests this assertion on his own and Morgagni's observations: he did not fall very short of the truth, and

* Albinus, Acad. Annot. Libr. vi. c. 9.

would have been quite correct if he had said, where there proceed hairs from the skin there are sebaceous glands. However, there are but few places in the integuments where sebaceous glands are found without hairs, as on the prepuce and glans penis. According to the description of Gurlt, the sebaceous follicles are of an oblong oval shape, and consist of cells, which when void of sebum are transparent. The excretory tubes of these cells open generally two in number, into a hair follicle. The sebaceous follicles are disseminated throughout the whole integuments of the body, with the exception of the palm of the hand and the sole of the foot. In some parts they are more easily discerned than in others; they are easily recognised in the integuments of new-born children, particularly of the scrotum, where the absence of fat under the corium prevents their being mistaken for little particles of that substance. As long as the lanugo has not yet fallen off, they are distinct also in other parts. But they are also seen very well in the adult, in the integuments round the mouth, about the nose, and in the axilla. If the epidermis is carefully raised from the corium (after the piece of integument has undergone some maceration) in the direction the hairs proceed from it, fine white threads are seen to go from the epidermis to the corium; these are the sheaths of epidermis that extend themselves into the hair and sebaceous follicles. The latter are, as was observed above, connected with each other, but the hair-follicles reach into the subjacent fatty cellular tissue, and the sebaceous follicles extend but a little into the corium. These organs can be very well seen at the same time with the sudorific glands next to be described, in thin perpendicular slices of integument, for the excision of which some make use of a knife with two blades fixed in a parallel together, which can be screwed more or less close to one another according to the thickness of the slices you wish to cut.

The sudorific glands have been described by Breschet and Gurlt; they often extend beyond the corium into the subjacent fatty cellular tissue, and are in different parts of a different size; for instance, in the palm of the hand they are larger, and of an oval, in the

integument of the head more of a long shape. In man they consist of a long manifold-twisted colourless transparent tube. The continuations of these glands or the excretory ducts are wound in form of a spiral as they proceed through the corium; the thicker the latter, the greater the number of windings. For a clear view of these organs, as well as of the preceding, I refer to the translation of Rudolph Wagner's Physiology, by Dr. Willis.

The papillæ of the corium consist, as has already been mentioned, of tortuous vessels and loops of nerves. In parts where sensation is more acute, these papillæ are more numerous, and show a peculiar arrangement. Whether the skin receives motor nerves or not, is not clearly ascertained. Carus is of opinion, that the peripheric nervous loops are formed by the union of a motor and a sensitive nervous fibre. However, there are not sufficient grounds to set up such an opinion; besides, the auditory nerve presents also such loops at its places of distribution. If it was certain that the skin received only sensitive, and the muscles only motor nerves, this would assist us to decide the question: but Rudolph Wagner observes, that the skin possessed some contractility dependent on nervous influence, and that the muscles were not entirely exempt of sensation, as the pain attending spasms evidently proved. Supposing that the skin received both motor and sensitive nerves, a question not less difficult, perhaps, to decide than the preceding, would arise —if the nutrition of the skin depended on the former or the latter? Johannes Müller says, of such an influence of the nerves in general on nutrition, that we are much in the dark about it. Morbid affections, or an undeveloped state of the nervous centres, are not always attended by changes in nutrition: in other cases the extremities are flaccid and withered, and, what Müller considers a principal proof of the dependency of nutrition on nerves, there is a greater disposition to gangrene. Schröder van der Kolk observed, that in paralyzed limbs the muscular tissue was sometimes displaced by a fatty substance, and the arteries ossified. In cases where, from a defect in development, the nerve destined to supply an organ was wanting, this organ was observed to be wanting also. However, it seems that the nerves are not indispensably necessary for nutrition, as is seen in the evolution of the ovum. But a nervous influence on nutrition is also not to be denied, as the experiments of physiologists, and daily experience, show. The question whether cerebro-spinal or sympathetic nerves possessed this influence is yet undecided : Müller says we know nothing to elucidate it, but that nutrition was not interfered with when cerebro-spinal roots were divided. Valentin says, in his Repertorium, 1838, that we know nothing certain about the influence of nerves on . nutrition. To support the opinion, that nutrition was independent of nervous influence, one might make the remark, that the bones received no nerves (although their nutrition was evidently proved by observations and experiments, as, for instance, those of Mr. James Paget*) if it was not likely that small nerves encircling the arteries of the bones accompanied them ; and this might lead them to the opinion, that since the sympathetic was the nervous system that supplied the blood-vessels, and the bones received only nerves with the latter, nutrition was regulated by the sympathetic. However, there is yet much to be investigated on this subject. Secretion and nutrition are evidently connected in one process. Müller says that few experiments had been tried for the direct proof of nervous influence on secretion, and confesses that we know little about it. He observes, that at first sight both cerebro-spinal and sympathetic nerves seemed to possess this influence.

The submaxillary and sublingual glands are supplied by the lingualis ; the tonsils by the glosso-pharyngeus; the capsule of the knee-joint by a branch from the tibial nerve; and the mamma is supplied by the third and fourth thoracic nerves. However, Müller considers it probable that the cerebrospinal nerves are accompanied by fibres from the sympathetic system. At all events, a dependency of the function of secretion on the nerves is evident in many cases of diseased brain or spinal cord : still, in hemiplegia of the one or the other of these nervous centres, the secretion of the skin is sometimes changed on one side of the body, but in others not. Those grey fibres found

by Remak in the sympathetic system, considered by him as nervous, were admitted as such by many physiologists, and amongst these by Müller, Schwann, and Henle, who went even so far as to consider them to be the nerves that rule the vegetative functions of the body. However, it is doubtful whether this structure is nervous at all. Valentin was the first who expressed himself against it; Volkmann and Bruns have latterly also denied their being a particular element of the sympathetic, and Rudolph Wagner seems convinced by their reasons. Valentin asks, if any one had ever seen grey fibres in the extremities of the adult. (Repertorium, 1840, Abth. i. p. 84.) And Henle, who, as we just mentioned, formerly adopted the nervous nature of these fibres (Pathologische Untersuchungen, 1840), has since changed his opinion, because they had no peripheric ends. If these fibres have no central (Valentin) and no peripheric ends, their nature must certainly remain problematical. Those who considered them nervous admitted only that they were nervous fibres different from others, perhaps less developed ; and on this hypothesis was built another : this undeveloped state was to explain why volition had no power on the vegetative organs, and sensation in them was incomplete. Considered as the nerves for the vegetative functions of the body, they were called organic fibres; Krause called them fibrillæ nodulosæ, after their appearance. Rudolph Wagner declares them to be cellular tissue. It would lead us beyond our limits to treat here of the sense of touch ; we must refer, in this respect, to the works on physiology.

From the surface of the corium the cytoblastema is secreted, in which there appear first the nuclei, and then the cells of the epidermis, as has already been described. The cells undergo a series of changes in form and structure till they are ultimately cast off. These changes cannot be considered but as taking place under the government of life, but they take place without assistance of vessels or nerves; they are in some degree, therefore, independent of the life of the individual ; they remind one of the changes the cells of the yolk in the ovum undergo. The layer of epidermis next to the corium is

* Froriep's Notizen, 1839, 1840.

commonly called the rete Malpighi; and it contains, besides those nuclei and cells known as those of the epidermis, which are cast off, others that contain pigment, are of a peculiar form, and of which it is not quite certain whether they are cast off or not. This layer is as if interrupted in its continuity by the elevated papillæ of the corium, and hence the term "rete" for it.

[To be continued.]

ON THE
INHALATION OF AMMONIA GAS
AS A REMEDIAL AGENT.

By Alfred Smee, F.R.S.

Surgeon to the General Dispensary, to the Bank of England, &c. &c.

(*For the London Medical Gazette.*)

Of all the physical states in which bodies are known to exist, substances in the form of vapour or gas are most readily absorbed by animal membranes, producing rapid and powerful effects from very small quantities. As a mass, we are but little acquainted with the properties of gases upon the animal economy, and the little we do know is principally due to the persevering inquiries of Sir Humphry Davy. The rapidly deleterious effects of minute quantities of the vapours of hydrocyanic acid, of bromine, of sulphuretted hydrogen, and even of many other gases, exemplify well their powerful action on the animal economy. At present gases are almost entirely discarded as remedial agents, but doubtless there are numerous cases where substances may be advantageously employed as remedial agents in their gaseous or aëriform state. Without wasting time upon general remarks, let me at once call the attention of the profession to a simple remedy of this nature, namely, the value of diluted ammonia gas for stimulating the mucous membrane of the mouth, fauces, trachea, and bronchi. By its local administration it may exercise its power over the whole system, as this gas may either be made to have a topical or general influence, according to the extent of its application.

The inhalation of so stimulating a gas as ammonia is well known to be, at first sight, perfectly startling to those who have never either tried it on their own persons or never seen it applied by others, but it is really, in many cases, with proper management, a simple and one of the most delightful remedies that can be employed. If a bottle, containing a solution of the gas, as the common liquor ammonia or hartshorn, be opened, part of the gas escapes. If this comes in contact with the conjunctiva it stimulates it and causes much fluid to be poured from its secreting surface, and its influence on the delicate lining membrane of the nasal cavities is not less powerful. In fact, this vapour appears immediately to cause a secretion of fluid from the parts with which it comes in contact.

When this gas is absorbed by the mouth in far larger quantities, it appears to cause in a similar manner an increase of the watery part of the secretion, usually passing from all the several parts with which it there can come in contact. *A priori* it might be expected the glottis would resist the intrusion of the gas, but this is by no means found to be the case when in a diluted state, as it apparently readily passes into the innermost recesses of the lungs, and instead of producing disagreeable effects, causes sensations which are extremely grateful and agreeable. The gaseous nature of ammonia allows it to come in contact with every chink of the air-passages, and even the upper and back parts of the pharynx, which from its peculiar construction resists the application of other topical remedies.

The immediate effect of the inhalation of this gas is to cause the fauces and pharynx, before dry, and perhaps covered with inspissated adherent mucus, to force out a watery fluid to lubricate and relieve the membrane; the phlegm will then separate and come away, and a more or less instantaneous relief is frequently felt. We all know the expectorant qualities of ammonia, and the value of its sesquicarbonate, whenever the system will bear its administration, as a general remedy, but its qualities, when used as a local agent, seem to be more active in this respect than when used as a general remedy.

The most convenient mode of administering the ammoniacal gas is to use the vapour that spontaneously exhales from solutions of ammonia. Of these it is preferable not to employ a solution stronger than the liquor ammoniæ of the shops, or weaker than the same diluted to twenty or thirty times its quantity of water. For general purposes, perhaps, the usual liquor may be employed diluted with ten times its bulk of water, but the strength of the ammonia must be regulated by the medical practitioner according to the nature of the case, and the susceptibility of the patient, and even according to the strength of the original liquor.

The liquor ammoniæ, diluted according to the discretion of the medical attendant, may be placed in a common phial, and as much should be inserted as to occupy about the two lower inches of the bottle. The patient has only to apply his lips to the mouth of this homely contrivance, and draw in his breath, when he will inhale a certain quantity of the ammonia. Before the application of the mouth to the bottle the patient should take care that none of the liquid adheres to the aperture, which on coming in contact with his lips would cause them to smart, and being no part of the cure, the pain would be perfectly useless. The number of inspirations to be taken at one time may be determined by the strength of the water and the effect of the remedy. Two, three, or four inspirations, will in general be sufficient at one time, but this must be repeated three or four times during the day.

A more convenient apparatus than the simple one last described may be readily made and advantageously employed. A bottle may be selected, and a cork procured, bored with two holes. Into one a piece of bent glass tube may be inserted, having the other end dilated for the convenience of applying the lips. Into the second hole of the cork a tube should be thrust, within half an inch of the liquid, so that when the patient inhales, the ammonia passing from the liquor is taken into the chest, and this is perhaps to be preferred to drawing the breath itself through the solution of ammonia.

Though the last apparatus will answer the purpose more or less efficiently, I have yet to describe a far more elegant device to be employed as an inhaling apparatus. A two-necked bottle is procured, as in the annexed cut; into one mouth a tube is adapted (p), to serve as a mouth-piece. This tube is ground to fit the neck, and when not used is removed for the insertion of a common stopper (s), that the strength of the ammonia may be preserved. Into the neck another tube (t) is ground, into the inside of which another stopper is fixed (s). When the inhaler is in operation, this stopper is withdrawn to allow the air to pass into the bottle, but when not wanted it serves to close the apparatus. This inhaler is most admirably adapted for the desired purpose, and perhaps for gaseous inhalations cannot well be surpassed. The diluted liquor ammonia (a) is seen in the subjoined cut at the bottom of the vessel, extending to within half an inch of the tube.

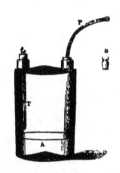

The vapour inhaled from the liquor ammoniæ does not seem to pass away immediately, but may be distinctly tasted for some minutes afterwards, even subsequently to the commencement of its beneficial action. The value of the local application of this gas is seen in cases of what is called dryness of the throat, which appears to arise from a deficiency of the secretion of the liquid which normally lubricates the mucous membrane. The mucus from that cause becomes dry, and causes much uneasiness to the individual. The common and popular remedy of applying hartshorn and oil to the throat for various affections is probably in great part owing to the inhalation of the vapour of the ammonia, which necessarily at the same time occurs, as it is impossible that this external application can be effected without a large quantity being imbibed at the same time.

Ammonia gas is also beneficial in chronic hoarseness, especially in that which is often left as a sequela of influenza.

This gas affords great relief and comfort to the relaxed, swollen, and apparently semi-œdematous state of the mucous membrane, which supervenes from remaining in crowded, overheated, and ill-ventilated rooms, where every person not only inhales his own breath over and over again, but is under the infliction of breathing his neighbour's also. In cases of incipient cynanche tonsillaris it appears to be of much value if used at the very commencement of the attack; the slight impediment to deglutition, which is generally the first premonitory sign, is sometimes removed by one or two inhalations. There are occasionally cases of syphilitic ulceration of the throat witnessed, where the patient suffers from such debility that the practitioner is afraid of applying any remedy capable of depressing the system, where the inhalation of the gas might probably be of great service, but as such a case has not occurred in my own practice for a long period, I am unable to speak practically upon the matter*.

In old standing cases of asthma, especially in those in which the medical man considers that the internal use of the sesquicarbonate of ammonia is indispensable, in which the extremities are cold, the pulse feeble, and the general vital powers depressed, the local application of ammonia is particularly grateful, the patients feeling, as they describe it, a glow after its exhibition, and the warmth first imparted to the lungs extending by degrees over their whole system.

In cases where the patient feels a peculiar sense of contraction upon passing into cold atmospheres, as though the lungs resisted the intrusion of so unpleasant an agent, the inhalation of ammonia seems to quiet the spasmodic action, relieve the breathing, and give a comfort to the whole chest, which is delightful to the feelings of the sufferer.

Perhaps it is almost needless to notice that this remedy would be deleterious when either special organs or the general system are attacked with acute inflammation, for there is but little doubt that the ammoniacal vapour is a decided stimulus, first locally in those parts with which it comes in contact, and, secondly, on the system in general, by its absorption into the circulation. As a stimulating agent it must obey the laws of stimulants generally. It should not, therefore, be employed when the part with which it comes in contact is inflamed, nor when a dry parched tongue, a full pulse, and a dry skin, denote a feverish system. In all chronic cases, or even occasionally with acute cases, with a feeble circulation, in fact, whenever the system is depressed, and stimulants are advisable, the inhalation of ammonia may be used with the greatest advantage and comfort to the patient.

I have made inquiries of those who have to deal with large quantities of ammonia, and are necessarily exposed to the inconvenience of a large escape of gas, but cannot find that even with extensive exposure it ever exercises poisonous or deleterious effects, nor does Ramazzini, in his curious little treatise on tradesmen's diseases, notice its action.

Not alone to the relief and cure of diseases is ammonia capable of lending its aid as a remedial agent, for it is an invaluable and effectual antidote to certain direct and powerful poisons. One of these poisons, the effects of which it thus counteracts, is bromine. This volatile fluid is perhaps one of the most deadly poisons with which we are acquainted. It lowers the circulation with great rapidity, and makes the action of the heart irregular, and unfortunately, from its volatile nature, cannot well be used without considerable escape. Its hurtful action on the animal economy is instantly counteracted by the vapour of ammonia, for when the two gases meet, dense white fumes are produced, when bromine probably ceases to exert its baneful influence, or at any rate only to a much less extent.* I

---

* The inhalation of ammonia might, perhaps, also perform the same good offices to syphilitic ulceration of the throat as cinnabar fumigation is known usually to effect. The use of the cinnabar, however, may be so much dispensed with by the antimonial and antimonio-ferruginous treatment which I have recorded (MED. GAZ), that the ammonia has not been used in any of these cases, but should further information be obtained upon this point, it will be the subject of a future communication.

* The production of these white fumes by the admixture of these two gases is interesting, and, so far as I know, has not been noticed by chemists, though I have myself long been in the habit of applying ammonia to distinguish between the fumes of bromine, iodine, and chlorine, the two latter elements having apparently not the same influence when brought into conjunction with ammonia. These white fumes are liable to be confounded with muriate of ammonia, if muriatic acid is present.

have known persons nearly poisoned by incautiously using this substance, and who have been quite at a loss to know how to proceed to neutralise its action. Those who have to deal with bromine would do well to have an open vessel of the liquor ammonia by their side, which is in general quite sufficient to prevent any unpleasant consequence, by combining with any bromine which may pass off in vapour.

Ammonia is also useful when prussic acid is floating in the atmosphere of a room, as in this case it not only neutralises the acid, but its stimulating properties are directly opposite to the depressing action of the acid.

As all bodies in burning give off ammonia, a consideration arises as to whether some of the effects of smoking may not be attributed to that agent independently of the active principles that substances used for smoking are known to contain. The possibility of such a thing has been suggested to me, but it is quite certain that only a small portion of the effects of smoking can be attributed to the ammonia. The presence of ammonia in a burning cigar may be shewn by collecting its vapour in a bottle containing a few drops of muriatic acid, when abundance of fumes arise. If liquor potassæ be added, the ammonia is again set free, and will again exhibit the white fumes if brought near muriatic acid.

There is an interesting physiological fact connected with the inhalation of ammonia, for in determining the lungs to increase their aqueous exhalation, it frequently at the same time causes a similar action on the skin by the exhalation of moisture from its entire surface. For the last two or three years I have occasionally been in the habit of inhaling ammonia as a luxury during the prevalence of the easterly winds, which by their action so dreadfully dry up and parch all living creatures.

The application of ammoniacal vapour, in the manner which has been already pointed out, is rather an agent of comfort, removing slight ailments and troublesome affections, than a remedy which is capable of saving life from violent diseases, except indeed when used as an antidote to certain poisons. Still, however, there is no complaint, however trifling, no system, however unimportant (if attended with discomfort and inconvenience to mankind), that it is not the duty of the medical man to endeavour to relieve or remove.

No. 7, Finsbury Circus, London,
          March 23, 1843.

ON

HÆMORRHOIDS OR PILES*.

By R. A. STAFFORD, Esq.
Senior Surgeon to St. Marylebone Infirmary, and Surgeon Extraordinary to H. R. H. the Duke of Cambridge.

(*For the Medical Gazette.*)

THE rectum (or straight gut, as it is termed) being the termination of the alimentary canal, and having the functional office of expelling the contents of the intestines after they have undergone the process necessary for the extraction of the nutritive matter to support the frame, is liable to many diseases, and these may be classed according to the structure in which they occur. The rectum is a continuation of the sigmoid flexure of the colon, and it is composed of two coats— the mucous or internal, and the muscular coat: at its superior part it is covered by a layer of peritoneum, but in the inferior portion it is not surrounded by that membrane, like the colon and the small intestines. It begins at and turns over the upper ridge of the sacrum, and at first is a little inclined from left to right, and then it becomes straight, and follows the hollow of the sacrum and os coccyx, being larger in volume at its termination. Its anterior portion is separated from the membranous portion of the urethra by a triangular space filled by cellular tissue, the superior portion of which corresponds with the prostate, and the inferior to the integuments of the perineum. The posterior surface of the rectum is covered by loose and fatty cellular tissue, which separates it from the levator ani and ischio-coccygeus muscles, and from the sacrum. The rectum is abundantly supplied by blood-vessels, there being large arteries going to it, and large veins returning from it, both of which are termed hæmorrhoidal. It has two muscles more particularly belonging to it—the levator ani, and the sphincter muscle.

* The substance of a lecture delivered at the St. Marylebone Infirmary.

The levator ani is destined to draw the rectum back after the expulsion of the fæces, and its fibres irregularly surround, and are attached to the gut, arising from the posterior part of the symphysis pubis, from the ilium above the obturator muscle, from the spine of the ischium, and from the fascia covering the obturator internus. The sphincter muscle surrounds the rectum at its termination at the anus, and arises from the fat and skin that surrounds the verge of the anus on both sides, nearly as far as the tuberosity of the ischium, and, by a narrow point, it is inserted into the perineum, acceleratores urinæ, and transversi perenæi muscles, and behind into the extremity of the os coccygis. Its office is to close up the rectum after the expulsion of the fæces.

Having, by way of introduction to my subject, given this brief account of the anatomy of the rectum and its appendages, I shall now speak of its diseases, and shall first treat on hæmorrhoids, or piles, the most common of them all.

Hæmorrhoids are an enlargement of the veins of the rectum, which become at first swollen and tense, and the blood contained in them remains coagulated, and thus a livid tumor is formed. At length, from the thickening of their coats, and from the coagulated blood contained in them becoming organized, they form excrescences on the internal surface of the gut, or at the verge of the anus. At first, their parietes are very thin, consequently they are apt frequently to burst, when they bleed very profusely, and are then termed *bleeding piles.* When they do not bleed, they have vulgarly acquired the name of *blind piles.* Hæmorrhoids are divided into internal and external, and they may be in various states of disease, each of which will require different treatment. They may be mere excrescences, when the only inconvenience they give will be their presence as foreign bodies : they may be inflamed, when they become very painful and swollen, looking not unlike a cherry ; they may be in a relaxed state, resembling a half-dried red grape, and they may be ulcerated.

The causes assigned for hæmorrhoids are many. People of sedentary habits are the subjects of them ; costiveness, by the pressure of the hardened fæces on the veins, will produce them ; and any thing that may irritate the rectum—for instance, a drastic purge, containing aloes, scammony, &c. I have known persons who have never had piles before take aloes and scammony, and they have been in such a state that they could hardly walk for them. Piles, I have no doubt, are, in some, constitutional and hereditary, and that they descend from father to son from generation to generation. I have frequently questioned those who suffer from them, and they have informed me that either their father or mother has been afflicted with them, and that the disease has been handed down to them as a family complaint. No doubt, in such instances, the rectum is naturally weak.

It has been observed that those who are affected by a disease of the liver are frequently the subjects of piles. This may be accounted for by the connexion the hæmorrhoidal veins have with the vena porta. The liver being diseased, the circulation of blood through this vessel is obstructed, and thus the hæmorrhoidal veins become congested. Any obstruction in the veins of the intestines will produce congestion of the veins of the rectum, and consequently hæmorrhoids : in short, whatever may impede the venous circulation of the viscera may give rise to this disease. Those who have diseases of the lungs, also, are frequently the subjects of hæmorrhoids and diseases of the rectum.

On examining many cases of hæmorrhoids which are presented to our notice, it could hardly be imagined that the excrescences which we see could ever have been connected with the veins; they are of so tough, hard, and even, in some instances, of almost a cartilaginous nature. I have seen piles so hard that their structure has resembled the gizzard of a bird when cut into ; or have been not unlike the texture of brawn. No doubt the constant irritation, and the repeated attacks of chronic inflammation of the part, bring them ultimately into this state.

When an individual is subject to hæmorrhoids, the first symptom he experiences is a sense of weight and fulness in the rectum. Heat and pain supervene, which is frequently followed by bleeding when he goes to stool. The piles now protrude at the anus, and are of a lesser or greater size, sometimes being inflamed, and sometimes not. When they are internal, there is pain in the sacrum, and a sense of weight and fulness high up in the gut. There is also considerable difficulty of voiding the fœces, constant straining, and tenesmus.

The treatment of piles varies according to the state in which we find them, and also whether they are internal or external. In simple piles, when they are external, and when there is no inflammation, laxatives internally, and astringents externally, are the best remedies. At first, perhaps, give a dose of castor oil, or an aperient of senna and manna, and sulphate of magnesia combined, or any other aperient, except aloes and scammony, which will answer the effect of relieving the bowels. After this order laxatives : such as the Confectio sennæ alone, or combined with potass. supertart, or sulph.sublim. and desire the patient to foment with the decoct. papaver alb. ; or sit over a bidet of warm water. Apply a solution of liq. plumb. acet. dil. Use a cooling ointment, such as cerat. plumbi acet., or if the hæmorrhoid requires being constringed, employ the ung. galli, the ung. oxyd. zinci, &c.; also, should they be in a relaxed state, desire the patient to use an injection of the decoction of the elm or oak bark, with the addition of alum in proper proportions.

In some cases it has been recommended by Sir Astley Cooper to puncture the pile with the point of a lancet, and squeeze out its contents. This should be done cautiously, for fear of hæmorrhage. In chronic piles the confectio piperis has been of great service, continued for some time. It appears to stimulate, and give a new action to the parts. If the piles are inflamed, then apply leeches upon them, or to the verge of the anus, using an evaporating lotion, a poultice, an opium injection, or an opium ointment, as the case may require, repeating all these remedies as often as they may be necessary. The diet is of great importance; it should be bland, and meat should be avoided. Gruel, arrowroot, puddings, macaroni, &c., is the best food.

The case before us is one of aggravated piles ; so aggravated, that when protruded at the expulsion of the fœces, they are retained by the sphincter of the rectum, and cannot return with the bowel by the action of the levator ani ; consequently they remain with that part

of the intestine to which they are attached external, and appear like prolapsus ani. In such a case as this none of the common remedies are of use. Aperients, laxatives, astringents, soothing ointments, Ward's paste, &c. may give temporary relief, but the only chance of cure is by their removal.

There are two methods of removing piles ; by excision, and by ligature. When the pile is not attached to the intestine by a broad base, or is not internal, then excision is the quickest method of relief, but when it arises by a broad base, or is internal, then the removal by ligature is preferable. In Elizabeth Brown's case—Female ward, No. 2— excision answered very well, as the piles were external, and attached by a pedicle, but in the present case, where they are of immense size, there would be great danger of hæmorrhage; hæmorrhage of so fearful a description that the death of the patient might be the termination. I have seen hæmorrhoids removed by excision, where the bleeding was so great, that the surgeon has been obliged to remain with the patient for hours, employing ice, pledgets of lint, and styptics of every description, and it has been with extreme difficulty the bleeding has been made to cease. I remember some years ago assisting a surgeon of great eminence, of this town, who is now dead, to remove some internal piles from a naval officer of distinction. The operation was effected with great skill, but hæmorrhage supervened. Without exaggeration, I may say that at least a moderate sized chamber-pot full of blood was lost before it could be stopped. The surgeon expressed to me that he was never more alarmed in his life; so little control, for hours, had he over the bleeding. At length, by ice, pledgets of lint, and the exhaustion of the patient, &c., the vessels became plugged up by coagulation. I acknowledge the fearful hæmorrhage in this case determined me never to remove piles by excision unless I was certain no bleeding of consequence could occur ; for although in six cases it might succeed, yet in the seventh the loss of life might be the result from this cause. Sir Astley Cooper, in his Lectures, mentions two or three cases where hæmorrhoids were removed by excision, and death from hæmorrhage was the result. One was in the person of a nobleman in whom two operations by excision were performed. The first succeeded, but in the second hæmorrhage followed, from which he died. Sir Astley relates his case thus:—

" Five years ago a nobleman applied to me with internal piles. I was upon my guard in this case, and said I did not like to remove the piles without a consultation. A consultation was held, and the removal by excision was agreed to; I accordingly removed them, and he was well in a very few days. Two years after he sent for me again, and said that he had some more of these piles, with prolapsus ani, and that he wished me to cut them off again; I did so, and as I advised the recumbent posture he went immediately to bed. As I was anxious about this patient, I did not immediately quit the room, but stood chatting with him for a short time, when he said, I believe you must quit the room, for I must have a motion. I went out of the room, and upon returning shortly after I found him trying to get into bed, and upon looking into the vessel I perceived a considerable quantity of blood in it. In a few minutes after, he said he must have another motion, got out of bed, and again discharged a considerable quantity of blood. This he did four different times; one of the hemorrhoidal arteries in the centre of one of the piles which had been removed was divided, and as I was determined he should not die of hemorrhage, I said I must secure the vessel which bled, and with a speculum ani I opened the rectum sufficiently to see the blood-vessel, took it up with a tenaculum, and put a ligature round it. On the following day I found the patient, who was much advanced in years, extremely weak; he had had a severe rigor, he grew gradually worse, and in four days after he died. On examination of the body there appeared to be some slight disease of the intestines, but not sufficient to account for death; he was seventy-four years of age."

In another instance, also, Sir Astley was asked to see a gentleman who had been operated on by another surgeon. The piles had been excised by the scissors, and the patient evacuated such a quantity of blood from time to time that he died in a few days afterwards.

He therefore, however the operation in some cases may be successful, was strongly against their removal by excision. From the experience I have

had I am of the same opinion. I have observed that when internal vessels are wounded, we have but little control over them; and this most probably arises from the warmth of the part, and their little power of contractility in comparison to vessels more external.

There are two modes of applying a ligature to hæmorrhoids; one by surrounding them at their base, the other by passing a double ligature through their centre, at their base, by a needle, and then tying each half separately. When the pile is not large, the first of these methods is best; but when it is the latter is preferable. Should there be any doubt whether the vessels supplying the pile can be strangulated by tying the whole base of the tumor, it is, better at once to use the double ligature. By doing so you will be certain of cutting off the supply of blood, and the hæmorrhoid must slough off; for by piercing the base at the middle with a double ligature, you immediately destroy the circulation through the vessels at the centre, and thus the death of the part is certain.

Before the operation is performed the patient should be desired to protrude the bowel, when the piles will be exposed. He will probably find it most convenient to lean forward on the edge of the bed, or to lie down on the side, to effect this object. Having ascertained the number of the tumors, and completely defined their base, you thread a curved needle, or a pile needle made for the purpose, with a double ligature. You then pass the point of the needle through the base of the pile: having done so, you cut the ligature and take the needle away, whereby you have two distinct threads through it: you now tie each thread tightly on each side of the base of the pile, and thus you completely strangulate the vessels supplying it. You treat each hæmorrhoid in the same manner, when in a few days they all slough off, and the bowel heals. Sometimes it happens that another crop of piles makes its appearance when the first you have tied disappears: this is owing to there being more left behind internally. Under such circumstances you must tie them in the same manner as the others were.

I shall now relate some cases.

W. Simmons, æt. 45, was admitted into this infirmary during the last summer, having a festoon of piles round the verge of the anus, and internal piles of so large a kind, that, when he evacuated his rectum, the gut remained like prolapsus ani, and he was obliged to return it with his fingers, or it would have continued down. He had been in this state for some years. None of the common remedies could have been of the slightest service; consequently, as you saw, I tied these piles (six in number), in the manner I have described, and in a week they all sloughed off, and in a few days afterwards the man went away quite well.

The second case, which occurred in Captain C., was even worse than the last. He actually, from this disease, had been obliged to sell out and leave his regiment. One of you assisted me in removing these hæmorrhoids; and so numerous were they, that when the first crop which I had tied sloughed off, a second made its appearance, and was removed in the same manner. This case did remarkably well. I have frequently heard from the gentleman, and he keeps in excellent health, and since is married.

The third case occurred in a Mr. W., who was in one of the government offices. Being constantly obliged to sit, he suffered the greatest agony: at length he began to feel that he must give up his employment. He was a friend of mine, and consulted me upon his case. I told him he might get rid of his annoyance with but little trouble and little pain. He consented that I should operate upon him; I did so. In a week or ten days all the piles, which had been a source of vexation to him for years, dropped off, and he has never since had any return of them.

The fourth case was in a gentleman who had also an affection of the lungs. Independent of a cough and short breath, he was teased to death with ulcerated piles—so much so that there were very few chairs he could sit down upon. He was perfectly miserable. He had but little idea that any thing could be done to relieve him, so long had he suffered. He consulted me, and was surprised when I told him that, with but little trouble, his disease might be cured. He allowed me to tie ligatures round his hæmorrhoids, and in a fortnight he was well.

I have known cases of hæmorrhoids so bad that they have been the cause of preventing the individual from walking or riding. In one instance, a gentleman was extremely fond of shooting, but after he had walked one day he was attacked by piles to such a degree that he was obliged to give up the sport and lie upon the sofa. This was a source of great vexation to him, for he enjoyed the amusement beyond anything, and had excellent manors. He had employed all the palliative measures over and over again, but they gave him no permanent relief. Each time he went out, the next day he was attacked, and at length was forced to relinquish his favourite pursuit. This he had done for a year or two when he told me of his distressing situation. On protruding the piles they were of immense size, four or five in number, and in two of them their base was as large as the circumference of half-a-crown. He told me that every morning after he had gone to the water-closet, he was obliged to sit for half an hour, or more, to return them back with his fingers, and that he really was most miserable. I gave him my opinion that, however severe the case might be, yet if he would consent to have them tied in the manner I proposed, I felt certain he might get rid of this annoyance. He readily agreed to my proposal. Having prepared him for the operation, by giving aperients, &c. and ordering him moderate diet, I accordingly tied the piles. Not so much pain was experienced as might have been expected. In five or six days they sloughed off, but the surface of the bases of them ware so great that it took some little time to heal them. In six weeks he returned home quite well. This was two or three years ago, I have both seen and heard from him frequently since, and he remains quite well, and pursues his favourite sport—shooting.

In another case, a gentleman of considerable consequence was excessively fond of hunting. He was, however, extremely afflicted with hæmorrhoids. Although he went out every day that he could with the hounds, he never returned home without being immersed in blood posteriorly from hæmorrhage; so much so, that it was remarked by the whole field. This state of things went on for a considerable time, when he consulted me. I found that the piles could be easily removed by ligature. The operation was performed, and in a few days he got rid of what had annoyed him for many years of his life.

It is unnecessary to relate any more cases. All of these some of you have seen, either in the infirmary or in my private practice. I have neglected to mention a few circumstances in the treatment of these cases. In the first place you must take care to have the bowels well opened before the operation, which will be best effected by castor oil, the compound senna draught, or perhaps a dose of jalap, or what may best suit the patient. When the operation has been performed, and you are certain that the piles are perfectly strangulated, there can be no objection, if they are very large, and obstruct the passage of the rectum, to cut off their upper portion; for then no bleeding can take place. If there is great pain, a poultice may be applied, in a simple form, with the addition of Tinct. Opii. Having well opened the bowels before the operation, it is not desirable to give any aperient until the piles have sloughed off.

RESEARCHES

TENDING TO PROVE THE

NON-VASCULARITY AND THE PECULIAR UNIFORM MODE OF ORGANIZATION AND NUTRITION OF CERTAIN ANIMAL TISSUES,

NAMELY,

Articular Cartilage, and the Cartilage of the different classes of Fibro-Cartilage; the Cornea, the Crystalline Lens and the Vitreous Humour; and the Epidermoid Appendages.

By J. TOYNBEE, Esq. F.R.S.

Surgeon to the St. George's and St. James's Dispensary.

(*For the Medical Gazette.*)

IN the Introduction to this paper the author first speaks of the process of nutrition in those animal tissues which are pervaded by the ramifications of blood-vessels, pointing out the circumstance that even in them there is a considerable extent of tissue which is nourished without being in contact with vessels. The knowledge of this fact leads to the study of the mode of

---

* This paper was published in the Philosophical Transactions for the year 1841, of which the present is a brief abstract.

nutrition in the non-vascular tissues, which are divided into the three following classes, viz. :—

The *first*, comprehending articular cartilage and the cartilage of the different classes of fibro-cartilage.

The *second* comprises the cornea, the crystalline lens, and the vitreous humour.

The *third* class includes the epidermoid appendages, viz. the epithelium, the epidermis, nails and claws, hoofs, hair and bristles, feathers, horn, and teeth.

The author then proceeds to show that the due action of the organs, into the composition of which these tissues enter, is incompatible with their vascularity. In proof of the non-existence of blood-vessels in these tissues, he states that he has demonstrated, by means of injections, that the arteries, which previous anatomists had supposed to penetrate into their substance, either as serous vessels, or as red blood-vessels too minute for injection, actually terminate in veins before reaching them; he also shows that around these non-vascular tissues there are numerous vascular convolutions, large dilatations, and intricate plexuses of blood-vessels, the object of which he believes to be to arrest the progress of the blood, and to allow a large quantity of it to circulate slowly around these tissues, so that its nutrient liquor may penetrate into and be diffused through them. The author states that all the non-vascular tissues have an analogous structure, and that they are composed of corpuscles, to which he is induced to ascribe the performance of the very important functions in the process of their nutrition, of circulating throughout, and perhaps of changing the nature of the nutrient fluid which is brought by blood-vessels to their circumference. The author then brings forward facts in proof of the active and vital properties of these corpuscles, and concludes his Introduction by stating, that it appears to him, that the only difference in the mode of nutrition of the tissues which contain blood-vessels and those which do not is, that in the *former*, the fluid which nourishes them is derived from the blood that circulates throughout the capillaries contained in their substance; whilst, in the *latter*, the nutrient fluid exudes into them from the large and dilated vessels that are distributed around them: and that in both classes, the particles of which the tissues are composed derive from this fluid the elements which nourish them.

The author then enters on an examination of the structure and mode of nutrition of the several tissues of each of these three classes.

In considering the First Class, the development of articular cartilage is described at great length during its various stages and at the different periods of life. Numerous dissections of the ovum and fœtus are given in detail to illustrate the *first stage*, during which it is shewn that no vessels enter into the substance of any of the textures composing a joint, but that the changes they undergo are effected by the nutrient fluid from the large blood-vessels, by which each articulation is surrounded. In the *second stage* of the development of articular cartilage it is shown that the epiphysal cartilage is gradually hollowed into canals, within which blood-vessels are extended, which converge towards the attached surface of the articular cartilage; in this stage vessels are also prolonged over a considerable portion of the free surface of the cartilage between it and the synovial membrane.

In the *third stage*, that which is exhibited in adult life, the epiphysal cartilage is converted into osseous cancelli. These contain large and very numerous blood-vessels, ramifying throughout the whole of their cavity, and are separated from the articular cartilage by a very fine but complete lamina of bone, the articular lamella, which is composed of corpuscles, and

A vertical section of the inferior extremity of the os femoris, highly magnified.

Fig 1.

A, The impervious layer of bone (articular lamella) to which the cartilage is attached, separating the latter from the cancelli.
B, The firm vertical fibres of the cancelli implanted into the upper surface of the articular lamella.

the author believes that the principal source of nutrition to the articular cartilage is the nutrient fluid eliminated by the large vessels of the cancelli, and which permeates the articular lamella. The free surface of adult articular cartilage is nourished by vessels which extend to a short distance over its margin, and between it and the synovial membrane.[*] It is quite certain that the

A section of part of the inferior extremity of the os femoris, showing the relation of the blood-vessels of a bone to the articular cartilage covering it.

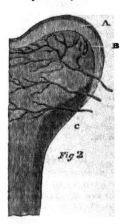

Fig 2

A, The articular cartilage.
B, The articular lamella.
C, The blood-vessels of the cancelli.

vessels thus situated do not enter the substance of the articular cartilage, inasmuch as the arteries terminate in veins at the circumference of the latter. In this situation the arteries become continuous with the veins in the following ways: firstly, by their all ending in a single vessel similar to the terminal sinus in the vascular area of the chick, from which the veins arise; secondly, the arteries terminate in dilated cavities, which give origin to veins; and lastly, the two sets of vessels are directly continuous by means of loops of various characters: the apparent object of all these modifica-

* It is very probable that synovia, a highly animalized fluid, has some share in the nutrition of articular cartilages, especially as it appears that false cartilages, without having any attachment to the synovial membrane, are developed and grow floating in it.

tions is to cause a considerable quantity of blood to circulate slowly in the vicinity of articular cartilage.

The author points out the presence of fine tubes which pervade the attached portion of articular cartilage : to these he ascribes the function of transmitting through its substance the nutritive fluid derived from the vessels of the cancelli, and he also shows that articular cartilage becomes thinner as man advances in life, and that this change is effected by its gradual conversion into bone, a process which is always going on.

Fibro-Cartilages constitute the second tissue of the first class : they are divided

Vessels situated between the synovial membrane and the border of the articular cartilage of the condyle of the os femoris at the period of birth.

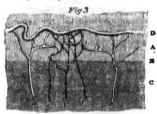

Fig 3

A, The articular cartilage ; B, its margin ; C, the synovial membrane ; D, the single vessel in which the arteries terminate ; a, artery ; v, vein.

by the author into two classes ; one comprising those which are not covered by a synovial membrane ; the other includes those which have each surface lined by it. The structure of fibro-cartilage is carefully investigated, and in order to arrive at some definite conclusions on this subject, whereon anatomists of all ages have so much differed, he made numerous dissections of fibrocartilages in the different classes of animals at various periods of their development, the results of which he details. He shows that this tissue is composed of cartilaginous corpuscles and of fibres ; the latter preponderating in adult life, the former in infancy ; and that during life the corpuscles are gradually converted into fibres. He enters at length into the question of the vascularity of these cartilages ; and from a careful study of many injected specimens of man and animals at various periods of their development, the particular results of which he relates, he states that bloodvessels are contained only in their

fibrous portion : these have the function of nourishing the part that is cartilaginous, which, being subject to compression and concussion, does not contain any.

The Cornea, Crystalline Lens, and Vitreous Humour, are included in the Second Class of extra-vascular tissues.

1. The structure of the *cornea* is described as being very lax, and containing corpuscles only in a small quantity, mixed with bright fibres. The opinions in favour of its vascularity are combated, and it is shewn that the blood-vessels which converge towards its circumference are disposed in two different

A portion of the internal semilunar fibrocartilage of the knee-joint.

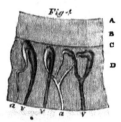

Fig 4

A, the free internal border of the fibro-cartilage ; B, the true cartilage ; C, the line of separation between the cartilage and the fibro-cartilage ; D, the fibro-cartilaginous portion ; a, the artery ; v, the vein.

Represents the vessels (sclerotico-corneal) situated in the substance of the sclerotic membrane, which approach the border of the cornea.

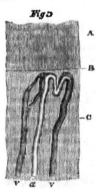

Fig 5

A, The cornea ; B, the line of separation between the cornea and the sclerotic ; C, the sclerotic ; a, artery ; v, vein.

ways: those which are the principal source of the fluid that nourishes it, and which from their position may be styled the sclerotico-corneal arteries, are large and numerous; they are situated in the substance of the sclerotic, and they converge to the point where this latter structure joins the cornea, in which position, without much diminution in their size, they suddenly become continuous with the veins that take a retrograde course.

A second set, the conjunctivo-corneal arteries, pass over a small extent of the surface of the cornea, where they form a narrow band: the arteries terminate by forming loops with the veins, and do not penetrate the substance of the cornea.

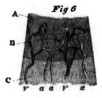

Fig 6

Represents the vessels (conjunctivo-corneal) which pass to a certain extent over the surface of the cornea, between it and the conjunctiva.

A, The cornea; B, the conjunctivo-corneal vessels; C, the sclerotic; a, artery; v, vein.

2. The *crystalline lens* is described as being composed of corpuscles of which the radiating fibres are constituted. The arteria centralis retinæ is the source of nutrition to this organ; it ramifies over the posterior surface of the capsule in the form of large branches; these pass round the circumference, upon the periphery of which they become straight, and terminate by forming loops with the venous radicles.

3. The *vitreous humour* does not present any traces of vascularity, and although many anatomists have in general terms represented the arteria centralis retinæ as giving off in its course through the organ minute branches into its substance, still those who have paid especial attention to this subject have not been able to find such vessels. The author believes that the nutrition of this structure is accomplished by the vascular ciliary processes of the choroid, and that the

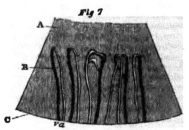

Fig 7

Represents the mode in which the blood-vessels are distributed that nourish the crystalline lens. Human fœtus.

A, The anterior surface of the lens; B, terminal branches of the arteria centralis retinæ; C, the circumference of the lens; a, artery; v, vein.

fluid brought by the latter is diffused through its substance by means of the corpuscles of which its membrane is composed, assisted by the semi-fluid character of the humour.

The Third Class of extra-vascular tissues comprehends the epidermoid appendages. The author describes them all as composed of corpuscles, which are round and soft where they are in contact with the vascular chorion, compressed and flattened where they are farther removed from it. He points out, in the substance of the hoof of the horse, the existence of fine canals, which he supposes to conduct fluid through its mass; and he states that the perspiratory ducts of the human subject possess a structure analogous to the spiral vessels of plants. The author describes each of the tissues of this class, and shows that the various modifications presented by the vascular system with which each is in contact have the sole object of enabling a large quantity of blood to approach and circulate slowly around them. He also points out, in connexion with this subject, the remarkable vital properties which are possessed by these non-vascular tissues.

In the conclusion to this paper, the author states that his object has been to establish as a law in animal physiology, that organs are capable of being nourished, and of increasing in size, without the presence of blood-vessels in their substance.

The application of the above-named law to the study of *Surgery*, in reference to the causes of the extension of vessels into the extra-vascular tissues when in a diseased state, and to the measures to be adopted for the prevention and cure of those affections which are dependent thereon ; and to *Pathology*, in the investigation of the nature of morbid structures, particularly of those classes which contain no blood-vessels, will, the author feels certain, be productive of scientific interest, and of practical advantage.

POST-MORTEM EXAMINATION IN A CASE OF SUDDEN DEATH.

To the Editor of the Medical Gazette.

SIR,

MY attention has been directed to some remarks that have been made in the public journals upon the case of sudden death that has recently taken place in this village, and in which an imputation has been cast on the good faith of the parties who examined the body. As one of these individuals, I forward to you a statement of the circumstances, and our notes of the examination, for the purpose of placing on record the facts of the case, which have not yet, as far as I am aware, been fairly placed before the public.

I was hastily summoned, on the morning of Saturday, the 4th of February, to the shop of Mr. Pledger, a druggist, whom I found on the floor, supported by one or two individuals residing on the spot; a slight examination convinced me that he was dead— no lingering trace of vitality remained. The thought passed through my mind that he might have destroyed himself, and on looking round I saw on the mantel-piece of the adjoining room a phial labelled "Ol. Ess. Amygd. :",but as I could detect no smell of it when I examined the mouth of the deceased, I concluded that he had died from an affection of the heart under which he had often told me that he was labouring.

On Tuesday the 7th, a jury assembled to inquire into the circumstances attending his death, but as no suspicion was created in their minds, they recorded a verdict of "Died by visitation of God." So suspicious, however, was one member of his family, that his death had not been a natural one, that an examination of the body was after-

wards required; and Mr. Baker, a friend of the family, but a perfect stranger to myself, was requested to undertake it. Mr. Baker called at my house on the evening of the day after the jury had returned their verdict ; and to his request, that I would assist him in the examination, I consented.

I enclose you the notes of the appearances we observed : they clearly reveal the cause of death, and are conclusive as to the object for which the investigation was undertaken. I pass no censure on the coroner and jury, but leave every man to judge for himself whether they performed their duty with intelligence and ability.

I am, sir,
Your obedient servant,
B. HANDS.

Hornsey, March 22, 1843.

Notes of the examination of the body of Mr. Henry Pledger, at Crouchend, Hornsey, on the evening of Wednesday, Feb. 8, 1843.

There was nothing peculiar in the external appearance of the body, nor any smell that excited suspicion. We reflected back the integuments in the usual manner, and, upon dividing the cartilages of the ribs, we first detected the smell of prussic acid; the further we proceeded in the examination the more obvious it became, till at length it was almost overpowering. The viscera of the chest were healthy. The heart particularly attracted attention, but nothing could be detected to account for his death.

The abdominal viscera were healthy ; there was no trace of disease ; and we remarked that, from the appearance of the organs, he might have lived to an old age. A ligature was placed around each orifice of the stomach, which was removed for further examination, though the odour given off left no room for doubt as to its contents.

The head was not examined.

Signed { James Baker.
{ Benjamin Hands.

We, the undersigned, certify that we were present at the examination of the body of Mr. Henry Pledger, that we were not aware of any peculiar smell when we entered the room where the body lay, but that whilst the examination by the medical gentlemen was proceeding, we became sensible of the smell of prussic acid; that it became more powerful as they proceeded, and that from what we saw and smelt of the contents of the stomach, we consider there can be no reasonable doubt that he died from the effects of poison.

Signed { Thomas Consfield—Brother-in-law to the deceased.
Benjamin Baillie—Medical pupil.

N.B.—The stomach and its contents are in the possession of Mr. Baker.

SULPHATE OF QUININE.

To the Editor of the Medical Gazette.

SIR,

I OBSERVE in the MEDICAL GAZETTE of 6th January last, the following paragraph, without any observations attached. "Sulphate of Quinine. According to a Parisian journal (the Examinateur Medical, of December 15th), serious symptoms, and even death itself, had lately followed the administration of large doses of sulphate of quinine in the hospitals." It would have been more satisfactory had an analysis of the salt been given, as we know that it is frequently adulterated. In confirmation, however, of the occasional poisonous properties of the sulphate of quinine, I find the following entry in my case-book, dated 1829. "Lloyd and Hackney, the one labouring under continued, the other bilious remittent fever. Exhibited the sulphate of quinine during the intermissions of the fever. In both cases an alarming syncope was produced; in the first after the exhibition of 48 grains, and in the latter of 42 grains. The average daily quantity given in both cases did not exceed 4 grains. The syncope easily yielded to cordials, and the usual means, but was attended with a peculiar feeling of annihilation. The drug was immediately omitted, and no evil consequence followed; on the contrary, health was rapidly established.

Of the influence of sulphate of quinine in producing the mercurial action.—John Pedley had suffered for 8 or 10 months previous to my seeing him, either from inflammatory action of the peritoneum, or some of the viscera of the abdomen, but I could get

no proper history of the case. He had been attended about three weeks by a medical gentleman, who, from the pain and tenderness of the belly, and white clayey colour of the stools, endeavoured, by rubbing in and otherwise, to bring on mercurial action, but with very partial effect, for two days only procuring a slight alteration of the stools. It was about five or six weeks after this I saw him—a most wretched object, worn almost to a skeleton. He had great pain, puffiness, and tenderness of the abdomen, particularly in the region of the liver and of the hypogastrium, with scanty, irregular, and clay-coloured stools, weak and feeble pulse, and, in short, the case was a most miserable and hopeless one. Recollecting a practice I often followed of exhibiting mercury to detect collections of matter in the liver, which, when this is present, seldom salivates, and always weakens and injures the patient, I thought it not unlikely that this patient might have had the injurious effects of an injudicious use of mercury added to his original ailments; and partly with a view to recover him from this, and partly to try to give him temporary relief, I ordered him the sulphate of quinine, conium and hyoscyamus, with a little carbonate of soda, in the usual doses, three times a day. In the course of twenty-four hours his sufferings were greatly alleviated, and he began to part with large and copious stools, quite altered in appearance, being loaded with bile, fæculent, and lumpy. In a short time his mouth became sore; and from this and a great degree of faintness and exhaustion coming on, his pills were refused, and consequently omitted. Whether to attribute the faintness and exhaustion to the quinine, or the narcotics prescribed with it, I can scarcely decide; but the quantity of quinine taken was 60 grains (about four grains daily on the average) and the symptoms very similar to the above-noted cases. In the 3rd vol. of the Edin. Med. Journ., there are some remarks by Dr. Hardy on the same influence of quinine in promoting the mercurial action. It is to be remarked, in the above case, that a mercurial action, at least the specific action of mercury on the system, could not be obtained at the time mercury was exhibited, but that, a long time after, effects the same as those prod uced by mercury were obtained.

I have reason to believe the sulphate of quinine employed by me was perfectly pure.—I am, sir,

Your obedient servant,
JAMES RANKING, M.D.

Ayr, N. B. March 28, 1843.

SPERMATOZOA OBSERVED A SECOND TIME WITHIN THE OVUM.

BY MARTIN BARRY, M.D. F.R.SS. L. & E.

(*For the Medical Gazette.*)

SEVERAL months since I communicated to the Royal Society the fact that I had observed, and shown to Professor Owen and others, spermatozoa *within* the mammiferous ovum. The ova were those of the rabbit, taken twenty-four hours *post coïtum* from the Fallopian tube[*].

I have this day confirmed the observation; several ova from the Fallopian tube of another of these animals, in a somewhat earlier stage, having presented spermatozoa in their interior, *i. e.* (as in the first observation) within the thick transparent membrane ("*zona pellucida*") brought with the ovum from the ovary.

London, 31, iii. mo. (March) 1843.

MEDICAL GAZETTE.

Friday, April 7, 1843.

" Licet omnibus, licet etiam mihi, dignitatem *Artis Medicæ* tueri; potestas modo veniendi in publicum sit, dicendi periculum non recuso."

CICERO.

POPULATION OF ENGLAND.

THE fourth annual Report of the Registrar-General to the Secretary for the Home Department contains an immense mass of interesting and important statistical information. The portion of these documents on which we purpose making some remarks relates to the progress of population, as shewn

---

[*] See " Proceedings of the Royal Society, Dec. 8, 1842."

by the registration of births, deaths, and marriages, in the various districts of England. And we may here remark, that the kingdom has been divided into 619 districts, and these again subdivided so as to form 2184 minor portions, affording great facilities in conducting statistical inquiries.

The births and deaths are registered according to districts, and the calculations as to the increase or decrease of population made from the documents thus formed. The result of this arrangement according to districts is, that those interested may form tables of mortality, and estimate the mean duration of life in any particular situation. By these means the residents in any district or locality may accurately determine the salubrity or insalubrity of the place, and compare the results with those obtained in any other part of the kingdom. Information of this kind comes home to the feelings of every one, and will in all probability lead to beneficial results, by directing attention to the causes of disease, and the means of their removal. The value of human life, too, differs so considerably in different situations, that insurance companies and friendly societies will probably find the facts thus laid open to them of much assistance in regulating their premiums and subscriptions: nor is it easy to estimate the extent to which the information thus obtained may influence the operations of such bodies.

Much statistical information of another kind is also conveyed—such as the number of marriages, the ages of the parties, their amount of education, and various other important points. It is scarcely possible for us to do more than allude to the countless accumulation of facts which are thus brought together; but of the more interesting we select a few as specimens.

The marriages appear to have been

nearly 1 in 127; the births 1 in 32; and the deaths 1 in 45, of the whole population. This, we believe, is rather under the usual calculation as to marriage; and it is curious to observe, that the marriages in the last year were nearly 3 per cent. less than the preceding, relatively to the female population; the decrease having been most conspicuous in some of the northern divisions of the kingdom. The greatest number of marriages relatively takes place in the metropolis, a circumstance which seems to arise, in great measure, from a considerable number of persons who are usually resident in the country coming to London on the occasion of their wedding. It is thought, however, that after making due allowance for this, the number of marriages is still somewhat greater proportionally in the capital than elsewhere.

Considerable difference is observed, as might be expected, in reference to age. The proportion of women who marry under age is nearly as 3 to 1 when compared to the men, and in London is so high as 4½ to 1. More than half the males were married between 20 and 25 years of age; and nearly the same holds good with regard to the females; but of the latter, (as may be gathered from what we have above stated), a considerable number were under 20, while comparatively few of the men were so. Yet the average age of marriage, on the great scale, is less different on the two sexes than the preceding statements might lead us to expect, being 25·5 years for the men, and 24·3 for the women.

The registration of births seems to be conducted in an unsatisfactory manner, the omissions amounting to not less than "several thousands." The proportion of births is above the average in the northern and western districts, and below it in the Welch,

eastern, and metropolitan districts. There is a slight excess of boys over girls; and this excess is greatest in the northern, and least in the southern parts of the kingdom. The greatest number of births take place in winter and spring; and it is remarkable that, during those times, the excess of males over females is also most conspicuous. But this excess does not endure more than the first twenty years of life, by which period the sexes are nearly equal, owing of course to the greater mortality of the males. More deaths appear to have occurred in 1841 than in any other year of the period, the number having exceeded that of some of the previous years by nearly 25,000.

It has long been known that the mortality is greater in cities than in the country; and the causes of this constitute a very interesting subject of inquiry, with reference more especially to their removal; and we are glad to learn that, in some of the provincial towns of England, they are undergoing rigid examination. One point clearly made out, and corresponding with what might be expected, is, that the mortality in towns increases, as a general rule, with the density of the population, owing in great measure to the comparative neglect of sewerage and purification in the poorer districts.

Another very interesting point is the mortality at different periods of life; but it is too intricate, and involves too many figures, for us to do more than allude to it. One general fact may be stated, that, under ordinary circumstances, an increase of mortality is chiefly observable among those under puberty, and among the aged; the number of deaths between 20 and 60 varying but very little.

Yet another curious point, illustrated by the marriage registers, is the state of education. The parties are required to sign their names; and it appears that, on the average of three years, 33 men and 49 women per cent. could not do so, but merely put a *mark*. Now, taking the average ages of those who marry at 25, this test shews us the state of education from ten to twenty years ago, when it appears that, among women, very nearly one half were unable to write their own names. But there exists a great difference as to the amount of education in different parts of the kingdom. Thus, in Cumberland, only 16 in 100 signed the register with marks, while in Bedfordshire there were 52 who did so !

At the conclusion of the report a hope is expressed in which we cordially concur—namely, that the registrars will attend to the classification of fatal diseases, and that the members of the medical profession will assist, as in fact they alone can furnish correct information on the subject.

ROYAL MEDICAL & CHIRURGICAL SOCIETY.

March 28, 1843.

THE PRESIDENT IN THE CHAIR.

On two remarkably similar cases of osteo-sarcoma of the thigh bone, requiring amputation in both instances. By R. A. FROGLEY, Esq., of Hounslow, in whose practice they occurred. — Communicated by SAMUEL LANE, Esq.

THE first case is that of a female, æt. 26, who had a tumor of the thigh, which measured in its greatest diameter 35½ inches, and reached from within an inch of the trochanters to the knee-joint. It began in the summer of 1829, with a pain in the condyle of the femur, and in May of the following year a tumor had formed of the size of the half-closed hand. It continued gradually to enlarge, without pain, or discolouration of the skin, or materially impeding the motions of the limb, till March 1843, when the limb was amputated. Owing to the close proximity of the upper part of the tumor to Poupart's ligament, it was anticipated that it might be necessary to disarticulate the bone at the hip-joint; but in the course of the operation, when the two lateral flaps had been made, the femur

was found in a healthy condition below the lesser trochanter, and it was sawn through at this joint. Mr. Lane, who assisted, commanded the blood-vessels by pressure with his fingers on the external iliac artery, so that scarcely any arterial hæmorrhage took place. What little occurred was immediately arrested by another assistant grasping the flap until as many as ten ligatures were applied. After the operation the patient caused much alarm by falling into a faint, in which she gasped as *in articulo mortis*; but she was soon restored from this condition. The stump healed favourably, and there has been no return of the morbid growth. A longitudinal section having been made of the thigh bone and tumor, it was seen to consist chiefly of a whitish, elastic, hard tissue, resembling cartilage, but rather more transparent. There was very little deposit of osseous structure in it, and the tumor appeared more connected with the periosteum than with the bone itself, which could be readily distinguished in the morbid mass, from preserving its sound condition: numerous cysts communicating with each other, and with a large central cavity, were developed in the tumor, and these contained several pints of a yellow tenacious honey-like fluid.

The second case is that of a married lady, æt. 37, who had also a tumor of the thigh. The swelling was first observed eleven years ago, as a hard lump, about the size of half a walnut, situated on the inner condyle of the femur. When seen by Mr. Frogley, five or six years after its commencement, it had not increased perceptibly in size; but in five years more it had acquired considerable magnitude, and had extended up the thigh. Finding that it made more rapid progress, so that it measured at its largest part 20½ inches in circumference, while the thickness of the limb below was only 12 inches, she consented to undergo amputation, which was performed in August 1842, and the stump healed by the first intention. Upon making a section of the thigh-bone and tumor, it was remarked that the morbid growth, although smaller than in the preceding case, presented the identical appearances, both in position and structure, which have been described in this case. Casts, drawings, and preparations of the tumors in both patients, were exhibited.

Remarks on Gangrene of the Face, and its Treatment. By HENRY OBRE', Esq.

The author commences with some observations on the condition of the system in children, in which this disease is most liable to occur ; dwelling on the ravages it produces, and its usually intractable nature. He then gives the result of his treatment of the complaint, by applying the actual cautery to the sloughing surfaces, as recommended by some continental writers, and describes the success which he has met with. He relates two cases where he adopted the plan. In the first, the gangrene came on after typhus fever, and it proceeded rapidly to destroy a large extent of the cheek. Having tried various other applications unsuccessfully, he had recourse to the actual cautery, and immediate amendment followed, so that the edges soon healed. The appearances before and after the case were illustrated by coloured wax casts taken from the patient. In the other case, the disease was so extensive, and the child so much debilitated, that the author did not succeed in saving the patient's life; but manifest advantage was gained by the use of the cautery, so as to convince him of its beneficial influence in the treatment of the disease.

Remarks on Cancrum Oris, and Phagedæna of the Cheek, and on the Effect of the Chlorate of Potash on those Diseases. By HENRY HUNT, M.D.

The author describes these diseases as being identical, varying only in the degree of severity—both commencing by ulceration of the mucous membrane of the cheek, or where it joins the gums, and that the external eschar is the consequence of the internal ulceration. He considers them to proceed from a cachectic state of the system; that they occur more commonly in cold and wet weather—sometimes attacking several members of the same family simultaneously, and occasionally prevailing almost like an epidemic. The author has treated them very successfully by a free exhibition of the chlorate of potash, the beneficial influence of that salt being generally apparent within forty-eight hours of its being given, that it seldom fails to arrest the progress and to effect a cure, if administered prior to the patient being very much exhausted. The quantity of the salt he has been in the habit of prescribing varies from Ɉj. to Ɉij. in twelve hours, according to the age of the child. Two cases are related in corroboration of the foregoing statement.

MEETING OF THE PROFESSION IN WORCESTERSHIRE.

A HIGHLY respectable meeting of the profession of the above county was held on Tuesday last (the 4th) in the Council-Room of the Worcestershire Natural History Society, to consider the propriety of petitioning Parliament on the measures now in contemplation for regulating the medical profession. Jonas Nalden, M.D. was called to the chair, and, after apologising for the absence of Dr. Hastings, who had been urgently called out of town, he briefly, but suitably, addressed the meeting upon the subject for which it had been convened. It was then proposed by R. J. N. Streeten, M.D., of Worcester; seconded by Anthony Martin, Esq. of Evesham; and resolved unanimously,—

That a petition be sent to both houses of Parliament on the contemplated legislation respecting the medical profession, and that the following petition to the House of Commons be adopted :—

To the Honourable the Commons of the United Kingdom of Great Britain and Ireland, in Parliament assembled.

The humble petition of the undersigned members of the medical profession, residing in the county of Worcester.

Sheweth,

That your petitioners, understanding that measures are in contemplation for reforming and regulating the profession generally, beg to represent to your Honourable House, that no reform can be effectual or permanent unless it provide for the efficiency and respectablity of the whole profession, by securing uniformity of the primary qualification, tested by sufficient examination, equal right to every member to practise throughout her Majesty's dominions, and the adoption of the representative system in the formation of the councils or governing bodies.

That the supply of an adequately qualified class of general practitioners is of national importance, and that a legislative re-organisation of the whole profession has become of indispensable necessity, from several causes; and, among others, from the various and incongruous modes by which medical practitioners procure admission into the profession; there being no less than sixteen different sources from which certificates of qualification may be obtained.

Your petitioners therefore pray, that your honourable house would cause inquiry to be made into the present state of the medical profession, delaying any legislative measure which might lead to the granting of new charters to the Colleges of Physicians and Surgeons until the whole subject of medical regulation and reform has been well and thoroughly investigated by a committee of your honourable house, and has undergone adequate discussion in Parliament.

And your petitioners will ever pray, &c.

Proposed by James Lewis, Esq., of Hanley; and seconded by G. M. Pritchett, Esq., of Kempsey, and resolved unanimously,—

That a similar petition be adopted for presentation to the House of Lords.

Moved by Paris Dick, M.D., of Tewkes-bury; and seconded by J. H. Walsh, Esq., of Worcester, and resolved unanimously,—

That the right honourable Lord Lyttelton, Lord Lieutenant of the county, be respect-fully requested to present the petition to the House of Peers.

Moved by William Cooper, M.D., of Ink-berrow; and seconded by Henry B. Marsh, Esq., of Upton-on-Severn, and resolved unanimously,—

That General the Honourable H. B. Lygon be requested to present the petition to the House of Commons, and that the other members for East and West Worcestershire, the members for the City of Worcester, and for the Boroughs of Bewdley, Droitwich, Dudley, Evesham, and Kidderminster, be also requested to favour the petitioners with their support on the occasion.

Moved by W. Doughty, Esq., of Kidder-minster; and seconded by David Everett, Esq., of Worcester, and resolved unani-mously,—

That it appears desirable, that at the present juncture the sentiments of the mem-bers of the medical profession should be made known to the legislature; and it is therefore suggested, that meetings similar to the present, and to that which has taken place in the County of Surrey, should be called in other Counties; and it is also re-commended that medical practitioners should severally, to the extent of their personal in-fluence, endeavour to call the attention of members of both houses of Parliament to the subject of the legislative regulation of the profession.

A vote of thanks was passed to the chair-man, and the petitions being signed by all present, the meeting broke up.

MEDICAL REFORM.

Sir James Clark has just published a Second Letter upon this subject. It extends to forty pages; but his views will be found embodied in the three short extracts which we subjoin, and to which we prefix headings for the convenience of our readers :—

Uniformity required in medical educa-tion.—For these and other reasons, there should, I think, be but one *prescribed* course of medical education exacted by the state; it should comprehend what is necessary for every medical practitioner; and it should be the same throughout the empire. This I consider the fundamental principle upon which a legislative enactment on the subject of Medical Education should be based. Whatever department of the profession the

medical man may choose as the field of his practice, to practise that part properly he must be acquainted with the whole. When possessed of such general knowledge of his profession, the practitioner may, by devoting his attention to one department chiefly, be fairly supposed to excel, and generally will excel, the man who practises them all. Thus one man by directing his principal at-tention to the investigation and treatment of diseases affecting internal organs and the general system, another by directing his chief attention to the diseases and injuries of the external organs and the operations and mechanical appliances required for their cure, may each attain, in their respective departments, a degree of perfection which cannot be expected of him whose attention is divided among the whole range of human infirmities and accidents. Hence there will always be Physicians and Surgeons who, in addition to their individual practice, will be consulted by the General Practitioner in all dangerous and obscure diseases; and every honourable inducement should be held out to encourage men to qualify themselves for such responsible positions by a higher pre-liminary education, and a more extended course of professional instruction, than could be laid down as the rule for all medical practitioners. But, as Dr. Thomson has justly remarked, " It is in the proper edu-cation of the whole body of the members of the medical profession, and in the experience which particular individuals may acquire by extensive private practice, or by attendance in dispensaries or hospitals, that the public have their best, and indeed their only securities for an adequate supply of intelligent and experienced Consulting Practitioners. The Legislature, therefore, will have per-formed its duty when it shall have taken care that no one can be licensed to enter on the practice of medicine without such pre-paration as a thorough preliminary and pro-fessional education can afford. Beyond the requirements necessary to obtain a license which should entitle the possessor to practise any and every branch of his profession—to qualify, in short, for a General Practitioner—the Legislature need not, perhaps ought not, to interfere with Medical Education or Medical Degrees. The regulations respect-ing honorary Degrees in Medicine may be safely left to the Universities and Medical Colleges.

Although medical education in this coun-try is much superior to what it was, even a quarter of a century ago, it is still defective in all classes. The education of the Physi-cian is defective, inasmuch as he is not generally instructed in all the departments of his profession. That of the Surgeon is still more limited. He has, in truth, been hitherto educated almost exclusively in surgery, whilst his practice is as much in medical as in surgical diseases : his knowledge of medicine is therefore generally acquired during the first years of his practice ; and, moreover, the confined range of his medical education is unfavourable to his ever becoming a good Physician. The education of the General Practitioner, although much superior to what it was, has not by any means kept pace with the increase of his professional responsibilities. It is defective in several ways, but more especially in its preliminary or general part—in those departments of science a knowledge of which is necessary to prepare him for entering on his more strictly professional studies. To bring the education of the General Practitioner up to the standard of his responsibilities it is that a legislative enactment is required.

Necessity of having an Educational Board independent of the Medical Corporations. — When the standard of medical education has been raised to what it ought to be, the next point for decision will be the formation of a body to whom is to be delegated the power of carrying out the principles of education laid down by the government. That power should, in my humble opinion, be intrusted only to an independent body, unconnected with the educating institutions on the one hand, and the medical corporations on the other ; a body responsible to the government for its acts, having no collateral interests to divert its attention from carrying out in the fullest manner the principles embodied in the legislative enactment. But I have stated my views on this subject in my former letter, and further reflection has only tended to confirm my opinion,— that this important trust should be vested in a body in each division of the kingdom, appointed by Government, for the exclusive purpose of regulating the course of education, preliminary and professional, and of testing candidates for licenses to practise.

Unless the regulation of medical education is intrusted to such a body, it will be in vain to expect well-educated medical men. The subject of education must be taken up as a whole, and directed upon a well-devised system, otherwise it can never be successful. It has been because the regulations respecting the education of medical men have been intrusted chiefly to the Medical Corporations that the preliminary education has been so totally neglected. Such bodies are not qualified to test candidates on their scientific acquirements. It is not their province, and in no other country, I believe, is such a duty intrusted to them. If the Colleges of Physicians and Surgeons are to have any share in examining candidates, it should be restricted entirely to testing their practical knowledge. The selection of a proper body for this purpose, for regulating the education and testing the qualifications of medical men, appears to me, in point of importance, and in the accomplishment of a sound reform of the medical profession, second only to the establishment of a good preliminary and medical education to be required of every member of the profession as a condition of his receiving a license to practise.

Necessity of Separating Pharmacy from Medicine. — In thus advocating a liberal education for the General Practitioners, as the only means of insuring their respectability as a body, and giving them a status in their profession, it must be evident to themselves that so desirable a change in their position cannot be effected until the dispensing of medicines ceases to be a part of their duty—until the practice of Pharmacy is separated from that of Medicine. In towns the separation may be effected without difficulty. In Edinburgh it may be said to be already accomplished. It is true that in villages and country districts the Practitioner would require to keep such medicines as were necessary for immediate use, more especially in the treatment of acute diseases. In such cases, however, the medicines ought not to form a separate charge, but be included in that for attendance, being considered in the same light as surgical instruments. But until the practice of Pharmacy is separated generally from that of Medicine, General Practitioners cannot attain that position in their profession, nor hold that station in society, which they ought. The influence which such an arrangement in the practice of Medicine would exercise on the position of Medical Practitioners generally, must be sufficiently obvious to every one who gives the subject a little consideration ; but the far greater benefits which the public would ultimately reap from it can only be known to those who are acquainted with the present state of medical practice in this country.

Difficulties will, no doubt, present themselves to the establishment of a uniform scheme of medical education ; but these difficulties are really less formidable than they at first sight appear to be.

The present Medical Corporations and the English Universities may oppose such a measure. The opposition of either ought to have little weight, if it can be shown to be unreasonable and opposed to the public weal ; and assuredly whatever is opposed to the improvement of Medical Education and to the character and respectability of the great body of Medical Practitioners is so.

FATAL EFFECTS OF HOMŒOPATHY.

To the Editor of the Medical Gazette.

SIR,

ANOTHER victim is added to the lengthening list of homœopathic deaths. The obituary of to-day announces the decease of a lady of rank, a believer and follower of homœopathy.

In a former communication to you touching the melancholy death of another lady of rank, I elicited two charming productions in the shape of a vindication of the homœopathic treatment, and which pretty clearly verified the adage, which I must only hint at—it was a quarrel between two culinary friends as to which was the blackest. Now I wish to reverse the matter, and ask for the doctor's version of the case before I send you my account of it ; and as I love the science of medicine, *especially that of homœopathy.* I would beg Dr. C——, the attendant on the late Lady L—— D——, to give us the particulars of the failure of the remedies used ; *known as certain preventives of the contagion of scarlatina,* and from what circumstances a *fatal* instead of a *favourable* issue resulted. I have no doubt but that it will be greatly conducive to extending the belief in, and practice of homœopathy, to know if in this case the patient was lost from *broth! brandy ! !* or *belladonna ! ! !* It is to be hoped that Dr. H. D—— was also in attendance, and will favour the medical men "who will take the trouble of calling on him" with *his* statement of the case, as between their *conflicting* accounts the truth may be rendered visible to people of plain common sense.

Dr. Curie, in his letter (see MEDICAL GAZETTE, 3d February, 1843), alludes to his great patron, thus : "Like a noble earl well known for the interest he takes in medical science, who has not thought it beneath him, in order to complete his general education, to take his place upon the benches of a surgical class." Now in these days our aristocracy are doubtless very learned and scientific men, but I would suggest that the ability of this noble earl must be more than gigantic, when a single course of lectures shall enable him to judge, and lead others into the belief, of a system, which is pronounced by men whose years of experience greatly outnumber those of the noble earl's age, to be based on a foundation of absurdities, and dangerous in its practice. May we ask, with that deference which becomes us in approaching a person of such transcendant powers, what his feelings are, if he deign to reflect on the awful results of his recommendation.—I am, sir,

Your obedient servant,

M.D.

ON

THE PHOSPHATES IN POTATOES.

To the Editor of the Medical Gazette.

SIR,

IN Dr. Golding Bird's lecture, contained in the last number of the LONDON MEDICAL GAZETTE, is a table showing the "proportion of phosphates in articles of diet." In this table Dr. Bird states, on the authority of Liebig, that one ounce of potatoes contains 23·56 grains of phosphates ; and he goes on to show, that if a person take three ounces of potatoes at a meal, he consumes 94·24 grains of phosphates.

Now, according to Cocker, if one ounce of potatoes contain 23·56 grains of phosphates, three ounces must contain 70·68, not 94·24 grains.

But I should be glad to be informed in what part of Liebig's writings does this distinguished chemist state that an ounce of potatoes contains 23·56 grains of phosphates? At page 285 of his Animal Chemistry he quotes the following analyses of Boussingault and Bœckmann :—

Potatoes.

	Boussingault.	Bœckmann.
Water	72·2	73·2
Dry matter . .	27·8	26·8
	100·0	100·0

And in the same page it is also stated, that 100 parts of potatoes [*thus dried*] contain, according to Boussingault 5·0, according to Bœckmann 4·915 per cent. of ashes. Consequently, in 100 parts of undried potatoes, there would be, according to Boussingault, 1·39 parts of ashes ; and assuming these to consist entirely of phosphates (which they do not), one ounce Troy of potatoes would contain 6·672 grains of phosphates, instead of 23·56 grains as stated by Dr. Bird ; and, therefore, if a man took at a meal three ounces of potatoes, he would consume 20·016 grains, not 94·24 grains, of phosphates.

In these calculations I have followed Boussingault's analysis, as quoted by Liebig, since it is the most favourable to Dr. Bird's statement. But his later analysis* is more unfavourable, since it shows that one ounce of potatoes really yields only 4·6272 grains of ashes.—I am, sir,

Your obedient servant,

A CONSTANT READER.

* Mémoires de l'Académie Royale des Sciences, t. xviii. 1842.

FŒTAL CIRCULATION.

To the Editor of the Medical Gazette.

SIR,

SINCE the appearance of the last number of the GAZETTE, I have received a note from Dr. Carpenter, of Bristol, directing my attention to the circumstance that I had committed an error in my paper on the Fœtal Circulation, published in your last number, in ascribing to *him* the paternity of the notion which regards the red particles of the blood in the light of glandular agents destined to convert the simpler or least organized elements which enter, from various sources, the current of the circulation, into its higher and more animalized principles. Some time had elapsed since I had read his admirable article on the Physiology of Cells, published in Forbes's Foreign Review for January 1843. On again referring to the same source, I find that Dr. Carpenter contends against, rather than advocates, this view, which, on the contrary, is entertained by Wagner, Henlè, and Wharton Jones.

He maintains the somewhat modified doctrine, that since the blood of invertebrata is altogether destitute of *coloured* corpuscles, while it abounds in the *colourless*, united to the fact, that, like the changes which are perpetually being kept up in the blood of the vertebrate animal, the albuminous principles in their blood must be continually undergoing similar transformations into the more elaborate fibrinous products, this mysterious catalysis is a duty which must devolve rather upon the *colourless* than the *coloured* corpuscles of the blood. I think now that I have rectified the mistake, and placed the pleasing fabric of this sweet-sounding theory upon the merited eminence of a " cloudless vantage ground :" those who desire further information upon the subject I must refer to the valuable and superior paper of Dr. Carpenter.—I am, sir,

Your obedient servant,
THOMAS WILLIAMS.

15, Duke Street, London Bridge,
April 5, 1843.

ROYAL COLLEGE OF SURGEONS.

LIST OF GENTLEMEN ADMITTED MEMBERS.

Friday, March 31, 1843.

J. N. Watters.—C. Irving.—J. W. James.—N. J. Highmore.—J. Harrison.—J. H. Stallard.—F. H. Green.—H. M. Cannon.—J. M. Hudson.—J. Paley.—T. Smith.—G. Taylor.—G. P. Dale.—G. W. Timms.—J. T. W. Bacot.

BOOKS RECEIVED.

Lectures on the Eruptive Fevers, delivered at St. Thomas's Hospital in January 1843. By George Gregory, M.D. &c. &c.

A Lecture on Quack Medicines, delivered to the Wakefield Mechanics' Institution, Feb. 20, 1843. By T. G. Wright, M.D.

On Feigned and Factitious Diseases. By Hector Gavin, M.D. &c. &c.

A TABLE OF MORTALITY FOR THE METROPOLIS,

Shewing the number of deaths from all causes registered in the week ending Saturday, March 25, 1843.

Small Pox	5
Measles	22
Scarlatina	23
Hooping Cough	36
Croup	3
Thrush	2
Diarrhœa	6
Dysentery	3
Cholera	0
Influenza	6
Typhus	50
Erysipelas	4
Syphilis	2
Hydrophobia	0
Diseases of the Brain, Nerves, and Senses	170
Diseases of the Lungs and other Organs of Respiration	282
Diseases of the Heart and Blood-vessels	22
Diseases of the Stomach, Liver, and other Organs of Digestion	68
Diseases of the Kidneys, &c.	6
Childbed	3
Ovarian Dropsy	1
Disease of Uterus, &c.	6
Rheumatism	1
Diseases of Joints, &c.	6
Ulcer	1
Fistula	0
Diseases of Skin, &c.	0
Diseases of Uncertain Seat	134
Old Age or Natural Decay	72
Deaths by Violence, Privation, or Intemperance	42
Causes not specified	4
Deaths from all Causes	986

METEOROLOGICAL JOURNAL.

Kept at EDMONTON, *Latitude* 51° 37' 32"N.
Longitude 0° 3' 51" W. *of Greenwich.*

March 1843.	THERMOMETER.		BAROMETER.	
Wednesday 29	from 27 to 52		29·85 to 29·95
Thursday . 30	40	54	29·80	29·81
Friday . . . 31	45	57	29·44	29·35
April.				
Saturday . 1	47	56	29·46	29·48
Sunday . . 2	48	59	29·43	29·61
Monday . . 3	48	61	29·73	29·63
Tuesday . 4	45	55	29·32	29·46

Wind, N.E. on the 29th; S.E. and S. on the 30th and 31st ult. S. on the 1st; S.W. on the 2d and 3d; S.E. and S.W. on the 4th instant.

Since the 29th ult. generally cloudy, with frequent rain.

Rain fallen, ·6 of an inch.

CHARLES HENRY ADAMS.

NOTICE.

We regret that we cannot make room for Dr. Marshall Hall's letter. As we did not insert the attack to which he alludes, it would be contrary to usage to publish his answer to it.

WILSON & OGILVY, 57, Skinner Street, London.

THE

LONDON MEDICAL GAZETTE,

BEING A

WEEKLY JOURNAL

OF

Medicine and the Collateral Sciences.

FRIDAY, APRIL 14, 1843.

LECTURES

ON THE

THEORY AND PRACTICE OF MIDWIFERY,

Delivered in the Theatre of St. George's Hospital,

BY ROBERT LEE, M.D. F.R.S.

LECTURE XXIII.

Protracted and difficult labours, from rigidity and premature rupture of the fœtal membranes; over-distension of the uterus; and unusual size and presentation of the head of the child.

VENESECTION, as recommended so strongly by Mauriceau, is undoubtedly the most important remedy which can be employed in cases of protracted labour from rigidity of the os uteri and other soft parts, especially where there is fever with determination of blood to the head. But it is not generally necessary to take away more than twelve or fourteen ounces of blood from the arm, or twenty in very robust plethoric persons, and I have seen no cases in which the abstraction of forty or fifty ounces at a time was required, or would have been justifiable. In America, women have been bled to this, or to a still greater amount, to promote general relaxation of the system, and of the parts. But, like other powerful remedies, as Dr. Merriman observes, "this has sometimes been carried to excess, so as to be injurious to the patient during parturition, and rendering her recovery tedious, if not doubtful." A woman with rigid os uteri during labour does not require the same quantity of blood to be taken away which it would be necessary to remove if she were labouring under pneumonia or peritonitis. The results of my experience on this point are very different from those of Dr. Hamilton, who says,

"hitherto, in a very large proportion of the cases of protraction from this cause, he has found copious blood-letting rapidly promote the dilatation. By copious blood-letting he means, abstracting as much blood by one venesection as he should direct in a patient of a similar constitution, if she were labouring under an acute inflammatory disease." He admits, however, that "in cases of relaxed debilitated women, with *toughness* of the os uteri, venesection cannot be ventured upon, and it becomes necessary to administer an opiate enema. The author had recourse to this practice, he must confess, with great reluctance, having seen many cases where the administration of opiates had been prejudicial. But he can now say that, under proper management, the practice is safe. The utility and safety of the practice are mainly influenced by the time at which it is adopted. If strong and frequent pains, continued for six or eight hours, do not decidedly promote the dilatation, the opiate enema should be had recourse to, and it will seldom disappoint the expectation of the practitioner. But if the first stage, with strong and frequent pains, be allowed to go on for twelve hours or upwards, without having completed the dilatation of the os uteri, there is the risk that the opiate will so far interfere with the progress of the labour that instrumental delivery shall become necessary." "In some instances," says Dr. Collins, "especially with first children, the mouth of the womb continues rigid and hot, with little tendency to yield under uterine action, accompanied not unfrequently by considerable irritation. In such, bleeding to the extent of ten or twelve ounces, and keeping the patient under the influence of slight doses of tartar emetic, to which a small quantity of opium should be added, will be found to promote relaxation, and thus be productive of the best effects." Spontaneous vomiting is often followed by relaxation of the os uteri, but I have never ventured to prescribe an emetic to any woman in labour.

Dr. Lowder says that he seldom found benefit from their exhibition, though he has frequently seen them used. The warm bath was employed in America, but excessive hæmorrhage so often followed it, that the practice was abandoned. Dr. Merriman states that he has seen good effects produced from the warm or tepid hip-bath, in relaxing the soft parts. " Upon the same principle of inducing relaxation and consequent dilatation of the os uteri, he says clysters of tobacco were recommended in America : but the alarming symptoms which followed in the single case where tobacco was thus employed, will I trust prevent a repetition of this experiment."

In some cases, after the labour has continued many hours, the os uteri is so thick, hard, smooth, and polished, and so little dilated, that you might be induced to believe that the head would never pass, but it is astonishing how it will yield in time if you have patience, and employ the proper measures to prevent exhaustion and fever. These means will not, however, invariably succeed, and artificial delivery sometimes becomes imperative, and from all that has fallen under my observation I am convinced that there is far less danger from premature interference, than from delaying too long to deliver artificially. In the eleventh volume of the Medico-Chirurgical Transactions, Mr. P. N. Scott, of Norwich, one of the most judicious and experienced practitioners now in Britain, has recorled the following very remarkable case of extreme rigidity of the os uteri, in which the separation of the inferior segment of the uterus took place during labour, and the patient recovered. " On Sunday, the 29th of October, at seven o'clock in the evening, I was requested by Mr. Keymer, a respectable surgeon of this city, to visit Mrs. Hall, a married woman, aged 36, who was in labour of her first child. He stated to me that he had been in attendance for sixteen hours, that labour had commenced about six o'clock on the Saturday evening, when he first saw her, and that though the liquor amnii (as he was informed by the nurse), had escaped some hours previous to his first visit, there had been but little progress made towards delivery. Mr. Keymer is a gentleman of very extensive experience, having been above fifty years in large practice, particularly in this branch of the profession, but he assured me that he had never seen a case in which the sufferings of the patient were so extreme, and in which the os uteri was so tense and rigid. On seeing the patient, I found that her sufferings continued unabated, that the os uteri was not dilated to more than the size of a half-crown piece, and that it was principally of a thick, unyielding, but, at a small portion of its

extent, of a somewhat spongy texture. As Mrs. Hall was of a very thin, spare, delicate habit, I thought it improper to bleed her, and therefore recommended warm fomentations, and other means to allay irritation. The following morning, at eleven o'clock, I again visited her with Mr. Keymer; she had passed a restless night, distressed with most violent and constant pains, continually exclaiming that she was certain she would burst. I found her in a most alarming state, and she appeared to be rapidly sinking : she with difficulty told me, that two hours before, during a most severe pain, she felt something snap, and to use her own words, ' the web of her body had given way ;' the noise of which one of her attendants declared she heard ; the pains had then suddenly ceased, attended with a discharge of blood, fainting, cold sweats, feeble pulse, and a vomiting of a brownish fluid. On introducing my hand under the bed-clothes, I found there had been a very considerable hæmorrhage, and among the coagula I discovered a substance which I put aside for future examination. At this time I found the head of the child so low as to enable me to accomplish delivery speedily with the vectis. The child was living, and the placenta was expelled without any difficulty. After waiting some time, by the use of light cordials the patient appeared to revive, but there was a singular fulness and tension of the abdomen, such as I had never before witnessed. It appeared to me to be a hopeless case, and I left the patient, fearing she could not long survive. On the Tuesday morning her abdomen was swelled to an enormous degree, much larger than previous to her delivery, and for ten days it remained very tense and tender : the pulse was at the same time exceedingly rapid and feeble, skin hot, and tongue furred. I drew off between three and four pints of urine in a very fœtid and acrimonious state, and had occasion to repeat this operation three or four times in as many days. In a week the bowels required large doses of calomel, Epsom salts, senna, &c. &c. to relieve them, and for a month the patient was feverish, and excessively weak and languid. During this time several large coagula were expelled, and the body regained its natural size. She was much emaciated, but by the use of light tonics and nutritious diet she gradually recovered her strength. Her health is now much re-established, but she has always suffered considerable inconvenience from a slight prolapsus uteri, which still continues. There is very considerable tenderness in the pudenda, and at the last examination per vaginam, which was about three weeks after the delivery, I found a continuous cavity, without any distinction between vagina and uterus. The catamenia appeared about five weeks ago; they were preceded by pain in the back, and continued in very small quantity for two days. The child is in good health, and the mother has a plentiful secretion of milk. The appearance presented by the os uteri, and an irregular part of the cervix surrounding it, has been represented in *this* coloured engraving [shewing it] which precedes the paper. I had an opportunity some years ago of seeing the preparation of the parts at the Middlesex Hospital, in the collection of Dr. Merriman, which passed into the possession of Dr. Hugh Ley, and since his death into that of Dr. Bull. I could not obtain permission to remove it from the spirits to ascertain if the Nabothean glands and penniform rugæ were visible, but the whole history of the case, and the appearance of the preparation, leave no doubt that the os uteri and cervix had been torn away from the body of the uterus. A great many anatomists and surgeons who examined the part in the recent state formed this opinion. Mr. Scott concludes this communication with the following explanation of the manner in which the accident occurred. " It has appeared to me, as Dr. Merriman suggested, that the head of the child passed through the superior aperture of the pelvis, carrying the uterus before it with the os uteri very little dilated, and that in this way the dilatation of the uterus was prevented by the head pressing it firmly against the sides of the pelvis, so as to prevent the action of the uterus from being exerted on the cervix. The great force of the uterus acting on the body of the child might thus produce the separation of the circular portion exhibited." I saw a case in consultation with Mr. Owen, of Holborn Bars, where the os uteri was thick, hard, smooth, and so little dilated, and pressed so close to the outlet of the pelvis after labour had continued for thirty hours with great severity, that it seemed probable an accident similar to that described would take place, but the labour was at last safely effected. After venesection, an opiate enema, and artificial dilatation, had been employed.

Oblique position of the os uteri has been enumerated by Dr. Denman among the causes of difficult labour depending on rigidity of the parts to be dilated, and Daventer erroneously attributed nearly all difficult labours to obliquities of the uterus. Where great relaxation of the abdominal parietes exists, the fundus uteri sometimes falls forward, and the os uteri is consequently thrown upward and backward in an unusual degree, but this cannot be regarded as a common cause of difficult labour, and where it occurs it is readily relieved by applying a bandage firmly around the body, and by

keeping the patient during the first stage of labour upon the back with the shoulders slightly depressed. Daventer, Baudelocque, and Desormeaux, have all attributed an undue degree of importance to obliquities of the uterus, and have recommended passing the fingers, or even the whole hand, into the vagina to push the head of the child above the brim of the pelvis, and also the lower part of the uterus, and with the extremities of the fingers to drag forward the anterior lip of the os uteri to the centre of the pelvis, and to keep it there until complete dilatation has taken place. This is one of the numerous and dangerous manœuvres described by writers, which ought never to be thought of. " Cases have been recorded," says Dr. Denman, " in which it was said that the os uteri was perfectly closed, and in which it has not only been proposed to make an artificial opening, instead of the closed natural one, but the operation has actually been performed. I do not know that I should be justified in saying that such cases have never occurred in my practice, but I am persuaded that there has been an error in this account, and that what has been called a perfect closure of the os uteri has not been such, but that we have been unable to discover it by reason of its obliquity."

Dr. Merriman is of opinion that the cases of difficult labour from the os uteri being projected above the symphysis pubis, described by Daventer and other writers, were instances of retroversion of the uterus at the full period. I have met with no cases tending to confirm or refute this opinion. Sometimes the os uteri descends with the head to the outlet of the pelvis, or actually passes through it at the commencement of labour: where this happens, the patient should be placed upon the back, with the pelvis elevated and the shoulders depressed, and the prolapsed uterus returned to its natural situation by long-continued gentle pressure with the expanded fingers. In some cases the anterior wall of the vagina and neck of the bladder are pushed down even through the external parts during labour, before the presenting part, and sometimes the posterior wall. In one case the latter was mistaken for the fœtal membranes, and an unsuccessful attempt was made to perforate with the finger the back part of the vagina. Where this accident occurs the protruded part of the vagina and bladder should be pressed up and supported by the fingers during the pains, that the head of the child may escape. Dr. Merriman relates a case in which the bladder distended with urine filled up the anterior part of the vagina, and was punctured and afterwards sloughed. The practitioner supposed that it was the child's head enlarged by hydrocephalus.

3. *Of protracted and difficult labours from rigidity of the fœtal membranes—their premature rupture—imperfect discharge of the liquor amnii—over distension of the uterus by dropsy of the amnion and a plurality of children.*

The membranes not unfrequently burst spontaneously, and the liquor amnii begins to escape before the commencement of the labour pains and the dilatation of the os uteri. One, two, or three days, or only a few hours, may elapse after the water begins to flow and uterine action occurs. The nature of the presentation should be ascertained as soon as possible by an internal examination, in all cases of premature rupture of the membranes.

The early rupture of the membranes is almost a diagnostic sign of preternatural presentations. The whole liquor amnii may be quickly discharged, or if the opening in the membranes be small, and at a distance from the cervix uteri, or the head of the child lies over the aperture, it may escape in small quantities at a time, or it may ooze out slowly, and keep the patient during a long period in a very uncomfortable state. When active uterine contractions take place, whether it be a first or subsequent labour, the process often goes on as safely and expeditiously as if nothing unusual had occurred, and no interference is necessary or proper. It is only in cases of labour protracted by feeble uterine action, from imperfect discharge of the liquor amnii, or, as it has been called, dribbling of the waters, that any thing is required to be done, and then the membranes should be freely torn open, and the head of the child held up or pressed towards the sacrum between the pains, and the os uteri, if not rigid, very gently dilated with the fingers. Unusual rigidity or thickness of the fœtal membranes, with or without an excessive quantity of liquor amnii, is a much more common cause of protracted labour than their premature rupture, and their artificial rupture is often followed by strong and regular contractions, and the safe and speedy termination of the labour. If the perineum and os uteri are rigid, and the head is high up, and it is the first child, it is seldom necessary to have recourse to rupturing the membranes before the first stage of labour is nearly or fully completed. When the first stage is far advanced, the parts yielding, yet the pains are feeble and ineffective for several hours, then you may rupture the membranes. Where there is a great quantity of liquor amnii, or the uterus is over distended by twins, it has not the power to contract upon its contents with sufficient force to rupture the membranes, and it may become completely exhausted if this is not done artificially. The uterus, as Smellie states, cannot come in contact with the body of the child, and press down the head, until the membranes are pushed a considerable way before it into the vagina, nor even then until they are broke. Where there is a considerable quantity of fluid between the head and membranes, and the pains are sufficiently strong to render them tense, there is usually no difficulty in perforating them with the point of the finger sharply forced against them; but where the pains are feeble, and the membranes are in contact with the head, very great difficulty is often experienced in opening them. The best and safest method is to pass the nail of the fore-finger backward and forward over the membranes like a saw, till the liquor amnii is felt escaping. I have never found it necessary to use a probe, or any other instrument than the finger, for this purpose.

4. *Of protracted and difficult labours from shortness of the umbilical cord, in consequence of being twisted once or several times around the neck and trunk of the child.*

Sometimes the umbilical cord is so short, without surrounding the neck of the child, that it is torn during the expulsion of the trunk and lower extremities, or it is necessary to tie and divide it before they can be extracted. Much more frequently the cord is twisted once or oftener around the neck, and during both the first and second stages of labour the head is in consequence not only retracted upon the declension of every pain, but during the pains it is not pushed forward with the usual force, and the labour is protracted. In some cases the head is held up so high by this twisting of the cord around the neck that the nature of the presentation cannot be positively ascertained till the first stage of labour is nearly completed. You may suspect it to be an arm presentation, because no part of the fœtus can be touched when the os uteri is fully dilated; and yet, when the hand is introduced to turn, and the membranes are ruptured, the head presents, and is prevented from descending in the ordinary manner from the shortness of the cord. In the second stage of labour, when the head is in the cavity or pressing against the parts at the outlet of the pelvis, you may suspect that the cord surrounds the neck, by the head receding in an extraordinary manner after each pain goes off. There is no rigidity of the parts, nothing unusual about the size and position of the head, no deficiency of uterine contractions, yet the head does not pass for many hours; not, indeed, till your patience and the woman's strength are both very nearly exhausted. You may be certain that this is the cause of the delay by passing up two fingers, or the whole hand as high as possible between the symphisis pubis and head, and feeling the cord surrounding the neck. If it pulsates strongly I entreat you to have patience, to leave the case to nature if immediate delivery is not necessary on some other ground, and to abstain from exhibiting ergot of rye or applying the forceps. But if the pulsations were becoming gradually feebler, and you had proofs of the fœtal circulation being interrupted, and the labour were greatly protracted, the best practice certainly would be immediately to deliver with the forceps. In a case of tedious labour, which I lately saw in consultation with Mr. Russel, of Broad Street, I declined at first employing the forceps, because the cord was around the neck and was pulsating vigorously, and the mother was not exhausted; but after some hours the pulsations in the cord had become extremely weak, and the child would probably have been destroyed in a short time had we not interfered. The blades of the forceps were easily applied, and the child was soon extracted alive and uninjured.

The operation of turning was sometimes had recourse to by Smellie in these cases.

"In June 1751," he says, "I was called by a midwife to a woman who had been many hours in labour, and found, that after the discharge of the waters, the head was forced low down by every pain, but afterwards drawn up again. I was likewise informed, that formerly she used to have large children and quick labours. Encouraged by this information, I tried to turn the child, but was prevented by the strong contraction of the uterus; but in making this trial, and raising the head, I not only found the funis surrounding the neck, but likewise the uterus contracted before the shoulders. This last I dilated with my fingers as much as possible, then withdrawing my hand, applied the forceps and delivered the child, which had been dead for some days. The funis was three times round the neck, being much tumified and of a livid colour." Smellie made two capital mistakes in the treatment of this case; the first was in attempting to deliver by turning the child, which ought never to be done under similar circumstances, and which I hope the uterine contractions will also prevent you from carrying into effect should you make the attempt. The next practical mistake was in delivering with the forceps, when he knew, or ought to have known, that the child was dead.

5. *Of protracted and difficult labours from unusual size and ossification of the head of the child. Hydrocephalus — the forehead situated under the arch of the pubes—presentation of the face—one of the arms with the head—death of the child, and the distension of its abdomen with air or fluid.*

If the pelvis is not above the average size, and the head is unusually large and hard, it will pass through the apertures with difficulty, or be arrested in them. The progress and termination of these cases is similar to those in which the pelvis is small or distorted, and the head does not exceed the ordinary size. If the disproportion between the head and pelvis is inconsiderable, the labour is protracted, but if time is given, and no improper treatment be employed, it is at last completed without artificial assistance, and the child's life is preserved. But where the head is much too large to pass, it becomes arrested and impacted in the brim; the bones are gradually compressed, so as to ride over one another between the pains, and it becomes swollen and elongated in a remarkable manner, where the head has been allowed to remain long strongly compressed either in the brim, cavity, or outlet of the pelvis; the child is usually destroyed by the injury inflicted on the brain, and the soft parts of the mother suffer from the long-continued pressure. The symptoms which here indicate the necessity for artificial assistance have already been fully described, and the safety both of the mother and child will generally, I am satisfied, be best secured by interposing as soon as it is evident that the natural powers are insufficient for the expulsion of the head.

Hydrocephalus in the child is not a common cause of protracted labour; but the diagnosis is very difficult, and if the nature of the obstruction be not early ascertained the result has generally been unfortunate; the os uteri dilates or is dilatable; but the head, if much distended with fluid, cannot enter or pass through the brim of the pelvis, and exhaustion or rupture of the uterus takes place. Where the affection is in a slighter degree, or if the pelvis be very large, the head is expelled by the pains undiminished. "I have known," says Dr. Merriman, "one hydrocephalic fœtus pass entire, the circumference of whose head was seventeen inches; another passed alive, and lived an hour, whose head measured in circumference twenty-two inches; both the above labours were long and painful." Where the cause of the difficulty is clearly ascertained, by feeling the bones of the fœtal head widely separated from one another, and a sense of fluctuation is also perceived, and where the os uteri is dilatable, and the pains have continued strong for some hours, and the head has not entered the brim, the perforator should be employed without loss of time. The following cases which have come under my observation will convince you that congenital hydrocephalus is detected with great difficulty during labour, and that it is often followed by the most fatal consequences. Every case of this kind which I have seen has terminated fatally, and in the greater number of them the cause of the difficulty was not ascertained till it was too late.

In 1834, I was called to a woman in

Warwick Street, who had been in labour nearly 60 hours. It was the first child. The head had not entered the brim, and it had not been discovered that the head was enormously distended with fluid. The delivery was easily effected by the perforator and crotchet; but inflammation of the uterus took place, which proved fatal in a few days. On the 14th of July, 1829, the late Dr. John Prout called me to see a woman, æt. 31, residing at No. 6, Draper's Place, Euston Square. She had been long in labour with her first child, and the presentation could not be positively determined. After the escape of an immense quantity of liquor amnii, and the complete dilatation of the os uteri, the presenting part remained entirely above the brim of the pelvis. It was not till I introduced the hand into the uterus, to deliver by turning, that I knew with certainty that the head presented, and that it was distended with fluid. Instead of turning, the hand was immediately withdrawn on the nature of the difficulty being ascertained, and the perforator employed, when several pints of a bloody fluid gushed out. The head was readily extracted, but she had a violent fit of cold shivering immediately after, and had nearly died from exhaustion. She was ultimately destroyed by uterine phlebitis and gangrene of the lungs. On the 12th of March, 1828, I saw another case of hydrocephalus in the fœtus with dropsy of the amnion, where the nature of the difficulty was not ascertained in time to be of any use to the patient, who was left too long in labour, and afterwards died from inflammation of the muscular structure of the uterus. But the two most unfortunate cases of difficult labour from hydrocephalus that I have ever seen occurred last summer, and within a week of one another. Their histories are the following :—

A woman near the full period, residing at No. 9, Castle Street, St. Martin's Lane, was seized with slight labour-pains on Saturday, June 18, 1842. The liquor amnii soon after escaped. The pains continued during the 19th and 20th at long irregular intervals, and had little effect on the os uteri. Early on the morning of Tuesday, the 21st, they were stronger and more frequent, and the midwife thought the labour would soon be finished. Suddenly a violent pain, like spasm, was experienced in the epigastric region, and soon after, sickness, faintness, hurried breathing, and coldness of the extremities, took place. Mr. Tucker was called to her about two hours after the occurrence of these symptoms, and found the placenta filling the os uteri, which was considerably dilated, and some hæmorrhage going on. I saw her not long after, and thought she would probably die before the delivery could be completed. The hand passed readily into the uterus, and, there

being no pain, came in contact with what seemed at first the bodies of two children. It was passed on to the fundus, where there was a foot felt. I grasped this, and, without the slightest exertion, brought it down and extracted the trunk and extremities of the child, but the head would not follow. I perforated the back part of the head with the scissors, when there escaped a very large quantity of fluid, and it was not till this began to flow that I properly understood the cause of the difficulty. With the crotchet passed into the opening, the head was easily drawn through the pelvis, and the placenta being loose was soon removed. Little hæmorrhage took place, and for twenty-four hours the symptoms were so favourable that it appeared she might recover. The sickness, however, never subsided, and she died suddenly forty-eight hours after being delivered. I examined the body the following day with Mr. Tucker, and we found all the coats of the uterus torn from the fundus to the orifice on the anterior part. (The uterus is in my possession, and you shall have an opportunity of seeing it.) There were ℥ij. of blood in the peritoneum. The bones of the head were at least twice the natural size, the ossification, particularly of the parietal bones, having kept pace with the distension of the head from the fluid. The skull has been dried, and you see it is nearly as large as the head of an adult.

Mrs. G——, æt. 30, 96, Drummond Street, Euston Suare. Being at the full period of pregnancy, the liquor amnii began to escape at 6 P.M. 22d June, 1842. Labour pains commenced at 1 A.M. of the 23d, and Mr. Kennedy, of Tavistock Square, saw her at 3 A.M. The pains were feeble till 11, and then for several hours after they became more active and frequent. At 3 P.M. a small loop of the funis, along with the head, was felt at the brim of the pelvis. The pains gradually ceased after 3, and she complained of cramps about the stomach. At 6, there was no dangerous symptom; but at 8, violent pain was felt at the fundus uteri. At 10 P.M. I first saw her with Mr. Kennedy; she was then sitting up in bed, supported by pillows, the breathing hurried and pulse feeble, with sickness and vomiting. She complained of excruciating pain in the upper part of the uterus, which she could not bear to be touched, and which felt remarkably hard and irregular. Slight hæmorrhage from the uterus; the funis still felt, but the presenting part had receded beyond the reach of the finger. I passed the hand into the uterus and felt the placenta adhering to the posterior wall, but could feel no part of the child. So violent was the pain produced by the hand, that I withdrew it without making any attempt to pass it through the opening in the uterus to extract the child. A large opiate was given, and she fell asleep for a short time. Feeling anxious that she should not die undelivered, we resolved to make an attempt to extract the child. I again passed the hand into the uterus, carried it forward through a great rent in the fundus, when it came immediately in contact with one of the feet, which I seized and brought back into the uterus. I had little difficulty in extracting the trunk and extremities of the child, but the head would not follow, though great force was employed, till perforated behind one of the ears, and then several pints of fluid escaped. Abdominal inflammation followed, the acute symptoms of which yielded to treatment; but fifteen days after delivery fæculent matter began to pass by the vagina, and the whole continued to escape through the vagina for thirteen days after, when she died. The omentum and all the parts around the uterus were glued together. The lower part of the ilium adhered firmly to the fundus uteri. On separating the ilium, a large irregular opening was seen in the uterus, the edges of which were in a black sloughing state. The ilium was perforated in the part corresponding with the rent in the uterus, and through this opening the fæculent mettar had passed from the ilium, through the cavity of the uterus, into the vagina. Had the cause of the difficulty been ascertained sufficiently early in this and the four preceding fatal cases of hydrocephalus in the fœtus, it is impossible to doubt that several of them, if not all, would have ended favourably.

In a case of difficult labour from hydrocephalic fœtus, recorded by Perfect, the woman died in two hours after being delivered. The head was twenty-four inches in circumference.

Smellie has related four cases of hydrocephalus, one of which occurred in 1747, and he states that after the orifice of the uterus was largely dilated, the head continued long high up at the brim, and felt in such an uncommon manner that he was for some time uncertain whether it was the head or breech, but the waters being discharged it was pushed a little lower down; then he felt the hairy scalp, and perceived the head was dropsical from the looseness of the bones, and the great distance between them. The head was expelled without artificial help. Another case occurred in 1753. It was the first child. The membranes and waters opened the os uteri in a very slow manner, and when they came down to the middle of the vagina, felt as if there had been one set of membranes within another, though the internal seemed to be much thicker than the external. But before the os uteri was fully opened, the membranes broke, and then I discovered the other was the hairy scalp,

pushed down by water contained in the skull. This the pains forced down lower and lower, so that the os internum being fully opened, it stretched the vagina and the os externum in the same manner as they are commonly dilated by the membranes and waters of the secundines; and he says, I felt the bones of the skull loose and riding one over another. The head was expelled without assistance, but a good deal of force was required to extract the body and shoulders, because the abdomen was swollen. The child had been dead ten days. These cases prove that the diagnosis is sometimes most difficult in protracted labour from an hydrocephalic state of the fœtus, and that it has often terminated fatally. I have related these and the following cases with the view of rendering you cautious how you employ ergot of rye, or any other means, to excite strong uterine contractions before the presenting part has been clearly ascertained.

Smellie mentions another case in which flooding took place before delivery, and all his efforts to extract the head after turning were useless in consequence of hydrocephalus. He exerted great force, and continued to increase it till he found the neck and mouth to give way. A curved crotchet was then passed up along the child's head to the upper and convex part of the forehead, and, on pulling forcibly, the bones of the skull collapsed, and a quantity of water escaped. The head was about a third larger than common, and the woman died 18 or 20 days after. The delivery would have been more easily effected by perforating the back part of the head, and then extracting it with the crotchet, which he did in another case. In the 4th vol. of the Medico-Chirurgical Transactions, Sir C. Bell relates a case of hydrocephalus in which the uterus was ruptured. Dr. Ramsbotham relates three cases, two of which terminated fatally.

Ascites in the fœtus is a still more rare disease than hydrocephalus, and it may prevent the body of the child following the head through the pelvis. The same effect is produced by distension of the abdomen with air where the fœtus is dead, and where the kidneys and bladder are distended with urine in consequence of the urethra and ureters being impervious. In all these cases, where any difficulty arises in extracting the trunk of the child, the perforator should be passed up, and the air and fluid in the abdomen should be evacuated.

(Continued from page 54.)

CASE OF

DIABETES MELLITUS,

WITH NUMEROUS OBSERVATIONS,
AND A REVIEW OF THE PATHOLOGY AND
TREATMENT OF THIS DISEASE.

By JOHN PERCY, M.D. (Edin.)

Physician to the Queen's Hospital, and Lecturer
on Organic Chemistry at the Royal School of
Medicine and Surgery, Birmingham.

*Record of Chemical observations made
in respect to Merchant.*

I EXAMINED the urine at repeated intervals, from the time of his admission to that of his death. It had the ordinary properties of urine in diabetes mellitus. Colour pale straw. Without sediment. Delicate mucous cloud. Odour *sui generis*, and not urinous. Acid. It furnished well-crystallized grains of grape-sugar, by exposing the syrup obtained by evaporation over the steam-bath to the air for several days. Crystals of uric acid were separated by the addition of hydrochloric acid. At first, I was unable to detect urea, but afterwards I was enabled to separate well-formed crystals of nitrate of urea. The specific gravity will be found by reference to the table. In respect to the proximate analysis of diabetic urine, there are three points on which I shall offer some observations, viz. the determination of the *water*, of the *sugar*, and of the *urea*.

1st. *Of the dermination of the water.* —The amount of water is usually estimated by evaporation over the steam-bath; and the data upon which the well-known table of Dr. Henry is founded were obtained in this manner. The loss occasioned by such evaporation is regarded as water. For practical purposes merely, this truth is sufficiently accurate; but it is not satisfactory to the analytical chemist. The following comparative experiments, performed with the greatest attention to accuracy, will shew that at the temperature of boiling water decomposition of the organic matter of the urine is effected. Even in vacuo, decomposition in a slight degree takes place; and if diabetic urine be evaporated over strong sulphuric acid, in the receiver of the air-pump, the acid acquires a pale brown colour.

I evaporated 500 grains of diabetic urine, sp. gr. 1035·3· 62°F, over strong sulphuric acid in the exhausted receiver of the air-pump, April 22d, 7 P.M.

Weight, May 3d, 7 P.M.   46·3.
Ditto.   May 7th, 1 P.M.   46·3.

The desiccation in this case must have been complete. The extract was nearly colourless, and was full of small bubbles.

500 grains of the same urine were evaporated over the steam-bath, April 23d, 11 A.M. The bath consisted of a tin vessel, the cover of which contained a circular aperture just sufficient to receive a Berlin capsule.

Weight at 4½, P.M.   48·7
   „   6½   „   46·6
   „   9½   „   45·1

The desiccation was continued on the following morning,

Weight at 12 A.M.   44·7
   „   2½ P.M.   44·1
   „   8½   „   43·5

The residuum was hard when cold, and had a dark brown colour.

Evaporation in vacuo   46·3
   "   over steam-bath   43·5
                        _____
      Difference   2·8

Again, evaporation of diabetic urine, sp. gr. 1027°, continued for many hours over the steam-bath. 200 grains employed.

1st weighing   13·2
2d   „   12·2
3d   „   11·7
4th   „   11·6
5th   „   11·4

It was not ascertained whether 11·4, the result of the fifth weighing, was the quantity which would not admit of further diminution in weight by continued evaporation. The same objection, on the ground of accuracy, will also apply to the drying apparatus of Berzelius, represented and described in Plate 7, Fig. 31, Tome 8ième, Traité de Chimie. From the specimens of diabetic urine subjected to experiment, I obtained well crystallized grape-sugar.

Again, evaporation of 200 grains of urine, containing an excess of urea, over the steam-bath, sp. gr. 1027°.

1st weighing	12·5	6th weighing	10.2
2d „	11·7	7th „	10 1
3d „	11·0	8th „	10·0
4th „	10·6	9th „	9·8
5th „	10·3	10th „	9·6

The experiment was begun at 11 A M. and continued until 10 P.M. of the same day. The preceding experiment, together with numerous others of a similar kind, have induced me always, in delicate analyses of the urine, in which I wish to attain extreme accuracy, to determine the amount of water by evaporation in vacuo over strong sulphuric acid at the ordinary temperature. 500 grains of Merchant's urine, sp. gr. 1040°, left, after exposure to the influence of strong sulphuric acid in vacuo for nine days, 51·63 of pale brownish yellow frothy extract. Now, a wine pint of diabetic urine, of sp. gr. 1040°, = 7581·3 grains; and, according to Henry's Table, should contain 766·4 of solid matter. Therefore, 1000 grains of such urine should furnish 101·08 of solid matter. However, by desiccation in vacuo, as mentioned above, I obtained from 1000 grains of such urine 103·26. Excess in the latter amounts to 2·18 grains.

2d. Of the determination of the sugar. In order to procure crystallized grape-sugar from diabetic urine, it is essential to leave the brown syrup obtained by evaporation over the steam-bath, exposed to the air, sometimes for several days. In this case the crystallization does not depend upon any further degree of evaporation, which may be effected by such exposure, but is connected with a molecular change, which, when once excited, proceeds with considerable rapidity. The attraction of cohesion in the syrup interferes with the freedom of molecular motion essential to rapid crystallization. I have had syrup of diabetic urine, which has not crystallized in less than a fortnight.

I have obtained beautiful and almost colourless grains, composed of minute and perfect crystals, by exposing the syrup left by evaporation in vacuo. In the estimation of the quantity of sugar I have resorted to the process of fermentation.

Oct. 26th.—To f3iij. of Merchant's urine, sp. gr. 1036°, I added a minute quantity of yeast. The gas evolved was first passed over chloride of calcium, and then into Liebig's potash bulb apparatus, just as in ordinary organic analysis. The urine was contained in a two-necked bottle, one neck of which was connected with the chloride of calcium tube, whilst the other received a small tube, drawn out to a capillary extremity, which was introduced below the surface of the urine, the other extremity communicating with the atmosphere. By this arrangement, I could, as in an organic analysis, cause the carbonic acid remaining in the bottle after fermentation to pass into the potash apparatus, by inhaling in the usual way with a pipette. Fermentation was soon established, and the gas was disengaged with regularity. The corks used in adjusting the tubes to the two-necked bottle were varnished. When the gas ceased to be evolved, as indicated by the rising of the solution of potash, the potash apparatus was detached and weighed, the carbonic acid remaining in the bottle and chloride of calcium tube having been previously displaced by air, in the manner described.

After fermentation . .	769.94
Before „ . .	737·02

Increase, due to carbonic acid. 32·92

One atom of grape sugar ($C_{12} H_{14} O_{14}$) 199·44* (C = 6·12.)
One atom of ditto by fermentation, yields $4CO_2$ = 88·48

$$\therefore 88·48 : 199.44 :: 32·92 : 74·203.$$
$$\therefore f. 3iij : 74·203 :: f. 3xvj : 395.749 \text{ grains of grape-sugar in a wine pint of urine.}$$

Now, according to Henry's Table, one pint of such urine contains 689.6 of solid matter. Hence, in this quantity we should have 689·6 — 395·749 = 293·851 of *organic* and *saline* matter, besides *sugar*.

Nov. 9th.—In precisely the same manner, I fermented 1000 grains of Merchant's urine, sp. gr. 1040°.

---

* At 212° it loses 2HO.

Potash apparatus, after fermentation, weighed   810·62 grains
Ditto   before   Ditto   Ditto   781·91
Increase, carbonic acid   .   .   .   .
                                              28·71

Hence, this quantity of urine contained 64·714 grains of grape-sugar. 1000 grains of this urine, we have seen, furnished, by complete desiccation *in vacuo*, 103·26 grains. A wine pint would contain 471·765 grains of grape-sugar. Now, a wine pint of Merchant's

urine of sp. gr. 1036°, contained 395·749 grains. We have, then, in a wine pint of urine of sp. gr. 1040°, 76·016 grains of sugar more than in the same measure of urine of sp. gr. 1036°. Now from Henry's Table we learn, that a wine

pint of urine, sp. gr. 1040°, contains, of solid matter   .   .   766·4 grains
and   Ditto Ditto 1036°,   Ditto   Ditto   .   .   .   689·6

                                              ·Difference   76·8

This excess, then, would appear to be entirely grape-sugar, as will be seen from the statements immediately preceding. 76·8—76·016=0·784.

In regard to the method of estimating the quantity of sugar in diabetic urine by the process of fermentation, it is alleged that two sources of error exist, viz. the production of carbonic acid from the yeast, and the resolution of the urea which may be present into carbonate of ammonia. I admit this allegation in a strictly chemical point of view; still, I am convinced that the absolute amount of error from these sources is exceedingly small, and may generally be safely neglected. In the first place, a minute quantity of good yeast is sufficient to excite fermentation; and, from experiments performed over mercury with a view to estimate the amount of carbonic acid evolved from the yeast alone, I am satisfied of the truth of what I have just advanced. Concerning the second source of error, I may state, that, in the case of Merchant, it must, indeed, have been small, for urea existed only in minute proportion, as will hereafter be clearly seen in the detail of an ultimate organic analysis of the residuum obtained by evaporation *in vacuo*. Besides, all the carbonate of ammonia generated and dissolved in the urine would not readily pass over with the carbonic acid. Dr. Christison states that the test of fermentation is so delicate, that one part of diabetic sugar in 1000·0 of healthy urine, sp. gr. 1030°, may be detected by it, the carbonic acid evolved being collected over mercury in a graduated receiver.—(Library of Practical Medicine, vol. iv. p. 249.)

3. *Of the determination of the urea.* —This principle, frequently, cannot be detected in diabetic urine in the usual manner, by evaporation and the addition of nitric acid; the sugar preventing the precipitation of the nitrate of urea, or the urea existing only in small quantity. At one time the opinion prevailed that urea was generally absent from diabetic urine, but this opinion has, of late, been proved to be erroneous. To Dr. Kane we are indebted for the knowledge of the fact, that, when nitric acid fails to precipitate the urea in the state of nitrate, at the ordinary temperature, this salt is readily separated at a very low temperature. Accordingly, by the aid of refrigerating mixtures, urea may always be precipitated by the addition of nitric acid, in excess, to diabetic urine, reduced sufficiently by evaporation. Sometimes, however, a considerable time is required in order to effect this precipitation of nitrate of urea.

The following experiments were carefully made upon this subject:—

1. To f℥ss. of Merchant's urine, sp. gr. 1040°, I added, f℥ss. of nitric acid, diluted with the same measure of water. I introduced the mixture, contained in a thin glass-tube, into a mixture of snow and dilute sulphuric acid for three-quarters of an hour, the thermometer indicating — 2 F. No crystallization of nitrate of urea occurred, nor was the transparency of the liquid in the least degree disturbed.

2. I then exposed a mixture of f℥j. of this urine, and f℥ij. of the strongest and pure nitric acid, to the same temperature for the same period, and with the same result.

3. I mixed fʒij. of healthy urine with an equal bulk of the same nitric acid, and exposed the mixture to the same circumstances. A considerable quantity of beautiful and nearly colourless crystals of nitrate of urea was separated, and remained on the following day.

4. I washed the residuum from 500 grains of Merchant's urine, evaporated over steam-bath, with cold rectified spirit. I evaporated the spirituous solution to a syrup, to which I added a small quantity of distilled water. I thus obtained fʒij. of solution, which, mixed with fʒij. of strong nitric acid, and left in the same frigorific mixture all night, presented, on the following morning, beautiful crystals of nitrate of urea.

Occasionally, urea may be readily separated in the state of nitrate by washing the extract of diabetic urine with cold rectified spirit, evaporating the spirituous solution, re-dissolving the residuum in a small quantity of water, and then proceeding in the ordinary way. Sometimes the urea may be separated at once, as nitrate, by the addition of nitric acid to the syrup. A short time ago, I succeeded in this manner in separating urea from diabetic urine of sp. gr. so high as 1045°. I could not detect a trace of urea by acting upon the residuum of Merchant's urine with common æther; though from the residuum of healthy urine this menstruum readily dissolves out the urea, and, by evaporation, leaves long and beautiful crystals. One part of pure urea, I find, dissolves in 63 parts of common rectified æther (of sp. gr. 759·3 59° F.), at 49° F. The usual mode of estimating the quantity of urea is, I am persuaded, from numerous experiments, incorrect in a very appreciable degree. I have ascertained the amount of error, but, on the present occasion, it would be superfluous to enlarge upon this subject. The absolute amount of urea may, probably, be inferred from the ultimate analysis, to which I have before alluded, and which will be found in the sequel.

The determination of the fixed saline ingredients of diabetic urine, by the process of incineration, is tedious, and requires considerable attention. The residuum of evaporation swells up exceedingly on the application of heat, so that a large platinum crucible must be employed. The carbon gradually burns away, and leaves a delicate skeleton of saline matter, from which any remaining portion of carbon may be removed by the very cautious addition of nitrate of ammonia. To prevent any loss by projection, it is advisable to replace the cover of the crucible immediately after the introduction of each particle of nitrate of ammonia. I have, previously to incineration, sometimes destroyed the sugar and similar organic matter, by evaporating the urine with nitric acid. One source of error, in this mode of determination, may be the volatilization of a minute quantity of chloride.

Analysis of 1000 *grains of diabetic urine, sp. gr.* 1040°.

Water	896·740
Sugar . . .	64·714
Urea, uric acid, colouring matter, volatile saline matter, and other organic constituents	32·746
Chlorides . . .	2·5
Sulphates . . .	1·5
Alkaline carbonate, probably derived from the decomposition of an organic salt	0·5
Phosphates of lime and of magnesia	1·3
	1000·000

Ultimate analysis of the residuum of diabetic urine of sp. gr. 1036°. I believe this was the sp. gr., though I cannot be certain to two or three degrees.

The residuum was obtained by evaporation *in vacuo*, and then allowed to crystallize completely by exposure to the air. Thus crystallized, it was again desiccated *in vacuo* over strong sulphuric acid, for several weeks. The nitrogen was determined by the ingenious method of Varrentrapp and Will, described in the Philosophical Magazine, Vol. 20, p. 216. Two analyses were made, with the greatest attention to accuracy, with chromate of lead. The amount of fixed saline constituents was determined by incineration.

Hydrogen . . .	6·360
Carbon . . .	39·594
Oxygen . . .	49·114
Nitrogen . . .	1·179
Residuum . . .	3·753
	100·000

The weighings extended to thousandths of a grain. Dividing by the respective atoms (C estimated as 6·125, and N as 14·186, Berzelius), we have—

Hydrogen	.	.	6·360
Carbon	.	.	6.454
Oxygen	.	.	6·139
Nitrogen	.	.	0·083

Hence, it is clear that, even admitting all the nitrogen to have existed in the state of urea, only a very small proportion of this constituent was present. In 100·0 parts of organic matter, exclusive of fixed saline matter, we should have—

Hydrogen	.	.	6·607
Carbon	.	.	41·137
Oxygen	.	.	51·029
Nitrogen	.	.	1·224

By comparing these results with those obtained by our honoured countryman, Dr. Prout, we find that the organic matter of Merchant's urine, exclusive of sugar and azotised matter, has nearly the composition of grape-sugar. Thus,—

Dr. Prout's Analysis of Diabetic Sugar.

Hydrogen	.	.	6·67
Carbon	.	.	40·00
Oxygen	.	.	53·33

Of the indeterminate organic matter of urine there is little of a satisfactory kind at present published. We can conceive that, generally, it may vary much in respect to ultimate composition, according to variation in diet. In diabetes mellitus, however, its composition is, probably, less liable to variation; for we know that specimens of urine, in this disease, and from different patients, closely resemble each other in physical as well as chemical properties. I make this remark with due regard to exceptions.

There does not appear to have been great variation in the absolute amount of fixed saline matter in Merchant's urine. Three incinerations were carefully made, and the results are as follow :—

1. 1000·0 grs., sp. gr. 1036°, furnished 4·6
2. Do. do. do. do. 3.753
3. Do. do. 1040° do. 5·8

There is only one analysis of diabetic urine in the "Chimie Pathologique" of L'Héritier, p. 558. It differs considerably from my own, and the quantity of sugar is not clearly estimated.

L'Héritier's Analysis of 1000·0 parts, of sp. gr. 1042°.

Water	.	.	931·200
Urea	.	.	7·600
Uric acid	.	.	0·080
Organic matters	.	.	52·575
Inorganic salts	.	.	8·545
			1000·000

Of the 52·575 parts of organic matter, L'Héritier ascertained, by another analysis of the same urine, that 46·936 were sugar. The mode in which the sugar was determined is not mentioned. We are indebted to Dr. Christison for some valuable observations on the urine of diabetes, published in the Edinburgh Monthly Journal of Medical Science, No. 4, April 1841, pp. 233 et seq. They are as follow :—

Feb. 13th.—1000·0 grains, of sp. gr. 1048·5, contained 57·7 of sugar, and 12·6 of urea.

March 13th.—1000·0 grains of urine, from the same patient, contained 101·6 of solid matter, of which 69·9 were sugar, and 14·0 urea.

March 13th.—1000·0 of urine, of sp. gr. 1038·0, of another patient labouring under diabetes, contained 84·74 of solid matter, of which 50·5 were sugar, and 23·22 urea.

1000·0 grains of urine, in another diabetic case, of sp. gr. 1033°, contained only 2·0 grains of urea. The urine of the same man, four days afterwards, sp. gr. 1035°, contained 81·5 parts in 1000·0, of which 4·63 were urea. The urine of the same individual, two days afterwards, its quantity having increased, had sp. gr. 1032°, and contained, in 1000·0 parts, 40·8 of sugar, and 13·9 of urea.

Miscellaneous Observations on Merchant's Urine, sp. gr. 1040°.

1. By boiling for a few minutes, it became turbid, and greyish flocculent matter subsided. The turbidity was almost entirely removed on the addition of nitric acid.

2. Tincture of galls gave a flocculent lemon-coloured precipitate.

3. Boiled with bichromate of potass, green oxide of chromium was liberated (? with formation of oxalate of potass).

4. Sulphate of copper, boiled for some time with this urine, produced a dirty-greenish precipitate, and the supernatant liquid had a clear apple-green colour.

5. Nitrate of silver, heated with this urine, was decomposed, with the liberation of metallic silver.

In the last stage of the disease, as is usual, the sugar disappeared from the urine, which contained an abundance of urate of ammonia, and of deep brownish-red crystals of uric acid.

Dec. 29th.— Urine passed on the morning of the 28th. Sp. gr. 1025°. Brown. Copious deposit, on cooling, of amorphous sediment, immediately soluble in hot water (urate of ammonia). Filters clear.

31st.—Precisely similar in appearance to that passed on the 28th. Odour urinous. Reddens litmus. Sp. gr. 1013°. Copious deposit of urate of ammonia and crystals of uric acid. 500·0 grains, evaporated over the steam-bath, left 24·3 of brown urinous syrup. This urine, simply by careful evaporation, furnished, on cooling, long and beautiful crystals of urea. The syrup, on the addition of nitric acid, became a solid crystalline mass. To 500·0 grains of this urine I added, without previous evaporation, f3vj. of strong nitric acid. On the following day an abundant crop of crystals of the nitrate of urea had separated. I fermented f3viij. with yeast. Three days afterwards I distilled over f3vj., which I mixed with carbonate of potass, and then redistilled. The product was received in a small tube, containing carbonate of potass. Instantly, after agitation, was separated a stratum of alcohol, which burned with a blue flame.

Jan. 2d. — Merchant's last urine. Brown. Slightly turbid. Acid. Sp. gr. 1020°. With pale brown deposit of urate of ammonia. No sugar was detected by fermentation. Long and beautiful crystals of urea were readily obtained by treating the evaporated urine with cold æther.

Analysis of 1000·0 *grains.*

Water	954·4
Urea	23·77
Uric acid, colouring matter, and indeterminate organic matter }	18·33
Salts soluble in water . .	3·1
Insoluble phosphates . .	0·4
	1000·00

Examination of Merchant's Breath, in respect to Moisture.

Nov. 11th.—He came in a car to my house, this morning, at 10¼ A.M. I caused him to expire very carefully through one of Liebig's chloride of calcium tubes, filled with chloride. What he expired was passed into a graduated receiver over water, so that the volume of breath could be precisely ascertained. I allowed him only to expire a small quantity through the tube at a time; and, during the experiment, he breathed out freely several times. I weighed the tube after the passage through it of fifty cubic inches. I obtained 0·41 increase. Mr. Clay, one of the pupils of the hospital, was then made the subject of a precisely similar experiment, and the same quantity of increase occurred. The temperature was 54° F., and the weather appeared to be damp.

[To be continued.]

THE

HUMAN SKIN AND ITS PATHOLOGY.

By OTHO WUCHERER, M.D.

Member of the Royal College of Surgeons in London; Rua de Boa Vista, Lisbon.

(For the Medical Gazette.)

(Concluded from page 59.)

THAT the secretions of the skin are necessary for the maintenance of a healthy composition of the blood seems to be proved sufficiently by physiological and pathological facts. The importance of these secretions in that respect might be inferred already from the considerable quantity of matter secreted, and from the antagonism between the skin and inner organism in respect to their secretions.. In the skin two secretions are said to take place, that is, besides that of the cytoblastema, in which the cells of the epidermis originate, viz. that of a sebaceous kind by the sebaceous follicles, "and that of the sudorific glands, commonly termed perspiration, when it takes place more profusely and visibly, for generally it is of a vaporous kind, and therefore not perceived: hence the term insensible perspiration, so frequently found in works on pathology. A secretion that is also vaporous, and shows in other respects analogy to that called perspiration, is that of the lungs. For detailed accounts of these secretions we refer to Johannes Müller's Physiology; and of their chemical composition to the 9th vol. of Berzelius's Chemistry. Müller says, that the chemical analysis of these secretions had as yet not cast any light on their value. The serum secreted by the follicles is supposed to be designed to make the skin soft and pliable. Perspiration is known to answer the purpose of regulating the temperature of the body. At the same time, it depends on the temperature of the atmosphere, as well as on the quantity of water which the latter contains suspended or dissolved. If the atmosphere is warm, the skin secretes freely; if cold, it secretes less. But when the skin secretes freely, the kidneys secrete less; and when it secretes little, the kidneys secrete more; so that both organs are capable of taking, to some degree, one another's place. This may explain the greater frequency of cutaneous diseases in warm climates, and the comparatively less frequency of diseases of the urinary organs in those parts; whilst cutaneous diseases were observed to be less frequent in cold climates. If perspiration is prevented to some degree in an individual at the same time that his body attains higher temperature, as by exercise, he feels uncomfortable, and considerable anxiety may be the consequence in some persons. I have heard several complaints in this country that the Indian-rubber cloaks had this effect, and that Indian-rubber shoes made the feet feel hot and uncomfortable. The skin stands in sympathy with many internal organs, as observed in daily experience; and, as Müller remarks, it presents an extensive field from which to act on the nervous centres in their morbid affections. We refer to his work for detailed accounts of these sympathies. The different parts of the skin show a consensus with one another, which seems explicable only by action of nerves. Henle says, in scabies, parts of the skin have pustules to which the acarus has not reached. A blister does not act solely on that part of the skin it occupies, and it is often used to augment the secretion of the whole skin. If tartar emetic ointment is rubbed in a part of the skin, there often appear pustules in other parts of the skin. The influence of nerves on the skin and its secretions is evident in diseases of the mind, or nervous centres, but also in affections of other organs; and very often we draw conclusions from the state of the skin on that of the powers of a patient, &c.

That the temperature of the skin depends in part on nervous influence is shown by experiments, and seen in many diseases. But it is needless to quote more striking proofs of the dependency of the skin and its secretions in particular on nerves. Many facts that show this connexion exhibit at the same time the laws of reflex function discovered and illustrated by Marshall Hall and F. Müller.

The description of the epithelia we gave after Henle, and did not mention at the same time some observations by Reichert, which seem to prove a material difference in respect to manner of development and functions between the epithelium of the skin and the so-called epithelium of the intestinal canal. Burdach says somewhere, that the nervous system served often as an asylum for our ignorance, and that to it all changes were attributed which we were otherwise unable to explain. It is remarkable, that about the same time, when numerous physiologists were employed to elucidate the functions of the nervous system by experiments, the independency of cells from nervous influence should have been so clearly and universally illustrated. The cylindrical or conical cells that cover the inner surface of the intestines, regarded by Henle as a kind of epithelium, Reichert has endeavoured to prove to be the mucous membrane of this canal, at least the membrane which possesses the property of absorption. His reasons for this opinion are the following: —In the first place, the structure described by Henle as an epithelium is deposited by the yolk of the ovum on the inside of the intestinal tube, and is no secretion like the epithelium of the skin. Besides, Reichert observes that in the frog the intestinal canal consists only of a muscular membrane and the layer of cells corresponding to the membrane now in question. If this is not the organ of absorption, which then? Reichert could find no blood-vessels or nerves in this structure, but this cannot diminish our opinion of the importance of the cells; it serves us only as a proof of the important properties of cells in general; for the knowledge of which we are indebted to Schwann in the first place, and also to Müller, Reichert, and others. Müller considers Schwann's discovery the greatest made in physiology for a long period. After having given the description of the formation of the mucous membrane, taken from Reichert's manuscript, Müller says he avoided the scrupulous term "epithelium," because this structure might have a higher importance than was generally supposed; and he seems induced to this opinion by Reichert's ingenuous observations. The independency of the cells that compose the absorbing tunic of the digestive tube reminds one forcibly of that possessed by the cells of the yolk in the ovum to develope themselves, tending to form the organs of the embryo. It shows, at the same time, a striking analogy to the properties of the cells in plants, and gives a proof of the correctness of Schwann's opinions, If Reichert is right in considering the cellular covering of the digestive tube as the organ of absorption, there is a great difference in its designation and that of the epidermis, supposed to be principally intended as an envelope for the body, which, in one or the other form, all living bodies seem to possess, and by which they exclude themselves from foreign influences. However, these foreign influences cannot be entirely overcome—they would act on the body if the latter did not pay a tribute; this tribute is the epidermis, which is composed of cells, the lowest order of organic development, nature thus avoiding the sacrifice of more developed orders. Before Schwann's discovery, the vibratory epithelium was found out; and it gives another example of vital motion without nerves. For accounts of it, as well as of the purpose it is said to answer, I refer to the works on physiology by Müller and R. Wagner. The latter treats of analogous vital motions observed in plants and animals, and observes that he intends to publish a separate work on these phenomena.

If you consider that the skin is so accessible to anatomical investigation, and that its diseases are so open to view, it must appear remarkable that our knowledge of its anatomy and pathology should have remained so long imperfect. The fact that diseases, which present themselves in other organs in such a number of various symptoms, caused but a limited number of changes in the skin, might have led to an inquiry into the structure of the skin, particularly since it made the

classification of these affections so difficult. Already, Lorry, and many other authors on cutaneous affections, considered the sebaceous follicles a frequent seat of those diseases which appear as circumscribed inflammations of the skin. One author after the other copied this remark, without inquiring further into the subject. Even Schönlein, who endeavoured to construct a natural system of diseases, gave very artificial diagnostic signs for the discrimination of cutaneous diseases. He calls the halo (which term he censures) at the base of the pustules, vesicles, &c. pericarpium; and distinguishes a pericarpium simplex, bearing only one pustule, vesicle, &c. called the fruit, and a pericarpium commune, bearing several fruit. But he mentions nowhere that observation in respect to the sebaceous follicles made already by Lorry (Dr. F. L. Schönlein's Allgemeine und specielle Pathologie und Therapie, St. Gallen. Im Litteratur Comptoir, 1839). An opinion formerly entertained (Peter Frank), that the seat of cutaneous diseases could never be sought in the epidermis, since it had no vitality, possessing no vessels and nerves, can of course no longer be admitted since Schwann's discoveries. And Schwann's assertion, considering the origin of all tissues in the healthy animal body from cells, has been shown by J. Müller to be equally true for morbid tissues (see the translation of his work, Ueber den feineren Bau und die Formen der krankhaften Geschwülste, Berlin 1838). According to Henle, the following changes may take place in an effusion of lymph consequent on inflammation or other causes.

1. There appear cells, which develope themselves in the same way as those of the tissue surrounding the effusion, and this is the process of regeneration and hypertrophy.

2. The cells do not develope themselves in the manner of those of the tissue into which the effusion took place, but in that corresponding to the manner of development in cells of some other tissue in the body, as in ossification, induration, &c.

3. The cells develope themselves in a manner altogether strange to the body; and here their development, independent of the latter, is particularly evident, since the structures formed by these cells tend to dispossess the an-

nexing tissues: hence they are often called parasites.

These cells, if deposited in another part of the body, develope themselves always in this peculiar manner. Even if removed to other bodies, they develope themselves to constitute the same structures, as shown by Langenbeck's interesting experiments. He brought cells from a cancer of one body into the circulating system of another, and the disease appeared in the latter. This fact supports an opinion, defended by Henle, that the contagium of diseases is not their mere cause, but their actual germ. His reasons for this supposition are the following. Only living beings possess the capability of increasing by assimilation of strange matter: fermentation has been adduced as a proof against this law; but as the observations of Cagnard, Latour, and Schwann show, fermentation depends on the propagation of organic bodies of plants (Torula cerevisiæ, Turpin; the sal aceti of Leeuwenhoeck). A single cell of these bodies is sufficient to cause the development of an infinite number if brought into a substance favourable to their propagation. In like manner but a minimum of contagion is necessary to carry the disease from one individual to another. Harvey's sentence "omne vivum ex ovo," so frequently assailed for so many years back, seems to be true after all, according to the convincing experiments of Schwann, and Ehrenberg and Eschricht's observations; and if it is true, it supports the opinion adopted by Henle. It has often been observed that no one had ever seen a contagium however, besides the analogy of fermentation, organic bodies resembling the lowest orders of plants and animals have been observed by Bassi, Audouin Balsamo, Lomeni, and Montagne, to be the cause of a disease, on silkworms, the bearers of the contagium, or rather the contagium itself, a single cell taken from one animal being sufficient to produce the disease in another. Similar observations have been made by Hannover and Henle in respect to Triton cristatus, on which they found vorticellæ to form a destructive disease; by Ehrenberg in respect to fishes. Besides, there seems to exist a great analogy between the cutaneous diseases of animals and plants, the latter being caused by living bodies of the lowest

orders, as shown by Uenger. But as yet we are convinced of the existence of only one living contagium for the human body, the acarus known to cause the itch. A similar animal was found in syphilitic ulcers, but its relation to the contagiosity of the disease is yet dubious. Henle has collected many facts besides to defend his opinion, for which we must refer to his work, "Pathologische Ucntersuchungen, 1840." All these observations concerning the living contagium well deserve the attention of the profession, even if the conclusions drawn from them till now should appear problematical.

A structure I have not hitherto mentioned is the subcutaneous cellular tissue. Its contraction is considered to cause the cutis anserina. The elevations that appear in this case are formed by the sebaceous follicles. From each of these elevations remarked in cutis anserina you observe to proceed a hair. The contraction of the subcutaneous cellular tissue may also be regarded as the cause of an erection of the hairs observed in some cases. This erection of the hairs depends besides on the contraction of the cellular tissue, on their piercing the skin in an oblique direction, and their extending with their fixed ends into the cellular tissue. If the latter contracts itself, it moves the end of the hair, which having its hypomorhlion in the opening of its follicle, is erected. That a single hair proceeds from each nodule in rubeola was already observed by Wedekind; Willan describes a lichen pilaris. Sometimes the hair is only visible by means of the magnifying glass. On the skin of almost all persons you perceive slight elevations, of a white, or when rubbed of a reddish colour: they consist of a crust of almost pellucid substance. If you lift this crust off, you perceive an elevation on its inferior surface, which corresponds to a depression on the spot of the skin from which it was taken. In the depression you observe a hair, folded up in a tortuous manner, which proceeds from an opening at the bottom of the depression. If the crust is moistened in water, and brought under the magnifying glass, you perceive it to consist chiefly of epithelium cells. To explain the formation of these elevations, and what is evidently their consequence, the folding up of the hair, we must suppose that, first, the hair of each of these thus affected follicles had fallen out; perhaps the secretion of the sebaceous follicles was at the same time altered, so as to obstruct the opening of the follicle, through which then the new hair could not pass, and continuing to grow, it became folded in that manner. Whether these elevations can be the cause of any inconvenience I do not know; perhaps, however, some species of prurigo might find in them their explanation. That the disease called acne depends on an obstruction of the opening of these follicles is well known; in the white matter you can often press forth from these follicles, you generally find one, seldom two small hairs. If the white substance is moistened in water, you find it to consist of cells of epithelium when you regard it under the microscope. The follicles may be extended by their secretion, if its passage outwards is prevented, to an enormous size, and form thus, according to some, bodies that have great resemblance to those encysted tumors known under the name of atheroma. From the middle of variola pustules you often find to proceed a hair, but the peculiar cellular structure of these pustules is not satisfactorily explained. Miliaria, Rosenbaum (see the article Miliaria, in Blasius Handwörterbuch der Chirurgie. Berlin, 1838) has declared to be an affection of the sudorific glands, which, he says, become inflamed, and form slight elevations over the surface of the skin. The swelling of the glands he considers the cause of obstruction in their secretory ducts, which is a new cause of enlargement of the glands. The vesicles that appear on the skin he declares to be the extended secretory ducts of the glands. And so almost all cutaneous diseases have been regarded of late as affections of one or other organ in the skin; but every one must acknowledge that, as yet, very little is known of the pathological anatomy of these affections: before a positive foundation is layed herein the classification will remain difficult and vague. Almost every year there appear new works on the subject, and every author thinks himself justified to produce a new system of cutaneous affections, and to invent new names, of which there is already such a superabundance. The observations of Breschet and R. de Vauzeme, of Gurlt,

Helwig, Berres, Zeis, Henle, Müller, and Bidder, have enlightened our knowledge of the healthy state of the skin; and it is to be hoped that their discoveries will lead to a more successful investigation of cutaneous diseases.

CASE OF

PERFORATION OF THE STOMACH,

AND CONSEQUENT PERITONITIS.

To the Editor of the Medical Gazette.

Sir,

WILL you oblige me by publishing the following case in your valuable journal.

Thomas Hayes, æt. 52, a porter, had been in delicate health five or six months, and had been observed of late years "to age" very much. For some weeks past he complained of frequent griping pains, loss of appetite, looked care-worn, had slight cough; he was not evidently ill, and continued at his work. He returned home on the evening of Thursday the 30th of March, apparently not worse than usual.

About half-past seven he complained of being very poorly, was cold, and shivered; he got some warm tea, and went to bed. In about an hour an alarm was given that he was very ill, and a neighbour who went in found him at the bed-side vomiting violently, and complaining of great pain in the belly. The matter ejected is said to have been very offensive, dark coloured, and frothy, but contained no blood. After a while he felt a little relieved, got into bed again, and did not agree to the proposal of sending for a doctor, as he thought he should soon be better.

He passed a very bad night, but I could not learn the particulars. In the morning, Mr. Hatton, surgeon, saw him, and considered him sinking. Mr. Strickland, house-surgeon of the Chorlton - upon - Medlock Dispensary, who saw him also, found him nearly pulseless, the countenance expressive of exhaustion rather than of pain; the eyes were sunk; the extremities cold; voice just audible. The belly was very tense, but he did not complain of pain when it was pressed; in fact, he was just dying, and nearly insensible. He gradually sank, and died at 11 A.M. on Friday, seventeen hours after the *apparent* commencement of the disease.

H

The imperfect account which I have been able to gather clearly justified suspicion that it might be poison. They were just those symptoms of irritant poisoning which a non-medical observer would be likely to remark: vomiting, pain, and exhaustion quickly following the taking of food, constancy in the character of the symptoms, and rapid progress to a fatal termination. There were no moral circumstances to lead to such a surmise; but a case so ambiguous required further investigation. By Mr. Strickland's kindness I was enabled to witness the inspection, about fifty hours after death.

Externally we observed nothing remarkable, except lividity of the organs of generation. The man looked considerably older than he was reported to be; his features were contracted and sharpened; his teeth very much decayed.

The abdomen was tympanitic, and, when opened, the whole peritoneal surfaces were found crimsoned with inflammation; the intestines glued together, though not firmly, with recently effused lymph; about two quarts of serous purulent fluid, of very offensive smell, was in the peritoneal cavity. This fluid caused sharp smarting of my hands (my skin is very thin and tender); in it were observed a few currants, which had escaped, together with a few ounces of greenish-yellow bile, from the stomach. Between the stomach and liver, and especially behind the stomach, firmer adhesions had formed, but they were easily torn through; when we saw a perforation both on the anterior and posterior surface, just at the edge of the lesser curvature, about two inches from the cardiac orifice.

On removing the stomach and opening it, we could find no trace of ulceration or softening, or any disease of its mucous membrane, except a little reddening, and that probably cadaveric. At the lesser curvature there was an irregular-shaped hardened mass, about an inch and a half thick, very firm, and studded with tubercular matter. In the middle of this mass was a cavity, apparently the empty sac of an abscess, which communicated with the stomach by an opening of nearly an inch diameter, with irregular edges, not evidently ulcerated. It communicated also with the peritoneal cavity by

the two openings already mentioned, which were each not quite large enough to admit the little finger, and had hard thick edges.

The stomach, although there had been violent vomiting, was not empty; it contained about half a pint of pultaceous matter, consisting principally of half-digested potatoes. The intestines, though highly injected externally, showed no disease within. There was an unusual quantity of chyme in the small, and of fæces in the large intestines. The colon was much distended with air.

It was reported that this man had had long-continued suppression of urine; this is not probable, for the bladder was nearly empty, and the kidneys appeared quite healthy. The liver was rather hardened on its surface, but appeared healthy within.

The heart and lungs were healthy; the latter were congested, but this was probably a cadaveric appearance. The abdominal vena cava was remarkably empty; the right side of the heart, however, contained its usual quantity of semi-coagulated blood.

I presume there can be little doubt about the nature of this case. It is evident that the disease was of long standing, and of insidious progress. I think it probable that a tuberculous abscess had formed, that it opened by ulceration, and allowed the escape of the gastric contents into the abdomen on the evening preceding death; that the sensation of cold complained of was a rigor previous to the giving way of the abscess, and that the peritonitis was excited by the irritation of the escaped bile and other contents of the stomach.—I am, sir,

Your obedient servant,
P. H. HOLLAND, M.R.C.S.L.
Manchester, April 4, 1843.

R E M A R K S
ON
CERTAIN DISEASES OF THE EYE.
By JOHN CHARLES HALL, M.D. F.L.S.
Member of the Royal College of Surgeons, London.

(For the London Medical Gazette.)

Pterygium.

THE name of this affection of the eye is derived from πτέρυξ, *a wing*. It is seldom seen by the surgeon in its incipient state, and very frequently acquires a considerable magnitude before the patient solicits relief. It arises without pain, and is of very slow growth. In the end, however, it creeps from the corner of the eye over the whole cornea, and the vision becomes impaired, and at length altogether obscured. Unless affecting the conjunctival covering of the cornea, the disease only produces a trifling deformity, and does not occasion any impediment to vision. It always assumes a triangular form, which, says Scarpa, " ought to be referred to the adhesion of the lamina of the conjunctiva becoming stronger as it advances from the circumference towards the centre of the cornea." It is a disease which generally makes its appearance at or beyond the middle period of life : it has, however, been noticed shortly after birth ; and I have at this moment two cases of it under my care—one in a young lady of seventeen, the other in a boy of twelve. In the boy it followed an attack of inflammation, induced by some lime which had been thrown into the eye ; and this certainly strengthens the opinion of Beer, who believed that lime or stone dust produced pterygium, as he most frequently saw it in masons' labourers. The varieties of pterygium are three—

1. The adipose.
2. The fleshy.
3. The membranous.

The first is of a white soft texture, something like dirty fat ; the second resembles muscular fibre ; and the third variety exhibits a partial thickening of the ocular conjunctiva, with two or three large vessels meandering upon the diseased mass.

These are the only varieties I shall notice. I have never seen a carcinomatous or malignant pterygium, and in all probability never shall. Beer remarks, " that Scarpa's belief in the existence of cancerous pterygium requires confirmation." Mr. Travers does not even mention this form of the disease, and Mr. Middlemore " is not inclined to admit the existence of such a variety." Of course no one attempts to deny that this, in common with many other morbid growths, however simple at first, may become malignant from improper management.

Treatment.—In the treatment of this disease astringents and escharotics are of little use, and frequently do more harm than good ; much time is lost by their employment, during which the disease daily advances, and in the end it is discovered that it ought to have been removed at once, instead of wasting weeks, perhaps months, in such inefficient trifling. The removal of the diseased part ought at once to be recommended ; this caution is, however, necessary, viz. that the part of the morbid growth extending over the cornea must not be incised. Should the surgeon incautiously do this, during the healing of the divided parts an opaque deposit will take place, which may prove even worse than the original disease.

CASE.—Miss U., residing near Tuxford, consulted me for a pterygium growing from the outer cornea of the right eye, and extending over two-thirds of the cornea. This young lady was requested to sit on a chair, and whilst an assistant separated the lids, I passed a narrow-bladed knife, having its back towards the cornea, between the pterygium and the sclerotic coat. The pterygium was then separated from the sclerotic as far as the margin of this transparent structure, and the flap thus formed was raised by a little hook, and cut off with a pair of scissors. The eye was washed with warm water, and after a day or two with mild astringent lotions. Some ragged portions of the conjunctiva were afterwards removed with the scissors, which I think a better and far less painful plan than attempting to destroy them by powerful caustic substances.

After the operation the eyelids must be closed, but not tightly fixed upon the globe, with a bandage. The granulations must be encouraged or repressed, as circumstances may point out, and care taken that the eyelid does not become adherent to the eyeball.

There are other modes of performing this operation. Mr. Middlemore employs both a scalpel and probe-pointed scissors ; others pass a curved needle and ligature beneath it, and obviate the risk of wounding the eyeball. In this, as in every other operation, many plans have been proposed. Knives, concave and convex, blunt and sharp, spear and probe-pointed lancets and scissors, needles and ligatures, have all their respective advocates ; but the plan I have ventured to propose is very simple, and can be very easily performed if the hand is steady; and if it is not so, the sooner a man gives up operating the better, both for his own sake and also for that of his patient.

Pterygia are more frequent in warm climates than in this country. It very often happens that the disease which has been advancing slowly for years stops at the edge of the cornea, and spreads no further during the life-time of the patient. Under such circumstances I strongly advise that no operation should be performed. As the disease gives no trouble it ought to be left to itself, an operation only being required when it encroaches on the transparent portion of the eye.

Grove Street, East Retford,
March 27, 1843.

A NEW KIND OF PESSARY.

To the Editor of the Medical Gazette.

SIR,

I SHALL be obliged if you will allow me, through your pages, to call the attention of the profession to a pessary I have invented, which I believe to be preferable, in most respects, to all the various kinds at present in use. It consists of a piece of sponge cut into the form of a sphere, or, what is better, of an oblate spheroid, and tied up, by means of small twine or silk thread, in a circular piece of oil-skin, in such a manner that a small stem or tail is left half or three-quarters of an inch in length. The firmer kinds of sponge, which possess a good resiliency, are best; and the oiled silk is closed as firmly as it can be by tying, but no extraordinary means are used, by cement or otherwise, to make it completely impervious to air.

When this pessary is compressed in the hand, the air contained in the cells of the sponge is gradually forced out at the neck, between the folds of the oil-skin. In this form it can be very easily introduced; and when passed above the narrow part of the vagina and left at liberty, the elasticity of the sponge, and the pressure of the atmosphere together, cause air to re-enter the instrument, and it assumes its expanded form. The small tail hanging downwards will facilitate its removal at any time.

The chief advantages of this pessary are, I consider—

1. Its capability of being diminished in size during its introduction and removal.

2. Its softness, which is such that it can scarcely cause any of the effects of a foreign body.

3. Its small weight.

4. The tendency of its elasticity to keep it in its position; for any sudden pressure of the viscera above will be spent in overcoming this elasticity, instead of forcing the instrument through the external parts; and, moreover, such pressure will flatten it and make it wider, and thus render its extrusion the less possible.

As additional advantages I may mention its cheapness and its durability, which will be as great as that of the oil-skin; and this, if requisite, can be applied double.

I have applied this pessary with perfect success up to this time, in three cases in which the uterus, except in the recumbent posture, had protruded entirely beyond the external parts for a number of years; and in two of these cases various other pessaries had been tried, but in one case would not remain, and in the other could not be borne. As it is only about two months since I first applied these instruments, I will postpone any more particular account of the cases till another time.

Sponges are occasionally used as pessaries; but as they become charged with mucus and other fluids, and soon decay or become offensive, and a source of irritation, they are only resorted to as a temporary expedient. A small sponge dipped, from time to time, in some astringent fluid, and applied in the beginning of prolapsus uteri, when it is yet but slight, as Dr. Denman suggested with the object of performing a cure, may, I believe, often fulfil that desirable intention. The pessaries which I have hitherto used I have made myself; but I have now got Mr. Read, of Regent Circus, to make some, and he can supply them to medical gentlemen. Of course care will be required in adapting the size of these as well as other pessaries: when expanded these should be somewhat larger than a rigid pessary for the same patient.

I remain, sir,
Your obedient servant,
JOHN SNOW, M.R.C.S.

Frith Street, Soho Square,
April 7, 1843.

ANALYSES AND NOTICES OF BOOKS.

—

"L'Auteur se tue à allonger ce que le lecteur se
tue à abréger."—D'ALEMBERT.

—

*Dr. Hooper's Physician's Vade Mecum;
or, a Manual of the Principles and
Practice of Physic. A new edition,
considerably enlarged and improved;
with an Outline of General Pathology
and Therapeutics.* By WILLIAM AU-
GUSTUS GUY, M.B. &c. London,
1842. pp. 492.

THE late Dr. Hooper was a most successful author, and his works always
enjoyed a high degree of popularity.
This was especially the case with the
present one, which possessed considerable merits of a peculiar kind. A plain
enumeration of the most prominent
and ordinary symptoms of a disease,
with a brief notice of its causes, diagnosis, and prognosis, was followed by
a detail of the most obvious and rational indications for treatment, and
by rules for practice, and copious prescriptions, which were generally valuable, inasmuch as they emanated from
the author's practical experience, and
were not mere theoretical compositions, framed in the closet, in accordance with some chemical idea of what
the action of medicines ought to be.
Thus the work formed a guide to the
treatment of disease, which might
safely be trusted as far as it went, and
which was admirably adapted for a
large class of practitioners whose education had led them to be more solici-
tous about results than about the reasonings which lead to them; and who
were, properly enough, desirous to
know the easiest and quickest way of
removing palpable symptoms; which
is, in fact, no small portion of the
practice of physic.

The present edition has received
some very valuable additions from the
pen of Dr. Guy, who has prefixed about
150 pages of introductory matter, including a scheme of medical study,
directions for taking cases, and a brief
but exceedingly well-digested outline
of general physiology, pathology, and
therapeutics. He has also added to the
whole work whatever was necessary to
bring it to the modern standard. Perhaps it would have been better had he
adhered more strictly to the author's
original model; preserving the con-

cise, detached, aphoristic style and
regarding the book rather as a guide
to the *practice* than to the *study* of
medicine; for which latter purpose,
however, Dr. Guy's introductory chapters are well adapted.

*On the Theory and Practice of Mid-
wifery.* By FLEETWOOD CHURCHILL,
M.D. M.R.I.A. Illustrated by upwards of one hundred highly-finished
wood engravings by Bagg. London,
Renshaw; Dublin, Fannin. 1842.
8vo. pp. 479.

DR. CHURCHILL tells us in his preface
that he undertook this work at the
request of the publishers, who wished
" to offer to the student in midwifery a
work embracing the modern discoveries in the physiology of the uterine
system, with all the recent improvements in practice, in a condensed form,
amply illustrated, and at a moderate
price." It is certainly a matter of congratulation that modern publishers find
it worth their while to present us with
books of so luxurious a character, and
yet so cheap as the one before us, the
thick smooth paper and clear distinct
type of which will be duly appreciated
by all who read by candle-light; whilst
the numerous and exquisite woodcuts
by Mr. Bagg add both to its ornamental
effect, and to its utility to the student.

With regard to the literary portion,
it is no small praise to Dr. Churchill
to say, that this production deserves to
rank with the recent works of Dr.
Ramsbotham and Dr. Rigby. The
introductory chapters contain a full
account of the physiology of utero-
gestation, and the development of the
fœtus, according to the most recent
researches of Barry, Wharton Jones,
and the continental physiologists, who
have built up the modern science of
embryology; whilst the body of the
work, relating to the history and treatment of the different varieties of labour, and to the diseases of parturient
women, leaves nothing to be desired
for clearness of description and judicious rules for practice. It is, moreover, illustrated with copious statistical tables, shewing the success or
fatality attending the treatment of the
various deviations from natural labour,
and intended to afford a numerical estimate of the value of various operations.
We are aware that objections have

been raised to the correctness and impartiality of some of these tables; but this is a point on which it is not our province to decide at present. The parties interested in the dispute have published their statements in the pages of the GAZETTE, and the public must be the judge: at all events, we believe that no objection has been raised against their practical usefulness.

We must observe, that we think Dr. Churchill ought to have included some account of the management of pregnancy, and of its diseases—a subject much more strictly belonging to a treatise on midwifery than the disorders of menstruation, to which he has devoted a long chapter. We must also complain of the meagreness of the index; although we are ready to admit, in extenuation, that a copious index, however useful to the reader, is a most tedious and ungrateful addition to the toils of authorship.

MEDICAL GAZETTE.

Friday, April 14, 1843.

"Licet omnibus, licet etiam mihi, dignitatem *Artis Medicæ* tueri; potestas modo veniendi in publicum sit, dicendi periculum non recuso."
　　　　　　　　　　　　　CICERO.

MEDICAL EDUCATION.

THE Abbé Sieges, it is said, carried in his pocket several plans of constitutions duly matured, and ready to be produced and acted upon at a moment's warning; and such a councillor must have been useful, and the commodity he possessed must have had much chance of being in request, at a time when new monarchies and republics were being formed to supply the place of those overthrown by the daring genius of Napoleon. Very few indeed, however, have been the occasions when opportunities for constructing such fabrics have arisen, and still fewer the opportunities for a patient and long-continued trial of their working qualities. The adoption of new systems is

generally slow and almost imperceptible. As old things become unfit for present purposes, new ones gradually take their place, but this is done only by degrees; the old usages become first unfit, then burdensome, and lastly intolerable, and those who perceive existing evils are seldom permitted to see the full effects of their labours for their removal. But when this ordinary course of change is departed from, when the agitating and destructive energies have wrought with such unusual force that remodelling and reconstruction have become absolutely necessary for carrying on the daily business of life, the new machinery has rarely indeed been found to answer the intended purpose, and the defeated minority has either gathered strength to reproduce much of the old form, or at least greatly to impede the working of the new. When reformers of the destructive class have succeeded in hurrying on their gigantic experiments, their full trial has nearly always given occasion to exhibit their inefficiency. The mistakes of Calvin had time to exhibit themselves during his life-time, and to convince the world that the religious tyranny of Geneva was no more fitted for civil government than the abominations which it had cast out: so also the despotic power which enabled Cromwell to try his well-meant experiments in England, gave full proof to the world of their entire failure. What wonder, then, if studious and thinking men, either steadily resist all novelty as pernicious, and all change as perilous, or lapse into a state of quietism and indifference more provoking to the ardent reformer than more determined resistance? Though these are times of remarkable change, this is not a country in which a new plan can be universally approved nor quickly adopted, and the reformer who loses his rest in planning, and his temper in urging any favourite scheme for making mankind happy, will wear out his life before he sees the experiment tried.

Most men who, in after life, find their powers and acquirements unequal to their desires, complain bitterly of the defects in their education; and from this weakness the greatest and best of men, men at whose deeds the world admires, are not exempt, any more than those who have just enough of energy to attempt great things, or just enough of intelligence to perceive their deficiency; and those who are doomed to listen to such complaints are seldom reasonable enough to see, or faithful enough to acknowledge, that the neglect of opportunities that might have been enjoyed has been more in fault than their actual deficiency. It is especially when men who have risen to considerable eminence complain of their own disadvantages, and strive eagerly to remedy this defect in those who are to come after them, that the suggestion arises—How, then, do you hold your present position? Either your own opportunities have been great, and you have but reaped the advantages naturally to be expected from them, or your diligence, perseverance, or more brilliant qualities, have surmounted real disadvantages. From such good qualities, happy results may fairly be expected, in spite of the very greatest disadvantages.

The last writer of eminence on medical education seems to stand very much in this position. Beginning life in a situation which experience proves to be more than most others conducive to mediocrity, he is the favoured medical councillor of his sovereign, the medical chancellor of England, and is exercising a wide and beneficial influence on the sanatory condition of his country; and it may fairly be left to his own candour to determine whether this eminent position be the result of ex-

isting medical institutions, or of such faculties as, if well exerted, could not fail of raising their possessor to eminence. No one who has read the second letter of Sir James Clark to the Home Secretary can fail to agree with the writer on the extreme desirableness of an extended course of philosophical education, nor to deplore the lamentable deficiencies in the most common requirements of a gentleman, observed in candidates for licenses to practise, which their professional acquirements make it impossible to withhold from them.

Nor can any very reasonable objection be found against the kind or amount of preliminary education suggested as a remedy for these deficiencies.

The principal doubt that arises will be as to their practicability; not that they are unattainable by the few, but by the many. The worthy Baronet's hope that this may cease to be an obstacle, that the many may become few, is indeed benevolent, *faxit Deus!* but will it be realized, and when? Are these Deuteronomic blessings for us or for our children? How long will it be before parents will cease to condemn their sons to the practice of physic, and the public to countless doctors. The London Directory gives the names and addresses of 320 physicians, 1400 surgeons, 10 apothecaries who are not surgeons, and 600 chemists and druggists, who, it is to be feared, are both *tant soit peu*, making a gross total of 2330. Do we find much thinning out of the young plants, hardy and hot-house, raised every year at those goodly *pepinières*, the medical schools; and do those transplanted to different parts of the kingdom seem to thrive? It is to be feared not.

There is a great fact which must not be lost sight of in legislating for the medical profession. We have

to lay up a good general education, that we may be capable of
profitably learning a science, and we
learn the science of medicine that
we may live by practising the art.
Now this, in spite of all legislation and
all theory, divides the members of the
profession into two great natural orders;
those namely, who can afford to wait,
and those who cannot. To one or other
of these two groups all who enter the
profession belong. But if every existing chartered or corporate body were
at once abolished, these two classes of
persons would have to be cared for.
And the existing corporate bodies, however faulty in their principles or details,
do at present care for them, and legislate for them more or less efficiently.
The first class, those who can afford to
wait, living on their capital and
private resources until they can realize
a professional income, are cared for by
the College of Physicians. This class,
and the body which rules it, gives but
little trouble to the state—its police is
internal rather than external, private
rather than public. In its earliest days
it undertook to secure the learning, the
" mores," even the piety of its members,
and though empowered also to act on the
offensive and defensive against all unqualified attempts on the health of the public
it soon gave up this disagreeable duty,
and merely insisted that the conduct of
its members, while unemployed, should
be inoffensive, and when employed
honest and of good report. The Censors
left off emptying the gallipots of unprincipled apothecaries into the kennel,
and gave their dignified attention to
the new office of guarding their College
from the admission of the unorthodox,
and the correction of the contumacious
members.

The apothecaries practising without
license from the College of Physicians
soon required a very different kind of
police ; and the charter of the Apothe-

caries' Company was intended to supply that want. Entrusted with the
power of granting licenses to practise,
the company soon conferred their
privileges on a very numerous body,
and occupied itself diligently in fenc-
ing the approaches and guarding the
outworks of medicine. For internal
police they had no time, no taste, or no
powers : whoever obtains their license
may practise where he likes and how
he likes—may get a high price for his
skill and acquirements, or may compete
with the neighbouring grocer in the
selection and display of his wares.

FELLOWES' CLINICAL PRIZE REPORTS.

By Alfred J. Tapson.
University College Hospital, 1842.

[Continued from p. 940 of the preceding volume.]

Case IX.—*Erysipelas of the face, followed
by scarlatina and an abundant minute
vesicular eruption ; cured by aperients,
antimonials, &c.*

Thomas Bateman, ætat. 32, admitted
April 30th, 1842, under Dr. Williams. A
large stout man of a full habit of body, and
sanguine temperament ; is married, but has
no children ; is a footman, and has been in
the habit of drinking about three quarts of
beer daily, often more, sometimes getting
drunk. Has no hereditary predisposition to
disease ; his general health has been good.
About fourteen years since he had a severe
attack of brain fever, and has ever since
been subject to giddiness on stooping, &c.
Four years ago he had an attack of rheumatism in the right knee which laid him up for
two months ; has had a cough for the last
three or four months, and says he has got
much thinner, but he still has plenty
of fat.

The *present attack* commenced two days
since ; he had been walking several miles
and got very hot, and returned home in the
evening when it was cold, and drank three
glasses of rum and water, which he is not in
the habit of drinking at all. Soon after he
arrived home he felt shivered very much,
and the left side of the lower jaw felt painful,
and the teeth ached ; swelling speedily came
on about the angle of the jaw, and by the
next morning had extended all up that side
of the face, partly closing the left eye ; the
swelling was red and shining, there were no
vesicles on it ; at this time he felt very sick,

and vomited whatever he took; he, however, managed to keep down one dose of pills which purged him freely; the vomiting continued all the day; he was very hot and perspired abundantly.

Present symptoms.—The swelling has now extended to the right side of the face and nose; it does not pass up over the scalp, but the redness terminates by an abrupt margin near the scalp; the swelling is hard, red, and shining, not very painful; but the face feels stiff; the skin is hot; pulse about 100, and full; has a slight headache; no difficulty of breathing; the tongue is furred a good deal, and he has a bad taste in the mouth, and is thirsty; urine scanty, and high coloured.

Foveatur facies aquâ calidâ frequenter. Low diet.

℞. Ext. Col. Comp. gr. x. omni nocte sumend.

℞. Antimon. Potassio Tart. gr. ⅓.; Acidi Hydrocyan. dilut. ℳv.; Sodæ Tart. ʒss.; Aqua, ℥i. M. f. haust. ter die sumend.

May 1st.—The swelling has increased in the lower part of the face, and has extended down into the neck; it itches very much; the vomiting has ceased; there is no delirium.

2d.—Swelling much the same; bowels confined.

℞. Haust. Sennæ Comp. cras mane.

3d.—The swelling is very much reduced, and he feels much easier. The urine increased in quantity, and paler. Towards the afternoon shivering came on with slight soreness and dryness of the throat, cough, and a little mucous expectoration; the shivering continued for some hours, and in the evening a slight redness was observed on the chest and side, and the urine was again scanty and high coloured.

4th.—The swelling of the face and neck is almost gone, and the cuticle is desquamating all over the face. The redness that commenced yesterday is gradually extending over the trunk and extremities: he is still shivered at times, and has some headache; the bowels are open; the urine high coloured, not albuminous; the tongue is much cleaner than it was, and there is less thirst.

5th.—During the night the skin has become of a bright scarlet all over the body; the redness is not like that of erythema, being in points, and not diffused; it is removed by pressure, but quickly returns; the skin feels hot and rough to the touch, and the roughness is found on close examination to depend on an umber of minute distinct vesicles containing a turbid serum (as was ascertained by puncturing some of the larger of them); they are scattered very thickly all over the surface of the trunk, and also at the bend of the elbows and in the groins. He complains of a " smarting kind of soreness" all over the body, but especially at the joints, and the palms of the hands are rather hot and tender; there is no swelling except about the feet and ankles, which are slightly œdematous, and pit on pressure. The uvula, fauces, and tonsils, are red and sore, and the tongue is now morbidly clean, very red and rather dry; the surface of it is totally smooth, and the papillæ are not enlarged, or only very slightly so indeed; there is no running at the eyes and nose; pulse 86, regular, &c.; bowels open; urine free, lighter coloured than it was, sp. grav. 1020, not albuminous by heat and nitric acid.

6th.—The redness is faded considerably, and most of the vesicles have disappeared, and the cuticle is beginning to desquamate at the bending of the joints, also in the hollow of the back and over the shoulder; it comes off in large flakes, and is not therefore merely the desquamation of the vesicles. The flakes when examined by the microscope are seen to be composed of a single layer of the scales of the epidermis, each more or less regularly hexagonal in form. The skin is still rather above the natural temperature; the tongue and fauces are less red, and more comfortable; the thirst less. On the shins there is a deeper redness, which is not removed by pressure, and indeed, in those parts of the body where the redness is removed by pressure, the skin is observed to have a yellow tinge, depending probably on some alteration of the colouring matter of the blood. The eyes feel weak, and there is a little running from them; there is not much swelling of the ankles; urine still high coloured, but not albuminous.

7th.—Much better altogether; the skin is desquamating generally over the surface of the body, and there is very little redness remaining, excepting on the shins; the throat is not sore now; tongue still red; appetite returning, no running at the eyes or nose; pulse 85; bowels open; urine abundant, less high coloured; reaction neutral, sp. grav. 1020, not albuminous.

Omittatur Mistura. Middle diet.

9th.—Nearly convalescent; feels stronger; appetite good; tongue clean and natural; no thirst; the redness is almost gone from the shins. Bowels open; urine plentiful: on heating it, and then adding nitric acid, slight cloudiness is produced, but scarcely enough to prove the existence of albumen.

10th.—The swelling is quite gone from the ankles, and the colour of the legs is almost natural; desquamation is still proceeding ; urine natural ; reaction acid ; sp. gr. 1018, not at all albuminous.

11th.—Urine not albuminous.

13th.—Slight desquamation taking place from the legs.   Urine not albuminous.

15th—Discharged cured.

REMARKS.—After reading the preceding report, it is pretty apparent that he came into the hospital with erysipelas, and that when he was recovering from this he was attacked by scarlatina. Both the diseases proved slight, and he was discharged cured in a little more than a fortnight from the time of his admission.

The symptoms under which he laboured on his admission were so obviously those of erysipelas, that no doubt could be entertained of the nature of his disease. 1st, The characters of the swelling itself—its red, smooth, and shining surface, bounded by an abrupt margin, and its tendency to spread. 2d, The symptoms attendant on its development—the shivering, quick pulse, and gastric disturbance, amounting to vomiting, which lasted till the swelling had attained almost its full extent ; and also, 3d, The mode of its departure—a gradual subsidence of the swelling, followed by desquamation of the cuticle. Again, the subject of the attack, and the circumstances preceding its appearance—the patient being a man of a full habit of body, in the habit of drinking freely, and whose kidneys, therefore, may be imagined to be somewhat impaired in function, and unable to carry off any noxious or superfluous matters when the excretion by the skin was arrested, as probably it was here, by the exposure to cold after active exertion, and then the fact of his drinking several glasses of rum and water, a liquid to which he is not accustomed—all of these would favour the occurrence of such an attack, especially as it appears his health has been suffering ever since Christmas ; and the wonder is, that as the part attacked was the face, and he had previously had brain-fever, and determination of blood to the head since, that there were no cerebral symptoms produced.

The treatment indicated was to set the secretions free, especially those of the bowels and skin, and this was effected by a combination of aperients and antimonial salines, and warm fomentations were applied to the part to soothe the irritation and promote perspiration. The cause of the erysipelas was apparently not of a specific nature, and the attack was probably produced by the combination of circumstances above mentioned.

The prognosis was favourable from the attack not being very severe, and the constitution naturally good.

Next, with respect to the second attack of feverishness and the accompanying eruption,

there are a few points deserving attention. First, as to the *diagnosis :* if we look merely at the general features of the case, we shall have very little hesitation in pronouncing it to be scarlatina simplex : it commenced with feverishness, pain in the head, slight sore-throat, scanty high-coloured urine, &c., followed by a rash, which at first was of a pale red colour, spreading over the whole body by the third day, and becoming of a scarlet or crimson colour, and attended with smarting—the redness beginning to fade on the fourth day, and ending in universal desquamation of the cuticle by the sixth or seventh day. The only symptom of scarlatina that was not well marked, was, that the papillæ of the tongue were scarcely, if at all, enlarged, though the tongue was very red. This might be partly due to the age of the individual, rendering the tongue less readily affected than it is at the age at which we most commonly see scarlatina ; and it is certain that in children the papillæ of the tongue are more readily affected by other causes than in adults ; and also the enlargement of the papillæ is less marked in scarlatina simplex than in scarlatina anginosa.

In addition, however, to the usual symptoms of scarlatina, there was, in this case, a remarkably abundant vesicular eruption at the time when the rash was most vivid, and this caused a little perplexity as to whether the disease really was scarlatina ; but we know that a vesicular eruption is not a very uncommon occurrence in scarlatina, and in some other fevers, and the fact of its being so much more abundant here than usual cannot be of much importance ; and besides, the redness was quite characteristic of scarlatina, both in intensity and in tint ; and also it was in points which distinguish it from erythema læve, the only other disease with which it was at all likely to be confounded. Had the vesicular eruption occurred with less redness it might have been called miliary fever.

The indications of treatment were much the same as for the erysipelas, and the same remedies were continued—and the early disappearance of the vesicles and redness, and the rapid decline of all the symptoms, confirmed the idea that had been held respecting the nature of the disease, viz. that it was scarlatina simplex, accompanied by an accidental miliary eruption.

The cause of the attack is not evident ; but considering that scarlatina was prevalent at the time, and that he had only been in the hospital three days before the symptoms of it came on, we conclude that notwithstanding he is not aware of having been near any one with scarlatina, he must have been exposed to it in some way or other, and that recently before his admission. It may be mentioned that he had never had scarlatina before. With regard to the urine, it is stated by Chevreul that this generally contains albumen at the period of the desquamation of the cuticle in scarlatina; in this case the urine was carefully examined every day about this time, and on no occasion was there any decided evidence of albumen in it, and there was only a slight amount of anasarca, The age of the patient was probably the chief cause of this, for Dr. Prout remarks that "anasarca and albuminous urine are much more rare as a sequela of scarlet fever in adults than in children, and the severity is in the inverse ratio of the eruptive fever and sore-throat." As none of the sequelæ had appeared before he left the hospital, it is most likely that he will escape them.

ON THE
SPECIAL FUNCTION OF THE SKIN.

By R. Willis, M.D.

The purpose which is answered in the animal economy by the function of the skin has not yet been precisely indicated by physiologists. It is universally acknowledged of immense importance to the health; but no one has said how or wherefore it is so. The chemical analysis of the sweat is acknowledged to throw no light on the ends for which it exists; and the principal matter excreted from the skin is water: sweat contains about 99 per cent of this fluid. The author of this paper considers the water as the essential excretion; not, however, in the usual sense in which the word excretion is used, nor yet as a means of regulating or reducing temperature. In the means which nature takes to preserve the lower animals from the effects of loss of heat by sending them into the world ready clothed, and in the uniformity with which man contrives to clothe himself over so large a portion of the earth's surface, he sees that the object is generally to economise heat, not to dissipate it. He says there is even something like an absurdity involved in the invocation of a system to cool the body, seeing that one great business of life, in all the temperate and cold countries of the world, is to guard against the loss of heat. Heat is lost, indeed, to a great extent, in converting the product of the sudoriparous glands into vapour; but the loss here was unavoidable; it is not the end. In spite of all the sudoriparous glands can do, also, the experiments of Delaroche and Berger have shown that the heat of the body rises considerably above the standard when exposed to temperatures somewhat higher than itself. In chambers heated to 120° and 130° Fahr. the tempera-

ture of animals rises, within an hour, to from 11° to 16° above what it had been before, and life is destroyed. And then the suppression of the cutaneous exhalation is by no means followed by a rise in the temperature of the body. In general dropsies, which are attended with a remarkable diminution of this secretion, an icy coldness usually pervades both the body and the limbs. A great fall in the animal temperature was likewise found by Fourcault and Becquerel and Breschet to be the effect of covering the body with a varnish impervious to perspiration; and so serious was the general disturbance of the functions in these circumstances, that death sometimes ensued in the course of from three to four hours. Delaroche and Berger had also found that confinement in an atmosphere of no higher temperature than the body of an animal, but saturated with moisture, was rapidly fatal; animals scarcely resisted such an atmosphere for an hour before they were reduced to extremity. Whatever prevents the skin from performing its function, i. e. from throwing off a little water, is very speedily fatal.

How may this effect be produced ? How does it happen that health and even life can be so immediately dependent, as they certainly are, on the elimination of some thirty-three ounces from the general surface of the body in the course of the twenty-four hours ? To this the author answers,—by securing the conditions which are necessary for the endosmotic transference between arteries and veins of the fluids that minister to nutrition and vital endowment.

It is admitted by physiologists that the blood, while still contained within its conducting channels, is inert with reference to the body, no particle of which it can either nourish or vivify until that portion of it which has been denominated the *plasma* has transuded from the vessels and come into immediate contact with the particle that is to be nourished and vivified: but no physiologist has yet pointed out the efficient cause of these tendencies of the plasma, first, to transude through the wall of its efferent vessels, and secondly, to find its way back again into the afferent conduits. The explanation given by the author is that, in consequence of the out-going current of blood circulating over the entire superficies of the body perpetually losing a quantity of water by the action of the sudoriparous glands, the blood in the returning channels has thereby become more dense and inspissated, and is brought into the condition for absorbing, by endosmosis, the fluid perpetually exuding from the arteries, which are constantly kept on the stretch by the injecting force of the heart.

Repeated experiment has demonstrated the fact that the blood in the veins is of somewhat greater density than that in the arteries. If the specific gravity of arterial blood be allowed to be 1,050, that of venous blood in the mean will be 1,503.

In an appendix to the paper, the author points out a few of the practical applications of which the above-mentioned theory is susceptible. Interference with the function of the skin, and principally through the agency of cold, he observes, is the admitted cause of the greater number of acute diseases to which mankind, in the temperate regions of the globe, are subject. He who is said to have suffered a chill, has, in fact, suffered a derangement or suppression of the secreting action of his skin, a process which is altogether indispensable to the continuance of life; and a disturbance of the general health follows as a necessary consequence. Animals exposed to the continued action of a hot dry atmosphere die from exhaustion; but when subjected to the effects of a moist atmosphere of a temperature not higher than their own, they perish by the same cause as those which die from covering the body with an impervious glaze; for, in both cases, the conditions required for the access of oxidized, and the removal of deoxidized plasma, are wanting, and life necessarily ceases. The atmosphere of unhealthy tropical climates differs but little from the vapour-bath at a temperature of between 80° and 90° Fahr.; and the dew point in those countries, as for example on the western coast of Africa, never ranges lower than three or four degrees, nay, is sometimes only a single degree, below the temperature of the air. Placed in an atmosphere so nearly saturated with water, and of such a temperature, man is on the verge of conditions that are incompatible with his existence: conditions which may easily be induced by exposure to fatigue, to the burning sun, or other causes which excite the skin while the circumstances necessary to the exercise of its natural function are wanting. The terms *Miasma* and *Malaria* may, according to the author, be regarded as almost synonymous with air at the temperature of from 75° to 85° Fahr., and nearly saturated with moisture.

The secretion of the skin otherwise suppressed is attended with no less fatal consequences. What kills a patient within the first 48 hours of a bad attack of scarlet fever? The autopsy shows nothing amiss. He dies undoubtedly from the complete suppression of the function of the skin. Restore this and he will do well; all the stimulants in the world will not rouse him if the function of his skin be not restored.—*Proceedings of the Royal Society*, March 2d and 9th.

THE TWENTY-SIXTH REPORT OF

THE AYR, NEWTON, AND WALLACE-TOWN DISPENSARY,

1843.

Now that there is a government commission appointed to inquire into the operation of the Poor Law of Scotland, all matters connected with the poor are of course excited at present a high degree of interest in that country, and we trust that the commissioners will not only direct especial attention to the state of the medical charities presently in active operation, but that they will devise some means of more perfectly providing for the sick poor in rural districts as well as towns. The excellent and interesting report now before us proves in an eminent degree the necessity there exists for great alterations being made with a view to ameliorate the condition of the sick poor. It appears that this Institution extends its beneficial operations over a locality which comprises a population of 14,285. "To keep up," says the reporter, "the dispensary, £95 is paid annually by 150 subscribers, which is an average payment of 12s. 8d. each!"

If the only medical charity available (we are aware that a Fever Hospital is in progress of erection) to the destitute sick, of a population of 14,285, can be kept up by an annual expenditure of £95, we should have declared ourselves utterly unable to guess by what even *canny* management an efficient Institution for such a district could be *kept up* with means so apparently insignificant, had we not observed some time ago, in a report furnished to the Poor-Law Commissioners by Dr. Sym, of Ayr, the following statements:—"The poor are humanely attended, and their diseases skilfully treated, by five dispensary surgeons, who divide the town into districts and visit the patients in their own houses;" "the *expenses are defrayed* by an annual subscription" (£95!) "The surgeons receive a trifling sum, (£5 annually, each, we believe) not as a remuneration for their services, but as a token of gratitude for the sacrifices they make for the good of the community."* What, we would ask, would a surgeon of any of our English Unions think, if he were to receive the gratifying assurance that he might calculate on £5 after a year's most toilsome and disagreeable labour! which he is most benevolently requested by no means to look upon as a remuneration for his services, but as a token of gratitude for the sacrifices he has made for the good of the community?"!!!

We can scarcely suppress a smile when

the talented reporter, in the face of this, can only summon up courage to enable him " to *venture* to express *a hope* that the Commissioners recently appointed to enquire into the state of the poor in Scotland will take into consideration the propriety of supporting medical charities by assessment."*

MEDICAL REFORM.

To the Editor of the Medical Gazette.

SIR,

As it appears to be the intention of the government to bring forward some measure on medical reform, and believing it to be their anxious desire to be guided by the soundest judgment and discretion, permit me to state, through the medium of your columns, those results at which long experience has enabled me to arrive on this important question.

No reasonable being can suppose or expect that the government should so interfere with any other view than that of securing the greatest amount of public security and of public good.

Called upon, as it now is, to interpose its influence, by the obstinate refusal of all reasonable concessions on the one hand, and, on the other, by extravagant demands, it seems to me important to direct attention to the following facts.

Although it is imperatively necessary to establish the most efficient forms of examination, so as to secure fitly educated men for so responsible a station in life as that which all medical practitioners necessarily occupy, I am quite satisfied that the plans hitherto adopted have totally escaped that attention which they so seriously demand from the public at large.

We must all feel, that a diploma granted upon oral or written examination, on "*professional qualification or power*" can afford no real safeguard to the public, nor any evidence of the candidate's fitness to practise in any branch of his profession. I declare that a diploma granted upon such evidence conveys to the public mind a fallacious and dangerous claim to confidence and skill.

Let me illustrate this assertion by evidence, in its most glaring shape. Is it not the universally received opinion of mankind, when they see the title of "Doctor," or "M.D." appended to a name, that they implicitly, yet ignorantly, conclude this man to possess superior skill, and to carry with him a proportionate degree of security by his attendance? Can any thing be more deceptive or more dangerous? I assert, and defy

* We should be glad to receive the other communications alluded to by our correspondent.
ED. GAZ.

contradiction, that there are many members of the College of Physicians, and not a few of these backed by an Oxford or Cambridge Degree, totally devoid of all practical knowledge, and whose minds are unfitted to acquire it. I say not this with any feeling of intentional disrespect; my only object is to show the naked truth, and, in doing so, to prove the absurdity of those artificial distinctions which at present exist, and to point out that change which I believe alone capable of remedying the evils complained of, so far as it may be practicable to do so.

It seems that the government is now pausing whilst the Colleges of Physicians and Surgeons reconcile some conflicting opinions; but if Parliament seriously keep in view the public welfare, and legislate, as it is in duty bound to do, for the promotion of *this one great object*, I deem it absolutely necessary to throw overboard the entire corporate and chartered privileges of the Colleges of Physicians and Surgeons, and of the Apothecaries' Company also.

Having already offered indisputable evidence against the present system of examination affording to the public a greater extent of protection through the College of Physicians itself than through either of the other two licensing bodies, I maintain that if one Faculty or College be instituted, such a system may be devised as will accomplish every useful and necessary purpose. I will leave the form of appointment of this one Faculty for the present untouched; I simply throw out the suggestion.

The examinations, academical and professional, should be the same for all candidates; but as the profession naturally subdivides itself into three separate states, viz. the physician, the consulting surgeon, and the general practitioner, every candidate, after his examination, should be required to take out his diploma for that branch of his profession which he intends to pursue. Each of the three branches should have the option to practise midwifery, and I would leave the public to determine every other point of respective right. I am positively convinced that no legislation can ever extinguish or amalgamate the three distinct divisions before stated.

Would Sir Benjamin Brodie attend a case of fever? Dr. Chambers a fractured limb? or would the public entirely repose their confidence in the hands of the most able general practitioner? or, indeed, would the practitioner himself desire it? Most certainly not. A plan might even be adopted by which the powers of this newly constituted body should be strictly confined to examination, and, having so satisfied itself of the candidate's due qualification, should remit him with its certificate to that body under whose diploma it is his intention to act.

The fees or exclusive rights of each of the three present corporations would then remain intact and perfect. As, however, unforeseen events and circumstances often blast the brightest prospects, or cause the dazzling glare of unlimited success and wealth to fall where least expected, I would reserve to every man, at any subsequent period of life, the power to exchange his diploma, for one of higher or lower degree, upon the production of such certificates of character, conduct, and motives, as the faculty should deem satisfactory. Hence the great utility of the examination being the same for all three departments : and as there are unquestionably many physicians and surgeons, who would, at this time, gladly avail themselves of pharmaceutical practice, if the Apothecaries' act did not prohibit them ; and as there are some few general practitioners, who, being fully qualified by experience and position, might choose to take out their diploma as physicians, I would make due provision for these purposes, on similar testimony to that required in cases of change of degrees.

It is desirable to put an end to all dissension, which I believe such a measure as I advocate is fully adequate to accomplish.

It does not destroy any peculiar powers contended for, either by one body or another. It does destroy all unjust claims of distinction between the physician, the surgeon, and the general practitioner. It provides for the public safety in a greater degree than has hitherto been done. It leaves all men free to act as they please for the future ; the possession of which power deprives every member of all ground of complaint, and at the same moment extinguishes every desire for that change after which the mal-content has been brawling during the greater portion of his life.

The same law ought to govern the three kingdoms, and one Pharmacopœia ought to be adopted. Every man practising without due license ought to be prosecuted by the licensing body; and with this provision, quacks and quackery may be safely left as sources of justifiable public amusement.

I am, sir,
Your obedient servant,
NEMO.

THE PHOSPHATES IN POTATOES.

To the Editor of the Medical Gazette.

SIR,

IN my last lecture, in the number of the MEDICAL GAZETTE for March 31, an error occurred, which has been alluded to by a correspondent in to-day's number. In the manuscript lecture "three" ounces of pota-

toes were inserted instead of four ; so that, in page 16, line 52 in the first column, for *three* ounces, *four* should be substituted.

The quantity of phosphates in potatoes I took from the table given in page 78 of the very interesting and talented work of Dr. Bence Jones, "On Gravel, Calculus, and Gout," 1842; where, on the authority of Liebig's work, he has stated 49·1 ashes to be present in 1000 grains of potatoes, equal to 23·56 in the ounce of 480 grains. On referring to Liebig's work, I find that Dr. Jones misplaced the decimal point ; so that, instead of 49·1, the quantity is really 4·91 grains = 2·356 in an ounce, and reducing the quantity of phosphates in my "imaginary" meal to rather more than 30 grains. I need hardly say, this error does not affect the argument.

In page 14, col. 1, line 7, an absurd error escaped correction: instead of " polarised light," it stands in the text " pulverised light."

I should have corrected these errata in a foot-note to the next lecture, had not they been noticed in the present number.

I remain, sir,
Your obedient servant,
GOLDING BIRD.

14, Myddelton Square,
April 7, 1843.

TREATMENT OF INSANITY.

THE Visitors, in complying with the annual custom of presenting a Report of the Asylum to the public, have still the satisfaction of referring to the successful treatment pursued in it, and to the increased domestic comfort which has been insured to the patients.

The system they reported last year as under trial, of introducing a limited number of students of each sex to an association with the patients of both sexes, and of employing females more freely to assist in the attendance upon the male patients, has been persevered in throughout the year, and has fully answered the expectations entertained. The patients being under the immdiate direction of educated persons, instead of being left to the care of servants, have been manifestly more comfortable, and that state of irritation and disquietnde, so often observed amongst the inmates of an Asylum, has been so generally removed, that the resident Physician has formed the first-class patients of both sexes, together with the students and the members of his own family, into one domestic party, and they daily assemble for meals and for amusement, in one or other of their respective apartments.

It is perhaps needless to allude to the effect of this friendly and domestic union upon the minds of the patients ; the advantages are manifest and numerous; but its influence in removing much of the pain of restricted liberty, and in shewing the patient, that though controlled by, he is still the companion of, his medical director, is worth an especial notice.

All mechanical restrictions upon the persons of the patients have continued to be disused during this year : the state of the house has, in its quietness and tranquillity, warranted this; and though occasional violence on the part of patients has, as formerly, occurred, a more judicious appeal to the moral instead of the physical powers of the attendants—a removal of the excited from the society of his comrades—or, a more complete seclusion in a well guarded chamber —have been found to subdue the violence, when mechanicallly confining the limbs might only have increased the irritation. But besides this, in the disuse of mechanical restraint *altogether*, the feelings of those whose quiet deportment would always have secured them from its application to their own persons, are saved the offence of witnessing its application to their less tranquil companions.

The employment of the patients has been very much increased. A resident tailor and a shoemaker have been added to the Establishment, and those of the patients who are, either from previous acquaintance with these trades, or from a desire to learn them, inclined to undertake work in them, are encouraged to do so; but our medical officers encourage more generally those employments which lead the patients from a sedentary state, and which will engage them in the open air; and for this purpose the greater attention is still given to the work of the garden.

To the accustomed round of balls, evening parties, &c. our Superintendent has for some time past added the Mainzerian system of singing for his patients, and of all the amusements calculated for a Lunatic Asylum, it is perhaps one of the best that could be devised. It may not be the most perfect mode of teaching *the art*—it may not be so essential to the individuals whose station in society, and whose means, may have enabled them to cultivate music on a more extended scale—but, to the less favoured, and the most numerous class of patients in the Asylum, it is the greatest treat ; and no evening in the week is looked forward to with so much pleasure as the "singing" one. It is valuable, not as an *amusement* only, but as an *occupation*—for the patient has something to do—something to prepare himself for—and many an hour in the week, which, perhaps, might have been painfully past, glides pleasantly away as he cons over his part for the ensuing concert. But this practice calls out also the kindler feelings of those patients,

to whom such a mode of singing is less acceptable for their own amusement ; it leads the better classes to enter into it, and to encourage it, because it gives delight to the poorer and less informed ; and thus the strongest feeling in insanity—*selfishness*—is in a material degree subdued and corrected in their minds.

This gradual advance which has been made in the improved treatment of the insane has necessarily led to an improved provision for them in the Asylum. For those of the first and second classes especially the accommodations have been made nearly resembling their homes : the wards of the Asylum have been assimilated to domestic dwellings, and the strangeness of a place of confinement as far as possible changed into the appearance of comfort and cheerfulness. This improvement in the treatment of the insane, and the quietness which ensues from it, together with that system of individual confidence, in which this Asylum ventures to claim a peculiar success, produce important consequences in point of economy. For a very great increase of pauper patients has been accommodated with but little expense in building, by the discovery that it is no longer necessary, as was formerly supposed, to have a separate sleeping cell for each patient, but that a proportion (at present, nearly *one-half*,) may safely be placed in dormitories containing four to sixteen beds, and in which they pass the night without even the presence of an attendant. This is not a saving which affects the weekly amount of charge for maintenance, but it much lessens the other head of charges, which must else have been thrown on the county.—*Report, Gloucester Lunatic Asylum.*

PAYMENT TO MEDICAL OFFICERS OF UNIONS.

To the Editor of the Medical Gazette.

SIR,

IN March 1842, I addressed a letter to the surgeons of the London Unions, who had called on me as the then President, and on the Vice-Presidents of the Royal College of Surgeons, stating my views respecting the medical order of the Poor Law Commissioners of the 12th of that month, regulating the payments to be made to the medical officers of unions for *extraordinary* services ; which letter you were pleased to publish. You also thought it right to make known a second letter I addressed to the same gentlemen, on the subject of an arrangement I hoped I had made with the Secretary of State and the Poor Law Commissioners, with respect to certain fixed payments for the ordinary services of the medical officers of Unions, and which I was led to apprehend, would have formed a part of the amended Bill about to be laid before Parliament.

The difficulties and alarm, under which the country, and particularly the agricultural part of it, have been for some time labouring, will I fear prevent the accomplishment of this object, which is so much desired by the members of the medical profession, unless the sense of the House of Commons should be strongly expressed upon it. In order to obtain this, it is necessary that a clear and accurate statement of the sufferings of the sick poor should be laid before it, and of the grievances which medical men sustain under the authority (but, I am firmly convinced, against the wishes) of the Poor-Law Commissioners, which prevent their being able to give these unhappy persons that assistance which their state demands and deserves at the hands of their more fortunate neighbours.

Colonel Wood (Middlesex) has moved for such returns (and will move for more if necessary) as will enable him to bring this matter under the consideration of the House of Commons as soon as the amended bill shall be presented. To enable him to do this effectually, a statement must be furnished to him of all the sufferings and grievances above alluded to; and if the members of the medical profession who have suffered, and are suffering, or are aggrieved, shall be pleased to address their statements to me, I will prepare such digest of them as will enable him and the House of Commons to understand this subject.

I shall be careful in alluding to the different facts confided to me, not to mention either names or places, and those who may think fit to send them may rely on my discretion.

I shall be obliged by your giving insertion to this letter, and have the honour to be, sir,

Your obedient servant,
G. J. GUTHRIE.

4, Berkeley Street, Berkeley Square,
April 11, 1833.

APOTHECARIES' HALL.

LIST OF GENTLEMEN WHO HAVE RECEIVED CERTIFICATES.

Thursday, April 6, 1843.

S. T. Smyth, Gorleston, Suffolk. — J. P. P. Chambers, Wolverhampton, Staffordshire.—G. Bowring, Stockport.—H. Gavin, London.—J. Ellam, Ashbourn, Derby.—E. P. Phillips.—Haverfordwest. —A. Fuller, Taunton. — William H. Pettigrew, London.—G. Sayle —Edward Hearne, Taunton.—J. J Fox, Falmouth.—James Palmer, York.—G. White, Tetbury, Gloucestershire.—J. Croft, London.—W. Mott Hancox, Bilston.

ROYAL COLLEGE OF PHYSICIANS.

LIST OF GENTLEMEN WHO HAVE PASSED THEIR EXAMINATION.

Friday, March 31, 1843.

Samuel Mason, 1, York Place, City Road. — James Atkinson.—Richard Dawson, Stockton.on-Tees.—W. Odlum, Antigua.—J. Lockyer Seale, Bath.

ROYAL COLLEGE OF SURGEONS.

LIST OF GENTLEMEN ADMITTED MEMBERS.

Friday, April 7, 1843.

J. R. Ashford.—V. Webb.—G. Moseley.—C. L. A lwork.—A. Heeley.—S. Barnett.—J. Simons.— C. Barrett.—M. S. Todd.—M. J. Taylor.—F. Wildbore.—J. Baber.

A TABLE OF MORTALITY FOR THE METROPOLIS,

—

Shewing the number of deaths from all causes registered in the week ending Saturday, April 1 1843.

Small Pox	8
Measles	17
Scarlatina	22
Hooping Cough	37
Croup	6
Thrush	5
Diarrhœa	9
Dysentery	3
Cholera	0
Influenza	2
Typhus	47
Erysipelas	3
Syphilis	0
Hydrophobia	0
Diseases of the Brain, Nerves, and Senses	142
Diseases of the Lungs and other Organs of Respiration	315
Diseases of the Heart and Blood-vessels	20
Diseases of the Stomach, Liver, and other Organs of Digestion	71
Diseases of the Kidneys, &c.	3
Childbed	10
Ovarian Dropsy	2
Disease of Uterus, &c.	1
Rheumatism	3
Diseases of Joints, &c.	1
Ulcer	0
Fistula	0
Diseases of Skin, &c.	1
Diseases of Uncertain Seat	119
Old Age or Natural Decay	98
Deaths by Violence, Privation, or Intemperance	26
Causes not specified	4
Deaths from all Causes	946

ERRATA —In our last number, the figures illustrative of Mr. Toynbee's paper were not properly arranged. Fig. 3, p. 69, should follow the word "cartilage," ending the first paragraph. Fig. 4, in the same page, should follow the first paragraph, ending with the word "any." Fig. 7, p. 70, should follow the word "radicles," ending the third paragraph of the preceding column.

WILSON & OGILVY, 57, Skinner Street, London.

THE

LONDON MEDICAL GAZETTE,

BEING A

WEEKLY JOURNAL

OF

Medicine and the Collateral Sciences.

FRIDAY, APRIL 21, 1843.

LECTURES

ON THE

THEORY AND PRACTICE OF MIDWIFERY,

Delivered in the Theatre of St. George's Hospital,

By ROBERT LEE, M.D. F.R.S.

LECTURE XXIV.

Protracted and difficult labours, from the forehead of the child being inclined to the symphysis pubis: presentation of the face and superior extremity with the head.

THE head may present, but the vertex may be in the hollow of the *sacrum, and the forehead turned or inclined towards the pubes.* If the head and pelvis are of the usual dimensions, and the uterine contractions strong, the forehead and face are in most cases gradually forced downward under the symphysis pubis, through the os externum, and the delivery is safely accomplished without any artificial assistance, or the nature of the presentation even being ascertained, till the occiput is found directed to the coccyx, and the face to the pubes, after the expulsion of the head. But if the head be large, the pelvis narrow, and the labour is in consequence protracted, the kind of presentation is discovered on making a more careful examination, by feeling the anterior fontanelle towards the symphysis pubis; or even the root of the nose and eyes may be touched, if the finger is passed sufficiently high up behind the symphysis. In these cases the presenting part is unusually flat towards the arch of the pubes, the parietal bones do not overlap one another in the ordinary manner, the swelling of the scalp does not form so speedily, and not only is the cavity of the sacrum imperfectly filled up with the occiput, but the sagittal suture may be distinctly traced

backward to the posterior fontanelle, if the head has not remained long in the pelvis and suffered much from pressure. When this is found to be the position of the fœtal head, it does not follow, as Dr. Denman observes, that any thing ought to be done; but we are to wait a longer time, because as experience has proved that the head in this position may be, and almost universally is, ultimately expelled by the natural efforts, so long as these are continued no artificial help should be given or attempted. But when the pains cease, or when we are fully convinced that they are unequal to the exigencies of the case, such assistance must be given as the situation of the patient may require and allow. With this position of the head, besides the greater length of time which may be required for moulding and expelling it, there will also be a greater distension of the external parts; because the hind-head cannot be cleared of the perineum before the chin has descended as low as the inferior edge of the symphysis of the ossa pubis; by which an inconvenience is produced equal to what an increased depth of the cavity of the pelvis would occasion, or a deficiency in the arch of the pubes. "This kind of labour," says Dr. Merriman, "is not in general very unmanageable. The head may be longer than ordinary in passing through the pelvis; but if this be well formed, and the pains are strong, it will be at length excluded, and in the majority of cases the child will be born alive." In the treatment of these cases, then, except guarding the perineum with more than common care while the head is passing through the outlet of the pelvis, nothing peculiar is required to be done. If the labour, however, is much protracted, the head of the child, as represented in the twenty-first table of Smellie, which I now show you (exhibiting it), becomes compressed into a longish form, with a tumor on the vertex, and the natural powers may be insufficient for its expulsion. Various methods have been recommended and adopted by

face being incapable of compression, or of being moulded into the form of the pelvis, like the bones of the cranium, and from the head occupying a greater space in the pelvis than natural. But the head nevertheless, in a great proportion of cases in which the face presents, passes through the pelvis without artificial assistance, and no unpleasant consequence is produced except a swollen state of the child's face from the long-continued pressure, but which soon disappears. Portal was the first who observed that cases of face presentation, though somewhat tedious, usually terminate without the assistance of art, and recommended them to be treated like cases of natural labour. Smellie, as I have already stated, had recourse to the operation of turning, and bringing down the feet in face cases; but I am satisfied that the practice is highly objectionable under any circumstances, and I have not seen a single instance in which it would have been proper. Dr. Merriman, however, seems rather to be of opinion that there are cases, although he does not state that he has actually met with them, in which it might be right to turn and bring down the feet. " I am quite convinced," he says, " that, as a general rule, it is wrong to turn in face cases : yet under some very favourable circumstances such an operation may perhaps be admissible. If, for instance, the head of the child were found lying above the brim of the pelvis, the membranes unruptured, the os uteri well dilated, and the vagina and the perineum in a state of relaxation, the probability of saving the life of the child would be considerable, and might justify the operator in having recourse to such a proceeding." My firm belief is, that the child, even under such favourable circumstances, would have a far better chance to be born alive if the labour were left wholly to nature, and, if the natural powers were inadequate, to extract it with the forceps. Professor Bang relates ten cases of face presentation; in three, the child was turned, and in every case was still-born. In four, after ineffectual attempts to turn, the children were at length expelled by the pains, and were all stillborn. In one, the forceps was used about 21 hours after the labour began. The child was dead. Two were left entirely to nature, and the children were born alive. In most of these cases, observes Dr. Merriman, turning seems to have been undertaken sooner than would allow the parts to be properly dilated. " In thirty-three cases," says Dr. Collins, " the face of the child presented; 4 of the 33 were still-born : with the first, the labour lasted 8 hours, and with the fourth 7 hours; all were delivered without assistance. In 12 cases the head presented with the face to the pubes; 6 of

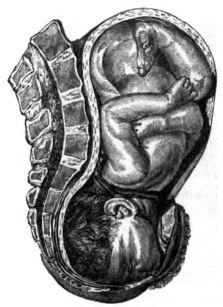

the 12 children were still-born ; with the first, the mother had been a considerable time in labour before admission ; with the second, there were three convolutions of the funis on the neck ; the labour lasted 16 hours, and the forehead suffered much from compression ; with the third, the mother was deformed, and the pelvis very defective ; with the fourth, the mother had been long in labour before admission ; this was her second pregnancy, and both deliveries were effected with the crotchet : the fifth was a woman with a deformed pelvis : with the sixth, the funis and hand descended with the head. The third, fourth, and fifth, were delivered with the crotchet. By reference to these cases Dr. Collins states that it will be clearly seen that the position of the child did not, in any instance, render artificial delivery necessary.

Smellie's twenty-third table shows, in a lateral view, the face of the child presenting, and forced down into the lower part of the pelvis ; the chin being below the pubes, and the vertex in the concavity of the os sacrum ; the waters likewise being all discharged : the uterus appears closely joined to the body of the child, round the neck of which is one circumvolution of the funis.

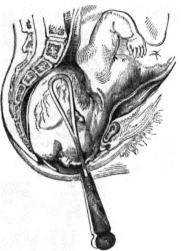

" When the pelvis is large," he observes, " the head, if small, will come along in this position, and the child be saved ; for as the head advances lower, the face and forehead will stretch the parts between the frænum labiorum and coccyx in form of a large tumor. As the os externum is dilated, the face will be forced through it ; the under part of the chin will rise upwards over the anterior part of the pubes, and the forehead, vertex, and occiput, turn from the parts below. If the head, however, is large, it will be detained either when higher, or in this position. In this case, if the position cannot be altered to the natural, the child ought to be turned, and delivered footling." " If the pelvis, however, is narrow, and the waters are not all gone, the vertex should, if possible, be brought to present : but if the uterus is so closely contracted that this cannot be effected, on account of the strong pressure of the same, and slipperiness of the child's head, in this case the method directed in the following table is to be taken." (See top of next column.)

This figure represents, in the lateral view, the head of the fœtus in the same position as in the former figure ; but the delivery is supposed to be retarded from the largeness of the head, or a narrow pelvis.

" In this case," says Smellie, " if the head cannot be raised, and pushed up into the uterus, it ought to be delivered with the forceps in order to save the child. This position of the chin to the pubes is one of the safest cases, where the face presents, and

is most easily delivered with the forceps, the manner of introducing which over the ears is shewn in this table. The patient must lie on the back, with her breech a little over the bed, her legs and thighs being supported by an assistant sitting on each side. After the parts have been slowly dilated with the hand of the operator, and the forceps introduced and properly fixed along the ears of the child, the head is to be brought down by degrees, that the parts below the os externum may be gradually stretched ; the chin then is to be raised over the pubes, whilst the forehead, fontanelle, and occiput, are brought out slowly from the perineum and fundament, to prevent the same from being hurt or lacerated. But if the fœtus cannot be extracted with the forceps, the delivery must be left to the labour pains as long as the patient is in no danger ; but if the danger is apparent the head must be delivered with the crotchet. When the face presents, and the chin is to the side of the pelvis, the patient must lie on her side ; and after the forceps are forced along the ears, the chin is to be brought down to the lower part of the os ischium, and then turned out below the pubes, and delivered in a slow manner as above. In these awkward presentations the delivery should be always trusted to the natural pains as long as the patient is in no danger." (See next page.)

This figure shows, in a lateral view of the right side, the face of the fœtus presenting as in the last two figures, but in the contrary position, that is, with the chin to the os sacrum and the bpr⸺ ⸺ubes. the waters evacuated, a ⸻A. The same treatm

different practitioners under these circumstances. Smellie was accustomed, in these and in all cases of face presentation, even when the liquor amnii was evacuated, the first stage of labour completed, and the head of the child was low in the pelvis, to attempt to force back the presenting part and bring down the feet. If you read the histories of some of the cases recorded in his third volume, you will find that, about the year 1746, this was his general practice, but that it was almost always unsuccessful. The operation of turning is never now employed in this country by experienced practitioners, where the membranes have been ruptured, and the head has passed through the os uteri into the cavity of the pelvis. Turning, where the head has advanced so far in the pelvis, is truly a most dangerous operation both for the mother and child, and should never be attempted. If the child cannot be delivered with the labour pains, or turned and brought footling, the forceps, says Smellie, are to be applied on the head as described in this figure, and brought along as it presents; but if that cannot be done without running the risk of tearing the perineum, and even the vagina and rectum of the woman, the forehead must be turned backwards to the sacrum. To do this more effectually the operator must grasp firmly with both hands the handles of the forceps, and at the same time pushing upwards, raise the head as high as possible in order to turn the forehead to one side, by which it is brought into the natural position. This done, the head may be brought and delivered as in natural labour. In several cases of this kind he was obliged to employ the crotchet after trying the forceps. With the short straight forceps, the head may be turned slightly round with safety and advantage, as you depress the handles and bring the forehead and face out under the symphysis pubis; but I believe it to be impossible to perform the operation here described by Smellie, with the long curved forceps represented in the figure, without destroying the child or lacerating the vagina.

"In this case," Dr. F. Ramsbotham correctly observes, "we have the choice of two methods by which to extract the head: we may either bring the face under the pubes, making a quarter turn of the half pelvis, or we may make a three-quarter turn, and throw it into the hollow of the sacrum. Of these modes I should certainly prefer that in which there is the least turn to be made, namely, with the face under the pubes, provided it could be effected; because we are less likely to do injury to the mother and also the child. If we make a three-quarter turn we may injure the mother's parts by bruising and perhaps by laceration; and we might even destroy the child; for if its body be strongly

embraced by the contracted uterus, and do not follow the extensive turn which we cause the head to make, we must infallibly twist its neck to a great extent, and we might dislocate the vertebræ to the destruction of its life."

A safer mode was sometimes employed by Smellie to turn the forehead round to the sacrum. In describing a case of this sort, he states that he "gently opened the os externum during every pain, raising the head a little when the pain began to abate, and moving the forehead to the left side of the sacrum, by which means he effected the delivery." Dr. Merriman says this appears to have been his common practice in such presentations, and that a somewhat similar manœuvre was recommended by Exton. "It is not a little extraordinary," he further observes, "that the late Dr. John Clarke was unacquainted with this direction of Smellie. In his paper on the management of cases in which the face of the child presents towards the os pubis, Dr. Clarke evidently thought that he proposed a novel practice, when he recommended to push the forehead round towards the sacrum. He says, "all the best writers upon the practice of midwifery have taken notice of this cause of difficulty in labours; but they have been contented with describing it, without suggesting any means more especially suited to this case." Dr. Clarke directs either one or two fingers to be passed up, between the left side of the head, near the coronal suture or the temple and the symphysis pubis, and steady pressure to be made during a pain against the frontal or parietal bone. Sometimes this method is attended with success, but it most frequently fails, and the head returns to its original position before the pressure was begun to be made. I cannot agree with Dr. Burns in thinking that it would be justifiable, where the presentation was discovered early, to rupture the membranes and turn the vertex round. From all that I have seen of these cases, I am disposed to believe that it is best to leave them to the natural efforts, and to avoid all interference,—all attempts to change the position, while the pains continue regular, and the head advances, however slowly. Dr. Merriman has very recently informed me that he entirely coincides in this opinion. If exhaustion should take place it will then become necessary to deliver artificially, in the manner which will afterwards be described.

This figure from Smellie's Engravings represents the vertex in the concavity of the sacrum, and the forehead turned to the pubes. When the head is small, he says, and the pelvis large, the parietal bones and the forehead, will in this case, as they are forced downwards by the labour pains, gradually

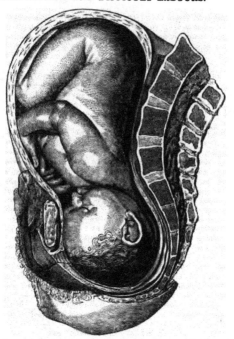

dilate the os externum, and stretch the parts between that and the coccyx in form of a large tumor, till the part come down below the pubes, when the head will be safely delivered. But if the same be large and the pelvis narrow, the difficulty will be greater, and the child in danger, as in the following figure, also copied and slightly altered from

Smellie; the short straight forceps being represented instead of the long curved forceps you have seen in the original engraving. By looking at this figure you will be able to form a good idea of the extent to which the neck of the child would be twisted by turning the face entirely round into the hollow of the sacrum.

Protracted and difficult labours from presentation of the face.

The face is readily distinguished from every other part of the foetus by the inequality of its surface, and by the eyes, nostrils, mouth, and chin. The mouth, as represented in the following figures from Smellie's Plates, may either be under the symphysis pubis, with the vertex occupying the hollow of the sacrum, or it may be situated close to the lower end of the sacrum and coccyx, with the vertex behind the symphysis pubis. The first of these positions is considered the most frequent and favourable; but the head, in a great proportion of cases, whether it be situated in this or in the second position, is expelled by the natural efforts, though a longer period than usual be required for the completion of the labour. The difficulty arises from the bones of the

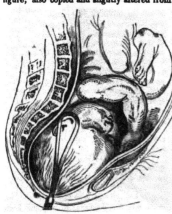

[left column largely illegible]

child were found lying above the brim of the pelvis. the membranes unruptured. the os uteri well dilated. and the vagina and the perineum in a state of relaxation. the probability of saving the life of the child would be considerable. and might justify the operator in having recourse to such a proceeding." My firm belief is. that the child. even under such favourable circumstances. would have a far better chance to be born alive if the labour were left wholly to nature. and. if the natural powers were inadequate. to extract it with the forceps. Professor Bang relates ten cases of face presentation : in three. the child was turned. and in every case was still-born. In four. after ineffectual attempts to turn. the children were at length expelled by the pains. and were all still-born. In one. the forceps was used about .. hours after the labour began. The .. was other. Two were left entirely to nature. and the children were born alive. In most of these cases. observes Dr. Merriman. turning seems to have been undertaken sooner than would allow the parts to be properly dilated. "In thirty-three cases." says Dr. ..... "the face of the child presented .. of the all were still-born : with the rest the labour lasted 5 hours. and with the ...... 7 hours. all were delivered without assistance. In 12 cases the head presented with the face to the pubes : 6 of

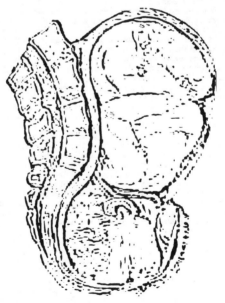

the 12 children were still-born ; with the
first, the mother had been a considerable
time in labour before admission ; with the
second, there were three convolutions of the
funis on the neck ; the labour lasted 16
hours, and the forehead suffered much from
compression ; with the third, the mother
was deformed, and the pelvis very defective ;
with the fourth, the mother had been long in
labour before admission ; this was her second
pregnancy, and both deliveries were effected
with the crotchet : the fifth was a woman
with a deformed pelvis : with the sixth, the
funis and hand descended with the head.
The third, fourth, and fifth, were delivered
with the crotchet. By reference to these
cases Dr. Collins states that it will be
clearly seen that the position of the child did
not, in any instance, render artificial delivery
necessary.

Smellie's twenty-third table shows, in
a lateral view, the face of the child presenting, and forced down into the lower part
of the pelvis ; the chin being below the
pubes, and the vertex in the concavity of the
os sacrum ; the waters likewise being all
discharged : the uterus appears closely joined
to the body of the child, round the neck of
which is one circumvolution of the funis.

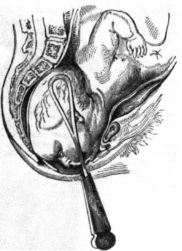

"When the pelvis is large," he observes,
"the head, if small, will come along in this
position, and the child be saved ; for as the
head advances lower, the face and forehead
will stretch the parts between the frænum
labiorum and coccyx in form of a large
tumor. As the os externum likewise is dilated, the face will be forced through it ; the
under part of the chin will rise upwards over
the anterior part of the pubes, and the
forehead, vertex, and occiput, turn from the
parts below. If the head, however, is large, it
will be detained either when higher, or in this
position. In this case, if the position cannot
be altered to the natural, the child ought
to be turned, and delivered footling." "If
the pelvis, however, is narrow, and the
waters are not all gone, the vertex should, if
possible, be brought to present : but if the
uterus is so closely contracted that this
cannot be effected, on account of the strong
pressure of the same, and slipperiness of the
child's head, in this case the method directed in the following table is to be taken."
(See top of next column.)

This figure represents, in the lateral view,
the head of the fœtus in the same position
as in the former figure ; but the delivery is
supposed to be retarded from the largeness
of the head, or a narrow pelvis.

"In this case," says Smellie, "if the
head cannot be raised, and pushed up into
the uterus, it ought to be delivered with the
forceps in order to save the child. This
position of the chin to the pubes is one of
the safest cases, where the face presents, and

is most easily delivered with the forceps, the
manner of introducing which over the ears
is shewn in this table. The patient must lie
on the back, with her breech a little over
the bed, her legs and thighs being supported
by an assistant sitting on each side. After
the parts have been slowly dilated with the
hand of the operator, and the forceps introduced and properly fixed along the ears of
the child, the head is to be brought down by
degrees, that the parts below the os externum
may be gradually stretched ; the chin then
is to be raised over the pubes, whilst the
forehead, fontanelle, and occiput, are brought
out slowly from the perineum and fundament, to prevent the same from being hurt
or lacerated. But if the fœtus cannot be
extracted with the forceps, the delivery must
be left to the labour pains as long as the
patient is in no danger ; but if the danger is
apparent the head must be delivered with
the crotchet. When the face presents, and
the chin is to the side of the pelvis, the
patient must lie on her side ; and after the
forceps are forced along the ears, the chin is
to be brought down to the lower part of the
os ischium, and then turned out below the
pubes, and delivered in a slow manner as
above. In these awkward presentations
the delivery should be always trusted to the
natural pains as long as the patient is in no
danger." (See next page.)

This figure shows, in a lateral view of the
right side, the face of the fœtus presenting
as in the last two figures, but in the contrary
position, that is, with the chin to the os
sacrum and the bregma to the pubes, the
waters evacuated, and the uterus contracted.
The same treatment is recommended.

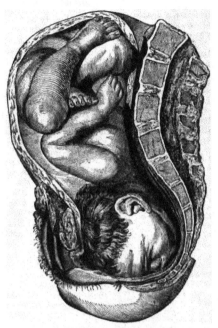

Labour is sometimes protracted and diffi-cult, from one of the extremities descending along with the head. The hand of the child may be felt closely applied, in some cases, to the side of the head, before it has entered the brim of the pelvis; and if the pelvis is large, and the uterine action strong, they may be expelled together without assistance. But, under the most favourable circumstances, the hand adds much to the size of the head; and if the pelvis be small or distorted, they become impacted in the brim or outlet. The difficulty is still greater if the arm descends along with the head or before it, and the natural efforts may be insufficient, in this case, for the completion of the labour. Whether it be the hand or arm which pre-sents along with the head, it is advisable in all cases to push it up beyond the head, and to hold it up until the head has come down so low as to occupy the brim of the pelvis completely, and it is impossible for the hand or arm again to descend by the side of the head or before it, and impede its pro-gress through the pelvis. You will not succeed in pushing the hand or arm above the head of the child unless you introduce the whole of your hand into the vagina, and partially through the os uteri, and with your fingers press up and hold up the hand or arm of the child between the pains, until the

head has sunk down so far as to be clear of the obstruction. In some cases, by doing this, a labour which has been protracted for many hours is brought, after a few pains, to a successful termination. Without intro-ducing your whole hand into the vagina, you will most frequently fail in obviating the difficulty, and you may be compelled to have recourse to the forceps, or to the perforator, if the head and arm should become jammed in the brim. In a case which I lately saw, in consultation with Mr. Taylor, of Leicester Square, the head, left arm, and funis of the child, without pulsation, presented; the membranes were ruptured, and the uterus closely contracted around the child. As the child was dead, I opened the head and drew it readily down before the arm and delivered. Had the cord been pulsating, the operation of turning, I suppose, would have been the proper practice, though, under the un-favourable circumstances, there would have been little or no chance of preserving the child's life, and the uterus might have been injured in the delivery.

A foot may present along with the head, and obstruct its progress through the brim of the pelvis. On the 1st of June, 1842, at mid-day, I saw a case in Buckingham Place, Fitzroy Square, in which the head, the funis, and a foot presented. Labour began the previous afternoon : at 5 o'clock the liquor amnii escaped, and the midwife felt the head, a foot, and a great loop of the funis presenting. She thought the proper practice was to put back the foot, and this she attempted to do for six hours. At midnight she requested a surgeon to see the case, and deliver the woman, but he did nothing except administer two doses of the ergot of rye. In this condition the patient remained till 12 o'clock the next day, when I saw her. As there was no pulsation in the cord, the only subject for consideration was, how the patient might be relieved with the least risk. I passed up my hand into the vagina, grasped the foot, and brought down the nates, while, at the same time, I pushed the head aside and easily delivered. If the head had not gone up by the pressure, I would have opened it, and delivered with the crotchet, without paying any attention whatever to the foot. In a protracted labour which came under the care of Dr. John Ramsbotham in 1820, he found the head above the brim of the pelvis with the foot down by its side. Without withdrawing the hand, which had been passed into the vagina, he pushed up the foot, and at that moment a strong uterine contraction coming on, the head was brought down into the brim, so that the foot was left above. Keeping the hand in that situation till another pain came on, he found the head descend without the foot. In pushing up the foot a hand also was felt just by the side of the head. The case was then left to the natural action of the uterus, and in about two hours a living child was expelled.

CASE OF

DIABETES MELLITUS,

WITH NUMEROUS OBSERVATIONS,

AND A REVIEW OF THE PATHOLOGY AND TREATMENT OF THIS DISEASE.

By JOHN PERCY, M.D. (Edin.)

Physician to the Queen's Hospital, and Lecturer on Organic Chemistry at the Royal School of Medicine and Surgery, Birmingham.

[Continued from page 93.]

To the inquirer of chemical pathology, there is no disease more deeply interesting than diabetes mellitus. The formation of grape-sugar in the system in large quantity, and its elimination by the kidneys, are facts well calculated to arrest the attention of the reflective mind; and, accordingly, we find that the disease in question has frequently been made the subject of minute investigation, as well as fanciful speculation; and yet its pathology continues to be involved in considerable obscurity. To our countryman, Dr. Prout, not less distinguished as a philosophic and practical chemist than as a philosophic and practical physician, we are indebted for much valuable knowledge concerning diabetes. And I may avail myself of this opportunity of expressing my satisfaction that the labours of that correct and discriminating mind in respect to the very foundation of chemical science have at length begun to receive remarkable confirmation from other chemists; and, by way of illustration, I may mention the beautiful results recently obtained by Messrs. Dumas and Stas in the determination of the atomic weight of carbon. It is not my intention, in the following pages, to present an elaborate detail of the various opinions which have been entertained from remote antiquity to the present day respecting the nature and cause of diabetes; for laborious details of this kind may be found in numerous monographs and treatises, and of these I may mention especially the treatise of Dr. Latham (London, 1811, pp. 244). I propose, so far as my humble ability will permit, carefully to review the well-ascertained *facts* of diabetes, and those of physiology relating to the subject, with a view to arrive at such conclusions as appear to be warranted by the present state of our knowledge. I have performed numerous physiological experiments, which have been suggested either by reflection or by the statements of physiologists, and I have obtained results diametrically opposed to some of these statements. I am deeply sensible of the responsibility imposed upon the man who appeals to nature in the way of experiment; for any erroneous conclusion, whether the effect of inadvertence or inaccuracy in experimenting, is worse than ignorance, inasmuch as it is positive error. I hope that I have attempted in this, and shall ever continue, in similar investigations, to dispossess my mind of every thing but an honest desire to discover truth. I shall relate minutely each experiment, that the reader may be enabled to judge how far my results are worthy of his confidence; and this must be my ground of apology for what might appear to be tedious and superfluous detail. There is one point on which I am especially anxious to offer a few observations, and that is, the extreme difficulty, not to say impossibility, of acquiring comprehensive information in any scientific department in a provincial town. A man, before he sits down to write on any particular subject, should be acquainted with all that has been previously written upon this subject; but if this condition were absolutely indispensable and imperative, few men in the provinces would be found qualified to write. There are numerous papers relating to diabetes in various periodical works, French and German, which I have been extremely desirous of consulting, and which desire it has been impossible for me to gratify; for Birmingham cannot at present boast of an extensive medical library. If, then, I should be found to betray ignorance in some respects of the labours of continental writers, it will, I hope, be charged, not to wilful negligence on my part, but to the impossibility of my obtaining access to their writings where I now reside.

OBSERVATIONS AND EXPERIMENTS CONCERNING DIABETES MELLITUS.

1st. *Of the formation of grape-sugar, and its elimination by the kidneys.*— The question which is first suggested by this part of the subject is, whether grape-sugar is produced in the healthy system? Let us first examine recorded observations. "*Sugar* is not found in the blood in a state of health, but has been many times distinctly recognised in the blood of diabetic individuals, where it probably always exists in a greater or less degree. Sugar, also, is not a natural ingredient of the urine, but is found in large quantities in that fluid in the disease just mentioned (diabetes). I am not aware that sugar has been ever found in the blood, or even in the urine, of any inferior animal, which may be considered a remarkable circumstance." (*Stomach and Urinary Diseases*, Dr. Prout, 3d edit. Introduction, p. xciii.) " Now the reduction of all the forms of the saccharine principle appear to be accompanied by the development of a *low* sugar; which low sugar, in the healthy condition of the stomach, is speedily *converted* into albuminous and oleaginous matters. Hence, as the existence of sugar in the stomach is only momentary, or, as it were, a point

in transitu, its presence in the healthy organ is with difficulty detected • • The first step in the derangement, therefore, producing the disease called diabetes, does not consist, as some have supposed, *in the development of the sugar in the stomach, which is a natural process.*" (Dr. Prout, op. cit. p. 16). From these statements, then, we conclude that Dr. Prout admits the formation of *a sugar* in the stomach as a process of healthy digestion. Tiedemann and Gmelin found that " boiled starch (in the stomach of a dog) was, in the course of a few hours, converted into gum of starch and sugar." (*Müller's Elements of Physiology*, translated by Baly, vol. i., p. 578.) Saliva has the property of converting starch into sugar. *Müller, op. cit.* p. 577; *Dr. Wright on the Saliva, Lancet,* 1842) " Thus, amylaceous matters (in digestion) are converted into gum and sugar; the saccharine matters are absorbed." (*Dumas, Essai de Statique Chimique des Etres Organisés,* 1842, p. 41). Probably, numerous other authorities might be cited in answer to the question proposed, but the preceding suffice to show that the conversion of starch into sugar in the stomach is generally admitted to occur in the condition of health. Now, before proceeding to the detail of direct experiments on this point, so deeply interesting and important, let us inquire concerning the introduction of *saccharine* matters into the stomach, with a view to ascertain whether such matters can be *directly* absorbed. Magendie fed dogs exclusively upon sugar and water, and the urine of these animals was examined by the accurate and laborious Chevreul. It was "found to be alkaline, as in herbivorous animals, and to contain no uric acid or phosphates." (Müller, op. cit. vol. i., p. 526). No mention is made of the existence of sugar in such urine. " We know that the urine of dogs, fed for three weeks exclusively on pure sugar, contains as much of the most highly nitrogenized constituent, urea, as in the normal condition." (*Marchand*, Erdmann's Journal für praktische Chemie, xiv. p. 495; *Animal Chemistry, &c.* Liebig, pp. 61-62.) No mention is made of sugar. Neither does the martyr, Dr. Stark, appear to have observed any saccharine condition of his urine when subsisting principally on a diet of saccharine matter, although his urine was occasionally, during this period, much increased in quantity. (*The Works of the late William Stark, M.D. &c.* Lond. 1788, 4to. pp. 131, 163, &c.) On the other hand, on the authority of Dr. Krimer, " When diabetic urine is introduced into the stomach of an animal, we find, on the following day, saccharine matter in its urine, and continue to do so so long as we administer this substance, and even some days after we have ceased to inject it." (*Bell's Essay on Diabetes. translated by Markwick*, p. 48.) I have made several experiments on this subject. I proceeded first to ascertain whether direct absorption of saccharine matter in the stomach would occur when the most favourable conditions of absorption were presented, namely, *fasting* and the *abstraction of blood*.

Experiment I.—March 14th. I selected a small mongrel dog, which had not been fed since the 11th, although it is probable that during this interval he picked up scraps of food. He was fat, and in good condition. He ate the sugar of raisins, crystallized, and in the state of thick paste; he drank water afterwards. In the course of half an hour I injected into the stomach about the same quantity as he had eaten, dissolved in water. I suppose that altogether he must have had about three ounces, although I did not ascertain the precise amount, of dry sugar. In another half hour, I opened the right jugular vein, and collected the blood. No urine was evacuated. I then destroyed the animal with strong hydrocyanic acid, which occasioned vomiting and slight general convulsive action. No urine, however, contrary to what is the usual effect of the poison, was voided. As soon as the heart ceased to beat, I removed the bladder, which was distended by limpid urine. The stomach contained solution of sugar, as manifested by the odour and appearance, and a few pieces of straw were also observed. I added a small quantity of yeast to the urine, which was introduced into a graduated receiver over mercury; it occupied the volume of 1·2 cubic inch. Late in the evening, about two hours after the experiment was arranged, I observed that gas was sensibly evolved. On the following morning the tube was completely

filled with gas, all the liquid having been forced out; and the gas was under considerable pressure, as the tube, of which the capacity was 2½ cubic inches, was retained midway in mercury. All the gas was immediately absorbed by solution of caustic potash. I had not expected this striking result; otherwise I should have employed a graduated receiver of much larger capacity. The blood was examined with a view to the detection of sugar, but, owing to an accident, the result is not satisfactory.

Experiment 2.—March 24th. Since the 18th, a middle-sized mongrel dog was fed exclusively on common brown (cane) sugar and water. Altogether, he had taken 4 lbs. avoirdupois. He drank freely of cold water. He was observed occasionally to have fits, during which he turned round and foamed at the mouth: fits of this kind not unfrequently occur during the distemper. These fits were not noticed previously to his feeding on sugar, although it is possible he might have had them. He appeared tolerably lively, and was daily led about for exercise. On the 23d, he was carefully watched for ten hours in succession, in order to collect any urine which might be voided, but without success, as no urine was passed during this period. He was much purged,· and the fæces were liquid and dark. This morning (24th), at half-past 10, he ate about ¼ lb. of sugar, and afterwards drank water. He was again watched until 2 P.M when, having passed no urine since half-past 10, he was destroyed by hydrocyanic acid. During the convulsive action which followed, he evacuated only a small quantity of urine, which I collected; some brown liquid escaped through the nostrils. I immediately opened the body, and collected what urine remained in the bladder by pressing this viscus. Here I may relate the post-mortem appearances, as illustrating, in a certain degree, the influence of an exclusively saccharine diet.

Chest : the *lungs* did not much contract. They were gorged with frothy colourless liquid; I think I never saw before so large a quantity of liquid escape from the trachea and bronchi. The *liver* was large, and apparently healthy. *Abdomen :* the *spleen* contained minute light-coloured specks, such as I have before occasionally seen in the spleen of dogs. The *kidneys* were natural. In the *stomach* was a small quantity of brown liquid, mixed with dark flocculent matter, and having the smell of brown sugar; I found, also, some small pieces of straw. Except in the vicinity of the pylorus, the mucous membrane presented the usual light plum-tint. The summits of the rugæ throughout had a red blush; the intervals were pale. The *intestines* contained liquid brown fæculent matter; which, in the rectum, was pasty, and similar to that evacuated during the action of the hydrocyanic acid. The odour of the fæces was not particularly fœtid. The contents of the stomach and intestines had a decided acid reaction.

Urine : taste *salt*, and not in the slightest degree *sweet*. I collected f℥ss. precisely. Pale straw. Strongly acid, immediately reddening litmus; sp. gr. more than 1040°. I mixed f℥ij. with a minute quantity of fresh yeast in a graduated jar over mercury; distilled water was added. The volume occupied by the liquid was 1·4 cubic inch: 2·6 cubic inches of gas were evolved, and instantly absorbed by caustic ley. I then distilled the fermented liquid with carbonate of potass in the chloride of calcium bath. I obtained only a minute quantity of incombustible liquid, which had a decided ammoniacal odour, and immediately restored the colour of reddened litmus. To the product I added carbonate of potass, when a supernatant stratum, a quarter of an inch in depth, was formed. By means of an extremely fine pipette, I removed some of this stratum, and found it to burn readily with a blue flame. I have preserved this specimen in a hermetically sealed tube.

The remaining f℥ij. of urine were evaporated over the steam-bath. I obtained a clear brown syrup, to which I added nitric acid in excess, and stirred well. March 25th.—No crystallization of nitrate of urea. 30th.—Still no crystallization. I then evaporated in order to ascertain whether *oxalic acid* would be produced. I procured minute and distinct colourless crystals, which occasioned a precipitate in a solution of chloride of calcium, insoluble in acetic acid. I should be inclined to infer, from the small quantity of gas evolved by fermentation,

and the quantity of oxalic generated, that this acid was probably derived in part from the *colouring* or other *organic matter* of the urine besides true *sugar.*

Experiment 3.—March 29th. Since the morning of the 27th, a large bull-terrier dog was fed entirely on common brown (cane) sugar and water. At first, he ate freely ¼lb. Altogether, he took 2lbs. Yesterday, and early this morning, he evacuated light brown, watery, and offensive fæces. At ¼ before 8 this morning, he ate ¼lb. of similar sugar, and drank ½ pint of water. At 10 A.M. he freely passed urine : f℥v. were collected. Colour brown. Odour peculiar. Feebly reddened litmus. Taste *not* sweet even in the slightest degree. Surface covered with minute and peculiar crystals, not resembling in form the ordinary ammoniaco-magnesian phosphate. I examined these crystals minutely, but, in this place, I need not describe them. Filtering paper was stained yellow by this urine. I mixed 1·2 cubic inches of the urine with a minute quantity of fresh yeast over mercury in a graduated receiver. April 1st, 9½ P.M. Temp. 59° F. Barometer not observed. I measured 5 cubic inches of gas. The fermented urine was then distilled for a few minutes *per se*, and to the product was added carbonate of potass. I obtained a supernatant stratum of spirit ₁₋₂ inch in diameter, and ₁₋₂ in depth. It burnt with a blue flame. The specimen is preserved.

I evaporated over the steam-bath 500·0 grains of urine, and obtained a brown syrup, having a strong smell. On the addition of nitric acid, crystals of nitrate of urea were separated in *small* quantity. No coagulation was produced.

From these experiments, then, we are justified in concluding that *sugar* existed in the urine, after its introduction into the *stomach*. In the first experiment sugar was found in the urine, in a very short time after the animal had received sugar by the mouth. We shall also be justified in concluding that in these cases the sugar passed directly into the blood, and was simply eliminated by the kidneys; provided we ascertain by experiment that the urine of a dog, which has not taken sugar, does not undergo fermentation by the addition of yeast. Accordingly, the following experiment was made.

Experiment 4.—April 3d. The dog which was the subject of Experiment 3 was fed on horseflesh and potatoes since March 29th. The urine was readily collected this morning. Odour strong and peculiar. Reaction acid. Amber-coloured. Sp. gr. 1046°. I mixed 1·1 cubic inches with a small quantity of fresh yeast in a graduated tube over mercury. In the evening, no gas had been evolved. April 4th, *morning*. Not the slightest disengagement of gas; *evening*, 7½, still not the slightest evolution of gas. It must be remarked that, as nearly as possible, the same condition of temperature was preserved in all these experiments. One cubic inch of carbonic acid gas evolved corresponds nearly to one grain of grape sugar. In Experiment 2, then, we should have about 10 grains in the fluid-ounce, and 160 in the pint.

Now, in these experiments, it must be admitted that the conditions under which the absorption of sugar was effected were in a greater or less degree artificial, for sugar was present in the stomach in *inordinate* quantity, and the animals were exposed to peculiar circumstances. It is, however, probable, that, in the healthy state, when sugar is introduced into the stomach in small quantity, even supposing it to pass directly into the circulation by absorption, it is never eliminated by the kidneys, but supplies material either for assimilation of some kind or other, or for pulmonary oxidation. The following experiments concerning the injection of sugar into the veins relate directly to this part of the subject.

Experiment 5th.—March 22d. Into the right jugular vein of a large mongrel-mastiff dog, which had not been fed since the previous morning, I injected 200 grains of the crystallised residuum of Merchant's urine dissolved in f℥ij. of warm distilled water. No symptoms, except such as might be referred to the operation and consequent excitement, followed. In 1½ hour afterwards I poisoned the animal with anhydrous hydrocyanic acid, and collected 4½ fluid-ounces of deep amber-coloured urine, voided during the convulsive action. A small quantity escaped, and some also remained in the bladder, and was obtained by squeezing that viscus *in situ*. Odour peculiar. Sp. gr. 1040°. Reddens litmus. I mixed the whole quantity with a small

proportion of yeast, in a two-necked bottle, precisely as in the examination of Merchant's urine.

March 24th.—Potash bulb apparatus
after   585·22
March 22d.—Potash bulb apparatus
before   585·15
                              ·07

Here, the increase is so small, that it may be entirely neglected; and we may conclude that no sugar had passed into the urine.

Experiment 6.—March 29th. Into the right jugular vein of a powerful bull-terrier dog, I injected 500 grains of the residuum of Merchant's urine, dissolved in f℥iij. of warm water. Half an hour afterwards I destroyed him with hydrocyanic acid. No urine, however, was evacuated. The body was immediately opened, when the bladder, which was distended with urine, was removed. The stomach contained food. The heart was large. There was but little fat, and the muscular fibre was every where firm. The animal was in excellent condition.

Urine.—I collected 4 fluid-ounces and 1 dram. Colour brown. Taste not sweet, but saltish. Odour peculiar. Nitric acid added to this urine *cold* occasioned considerable effervescence, but no coagulation. Hydrochloric acid also produced effervescence. Sp. gr. 1041°. f℥iij. were mixed with a small quantity of yeast, and left to ferment in the usual manner.

April 1st, 9½, P.M.—Potash apparatus *after*   594·19
March 29th, 9½, P.M.—Potash apparatus *before*   585·21
                              8·98

The ley had risen in the large bulb, and the carbonic acid was displaced in the usual manner by atmospheric air. I evaporated some of the urine over the steam-bath; it evolved a peculiar and very disagreeable odour, not very unlike phosphuretted hydrogen. Considerable effervescence occurred on the addition of strong nitric acid to the syrup *cold*, and an abundance of almost colourless crystals of nitrate of urea was immediately separated.

Experiment 7.—March 2d, ½ before 5, P.M. Into the right jugular vein of a middle sized mongrel bitch, I injected a considerable quantity, probably an ounce and a half moist, of the sugar of raisins, dissolved in warm water. Urine was evacuated. The breathing became somewhat laboured, and the dog appeared drowsy. He was closely watched for 3¼ hours, with the intention of collecting his urine. During this period he vomited chyme, and, afterwards, tenacious mucus-like liquid. I then poisoned the animal with strong hydrocyanic acid. During the convulsive action I collected f℥vj. of clear brown urine, having an odour *sui generis*, and resembling that of the dog's hide. More urine was passed than I obtained.

Urine.—Transparent. Colour brown. Reddens litmus. Sp. gr. 1031°. Taste not in the least degree sweet. 500 grains were mixed with a small quantity of yeast.

March 4th.—Potash apparatus *after* fermentation   588·08
March 2d.—Potash apparatus *before* fermentation   585 81
                                            2·27

250 grains of this urine evaporated over steam-bath left 18·6 of dark brown extract.

Experiment 8.—In this experiment I was aided by my respected friend Dr. Wright. Into the right jugular vein of a middle-sized terrier, we injected at 11, A.M. in successive syringefuls, nearly 1500· grains of white (cane) sugar, dissolved in f℥iv. of warm distilled water. The act of injecting occupied 20 minutes. The heart's action at first became irregular and intermitting; then, strong, rapid, and regular; 180 in the minute, as nearly as I could count. This excitement, however, was only temporary, for the pulsations became irregular and intermitting, 92 in a minute. The respiration was somewhat laboured, and the dog appeared drowsy. At 20 minutes before 12, reddish, sweet, and turbid urine was passed, and continued to be voided almost continually, sometimes stillatim, and at other times copiously, until death at 12; life was nearly destroyed by bleeding from the jugular vein, and then completely extinguished by anhydrous hydrocyanic acid, of which the effect was neither so powerful nor so rapid as upon an animal in ordinary circumstances. During the bleeding, towards the last, general convulsive action occurred, with the evacuation of a small quantity of offensive fæces. We examined the body ¼ before 3, P.M.: lungs collapsed considerably.

Nothing abnormal in the thorax: no effusion. The intestines were pale and blanched. Half a fluid-ounce of clear serous liquid was collected in the peritoneal cavity; and on cooling, for the body was yet warm, it became thick, concreted into an albuminous mass like the white of egg, and presented a membraniform appearance. The kidneys appeared natural. The bladder was completely contracted, and contained a small quantity of coagulated blood. The mucous membrane of the viscus presented several bloody points. The sp. gr. of the urine first collected was 1046·7; sp. gr. of that collected towards the last was 1050. It contained blood, as the red particles subsided after a short time. 500 grains of the first urine left by evaporation 62·3 of crystallised sweet mass. I obtained beautifully perfect crystals of cane sugar, and have preserved them.

From the experiments which have now been related we learn the following facts:—

1. When grape-sugar is present in the blood in a certain quantity, a portion of it is speedily eliminated by the kidneys, and may be found in the urine.

2. When grape-sugar is present in the blood only in small quantity (Experiment 5), it does not pass into the urine in an appreciable degree. In this case it probably undergoes oxidation in the lungs.

3. When cane-sugar is present in the blood in a certain quantity, a portion of it passes into the urine as cane-sugar. It does not appear to be converted in the smallest proportion into *grape-sugar*, during its passage through the blood. (Experiment 8.)

4. When cane-sugar is present in the blood, in large quantity, (Experiment 8), it exerts a powerfully diuretic action, and the urine evacuated appears to be principally solution of sugar.

5. When grape-sugar is introduced into the stomach (Experiment 1), under conditions favourable to absorption, a portion of it is rapidly absorbed (possibly by the veins?) and passes into the urine.

6. When a dog is fed upon cane-sugar and water, a portion of the sugar may be found in the urine.

Before proceeding, it is proper to mention, that my results do not exactly accord with those previously published. It is stated, in the "Essay on Diabetes" (by Bell, translated by Markwick, p. 49), that " by injecting into the vessels a solution of cane-sugar, we do not find that the sugar passes into the blood or urine, but by the pulmonary transpiration. We know that cane-sugar, taken into the stomach in whatever quantity, never passes by the urine." The authority upon which these statements are made is not mentioned. There is, evidently, an error in the construction of the first sentence, which has, doubtless, escaped the attention of the translator, for it is impossible that sugar can be injected into the vessels (if blood-vessels be meant), and not pass into the blood. Again; Dr. Krimer, as I have already remarked, states, that " when diabetic urine is introduced into the stomach of an animal, we find on the following day saccharine matter in its urine, and continue do so as long as we administer this substance, and even some days after we cease to inject it." (Op. cit. p. 48.) When grape-sugar is introduced into the stomach of a dog, I have been unable to discover a trace of sugar in its urine on the following morning. The dog which was the subject of Experiments 3 and 4, ate 10 ounces of moist sugar of raisins at 9½, A.M. and drank a small quantity of water. On the following morning at 10½, his urine was collected. I obtained precisely ℥j. of a pale brown colour. In the evening, it was evaporated, and mixed, while yet warm, with a small quantity of yeast in a graduated receiver over mercury. The volume occupied by the liquid was 0·6 cubic inches. On the following evening, 7, P.M. not the slightest disengagement of gas had occurred.

I have not succeeded in detecting sugar in the urine of man after the introduction of grape-sugar into the stomach. I am not disposed to incur the risk of disordering my own stomach by experiments of this kind, and, therefore, I am unwilling to practise upon the stomachs of others. However, from the preceding experiments upon dogs, we shall, probably, not err in concluding that under similar circumstances similar results would be obtained with man. In my next communication I shall revert to the question at first propounded, concerning the formation of sugar in the system in a state of health, and shall then detail a variety of experiments performed in reference to this subject.

[To be continued.]

ESSAYS ON THE DISEASES
OF THE
HEART, GREAT VESSELS, AND
CIRCULATING FLUID.

BY R. WILLIS, M.D.

Lecturer on the Principles and Practice of Medicine in the Aldersgate Street School of Medicine, late Physician to the Royal Infirmary for Children, &c.

[Continued from p. 870 of preceding volume.]

SPECIAL PATHOLOGY OF THE HEART.

Malformations of the Heart.

THE heart is subject to a great variety of congenital affections, the majority of which, as they rather interest the morbid anatomist than the practical physician, do not require any particular notice in this place. Sometimes the heart is not in its usual situation ; it is contained in the abdomen, or in a pouch outside the thorax; or otherwise, and this is of much less importance, it is merely transposed, the apex of the organ being directed to the right instead of the left side of the chest. Such cases fall under the category of misplacements of the heart—ectopiæ cordis. Sometimes, again, the heart consists of but two great cavities instead of four, one representing the auricles, another the ventricles. Occasionally the arteries arise amiss, the aorta springing from the right, the pulmonary artery from the left ventricle, &c. These various states are by no means incompatible with life within the uterus ; but they are, for the major part, altogether inconsistent with existence apart from the body of the parent.

Cyanosis.

Among the most important of the congenital malformations of the heart with which we are acquainted, and which do really interest us as practitioners of medicine, are those with which the affection denominated cyanosis, or blue disease, in young subjects, is connected.

Cyanosis is characterized by the skin having more or less of a livid or blue colour, especially in those situations where the capillary vessels of the ge-

neral tegumentary membrane are most
conspicuous, or where this membrane
is most delicate, as in the lips, the
cheeks, and under the nails. The mucous membrane of the mouth and nostrils also presents a livid instead of its
usual bright scarlet tint. This livor of
the general surface is accompanied
by habitual dyspnœa, tumultuous action of the heart, irregularity and in-
termittence of the pulse at the wrist,
and an inferior capacity to engender
caloric. The dyspnœa and irregular
action of the heart, generally more or
less felt at all times, are greatly aggravated upon occasion. Slight efforts,
the act of coughing, of going to stool,
and the like, are apt to bring on fits of
suffocation, and, when the disease is
far advanced, attacks of leipothymiæ,
in one of which the patient commonly
expires.

Young subjects affected with cyanosis are extremely susceptible to cold.
They, in fact, scarcely maintain their
temperature at the 98° F., which is
held the standard for man in temperate
latitudes. It has been found three and
four degrees lower under the tongue.

Cyanosis is usually apparent from
the period of birth. The new-born
infant is familiarly known to have a
much darker colour than it acquires
immediately after the play of the lungs
is fully established, and the circulation
through the umbilical cord has ceased.
The colour can be observed brighten-
ing visibly. This is not the case in the
infant that is to be the subject of cyanosis. From the birth it presents a
livid or purple hue ; and if this be very
deep, it will in general scarcely survive
more than a few days or weeks. If
the livor be less, the child may struggle
on languidly for a longer time ; and if
still less, it may attain to maturity of
years. It is not, indeed, very rare for
children who have presented a decided
blue colour of the tongue and lips and
general surface from their birth, to
reach the period of puberty, when they
very commonly perish. Such children
have been observed to grow tall and
slender ; their muscular system is but
very slightly developed ; their extremities seem to consist of little more
than skin and bone ; they are fragile
beings, upon whose likelihood of long
life no venture can be made. Nevertheless, we cannot always say precisely
that cyanosis, even when pretty well

marked in infants, is necessarily to
continue and prove fatal in the end.
About a year and a half ago I was
consulted in regard to a *blue child*
about six weeks old. This infant had
all the usual indications of cyanosis
perfectly well marked ; the whole surface was of a pale livid hue ; the tongue
and lips and finger-nails were purple.
It did not seem to suffer any inconvenience, however, and I was assured by
the nurse and the parents that the
colour was now lighter than it had
been. I recommended that the infant
should be kept very warm, and particular attention paid to the nursing;
and ventured to express a hope that,
as matters had mended to a certain
extent, they might improve still farther. And this has actually taken
place ; the infant throve amain ; the
livor of the surface and mouth became
less and less conspicuous, and at the
present time the child would not be
remarked as differing from other children of the same age. Such cases I
can imagine to be more frequent than
is generally supposed.

The occurrence of cyanosis appears
to have been connected at an early
period in modern pathological inquiry
with an imperfect condition of the partition between the right and left auricles of the heart. Morgagni and
Senac, however, were the first who
particularly fixed the attention of physiologists upon this state as explaining
the phenomena of the disease, which,
as may be anticipated, were attributed
to an admixture of the venous and
arterial blood, and the circulation of an
imperfectly aerated fluid. A patent
state of the foramen ovale, a normal condition in the fœtus, was long universally received as the cause of cyanosis.

There can be little doubt but that
cyanosis is frequently connected with
such a state of the inter-auricular septum ; but the celebrated Corvisart, and
then Dr. Crawford, of Dublin, showed
that cases of cyanosis occurred which
were not referable to any such organic
imperfection ; and, on the contrary,
many cases are now on record in which
the freest communication between both
auricles, and even between both ventricles, has been discovered, without the
fact having been proclaimed during
life by a single symptom of cyanosis.
In one very remarkable instance, the
particulars of which are contained

in the Transactions of the King's and Queen's College of Physicians of Dublin, the communications between the two sides of the heart were so large that the organ might have been considered as single, or as consisting of but one auricle and one ventricle. Other cases nearly similar have been met with. It would appear, therefore, that very ample communications between the right and left sides of the heart, conditions which we should say admitted of the freest admixture of the black with the bright blood in the heart, occasionally occurred without cyanosis being the consequence. Some have therefore maintained that the essence of cyanosis consists in a stasis of blood in the capillaries of the body generally, and not on any admixture of unoxygenated with oxygenated blood.

I find it difficult, for my own part, to agree to this without some limitation; the livor in cyanosis is not precisely of that kind which we observe in connexion with impediments to the access of venous blood at the heart; in cyanosis there is no unusual development of the minute blood-vessels and intermediate vascular rete; the livor is precisely that of asphyxia, in which we know that black blood is circulated. Nevertheless, it must be confessed that the pathological condition which has been found accompanying most of the cases of cyanosis that have been recently examined has been, not a patent condition of the foramen ovale, or imperfection of the inter-ventricular septum, but a dilated and thickened state of the right cavity of the heart. Organic affections of the right side of the heart occurring in riper years are particularly, and at a very early period, proclaimed by a livid or violet colour of the face and extremities. The systemic venous circulation is greatly under the control of the right side of the central organ of the circulation, and implication of this is always accompanied by a retarded movement in the capillaries—hence the blue colour of the skin. The only explanation that could be given of the absence of cyanosis in those cases in which imperfections of the auricular and ventricular septa have been discovered, would be grounded on the accurate maintenance of the proportion between the powers of each side of the heart, and the resistance which it has to overcome. The

tension upon every part of the vascular system, I apprehend, must be the same; and as streams of like magnitude meet and roll their tides for many miles without mixing, so may the tides pertaining to the right and left sides of the heart be forced along their appropriate channels without becoming commingled in the heart.

With regard to the *treatment* of cyanosis, this must be entirely palliative. We cannot hope to remove by any medicine the organic imperfections or lesions on which it depends. Still, from what I have already said, it will be seen that no case should be abandoned as utterly hopeless. In infancy unusual care is required; engendering caloric less abundantly than other infants, the blue child is to be kept wrapped up in blankets frequently warmed, and should be supplied with the only nutriment that is adapted to its tender age, made additionally tender by its disease — mother's milk. By and by the food should be unstimulating, but nourishing, and never given in large quantities at a time. In the paroxysms of dyspnœa that are so distressing in cyanosis, after the first years of life have been passed, we sometimes feel strongly tempted to abstract a little blood; and, indeed, to relieve the labouring ventricle, we are sometimes forced to have recourse to the lancet. But this should always be done with great discretion; the loss of blood in such circumstances is ever followed by great prostration. Absolute repose, cool air, the application of cloths dipped in cold vinegar and water to the region of the heart, cold drinks or ice internally, and some sedative, such as hyoscyamus or opium—digitalis is too tardy in its action to be of service here—generally suffice to allay the paroxysm. When the disease towards its termination is attended with dropsical effusions, particular attention must be paid to the action of the bowels and kidneys; diuresis is less depressing than purging, and, therefore, preferable to it. When the strength is greatly reduced and the circulation extremely languid, we have recourse to tonics and even to direct stimulants, such as ammonia and wine, to keep the heart moving. This system of medication of course can only be pursued for a time; the powers of life fall lower and lower by degrees, and the organs finally failing to be influenced by our stimulants, they cease entirely from their functions, and the patient is lost.

Inflammation of the heart, and of its internal and external investing membranes—Carditis, Endocarditis, and Pericarditis.

Carditis, Myocarditis. — There can be no doubt of the occasional though rare occurrence of inflammation of the muscular substance of the heart, apart from implication either of its external investing or internal lining membrane. It is infinitely more common, however, to find distinct traces of inflammatory affection of one or other, or of both these serous coverings, along with evidences of inflammation of the proper substance of the heart. Corvisart believed that carditis could not be distinguished during life from pericarditis, and Laennec maintained that carditis had never been observed otherwise than in connection with this disease or with endocarditis. We have, in fact, no signs pathognomonic of carditis existing *per se*. Unfortunately, in that which is held to be one of the most satisfactory instances on record of acute inflammation affecting the entire substance of the heart, the disease was complicated with an affection of the brain, which probably masked the symptoms, or at all events called off attention so completely from the central organ of the circulation, that the changes which it was found to have undergone in consequence of acute inflammation were not once suspected during the life of the patient. The particulars of this case may be found recorded at length in the seventh volume of the Medico-Chirurgical Transactions, by Mr. Stanley. The subject of it was a boy, twelve years of age, belonging to Christ's Hospital. He was apparently well on Saturday, April the 20th, after having visited one of his relations. Next morning, Sunday, April the 21st, he was brought to the infirmary of the establishment extremely ill. The symptoms were those of general acute fever; the skin was hot; the pulse was quick; the tongue was dry, &c. On Monday the fever had increased in intensity. The only pain complained of, however, was in the left thigh and knee, and had ceased before night. In the afternoon

he became affected with delirium, and had no sleep during the ensuing night. On Tuesday the delirium still continued; the pupils were dilated, and did not contract under the influence of light. The patient still made no complaint of pain; but when pressed on the subject he pointed to his forehead. In the afternoon he had a convulsive fit. Every symptom became greatly aggravated. The night was passed as usual without sleep. On Wednesday morning the patient was greatly exhausted, and the breathing was now for the first time observed to be difficult. He was sensible in the morning, but sank into a state of insensibility as the day advanced, and continued to decline till two o'clock in the afternoon, when he died. He had never complained of pain in the chest, and no irregularity had been noted in the action of the heart or pulse at the wrist. It is not stated particularly that the chest was examined; the stethoscope was not then known. On examining the body after death, the skull was found very thick and heavy; the bones showed no diploe, but were dense and solid throughout. The sutures were obliterated. The vessels of the brain were congested, but not in a very striking degree. In the thorax, the lungs were healthy. On laying open the pericardium, it was found to contain between four and five ounces of turbid serous fluid, with flakes of coagulable lymph which floated through it. The internal surface of the pericardium, both where it constitutes the containing pouch, and where it is reflected upon the heart, was covered in various places with a thin layer of lymph, having a reticulated appearance. The heart itself was natural in point of size, but upon cutting into its substance the muscular fibres were found exceedingly dark coloured, almost black, and very soft and loose in their texture, easily separable, and readily crushed between the finger and thumb. On looking attentively at the cut surface of the ventricles numerous small cells full of dark-coloured pus were visible in distinct points among the muscular fibres. Some of these points of pus were situated deeply near the cavities; others lay more superficially, so as even to raise the reflected pericardium. The muscular fibres of the auricles were likewise soft and dark coloured, but they did not appear to contain any purulent points. The endocardium was judged to be healthy, as were the valves, save that the vascular ramifications upon these parts were more distinct than usual.

This case is frequently referred to in works on diseases of the heart; but, strange to say, it is seldom quoted correctly. Dr. Latham, for instance, citing it as a case of disease of the heart simulating disease of the brain, says, " not a vestige of disease was found within the cranium." But I have quoted immediately from the reporter, and shown that he speaks of congestion of the brain, and of an eburneous state of the skull, with obliteration of the diploe and sutures; a state which very certainly cannot be called healthy in a boy of 12 years of age. Neither is there generally any mention made of the evidences of inflammation of the pericardium which were discovered; the case after all was not one of pure carditis, but of carditis complicated as usual with pericarditis.

In discussing the symptoms of carditis, we are reduced to indicate phenomena which from analogy we should anticipate, rather than able to speak of any which have been positively observed. Where the attack is slight, it is presumed that there would be pain of greater or less severity, and in all probability occurring suddenly in the region of the heart; disturbance in the action of the heart, at first violent, but speedily becoming feeble, (for the invariable and very rapid effect of inflammation affecting the muscular substance is to paralyse it), and as in all inflammatory diseases, the symptoms of general fever. The attack being graver in its character would be marked by the occurrence of pain of a severer description, of an oppressive and stringent kind, referred to the heart; by violent palpitation, tumultuous and irregular action of the heart, accompanied by a sense of anguish, of alarm, and of imminent dissolution. I cannot imagine that any peculiar bellows sound need necessarily accompany the disordered action of the heart in simple carditis. The pulse at the wrist under such circumstances can only be expected to have volume and power in the very beginning of the attack; it would soon become small and fluttering, and be unrhythmical, in accordance with the character presented by the action of the heart. The respiration would be accelerated, but not otherwise peculiarly affected, unless congestion of the lungs were superinduced. The alimentary canal, save in connexion with the general pyrexia, would not be affected. The extremities would be cold; the expression of countenance, as in heart diseases of the gravest kind, would be that of great distress. The functions of the brain and nervous system would appear occasionally to be very seriously implicated in carditis; delirium, convulsions, and coma, have been indicated as frequent sympathetic consequences of the disease. Carditis would, in fact, appear occasionally to have existed, and even gone on to a fatal termination, altogether unsuspected, because of the severity of the symptoms referable to implication of the brain. Both M. Andral and Dr. Latham have given cases of fatal cardiac and pericardiac disease, where during life the symptoms were all referred to the centre of the nervous, not of the circulating system; and in a remarkable instance, which I have quoted after the report of Mr. Stanley, the same circumstance occurred. In one of M. Andral's cases there was delirium, general convulsive movements, and twitchings of the tendons, for three days; on the fourth day the delirium ceased, but the convulsive motions continued, and the arms were from time to time thrown into a state of positive tetanic spasm. On the fifth day the delirium returned, and the upper extremities became paralytic. The patient then fell into a comatose state, and died. On dissection neither the brain nor the spinal marrow, nor the membranes, presented the slightest trace of disease; neither did any other organ of the body, except the heart, show evidences of having been the seat of morbid action. Upon the surface of the pericardium, however, there was a copious deposit of lymph, and into its sac an effusion of serous fluid. So also in a case of acute rheumatism, which was under the care of Dr. Latham, in St. Bartholomew's Hospital, the whole force of the treatment was directed to the head, under the impression that the brain was inflamed, the symptoms being those that usually accompany and proclaim phrenitis. Upon dissection, however, the brain and its coverings were found in a perfectly healthy state; but in the pericardium, towards which there had been no symptom to direct suspicion, unequivocal marks of recent and acute inflammation were discovered.

For my own part I always hear of such cases as those just referred to with regret, especially where they are dwelt upon as matters of mystery. According to my interpretation, they are, in the great majority of instances, but evidences of our carelessness or of our want of accurate knowledge. Probably the blood being irregularly distributed to the brain in such circumstances, its functions are interfered with: the sentinel, pain, goes to sleep, and gives no information of the enemy that is knocking at the gates, and then we are left in a state of delusive security as to the actual circumstances of the case before us, a security which more careful examination would almost certainly dissipate. We are now generally aware of the necessity under which we lie of examining all the organs in every case of disease. We do not at present commonly content ourselves by exploring the pulse at the wrist: we also ascertain the state of the heart, &c. Were this practice to be followed invariably, such anomalous cases as those I have just referred to would certainly occur more rarely than they do. Effusion cannot take place into the pericardium without the fact being proclaimed by unequivocal physical signs, carefully looked for, it will certainly be discovered in every case to which it happens: what I see obscurity hung over the cases just quoted, in the first instance, therefore, might to have been removed at a later period.

The appearances presented by the heart in fatal cases of acute carditis have been in some sort anticipated in the account hitherto have been given of those of the body fresh applying but had a Hospital. It has been compound with softening upon of the patho-genic months along of the substance of cardiac inflammation of all stops the muscular substance of the heart of of the pericardium of the heart the do of the post of the inflammation of the heart to the inflammation of the heart the post of the inflammation ...

of the heart, and especially its lining membrane, and stains the entire organ of a deep red colour. In such circumstances there is simple dyeing of the textures; the blood is obviously not included within the delicate vessels; the redness is uniformly diffused, or it occurs in marbled stains. There is this difference also in the characters of the redness induced by inflammation, and that which results from sanguineous penetration, that, when it is due to the former, the shade of colour is uniform, when to the latter, the tint is usually notably darker or browner on the right than on the left side of the heart. Farther, inflammation of the muscular tissue that has continued even for a very short time is attended with softening, first in points and then more extensively: the fibres disappear, and are resolved into a kind of gelatinous pulp of a dark red colour; by and by, purulent matter is produced. If we find the substance of the heart preternaturally red and soft at the same time, without any trace of commencing decomposition, we should be warranted in ascribing the change to antecedent inflammation.

The causes of carditis are obscure; those that have been most insisted on of late years are such as are acknowledged favourable to the development of rheumatism in the muscular and fibrous systems generally. Intemperance in the use of spirituous liquors seems to predispose to carditis as well as to various other acute and passive diseases of the circulating system. Organic affections of one or other of the parts of the heart—its valves, its orifices—seem also to predispose, in a marked degree, to acute inflammatory affections of its substance and their consequences—abscess, ulceration, and rupture—which I shall have occasion to illustrate by and by.

Acute carditis is a most dangerous, probably it is always a fatal disease when it occurs. The prognosis is therefore invariably unfavourable. The difficulty of detecting the disease may readily be conceived as adding very materially to its danger. Whoever is attacked with carditis certainly runs no small hazard of losing his life.

The treatment of acute carditis must ... upon what are called antiphlogistic principles of the strictest ... to the patient whose medical adviser, alarmed by the smallness and want of rhythm in the pulse, neglects venesection in the earliest period of the disease! If this fatal error be committed, all else will be in vain. Bloodletting is the only means that can be relied on, the only remedy competent to cut short so formidable a disease as carditis, whether its immediate tendency, or its consequences, should it not destroy the patient at once, be considered. General blood-letting, then, in the first instance, followed by local depletion, each repeated again and again in proportion to the violence of the symptoms rather than the estimated strength of the patient, is what we have to rely upon for the cure of inflammation of the heart. Along with this powerful means it is at the same time proper to call in the depressing effects of antimony and opium, or digitalis, and, farther, to use every effort to get the system under the specific influence of mercury, administered by the mouth and by inunction simultaneously. The patient should of course be kept in a state of the most perfect quietude, and allowed nothing but a little cold or iced drink to quench thirst and allay excitement.

[To be continued.]

EFFICACY OF CARBONIC ACID GAS IN GOUT.

To the Editor of the Medical Gazette.

SIR,

IN a work that I recently published, with the express object of recommending a particular remedy for the cure of that intractable and painful malady, gout, it was stated that, as far as my experience went, the remedy in question—carbonic acid gas—shortened the paroxysms, and lengthened the intervals of the attacks, to a greater extent than any other with which I was acquainted; so that attacks, which before lasted two or three months, were reduced in the end, and after the lapse of some years, to as many weeks or days; while the disease itself, instead of returning twice or three times every year, was only experienced every second, third, or fourth year. Two cases only were then given as illustrative of its efficacy; one shewing the effect of the medicine during the paroxysm, and the other its ultimate result. I was in

hopes, however, that some of my professional brethren would, ere this, not only have given the remedy a fair and proper trial, but, at the same time, have been induced to make the result of that trial public; for it was in this hope and expectation that I published the work in question. Being disappointed, however, in this respect, and having received several private communications on the subject, I have selected the following case, from among several others, thinking that it may not be uninteresting to the readers of the MEDICAL GAZETTE. The particulars were forwarded me a short time since from Barcelona, where my work is about to be published in Spanish, Dr. Fritz being now engaged in translating the same.

The writer is an English gentleman, who, having experienced an attack of gout last spring, wrote to me for directions respecting his own case, and subsequently for that the history of which I am about to relate.

After speaking of the satisfactory state of his own health, the writer thus continues:—"You must know, then, that your remedy appears to have effected a *radical cure* in the patient, who has been under our care since last June. It is such a striking case of the success of your treatment, that it really deserves to be added to the work; and I regret very much that I am so little qualified to draw up a report for that object. I could, however, get something like a deposition from the patient, attested by respectable witnesses, if such a document could be of any service in making known the wonderful effect of *carbonic acid gas*.

"The person in question (a Spaniard) is about 40 years of age, and has suffered very severely for about fifteen years with three or four attacks every year of the most severe kind; the disease generally commencing in the hands or feet, and extending itself to the elbows, knees, shoulders, &c.; and on one occasion to the testes. He describes the agonies he used to suffer as so great, that he has frequently called on those about him to put an end to his existence. His fingers are distorted and crooked; and, in short, although it may be an improper remark on such a serious subject, he went by the nick-name of 'Commander of the Gouty Legion.'

" The draughts (effervescing) were administered to him, in the first instance, at the onset of an attack in the right hand, brought on, as he supposed, by a fit of passion the preceding day. The inflammation subsequently reached the elbow, but went no further. He complained, however, of the pain this time being even greater, if possible, than he had ever suffered; and, being an ignorant man, had got it into his head that it was owing to the disease not being able to spread as usual, by which all its malignity was concentrated in one spot. I made him take the draughts every three hours, supplying him out of my own stock of French soda, not trusting to the Spanish, which, you know, is inferior. In three days he came round, the violence of the pain and inflammation having entirely subsided; after which he only took the draughts three times a-day, until all symptoms of the attack had disappeared.

" After this he continued quite free from the disease for three months, when symptoms of another attack were felt; but, full of belief in the efficacy of the remedy, he passed the first or better part of the night in taking a draught every two hours, or even more frequently, till at last sleep overcame him; and when he awoke late in the morning every symptom had disappeared, and he found himself as if he had been dreaming, and quite well. From that time down to the present day (now five months), he has had no signs whatever of the distemper.

" It is right to state that, in addition to the effervescing draughts, I advised the patient, as soon as the intensity of the attack had subsided, and the inflammation had partially disappeared, to take a few grains of blue pill every other night, and in the morning an electuary, composed of sulphur and magnesia—a prescription I have found to suit the irritable and weak bowels of gouty subjects better than most others. When the latter combination was not found sufficient, an aloetic preparation was recommended to be added to the blue pill, and a slight aromatic tonic during convalescence."

In closing these remarks I am bound to add, that the result obtained in so old and severe a case would appear to be greater than that which I have myself hitherto experienced; and I am induced, therefore, to ascribe the difference to a circumstance that has been before dwelt upon by me, viz. that in Spain many diseases are milder and less complicated than in this country[*]. Not that I concur in the opinion expressed by the narrator of the present case, that a radical cure has been effected, if, by radical cure, be meant a total exemption in future from attacks of the disease. Such a result ought not, and cannot be expected; for if the remedy in question acts only, as I presume, by removing the cause—no matter what that cause is, whether external or internal—the individual must always be liable to be again brought under its injurious operation, the same as before the first attack of the disease. If, however, gout be produced, as I infer, from the presence of a morbid matter in the blood; and if, as I still further conclude, we possess an agent capable of combining with it, and rendering it innocuous, all that we require is a certain amount of time, (varying, of course, according to the severity of the disease), and the duration of the attack and recovery of the patient, instead of depending, as heretofore, on the efforts of nature, or the as uncertain efforts of art, may then be calculated on with something like a certainty; while the attacks themselves, instead of continuing for months, and returning two or three times every year, will only be experienced once in two or three years, and then only continue for a few days or weeks. I, of course, except those cases, too frequent, alas! in which structural or organic alteration has taken place in any vital or important organ, produced not only by the injurious but the long-continued operation of a cause, that the science of medicine has hitherto been unable to remove with certainty and with safety.

Trusting that the history of the preceding case will prove interesting to the readers of the MEDICAL GAZETTE, and that the result of the treatment may induce some of your numerous subscribers to give the remedy in question a fair trial, I have only to add that, whatever the result of the trial may be, it will, I hope, be made public; not for my satisfaction, but for that of a large class of sufferers who,

* Vide Lancet, May 12, 1838: On the State of Medicine in Spain.

at present, are too generally sceptical of the efforts of art in the cure of their complaint.—I am, sir,

Your obedient servant,

J. PARKIN.

18, Dover Street, April 3, 1843.

SEVERE AFTER-PAINS FOLLOW-ING LABOUR,

TREATED SUCCESSFULLY BY BELLADONNA PLASTERS.

To the Editor of the Medical Gazette.

SIR,

SHOULD the following case be deemed sufficiently interesting, its insertion in your columns will oblige, sir,

Your obedient servant,

ROBERT NIXON.

Wigton, April 1, 1843.

Mrs. B., aged 28, a lady of cultivated and lively turn of mind, but of a marked leucophlegmatic temperament, and who had experienced a severe hysteric seizure, the consequence of prolonged uterine hæmorrhage during a former puerperal confinement, was taken in labour on the 27th of October, 1842, of her third child, which was born with comparatively trifling suffering. The placenta came away spontaneously, and all went on favourably until the morning of the 29th, when the after-pains, which had previously been slight and not frequent, became so distressing, that a table-spoonful of the following mixture was ordered every half-hour till relieved.

℞ Solution. Morphiæ (equal to Laudanum) ʒiv.; Aquæ Destillatæ, ʒiiiss.

Nine hours elapsed ere I could again visit my patient; and notwithstanding that the morphia had been persevered in, the lady's pains were much increased. Tossing in bed, she caught at every thing for a fixed point to cling by; her moanings were heart-rending; her countenance anxious, and indicative of great suffering; the pulse, naturally feeble, was hurried and thready, and the extremities were cold. Some hot brandy and water was given; friction, hot water, and stockings filled with heated salt, were applied to the legs and feet. A starch enema was substituted for the anodyne mixture, containing a tea-spoonful (ʒiss.) each of laudanum and solution

of morphine, and was repeated every half hour until nine had been given, and they were all retained. Thus gr. v. of morphia were taken into the stomach, and an equivalent to gr. xvj. and a fraction passed into the rectum, without the slightest alleviation to her dreadful agony, the pains continuing as obstinate as before. Laying aside other remedies, I now covered the entire hypogastric region with a belladonna plaster, made by spreading the extract thickly upon linen, and waited the result. In an hour and a quarter the pains were much diminished in violence, occurred at longer intervals, and finally altogether ceased; but she complained of a prickling sensation over the body, especially the face, across which she rapidly, apparently involuntarily, passed her hand. The plaster was now removed, and some time afterwards she complained of the closeness of the apartment, and was obliged to be fanned. Suddenly she started up in bed, gasping and shivering most violently. A wine-glassful of brandy and water happening to be at hand, she drank it with difficulty and danger of breaking the glass from spasmodic action of the muscles of the jaws and face. Active friction was again made use of to the hands and feet, which were still cold; a few tea-spoonfuls of very strong coffee having been given, in about twenty minutes she expressed herself better, and quietly laid down in bed, when gentle perspiration came on, and was succeeded by five hours' sleep. She awoke in the morning much refreshed; but during the day there was a return of the after-pains, which, towards night, became more severe. Bladders, partially filled with hot water, were applied over the womb for about two hours, when they were gradually mitigated, but recurred at intervals for several days afterwards. Slight hæmorrhage was observed after the application of hot water, which continued about a week, and materially contributed to reduce the sufferer, who, however, was convalescent in four weeks.

REMARKS.—It may be asked, why not have had recourse to the application of hot fomentations when the failure of morphia was clearly ascertained? The dread of inducing hæmorrhage, the effects of which had nearly proved fatal to the lady during a previous delivery, alone deterred me. The result of the experiment made in the present instance, when a relapse occurred, sufficiently points out the danger of such a procedure. With the concurrence of my experienced friend, Dr. Rigg, of Woodrow, I was induced to follow up the exhibition of morphine and laudanum until 21 grains of the salt were administered, as already detailed, without the slightest manifestation of change, the intensity of the pains being in no degree abated. The relief afforded by the application of belladonna was very decided, and contrasted strongly with the inadequate powers of opium and its preparations. Indeed, the marked success witnessed in this instance, without presuming too much upon an individual case, warrants me in recommending a further trial of it by the profession, believing it may become a powerful auxiliary in the treatment of this extraordinary kind of after-pain, fortunately not often met with in these latitudes.

What is the pathological condition of the uterus, which either completely nullifies the effects of poisonous doses of morphia, or apparently in precisely similar circumstances allows this organ to be brought under its immediate control by very minute quantities?

Note.—I may mention the solution of morphia was prepared from the muriate manufactured by Mr. M'Farlane, of Edinburgh.

INTRA-THORACIC TUMOR.

To the Editor of the Medical Gazette.

Sir,

As the subject of intra-thoracic cancer affords at the present time an interest to your readers, from a case lately related by Dr. Maclachlan, allow me to offer you some account of a similar instance of that disease—no less terrible to the patient, than, when observed for the first time, it is puzzling to the practitioner.

Having mislaid my notes, made during the progress of the case, I am under the necessity of writing from memory; and although, from this circumstance, I cannot undertake a very particular description of the advent and march of the symptoms, these are, from the intense suffering of the patient, which I never can forget, and from the speculation they excited in my own mind in reference to their probable cause, sufficiently imprinted there to enable me to give a true though brief sketch.

I think it better to divide my description of the case into three parts; not that such a division is warranted by any change in the character of the disease itself, which is uniform and progressive, but because, in proportion as it advanced, it encroached upon important organs, and thereby impressed the aspect of the case with new features and distinct points of interest.

M. L., male, æt. 45, with dark hair, pale complexion; of square build, muscular, with well-developed chest, and always having enjoyed good health, was attacked, in the year 1838, with severe intercostal neuralgic pain of the right side. This was considered to be rheumatic, and was treated accordingly, with apparent benefit. The patient had many relapses of the pain, but being much exposed to draughts, and the damp atmosphere of a chilly season, no surprise was occasioned.

In this first division of the case, the nerves only were embarrassed. In the second the respiration and circulation became affected; for there were cough, dyspnœa, rapid pulse, and hæmoptysis; the physical signs elicited being partial suppression of the respiratory murmur, and dulness of sound on percussion. At this period the opinion of the late Dr. Thomas Davies was sought, which, though not explicitly conveyed to me, I judged, from the character of his prescription, and the tenor of his directions to the patient, that experienced physician considered the case one of tubercular degeneration or hardening of the lung.

In the third stage the pain and cough were almost ceaseless, and the hæmoptysis more frequent and abundant. The right side of the chest was enlarged, distended, and immoveable. The respiratory murmur, last heard about the scapular region, could now nowhere be detected. The sternal region was insonorous, as also was the subclavicular region of the left side. The apex of the heart was observed pulsating two inches to the left of its original position, and the edge of the liver was felt some distance below the costal margin. There was general venous congestion, marked by a livid surface, distended jugulars, immense hæmorrhoids, and anasarca, more especially of the face and upper extremities.

The patient died suffocated in about five or six months from the first attack of neuralgic pain.

Post-mortem appearances.—The sternum and cartilages of the ribs having been removed, an immense tumor was exposed, entirely filling up the right pleuritic cavity, both mediastina, and the upper third of the right pleuritic cavity. It was everywhere firmly adherent, except where intruding on the left side. It was a fine specimen of " medullary sarcoma," consisting of hard, irregular, scirrhous portions and septa, inclosing lobulated masses of various size, and of brain-like appearance and consistence. It must have weighed from twelve to fifteen pounds. On removing it from its bed, the remains of the lung were found adhering to the posterior wall of the chest, compressed to the exclusion of all air, and about one-third of an inch only in thickness. From this latter circumstance, and from its apparently complete immunity from cancerous disease, I was led to consider the case one of cancer of a bronchial gland.

Your obedient servant,
WILLINGTON CLARK.

Sutton, Surrey, April 12, 1843.

MEDICAL GAZETTE.

Friday, April 21, 1843.

" Licet omnibus, licet etiam mihi, dignitatem *Artis Medicæ* tueri ; potestas modo veniendi in publicum sit, dicendi periculum non recuso."
CICERO.

LUNATIC ASYLUMS IN ENGLAND AND IRELAND.

DR. HARTY, on whose pamphlet we touched a few weeks ago, is fertile in objections to the Act passed last session for the regulation of lunatic asylums in Ireland. Many of his censures are well founded, the Act having been so hastily passed as to be frequently inconsistent with itself; while others are eminently hypercritical, and could scarcely be obviated, unless we repealed not only Acts of Parliament, but human nature itself.

Thus, " Section 7 enacts, that the license shall be signed by *two* or more Justices, while Section .) says, that it shall be under the hands and seals of *three* or more."

This is a gross inconsistency ; but to show how easily even critics may err in a matter of figures, we will just mention that two pages afterwards, Dr. Harty himself dates a letter September 20th, 1843.

Again, while the English Act ordains that no person shall be received into a licensed house without a written order from the person sending the patient, and two medical certificates, the Irish Act adds the words " or detained" after " received."

It is obviously desirable that certificates should be renewed from time to time, and that no man should be indefinitely detained on the strength of an old certificate ; but from the imperfections incident to Acts passed in August, a literal compliance with the requisitions of the statute is impossible. Thus it is enacted that the order for the detention of the patient shall be under the hands of the person by whom he was originally sent; whereas, in many cases, the original applicant has gone to that bourne from which no signatures can be sought.

We will not do more than mention a certain Schedule (H.) rich in blunders from beginning to end; nor will we insist on the fact, that while in Ireland the penalties imposed by the Act may be recovered by any person who sues for them, in England the transgressor is protected against common interlopers, for no suit can be brought under the Act, except by order of the Commissioners, or Justices, nor can penalties be sued for except by the Clerk of the Commissioners, or the Clerk of the

Peace. Dr. Harty thinks the Irish Act too severe on Irish offenders; perhaps, it is the English Act which is too hard upon English lunatics. From Dr. Harty's observation on the machinery of the Act, we learn that the Irish proprietors of lunatic asylums are a very different class from those of England. It appears that in the extra-metropolitan districts of England and Wales, " of 85 houses, containing nearly 3000 inmates, many are kept by women, and 30 only by members of the medical profession; and from the second return, embracing the metropolitan district, it appears that of 41 houses, containing upwards of 2000 inmates, six only were kept by physicians; whereas in Ireland all the proprietors of private Asylums are physicians, with two exceptions only, one being an apothecary, and the other a gentleman not professional."

Dr. Harty very reasonably proposes that if an asylum has but one proprietor, he should always be a member of the medical profession; or, if there are several, that one at least should have this qualification. For, since an asylum is an hospital for the cure of patients who want medical treatment, it is obviously absurd to neglect so great a step towards the thing required. In an asylum where the patients do not exceed ten in number, both the English and Irish Acts allow them to be visited by their medical attendant as seldom as once in four weeks! These "angels' visits, few and far between," may satisfy the law, but will be highly inefficient in physic. Dr. Harty attributes this inconsiderate legislation to the strange evidence tendered to select committees, and received by them, he says, " almost without comment." Now, the fact is, that select committees, like all other collectors of evidence, are obliged to take it as it is to be found, *i. e.* with an ample leaven of spleen, ignorance, and

exaggeration; did they refuse to hear any but philosophic witnesses, their labours would be brief indeed. It is their business, *ex Ennii stercore suum colligere;* to separate golden suggestions from the rubbish in which they lie buried, and extract something valuable even from the anger of Mr. Edward Wakefield. This noted land-agent had a prejudice against our profession, amounting, as we should now say, to a monomania; for, in his evidence before the Committee of 1815, he fancied that medical practitioners, and particularly the College of Physicians, were, of all persons, most unfit for inspectors of madhouses. This singular delusion, however, did not prevent the Committee from separating a portion of *aurum* from the *stercus,* and the improved state of madhouses is, no doubt, due, in some degree, to the zeal of this ardent reformer. We do not think, however, that the rareness of medical visits permitted by the legislature at the smaller asylums arises from Mr. Wakefield's hallucination, but rather from a disinclination to deal harshly with vested interests. As every lunatic asylum is an hospital, a practitioner ought to reside in each and every one; but as the profits of the smallest asylums could not afford the expense, such an enactment, though just in itself, would be equivalent to an Act for the abolition of small mad-houses. There is one point, on which Dr. Harty touches more than once, which can never be cleared up till lawyers and doctors can define the limits of eccentricity and madness—in short, can measure metaphysical difficulties with mathematical nicety. Till this be done, there will be many men at large whom some of their neighbours pronounce to be mad, which is surely better than that others should be confined whom their neighbours believe to be sane.

An M.D., however, who is on the confining side of the question, writes a long letter to Dr. Harty, complaining of the difficulty of immuring a supposed monomaniac, whose case he details. This eccentric gentleman forms wild speculations, and obtains money on the strength of these castles in the air, which he spends in drink and driving. In the words of the discontented M.D., "he is seized at times with the most irresistible desire for rapid motion, and will hurry about in all directions on hired cars, without any definite purpose." Even the sober Dr. Johnson thought hand-driving in a post-chaise the finest thing in life, and, in our age of railways, we cannot accept a love of rapid motion as a proof of insanity*. But the most curious complaint in the letter is, that the monomaniac carries the new Act about with him as his safeguard. On us this makes a different impression. In Ireland, where the bludgeon and the blunderbuss are the common referees on all occasions, and the still small voice of reason can scarcely be heard amid the cries of party, it is cheering to see an insane man appealing to parliament for protection, and asking no other ægis but the law.

We might comment on some other points in Dr. Harty's useful essay, but our limits warn us to pass on to the pamphlet which we alluded to in our last article on this subject; we mean the Report of the Visiting Justices of the Surrey Lunatic Asylum.

Springfield Asylum, which is a very handsome building, is situated between Wandsworth and Tooting, and is capable of accommodating upwards of 350 patients. Its total cost, including the purchase of land, furniture, &c. was £85,000. It was opened in June 1841; and the number of patients admitted up to September 23d, 1842, was 389. Restraint, though not wholly abolished at the Surrey Asylum, is but rarely resorted to. Omitting the confinement of patients to their bed-rooms, which, in this Report, is called restraint by seclusion, the whole number of patients restrained, from January 1st to September 23d, 1842, was but 11. Four of these had extensive sloughing sores, and their hands were bound by handkerchiefs to prevent their taking off the poultices, and irritating the sores. No strait waistcoat appears to have been employed in any case. The Committee, who say that they feel the importance of obtaining respectable and trustworthy attendants, assert that their remuneration has been fixed on a liberal scale. On turning, however, to table iij. we find that, of nine female attendants, three have £16 a year each, three £15, and three only £12. These salaries are less than the wages of upper servants in private families, and, in fact, less than what is given to the cook, bakeress, and laundress, in this very establishment. Considering the immense power for good and for evil of the nurses in a mad-house, this is certainly a false economy. As their remuneration is to increase annually during the first five years of service, this error will be mitigated, but, we apprehend, not entirely remedied.

The average number of males employed has been sixty-three; of females, ninety-two. The former have been employed in the garden, the farm, their several trades, the kitchen, and the wards; the latter in the laundry, kitchen, sewing, knitting, straw work, and the wards.

One hundred and twenty-three patients, on an average, have attended chapel.

---

* We have sometimes thought that a railway is a poor man's hunting field, where he may enjoy the pleasures of the chase, namely, rapid motion, with a spice of danger, at a trifling expense. The absence of a fox, which is to be killed, or a stag, which is not to be killed, can make no material difference.

Nor is amusement for mind and body forgotten.

" In the way of recreation, a bowling-green has been prepared, and a library commenced, which already contains about eighty volumes of useful and entertaining knowledge, together with the Saturday and Penny Magazines, and Chambers' Journal; draft-boards, and other means of amusement, are permitted; and the patients are indebted to the kindness of a member of the Committee for a pianoforte, which has been a source of much pleasure."

We will conclude by mentioning a useful and benevolent provision. The visiting Physician furnishes patients, on leaving the Asylum, with such rules as he considers best adapted to prevent a relapse. Sir Alexander Morison, fills this office.

TWO CASES

OF POISONING BY LEAD, IN MACCUBA SNUFF.

Communicated by Professor Otto, of Copenhagen.

Two cases of poisoning, probably by Maccuba snuff containing red lead, have excited universal attention in Copenhagen. In the spring of 1842, M. Dreyer, highly esteemed as a scholar and botanist, died there after four months' illness, the symptoms having been doubtful, and their cause difficult to ascertain.

The deceased was much lamented, but his death had been almost forgotten, when his friend Dr. Bramsen read in a journal that red Maccuba snuff was sometimes adulterated with red lead. On this, he imagined that his deceased friend, who took a great deal of this snuff, might have been poisoned by it. He therefore bought some at the shop where the deceased used to buy his, and found that it was mixed with a number of large and small grains, which looked like minium; and, on chemical examination, he discovered that the snuff contained from 16 to 20 per cent. of lead.

After this discovery, Dr. Ahrensen, the physician of the deceased, did not doubt that Dreyer had been killed by the lead contained in the snuff; and this opinion seems fully confirmed by the course of the symptoms.

The patient, who was always rather pale, but who had almost always been well, with the exception of some unimportant chest symptoms, fell ill in the autumn of 1841. He had the common symptoms of dyspepsia with costiveness and a muddy complexion. As he lived a sedentary life, and devoted himself with great diligence to scientific pursuits, exercise was advised, and bitter and laxative pills were described. After this, he felt a little better, when, a few days before Christmas, he was suddenly attacked by violent colicky pains, which made him scream loudly, and throw himself from one side of the bed to the other. The pulse was natural, the tongue clean, the abdomen normal on percussion, and not painful on pressure. The bowels had been open the day before. The laxatives which had been prescribed were omitted; but some clysters, containing a grain of opium, diminished the attacks, and at last removed them entirely. The course of the symptoms, the effect of remedies, and the absence of all indications of disease in the viscera of the abdomen, excited, even then, suspicions of lead colic; and it occurred to Dr. Ahrensen that the red wine which he had recommended the patient, and which was very cheap, might possibly contain lead; but the examination of the wine, as well as of the vessels in which the patient's food was prepared, gave only negative results.

His improvement was of short duration; evacuations from the bowels were extremely rare, and when there had been none for a couple of days, from the omission of the medicines, the colicky pains returned, combined with cardialgia, and sometimes so violently, that the patient seemed to be in the greatest danger. He had four of these attacks during the winter, which were removed, partly by cathartics, partly by opiates. In one paroxysm alone, the pulse was rather quick, and somewhat tense, and the abdomen tender on pressure; so that Dr. Ahrensen, to face the possibility of an inflammatory complication, bled once, and added calomel to the opium. As he could not discover any other cause for the symptoms, he supposed that a stricture of the colon existed, as well as a dilatation above it; a supposition which was confirmed by the evacuation of a large mass of round hard fæces during the last attack, after which the patient felt pretty well. Though he had become very thin, and his complexion was still dull and yellowish, he now began to attend to business; but, a week afterwards, he was suddenly attacked by violent headache, which he ascribed to catching cold. Dover's powder, and elder tea in the evening, relieved him on the following day, but in the afternoon the attack returned with increased vehemence, and, as the pulse at the same time decreased in frequency, and he fell into a comatose state, it could no longer be doubted that the brain was attacked. After being fruitlessly treated with leeches, blisters, and strong purgatives (croton oil), he was taken to the hospital, where the symptoms remained unchanged, and were terminated by death two days after his admission, six days after the commencement of the cerebral affection, and about four months after the first attack of colic.

On dissection, nothing abnormal was found in the abdomen, except a trifling enlargement of the colon, probably caused by the frequent clysters; the brain, too, was healthy, except a slight injection of the membranes.

The striking resemblance of the first symptoms of the disease to lead colic, the agreement of the cerebral symptoms with those which occur in the comatose form of the *Encephalopathia saturnina* described by Tanquerel de Planches, the negative results of the dissection, and the patient's almost constant complaints of colicky pains, which were present during the whole course of the disease, make it highly probable that the fatal event was caused by the adulteration of the snuff with red lead.

These circumstances have made the case of another patient, a young physician, who is still alive, very conspicuous. He has suffered for a year from an affection of the abdomen, characterized by colicky pains and obstinate costiveness during which he has become extraordinarily thin. This patient is also a great snuff-taker, and long used the same snuff as the deceased patient. As he has now left it off, it is to be hoped that his malady will be cured. The tobacconist has been cited to answer for his misdemeanor. —*Zeitschrift für die gesammte Medicin,* March 1843.

MEDICAL REFORM.

To the Editor of the Medical Gazette.

SIR,

SOME months have now elapsed since my last letter to you on the subject of medical reform*. This delay, which has been almost unavoidable on my own part, is of the less consequence, inasmuch as it was generally known that the last session of Parliament would be closed without any measure being adopted for the alteration of our professional constitution.

---

* See MED. GAZ. for July 15, July 29, Aug. 26, 1842.

The basis on which I had proposed to form the whole medical profession consisted of three corporate bodies—two already in existence.

1st, The College of Physicians,
2d. The College of Surgeons, and the
3d, A College or Society of Pharmacy.

This division of the profession I endeavoured to show was founded on the *nature* of our occupations, and calculated by certain combinations of their diplomas to meet every necessity arising out of the application of its services to the public good.

It remains now to be considered how this plan might be carried out; which, supposing it to meet the approbation of the majority of the profession, would be of no great difficulty in its accomplishment.

The Colleges of Physicians and Surgeons being already established, it would only remain so to alter and enlarge their statutes as to meet the case. The establishment of a new Society or College of Pharmacy, with appropriate charters, would not be difficult; and indeed the efforts of many of the best and most respectable chemists of the present day have long been tending in that direction. So far as regards doing : but there remains one little task of undoing : would that all reformers could be persuaded to allow their undoings to bear an equally small proportion to their doings! To this plan of medical reform the Company of Apothecaries, as a Company, must yield—must cease to exist! It is probable that a greater resistance to this proceeding would be made by the ruling powers amongst this Society than by the members generally. To these gentlemen, therefore, I would say most respectfully, as well as most sincerely, that I am by no means insensible of the debt of gratitude we all, as a public, owe them for their past services and zeal : to them, in great measure, we owe it that the general practitioners of later years have been so much higher in character, and so much better practitioners. But I need hardly remind them that it is the true characteristic of greatness to hold power no longer than it is required for the public good ; so soon as the necessity ceases, so soon will a truly greatminded man yield his power. If, then, it can be shown to their dispassionate judgment that the usefulness, the comfort, and the high character of our profession, may be raised by their relinquishment of power, and the establishment of a different regulation of our profession, I need hardly remind them that it is their duty not only to resign that power, but cheerfully to cooperate in promoting the public good and the advancement of that profession of which they have been no idle ornaments : I would conjure them to consider the arguments adduced, and to be adduced, and especially those directed to the general mass of apothecaries of which they are the head.

To the general practitioners as apothecaries I would say :—You have been the loudest declaimers for reform ! and with great justice. You have complained of want of protection both from the wolves within and without the sheep-fold. Those privileges which have cost you dear in time, in study, and in money, have availed you nothing. The impudent quack from without, the hungry foreign doctors, and the pert chemists, from within, have eaten the bread for which you have not only toiled but paid a premium.

It is evident, therefore, that the system under which you live avails you nothing ; the body corporate which has been supported and maintained by your labours and your purse, has had no power to defend you in the enjoyment of those privileges which it professes to have given you. You complain, with justice, of an equivocal social position. When that portion of your youth which should have been dedicated to the acquirement of useful general knowledge has been devoted to a slavish apprenticeship to the pestle and mortar, how can it be otherwise ? When, in after life, your usefulness as professional men, your improved manners from mixing with the world, your minds stored with no mean share of general knowledge, and probably with a vast knowledge of human nature, how can you expect to hold that position which your merits deserve ? When, to the most beneficent and high-minded avocations of your profession, you add that of a retailer, if I may so say it, in drugs, and, instead of demanding from the wealthy that sum which your services deserve, you call upon him for payment for a draught, a powder, or a pill ? If, then, this plan of reform were carried out, it would be only necessary that all members of the Apothecaries' Company should at once be registered as "Members of the College of Physicians," either gratuitously or on the payment of a small fee. As most of them are already Members of the College of Surgeons, they would incur no trouble of change as regards that corporation. In carrying out such a measure of reform I should strongly urge its being done with the utmost liberality to all existing qualified practitioners ; and as there are at present several Members of the Apothecaries' Hall who, though practising upon no other qualification, have yet probably, with a just appreciation of their merits, obtained so high a share of public patronage and opinion, as, in fact, to assume the characters of physicians by practising for fees and in consultation, I would advise that the *Fellowship* of the College of Physicians should at once be offered to them on the payment of the proper fees. For the future,

however, no such irregularities should be allowed. I need not, of course, say that under this system of reform the *Fellowship* of the College of Physicians should at once be conferred upon such of its present Licentiates who may wish to continue their career as pure physicians ; some might, perhaps, under these alterations, wish to fall into the order of general practitioners—such a change might be easily provided for.

As it is possible that in the first setting out of such a system of medical reform many existing general practitioners would be found unwilling to forego the profits accruing from the sale of drugs, it would be desirable that the Society of Pharmacy should, upon the payment of a smaller fee, admit such persons as members of their Society.

It now comes to be considered whether the College of Physicians should have the power of conferring degrees, as well as granting diplomas. I cannot see any direct good to be gained by this, and if it were granted to the College of Physicians it must also be granted to the College of Surgeons.

The power of granting degrees seems rather to belong to Universities ; and I have before shown that a College of Medicine or of Law, or any one science or profession, cannot with propriety be called a University. The degrees of M.D., LL.D., D.D. of the Universities, implies, or ought to imply, that their possessors have undergone that general system of liberal education which is peculiar to these Universities with credit and respectability ; but have more especially dedicated their studies to that branch of learning which such degrees imply. The degree of LL.D. probably, as less necessarily pointing out any professional distinction, is the one which is usually conferred as a distinction of honour upon eminent men unconnected with the universities.

As the prolonged course of study required of a person to enter the field as a physician affords a greater amount of leisure time, it is probable that the majority of those who commenced life as physicians would have obtained some university degree before becoming Fellows of the College of Physicians. This probability would be still further increased by the fact of their having to wait till a more advanced age before the acquiring any considerable amount of private practice. Latterly some few members of our English universities have entered the College of Surgeons ; and it is likely that still larger numbers would enter it as Fellows of that College.

Again, the power of conferring degrees by the Colleges of Physicians and Surgeons might cause some little jealousy in the universities, a circumstance the rather to be avoided as the carrying out this plan of reform must necessarily demand a small sacrifice on their parts, which it is reasonable to hope and expect they would willingly yield for the public good.

Hitherto the power of the College of Physicians, though nominally extended to the whole country, has been virtually limited to London and its environs; and even within these scanty limitations has been barely able to maintain its powers. Now, should the power of the College be extended, as appears to me most desirable, to the whole of England, it would require of the Bachelors and Doctors of Medicine, even of our English universities, to seek and obtain its diploma before they could enter into practice.

It may be said this plan of medical reform applies only to England; how are the difficult'es with respect to Scotch, Irish, and foreign degrees to be got over? With respect to Scotland and Ireland I would answer, why not carry out there also the same measures? If not, for these and all other degrees, we have only to deal with them in this way. Our medical corporations require such and such an amount of professional education as a qualification for examination at their board. A candidate has only to bring certificates of such qualifications, and having creditably passed his examinations, will be admitted a practitioner. Failing to bring such qualifications, and not duly passing such examinations, he cannot become a qualified practitioner.

Much has been written and said on the subject of medical education. No doubt professional education is a subject of vast importance, both to the profession itself and to the public generally; but it is questionable in my mind, in a profession like our own, in which so much competition exists, and where individual success can only be fairly hoped for and expected in proportion to individual labour and exertion, whether professional education is not safer in the keeping of the heads of that profession than in a government, however well disposed and constituted. It is my humble opinion, therefore, that we only need the assistance of government to put our professional institutions on a proper footing, and to afford them that protection which is alike due to them and really useful to the community; and that we shall be found competent in ourselves so to regulate professional education as to send into the world a class of medical practitioners who shall, as a whole, richly deserve the gratitude and protection of the country, and do honour to the bodies corporate of which they are members.

Medical education, indeed, so far as the mere amount of knowledge is concerned, has of late years kept pace with the vast strides of the march of intellect. No great cry for medical reform has been uttered

throughout the country from without, on the plea of the ignorance and disqualification of medical men. No! the public are contented, and justly contented, with the amount of medical knowledge, and for the rest, are unfortunately not sufficiently interested in our existence as a learned body, devoting our best energies to the public good, to care much about us.

Passing over, therefore, briefly, the subject of medical education, as being but slightly connected with the first steps in medical reform, and as being a matter rather to be left to the profession itself, whether it shall experience these alterations, or whether it be destined to remain exactly in its present state, I may yet perhaps be pardoned for throwing out a few hints to those powers who now regulate, or in future may regulate, this important subject.

The best general education will always be found the best and surest foundation for a professional one. A good general education should, therefore, not only be encouraged, but even required, previously to entering upon professional studies. In conducting professional education, the great object to be attained should never be lost sight of. Now, as the great bulk of medical students are destined to be practitioners, their education should be eminently practical; it is therefore most desirable that, both in their education, and in their examinations, which are intended to test the effects of that education and their qualification to enter upon the duties of their profession, this point should never be lost sight of.

The importance of anatomical studies cannot be too strongly insisted upon, both in the education of the physician and the surgeon; for how can the physician otherwise read those symptoms of disease which are only explicable by the aid of anatomy and physiology, or how discern the slighter, or even coarser shades of disease in structures of whose healthy appearance even he is ignorant? and how can the surgeon direct his knife through a labyrinth of delicate structures, of whose relative position he knows nothing? Anatomical studies should therefore be commenced with in the first stage of medical education, and continued throughout its progress; the more so, in that opportunities are at this season offered to the student which but few will have the privilege of enjoying in after life.

In the universities, and other large schools of learning, it has long been observed that a series of minor examinations, at short intervals, greatly promote the acquirement and retention of knowledge, and it is with no small satisfaction that I have seen this hint adopted in some of our large hospitals. Such a plan might be advantageously instituted in the proceedings of our present or future boards of examiners for medical diplomas. A person is less likely to cram for a series of minor examinations than for one grand climacteric effort, with the over-coming of which the idler thinks his labours are to close. This plan might, with especial advantage, be applied to anatomical studies. Anatomy may be said to be learnt by the head and the eye; it does not require, therefore, great mental powers to acquire, but is difficult of retention. Now as anatomy is readily divisible into certain portions, it would be easy to examine the student the first year in one branch of anatomy, the second year in another branch, and finally in the whole subject.

One useful hint, which, if my memory serves me right, has been suggested by your-self, towards the rendering of the examination more practical, is, that the pupil to be examined might be left to investigate several cases, and then to put down on paper his diagnosis, prognosis, and the plan of treat-ment he would adopt.

I have now completed, as far as is in my power, a general outline of my views re-specting medical reform; I shall, however, beg your indulgence for one more letter upon a few more general subjects connected with our profession; and in the meanwhile believe me to remain, sir,

   Your obedient servant,
     PHILOMATHES.

April 5, 1843.

- - - - - - - - - - - - - - - - -

THE PHYSICIANS OF DANTZIC SIXTY YEARS SINCE.

THE character of our Danzig physicians of that day left my father not the faintest hope of effecting his purpose by their means. In the first place, they were all and several ex-tremely old, and petrified in obstinate pre-judices. Whether they had ever been young, where they had lived, and what they had done in their youth, I know not; but I can affirm, that up to the twelfth or fourteenth year of my life, I had never seen nor heard of a young physician. These reverend gen-tlemen enjoyed the title of excellency, and not only in their own houses and from their own servants, but in society generally; only very intimate friends could sometimes ven-ture on a respectful " Herr Doctor." Their head was covered by a snow-white, pow-dered, full-bottomed periwig, with three tails, one of which hung down the back, while the others floated on the shoulders. A scarlet coat embroidered with gold, very broad lace ruffles and frill, white or black silk stockings, knee and shoe buckles of sparkling stones, or silver gilt, and a little, flat, three-cocked hat under the arm, com-pleted the toilette of these excellencies. Add to this a pretty large cane, with a gold head, or mermaid carved in ivory, upon which, in difficult cases, to rest the chin—and cer-tainly every one will admit the impossibility of so much as thinking of an innovation in their presence.—*Edinburgh Review*, Feb. 1843, from Mad. Schopenhauer's *Jugend-leben.*

[The innovation alluded to is inoculation of the small-pox.]

- - - - - - - - - - - - - -

ANEURISM BY ANASTOMOSIS—LIGATURE—CURE.

A FEMALE child, ætat. three months, was brought to the hospital on the 14th Febru-ary, with an aneurism by anastomosis of moderate size, seated a little in front of the anterior fontanelle. The mother stated that at birth it was but just visible, that its growth latterly had been rapid, and that it was daily increasing. Two needles were passed transversely beneath the base of the tumor, taking care that they should enter, and pass out a little distance beyond the diseased structure, after which a ligature was drawn around its base sufficiently tight to strangulate it. Two days afterwards the pins were removed, and a poultice of slippery elm applied to hasten the separation of the slough. This came away on the following day, leaving a healthy ulcerated surface, which in a short time was completely cica-trised.

The mode of procedure adopted in the above case of transfixing the tumor by means of needles passed beneath it, at right angles with each other, and securing a liga-ture tightly around its base, is that which I usually employ, and is well adapted for the removal of all tumors of this kind, of mo-derate size; the operation being safe and quickly performed, and the pain caused by it but of short duration. The double liga-ture passed through the base of the tumor, which is often employed, may be followed by some hæmorrhage after the tightening of it, from the separation of the surfaces through which the needle is passed; besides which, the shape or situation of the nævus may be such, as to make it very difficult to fasten the ligature on either side around its base, entirely beyond the limits of the affec-tion. A single needle placed under the centre of the tumor is also generally insuf-ficient to procure the enclosure of all the diseased part within the loop of the ligature. —*American Journal.*

STATISTICAL ACCOUNT OF THE ACCIDENTS BROUGHT TO THE LONDON HOSPITAL DURING THE YEAR 1842.

Admitted as In-Patients...1783 In-Patients—Male...1273 Out-Patients—Male...2522
Treated as Out-Patients...3720 Female. 510 Female .1198

Total during the year.. 5503 Total In-Patients...1783 Total Out-Patients...3720

Consisting of the following Cases :

		IN-PATIENTS.			OUT-PATIENTS.		
	No.	Male.	Female.	Total.	Male.	Female.	Total.
‡ Fractures	840	314	100	414	270	156	426
Wounds	1042	180	63	243	574	225	799
Contusions	2141	417	160	577	1087	477	1564
Sprains	567	96	45	141	246	180	426
Burns	265	67	66	133	68	64	132
Dislocations . . .	97	17	5	22	61	14	75
Hernia	75	32	18	50	18	7	25
Bites of Dogs . . .	58	4	1	5	42	11	53
Concussions . . .	52	29	10	39	7	6	13
Attempts at Suicide .	38	19	19	38	..	...	...
Various	328	98	23	121	149	58	207
Total . .	5503	1273	510	1783	2522	1198	2720

Report of 1783 *In-Patients.*   ‡ *The Fractures consisted of the following.*

	Dis-charged Cured.	Re-main in Hos-pital.	Died.	Total.
Fractures . . .	379	24	11	414
Wounds	237	4	2	243
Contusions . . .	571	3	3	577
Sprains	140	...	1	141
Burns	95	33	5	133
Dislocations. . .	22	...	...	22
Hernia	42	8	...	50
Bites of Dogs . .	5	...	...	5
Concussions . .	37	2	...	39
Attempts at Suicide	33	5	...	38
Various	111	8	2	121
Total...	1672	87	24	1783

	In-Patients	Out-Patients	Total.
Skull . . .	18	...	18
Face . . .	10	2	12
Spine . . .	3	...	3
Ribs . . .	125	50	175
Pelvis . . .	4	...	4
Thigh . . .	53	4	57
Patella . . .	10	...	10
Leg . . .	128	5	133
Foot . . .	5	3	8
Shoulder-bone	5	9	14
Collar-bone .	7	122	129
Arm . . .	27	43	70
Fore Arm . .	12	141	153
Hand . . .	7	47	54
Total..	414	426	840

London Hospital, 16th February, 1843.

PARALYSIS IN TEETHING CHILDREN.

WHILST on a visit to the parish of West Feliciana, La., in the fall of 1841, my attention was called to a child about a year old, then slowly recovering from an attack of hemiplegia. The parents, (who were people of intelligence and unquestionable veracity,) told me that eight or ten other cases of either hemiplegia or paraplegia, had occurred during the preceding three or four months within a few miles of their residence, all of which had either completely recovered, or were decidedly improving. The little sufferers were invariably under two years of age, and the cause seemed to be the same in all—namely, *teething.*—Mr. G. Colmer, in *American Journal.*

MEDICAL REFORM.

NORTH OF ENGLAND MEDICAL ASSOCIATION.

At a meeting of the Council of this Association, held at Newcastle-on-Tyne, Wednesday, April 12, 1843 (Dr. Headlam, president, in the chair), it was resolved unanimously, on the motion of Dr. Brown, of Sunderland, seconded by Dr. Charlton, of Newcastle :—

" That the cordial thanks of this meeting be given to Sir James Clark, Bart. for the able manner in which he has advocated the welfare and improvement of the medical profession, in the letters recently addressed by him to the Right Honourable the Secretary of State for the Home Department."

Resolved, on the motion of Dr. Knott, of Newcastle, seconded by T. M. Greenhow, Esq. :—

" That the foregoing resolution be forwarded to the Editors of the Lancet, Medical Gazette, and Provincial Medical Journal, with a request they will cause it to be inserted in their respective periodicals."

DR. RICHARD BUDD.

This gentleman, a brother of Dr. Budd, of King's College, has just been elected Physician to the North Devon Infirmary, in the room of Dr. Britton, resigned.

ROYAL COLLEGE OF SURGEONS.

LIST OF GENTLEMEN ADMITTED MEMBERS.

Friday, April 12, 1843.

T. Morris.—J. Kilner.—J. Machen.—J. Stevens.—A. Eccles.—A. W. Williams.—J. Whitterow.—H. H. Radcliffe.—F. P. Bowen.

APOTHECARIES' HALL.

LIST OF GENTLEMEN WHO HAVE RECEIVED CERTIFICATES.

Thursday, April 13, 1843.

A. Lloyd.—T. B. Stone, Leighton Buzzard.—E. H. Peters, Fairford.—E. Jones, Dolgelley.—R. Brown, Cobham.—H. Callaway, Tottenham.—T. Graham, Pinner, Middlesex.—R. Worsley, Blandford. — B. V. Asbury. — T. H. Baker, Kirkby de la Parks.—T. B. Oldfield, Warley, Yorkshire.—J. A. Carr.

A TABLE OF MORTALITY FOR THE METROPOLIS,

Shewing the number of deaths from all causes registered in the week ending Saturday, April 8, 1843.

Small Pox	9
Measles	20
Scarlatina	21
Hooping Cough	45
Croup	7
Thrush	3
Diarrhœa	5
Dysentery	2
Cholera	1
Influenza	1
Typhus	56
Erysipelas	3
Syphilis	0
Hydrophobia	0
Diseases of the Brain, Nerves, and Senses	154
Diseases of the Lungs and other Organs of Respiration	242
Diseases of the Heart and Blood-vessels	20
Diseases of the Stomach, Liver, and other Organs of Digestion	54
Diseases of the Kidneys, &c.	6
Childbed	4
Ovarian Dropsy	0
Disease of Uterus, &c.	0
Rheumatism	3
Diseases of Joints, &c.	4
Ulcer	0
Fistula	0
Diseases of Skin, &c.	0
Diseases of Uncertain Seat	84
Old Age or Natural Decay	83
Deaths by Violence, Privation, or Intemperance	24
Causes not specified	1
Deaths from all Causes	855

METEOROLOGICAL JOURNAL.

Kept at EDMONTON, *Latitude* 51° 37' 3$_2$"N. *Longitude* 0° 3' 51" W. *of Greenwich.*

April 1843.	THERMOMETER.		BAROMETER.	
Wednesday 5	from 39 to 55		29·62 to	29·85
Thursday . 6	35	56	29·82	29·63
Friday . . 7	50	57	29·51	Stat.
Saturday . 8	46	56	29·44	29·53
Sunday . . 9	48	39	29·55	29·63
Monday . 10	29	51	29·81	29·85
Tuesday . 11	24	46	29·88	29·93
April.				
Wednesday 12	from 23 to 46		29·87 to	29·83
Thursday . 13	29	46	29·72	29·86
Friday . . 14	26	53	29·81	29·94
Saturday . 15	43	60	30·04	30·02
Sunday . . 16	47	60	29·90	29·78
Monday . . 17	43	63	29·79	29·99
Tuesday . . 18	32	62	30·04	30·01

Wind, very variable ; S.W. prevailing. 5th, clear. 6th and 7th, cloudy, with a little rain. 8th, clear. 9th, cloudy till the evening. 10th, 11th, and 12th, generally clear. 13th, generally cloudy, snow in the morning. 14th and 15th, generally cloudy. 16th, 17th, and 18th, generally clear.

Rain fallen, ·36 of an inch.

CHARLES HENRY ADAMS.

WILSON & OGILVY, 57, Skinner Street, London.

THE

LONDON MEDICAL GAZETTE,

BEING A

WEEKLY JOURNAL

OF

Medicine and the Collateral Sciences.

FRIDAY, APRIL 28, 1843.

LUMLEIAN LECTURES

DELIVERED AT THE

COLLEGE OF PHYSICIANS,

MARCH 1843,

BY GEORGE BURROWS, M.D.
Physician to St. Bartholomew's Hospital.

——

LECTURE I.

Introduction. Modifications which the circulation within the cranium is capable of undergoing in health and disease. Opinions of Abercrombie, Kellie, Clutterbuck, Watson, and others, on the peculiarities of the circulation within the cranium. Quantity of blood within the cranium said to be nearly invariable. Experiments of Dr. Kellie to show that hæmorrhage does not deplete the vessels of the brain. Repetition of the experiments; whence it appears that anæmia of the brain is induced by fatal hæmorrhage. Experiments to show the striking effects of posture and gravitation on the quantity of blood within the cranium. Pathological and practical inferences from the foregoing experiments. Observations and experiments to determine the amount of congestion of the brain, when death takes place by Apnœa. Absence of cerebral congestion in some cases of death by suspension. Explanation of the anomaly.

IN addressing you, Sir, and the members of the College, on the present occasion, I think it is due to you and myself to premise, that, when the president, last autumn, did me the honour to select me as the Lumleian lecturer, I accepted the office with considerable reluctance, from the apprehension that my public duties during the winter months would unavoidably prevent the preparation of any thing worthy of being delivered from this chair, and before such an audience. It

is a bold attempt, and one of no ordinary difficulty, to satisfy the expectations of the learned, who have assembled here to listen to a dissertation on a subject with which they are already familiar; perhaps more so, than he who addresses them, *ex cathedrâ*.

We learn from the first oration of Demosthenes against Philip of Macedon, how much difficulty that great orator experienced in commanding the attention of his gifted countrymen, when their vital interests were at stake; and he thus describes the Athenians of his time—" περιιόντες αὑτοῦ, πυνθάνεσθαι, κατὰ τὴν ἀγορὰν, λέγεταί τι καινον;" no doubt most of you have hesitated before you would sacrifice this hour, and have as you passed " κατὰ τὴν ἀγορὰν," enquired λέγεταί τι καινόν; will he tell us any thing new? That it was only with such temptation of novelties that Athenians willingly spent their time, we learn from a higher authority. When St. Paul visited Greece, he found the Athenians so superior in intellectual acquirements to all their contemporaries, " εἰς οὐδὲν ἕτερον ἐυκαίρουν, ἢ λέγειν τι καὶ ἀκούειν καινότερον." Well do I understand that you do not willingly give your attendance here, unless it be to hear (τι καινότερον) " something rather novel." How shall I attempt to satisfy your expectations in this respect? I will at least endeavour to perform the duties of a pioneer, and remove some errors which have long tended to obstruct our advances in the pathology of a most important organ—the brain.

The pathology of the brain and spinal cord has, indeed, of late years derived great and valuable elucidation from the improved physiology of these nervous centres. The functions of particular parts of the cerebro-spinal system have been clearly pointed out by a succession of experimentalists following in the path which was first so successfully trodden by our distinguished countryman, the late Sir Charles Bell. But the simplification of the pathology of many complex affections of these organs, which, although

804.—XXXII.

L

bearing considerable resemblance in their symptoms, are in essence very different, "facies non omnibus una, nec diversatamen:" this has I believe been effected principally by Dr. Marshall Hall. While great progress has been made in the diagnosis of nervous affections, particularly in reference to the real source of irritation to the nervous centres, it appears to me that there has not been a corresponding advance in our pathology of affections of the brain depending on the state of the circulation in that organ.

I therefore propose, in this and the succeeding lectures, to inquire, first; what modifications the circulation in the brain is capable of undergoing in health and disease: secondly; how far the central organ of the circulation, the heart, when its circulating powers are increased or diminished, is capable of disturbing the functions of the brain, and in what manner these changes in the circulation affect the brain : and thirdly ; I shall call your attention to a class of diseases of the heart, which are often overlooked, and which create great disturbance in the functions of the brain, or rather of the cerebro-spinal system.

Many physicians of high philosophical attainments have directed their attention to the peculiarities of the circulation within the cranium ; and they, from experiments, and reasonings founded on the mechanical construction of the cranium, have arrived at the conclusion, that the absolute quantity of blood within the cranium is at all times nearly the same.

Pathologists, in apparent opposition to this conclusion, are in the habit of describing congestions of the blood-vessels of the brain, states of hyperæmia of that organ, and so on; while practical men are continually speaking of determination of blood to the heart, of plethora of the cerebral vessels; and assuming that such states actually exist, they employ various remedies to diminish these supposed conditions of repletion.

It will, I think, be not without interest and instruction, if we more closely investigate on what grounds the brain has been supposed to be exempted from these variations in the quantity of blood in its vessels, which are generally admitted to be such frequent pathological conditions of the vascular system in other organs.

This doctrine of the invariable quantity of blood within the cranium, was first asserted, as far as I can ascertain, by the second Monro, at Edinburgh. His opinions on this subject are recorded in his work on the Brain and Nervous System. He observes,[*] " as the substance of the brain, like that of the other solids of our body, is nearly in-

compressible, the quantity of blood within the head must be the same at all times, whether in health or disease, in life or after death, those cases only excepted in which water or other matter is effused or secreted from the blood-vessels ; for in these cases, a quantity of blood, equal in bulk to the effused matter, will be pressed out of the cranium."[*] Such was the opinion of Monro : others who have followed him have pushed this doctrine to a much greater extent.

Monro used to illustrate this doctrine by exhibiting a glass-ball filled with water, and desiring his pupils to remark that not a drop of the fluid escaped when its aperture was inverted.

In an appendix to Dr. Abercrombie's admirable work, entitled " Pathological and Practical Researches on the Brain and Spinal Cord," he has given, under the modest title of " Conjectures in regard to the Circulation in the Brain," some most interesting and original views on this point of physiology. Dr. Abercrombie informs his readers that his views are primarily founded on the appearances of the brain in animals which have been bled to death. " While in such animals all the other organs have been completely drained of blood, the brain has in general presented, in this respect, its usual appearance, and in some cases the superficial cerebral veins have even been found distended."

On the other hand, when similar experiments were repeated on other animals after a small opening had been made in the cranium by the trephine, the brain was found as much drained of blood as any other part of the body. Dr. Abercrombie quotes as his authority for these remarkable conditions of the brain, the experiments of Dr. Kellie, detailed in Vol. I. of the Transactions of the Medico-Chirurgical Society of Edinburgh.

These unexpected phænomena may, according to Dr. Abercrombie, be explained by reference to the peculiarities in the structure of the head. " The cranium," he observes[†], " is a complete sphere of bone, which is exactly filled by its contents, the brain, and by which the brain is closely shut up from atmospheric pressure, and from all influence from without, except what is communicated through the blood-vessels which enter it. In an organ so situated it is probable that the quantity of blood circulating in its vessels cannot be materially increased, except something give way to make room for the additional quantity, because the cavity is already completely full; and it is probable that the quantity cannot be ma-

---

* Observations, &c. on Nervous System. Alexander Monro, M.D. 1783.

* Medico-Chirurgical Transactions of Edinburgh, vol. i. p. 2.
† Op. cit. p. 302.

terially diminished except something entered to supply the space which would become vacant. Upon the whole, then, I think we may assume the position as being in the highest degree probable, that, in the ordinary state of the parts, no material change can take place in the absolute quantity of blood circulating in the vessels of the brain."

The accuracy of the experiments of Dr. Kellie, and his inferences from them, have not only been adopted by Dr. Abercrombie, and explained by arguments founded on the immutable laws of physics, but they have also been sanctioned by some of the first medical authorities of the present day.

Dr. Watson* entertains the opinion that the brain is the only organ which, under the ordinary state of the parts, contains at all times the same quantity, or very nearly the same quantity, of blood. "This depends," remarks Dr. Watson, "upon the mechanical construction of the cranium, and is capable of explanation upon the known principles of hydraulics." "This conclusion, which would be arrived at by à priori reasoning, is confirmed by certain very curious experiments performed by Dr. Kellie, of Leith, from which we learn that, in animals bled to death, the brain presented its ordinary appearance, or even seemed to contain more blood in its superficial vessels than usual; and in one instance the sinuses were loaded with dark blood, and the pia mater injected with florid blood."

Other modern writers on the pathology of the brain have carried these theories of Dr. Kellie and Dr. Abercrombie still further. Thus we find it stated by Dr. Clutterbuck, in his article on Cerebral Apoplexy, in the Cyclopædia of Practical Medicine, " that no additional quantity of blood can be admitted into the vessels situated in the brain, the cavity of the skull being already completely filled by its contents. A plethoric state, or over-fulness of the cerebral vessels altogether, though often talked of, can have no real existence ; not, on the other hand, can the quantity of blood within the vessels of the brain be diminished. No abstraction of blood, therefore, whether it be-from the arm or other part of the general system, or from the jugular veins (and still less from the temporal arteries), can have any effect on the blood-vessels of the brain, so as to lessen the absolute quantity of blood contained within them."

Thus Dr. Clutterbuck not merely adopts the opinion of Dr. Abercrombie, that in the ordinary state of the parts no material change can take place in the quantity of blood in the vessels of the brain, but he maintains that no abstraction of blood can lessen the quantity of blood in them.

Dr. Kellie's experiments (as quoted by

* Lectures on Medicine, MED. GAZ. VOL. 27.

Dr. Abercrombie) are cited by Dr. Clutterbuck in support of his opinions.

Such, then, are the physiological doctrines with respect to the peculiarities of the circulation in the cranium, which have been promulgated by many distinguished writers and teachers of the present day.

One and all appear to refer to the experiments of Dr. Kellie, and to the mechanical structure of the cranium, in support of this theory of the invariable quantity of blood in the vessels of the cranium. Permit me, then, now to draw your attention to the experiments and conclusions of Dr. Kellie, as they stand recorded in the Transactions of the Medico-Chirurgical Society of Edinburgh, Vol. I. I am more strongly induced to give an abstract of these experiments, because I suspect that most writers on this subject, subsequent to the publication of Dr. Abercrombie's work, have been satisfied with his allusions to the experiments of Dr. Kellie, and that few have taken the trouble to analyse the original account of them in the work just alluded to. As I proceed with this abstract, I shall detail analogous experiments performed by myself. The physiological conclusions deduced from them will contrast very forcibly with the opinions on this peculiarity of the cerebral circulation which have been maintained by Dr. Abercrombie, Dr. Kellie, and other modern British authors.

Dr. Kellie performed a series of experiments, from which he inferred—

1. That a state of bloodlessness is not discovered in the brains of animals which have died by hæmorrhage ; but, on the contrary, very commonly a state of venous cerebral congestion.

2. That the quantity of blood in the cerebral vessels is not affected by gravitation, or posture of the head.

3. That congestion of the cerebral vessels is not found in those instances where it might be most expected ; as in persons who die by hanging, strangulation, suffocation, &c.

4. That if there be repletion or depletion of one set of vessels (arteries or veins) in the cranium, there will be an opposite condition of the other set of vessels.

I shall proceed, first, to detail a few of the experiments performed by Dr. Kellie, and from which he has concluded that, when death takes place by hæmorrhage, it has not the effect of depleting the cerebral vessels ; but, on the contrary, that in such cases the cerebral veins contain as much, or even more, blood than is usual.

Dr. Kellie's experiments are enumerated by letters. We will take the experiment E.

" In this experiment both carotids of a sheep were tied, and four minutes after the jugular veins opened. The quantity of blood lost was ℥xxxviij., when the animal died. The heart contained no appreciable quantity of blood. The sinuses of the brain were in their usual state; those at the basis contained less blood than had been found in similar experiments, and the veins on the hemispheres were less filled; the choroid plexus was pale and empty: the vessels on the basis of the cerebrum were better filled, and those on the basis cerebelli minutely injected."

EXP. II.—" A dog was bled to death from the carotids, having lost ℥xxxvij. of blood. The viscera in general were well drained of their blood. The dura mater contained little blood: the lateral sinuses were, however, well filled. On the pia mater were several vessels of a florid colour, but not turgid. This brain seemed upon the whole more depleted than usual."

Now contrast the appearances of the vascular system of the brain in the two foregoing experiments, where the animals died by hæmorrhage, with the condition of the brain in two other animals, where death was caused by other means.

EXP. L.—Both carotids and both jugulars were tied in a dog, an operation which it survived twelve hours. The vessels of the dura mater were remarkably turgid, and all the sinuses much loaded with blood. Both the larger and the smaller vessels of the pia mater were fully injected with red blood. Not only the pia mater through its whole extent, but the cineritious substance, had a suffused, reddened, and, as it were, bloodshot appearance. "In short," writes Dr. K., " this brain was gorged with blood in all its minuter vessels," and was obviously in a very different state of vascularity to those of animals bled to death in the experiments E and H.

Let us analyse another experiment (M). In this a dog was poisoned with prussic acid. "The sinuses and veins were found loaded and congested, and the brain was every where turgid with blood. It was quite evident (writes Dr. Kellie) that this brain, and that of the dog (L), contained, beyond all doubt or dispute, a much larger quantity of red blood than the brains of any of the animals which had been bled to death. These comparative experiments afforded us the most satisfactory proof that the other brains had been really depleted by bleeding, and their vessels drained of a very sensible proportion of the red blood usually contained by them." (Page 115, op. cit.)

The summary of these observations is thus stated: that though we cannot entirely or nearly empty the vessels of the brain, as we can the vessels of the other parts of the body, it is yet possible, by profuse hæmorrhage, to drain it of a sensible portion of its red blood. If, instead of bleeding usque ad mortem, we were to bleed animals more

sparingly but repeatedly, there is no doubt that we should succeed in draining the brain of a much larger quantity of red blood, although serous effusion would be increased.

It may, then, appear surprising that Dr. Kellie has been so often quoted as asserting the brain cannot be depleted by blood-letting, when we find him stating, his experiments satisfactorily proved that these brains had really been depleted by bleeding, and their vessels drained of a very sensible proportion of the blood usually contained in them. But in opposition to the conclusions drawn from these experiments, we find, in a subsequent communication to the Medico-Chirurgical Society of Edinburgh, Dr. Kellie affirming " that, in the ordinary state of the parts, we cannot lessen, to any considerable extent, the quantity of blood within the cranium by arteriotomy or venesection;" whereas, if the skull of an animal be trephined, then hæmorrhage will leave very little blood in the brain.

This apparent contradiction between the results of experiments and subsequent statements induced me to repeat the experiment of bleeding animals to death, and comparing the state of the cerebral blood-vessels in them and in animals which had died from other causes.

In justice to myself I wish to state that, if I could have found any series of experiments, performed by others, which corroborated or invalidated the opinions of Drs. Abercrombie and Kellie, I should have refrained from the needless repetition of similar experiments on living animals. I have, however, up to the present time, fruitlessly searched for any additional information on this interesting point in physiology, a point which has such direct bearings on practical medicine. I had anticipated finding in Dr. Marshall Hall's work "On the Effects of Loss of Blood," the desired information; but it does not appear that, at the time of the publication of that volume, the author had made any examination into the state of the blood-vessels of the brain after hæmorrhage; for he remarks " that we are altogether in want of a series of observations on the effects of loss of blood on the internal organs." Thus disappointed in my search for information on this subject, I determined to resort to fresh experiments.

On the 11th of January, 1843, I killed two well-grown rabbits. The one (A) by opening the jugular vein and carotid artery on one side of the throat; the other (B) was strangled. Each animal died violently convulsed. A ligature was drawn tightly round the throat of the rabbit (A) immediately it expired, to prevent any further escape of blood from the vessels of the head. The rabbits were allowed to remain twenty-four hours on a table resting on their sides.

While the blood was flowing from the rabbit (A), the conjunctiva was observed to become pallid, and the eyeballs to shrink within the sockets. Upon the examination of the head of this rabbit, the integuments and muscles appeared blanched and exsanguined. Upon removing the upper portions of the cranium, the membranes of the brain were found pallid, and scarcely the trace of a blood-vessel was to be detected on the surface of the brain. The longitudinal and lateral sinuses were nearly empty of blood, and their course was not denoted by any colour of blood. Upon making sections of the brain, the interior appeared equally exsanguined.

Soon after the cord was drawn tight round the throat of the rabbit (B), the conjunctiva became congested, the eye-balls turgid, prominent, and even projecting beyond the margin of their sockets. The integuments and muscles of the head were found full of blood. Upon opening the cranium, the superficial vessels of the membranes, as well as the sinuses, were full of dark liquid blood. The whole substance of this brain, and its membranes, appeared of a dark reddish hue, as if stained by extravasated blood.

The contrast between the two brains in point of vascularity, both on the surface and the interior, was most striking*. In the one scarcely the trace of a blood-vessel was to be seen; in the other every vessel was turgid with blood. It seems hardly necessary to bring forward further evidence to prove that death by hæmorrhage has a most decided effect in depleting the vessels, and reducing the quantity of blood within as well as upon the outside of the cranium.

I have, however, repeated the experiments with similar results†. In fairness to Dr. Kellie I should state, that I have attended at the slaughtering of sheep by butchers, and find the brains of those animals much less depleted than the brains of rabbits which have died by hæmorrhage. But these sheep did not die from simple loss of blood; but partly from division of the pneumogastric nerves, and cervical portion of the spinal cord. These lesions, no doubt, influenced the appearances.

Hence it is not a fallacy, as some suppose, that bleeding diminishes the actual quantity of blood in the cerebral vessels. By abstraction of blood we not only diminish the momentum of blood in the cerebral arteries, and the quantity supplied to the brain in a given time, but we actually diminish the quantity of blood in those vessels. Whether the vacated space is replaced by serum, or

resiliency of the cerebral substance under diminished pressure, is another question, into which I do not now enter.

2dly.—Dr. Kellie, assuming the cranium to be a perfect sphere, proceeds to show that the quantity of blood in the cerebral vessels is not affected by posture.

"I think," writes Dr. K. "it quite certain, at least in a previously sound and healthy condition of the brain and its vessels, no change of posture can impel into, or confine more or less blood within, those vessels than naturally belongs to them; though I am willing to allow that the general pressure of the circulating fluid may in this way be, under certain circumstances, increased or diminished, and the circulation through the head accelerated, retarded, or disturbed."

In order to ascertain, as far as such an experiment can do, the total effect of the gravitation of the blood upon the vessels of the brain, Dr. K., immediately after administering a destructive dose of prussic acid to two dogs, suspended the one by the heels, and the other by the ears. He allowed them to remain thus suspended for 18 hours, when they were taken down for examination.

The effects of posture on the parts exterior to the skull Dr. K. reports to be very great. In the former animal the integuments and their vessels were filled and congested to the greatest possible degree; the integuments of the head of the second dog were pale, and the vessels empty. "Within the head," continues Dr. K., "the contrast was but trifling. The sinuses beyond all doubt were loaded in the first case, and rather empty in the other; the difference of appearance in other parts of the brain was but little striking." Dr. Kellie's own words, as to the condition of the sinuses in the two animals, assured me that posture had a much greater effect on vascular congestion of the brain than he was willing to admit. I therefore repeated his experiment.

On the 28th of December, 1842, two full-grown rabbits were killed by prussic acid, and, while their hearts were still pulsating, the one (C) was suspended by the ears, the other (D) by the hind legs. They were left suspended for 24 hours; and, before they were taken down for examination, a tight ligature was placed round the throat of each rabbit, to prevent, as effectually as was possible, any further flow of blood to or from the head, after they were removed from their respective positions.

In the rabbit (C) the whole of the external parts of the head, the ears, the eye-balls, &c. were pallid and flaccid; the muscles of the scalp and bones of the cranium were also remarkably exsanguined. Upon opening the cranium, the membranes and substance of the brain were pallid, the sinuses and other vessels were exsanguined; anæmic beyond my expectation.

---

* Coloured drawings of the brains of these animals were exhibited.

† The craniums of these rabbits opened were exhibited for inspection.

In the rabbit (D) the external parts of the head, the ears, eye-balls, &c. were turgid, livid, and congested. The muscles and bones of the cranium were of a dark hue, and gorged with blood, which at some parts appeared extravasated. Upon opening the cranium, the membranes and vessels were dark and turgid with liquid blood ; the superficial veins were prominent, the longitudinal and lateral sinuses were gorged with dark blood, and there was staining of the tissues, if not extravasation of blood into the membranes. The substance of the brain was uniformly dark, and congested to a remarkable extent.

Dr. Kellie asserts, but I think his experiments do not support him, that the contrast in the appearances within the heads of the two animals was but trifling. In my analogous experiments the contrast was most striking. In the one was to be seen a most complete state of anæmia of the internal as well as external parts of the cranium ; in the other a most intense hyperæmia or congestion of the same parts ; and these opposite conditions in the vascularity of the brain induced solely by posture, and the consequent gravitation of the blood*.

If the cranium were the perfect sphere, as taught by Monro, and as subsequently maintained by Abercrombie and other distinguished writers on the pathology of the brain, these effects on its circulation (which I have now exhibited) ought not to have resulted from the force of gravity on the blood in the cerebral vessels.

From the foregoing experiments it would appear, that the principle of the subsidence of fluids after death operates on the parts contained within the cranium, as well as upon those situated in the thorax or abdomen.

It is well known that, in former times, the stains, or sugillations as they are technically termed, which are discovered on the integuments of the under parts of a corpse, were not unfrequently mistaken for the effects of violence done to the body during life. Within a more recent period the cadaveric congestions of the posterior part of the lungs and of depending convolutions of the intestines have been mistaken for the effects of inflammation. M. Orfila and M. Trousseau have done much to dissipate those pathological errors. In the article " Pseudo-morbid appearances," Cyclopædia of Practical Medicine, I find Dr. Todd gives a caution, that, in estimating the colour of the cerebral substance, allowance must be

made for the quantity of fluid blood in that viscus, as well as for the position in which the head of the corpse has been laid since death. I hence infer that this able anatomist coincides in the opinion that the quantity of blood in the brain varies during life, and is affected by posture after death. It may now be inferred that the encephalon is not exempt from this law in physics—the gravitation of the fluids to the lowest parts of the corpse.

The discovery of the operation of this force on the blood within the cranium after death, suggests a precaution very essential to be followed, when it is desired to ascertain the precise amount of congestion of the cerebral vessels at the time of death. In such cases a ligature should be placed around the throat of the corpse, and drawn sufficiently tight to compress the cervical vessels, and arrest all flow of blood through them. This precaution will be most required in the examination of bodies, where, from the kind of death, the blood may be suspected to remain fluid in the heart and great blood-vessels. The depending or elevated position of the head during the examination of the body will not then induce deceptive appearances, which mislead us in our conclusions as to the previous amount of congestion in the cerebral vessels.

The third argument against the occasional repletion of the vessels within the cranium is founded on the reported condition of these vessels in those kinds of death where cerebral congestion might have been fairly anticipated, as in death by hanging, suffocation, drowning, and so on ; or in death by asphyxia, as it was formerly termed, but more correctly by apnœa. In support of this position, that cerebral congestion is not discovered when death takes place by asphyxia or apnœa, Dr. Kellie adduces an account of the appearances in the bodies of two pirates, who were hung at Leith, and dissected by Monro and himself. The bodies were examined while yet warm ; the limbs were not rigid ; the countenances livid, and the eyeballs suffused. In each body, on the division of the scalp, blood flowed from its vessels in such quantity as to afford ample proof of congestion of the external parts of the head. The sinuses of the dura mater contained no extraordinary quantity of blood ; the large vessels on the surface of the brain were but moderately filled ; the pia mater was paler and less vascular than it is found in ordinary cases. No sooner was the brain removed from the skull, than the blood, yet warm, began to rise, and flow profusely from the divided sinuses and vessels at the base of the skull : about one pint of fluid blood thus escaped, and coagulated on the floor.

That the brain and its membranes are not necessarily congested in the bodies of those

* Coloured drawings of the brains of these animals were exhibited, as well as the craniums of two other animals killed in the same way, and then laid open for comparison. The effects of posture on the quantity of blood in the cerebral vessels were also exhibited by drawings made from the brains of animals killed by placing a ligature around the trachea, and then suspending the one animal by the ears, but leaving the other resting on its side.

who have died by hanging, is corroborated by the detail of the condition of these parts in the body of Bishop, the resurrection-man, who was hung for the murder of Carlo Ferrier, in Nov. 1832. Dr. Watson states[*], that the integuments of the head and face were turgid with blood ; the inner surface of the scalp and outer surface of the skull red and bloody ; very dark-coloured blood ran from the divided integuments ; but when the bones of the head were sawn through, and the skull-cap removed, the large veins of the brain did not appear unnaturally full.

One more instance, equally worthy of credit, may be cited in proof of this condition of the vessels of the brain of those who have died by hanging. M. Esquirol gives the following account of these parts in the body of a woman who hung herself, and was found suspended six hours after death. The face was livid and bloated ; the scalp was loaded with fluid blood, while the membranes of the brain were slightly vascular, and the brain itself natural.

The appearances in the brains of these persons who died by hanging would appear to support the opinion that the cerebral vessels are not congested or overloaded in those cases where such a condition might be fairly expected. But, in opposition to such a conclusion, it would not be difficult to cite numerous well-authenticated instances of death by hanging, where the brain and its membranes have presented all the usual appearances of congestion, and even of apoplexy, to a striking extent. In the late Dr. Cooke's learned work on Nervous Diseases (which was the substance of his Croonian Lectures, delivered at the College in 1819), there will be found some remarkable examples of this kind. Sir B. C. Brodie informed Dr. Cooke, that he found congestion and extravasation of blood to a large amount in the brain of a man who had been hanged. The late Dr. Hooper had in his collection the brain of a person who died by hanging, and which exhibited the effusion of a great deal of blood into the membranes. M. Portal reports that, upon the examination of the bodies of persons who had been hanged, and which were brought to him for anatomical purposes, at Paris, a large quantity of blood was found in the vessels of the brain, or extravasated into that viscus.

But I would fain relate the pathological appearances in one other case of death by suspension ; because, from the rank of the individual, and the peculiar circumstances under which he died, the examination of the body was made with the most scrupulous attention by several scientific men, well qualified for their task.

In the autumn of 1830, a few months after the French Revolution, the Duke de Bourbon, the last of the Condés, was found dead in his bed-chamber, suspended by a couple of cravats to the fastening of his window shutter. His toes were slightly resting on the floor, which posture of the body, together with the advanced age of the Prince, his known infirmities, and certain political reasons, led to the suspicion that he had been murdered, and afterwards suspended, to give the appearance of suicide. His body was carefully examined by MM. Marc, Marjolin, Pasquier, and others. They reported[*] that the vessels on the surface of the brain, especially on the anterior lobes, were gorged with dark *fluid* blood Three ounces of serum were found in the ventricles and membranes of the brain. The lungs were also gorged with black *fluid* blood. The cavities of the heart devoid of blood. It was their opinion that the Duke had destroyed himself by hanging, and that death was induced by the *accumulation* and stagnation of blood *in the brain* and lungs.

But let it not be supposed that I have adduced these examples of cerebral congestion and cerebral hæmorrhage, in individuals who have died by hanging, in support of the theory that in this kind of death life is destroyed by apoplexy. It is well ascertained that obstruction to respiration is the principal cause of death in such cases. I have adduced these examples of intense cerebral congestion, where death was caused by hanging, to contrast with those other instances which have been cited as proofs that cerebral congestion is not found after this mode of death.

That an intense congestion of the cerebral vessels is discovered after death, produced by various kinds of obstruction to respiration, is manifest from the experiments and drawings which I now offer to your notice by way of illustration[†]. But how are we to account for the undoubted occasional absence of this congestion of the cerebral vessels in those who have died by hanging?

When criminals are hung by the executioner, the knot of the rope is usually adjusted on one side of the neck ; and it is found, after death, beneath the ear, resting on the mastoid process. It has been often observed, in the dissection of such criminals, that the cheek and integuments on this same side of the head are not near so livid and congested as on the other side. The pressure of the rope has not completely obstructed the return of blood through the external jugular vein on the one side, although it has effectually stopped the current on the other. In such cases it is probable

* Annals d'Hygiène, Vol. 5.
† Drawings to illustrate—Death by strangulation ; death by ligature on the trachea ; death by drowning.

---

* Lectures on Medicine, MED. GAZ. Vol. 27.

that the deep-seated internal jugular vein on the one side has only been partially compressed, and has permitted to a certain extent the return of blood from the internal parts of the cranium.

But there is another still more efficient cause of this occasional absence of congestion of the cerebral vessels after death by hanging; it is the subsidence of the *fluid* blood after death, while the body is yet suspended, through the cervical vessels which are not completely obliterated by the pressure of the cord. And it should be recollected, there are some channels which are scarcely if at all affected by the compression of the rope. These other channels are the vertebral sinuses, and spinal plexus of veins, so ably delineated by M. Breschet. Well may we adopt the language of Haller, in describing this complex contrivance to carry off the blood from the nervous centres :—
" Magna pulchritudo est sinuum, qui duræ matri medullæ spinalis adcumbunt, venæque. potius sunt, quam sinus," writes Haller; and after describing the circular distribution of these vessels, and their free communication with the cervical, intercostal, lumbar, and sacral veins, he says, " Eorum annulorum supremus cranioque proximus, cum sinubus occipitalibus et cum fossis jugularibus unitur." From this description we learn that the sinuses of the cranium may be drained through these vertebral sinuses. (Illustrated by diagram.)

Having already directed attention to what extent gravitation alone can deplete the cerebral vessels after the heart has ceased to beat, it cannot now be a matter of surprise that, in some of those who die by hanging, and whose bodies remain suspended for a considerable length of time after death. the fluid blood should gravitate, and that the " large veins should not appear unnaturally full," or even less distended than in some ordinary cases.

But the true state of the cerebral vessels in the bodies of those who have died by hanging, is often incorrectly estimated, from the anxiety to examine the lesions produced by the compression of the rope on the larynx and trachea, as well as the condition of the heart and lungs. In making such examinations all the great vessels of the neck are usually cut across, and the thoracic organs removed from the body before the head is examined. While the head is elevated during the operation of removing the skullcap and examining the brain, the *fluid* blood gravitates from the cranium, and pours from the divided cervical vessels into the chest ; and then, to the surprise of the by-standers, " the sinuses of the dura-mater, and the larger veins on the surface, are found but moderately filled," or " do not appear unnaturally full."

That these, are the causes tending to diminish the congestion of the cerebral vessels, when death takes place by hanging, appears to me probable from the intense congestion of the same vessels discovered in other examples of apnœa, where life is annihilated by obstruction to respiration, and where gravitation has had no effect upon the blood in the cranium.

These appearances are exhibited in the drawings made from the brains of animals that died by strangulation and suffocation, and which are exposed for inspection.

The deductions from the foregoing experiments are supported by the authority of one of the best and most recent writers on asphyxia. Dr. Carpenter states,[*] that when death is produced by the forcible compression of a ligature round the neck, to such an extent as to impede or prevent respiration, the veins and sinuses of the head partake of the general venous congestion ; and in well-marked cases an unusual number of red points are seen on slicing the brain. An apoplectic extravasation is sometimes, though rarely, found in simple asphyxia, but is more frequent in death by hanging or strangulation.

" It can scarcely be doubted," writes Dr. Carpenter, " that these variations in the congestion of the brain depend principally on the mode in which the ligature is applied to the neck :" and from a series of experiments detailed in the Annales d'Hygiène, Vol. 8, it would appear that the apoplectic condition of the brain is less likely to be found in proportion to the proximity of the ligature to the lower jaw, which is its exact situation in death by hanging. Enough has been said on this point of the pathology of the brain, to prove that, in the majority of instances, when death takes place by strangling, hanging, suffocation, drowning, and so on, that a congestion of the cerebral vessels is found after death. The same condition of the brain is also found after death from those diseases which obstruct the return of venous blood from the brain. And where such congested state of the cerebral vessels is not marked in cases of death by apnœa, the absence of congestion may often be accounted for from the subsidence of the blood, which is facilitated by its fluidity, and the posture of the body after death.

I must now postpone the further consideration of this subject until the next opportunity of addressing you.

----

* Asphyxia: Library of Medicine.

LECTURES
ON THE
PHYSICAL AND PATHOLOGICAL
CHARACTERS OF URINARY
DEPOSITS,

Delivered at Guy's Hospital, London,

BY DR. GOLDING BIRD.

LECTURE VI.

Pathology of deposits of triple phosphate and phosphate of lime—fœtid urine—phosphates in old people—in irritable bladder—treatment—siliceous deposits—organized deposits—blood-discs; supposed filament in—pus—mucus—organic globules—ferment—torula cerevisiæ—epithelial debris—analytic table.

In my last lecture I described to you the general properties and chemical characters of the different forms of deposits in which phosphoric acid enters as a constituent*. I also, you will recollect, pointed out to you the probable origin of the phosphoric acid existing in these saline combinations, and demonstrated to you, from the most trustworthy analyses to which I could refer, the fact that more phosphoric acid was taken into the stomach with the food than was excreted in the urine. I have now to direct your attention to a brief view of the pathological conditions under which such deposits most generally occur.

One general law certainly appears to govern the pathological development of the phosphatic deposits; I allude to a constantly depressed state of nervous energy, often general, rarely more local, in its seat. Of the former, the result of wear and tear of body and mind in old people, and of the latter the effects of local injury to the spine, will serve as examples. It is true that, in the majority of cases in which phosphates are deposited, there may be much irritability present; you may find an irritable pulse, a tongue white on the surface and red at the tip and edges, with a dry, and perhaps occasionally hot, skin. Still, it is irritability with depression—a kind of erythism of the nervous system, if I may venture to use such a term.

Triple phosphates (neutral).—Where the deposit consists of this salt you will generally succeed in tracing its connection to some cause which has rendered the system morbidly irritable, at the same time that its tone or strength has been depressed. The simplest example of this kind that has occurred under my notice is in the case of individuals who have periodical duties to perform requiring extreme mental tension and bodily exertion. It has occurred to me more than once to notice this state of things in clergymen, especially in those who, from the nature of their secular engagements, have been accustomed to lead sedentary lives during the week, and to perform full duty on Sundays. One of the best examples I ever met with of this kind occurred in the person of a well-known and deservedly popular clergyman, who, from his connection with a public school, scarcely used any exercise during the week, whilst on Sunday he performed duty three times in his church. This gentleman was a tall, thin person, of dark complexion, and almost phthisical aspect. He was the subject of nearly constant dyspepsia. The urine passed by him on Saturday evening, as well as on Sunday morning, although repeatedly examined, appeared to be healthy, although of rather high specific gravity, generally containing a deposit of urate of ammonia. Before his Sunday duties were completed, he generally became the subject of extreme fatigue, with a painful aching sensation across the loins, in addition to the flatulence and epigastric uneasiness under which he generally laboured. The urine passed before going to bed, after the severe exertions of the day, was almost constantly of a deep amber hue, of rather high specific gravity, and deposited the triple phosphate in abundance. The urine of Monday would contain less of this salt, which generally disappeared on the following day, and again re-appeared on the following Sunday evening. This state of things I observed for several weeks, and it ultimately disappeared by the patient relaxing from his duties, and travelling for a few weeks.

It is not an uncommon thing to find an iridescent film formed of a thin layer, or pellicle, of crystals of triple phosphate, floating on the surface of urine passed by persons labouring under some form of irritative dyspepsia. This often presents the same brilliant colours as a soap-bubble, or thin layer of oil on water. It is clearly the result of imperfect assimilation, and, in all probability, is to be regarded as an attempt at getting rid from the system of an excess of the earthy phosphates which had been absorbed from the ingesta. In this form I have never seen a decided gravel or deposit.

---

* In my last lecture an important error in the amount of phosphates said to exist in the potato has occurred; it is stated to contain 23·56 grains in the ounce, instead of 2·356. This arose from the decimal point being misplaced in the table given by Dr. Bence Jones, (49·1 instead of 4·91) from whose work (on Gravel, Calculus, and Gout, p.78) I copied it. In the text, at p.16, *three* ounces has been placed for *four*; the meal I cited as an illustration would contain 30 grains of earthy phosphates instead of 114.

Four ounces of beef . . 1·52
" " wheat . . 19·08
" " potatoes . 9·42
―――――
30·02

produced, and I am inclined to consider that it is rather to be regarded as an index, and a valuable one, of the state of the assimilative functions, than as holding out any fear of the ulterior deposit of calculous matter.

I have not unfrequently met with deposits of the triple phosphates in very old people, in whom the state of decrepitude depending on senility had either become extreme, or been aggravated by low living and a want of the ordinary comforts of life. In several cases of this kind occurring in octagenarian dependents on parochial relief, I have found the urine very pale, of low specific gravity, subacid or neutral, and extremely foetid. The foetor, which was like that of stale fish, did not appear to depend upon the presence of free ammonia, but in all probability was a result of some slow decomposition of the organic constituents of the urine ; a decay depending on the depressed vital energy of the bladder.

I have before alluded to the fact, that a deposition of the triple phosphate is often observed to occur in cases where a blow had been received on the lumbar region, or where some strain has been experienced in that region ; a fact first observed by Dr. Prout. This effect of injury to the loins is frequently met with as a temporary result of even slight blows or strains, and disappearing in a few days. I once saw a copious deposition of triple phosphates occur in the urine of a young gentleman who exerted himself rather more than his strength could bear in a riding school. In fact, whatever chemical explanation may be given to the presence of an excess of phosphates in the urine, it is indisputable that in the very great majority of cases there is ample evidence of the existence of some cause producing, to say the least, a depressed but irritable state of the nervous energies in the neighbourhood of the injury. The symptoms observed in these cases are nearly all explicable on this state of the nervous system.

The most prominent symptoms observed in these cases are, great irritability of temper, extreme restlessness, mal-performance of the digestive functions, with such imperfect assimilation of the ingesta, that a certain and often extreme amount of emaciation is a constant attendant. The appetite is uncertain, occasionally being voracious. Fatigue is induced by the slightest exertion ; there is a remarkable inaptitude to any mental or bodily exercise. and the patient is often, from the exhaustion thus produced, unfitted for his ordinary duties. In acute cases these symptoms become aggravated by an excessive elimination of urea, which aids considerably in depressing the patient's strength.

Regarding the treatment of these cases, whilst we must allow that in many cases the administration of acids will cause the deposit of phosphates to disappear, yet it must be admitted that we are thus treating but a symptom, although an important one, of a serious malady. It is, perhaps, wise to administer acids, especially the hydrochloric or phosphoric, and thus endeavour to render the urine sufficiently acid to prevent the crystals of the phosphate concreting into a calculus ; but, at the same time, we must direct our treatment to the digestive organs, and endeavour to allay the morbidly irritable state of the nervous system. You will often find that it is no easy matter to render the urine acid in this manner ; I have, in several cases, administered the mineral acids regularly, and in as large a dose as the patient could bear, without increasing the action of the urine on litmus paper, whilst in others the urine has appeared to be readily affected. This capricious effect observed in the use of acids renders their administration much less to be depended upon than when alkalis are given in cases where too much acid is secreted in the urine. The best mode of treating these cases is to regulate the bowels by tonic aperients, and allay the morbid irritability present by the use of sedatives. For this purpose, the Mist. Gentianæ Compos. may be made the vehicle for the administration of dilute hydrochloric acid in doses of fifteen or twenty minims, with half a drachm of the tincture of henbane thrice a day. In protracted and severe cases, the use of opium in graduated doses has, in the hands of Dr. Prout, been of great service. In one very severe case which occurred to myself I thought I found much relief in the administration of iron in the form of the acetate thrice a day, with a sedative at night. The preparations of zinc and silver also hold out great probability of being of service, from their well-known power in allaying morbid irritability of the digestive organs, and perhaps of the organic system of nerves generally.

With regard to the *pathological* indications afforded by the deposits of phosphate of lime, they are analogous to those already pointed out to you as peculiar to the triple salt. Intimately related as these salts are chemically, their pathological indications might be expected to be analogous ; and such, indeed, is the case, if we except the not unfrequent excessive secretion of phosphate of lime as the result of disease of the mucous surface of the bladder. It is not uncommon to find both phosphates mixed in a deposit, which is thus readily fusible in the blow-pipe flame, unless too great an excess of either ingredient be present. These mixed deposits are not unfrequent in gouty people, and in such cases I have seen deposits of crystalline and amorphous phosphates alternate in the urine passed in the evening, whilst the morning secretion was loaded with urate of ammonia. So far as I have had an opportunity of watching the progress of cases where phosphate of lime is deposited (and they are by no means of frequent occurrence) I have generally fancied that they present more marked evidence of exhaustion, and of the previous existence of some drain on the nervous system, than where the triple salt alone existed.

Occasionally, some curious cases are met with, in which phosphate of lime has come away in the urine for a long period without apparently doing much mischief. A very remarkable instance of this kind occurred in this hospital some years ago among the out-patients, in the person of an old man under the care of Dr. Hughes. This patient had for many years passed almost milky urine, which by repose deposited such an enormous quantity of phosphate of lime, that he brought to me at one time upwards of an ounce of this calcareous salt. He had been under the treatment of half the hospital physicians and surgeons in London, during fourteen or fifteen years, but his urine remained unimproved. He afterwards came under my care, but I found all the remedial measures I adopted useless: at the same time, I may remark, this man's health appeared so good that there was scarcely an excuse for submitting him to any course of treatment beyond the apprehension of the possible formation of calculus.

I cannot quit this part of my subject without pressing upon your notice the value derived in many of these cases from injecting the bladder with a very dilute mineral acid. I am confident that an irritable condition of the bladder, highly favourable to the secretion of earthy phosphates and excess of mucus from its mucous membrane, has been in some cases kept up by retention of phosphates in that viscus. Certainly, I have now seen many cases where viscid ropy mucus, mixed with abundance of phosphates, both magnesian and calcareous, have been secreted, and where the distress of the patient has been extremely increased by intense irritability of bladder. And in these, all plans of treatment have been unavailing, until the bladder has been carefully washed out by means of warm water, and an injection, consisting of half a dram of dilute hydrochloric acid, with a dram of vinium opii in half a pint of warm barley-water, has been thrown in by means of a double catheter, in the manner described by Sir B. Brodie. I had a case under my care last year, in consultation with a most excellent and talented provincial physician, Dr. Baker, of Maldon, in which the irritability of bladder was so intense that there was almost constant desire to pass water, attended with horrible suffering. The urine often contained blood, and rapidly underwent decomposition; it presented a copious dense deposit of puriform mucus, mixed with an enormous quantity of triple phosphate in very large

crystals. The state of distress to which this lady was reduced by the disease rendered her life a complete burden. On examining the urine carefully, I could detect no true pus; it did not coagulate by heat, and much of the opacity presented by the mucus was owing to the presence of the triple phosphate. I suggested the use of a solvent injection analogous to the one just described. Great difficulty was experienced in the use of the catheter, in consequence of the excessive suffering it produced. Ultimately the injection was very effectually administered by Mr. May, of Maldon, and the effect was most remarkable; the irritability of bladder rapidly subsided, and by repeating the injection it was completely removed, and on being called into Essex to a case in the neighbourhood some time after, I had the pleasure of seeing this lady apparently well.

Although it is not now my duty to point out to you the treatment of calculous affections, I felt anxious to draw your attention to this class of cases, on account of their great importance, and of the little notice taken of them by most writers, being generally confounded with the cases included under the general category of *catarrhus vesicæ*, or of irritable bladder.

I have little to say regarding the last ingredient of deposits made up of inorganized ingredients, viz :—

Silica, or silicic acid.

This substance exists in infinitessimally small quantities in some of the animal fluids, and therefore may by possibility be met with as an urinary deposit. I have, however, never met with an unexceptionable instance of its occurrence. It has been found in a calculus by the late Dr. Yelloly, and some others have recorded instances of its occurrence. Lassaigne[*] found a calculus consisting of nearly pure silica in the urethra of a lamb, and Wurzer[†] gives the analysis of a calculus removed from an ox, in which silicic acid existed to the amount of 38 per cent. You must, however, be on your guard regarding silicic concretions, for as there is a popular notion that calculous matter is *bonâ fide* gravel, whenever an imposition is intended a siliceous pebble is usually chosen to deceive the medical attendant. I have met with repeated instances of this kind, in which common rolled pebbles of quartz have been placed in my hands with the assertion that they were actually passed from the bladder. This has usually occurred in hysterical girls, who have laboured under that most unintelligibly morbid desire of deceiving the doctor, by representing themselves as afflicted with some ailment of the genito-urinary organs. I have heard of in-

---

[*] Recueil de Médecine Veterinaire, p. 445.
[†] Gurlt's Pathologische Anatomie der Haus-Sangethiere, B. 1. 840.

stances in which such pebbles have actually been thrust into the urethra by a girl, and thus have really reached the bladder. In a case mentioned to me by Dr. Christison, a piece of chlorite slate was found forming part of the supposed calculus, at once attesting its true origin, notwithstanding the positive assertions of the young woman who was said to have passed it, to the contrary. You have, I dare say, all heard of the case which occurred many years ago in this hospital, in which the late Mr. Cline operated, and removed from the bladder a quantity of common coals which had been introduced by the patient.

As, however, silica has been found in calculi by such excellent observers as the late Dr. Yelloly and Dr. Venables, and as the ox and lamb, mentioned by Wurzer and Lassaigne, could hardly be supposed to have put the silica into their own bladders, we must admit its possible occurrence in calculi. Still, that it is extremely rare, all experience has proved, as indeed might be anticipated, from the chemical relations of this most refractory substance.

I have next to direct your attention to a brief notice of

Deposits consisting of organised products.

Most of these have been carefully studied and well understood, but concerning some very little is known, and that little is anything but satisfactory.

Blood-discs.—Whenever a deposit consists wholly, or chiefly, of blood-particles, the urine generally possesses a tint which at once leads us to suspect the presence of some of the elements of blood. This tint varies from a pale dingy hue to a reddish brown, or, if the urine has become alkaline, a deep greenish colour is not of unfrequent occurrence. You will recollect that in my first lecture I pointed out to you the most prominent characteristics which distinguish urine containing blood-discs in diffusion.

Perhaps the best mode of detecting blood-discs in urine is to agitate it violently, and place a drop on a piece of glass; cover it with a piece of thin glass or mica, and examine it with a microscope furnished with a good object glass of ⅓ or ¼ inch focus. If the urine has not been passed too long, you will find the blood-discs scarcely changed, except that they generally have their margins more sharply defined, and the surface more concave than usual. This arises, in all probability, from the sac of the blood-disc becoming partly emptied by exosmosis, in the manner so clearly and satisfactorily pointed out by Dr. Rees *. The peculiar appearances described by Dr. Martin Barry as indicating the existence of a

* Guy's Hospital Reports, October 1841, and April 1843.

band or filament in the blood-disc is generally most beautifully marked in particles obtained from bloody urine, especially if it has been gently warmed, so as to facilitate the deposition of the discs before submitting them to the microscope. I have placed a specimen of some thus procured from bloody urine, preserved in dilute alcohol, in the collection of microscopic specimens, to which I have before alluded. These present the appearance of a spiral filament contained in the sac of the blood-disc. I confess I consider this appearance as a mere illusion, depending on the emptying of the sac by exosmosis, and the membranes consequently becoming congested in circular folds, thus producing the appearance of a spiral thread; and I believe an analogous explanation applies to all the cases of the supposed existence of filaments in blood, described by Dr. Barry. If blood-discs have long existed in urine they often become partly disorganised, their margins becoming irregularly crenate, and their whole form more or less irregular. You will find, however, notwithstanding the various changes produced in blood-discs by the action of urine, that they are seldom sufficient to alter it so as to prevent their ready recognition by microscopic examination.

Pus.—Whenever urine contains pus, it is always more or less coagulable by heat, as the pus particle is never secreted without its concomitant drop of serum, or *liquor puris*, in which it floats. Hence (at least if this view is correct) albuminous urine necessarily occurs when pus exists. Pus in urine, retaining its normal acidity, forms a cream-like layer at the bottom of the vessel, so closely resembling the fluid contents of an abscess, that there can be no great difficulty in identifying it. Here, however, a serious source of fallacy, to which I have alluded in my last lecture, exists, founded on the remarkably puriform appearances presented by some deposits of phosphates. The solubility of the latter in nitric acid will at once remove any difficulty in the diagnosis, unless puriform mucus exists with the phosphate, in which case the microscope can alone remove the difficulty.

If pus has remained long in the urine before it is submitted to examination, it will undergo certain changes which materially interfere with its generally recognised physical characters. It will undergo a change analogous to that produced by digesting pus in solution of common salt, as hydrochlorate of ammonia, described by Dr. Babington *, becoming in fact a ropy tenacious magma, more like purulent mucus than pus. This change is greatly accelerated, and, indeed, often produced immediately, if the urine is ammoniacal. The albuminous character of

* Guy's Hospital Reports, Oct. 1837.

the urine, and microscopic examination of the deposit, will even then generally remove all doubt as to its true character.

The true pus particle strongly refracts light, and, being roughly granular on its surface, often appears coloured, unless the achromatism of the object-glass is perfect, and the illumination well arranged. These particles vary in size; on an average, however, it may be stated that they nearly correspond to the blood-disc in diameter. If a drop of acetic acid be mixed with a purulent deposit, and carefully examined after covering it with a thin plate of glass or mica, the compound structure of the pus particle will become obvious. The particles will present the appearance of being broken up or disintegrated, leaving numerous extremely minute transparent bodies of a tolerably regular spherical form, and about one-fourth the size of the original particle. These bodies are probably arranged as symmetric nuclei in the original particle, for certainly at least two or three exist in each before the addition of the acid.

Mucus.—Whenever a preternatural quantity of mucus is poured out by the lining membrane of the bladder, it is voided with the urine, and forms a deposit in the latter by repose, which is generally sufficiently characteristic to allow of its being readily recognised. Mucus generally forms a semi-translucent, somewhat gelatinous deposit, which, when the urine is decanted, falls from the vessel in the form of a tenacious rope, often of considerable length, sometimes so tough as to be actually sectile. Urine of this kind generally passes with great readiness into decomposition, and becomes alkaline, the mucus acting as a ferment, determining a molecular change of the fluid in which it is immersed without itself undergoing any manifest alteration. Urine containing any marked excess of mucus is generally alkaline, but if very recently voided is sometimes neutral and very rarely sub-acid, in which case if a piece of reddened litmus paper be immersed in the mucous deposit, it always evinces the presence of alkaline properties in the latter. Even when a very small quantity of mucus exists in urine, its presence may be made out by microscopic examination. Sometimes a kind of web presenting the rudiments of an imperfect globular structure is observed floating in the drop of fluid examined. When this is the case it is not unfrequent to find crystals of the triple phosphate or of uric acid entangled in the web of mucus. More frequently, however, globular particles of mucus are found free and floating in the urine.

True mucous globule.—This is generally somewhat smaller than the pus particle, being about one two-thousandths of an inch in diameter. With a low magnifying power, as with an object-glass of half an inch focus the globules appear smooth and diaphanous, but with a glass of one-seventh or one-eighth of an inch, the surface of the particle appears distinctly granular, although not in so marked a manner as the pus particle. It is extremely difficult to distinguish the pus from the mucous particle, and even by comparison it is not easy, and certainly in many cases quite impossible, to distinguish between them. The fact of the urine not being albuminous, and of the particles not so readily evolving their nuclei when treated with acetic acid, nor of being dissolved on the addition of ammonia, will help in distinguishing between the pus and mucous particles.

Organic globules.—I have, in a paper giving a brief description of the globules found in urine (Guy's Hospital Reports, October 1842), ventured to give this name, as a generic term, to a series of very ill-defined and difficultly-discriminated globules occurring in urine. These appear to present certain differential characters, which prevent their being classed with pus and mucus, but which are not so well marked as to enable us to pronounce definitely on their nature.

Large organic globule.—A globule of frequent occurrence, especially in the urine of pregnancy, of irritable bladder, and of granular degeneration of the kidneys (morbus Brightii). It seldom forms a visible or distinct deposit, but is more generally scattered in the urine so sparingly that not more than a dozen or two are at once visible in the field of the microscope. These are distinguished with great difficulty from the two last-described globules, and perhaps are best known by their not presenting so distinctly a granular exterior, nor so readily evolving their nuclei on the addition of acetic acid. I suspect that this globule is identical with the one described by the French writers as muco-pus. There is a peculiarity in these globules which serves practically to distinguish them from other analogous bodies; depending upon their not undergoing any marked change when the urine is warmed. Thus, if a small quantity of urine containing them is gently warmed in a watch-glass, and a rotatory motion be given to the latter, the organic globules will collect at the bottom, forming a white deposit, which, when the supernatant urine is replaced by water, presents a remarkably glistening, or even crystalline aspect, like a deposit of oxalate of lime. On examining a portion of this by the microscope, the globules will be found unaltered by the heat, and perfectly free, so as to roll over each other on inclining the glass on which they rest.

I have occasionally observed a variety of this globule which differs in its behaviour with acetic acid from that just described. In its granular exterior, and in most of its pro-

... bark yields to wax ... more ... and less inert matter than when finely powdered (exp. 19.)

2. The inf... is separated from subpulverised bark with much greater facility, pressure not being employed for this purpose.

3. The additional expense of ... powdering is avoided.

4. A smaller quantity of water is sufficient.

The period of 24 hours is adopted as a matter of convenience. It will be shewn in a subsequent experiment that the bark yields to cold water in ... hours all that can be taken up in a single maceration.

The object of using so ... a quantity of water as *twice the* ... is to avoid taking up the ... matter, which being for the ... a constituent of the *tissue*, is ... than the secretions contained in ...

The specific gravity of the ... of different samples I have ... 1022 is the highest I have ... was more frequently 1010 or ...

For 1. *continued.*—The ... was ... in a ... flask over a water-bath, to ... ture of syrup ... g. 1200 ...

Pharmaceutical Analysis of Yellow Bark.

Exp. 1. 1st *Maceration.*—28 the (avds.) Howard's yellow bark imported in 1837, were subpulverised and macerated 24 hours in twice the weight (24 pints) of cold distilled water. The infusion was transparent, of a beautiful deep amber colour, aromatic and very bitter, acid to litmus paper. (s. g. 1024).

2d *Maceration.*—The same bark, not ... been deprived by pressure of the ... was ..., was again macerated ... in 24 pints of cold distilled ... The second infusion ... of the first, ... s. g. 1010.

In the same quantity ... infusion 1007.

perties, they cannot be distinguished, but when acetic acid is added the globules become more translucent, and the presence of two nuclei is readily demonstrable. These nuclei are not globular, as in the last described bodies, but are crescentic, with their concavities opposed, so that they resemble two menisci seen in section. I confess that I have been inclined to refer these organic globules to the same class as the colourless particles of the blood, in which, from the observations of Mr. Wharton Jones, the character of the nuclei I have described appears to be well marked.

Small organic globules.—I have occasionally discovered in urine, when gently warmed in a watch-glass, a white lustrous but scanty deposit, which, when examined under a power of one-eighth inch, appears to be composed of myriads of absolutely spherical globules, free from all asperities or irregularities of surface. Acetic acid, even on the application of warmth, produces no change in these globules. They are smaller than blood-discs, and very closely resemble in appearance the transparent nuclei of pus particles. Whether this, however, is their true nature, I am quite unable to state.

These minute globules I have but rarely met with ; they occurred in the urine of women who were menstruating, and were but transitory phenomena, as they were seldom present in a second specimen.

I have described to you these forms of organic products chiefly for the purpose of drawing your attention to what has been already observed with regard to them. The indications afforded by what I have termed " organic globules" are as yet scarcely known, and probably will remain in an exceedingly unsatisfactory state, until we acquire better means of distinguishing them than we at present possess.

Among the many microscopic phenomena presented by urine, few are more interesting than some observed in diabetic urine. If the urine passed by a diabetic patient be set aside in a tall vessel for a few hours, and the lower layers be examined between plates of glass under a good object glass of 1-8th inch focus, numerous ovoid vesicles will be observed floating in the fluid. These are free from all asperities, and are distinguishable by their oval form from other organic deposits. These are what are termed globules of ferment, analogous to those found in all fermenting fluids ; and are readily detected in the urine within eight hours of its being passed, if it be placed in a tolerably warm place. Whenever you meet with these oval bodies, you may be confident that the urine contains sugar. They are in fact spores of a peculiar confervoid organism, which is rapidly developed in saccharine fluids about

to undergo various fermentation. In 24 hours after diabetic urine is passed, a cloud rises to the surface, and soon after a distinct pellicle is formed : if this be examined under the microscope you will find it composed of the ovoid bodies referred to, mixed with minute jointed, single, or branched tubes. These are the young plants of a minute conferva, the torula cerevisiae.

Fig. 19.

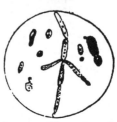

In a day or two this torula undergoes a change ; the tubes break up, and a copious deposit of fresh spores forms on the sides and bottom of the vessel. If these be placed in a solution of sugar, they will rapidly germinate, and produce fresh crops of confervæ. Cotemporaneously with the development of these minute conferve the elements of the sugar and of water undergo a metamorphosis, and alcohol with carbonic acid are the results.

You will very frequently, in your microscopic examination of urine, meet with certain organised particles, which are derived from the epithelial layers of the mucous membrane of the urinary passages. These are sometimes merely an amorphous debris, in which any definite structure is made out with great difficulty. You will scarcely, however, meet with a specimen of this kind in which you will not succeed in detecting epithelial cells, cylinders, or scales, sufficiently perfect to permit their being readily identified. Of the various forms of epithelial tissue, the most frequently met with is, perhaps, the oval nucleated cell; this often appears well defined, and is a very beautiful object, resembling in outline a shield with a central boss. I have found, mixed with these, roundish cells of considerable size, distended with fluid, and appearing perfectly distinct under a low power (½ inch focus). You will scarcely examine a specimen of urine passed in the morning on rising from bed in which you will fail to detect some debris of epithelium, and this becomes greatly increased if the patient is labouring under any inflammatory or irritable state of the mucous membrane of the urinary passages.

I have thus, gentlemen, brought to a close my remarks on the chemical and pathological characters of urinary deposits : I might have occupied your time during several more lectures, had I not wished to avoid making the subject tedious to you by being too prolix. I have endeavoured to point out to you those characters by which you will readily succeed in distinguishing the different deposits which are met with in urine, and which are no longer to be regarded as a mere piece of idle curiosity, but really of great importance in directing our diagnosis and treatment of some of the most important diseases to which our race is subject. In conclusion, I wish to direct your attention to a tabular analysis of the most prominent characters presented by the saline urinary deposits, including all those in the first two classes which have fallen under my own observation. This will, I hope, serve as a useful index to the detailed account of the deposits contained in these lectures, and assist you in their discrimination of them at the bed-side.

ON YELLOW BARK.

(To Sir Henry Halford, Bart.)

SIR,

I AVAIL myself of the kind permission you have given me on former occasions to address to you some observations on yellow bark, and on the concentrated cold infusion which I have for many years prepared under the name of *Liquor Cinchonæ cordifoliæ*, trusting that you will not consider I trespass too much on your indulgence.

Five years ago I had the honour of presenting to the Royal College of Physicians a paper, which was read on the 4th of May, 1838, containing some remarks on this subject.

The repeated assurances I have received from high medical authorities of the superiority of the concentrated cold infusion, and my own analyses and observations, have long satisfied me that it is a more perfect and efficient preparation of cinchona than any other now in use.

The value of yellow bark has been too generally and too exclusively attributed to the quinine it contains. It has ever been an object with me to *preserve unbroken that natural union by which several active principles are often combined in the same plant.* Every day's experience convinces me that neither the separation of certain principles, nor the more ordinary pharmaceutical operations by decoction, infusion, and spirituous digestion, furnish us with medicines of equal value with those which are obtained by simple maceration in *cold distilled water*, which takes up from plants, with few exceptions, all their medicinal properties, whether acid or alkaline, gummy or resinous, bitter or astringent.

Yellow bark is produced by an undetermined species of *Cinchona*. In the London Pharmacopœia it is still ascribed to the *Cinchona cordifolia*, a native of Bogata, the bark of which was erroneously supposed by Mutis to be identical with it. Genuine yellow, or as it is sometimes termed royal yellow bark, is not a native of Spanish Guiana, but of the provinces of La Paz and Potosi in Bolivia, or Upper Peru, and is brought to us not from Carthagena, but from Arica and Lima.

The drug merchants at Cadiz state that it is not conveyed to Lima by sea, like the other barks, but is found only at the distance of two or three hundred leagues from the capital, and conveyed over steep and almost inaccessible mountains. (Relph's Inq. into the Med. Efficacy of Yellow Bark, 1794, p. 69.)

The earliest notice that I am acquainted with of this bark is to be found in Pomet's History of Drugs, written in 1694. This old but valuable author mentions another kind of quinquina, or Peruvian bark, which comes from the mountains of Potosi, and is browner, more aromatic and more bitter, than the barks about Loxa, but abundantly scarcer than any of the rest.

It seems, however, to have fallen into disuse, and to have been forgotten, till about 1788 or 9, when a parcel having arrived at Madrid, and having been found on trial more efficacious than the pale sort, was immediately bought up by the king's order for the use of the Royal Family, and hence was distinguished by the name of royal yellow bark. Further experiments in Spain and France were attended with the same success. Murray, in his Apparatus Medicaminum, published at Göttingen in 1792, mentions (Vol. 6, p. 180), that a bark had recently been brought from London under the name of *cortex chinæ vel chinchinæ regius :* that he was unacquainted with its native country, but that in the year 1790 he had seen it at Frankfort on the Main, where it was sold for 16 dollars the pound, and subsequently at Wisbaden. He had also received the same bark from another quarter under the name of *cortex chinæ flavus*, and had seen specimens from Amsterdam, where it bore the name of royal yellow bark. *Cortex chinæ regius flavus.* Murray's description corresponds with our yellow bark, and he adds that the Frankfort physicians found it very superior in efficacy to the common Peruvian bark, especially in intermittents.

In 1793 the Spanish register ship St. Jago, having been captured by a French privateer, was retaken by Admiral Gell's squadron off Cape Finisterre in the Bay of Biscay, and on its arrival in England was found to contain a great many chests of this bark of first rate quality. The following year it was strongly recommended by Dr. Relph, of Guy's Hospital, as promising to surpass all the other kinds of Peruvian bark then employed in medicine."

Pharmaceutical Analysis of Yellow Bark.

EXP. 1.— *1st Maceration.* — 28 lbs. (avds.) Howard's yellow bark imported in 1837, were subpulverizised and macerated 24 hours in twice the weight (56 pints) of cold distilled water.

The infusion was transparent, of a beautiful deep amber colour, aromatic and very bitter, acid to litmus paper, and of s. g. 1020.

2d Maceration.—The same bark, not having been deprived by pressure of the water absorbed, was again macerated 24 hours in 24 pints of cold distilled water. The second infusion possessed the properties of the first, but in a far less degree. S. g. 1010.

3d Maceration.— In the same quantity of water. S. g. of the infusion 1007.

4th Maceration.—S. g. of infusion 1004.

5th Maceration.—S. g. 1000. This infusion was nearly colourless, and possessed scarcely any aroma, bitterness, or astringency.

OBS.—The method adopted in this experiment is the same which is invariably employed in making the cold infusion from which the liquor cinchonæ is formed, except that to form the liquor the operation is not continued beyond the third maceration.

The bark which I employ is not *finely powdered*, but only *subpulverised*, for the following reasons:—

1. Subpulverised bark yields to water as much quinine and less inert matter than when finely powdered (exp. 19.)

2. The infusion is separated from subpulverised bark with much greater facility, pressure not being employed for this purpose:

3. The additional expense of finely powdering is avoided.

4. A smaller quantity of water is sufficient.

The period of 24 hours is adopted as a matter of convenience. It will be shewn in a subsequent experiment (18) that the bark yields to cold water in 3 or 4 hours all that can be taken up in a single maceration.

The object of using so small a quantity of water as *twice the weight* is to avoid taking up the gummy matter, which being for the most part a constituent of the *tissue*, is less soluble than the *secretions* contained in it.

The specific gravity of the infusion of different samples varies considerably; 1020 is the highest I have met with: it is more frequently 1010 or 1012.

EXP. 1, *continued.*—The first infusion was slowly evaporated in a Wedgwood dish over a water-bath, to the consistence of syrup, s. g. 1200; care being taken that the temperature did not exceed 140. During the evaporation, and towards the close, a dark granular matter separated, destitute of taste and smell. (A.)

The concentrated infusion separated and left at rest for more than a week, did not undergo the slightest change. It was aromatic and intensely bitter, and readily blackened a weak solution of tinct. ferri. mur.

The second infusion during concentration let fall much red granular matter (A), and subsequently, when left at rest, formed a gummy precipitate containing evident crystals. (B.)

The third infusion underwent similar changes, yielding after concentration a still larger quantity of gummy precipitate.

The three infusions concentrated to s. g. 1200, and separated from the gummy and red granular matter, were mixed, and weighed 5lbs. 11 ounces.

OBS.—A much larger quantity of red granular matter usually falls from the latter, than from the earlier infusions probably because that which is obtained from the tissue is less soluble than that which is contained in the cells and is taken up during the earlier macerations.

In the quantity of liquor, and the specific gravity of the first infusion, Howard's bark of 1837 is nearly equal to that taken from the St. Jago; but the quality obtained from barks imported in other years, equally good in *appearance*, and treated exactly in the same way, is much less.

Horner's bark, imported in 1834-6, yielded 4 lbs. 7 ounces, and a sample of my own of another importation yielded only 2 lbs. 9 ounces.

EXP. 2.—Two ounces of the concentrated infusion, s. g. 1200, were diffused in eight ounces of distilled water. The mixture was very bitter and aromatic. Tr. ferri mur. rendered it quite black. The mixture was acidulated with pure muriatic acid, and saturated with magnesia, and the precipitate was washed and dried. The supernatant fluid was scarcely bitter, and tr. ferri mur. produced very little blackness. The dried magnesian matter was boiled in alcohol, s. g. 815, and the solution decanted. The spirit was distilled off, except one ounce, which was left to evaporate spontaneously. The mass remaining at the bottom of the dish was dissolved by dilute sulphuric acid carefully added till it was in the slightest degree in excess. The solution was slowly evaporated, and crystals formed of sulphate of quinine. These crystals were dissolved in distilled water, and ammonia being added a white matter fell *(quinine)*, weighing 96 grains.

OBS.—It appears from this experiment that 5 lbs. 11 ounces of the concentrated infusion contain within a few grains 10 ounces of quinine, which is therefore the quantity taken up by cold distilled water from 28 lbs. of yellow bark.

EXP. 3.—1 lb. (avds.) of yellow bark subpulverised was macerated all night over a water bath in 4 pints of distilled water acidulated with sulphuric acid. The liquor was strained through gauze. The bark was then boiled half an hour in two successive portions of acidulated water, and the liquor strained, pressure being used to displace the fluid.

The three liquors were mixed and oversaturated with fresh slacked lime. The mixture was boiled and filtered, and the precipitate dried and boiled in two portions of spirit of wine; the filter and the matter remaining on it being also washed and boiled in an additional portion of spirit of wine. The spirit filtered and distilled left of *quinine* 229 grains.

The refuse bark was finally macerated several hours in water acidulated with acetic acid, to which it imparted no colour. The infusion was not precipitated, and only slightly coloured by the addition of ammonia.

OBS.—28 lbs. therefore contain about 14 ounces of quinine. Experiments 1 and 2 show that the liquor prepared from 28 lbs. contains nearly 10 ounces of this. The remainder of the quinine not taken up by the cold water may be subsequently separated by acetic acid (see experiment 13), and added to the liquor, which will then contain the whole of this constituent. But this addition will scarcely repay the expense of the operation.

The quantity of quinine in different samples varies considerably, but the reduction of the specific gravity of the liquor to 1200 ensures a *uniformity* in this respect which cannot be obtained by the simple infusion or decoction of a definite quantity of bark.

EXP. 4.—One ounce of the liquor was dried and incinerated; the incineration was slowly accomplished, the matter burning like leather. The ashes weighed 37 grains.

The 37 grs. were boiled in distilled water, and the nitrates of baryta and silver indicated the presence of *sulphuric and muriatic acids* in the solution. The residuum was further dissolved in distilled water, acidulated with pure muriatic acid; and ferrocyanate of potash, ammonia, and bicarbonate of soda, detected *iron, alumina, and lime,* The residuum was *silex.*

OBS.—I have generally found the muriates most abundant in inferior samples of bark.

EXP. 5.—120 grs. of the red granular precipitate (A), were macerated in 4 oz. of alcohol. The spirit was deeply tinged. A second portion was slightly tinged. The residuum dried weighed 73 grs., 47 grs. having been taken up by the spirit. The 73 grs. were placed in distilled water, and liquor potassæ was carefully added. Turmeric paper indicated no free alkali till the quantity added amounted to 2 drms. The alkaline liquor took up 33 grs., leaving 40 grains undissolved.

OBS.—This precipitate appears to consist chiefly of tannin.

M

EXP. 6.—One ounce of the same matter was incinerated; the ashes weighed only 19 grs. Ten grains of this being taken up by distilled water gave to the nitrates of silver and baryta traces of *sulphuric* and *muriatic acids*. The residuum, boiled in water acidulated with pure muriatic acid, gave to ferrocyanate of potash, ammonia, and bicarbonate of soda, a little *iron, alumina*, and *lime*.

EXP. 7.—The gummy precipitate (B) as it dried formed beautiful crystals in considerable quantity. A portion of it was washed in spirit of wine to remove the *tannin* and *gummy* matter. The remaining mass of crystals was of a pale yellow colour, in appearance resembling sulphate of quinine. The crystals were dissolved in distilled water, and oxalic acid carefully added caused an abundant white precipitate (L). The supernatant liquor was not disturbed by the further addition either of oxalic acid or of lime-water, and therefore contained neither. It was evaporated to the consistence of syrup, and gradually deposited crystals for many weeks. These crystals, consisting of the peculiar acid of bark commonly called *kinic acid*, are perfectly colourless and very acid. They dissolve quinine readily, even without heat, forming with it a salt which does not redden litmus paper.

The precipitate (L) was dissolved in pure muriatic acid, the solution filtered, and lime precipitated by carbonate of soda.

OBS.—Kinate of lime does not appear to be an important constituent of bark, for inferior bark contains much the largest quantity.

EXP. 8.—Another portion of the gummy precipitate (B) was placed in distilled water, and the clear fluid poured off. The insoluble residuum (C) was a light powder, of a brownish red colour, scarcely bitter, and almost tasteless. 20 grains of it were incinerated; the odour was very fragrant, and much resembled castor: 1¼ grs. only remained.

Another portion of C was almost entirely dissolved in liquor potassæ and liq. ammoniæ, and tinct. ferri mur. added to the filtered solutions, formed a deep green colour, which soon became black. The small portion not dissolved by the cold alkaline solutions was *waxy*. Boiling ether

dissolved it, and water precipitated it from its solution. The *waxy* matter readily inflamed, burning with much smoke.

EXP. 9.—All the precipitates from 28 lbs. of yellow bark were placed in dilute sulphuric acid for several hours, and a little heat applied. The filtered solution was saturated with lime, and boiled over a water-bath. The residuum was then dried, boiled in spirit of wine, and the spirit distilled off, excepting 2 drs. which, being evaporated to dryness, left of *quinine* 22 grs.

OBS.—The precipitates, therefore, contain *quinine* and *lime*, combined with *kinic acid, gummy matter, tannin*, and *wax*.

EXP. 10.—The cold infusions tested with iodine did not indicate a trace of starch. A portion of the residual bark exhausted by 5 cold macerations was placed in fresh distilled water, and heat applied.

The colours produced by the addition of tr. of iodine at the different temperatures were as follows:—

At 135 deg. red
    140 „   pale violet
    150 „   full violet
    160 „   deep purple
    170 „   the same.

The bark was now removed and washed; a fresh portion of water was added, and the temperature raised to 190°. Scarcely a trace of starch remained.

OBS.—The *starch* is taken up between 140° and 170°.

EXP. 11.—The residual bark, after 5 cold macerations (ex. 1), was boiled half an hour in *distilled water*; the fluid was turbid. While hot it was of a reddish yellow colour, but became milky when cold. A slight bitterness and acidity were perceptible, and a little blackness was produced by the addition of tr. ferri mur.; the specific gravity was ·999· One half of this fluid was acidulated with sulphuric acid and boiled, and continued acid after boiling. It was saturated with lime, boiled, and filtered; and the residuum boiled twice in spirit of wine. The spirit filtered and withdrawn left of quinine 56 grs.

The other half of the fluid was strained and evaporated. It continued turbid, but no precipitation took place. When reduced to a dry state, it curled up like a layer of starch, and weighed only 1½ oz.

1 oz. of this matter was incinerated without flame. A little aroma escaped. The ashes, 50 grains, were boiled in distilled water, which took up 16 grs., leaving 34 undissolved.

The solution, tested with the nitrates of silver and baryta, and tartaric acid, indicated the presence of *sulphuric acid, muriatic acid*, and *potash*.

The 34 grains were almost entirely dissolved in water acidulated with pure muriatic acid. Ferrocyanate of potash, ammonia, and bicarbonate of soda, indicated *iron, alumina*, and *lime*.

Obs.—The sp. gr. of the decoction after cold maceration is sometimes above, but more frequently below, 1000. When the sp. gr rises above 1000, it is chiefly owing to the presence of a little gum. The starch is lighter than water. The quantity of quinine taken up from 28 lbs. of bark by boiling distilled water, after 5 cold macerations, is 112 grs.

Exp. 12.—The residual bark from Exp. 11. was boiled half an hour in distilled water *acidulated with sulphuric acid.* To the strained liquor, still acid, was added new burnt lime in powder. The mixture was boiled half an hour, and the fluid strained off through hempen bags. The collected matter was thoroughly dried, and boiled half an hour in 12 pints of rectified spirit. The spirit was passed through paper, and the refuse washed with a second portion of spirit, which was added to the first. The spirit was then brought over by distillation, and left in the balneum 3 oz. 280 grs. of *quinine* resembling wax.

Exp. 13.—28 lbs. of yellow bark having been subjected to 6 macerations in cold water until the infusion ceased to gain any increase in specific gravity, were macerated in water *acidulated with acetic acid* (specific gravity of vinegar 1004).

In half an hour the sp. gr. of the fluid was 1001, and ammonia gave a large precipitate. In 1 hour the sp. gr. was 1006. In 4 hours it still remained at 1006.

The fluid was drawn off and a fresh portion of acidulated water added. This operation was repeated 3 times.

The fluids were mixed, and precipitated by ammonia. The precipitate was placed in dilute acetic acid, but a considerable portion, 370 grs. remained undissolved.

The acetic solution was carefully precipitated by oxalic acid, and the precipitate, when dry and burned, (lime) weighed 152 grs. The fluid from which the lime had been separated by oxalic acid was then precipitated by ammonia, and the precipitate, when dry, *(quinine)* weighed 2 oz. 300 grs.

The 370 grains not taken up by acetic acid were macerated 24 hours in 1 pint of cold rectified spirit, sp. gr. 838. The spirit took up 201 grains, and became of a dark colour, leaving 169 grains undissolved.

The 169 grs. were boiled in spirit 10 minutes. The filtered fluid was dark. The insoluble refuse weighed 114 grs., having lost 55.

The two portions of spirit were mixed, and the spirit being separated by distillation in a glass retort, left 3 dr. 3 grs. of a dark matter *(tannin)* which produced an intensely black colour with tr. ferri mur.

The insoluble refuse, 114 grs., was burned, and left 6½ grs. of ashes extremely light and bulky.

Obs.—Exps. 12 and 13 show that after cold water has taken up the whole of the quinine and other soluble matters deposited in the cells of the bark, there may still remain a further portion of quinine, together with lime and tannin, so intimately united with the tissue itself as to be only separable by means of acids.

This portion of quinine, when completely separated by sulphuric acid, amounted, in this instance, to 3 oz. 280 grs.

Acetic acid takes up this second portion of quinine less perfectly than sulphuric acid, but the quinine is separated from acetic acid with greater facility and less expense by means of ammonia without the use of spirit. The quinine thus obtained is generally combined with more or less tannin, which it is extremely difficult to remove from it. There is, however, no necessity to do this if the quinine is to be added to the liquor, of which tannin is an important constituent. The combination is easily effected by dissolving the quinine and tannin in a little dilute acetic acid. I have before alluded, under Exp. 3, to the expense of this part of the operation, and 1 may add that I have sometimes found that cold water has taken up *the whole, or nearly the whole,* of the quinine, so that the residual bark has yielded little or none to acetic acid.

I shall here introduce two experiments to show more clearly the power of acetic acid as a solvent of quinine.

EXP. 14.—2 oz. of Howard's yellow bark, subpulverized, were placed in 14 oz. of distilled water and 2 oz. of *distilled vinegar* for half an hour, and frequently stirred. The fluid was filtered through washed white paper, and precipitated with ammonia so long as a creamy separation took place. The precipitate was very abundant. The colourless supernatant fluid, being treated with more ammonia, gave a yellow precipitate resembling powdered gamboge. The two precipitates mixed, weighed, when quite dry, 25 grs.

The bark was again macerated for half an hour in 7 oz. of distilled water and 1 oz. of distilled vinegar, and the fluid filtered through washed white paper. Ammonia being added as before, a considerable precipitation ensued, but much less than the first. The supernatant fluid was red, and the precipitate was tinged with the same colour. It weighed, when dry, 7 grs.

A third maceration was made with 7 oz. of distilled water and half an ounce of distilled vinegar, and ammonia added to the filtered fluid as before. The precipitate was a deep red colour, as well as the supernatant fluid. The former, when dry, weighed 4 grs.

The same operation was repeated with 2 drs. of distilled vinegar. The precipitate and fluid were quite red. The former weighed 3 grs. A fifth maceration with 1 drachm of distilled vinegar gave only half a grain. A sixth maceration with half an ounce of distilled vinegar yielded 0. The residual bark was boiled ten minutes in water acidulated with sulphuric acid. The strained fluid was saturated with magnesia, and the magnesian matter dried and boiled in rectified spirits for several minutes. The spirit being withdrawn left of quinine quite dry, barely 1 gr.

The precipitates, 1-5, weighing 39½ grs. were placed in half a pint of distilled water, and acetic acid added to dissolve the quinine; the filtered fluid was carefully precipitated by ammonia, and the quinine, when collected and dried, weighed 23 grs., to which may be added 2 grs. for the quinine remaining on the filter—in all 25 grs.

The 23 grs. were incinerated with difficulty, burning like leather. Half a grain only remained.

The last experiment was repeated as far as the third maceration with 4 oz. of bark; and the quinine subsequently separated from the residual bark by sulphuric acid weighed 3½ grs., which nearly agrees with the former result.

EXP. 15.—2 oz. of Howard's yellow bark were boiled ten minutes in 1 oz. of distilled water acidulated with *sulphuric acid*. The fluid was strained, and the bark boiled ten minutes in a second portion of acidulated water. The decoction was fully saturated with magnesia, and the dried magnesian matter boiled ten minutes in two successive portions of rectified spirit. The solutions were mixed, and the spirit being withdrawn left 26 grs. of quinine.

OBS.—The colourless precipitate from the first acetic solution was quinine nearly pure; the second, of a gamboge colour, chiefly tannin; the subsequent precipitates consisted almost entirely of tannin. The quinine taken up by sulphuric and acetic acids was as 26 : 25.

EXP. 16.—2 oz. of yellow bark subpulverized were macerated several days in 1 oz. of spirit of wine. The spirit was brought over, and left a small quantity of dry *inflammable* extract, consisting of *resin* and tannin.

EXP. 17.—1 lb. of yellow bark was macerated in 1 gallon of distilled water 2 hours, and then placed in a still well luted, and water added to prevent burning. 1 gallon was brought over, sp. gr. 1000, yielding the *odour* of the bark, and a little *essential oil* was detected on the surface. When the still-head was removed, the odour was very strong.

It appears from these experiments that yellow bark contains—

A peculiar acid, Exp. 7.
Quinine, Exp. 2, 3, 9, 11, 12, 13.
Tannin, Exp. 1, 2, 5, 8, 13.
Aromatic principle (essential oil?), Exp. 17.
Lime, Exp. 4, 6, 7, 11.
Potash, Exp. 11.
Alumina, Exp. 4, 6, 11.
Muriatic and sulphuric acids, Exp. 4, 6, 11.
Iron, Exp. 4, 6, 11.
Silex, Exp. 4.
Wax, Exp. 8.
Resin, Exp. 16.

Gummy matter, Exp. 7.
Starch, Exp. 10, 11.
Woody tissue.

The following experiment was made to ascertain the length of time required for the cold infusion.

EXP. 18.—Half a pound of yellow bark subpulverized was placed in two pints of cold distilled water. In five minutes the fluid was acid to test paper. In twenty minutes it was manifestly acid to the taste.

In half an hour the filtered infusion was of a beautiful straw colour, fragrant, and agreeably bitter, sp. gr. 1004½. Tr. ferri mur. produced a delicate grass green tinge, and a little separation.

Tr. of galls gave a slight brownish white disturbance; tartarized antimony, a whitish precipitate: *oxalic acid, no perceptible change.*

In one hour the fluid was a deeper straw colour, more bitter, but not unpleasant. The bitter remained long upon the tongue, sp. gr. 1006¼. Tr. ferri mur. produced a deep green colour, and a larger precipitate; tartarized antimony and tr. galls a great disturbance; *oxalic acid no change.*

In two hours the bitter was much more intense, and the test paper was made quite red. Sp. gr. 1009. Tr. ferri mur. produced instantly an opaque green, and the subsequent precipitation was still greater. The effect of tartarized antimony and tr. of galls was much the same as before. *Oxalic acid produced a great disturbance.* The precipitated matter was a yellowish white.

In three hours test paper had the same appearance; the taste was very bitter and permanent; sp. gr. 1011½. Tr. ferri mur. produced the same effect as in the first trial. The other tests as before.

In four hours, sp. gr. had not increased. Tr. ferri mur. and the other reagents produced the same changes as in the last.

In five hours and a half, sp. gr. was still 1011½. Tr. ferri mur. produced a dull green, but very little precipitate.

In six hours, sp. gr. the same. Tr. ferri mur. gave a still paler green, and no opacity or precipitation.

Two pints of cold distilled water were now added, which reduced the specific gravity of the fluid to 1006. At the end of one hour, sp. gr. was still 1006. Nothing therefore had been taken up by the additional water.

OBS.—The quantity of water employed in this experiment was four times the weight of the bark, on account of the small quantity of bark experimented upon.

The most agreeable cold infusion, and that which is most likely to suit a weak stomach, is formed in the first half hour. The sp. gr. continues to increase to the end of the third hour, after which little or nothing is gained by continuing the maceration in the same fluid.

If the fluid is now poured off, and a fresh proportion of water added, the maceration may be repeated for the same time.

The acid, quinine, tannin, and aromatic principles, are taken up rapidly from the commencement of the operation ; *the lime somewhat later.*

The tannin taken up by the water apparently forms subsequently a new combination, which diminishes its effect on salts of iron; for after six hours' maceration, the infusion, which had previously given a copious precipitate with tr. ferri mur., ceased to do so, though it acquired the green colour.

EXP. 19.—1 lb. of *finely powdered* bark was macerated one hour in four pints of cold distilled water, and the infusion filtered. As the filtration proceeded, more distilled water was added four successive times, until the sp. gr. of the infusion was reduced to 1000.

The bark was then boiled ten minutes in *water*, and the strained decoction slightly acidulated with sulphuric acid and boiled. At the termination of the boiling the decoction was still acid. The fluid was again strained and saturated with lime; and the residuum dried and boiled fifteen minutes in half a pint of spirit of wine. The spirit being abstracted from the filtered fluid, left, of quinine, 4 grs.

The bark was next boiled twenty minutes in *water acidulated with sulphuric acid*, and the strained fluid saturated with lime. The residuum was dried and boiled in two successive portions of spirit. The spirit mixed, and brought over by distillation, left, of quinine, 59 grs.

The same operation was performed by cold maceration with 1 lb. of *subpulverized bark*, till sp. gr of infusion was 1000. The quinine subsequently taken up by boiling water weighed 4 grs.; and the quinine taken up by boiling water acidulated with sulphuric acid weighed 58 grs.

It follows, then, that the quinine taken up by cold infusion must also have been the same in the two cases, and consequently that no advantage is gained by reducing the bark to the state of powder.

The conclusions to be drawn from these experiments are—

1. Bark will yield to *cold distilled water* all its constituents except starch and woody fibre, some earthy salts, and a small portion of tannin and quinine, which can only be separated from the tissue by means of an acid.

2. 28 lbs. of good yellow bark will yield from 5 to 6 lbs. of concentrated liquor, sp. gr. 1200, containing about 10 oz. quinine; the aroma, and the greater part of the tannin and iron, and the peculiar acid of bark, of which only a small portion is lost, forming an inert salt with lime.

3. To form this liquor it is only necessary to subpulverize the bark, and macerate it from four to six hours in twice its weight of cold distilled water, repeating the process twice, or at most thrice: to concentrate the infusions over a water bath to sp. gr. 1200, and allow the liquor to deposit the gummy matter and so much of the tannin as it cannot retain in solution.

To separate any gum that may still remain in the liquor, and to prevent any decomposition, proof spirit is added to it, until the sp. gr. of the liquor is reduced to 1100. The quinine still remaining in the bark, may, if it be thought desirable, be separated by acetic acid, and precipitated from its solution by ammonia; and being redissolved in a small quantity of dilute acetic acid, may be diffused in the liquor.

The advantages of this medicine are—

1. That it contains not one, but all the active principles of yellow bark.

2. That the greater part of the quinine is preserved *in its natural state* in combination with the peculiar acid of bark, in which it is more soluble than in sulphuric acid.

3. That the active principles *have undergone no change*, either from exposure to too great heat, as in the decoction, &c. or by being brought into too close contiguity, as in the extract, in which secondary formations take place to so great an extent that water is incapable of redissolving it.

4. That, containing no starch and little gum, it will remain unaltered for a great length of time.

5. That the quantity of spirit contained in a dose is too small to be objectionable.

6. That it is a convenient, agreeable, and elegant medicine, miscible with wine or water in any proportion.

On its merits as a therapeutic agent I forbear to enter. I will only add, that whatever yellow bark can accomplish will be best performed either by the recent cold infusion or the concentrated liquor. The latter not only agrees with the stomach, when irritation and nausea are produced by the disulphate of quinine, but it not unfrequently succeeds in obstinate periodic and cachectic diseases when the disulphate of quinine has failed. But the liquor cinchona has been so long before the profession, and is so extensively employed, that it requires no observations of mine to prove its efficacy. My object, in the present paper, is rather to make more generally known the exact method of preparing it, and to direct attention especially to those peculiarities in the process on which its elegance and efficacy chiefly depend.

The above is offered as a *pharmaceutical* analysis of yellow bark ; a *chemical* analysis I hope to have the pleasure of presenting before long, as well as a similar series of experiments on the cinchona lancifolia.

RICHARD BATTLEY.

Laboratory, Ophthalmic Hospital, Moorfields, April 1843.

CASE OF ILEUS.

(For the London Medical Gazette.)

WE beg to offer the accompanying account of a case of ileus to the Editors of the MEDICAL GAZETTE, for insertion, if approved, in their periodical; for—

1st. We may learn from it the advantage of adopting, in cases in which no rational plan of treatment presents itself, the *methodus expectans*, or of husbanding up the vital powers to support any providential efforts at recovery which may be made in the system.

2dly. It was daily observed that, when the intestines were loaded to fulness, the *passio iliaca*, or reversed action of the intestines, was uniformly accompanied by spasm or cramp of those muscles forming the abdominal parietes; so that the external surface or skin was corrugated and irregular, in like manner as is visible on the larger muscles of the extremities when under the influence of cramp; and this continued until the fæcal matters were brought up by the stomach.

3dly. We learn the length of time the body can be supported by the absorption of its own substance, after so serious an attack of disease, and such complete obstruction, together with material derangement, of a vital function.

D. R. & DAVID R. M'NAB.

Epping, April 20, 1843.

A—— B——, has had occasionally, for the last five years, pain in the right hypogastric region; and three years ago had an illness, with griping pain in the abdomen.

March 12, A.M.—Has griping pain in the abdomen, sickness, and desire to go to stool.

℞ Hyd. Chlor. gr. iiss.; P. Opii, gr. ½, stat. sum.

℞ Haust. Rhei, et Mag. Carb. hor. j. post hac sum.

7 o'clock P.M.—No evacuation of the bowels.

℞ Haust. Sennæ Co. stat. sum.: vomited. Administ. Enema Salis et Sap.: with this came away much hard fæcal matter.

13th.—Pain violent; vomiting and constipation continue; abdomen tympanitic; pain rather relieved by pressure. During the paroxysms of pain the pulse very small, and extremities cold. Tongue milky and dotted.

Capiat. Mist. Ol. Ricini, ex mucilag.: vomited again.

℞ Ol. Ricini, ʒss. 6tis hor. sum.

℞ Hyd. Chlorid. gr. j. hor. ij. post Ol. Ricini, et 6tis hor. sum.

Balneum calidum bis terve die. Dry heat to the abdomen.

P.M.—Administratur enema Ol. Terebinth.

℞ Linim. Hyd. Co. abdom. infricand.

14th.—Abdomen tender and tympanitic; vomiting and constipation continue.

℞ Hirudin. xij. abdom. applicand. Baln. calid.

To allay the violent paroxysms of colic pains—

℞ Morphiæ Acet. gr. ½, 3tiis hor. ad tert. vic. sum.

P.M.—℞ Mag. Sulph. ʒj. 3tiis hor. sum.

15th.—Leeches were again applied to the abdomen, and a blister, with a repetition of blue pill and morphia.

16th.—Stercoraceous vomiting came on; and from 16th to 31st, to produce evacuation of the bowels, besides injections, the following were prescribed:—

1.—℞ Hyd. Chlorid. gr. x.; Morphiæ Acet. gr. j. M. ft. massa in pil. iv. div. cap. j. 6tis hor.

2.—Croton oil enema, and croton oil in the form of a pill, every four hours, by which increase of pain and sickness were produced, and the matter vomited was in colour dark-green.

3.—Ox gall, by injections and as pills, to ʒiss.

After which remedies the system was supported by occasional beef-tea injections, effervescing medicine, brandy and water, and yoke of egg, &c.

The abdomen was vastly distended and tympanitic; vomiting and constipation continued; emaciation extreme.

The tongue, at first milky and dotted, became gradually furred, till redness, appearing as a streak in the centre, spread over the whole tongue, which was moist and dry according to the morning and evening changes of the typhoid symptoms.

Pulse variable, as affected by the remedies.

Mind at first very collected, and perceptions unusually quick; latterly much sopor, after which delirium followed, until the senses could be quite roused.

April 1st.—Passed involuntarily a large quantity of urine.

2d, 5 P.M.—Tongue still dry; pulse quick and sharp.

6 P.M.—At length, after a period of twenty-one days, two evacuations were passed from the bowels, yellow, and of thick gruel consistence. Pulse much softer.

Admin. enema sap., which was followed by a large evacuation like the above.

℞ Haust. Sod. Tart. Efferv.

3d.—No sickness; appetite returned.

4th.—℞ Quinæ Disulph. gr. j. bis die sum.

8th.—Tongue paler and moist; pulse soft and quick. Diet: port wine or brandy and water, broth, mutton chops, eggs, bread and milk, &c.

Sleeps frequently night and day. Mind listless and dull. Temper cross and self-willed. He has continued to improve.

MEDICAL GAZETTE.

Friday, April 28, 1843.

" Licet omnibus, licet etiam mihi, dignitatem *Artis Medicæ* tueri; potestas modo veniendi in publicum sit, dicendi periculum non recuso."
                                          CICERO.

MEDICAL EDUCATION.

THE practical division of the profession into two great classes, those, namely, who can afford to wait, and those who cannot—adverted to in a former number—produces also a difference, chiefly as to literary qualifications generally attained by each; and all that the State seems bound to do is to fix a minimum of the required professional education. In contending for a high standard of general education for all who enter the profession, no new thing is imagined. An *equally* high standard for all would be new, but there would be no harm in the novelty What was the case formerly, and what is the theory at present ? Two neighbours of the middling class send their sons to the same school—Eton, Harrow, Westminster, or a good private establishment. One goes to College, graduates in arts, and subsequently in medicine; comes to London, and studies the practice of his profession in the hospital and the lecture-room; gets, it may be, appointed to a public institution; spends his leisure in the pursuits of literature, science, or travel, and in the society of the gentry who were his companions at school and college; takes not a single fee for five years or more, and then gets gradually into practice as a physician, occupying a place more or less distinguished, according to his talents or opportunities. The other leaves school at 14 or 16, is bound apprentice to a general practitioner, spends five years in dispensing; and if he have a good master, or watchful parents, in profitable study of elementary works. At 19 he comes to town; spends two or three years at the hospital and lectures; passes his examination at 22, and becomes a general practitioner. What has made the difference between these two young men? What has made the parents of the latter select for him this course instead of the other? Not the mere difference in expense between a College education and a high apprentice-fee; but the difference between the prospect of his getting profitable employment soon instead of late. The one could afford to wait; the other could not. But how was the immediate return obtained ? Partly, no doubt, at least in former times, by the sale of drugs; for in the most private shops there was formerly something of this kind—families were supplied by the family apothecary. Or he might earn a good salary, and hold a respectable station in society as an assistant; but his principal dependence was on dispensing the prescriptions of physicians, and on his practice amongst the middling classes. An apothecary, twenty years ago, could pay his expenses by the prescriptions of physicians; and he often obtained these from houses where he never prescribed himself for the heads of the family.

This source of income is now entirely gone, or very nearly so. The apothecary, highly educated, and no longer the mere dependent of the physician, has become, in fact, a substantive person; but has he, with the professional education of the physician, the means of waiting till these acquirements shall be demanded and paid for by the public ? If he has, then, let him be called what he will, his actual status is the same as that of the physician, and he has ceased to belong to the class who cannot afford to wait. If he has not, then let us see what are his resources. As an assistant, what will he get? For an answer see the advertisements in the medical and daily journals. A Union—he may live *with* that, but hardly *by* it. He must in self-defence open a shop. To do this successfully, he must compete in matter and in manner with the druggist and the grocer; and now of what use is his degree *in literis humanioribus*, his ancient and modern languages, his " treatises *de senectute* and *de amicitiá*, his shorter or longer oration," his philosophy (that, indeed, is wanted), his algebra? —elegant recreations, and useful withal to fill up the time, together with driving away the flies in summer, and the cold in winter!

It is all very well for men in large practice, where cathartic mixture is made by the gallon, and pills by the gross, to get paid for the medicine made in their shops—*non olet;* but it taints the whole man, inside and out, who has to take pence behind his own counter.

In these days we are not likely to meet with practitioners, empirical or regular, uniting the family experience of seven generations in their own persons, like the one mentioned by Lady M. Wortley Montague; but there are qualities sometimes found among the unlicensed and the unlearned, which command a success denied to the laureated possessors of diplomas. The greatest skill in the practice of our art, and the most substantial marks of public favour, are often found with persons who are wofully deficient in those qualities, whether natural or acquired, which most dignify and adorn the inner man.

Do we, then, undervalue the function of the druggist as such—or that of the apothecary of days long past? By no means. Still less do we think lightly of the qualifications that ought to be possessed by every one who practises medicine. We do not think one degree of knowledge good enough for the constitution of the poor, and another for that of the rich; but we do happen to know that the ignorant poor, as well as the ignorant rich, will not go exactly where the best knowledge and skill are to be procured. They will go where they please; and if a totally uneducated man can attract the public to his shop, not only for medicine but for advice, then we would say, that to insist on those who advise having some qualification instead of none, is wise and humane.

The new bill, it seems, proposes to allow those to practise who are already practising, and will insist on the qualifications of future candidates being sufficient to render their practice at least harmless. This seems to be pretty much what was done in the case of the apothecaries. The Apothecaries' Act let in all those who were in practice before 1815; subjected all future candidates for admission to the surveillance of the Worshipful Society: and whatever theoretical objections may be made to appointing a private corporation the guardians of public interest in so important a matter, it is notoriously matter of experience that the present false position of the apothecary is in great degree consequent on the high standard of education required for the license of the Worshipful Society,—a circumstance indicating no neglect, on their part, of the public health.

The principal remedy for the existing evils is to be found in the gradual and persevering exertions of the general practitioner to improve his acquirements and his position, to educate himself and all about him to the highest standard of real professional dignity that his present position admits of. Let him be paid for his time and skill, not for his physic; and we would add, let him not hold that time and skill too cheap—charge enough for them when they are required, but pay no more visits than are wanted.

The physician and pure surgeon must take care of themselves, to keep their acquirements so much above those of the majority that they shall be looked up to as advisers worth having. This their ample means, the prolonged and scientific studies which they can command, and the public appointments for which these may fit them, ought to enable them to do. If these opportunities do not make them superior, no legislation will do so. Of really consulting physicians or surgeons but few are required, and those few must be really the best.

It would probably not be expedient, as it assuredly is not practicable, for the general practitioner to give up at once the dispensing of his own medicines. The public are not educated up to this; the profession cannot afford it. It is an excellent guarantee for the goodness of the drugs, that they are furnished by a person deeply concerned for their efficiency; only, do not let them be the thing paid for. We have no great faith in public meetings, to do badly and with tumult what the same number of persons could better do quietly, or we could wish there were an association to settle a scale of charges, below which no member should practise under pain of expulsion; but unity, not uniformity—individual firmness, not united clamour, are what the circumstances require.

MEDICAL REFORM.

(HOUSE OF COMMONS, Tuesday, April 25.)

MR. MACAULAY wished to put a question to the right hon. baronet the Secretary of State for the Home Department respecting a very important subject—he meant the subject of reform in the medical profession. He wished to know whether those negotiations which he had been told were in progress some time ago on this subject, had been brought to such a termination as to enable the introduction of a bill into Parliament on the subject? He wished to know, secondly, whether there was any reasonable expectation of such an act being passed into a law this session? And thirdly, if the right hon. baronet felt that they could not expect to pass a general measure on the subject this session, whether he would have any objection to introduce into the Poor Law Act a clause to remedy the most pressing and crying grievances under which the medical profession now laboured, from the construction of the present law, in the exclusion of Scotch and Irish medical men from practising in the workhouses?

Sir J. Graham said, he had no hesitation in saying that the negotiations to which the right hon. gentleman referred had been so far successful as to leave no doubt on his mind that in a very short period he should be able to ask the leave of the house to introduce a measure with respect to the medical profession. As to the second question of the right hon. gentleman, whether there was any hope of passing such measure this year, that of course must depend on the reception given to it. He was disposed to think that the measure was worthy the attention of the house, and he should bring it forward in the expectation that it would pass this session. At the present time he felt certain he should be able, in the course of the present session, to bring forward a measure on the subject, and it was his confident belief that it would pass into a law this session. He should only advert briefly to the third point. He felt that the practitioners of Scotland and Ireland were subjected to great hardship by the interpretation put on the act with reference to English practitioners, and that some legislative measure was called for on that particular point.—*Times.*

WIDOWS AND ORPHANS SOCIETY.

DEATH OF THE DUKE OF SUSSEX, THE PATRON.

THE late lamented Duke of Sussex became the patron of this Society on the death of the Duke of Kent, in 1820.

As soon as the death of His Royal Highness, on Friday last, was made known, an Extraordinary Court of Directors was summoned, by requisition, to consider the propriety of postponing the Annual Dinner of the Society. The Dinner had been appointed to take place on Saturday, the 29th instant, and His Royal Highness the Duke of Cambridge had graciously consented to preside on the occasion. The postponement was unanimously resolved on.

No other day can with propriety be fixed until the termination of the Court mourning, when it is probable that the Stewards will again endeavour to obtain the gracious presence of the royal Chairman.

MEDICO-LEGAL EVIDENCE IN A CASE OF SUSPECTED POISONING.

To the Editor of the Medical Gazette.

SIR,

I FORWARD to you an outline of the trial of Mary Hunter, indicted for the murder of her late husband, by administering to him arsenic, which caused the disease of which he languished from the 25th to the 28th of November, and then died. She was also arraigned on the coroner's inquest.

When your readers are informed that this trial, which was brought to a premature close by the case for the prosecution breaking down under the able cross-examination of the witnesses against the prisoner, before anything was urged in her defence, they will at once see that it is alike impossible for you to publish, or for me to write, a full report of the whole case. I will therefore attempt no more than to state, in the most succinct manner I am able, what, to the best of my judgment, are the true facts, qualifying those which were stated in the prosecution by what I know would have been urged in defence. I intend, at the earliest possible opportunity, to prepare a full account, which, in consequence of my very intimate knowledge of the circumstances, I believe I can do more completely than any other individual; if any, therefore, suspect that the following account is a partial one, I entreat them to suspend their judgment until they see the whole.

I will not attempt giving an outline of the evidence of each witness, for that you can refer to the Liverpool newspapers (the Mail and the Albion contain the best reports I have yet seen, but very imperfect nevertheless): I prefer stating in the natural order the circumstances which I consider proved, and which would not have been disproved by the witnesses or arguments for the defence.

Mr. Wilkins and Mr. Monk appeared for

the prosecution, and Mr. Pollock, of Manchester, for the defence.—I am, sir,

Your obedient servant,
P. H. HOLLAND, M.R.C.S.L.

Manchester, April 10, 1843.

Character of the deceased.—It was clearly proved that the deceased, a mechanic, was a hard-working thrifty man, of steady habits: that he had laid by a considerable amount of money as provision for himself and for his family; that he was a kind husband and father; and those in most immediate connexion with the family believed that for ten years he had lived with the prisoner in peace and comfort.

Character of the prisoner.—The witnesses all agreed in saying that she was an attentive wife and kind mother: that she was remarkable for keeping her husband's house clean and tidy. The only fault ascribed to her was the unhappy practice of drinking. It did not appear that she was a positive drunkard, but certainly she drank much and often. An attempt was made to prove that a long time ago she stole money from her husband to pay her drinking debts, lest he should discover her bad behaviour; and mention was made of some indecent levity of which it was said she had been guilty nearly two years before; committed, however, in the presence of witnesses who themselves considered it a joke. May we not judge of the *animus* with which the prosecution was urged by the fact of these old stories having (even if true) been raked up against her?

Poison in possession of prisoner.—It was distinctly proved, and, though at first denied, afterwards acknowledged by the prisoner, that she had purchased two ounces of arsenic, as she said, to poison twitchclocks (blackbeetles) and mice. It was also proved that her next-door neighbour's house, and therefore probably her own, was infested with twitchclocks, and though no mice were found on searching the house, that is no proof they were not there.

An attempt was now made to show that the arsenic was bought *secretly*, but it signally failed. She says that she lost the arsenic on her way home, and a witness said that she had given her the same account a week preceding the deceased's illness; and it is most probable that this is true, for a most diligent search discovered no trace of arsenic in any part of the premises. If so much as two ounces had been put into the fire, its penetrating garlicky fumes would have been almost inevitably perceived; if put into the privy, almost as inevitably detected by the rigorous chemical analysis which was instituted.

Behaviour of the accused.—At the inquest the witnesses all agreed in saying that nothing in her behaviour had excited their suspicion. When her husband was taken suddenly ill, she quickly gave the alarm, and ran off herself to her usual doctor, and not finding him in went to a second; again failing, went to a third, whom her husband wished to have. She nursed him attentively throughout his illness; told Mr. Harrison, the surgeon, that she was sorry he had not come sooner, as she had expected. This readiness to put the case under medical observation looks very unlike conscious guilt. The only neglect attributed to her was allowing the water to escape from a bottle put to her husband's feet, by which the bed was wet, and was allowed to remain so. There was no hasty putting away of the matters purged or vomited; there was a very natural attempt made to avoid inspection and an inquest, and a hasty seeking to get possession of his property. This, she says, was because she thought his relations would try to prevent her getting it; a suspicion which events have shown was not entirely without foundation.

Previous health of the deceased.—This was stated to have been perfectly good, as he was never off his work from illness, and had made no applications for " sick money" from the club; but I believe that though never positively ill, he was rarely quite well, that he had recently had syphilis, and probably had had mercury, that he had habitually stinking breath, griping pains, uncertain appetite, and wind; for which he was in the habit of taking cayenne pepper.

History of the fatal disorder.—The deceased returned from work about 6 on Friday evening, the 25th of November last, in apparently good health; he took five or six spoonsful of porridge made with milk and meal, and *almost immediately* became violently sick, with vomiting and purging. The matter first vomited was large in quantity, frothy brown, and offensive, and appeared to contain pieces of carrot; no particular examination of it was made. He was apparently purged violently; the first stools were not observed; that which the surgeon's assistant saw was clay-coloured and not particularly offensive, but one of the attendants said one before was ragged, loose, of a foul colour, and very bad smell. The deceased became extremely exhausted, and in half an hour was unable to walk, and when he was taken by the arm to be assisted to bed he screamed from pain, probably from the abdomen being thereby stretched.

When taking the porridge he complained of its taste: said, "Mary, thou hast put summut in this porridge, either pepper or snuff:" it made his throat hot and painful. This heat of the throat seems to have been complained of for a very short time only. The accused said that she had that morning boiled some cayenne pepper in the pan in which the

porridge was made, and that perhaps she might have neglected to wash it out. If any thing was in the porridge it must have been something besides arsenic, as that has no taste, would not very quickly produce heat of the throat, which cayenne would, and the heat produced by arsenic would not be, like that produced by a small quantity of cayenne, temporary only. The vomiting and purging having continued violently for half an hour, gradually subsided, and after two or three hours entirely ceased, and did not again recur; the pain and tenderness also, which had been violent at first, were entirely absent afterwards: upon this point the surgeon speaks quite positively : " he had no pain or tenderness at all after the subsidence of the vomiting." This is exceedingly unlike the progress of fatal gastritis from arsenic : there are many fatal cases recorded of no pain having been complained of at all, cases in which the patient dies from the overpowering effect upon the nervous system— one such I have myself put on record in your pages—but has there been one single case of severe pain once excited ever subsiding, except for short intervals, unless, indeed, recovery has followed? I am sure it is extremely rare, if ever it happened at all.

The deceased was seen at 9 o'clock, about three hours after the apparent commencement of the disorder, by Mr. Willis, assistant to Mr. Harrison, who describes his state then as that of collapse—the pulse very weak, and the extremities cold : the stool which he saw was clay-coloured, and the vomiting not bilious. He was then retching violently, but there was no vomiting. Mr. Willis considered it a case of common cholera, and prescribed some calomel and opium, and effervescing draughts with ten minims of laudanum in each.

It is probable that the case was not at that time considered a serious one, for Mr. Harrison did not visit the patient till 3 P.M. the succeeding day, 23 hours after the commencement of the disorder: the wife, however, complained that he did not come before. He found the patient " still in collapse, pulseless, very weak, with difficulty of breathing, no particular pain nor tenderness on pressure, which he had expected after such violent vomiting :" the vomiting and purging had then entirely ceased, and did not recur : he subsequently became costive. He was not in a state of stupor, but indisposed to answer questions. He had no hoarseness or change of voice; no remarkable change of countenance : he looked merely anxious and sharpened. The eyes were a little sunk, but not red or bright, or otherwise remarkable. The questions by which all this was elicited so distinctly and so unequivocally were put by Mr. Pollock in a manner which showed that he was, as I know he is, quite conversant with the subject, and should be a warning to all members of our profession how they venture unprepared into a witness-box. As I differ from Mr. Harrison in the view which he takes of this case, I think it only just to say that I am sure but very few could have borne so well so stringent an examination; a hundred times more severe and searching than I got at either the College or the Hall, whatever the experience of others may have been. But to proceed with the history. On Sunday forenoon Mr. Harrison found the patient " in the same state;" " he was very restless, had great thirst and tightness across the chest, and suppression of urine." There being yet no reaction, he thought the man in great danger, and told his wife so. He ordered him a drop of prussic acid in the effervescing mixture, a blister to his stomach, a bottle of hot water to his feet, and a mustard bath (to his feet, as I understand). All these means were properly employed, except from the carelessness about the bottle of hot water, which might easily pass undetected without any culpable negligence, as the man was so nearly insensible; and it appeared to me ungenerous in Mr. Wilkins to urge it against the wife as a presumption of animal indifference to her sick husband's comfort and safety.

On Sunday night he was seen again, and remained still in the same state.

On Monday morning he had great thirst, could scarcely speak, and was evidently dying.

One of his fellow workmen is reported to have heard him express, on the Monday, a strong expectation of recovery: " he had been very ill, but would be at his work by the end of the week." I have not, however, verified this statement; I suspect there is some error as to the time at which it was said. He had cramp on the Monday evening, but no convulsions or paralysis. He died on Monday night, about seventy-five hours after taking the suspected article of food.

Though both he and the accused herself attributed his illness to the porridge, he does not appear to have himself entertained any suspicion of her intentions. The wife foolishly, but very naturally, threw away the porridge and basin, and the meal of which it was made, lest, as she said, somebody else should be made ill by them. Some porridge found in a broken basin, in the privy, supposed to be this, was analysed, and nothing found. The deceased told his wife that the porridge was not fit to eat, and she might give it to the dog. She replied, "nay, if it has hurt you it will hurt him, she would throw it away;" and who is there that loves a dog that would not have done just the same? Though these little circumstances have been dwelt upon after-

wards as presumptions of guilty knowledge, so little did this attract notice at the time that no suspicion whatever appears to have been excited, until it was learned, the day after the man's death, that the wife had purchased arsenic from the druggist who was accustomed to supply her with medicine, who she herself voluntarily told that her husband was sick to death, and that Mr. Harrison was attending him—a very extraordinary communication to make by a woman who had a guilty knowledge of *the cause* of that sick husband's illness! Suspicion, however, being thus excited, a coroner's inquest was summoned, and an inspection of the body ordered, which was made on Tuesday evening, by Mr. Harrison and Mr. Dyson, Surgeons.

Externally every thing appeared healthy. There was no blackness or lividity of the genitals; no eruption of any kind; the body was not at all supple, as it often is when blood is prevented from coagulating by arsenic. The *post-mortem* contraction of the muscles seems to be, like the coagulation of the blood, the last act of vitality, and appears to be prevented by the same circumstances, namely a rapid exhaustion of the vital powers before death.

On opening the cavity of the abdomen every thing appeared healthy, till, on " removing the stomach and intestines as far as the rectum, and laying them open, very considerable inflammation presented itself in the stomach in particular, and in patches throughout the intestinal canal to the rectum, where there was considerable irritation; patches of redness in the jejunum; great corrugation of the bladder." The stomach and bowels were found *empty*, except a piece of potatoe at the pylorus (it appears that the deceased had not eaten potatoes during his illness; the last time was on Friday at noon). Upon more particular inquiry Mr. Harrison said that there were about four ounces of reddish brown fluid, apparently coloured with blood, in the alimentary canal, which is consistent enough with the expression empty; whereas Mr. Dyson's account, that "there was a large quantity of bloody fluid," is not consistent with Mr. Harrison's and his own previous description.

The mucous coat was highly inflamed in distinct patches, with evident destruction of some portions of that membrane. The patches were brick red, rather than black or brown, in colour; did not look as if they were seared with a hot iron. Mr. Harrison is doubtful if there was any real ulceration, or any thing more than abrasion with softening. Mr. Dyson speaks positively to ulceration. I believe neither of these practitioners pretend to any great accuracy of knowledge in morbid anatomy; and we shall all acknowledge this is a point not always easy to determine. Mr.

Harrison said positively that there were no livid spots on the mucous membrane; Mr. Dyer says that there were spots of extravasated blood on various parts of the mucous membrane. These appearances were not mentioned at all by the examiners in their written report the day after the examination, and it is difficult to believe that so remarkable a circumstance could have been overlooked even by the most careless observer, which we have no reason for supposing Mr. Harrison to be.

Both of the surgeons state that, in their opinion, the appearances are strongly indicative of irritant poisoning. Mr. Harrison stated, with some natural hesitation, that he thinks no natural disease with these symptoms would produce them. Mr. Dyson rests his opinion, which he gave in the most confident manner, upon his assertion that there was "intense inflammation of the mucous membrane of the stomach and bowels; very great degree of softening of the same membrane; spots of extravasated blood on various parts; a great number of points of ulceration, which were most present in those parts of the intestines (the jejunum) which in natural disease are free; and the quantity of red sanguineous effusion throughout the stomach and bowels. That he had been engaged in six cases of poisoning by arsenic; that the appearances in this were similar to those, only more extensive and severe. That the rectum was much inflamed, and also the whole of the large intestines were inflamed; which, Mr. Dyson says, rarely if ever occurs in any natural disease. "The bladder was empty and firmly contracted, which is usual after arsenic;" and after any severe irritation of the pelvic viscera, ought to have been added.

Ulceration of the jejunum, which Mr. Dyson principally relied on for the proof of arsenic, is not frequent after either natural gastro-enteritis, or that from poison, but rather less unfrequent after the former than the latter. The extent of the inflammation, granting it to have been real inflammation, of which there may be not unreasonable doubts, is, so far as it goes, a presumption against, rather than for, the supposition of poisoning.

But the strongest point is still to come. The stomach and the bowels, with their contents, were given to Mr. Davies, an experienced and careful chemist, who made an elaborate analysis of the tissues, as well as of the contents of the alimentary canal, and discovered nothing. Now, no one will assert that arsenic may not have done all this mischief, and have been entirely discharged by two or three hours' vomiting and purging; but has one such case ever occurred? I cannot find one. The only one approaching to it is mentioned by Dr. Christison, and in that he discovered the

25th of a grain. My friend, Professor Moutagu Phillips, and I, discovered and verified, from an organic mixture, the one-thousandth of a grain, and procured by Marsh's process unequivocal traces from quantities far smaller. In this case, also, a piece of potatoe was not dislodged: does any one believe arsenic to be as easily dislodged as potatoe? But the arsenic, it has been urged, might have been all in solution; it was stated on oath, positively stated too, that five spoonfuls of milk would dissolve the whole of thirty grains. Mr. Phillips found, by experiment, that two ounces would dissolve half a grain; would half a grain produce this extensive inflammation? It was then urged that more was taken, and might have been removed by absorption. But where had it gone? Off by urine? But he had suppression of urine. By perspiration? His skin was dry. By pulmonary perspiration? Does arsenic volatilize at a blood heat? It was carried to the other parts of the body. Where is the evidence of any considerable quantity being so carried?

I think I need not trespass further upon your space: I hope, if any of your correspondents know of cases in which any of these unusual circumstances have happened, they will point out where they are recorded.

I am, sir,
Your obedient servant,
P. H. HOLLAND.

NON-MALIGNANT MAMMARY TUMOR
OF FOUR YEARS' STANDING—EXTIRPATION —CURE.

ELLEN CURTIS, ætat. 23, unmarried, from Gloucester county, New Jersey, was admitted February 17th, on account of a large tumor of the right breast. She states that some time in the winter of 1838, she first perceived a small, moveable tumor, situated apparently just below the skin, and on the inner side of the right mamma. This gave but little uneasiness, till it increased to the size of a walnut, when she received a kick on the part from a cow, after which it was at times slightly painful. She now covered it with a simple plaster, which treatment she continued till the month of May 1841, when she fell into the hands of a quack, applied a caustic plaster to the part the course of a short period of time, a lancet into the tumor at twelve different times. no discharge followed application of the sloughing of the skin left an ulcerated su

up to the present period. After this treatment the tumor slightly enlarged, and has since that time presented a more angry and inflamed appearance. Five weeks since, owing to a large venous trunk having been opened by extension of the ulceration, hemorrhage to a very large amount took place, which was arrested upon the occurrence of syncope ; and on the evening previous to her admission into the hospital a second bleeding to the extent of three pints had occurred, from the same cause, which was arrested by pressure.

The tumor is now of large size, is very heavy, and is observed to be strongly lobulated, deep depressions existing between the lobes. These lobes are hard and inelastic, and the whole tumor is loose and free from any attachment to the parts beneath. About one-fourth of the skin covering the breast is ulcerated, the parts below presenting the appearance of a healthy indolent ulcer, discharging laudable pus, and with nothing like a fungous growth protruding from it. No hemorrhage has ever occurred from the surface of the ulcer. The skin is reddened around the ulcerated part, but is at no point puckered, and the veins on the upper surface of the breast passing towards the neck are very much enlarged. The nipple is observable, below the ulceration, healthy in structure, though nearly obliterated ; at no time has there been any discharge from it. The tumor is not tender to the touch, neither is it painful, except on the approach, and during the continuance, of the menstrual discharge ; and with the exception of its weight and size, the patient, until within a short time, has experienced no inconvenience from it, and up to within two weeks of her admission into the hospital had been actively employed in the domestic duties of a farmer's family. The left breast is of normal size and appearance. Her general health is good, and there is no enlargement of the cervical glands, or of those in the axilla. She is not emaciated, and her skin is free from sallowness, though her appearance is that of a person debilitated from large losses of blood. Her menstrual periods, which on the first appearance of the swelling were irregular, both as to quantity and time, are now natural, and with the exception of some enlargement of the tonsils, she presents no mark of a scrofulous taint.

Upon the first aspect of this case it presented the appearance of, and might upon a superficial examination have been pronounced, a tumor of a malignant kind ; but the history of its rise and progress, as well as a careful examination of it, readily showed its true nature. The age of the patient, the want of sallowness in her skin, her comparatively good general health, and the slight pain she had suffered from it, were alone sufficient to lead us to suspect its freedom from malignancy ; and when taken in connection with the great weight of the tumor, its loose attachment to the surrounding parts, the slow progress and duration of the disease, the absence of glandular disease in its vicinity, together with the want of all fungous growth, and the discharge of laudable pus from its ulcerated surface, and its marked lobulated feel and appearance, proved conclusively that the character of this case had nothing in common with either cancer or fungus hæmatodes. The disease was looked upon as belonging to that class denominated chronic mammary tumors, and in the advanced stage in which it existed, evidently a proper case for the knife. It differed, however, from most tumors of this class in its great size, and a correct diagnosis of it was particularly important, as we could confidently predict for the sufferer freedom from any return after the operation.

In consequence of the occurrence of her menstrual period a day or two after her admission into the hospital, the disease was not extirpated till the 2d of March. The operation was done in the usual manner, the tumor being included in two elliptical incisions. The hemorrhage following it was not great ; a point of suture was inserted in the middle of the wound, and its sides, in addition, were brought together with two or three strips of adhesive plaster, after which the wound was covered with a little lint, and the arm supported by a sling.

Upon examination after removal, the tumor was found to be made up of a number of separate lobes, very closely connected together by cellular tissue. The structure of these lobes was very dense, and when divided presented very much the appearance of sweetbread. No vessels could be traced running through the tumor, which was completely surrounded by a covering of thick tendinous substance.

After the operation, she suffered from repeated attacks of erysipelas, as well around the wound as on the back, abdomen, legs, arms, and face. These were treated by a careful use of the blue pill and mild cathartics, together with neutral or effervescing mixtures ; the parts affected being bathed with soap liniment ; and in consequence of her great debility, tonics and nourishing food of an unstimulating kind, in such forms and quantities as her excessively irritable stomach would allow her to retain, were administered. The applications to the wound, after the first day or two, were principally the common mucilaginous or water dressing, an adhesive strap being at the same time applied, to favour cicatrization.

On the 25th of March a large abscess seated over the lower part of the back was opened. On the 31st, abscesses which had formed on both upper extremities above the elbows, were opened. By the 2d of April, the wound was completely cicatrized. On the 12th and 23d of April, other large collections of matter, resulting, as in the former instances, from erysipelas, were laid open, and on the 5th of May she left the hospital for Jersey, in good health.—*American Journal.*

MATERIA MEDICA.

Mr. BATTLEY requests us to announce that he has re-opened his Museum of Materia Medica at the Saunderian Institution, adjoining the Ophthalmic Hospital, Moorfields, and that he will also exhibit on a larger scale the articles of the Materia Medica, classed according to their operation on the human body.

The latter articles will be demonstrated and described on the second Friday of each month.

The class " Purgatives," now ready for inspection, and will be described on Friday, May 12th, at 4 P.M.

DECEASE OF DR. LATHAM.

" ON the 20th instant, at Bradwall Hall, Cheshire, in his 82d year, John Latham, M.D. F.R.S., formerly President of the Royal College of Physicians."

The preceding notice is copied from the newspapers; and we may add, that Dr. Latham was for many years a highly respected practitioner in London, but had latterly resided entirely at his place in Cheshire.

LITERARY INTELLIGENCE.

Mr. CHURCHILL will shortly publish the following Works :—

Dr. Prout, F.R.S.—On the Nature and Treatment of Stomach and Urinary Diseases. Fourth edition, with considerable additions.

Dr. Williams, F.R.S.—Principles of Medicine : comprehending General Pathology and Therapeutics.

Dr. Royle, F.R.S.—A Manual of Materia Medica, illustrated with wood engravings.

G. J. Guthrie, F.R.S.—On the Anatomy and Diseases of the Urinary and Sexual Organs. Third edition.

A. Taylor, F.L.S.—A Manual of Medical Jurisprudence.

G. Fownes, Ph.D.—A Manual of Chemistry.

Dr. Golding Bird, F.L.S.—Elements of Natural Philosophy. Second edition, with considerable additions.

Dr. Hall, F.L.S.—Clinical Remarks on Diseases of the Eye, and on Miscellaneous Subjects, Medical and Surgical.

J. Yearsley.—On the Enlarged Tonsil and Elongated Uvula, and other Morbid Conditions of the Throat. Second edition, with additions.

ROYAL COLLEGE OF SURGEONS.

LIST OF GENTLEMEN ADMITTED MEMBERS.

Friday, April 21, 1843.

C. R. Hatherly. — F. Manning. — G. P. H. Milsone. — A. W. Gabb. — S. Curtis. — R. H. Bradley.—J. Williams.—T. Pollard.—E. Dewes. —W. Pollard.—W. Millington.—C. Scaife.—T. Slater.

APOTHECARIES' HALL.

LIST OF GENTLEMEN WHO HAVE RECEIVED CERTIFICATES.

Thursday, April 20, 1843.

G. Taylor, Derby.—G. Dimock, Sussex.—S. Fenwick, Newcastle.—T. Young, South Shields. — E. J. Newcomb, Kidderminster. — H. H. Parrot, Yorkshire.—R. A. Lafargue.—R. Whitfield, Biddenden.

A TABLE OF MORTALITY FOR THE METROPOLIS,

Shewing the number of deaths from all causes registered in the week ending Saturday, April 15, 1843.

Small Pox	10
Measles	22
Scarlatina	21
Hooping Cough	49
Croup	4
Thrush	2
Diarrhœa	7
Dysentery	1
Cholera	0
Influenza	3
Typhus	59
Erysipelas	3
Syphilis	2
Hydrophobia	0
Diseases of the Brain, Nerves, and Senses	139
Diseases of the Lungs and other Organs of Respiration	228
Diseases of the Heart and Blood-vessels	15
Diseases of the Stomach, Liver, and other Organs of Digestion	62
Diseases of the Kidneys, &c.	6
Childbed	4
Ovarian Dropsy	0
Disease of Uterus, &c.	0
Rheumatism	6
Diseases of Joints, &c.	3
Ulcer	0
Fistula	0
Diseases of Skin, &c.	0
Diseases of Uncertain Seat	91
Old Age or Natural Decay	55
Deaths by Violence, Privation, or Intemperance	12
Causes not specified	2
Deaths from all Causes	816

NOTICE.

We shall be happy to hear again from △.

ERRATUM.—In our last Leader, p. 137, col. 1, line 16, for "hand-driving," read "hard driving."

THE

LONDON ·MEDICAL GAZETTE,

BEING A

WEEKLY JOURNAL

OF

Medicine and the Collateral Sciences.

FRIDAY, MAY 5, 1843.

LECTURES

ON THE

THEORY AND PRACTICE OF MIDWIFERY,

Delivered in the Theatre of St. George's Hospital,

BY ROBERT LEE, M.D. F.R.S.

LECTURE XXV.

ON PROTRACTED AND DIFFICULT LABOURS.

6. *Original smallness of the pelvis, distortion, exostoses, and other morbid conditions, are the most frequent causes of difficult labour.*

ABOUT one-sixth of all the cases of difficult parturition which I have observed in London depended upon narrowness of the pelvis, from arrest of development, and distortion. When the pelvis does not expand in the usual manner at the age of maturity, the brim, cavity, and outlet, remain through life smaller than in the ordinary standard female pelvis, without being distorted. In some persons there is no distortion, yet the distance between the base of the sacrum and the symphysis pubis does not exceed three inches, so that a fœtal head of the ordinary size cannot pass through it ; and all the consequences follow, in labour, which usually take place when a disproportion exists, from distortion or any other cause, between the dimensions of the pelvis and the head of the child. This original smallness of the pelvis exists in a considerable number of women, whose spinal column and long cylindrical bones are not unusually bent, and in whom there is no appearance of rickets, or symptom to excite a suspicion, before the commencement of labour, that the capacity of the pelvis is defective. The effects produced upon the pelvis by softening of the bones from rickets and malacosteon, you have

already seen in a variety of specimens of distorted pelvis, removed from the bodies of women who had died in consequence of the effects produced upon the soft parts from obstruction to the progress of the head of the child during labour.

In small or slightly distorted pelves, where the short diameters of the brim and outlet exceed three inches, and the long bones of the extremities are not bent, when labour comes on the os uteri dilates in the usual manner, and the head enters the brim, but it passes through with great difficulty. The parietal bones overlap one another, even in the intervals of the pains, and, if the labour is much protracted, a large swelling gradually forms under the scalp, and for hours it may be doubtful whether the uterine contractions will be sufficiently powerful to force the head into the cavity of the pelvis. When it has cleared the brim, if the outlet of the pelvis be less contracted, a few pains only may be required to complete the labour, and the child may be born alive without having sustained any injury. But when the contraction of the brim is greater, the head, after entering more or less deeply into it, ceases to advance, and becomes gradually more and more firmly compressed between the base of the sacrum and symphysis pubis, and at last so completely impacted, locked, or, as it has been expressively called, nailed in the pelvis, that the finger cannot be passed up around the head, and the pains, however violent, have no effect in moving it forward. This state has been termed enclavement or paragomphosis of the head, by foreign writers, and if it is allowed to continue many hours, and the uterus is acting powerfully, the most injurious consequences usually follow both to the child and the mother. In *this* fœtal head which I now shew you, the right parietal bone which was applied to the projecting base of the sacrum in labour has been depressed and fractured. Slighter compression of the head, long continued, usually destroys the life of the child before

N

the labour is finished. If it is born alive death soon afterwards takes place from extravasation of blood upon the brain, producing apoplexy and convulsions.

The soft parts of the mother surrounding the head become hot, dry, tumid, and inflamed, and all the injurious effects of pressure and interrupted circulation of the blood are sooner or later experienced. You cannot pass up the finger around the head without difficulty, and causing more or less distress to the patient; the discharges from the vagina become acrid and offensive; retention of urine takes place, from the pressure of the head on the neck of the bladder and urethra; the abdomen becomes tender; the tongue loaded with urgent thirst; the pulse rapid and feeble; and more or less general exhaustion ensues. In some cases rupture of the uterus takes place in the course of a few hours after the head has become wedged in the brim of a slightly distorted pelvis. Not unfrequently death follows artificial delivery in no long time, when the head of the child has been allowed to remain too long impacted in the pelvis, and still oftener sloughing of the vagina, bladder, and rectum, takes place.

In cases of slighter distortion of the pelvis, it is impossible to predict at the commencement of labour whether the head will pass or not, and while it continues to advance, and no unfavourable symptoms are present, you ought not to interfere—wait patiently, and see what nature can do. If the head descends so low into the cavity of the pelvis that an ear can be felt, and the os uteri is fully dilated, and there is room to pass up the blades of the forceps without the employment of much force, it is always proper, when delivery becomes necessary, to attempt to extract the head with the forceps. It is necessary, however, to remember that sloughing is apt to follow the use of the forceps, where the soft parts have been long pressed upon by the head, and that perforation of the head is a much safer operation for the mother, when the distortion is considerable.

The employment of the long forceps, in cases of distorted pelvis, has been recommended by Baudelocque, Boivin, Lachapelle, Capuron, Maygrier, Velpeau, and Flammant, whose works contain ample instructions for its use, before the head of the child has entered the brim of the pelvis; and the last of these writers has expressed his belief that the instrument is more frequently required while the head of the child remains above the superior aperture of the pelvis, than after it has descended into the cavity.

In this country there are no practitioners of judgment and experience who have frequent recourse to the forceps, or who employ it before the orifice of the uterus is fully dilated, and the head of the child has descended so low into the pelvis that an ear can be felt, and the relative position of the head to the pelvis accurately ascertained. The instrument is very seldom used in England where the pelvis is much distorted, or where the soft parts are in a rigid and swollen state, but it is had recourse to where delivery becomes necessary in consequence of exhaustion, hæmorrhage, convulsions, and other accidents which endanger the life of the mother. It is used solely with the view of supplying that power which the uterus does not possess.

Where the pelvis is distorted in a high degree, as in some of the specimens before you on the table, where the distance from the base of the sacrum to the symphysis pubis varies from an inch and a half to two inches and a half, the head of a full-grown child cannot enter the brim, however long the labour may be allowed to continue. The membranes burst, and the liquor amnii escapes as in natural labour, and the uterus closely contracts around the body of the child, and acts powerfully upon it, but the head presses upon the uterus at a distance from the orifice, and it is never completely dilated. In some cases, where the labour has lasted from forty-eight to sixty hours, the os uteri has not been more than half dilated, and the whole head of the child, swollen by the pressure, has remained entirely within the uterus above the brim, and pushed forward by the base of the sacrum over the symphysis pubis. This figure from Smellie's twenty-eighth table gives a side view of a distorted pelvis, with the head of a full-grown foetus squeezed into the brim, the parietal bones decussating each other, and compressed into a conical form. "This table shows," says Smellie, "the impossibility, in such a case, to save the child unless by the Cæsarean operation, which ought, however, never to be performed, excepting when it is impracticable to deliver at all by any other method. Even in this case, after the upper part of the head is diminished in bulk, and the bones are extracted, the greatest force must be applied, in order to extract the bones of the foetus and basis of the skull, as well as the body of the foetus." (See top of next page.)

The following figure from Smellie's twenty-second table gives a lateral view of a distorted pelvis, divided longitudinally, with the head of a foetus of the seventh month passing the same. "The head of the foetus here," he says, "though small, is with difficulty squeezed down into the pelvis, and changed from a round to an oblong form before it can pass, there being only the space of two inches and a quarter between the projection of the superior part of the sacrum and ossa pubis. If the head is soon deli-

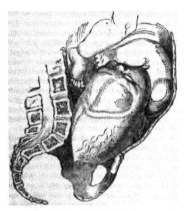

vered the child may be born alive; but if it continues in this manner many hours, it is in danger of being lost, on account of the long pressure on the brain; to prevent which, if the labour-pains are not sufficiently strong, the head may be helped along with the forceps." "This figure may serve as an example of the extreme degree of distortion of the pelvis, between which and the well-formed one are many intermediate degrees, according to which the difficulty of delivery must increase or diminish, as well from the disproportion of the pelvis and head of the fœtus—all which cases require the greatest caution, both as to the safety and management of the mother and child."

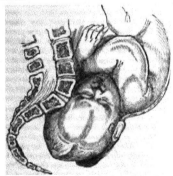

Where there exists a great degree of distortion of the brim of the pelvis, you may be unable to determine positively the distance between the base of the sacrum and symphysis pubis; and it is not necessary for practical purposes to do so with mathematical accuracy; but when it is under two inches and a half, you will readily discover,

if you have had considerable experience, on making the ordinary examination, from the unusual manner in which the sacrum projects, that it is impossible for a child at the full period to pass through it. If labour has commenced at the full period of pregnancy, and you discover before it has continued many hours that the pelvis is greatly distorted, and that the child cannot possibly pass alive, no advantage can result from allowing the labour to endure till the patient is exhausted, and you are satisfied that the difficulty cannot be overcome by the powers of the constitution. In such a case delay is dangerous, and there is nothing which can save the woman's life but opening the head of the child with the perforator, and extracting it with the crotchet. But this should never be had recourse to without a regular consultation of experienced practitioners, and before it has been placed beyond all doubt, by the most careful investigation, that the delivery can be accomplished in no other manner so as to preserve the mother's life.

In the greater number of cases of difficult labour from a high degree of distortion of the pelvis which have come under my observation, where it has been the first child, the process has been allowed to go on till the efforts of the patient were nearly discontinued, or had ceased entirely, and the favourable period for operating was lost. In some cases, even when the duration of the labour, and the local and constitutional symptoms, have made it manifest that such interference was justifiable and necessary, I have unfortunately delayed too long to deliver, in consequence of employing the stethoscope, and ascertaining that the child was alive. In cases of extreme distortion of the brim of the pelvis the proper practice is to perforate the head, as soon as the os uteri is sufficiently dilated to admit of the operation being done with safety, and afterwards leaving the patient in labour till the head has partially entered the brim, and the os uteri is considerably dilated. There can be no doubt that, in some cases, it is right to interfere before we certainly know that the child has been destroyed by the pressure; but we have nothing here to do with the question respecting the life or death of the child; our conduct will be biassed if we endeavour to solve this question. We have only to determine positively that delivery is absolutely necessary to save the mother's life, and that it is impossible for the head of the child to pass till its volume is reduced. Paré, Guillemeau, Mauriceau, Portal, Puzos, Levret, Smellie, and all the best accoucheurs who have since appeared in Britain, have performed the operation of craniotomy in many cases of distortion from rickets and malacosteon,

the labour is finished. If it is born alive death soon afterwards takes place from extravasation of blood upon the brain, producing apoplexy and convulsions.

The soft parts of the mother surrounding the head become hot, dry, tumid, and inflamed, and all the injurious effects of pressure and interrupted circulation of the blood are sooner or later experienced. You cannot pass up the finger around the head without difficulty, and causing more or less distress to the patient; the discharges from the vagina become acrid and offensive; retention of urine takes place, from the pressure of the head on the neck of the bladder and urethra; the abdomen becomes tender; the tongue loaded with urgent thirst; the pulse rapid and feeble; and more or less general exhaustion ensues. In some cases rupture of the uterus takes place in the course of a few hours after the head has become wedged in the brim of a slightly distorted pelvis. Not unfrequently death follows artificial delivery in no long time, when the head of the child has been allowed to remain too long impacted in the pelvis, and still oftener sloughing of the vagina, bladder, and rectum. takes place.

In cases of slighter distortion of the pelvis, it is impossible to predict at the commencement of labour whether the head will pass or not, and while it continues to advance, and no unfavourable symptoms are present, you ought not to interfere—wait patiently, and see what nature can do. If the head descends so low into the cavity of the pelvis that an ear can be felt, and the os uteri is fully dilated, and there is room to pass up the blades of the forceps without the employment of much force, it is always proper, when delivery becomes necessary, to attempt to extract the head with the forceps. It is necessary, however, to remember that sloughing is apt to follow the use of the forceps, where the soft parts have been long pressed upon by the head, and that perforation of the head is a much safer operation for the mother, when the distortion is considerable.

The employment of the long forceps, in cases of distorted pelvis, has been recommended by Baudelocque, Boivin. Lachapelle, Capuron, Maygrier, Velpeau, and Flamant, whose works contain ample instructions for its use, before the head of the child has entered the brim of the pelvis; and the last of these writers has expressed his belief that the instrument is more frequently required while the head of the child remains above the superior aperture of the pelvis, than after it has descended into the cavity.

In this country there are no practitioners of judgment and experience who have frequent recourse to the forceps, or who employ it before the orifice of the uterus is fully dilated, and the head of the child has descended so low into the pelvis that an ear can be felt, and the relative position of the head to the pelvis accurately ascertained. The instrument is very seldom used in England where the pelvis is much distorted, or where the soft parts are in a rigid and swollen state, but it is had recourse to where delivery becomes necessary in consequence of exhaustion, hæmorrhage, convulsions, and other accidents which endanger the life of the mother. It is used solely with the view of supplying that power which the uterus does not possess.

Where the pelvis is distorted in a high degree, as in some of the specimens before you on the table, where the distance from the base of the sacrum to the symphysis pubis varies from an inch and a half to two inches and a half, the head of a full-grown child cannot enter the brim, however long the labour may be allowed to continue. The membranes burst, and the liquor amnii escapes as in natural labour, and the uterus closely contracts around the body of the child, and acts powerfully upon it, but the head presses upon the uterus at a distance from the orifice, and it is never completely dilated. In some cases, where the labour has lasted from forty-eight to sixty hours, the os uteri has not been more than half dilated, and the whole head of the child, swollen by the pressure, has remained entirely within the uterus above the brim, and pushed forward by the base of the sacrum over the symphysis pubis. This figure from Smellie's twenty-eighth table gives a side view of a distorted pelvis, with the head of a full-grown fœtus squeezed into the brim, the parietal bones decussating each other, and compressed into a conical form. " This table shows," says Smellie, " the impossibility, in such a case, to save the child unless by the Cæsarean operation, which ought, however, never to be performed, excepting when it is impracticable to deliver at all by any other method. Even in this case, after the upper part of the head is diminished in bulk, and the bones are extracted, the greatest force must be applied, in order to extract the bones of the fœtus and basis of the skull, as well as the body of the fœtus." (See top of next page.)

The following figure from Smellie's twenty-second table gives a lateral view of a distorted pelvis, divided longitudinally, with the head of a fœtus of the seventh month passing the same. " The head of the fœtus here," he says, " though small, is with difficulty squeezed down into the pelvis, and changed from a round to an oblong form before it can pass, there being only the space of two inches and a quarter between the projection of the superior part of the sacrum and ossa pubis. If the head is soon deli-

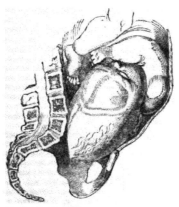

vered the child may be born alive; but if it continues in this manner many hours, it is in danger of being lost, on account of the long pressure on the brain; to prevent which, if the labour-pains are not sufficiently strong, the head may be helped along with the forceps." "This figure may serve as an example of the extreme degree of distortion of the pelvis, between which and the well-formed one are many intermediate degrees, according to which the difficulty of delivery must increase or diminish, as well from the disproportion of the pelvis and head of the fœtus—all which cases require the greatest caution, both as to the safety and management of the mother and child."

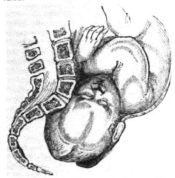

Where there exists a great degree of distortion of the brim of the pelvis, you may be unable to determine positively the distance between the base of the sacrum and symphysis pubis; and it is not necessary for practical purposes to do so with mathematical accuracy; but when it is under two inches and a half, you will readily discover,

if you have had considerable experience, on making the ordinary examination, from the unusual manner in which the sacrum projects, that it is impossible for a child at the full period to pass through it. If labour has commenced at the full period of pregnancy, and you discover before it has continued many hours that the pelvis is greatly distorted, and that the child cannot possibly pass alive, no advantage can result from allowing the labour to endure till the patient is exhausted, and you are satisfied that the difficulty cannot be overcome by the powers of the constitution. In such a case delay is dangerous, and there is nothing which can save the woman's life but opening the head of the child with the perforator, and extracting it with the crotchet. But this should never be had recourse to without a regular consultation of experienced practitioners, and before it has been placed beyond all doubt, by the most careful investigation, that the delivery can be accomplished in no other manner so as to preserve the mother's life.

In the greater number of cases of difficult labour from a high degree of distortion of the pelvis which have come under my observation, where it has been the first child, the process has been allowed to go on till the efforts of the patient were nearly discontinued, or had ceased entirely, and the favourable period for operating was lost. In some cases, even when the duration of the labour, and the local and constitutional symptoms, have made it manifest that such interference was justifiable and necessary, I have unfortunately delayed too long to deliver, in consequence of employing the stethoscope, and ascertaining that the child was alive. In cases of extreme distortion of the brim of the pelvis the proper practice is to perforate the head, as soon as the os uteri is sufficiently dilated to admit of the operation being done with safety, and afterwards leaving the patient in labour till the head has partially entered the brim, and the os uteri is considerably dilated. There can be no doubt that, in some cases, it is right to interfere before we certainly know that the child has been destroyed by the pressure; but we have nothing here to do with the question respecting the life or death of the child; our conduct will be biassed if we endeavour to solve this question. We have only to determine positively that delivery is absolutely necessary to save the mother's life, and that it is impossible for the head of the child to pass till its volume is reduced. Parè, Guillemeau, Mauriceau, Portal, Puzos, Levret, Smellie, and all the best accoucheurs who have since appeared in Britain, have performed the operation of craniotomy in many cases of distortion from rickets and malacosteon,

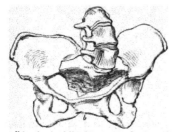

striking in the following case :—On Jan. 23, 1842, Mr. Kell, of Bridge Street, Westminster, requested me to see, with him and Dr. Hingeston, a woman, æt. 28, who was in the seventh month of her first pregnancy, and whose pelvis was greatly distorted by rickets. Some days before, Dr. Hingeston had passed a sound into the uterus, and detached the membranes from the lower part, but labour did not take place. I found the os uteri high up, and situated close behind the symphysis pubis. No difficulty was experienced in perforating the membranes in the usual manner, and the liquor amnii afterwards began to escape, and continued to flow till the evening of the 26th, when strong labour pains commenced. At 6 A.M. on the 27th, the os uteri was considerably dilated, and the nates were felt presenting. As it was obvious the breech would never pass through the brim, I brought down the lower extremities with the blunt end of the crotchet, and extracted the trunk without difficulty ; but I was obliged also to bring down the arms with the blunt hook. Afterwards I endeavoured to pass up the perforator to the back part of the head, and open it, but could not succeed in getting the point of the instrument beyond the upper cervical vertebræ. Being afraid of separating these, and detaching the head from the trunk, I gave up the attempt to perforate the back part of the head, and tried to draw the head through the brim of the pelvis with the crotchet, by fixing the point of the instrument over the bones of the face and forehead. After much exertion, continued for nearly two hours, the head was at last extracted, when completely torn to pieces. I believe it would have been impossible, in this case, to perforate the skull through the roof of the mouth, as has sometimes been done where similar difficulties have presented to perforating the back part of the head. The placenta was soon expelled, and the patient had a perfect and rapid recovery. It is impossible to doubt that the result of this case would have been widely different had the patient been allowed to go on without interference till the end of the ninth month. Being certain that a child of seven months could not pass through the brim of this pelvis, I resolved to induce premature labour at an earlier period, if

consulted in her subsequent pregnancy. On February 7, 1843, Mr. Kell again requested me to see this patient, who had completed her fifth month of gestation. The stiletted catheter was passed up readily into the uterus, but the liquor amnii did not escape. On the 10th, the point of the stilette having been sharpened, the instrument was again introduced, and the membranes readily punctured. The liquor amnii continued to flow till the 12th, when pains came on, and the child was expelled in a few hours, without artificial assistance. The head presented. The recovery was favourable. I was formerly of opinion that in no case of distortion, however great, could it be necessary to induce premature labour before the end of the fifth month of pregnancy, but in cases of extreme distortion from malacosteon, where the sacro-pubic diameter does not exceed an inch and a half, as in *this pelvis* which you now see, I think it would be advisable to put a period to the pregnancy before the fifth month, which can be done with perfect safety to the mother. The woman from whom *this distorted pelvis* was removed perished in consequence of the membranes not having been perforated sufficiently early. The following figure represents the appearance of a distorted pelvis in the possession of Mr. Barlow, and of the pelvis you now see.

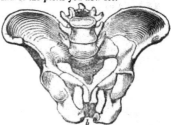

Ritgen has given a table of the period of pregnancy at which labour should be induced, according to the degree of narrowing of the sacro-pubic diameter. Labour, he thinks, should be induced at the twenty-ninth week, when the diameter of the pelvis is two inches and seven lines ; in the thirtieth week, when it is two inches and eight lines ; in the thirty-first, when it is two inches and nine lines ; in the thirty-fifth, when two inches and ten lines ; in the thirty-sixth, when two inches and eleven lines ; and in the thirty-seventh, when the sacro-pubic diameter is exactly three inches. When it is above three inches, the case must be left to nature.

Mr. Barlow has also published a synoptical table. In a well-formed pelvis, where the distance from the upper edge of the symphysis pubis to the superior part of the os sacrum, or conjugate diameter of the pelvis, is from five to four inches, delivery will take place, he says, by the efforts of nature alone where the conjugate diameter is from four or four to three or two inches and three quarters, the delivery may be completed by the efforts of nature, or assisted with the forceps or lever ; where from two and three quarters to two and a half inches, premature labour should be induced ; where from two and a half to one and a half inches, by embryulcia, or delivery with the crotchet ; and where the conjugate diameter of the brim is from one and a half inches to the lowest possible degree of distortion, by the Cæsarean operation.

Mr. Barlow thinks this table will facilitate further inquiry, although he justly observes that the practitioner should bear in mind the absolute impossibility of determining the mean degree of compressibility which the cranium of the fœtus may undergo by the efforts of the uterus ; and he very properly points out the necessity of making a very careful examination in each case before adopting any decided plan of treatment.

Baudelocque regarded the induction of premature labour as a useless, if not an injurious, operation ; and M. Dugès has recently characterised it as fatal to the mother, and the source of most frightful abuse. In the tables of the Maternité, by Baudelocque, Boivin, and Lachapelle, including nearly 60,000 cases of labour, there is no account of any case in which premature labour was induced. The last of these writers begins her strictures on the practice by declaring that she had never either employed "that method, or seen others have recourse to it." The propriety of inducing premature labour was brought under the consideration of the Academy of Medicine, Paris, in 1827, and they decided that the practice was unjustifiable under any circumstances.

The discordance which exists between Continental and British practitioners is also strikingly displayed respecting the Cæsarean section. The reports of 258 cases of this operation have been collected by Michaelis, 144 of which occurred in the last, and 110 in the present century. Of these cases, 140

proved fatal. Velpeau states that the operation was performed twenty-eight times between 1810 and 1820 ; and thirty-one times from 1821 to 1830. Dr. Churchill says the operation was performed 316 times between 1750 and 1841, and that the mortality was 52·8 per cent. for the mothers. I believe that it would have been much greater if all the unfortunate cases had been published, which has not been done. In Great Britain the reports of at least 27 cases have been published, and in 25 of them it was fatal to the mother. Other fatal cases have occurred which have not been recorded. I believe there is no practitioner of reputation now in this country who would recommend the operation upon the living body if delivery could be effected by the perforator and crotchet. Wherever the presenting part can be reached, to apply the perforator and crotchet, an attempt should always be made to deliver, and the Cæsarean operation reserved for those cases in which the distortion is so great that the os uteri and presenting part are entirely beyond our reach.

Most of you have already examined the following table, which has been published in the first of these clinical reports, exhibiting a comparative view of the frequency of forceps and craniotomy cases in some of the principal lying-in hospitals in Europe. It may be useful once more to compare the practice of different institutions, that you may be convinced that the first principles of operative midwifery have not yet been established, at least that they are not generally understood, and that there is no other branch of surgery at the present time in such a rude condition. In one hospital the forceps was employed once in every seven cases, and in another once only in 728 cases. How important it is that you should watch the progress of protracted and difficult labours, and discover the best method of treatment, and form correct opinions on the use of instruments, it is not necessary for me now to point out to you more particularly.

Hospitals.	Number of labours.	Forceps cases.	Proportion.	Craniotomy cases.	Proportion.
Dublin, Clarke.	10,199	14	1 in 728	49	1 in 248
Do., Collins.	16,654	27	1 in 617	118	1 in 141
Paris, Baudelocque.	17,388	31	1 in 561	6	1 in 2898
Do., Lachapelle.	22,243	76	1 in 293	12	1 in 1854
Do., Boivin.	20,517	96	1 in 214	16	1 in 1282
Vienna, Boer.	9,589	35	1 in 274	13	1 in 737
Heidelberg, Naegele.	1,711	55	1 in 31	1	1 in 1711
Berlin, Kluge.	1,111	68	1 in 16	6	1 in 185
Dresden, Carus.	2,549	184	1 in 14	9	1 in 283
Berlin, Siebold.	2,093	300	1 in 7	1	1 in 2093

Only a few cases have been recorded in which Exostoses, or Osteo-sarcomatous Tumors of the pelvis, have produced difficult

labour, and I have not met with any instance in practice.

Dr. M'Kibbin has related an example in

the Edin. Med. and Surg. Journal, April 1831, where the hollow of the sacrum and right side of the brim of the pelvis were occupied by an exostosis of a conical form. The woman had been in labour 50 hours, and the greatest space afforded for the passage of the child was on the right side, and it was only 1½ or 1¾ of an inch. From the apex of the tumor to the lower part of the symphysis pubis 1½ inch; from the brim of the pelvis on the right side, immediately over the foramen thyroideum to the lateral surface of the tumor at its widest part, 1⅝ inch; more posteriorly 1½ inch. The delivery was completed by the Cæsarean operation, but the child was dead, and the woman died after, the unsuccessful result being attributed to the delay. Dr. M. advocates the early adoption of the Cæsarean operation in all cases where uncertainty prevails as to the practicability of embryulcia, and where, he says, no two practitioners agree as to the actual space in the pelvis. " In short," he says, " where I was not satisfied that a passage existed for a full-grown fœtus of 2 inches in the short diameter, and 3½ in length, I should be inclined to adopt the Cæsarean operation in preference to embryulcia." I would draw an entirely different conclusion, and in all cases, whatever the degree of distortion might be either in the brim or outlet of the pelvis, attempt to deliver by embryulcia where the presenting part could be reached by the finger and the crotchet applied. Had the patient survived, and had impregnation again taken place, instead of repeating the Cæsarean operation, as he proposes, premature labour should have been induced in the early months of pregnancy. Dr. M. states, in the history of the case, that the patient suffered little or no inconvenience from this morbid growth during life, or the term of utero-gestation. At times she had colicy pains, and, on questioning her mother as to the probable cause of the exostosis, she admitted that her daughter had received a fall on the back when 6 or 8 years of age, which occasioned pain in the sacral region a short time afterwards.

In Dr. Haber's case of difficult labour from an exostosis of the sacrum, the history of which is contained in an inaugural dissertation published at Heidelberg, 1830, the disease also followed a fall upon the ice some years before, when the woman was carrying a heavy load upon the head. This accident was followed by pain in the back and pelvis, which gradually disappeared. She married, became pregnant, and during labour the whole cavity of the pelvis was found to be filled up with an osscous tumor which grew from the sacrum. The Cæsarean section was performed; but the child was putrid, and the patient died soon after the operation. The length of the tumor was seven inches,

and its greatest breadth six. The highest part of it hangs, as you will see by looking at *this* figure, over the place where the third vertebra of the loins is joined with the fourth. The lowest part of the tumor is distant about two lines and a half from the point of the sacrum. From the posterior surface of the body of the bones of the pubes the tumor is only one line and a half distant. Towards the anterior part, and downwards between the tumor and bones of the pubes, the space is eight or ten lines. The brim of the pelvis was almost completely filled up with the tumor. It appears from the history that there was no other method of delivering this patient but by the Cæsarean section. If the existence of the disease had been known during pregnancy, which however does not appear to have been the case, the induction of premature labour would have been proper in the early months, as soon indeed as the pregnancy was detected, which would have obviated the necessity for the operation. The same observation might be applied to the cases of osteo-sarcomatous tumors of the pelvis obstructing delivery, recorded by Grimmel, Stark, and others.

LUMLEIAN LECTURES

DELIVERED AT THE

COLLEGE OF PHYSICIANS,

MARCH 1843,

BY GEORGE BURROWS, M.D.

Physician to St. Bartholomew's Hospital.

LECTURE II.

Recapitulation. Disturbance of the cerebral circulation, by alterations in the relative quantity of blood in the arteries and veins. Reconsideration of the arguments upon which is founded the opinion that the quantity of blood within the cranium does not alter.

Pressure an important principle in sustaining and destroying the functions of the brain. Illustrations of vascular pressure on the brain in health and disease. Observations on the cephalo-spinal serum and its functions. Increased vascular pressure, and its effects. Diminished vascular pressure, and its effects. Syncope produced by insufficient vascular pressure, rather than by a diminished supply of blood to the brain. Examination and explanation of the phenomena of syncope produced under various circumstances. Cerebral disturbance in general anæmia attributed to insufficient vascular pressure more than to anæmia of the cerebral substance.

THE expiration of the hour allotted to a lecture, compelled me, on the former occasion, to conclude before I had completed a review of the subject which I brought before your notice. I must, therefore, be allowed briefly to recapitulate the points which then occupied our attention.

The subject of my former lecture was the modifications which the circulation within the cranium is capable of undergoing in health and disease, and the state of the circulation within the cranium after different kinds of death.

I quoted from the writings of many eminent physicians the opinions entertained by them on certain peculiarities of the circulation within the head. It appeared from this enquiry that an opinion was very prevalent, "that the quantity of blood within the cranium must be the same, or very nearly the same, at all times, whether in health or disease, in life or after death."

I informed you that this theory of the invariable quantity of blood within the head had been supported, 1st, by reference to certain experiments performed by Dr. Kellie, of Leith; and, 2dly, upon the supposition that the cranium is a complete sphere of bone, which is exactly filled by its contents, the brain, by which that organ is shut up from atmospheric pressure, and from all influence from without, except what is communicated from the blood-vessels which enter it.

I gave, in the first place, a concise analysis of the experiments from which it has been inferred that a state of bloodlessness is not discovered in the brains of animals which have died by hæmorrhage; but, on the contrary, very commonly a state of venous congestion. I then detailed some similar experiments of my own, the results of which were submitted to your inspection, and from which, I flatter myself, it appeared evident that the brains of animals bled to-death were deprived of their blood to the extent of rendering them pallid and anæmic. And from these experiments I inferred that it was not a fallacy, as some supposed, that arteriotomy or venesection diminished the actual quantity of blood in the cerebral vessels.

2dly, I detailed some experiments of Dr. Kellie, from which it was attempted to be proved that the quantity of blood in the cranium is not affected by the posture of the head. In opposition to this conclusion I exhibited to you the results of some analogous experiments, from which it was manifest that the quantity of blood in the head is affected to a most extraordinary extent by posture. I showed the effects of gravitation of blood to and from the head.

These results led me to suggest some practical rules which should be adopted in the examination of the cranium after death, where the blood remains fluid, if we wish to avoid being misled by pseudo-morbid appearances.

3dly, I pointed out how it had been attempted to support the opinion, that the quantity of blood in the cranium is invariable, by adducing the absence of congestion of the cerebral vessels in persons who have died by hanging. Admitting the accuracy of such statements, I related to you the appearances in other instances of death by hanging, which fully proved that not only congestion, but extravasations of blood, were often found in the brains of those that died by hanging. I then attempted to explain the occasional absence of congestion in these cases, (1) by the imperfect compression of all the jugular veins; (2) by the outlet afforded to the blood of the head through that beautiful plexus of sinuses which surrounds the spinal cord; also, (3) especially by the gravitation of the fluid blood during the suspension of the body; and, lastly, by the division of the cervical vessels before the head is opened. I also showed, by experiments, that when precautions were adopted to obviate the influence of such causes, then in death by apnœa there was intense congestion of the cerebral vessels.

Upon the present occasion I will complete my investigation of this interesting topic. And here I must remark, that those who maintain that the absolute quantity of blood in the cerebral vessels does not vary, admit a disturbance of the cerebral circulation in the following manner :—They point out the probability of a frequent alteration in the relative quantities of blood in the cerebral arteries and veins. Thus, they assert that those pathological states which have a tendency to cause influx of blood into the cerebral arteries, and accumulation in those vessels, will accomplish this change at the expense of the cerebral veins. Again, anything causing obstruction of the return of blood from the cranium will produce fulness of the sinuses and cerebral veins, but, at the same time, the quantity in the arteries will be equally diminished. They also maintain, if the quantity transmitted to the brain be lessened, the cerebral arteries will be comparatively empty; but there will be a corresponding fulness of the venous system within the cranium. These opinions of Drs. Abercrombie and Kellie are adopted by Dr. Watson, who supports them by similar reasonings. In states of anæmia, he informs us*, a diminished quantity of blood will be transmitted towards and into the cerebral arteries; but the whole volume of blood in the brain remains the same; therefore blood will accumulate more in the veins. "It is probably in this way that *the appearance of*

* Medical Lectures, op. cit.

the labour is finished. If it is born alive death soon afterwards takes place from extravasation of blood upon the brain, producing apoplexy and convulsions.

The soft parts of the mother surrounding the head become hot, dry, tumid, and inflamed, and all the injurious effects of pressure and interrupted circulation of the blood are sooner or later experienced. You cannot pass up the finger around the head without difficulty, and causing more or less distress to the patient; the discharges from the vagina become acrid and offensive; retention of urine takes place, from the pressure of the head on the neck of the bladder and urethra; the abdomen becomes tender; the tongue loaded with urgent thirst; the pulse rapid and feeble; and more or less general exhaustion ensues. In some cases rupture of the uterus takes place in the course of a few hours after the head has become wedged in the brim of a slightly distorted pelvis. Not unfrequently death follows artificial delivery in no long time, when the head of the child has been allowed to remain too long impacted in the pelvis, and still oftener sloughing of the vagina, bladder, and rectum, takes place.

In cases of slighter distortion of the pelvis, it is impossible to predict at the commencement of labour whether the head will pass or not, and while it continues to advance, and no unfavourable symptoms are present, you ought not to interfere—wait patiently, and see what nature can do. If the head descends so low into the cavity of the pelvis that an ear can be felt, and the os uteri is fully dilated, and there is room to pass up the blades of the forceps without the employment of much force, it is always proper, when delivery becomes necessary, to attempt to extract the head with the forceps. It is necessary, however, to remember that sloughing is apt to follow the use of the forceps, where the soft parts have been long pressed upon by the head, and that perforation of the head is a much safer operation for the mother, when the distortion is considerable. The employment of the long forceps, in cases of distorted pelvis, has been recommended by Baudelocque, Boivin, Lachapelle, Capuron, Maygrier, Velpeau, and Flammant, whose works contain ample instructions for its use, before the head of the child has entered the brim of the pelvis; and the last of these writers has expressed his belief that the instrument is more frequently required while the head of the child remains above the superior aperture of the pelvis, than after it has descended into the cavity.

In this country there are no practitioners of judgment and experience who have frequent recourse to the forceps, or who employ it before the orifice of the uterus is fully dilated, and the head of the child has descended so low into the pelvis that an ear can be felt, and the relative position of the head to the pelvis accurately ascertained. The instrument is very seldom used in England where the pelvis is much distorted, or where the soft parts are in a rigid and swollen state, but it is had recourse to where delivery becomes necessary in consequence of exhaustion, hæmorrhage, convulsions, and other accidents which endanger the life of the mother. It is used solely with the view of supplying that power which the uterus does not possess.

Where the pelvis is distorted in a high degree, as in some of the specimens before you on the table, where the distance from the base of the sacrum to the symphysis pubis varies from an inch and a half to two inches and a half, the head of a full-grown child cannot enter the brim, however long the labour may be allowed to continue. The membranes burst, and the liquor amnii escapes as in natural labour, and the uterus closely contracts around the body of the child, and acts powerfully upon it, but the head presses upon the uterus at a distance from the orifice, and it is never completely dilated. In some cases, where the labour has lasted from forty-eight to sixty hours, the os uteri has not been more than half dilated, and the whole head of the child, swollen by the pressure, has remained entirely within the uterus above the brim, and pushed forward by the base of the sacrum over the symphysis pubis. This figure from Smellie's twenty-eighth table gives a side view of a distorted pelvis, with the head of a full-grown fœtus squeezed into the brim, the parietal bones decussating each other, and compressed into a conical form. "This table shows," says Smellie, "the impossibility, in such a case, to save the child unless by the Cæsarean operation, which ought, however, never to be performed, excepting when it is impracticable to deliver at all by any other method. Even in this case, after the upper part of the head is diminished in bulk, and the bones are extracted, the greatest force must be applied, in order to extract the bones of the fœtus and basis of the skull, as well as the body of the fœtus." (See top of next page.)

The following figure from Smellie's twenty-second table gives a lateral view of a distorted pelvis, divided longitudinally, with the head of a fœtus of the seventh month passing the same. "The head of the fœtus here," he says, "though small, is with difficulty squeezed down into the pelvis, and changed from a round to an oblong form before it can pass, there being only the space of two inches and a quarter between the projection of the superior part of the sacrum and ossa pubis. If the head is soon deli-

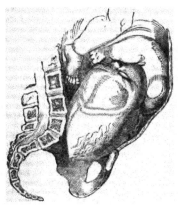

vered the child may be born alive; but if it continues in this manner many hours, it is in danger of being lost, on account of the long pressure on the brain; to prevent which, if the labour-pains are not sufficiently strong, the head may be helped along with the forceps." "This figure may serve as an example of the extreme degree of distortion of the pelvis, between which and the well-formed one are many intermediate degrees, according to which the difficulty of delivery must increase or diminish, as well from the disproportion of the pelvis and head of the fœtus—all which cases require the greatest caution, both as to the safety and management of the mother and child."

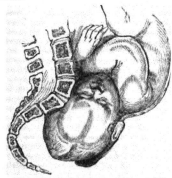

Where there exists a great degree of distortion of the brim of the pelvis, you may be unable to determine positively the distance between the base of the sacrum and symphysis pubis; and it is not necessary for practical purposes to do so with mathematical accuracy; but when it is under two inches and a half, you will readily discover,

if you have had considerable experience, on making the ordinary examination, from the unusual manner in which the sacrum projects, that it is impossible for a child at the full period to pass through it. If labour has commenced at the full period of pregnancy, and you discover before it has continued many hours that the pelvis is greatly distorted, and that the child cannot possibly pass alive, no advantage can result from allowing the labour to endure till the patient is exhausted, and you are satisfied that the difficulty cannot be overcome by the powers of the constitution. In such a case delay is dangerous, and there is nothing which can save the woman's life but opening the head of the child with the perforator, and extracting it with the crotchet. But this should never be had recourse to without a regular consultation of experienced practitioners, and before it has been placed beyond all doubt, by the most careful investigation, that the delivery can be accomplished in no other manner so as to preserve the mother's life.

In the greater number of cases of difficult labour from a high degree of distortion of the pelvis which have come under my observation, where it has been the first child, the process has been allowed to go on till the efforts of the patient were nearly discontinued, or had ceased entirely, and the favourable period for operating was lost. In some cases, even when the duration of the labour, and the local and constitutional symptoms, have made it manifest that such interference was justifiable and necessary, I have unfortunately delayed too long to deliver, in consequence of employing the stethoscope, and ascertaining that the child was alive, In cases of extreme distortion of the brim of the pelvis the proper practice is to perforate the head, as soon as the os uteri is sufficiently dilated to admit of the operation being done with safety, and afterwards leaving the patient in labour till the head has partially entered the brim, and the os uteri is considerably dilated. There can be no doubt that, in some cases, it is right to interfere before we certainly know that the child has been destroyed by the pressure; but we have nothing here to do with the question respecting the life or death of the child; our conduct will be biassed if we endeavour to solve this question. We have only to determine positively that delivery is absolutely necessary to save the mother's life, and that it is impossible for the head of the child to pass till its volume is reduced. Parè, Guillemeau, Mauriceau, Portal, Puzos, Levret, Smellie, and all the best accoucheurs who have since appeared in Britain, have performed the operation of craniotomy in many cases of distortion from rickets and malacosteon, without reference to the condition of the foetus. " True religion, and the common sense of mankind," observes Dr. Denman, " appear to have nothing contradictory. The doctrine they teach of its being our duty to do all the good in our power, and to avoid all the mischief we can, is applicable to the exigencies of every state, and we may be easily reconciled to it on the present occasion. In some cases of difficult parturition it is not possible that the lives both of the mother and child should be preserved. Of the life or death of the mother we can under all circumstances be assured : of the life or death of the child there is often reason to doubt, when we are called upon to decide and to act. The destruction of the mother would not, in the generality of cases which may bring the operation of which we are speaking under contemplation, contribute to the preservation of the child ; but the treatment of the child as if it were already dead, with as much certainty of success as is found in other operations, secures the life of the parent. It then becomes our duty, and is agreeable to our reason, to pursue that conduct which will give us the most probable chance of doing good : that is, of saving one life when two lives cannot possibly be preserved."

" The only means of effecting delivery," observes Dr. Collins, " where the disproportion between the head of the child and the pelvis is so great as to prevent us reaching the ear with the finger, is by reducing the size of the head and using the crotchet. This is, however, an operation that *no inducement* should tempt any individual to perform, except the imperative duty of saving the life of the mother when placed in imminent danger. I have no difficulty in stating, and that after the most anxious and minute attention to this point, that where the patient has been properly treated from the commencement of her labour; where strict attention has been paid to keep her cool; her mind easy; where stimulants of all kinds have been prohibited, and the necessary attention paid to the state of the bowels and bladder; that, under such management, the death of the child takes place in laborious and difficult labour before the symptoms become so alarming as to cause any experienced physician to lessen the head. This is a fact which I have ascertained beyond all doubt by the stethoscope, the use of which has exhibited to me the great errors I committed before I was acquainted with its application to midwifery, viz. in delaying delivery, often, I have no doubt, so as to render the result precarious in the extreme, and in some cases even fatal."

The operation of craniotomy is now performed by all British practitioners of reputation, whether the child be alive or dead, if the condition of the mother is such as to render delivery absolutely necessary, and the head of the child is beyond the reach of the forceps, or where, from distortion of the pelvis, or rigidity of the os uteri and vagina, it cannot be extracted if its volume is not reduced. This operation is performed from a conscientious belief and deep conviction that if neglected to be done at a sufficiently early period the mother's life will be sacrificed, and the life of the mother is considered as much more important than that of the child. Some continental writers affirm, but, I believe, unjustly, that in England we have frequently recourse to craniotomy without due consideration, and without proper regard to the life of the child ; and, whatever the state of the parent may be, they refuse to open the head till they can obtain certain evidence, which in some cases it is impossible to obtain, that it is dead. " Nothing could excuse the conduct of the practitioner," says Baudelocque, " who would perforate the head of a child without previously knowing with certainty that it was not alive, a circumstance which can alone authorize us to employ the perforator and crotchet." By following this erroneous principle, the lives of both mother and child would, I believe, in the majority of cases be sacrificed.

In numerous cases of distortion of the pelvis the induction of premature labour has been successfully employed in this country, and it is now ascertained that the operation, which will be described hereafter, is attended with little risk to the mother, and that nearly one half of the children are born alive, and continue to live, where it is performed after the seventh month of pregnancy. In cases of great distortion of the pelvis, the induction of premature labour at an early period of pregnancy, before the sixth month, is likewise known to be a safe operation, and to render craniotomy and the Cæsarean operation wholly unnecessary. The greater number of the best practical writers on midwifery in this country have considered the induction of premature labour applicable only to cases of slighter distortion, and have considered it improper in first pregnancies, and before seven complete months of utero-gestation have elapsed.

Little has been said by them respecting the safety and utility of the operation in cases of great distortion, to obviate the danger to the mother of fatal contusion or laceration of the uterus and vagina, which are always to be dreaded when much force is required after perforation to extract the head of the child. " If the pelvis be so far reduced in its dimensions," observes Dr. Denman, " as not to allow the head of a child of such a size as to give hopes of its living to pass through it, the operation cannot be attended with success. It is in those cases only in which there is a reduction of the dimension of the pelvis to a certain degree, and not beyond that degree, that this operation ought to be proposed or can succeed." "As the primary object is to preserve the life of the child," says Dr. Merriman, "the operation should never be performed till seven complete months of utero-gestation have elapsed." As early as 1769, it was proposed by Dr. Cooper to induce abortion in cases of extreme distortion of the pelvis. "Before I conclude," he remarks, in his history of a fatal case of Cæsarean section, "allow me to propose the following question, viz. 'In such cases where it is certainly known that a mature child cannot possibly be delivered in the ordinary way alive, would it not be consistent with reason and conscience, for the preservation of the mother, to produce an abortion?'"

I have met with two cases of such great distortion from rickets in the first pregnancy, that I have induced premature labour in the seventh month, and was enabled in consequence to complete the delivery with far less difficulty and danger than it could otherwise have been done. I shall read to you the details of these cases, with the view of impressing upon you the importance of the principle, and of inducing you to perform the same operation at an earlier period of the first pregnancy than the seventh month, if you should meet with any individual whose pelvis is so distorted that a child cannot then pass through it, or in whom the cavity of the pelvis is filled up with large exostoses and tumors. By having recourse to this operation in the early months, even before the fifth month, the Cæsarean operation can never be necessary except in those cases in which the condition of the pelvis has not been ascertained till the full period. In the case of extreme distortion from malacosteon, related by Sir Charles Bell, had the membranes of the ovum been perforated in the second or third month the necessity for the Cæsarean operation would not have occurred, and the progress of the disease would probably, for a time at least, have been arrested.

On Tuesday, January 9, 1838, Mr. Robertson, of Albemarle Street, requested me to see a woman whose pelvis and extremities were greatly distorted by rickets, and who was in the seventh month of her first pregnancy. From an examination of the pelvis, we thought the short diameter of the brim was considerably under three inches, and that a child at the full period could not pass through it without having the volume reduced by craniotomy, and that the operation would be attended by difficulty and danger. We resolved, in consequence, to induce premature labour, though it was the first pregnancy, and though a

rule had been laid down by the most judicious writers that the practice should never be adopted till experience had decidedly proved that the mother was incapable of bearing a full grown child alive. The os uteri was situated high up and directed backward, but I experienced no difficulty in introducing the stiletted catheter, and perforating the membranes. The liquor amnii began to escape immediately after, and continued to flow for three days, and labour pains then came on. For forty-eight hours they were feeble and irregular. Mr. Robertson then found the os uteri considerably dilated, and a foot of the child protruding through it. He extracted the breech and extremities without difficulty, but he could not succeed in drawing the head through the brim unto the cavity of the pelvis. I passed the point of the perforator up to the back part of the head without difficulty, and having made a large opening through the integuments and skull, the brain began to escape. The point of the crotchet was then introduced into the opening, and fixed upon the base; and by drawing downwards and backwards with the crotchet, and at the same time pulling upon the body of the child, the head soon passed through the pelvis, completely flattened on the sides. She recovered without a bad symptom. On the 17th of May, 1839, when the same patient had completed the seventh month of her second pregnancy, I punctured the membranes. The liquor amnii began immediately to escape, and continued to flow till the whole of the following day, and in the evening violent labour pains came on. The nates presented, and Mr. Robertson had no difficulty in extracting the child without perforation of the head. On the 19th, the usual symptoms of ruptured uterus soon appeared, and she died on the 22d. On the 24th, I examined the body with Mr. Robertson, and we found a large rent in the cervix uteri. This is the pelvis which you see now, and the following are its dimensions. The distance from the base of the sacrum to the symphysis pubis measures two inches and one line. The transverse diameter of the brim is five inches and three quarters. At the outlet, a line drawn between the tuberosities of the ischia measures four inches and a half, and another line, from the extremity of the coccyx to the lower edge of the symphysis pubis, three inches and a half. Had premature labour been induced at the end of the fifth month, or earlier, instead of the seventh, it is very probable the fatal accident which occurred would have been prevented.

The following figure gives a pretty correct view of the brim of this pelvis, although it was not taken from it. (See next page.)

The advantage obtained by inducing premature labour in a first pregnancy, where the pelvis is greatly distorted, was still more

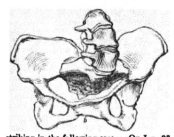

striking in the following case:—On Jan. 23, 1842, Mr. Kell, of Bridge Street, Westminster, requested me to see, with him and Dr. Hingeston, a woman, æt. 28, who was in the seventh month of her first pregnancy, and whose pelvis was greatly distorted by rickets. Some days before, Dr. Hingeston had passed a sound into the uterus, and detached the membranes from the lower part, but labour did not take place. I found the os uteri high up, and situated close behind the symphysis pubis. No difficulty was experienced in perforating the membranes in the usual manner, and the liquor amnii afterwards began to escape, and continued to flow till the evening of the 26th, when strong labour pains commenced. At 6 A.M. on the 27th, the os uteri was considerably dilated, and the nates were felt presenting. As it was obvious the breech would never pass through the brim, I brought down the lower extremities with the blunt end of the crotchet, and extracted the trunk without difficulty; but I was obliged also to bring down the arms with the blunt hook. Afterwards I endeavoured to pass up the perforator to the back part of the head, and open it, but could not succeed in getting the point of the instrument beyond the upper cervical vertebræ. Being afraid of separating these, and detaching the head from the trunk, I gave up the attempt to perforate the back part of the head, and tried to draw the head through the brim of the pelvis with the crotchet, by fixing the point of the instrument over the bones of the face and forehead. After much exertion, continued for nearly two hours, the head was at last extracted, when completely torn to pieces. I believe it would have been impossible, in this case, to perforate the skull through the roof of the mouth, as has sometimes been done where similar difficulties have presented to perforating the back part of the head. The placenta was soon expelled, and the patient had a perfect and rapid recovery. It is impossible to doubt that the result of this case would have been widely different had the patient been allowed to go on without interference till the end of the ninth month. Being certain that a child of seven months could not pass through the brim of this pelvis, I resolved to induce premature labour at an earlier period, if

consulted in her subsequent pregnancy. On February 7, 1843, Mr. Kell again requested me to see this patient, who had completed her fifth month of gestation. The stiletted catheter was passed up readily into the uterus, but the liquor amnii did not escape. On the 10th, the point of the stilette having been again sharpened, the instrument was again introduced, and the membranes readily punctured. The liquor amnii continued to flow till the 12th, when pains came on, and the child was expelled in a few hours, without artificial assistance. The head presented. The recovery was favourable. I was formerly of opinion that in no case of distortion, however great, could it be necessary to induce premature labour before the end of the fifth month of pregnancy, but in cases of extreme distortion from malacosteon, where the sacropubic diameter does not exceed an inch and a half, as in *this pelvis* which you now see, I think it would be advisable to put a period to the pregnancy before the fifth month, which can be done with perfect safety to the mother. The woman from whom *this distorted pelvis* was removed perished in consequence of the membranes not having been perforated sufficiently early. The following figure represents the appearance of a distorted pelvis in the possession of Mr. Barlow, and of the pelvis you now see.

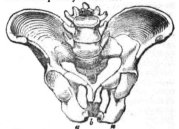

Ritgen has given a table of the period of pregnancy at which labour should be induced, according to the degree of narrowing of the sacro-pubic diameter. Labour, he thinks, should be induced at the twenty-ninth week, when the diameter of the pelvis is two inches and seven lines; in the thirtieth week, when it is two inches and eight lines; in the thirty-first, when it is two inches and nine lines; in the thirty-fifth, when two inches and ten lines; in the thirty-sixth, when two inches and eleven lines; and in the thirty-seventh, when the sacro-pubic diameter is exactly three inches. When it is above three inches, the case must be left to nature.

Mr. Barlow has also published a synoptical table. In a well-formed pelvis, where the distance from the upper edge of the symphysis pubis to the superior part of the os sacrum, or conjugate diameter of the pelvis, is from five to four inches, delivery will take place, he says, by the efforts of nature alone where the conjugate diameter is from four or four to three or two inches and three quarters, the delivery may be completed by the efforts of nature, or assisted with the forceps or lever ; where from two and three quarters to two and a half inches, premature labour should be induced; where from two and a half to one and a half inches, by embryulcia, or delivery with the crotchet; and where the conjugate diameter of the brim is from one and a half inches to the lowest possible degree of distortion, by the Cæsarean operation.

Mr. Barlow thinks this table will facilitate further inquiry, although he justly observes that the practitioner should bear in mind the absolute impossibility of determining the mean degree of compressibility which the cranium of the fœtus may undergo by the efforts of the uterus ; and he very properly points out the necessity of making a very careful examination in each case before adopting any decided plan of treatment.

Baudelocque regarded the induction of premature labour as a useless, if not an injurious, operation ; and M. Dugès has recently characterised it as fatal to the mother, and the source of most frightful abuse. In the tables of the Maternité, by Baudelocque, Boivin, and Lachapelle, including nearly 60,000 cases of labour, there is no account of any case in which premature labour was induced. The last of these writers begins her strictures on the practice by declaring that she had never either employed "that method, or seen others have recourse to it." The propriety of inducing premature labour was brought under the consideration of the Academy of Medicine, Paris, in 1827, and they decided that the practice was unjustifiable under any circumstances.

The discordance which exists between Continental and British practitioners is also strikingly displayed respecting the Cæsarean section. The reports of 258 cases of this operation have been collected by Michaelis, 144 of which occurred in the last, and 110 in the present century. Of these cases, 140

proved fatal. Velpeau states that the operation was performed twenty-eight times between 1810 and 1820 ; and thirty-one times from 1821 to 1830. Dr. Churchill says the operation was performed 316 times between 1750 and 1841, and that the mortality was 52·8 per cent. for the mothers. I believe that it would have been much greater if all the unfortunate cases had been published, which has not been done. In Great Britain the reports of at least 27 cases have been published, and in 25 of them it was fatal to the mother. Other fatal cases have occurred which have not been recorded. I believe there is no practitioner of reputation now in this country who would recommend the operation upon the living body if delivery could be effected by the perforator and crotchet. Wherever the presenting part can be reached, to apply the perforator and crotchet, an attempt should always be made to deliver, and the Cæsarean operation reserved for those cases in which the distortion is so great that the os uteri and presenting part are entirely beyond our reach.

Most of you have already examined the following table, which has been published in the first of these clinical reports, exhibiting a comparative view of the frequency of forceps and craniotomy cases in some of the principal lying-in hospitals in Europe. It may be useful once more to compare the practice of different institutions, that you may be convinced that the first principles of operative midwifery have not yet been established, at least that they are not generally understood, and that there is no other branch of surgery at the present time in such a rude condition. In one hospital the forceps was employed once in every seven cases, and in another once only in 728 cases. How important it is that you should watch the progress of protracted and difficult labours, and discover the best method of treatment, and form correct opinions on the use of instruments, it is not necessary for me now to point out to you more particularly.

Hospitals.	Number of labours.	Forceps cases.	Proportion.	Craniotomy cases.	Proportion.
Dublin, Clarke.	10,199	14	1 in 728	49	1 in 248
Do., Collins.	16,654	27	1 in 617	118	1 in 141
Paris, Baudelocque.	17,388	31	1 in 561	6	1 in 2898
Do., Lachapelle.	22,243	76	1 in 293	12	1 in 1854
Do., Boivin.	20,517	96	1 in 214	16	1 in 1282
Vienna, Boer.	9,589	35	1 in 274	13	1 in 737
Heidelberg, Naegele.	1,711	55	1 in 31	1	1 in 1711
Berlin, Kluge.	1,111	68	1 in 16	6	1 in 185
Dresden, Carus.	2,519	181	1 in 14	9	1 in 283
Berlin, Siebold.	2,093	300	1 in 7	1	1 in 2093

Only a few cases have been recorded in which Exostoses, or Osteo-sarcomatous Tumors of the pelvis, have produced difficult labour, and I have not met with any instance in practice.

Dr. M'Kibbin has related an example in

the Edin. Med. and Surg. Journal, April 1831, where the hollow of the sacrum and right side of the brim of the pelvis were occupied by an exostosis of a conical form. The woman had been in labour 50 hours, and the greatest space afforded for the passage of the child was on the right side, and it was only 1½ or 1¾ of an inch. From the apex of the tumor to the lower part of the symphysis pubis 1½ inch; from the brim of the pelvis on the right side, immediately over the foramen thyroideum to the lateral surface of the tumor at its widest part, 1⅜ inch; more posteriorly 1½ inch. The delivery was completed by the Cæsarean operation, but the child was dead, and the woman died after, the unsuccessful result being attributed to the delay. Dr. M. advocates the early adoption of the Cæsarean operation in all cases where uncertainty prevails as to the practicability of embryulcia, and where, he says, no two practitioners agree as to the actual space in the pelvis. "In short," he says, "where I was not satisfied that a passage existed for a full-grown fœtus of 2 inches in the short diameter, and 3½ in length, I should be inclined to adopt the Cæsarean operation in preference to embryulcia." I would draw an entirely different conclusion, and in all cases, whatever the degree of distortion might be either in the brim or outlet of the pelvis, attempt to deliver by embryulcia where the presenting part could be reached by the finger and the crotchet applied. Had the patient survived, and had impregnation again taken place, instead of repeating the Cæsarean operation, as he proposes, premature labour should have been induced in the early months of pregnancy. Dr. M. states, in the history of the case, that the patient suffered little or no inconvenience from this morbid growth during life, or the term of utero-gestation. At times she had colicy pains, and, on questioning her mother as to the probable cause of the exostosis, she admitted that her daughter had received a fall on the back when 6 or 8 years of age, which occasioned pain in the sacral region a short time afterwards.

In Dr. Haber's case of difficult labour from an exostosis of the sacrum, the history of which is contained in an inaugural dissertation published at Heidelberg, 1830, the disease also followed a fall upon the ice some years before, when the woman was carrying a heavy load upon the head. This accident was followed by pain in the back and pelvis, which gradually disappeared. She married, became pregnant, and during labour the whole cavity of the pelvis was found to be filled up with an osseous tumor which grew from the sacrum. The Cæsarean section was performed; but the child was putrid, and the patient died soon after the operation. The length of the tumor was seven inches,

and its greatest breadth six. The highest part of it hangs, as you will see by looking at this figure, over the place where the third vertebra of the loins is joined with the fourth. The lowest part of the tumor is distant about two lines and a half from the point of the sacrum. From the posterior surface of the body of the bones of the pubes the tumor is only one line and a half distant. Towards the anterior part, and downwards between the tumor and bones of the pubes, the space is eight or ten lines. The brim of the pelvis was almost completely filled up with the tumor. It appears from the history that there was no other method of delivering this patient but by the Cæsarean section. If the existence of the disease had been known during pregnancy, which however does not appear to have been the case, the induction of premature labour would have been proper in the early months, as soon indeed as the pregnancy was detected, which would have obviated the necessity for the operation. The same observation might be applied to the cases of osteo-sarcomatous tumors of the pelvis obstructing delivery, recorded by Grimmel, Stark, and others.

LUMLEIAN LECTURES

DELIVERED AT THE

COLLEGE OF PHYSICIANS,

MARCH 1843,

BY GEORGE BURROWS, M.D.
Physician to St. Bartholomew's Hospital.

LECTURE II.

Recapitulation. Disturbance of the cerebral circulation, by alterations in the relative quantity of blood in the arteries and veins. Reconsideration of the arguments upon which is founded the opinion that the quantity of blood within the cranium does not alter.

Pressure an important principle in sustaining and destroying the functions of the brain. Illustrations of vascular pressure on the brain in health and disease. Observations on the cephalo-spinal serum and its functions. Increased vascular pressure, and its effects. Diminished vascular pressure, and its effects. Syncope produced by insufficient vascular pressure, rather than by a diminished supply of blood to the brain. Examination and explanation of the phenomena of syncope produced under various circumstances. Cerebral disturbance in general anæmia attributed to insufficient vascular pressure more than to anæmia of the cerebral substance.

THE expiration of the hour allotted to a lecture, compelled me, on the former occasion, to conclude before I had completed a review of the subject which I brought before your notice. I must, therefore, be allowed briefly to recapitulate the points which then occupied our attention.

The subject of my former lecture was the modifications which the circulation within the cranium is capable of undergoing in health and disease, and the state of the circulation within the cranium after different kinds of death.

I quoted from the writings of many eminent physicians the opinions entertained by them on certain peculiarities of the circulation within the head. It appeared from this enquiry that an opinion was very prevalent, "that the quantity of blood within the cranium must be the same, or very nearly the same, at all times, whether in health or disease, in life or after death."

I informed you that this theory of the invariable quantity of blood within the head had been supported, 1st, by reference to certain experiments performed by Dr. Kellie, of Leith; and, 2dly, upon the supposition that the cranium is a complete sphere of bone, which is exactly filled by its contents, the brain, by which that organ is shut up from atmospheric pressure, and from all influence from without, except what is communicated from the blood-vessels which enter it.

I gave, in the first place, a concise analysis of the experiments from which it has been inferred that a state of bloodlessness is not discovered in the brains of animals which have died by hæmorrhage; but, on the contrary, very commonly a state of venous congestion. I then detailed some similar experiments of my own, the results of which were submitted to your inspection, and from which, I flatter myself, it appeared evident that the brains of animals bled to death were deprived of their blood to the extent of rendering them pallid and anæmic. And from these experiments I inferred that it was not a fallacy, as some supposed, that arteriotomy or venesection diminished the actual quantity of blood in the cerebral vessels.

2dly, I detailed some experiments of Dr. Kellie, from which it was attempted to be proved that the quantity of blood in the cranium is not affected by the posture of the head. In opposition to this conclusion I exhibited to you the results of some analogous experiments, from which it was manifest that the quantity of blood in the head is affected to a most extraordinary extent by posture. I showed the effects of gravitation of blood to and from the head.

These results led me to suggest some practical rules which should be adopted in the examination of the cranium after death, where the blood remains fluid, if we wish to avoid being misled by pseudo-morbid appearances.

3dly, I pointed out how it had been attempted to support the opinion, that the quantity of blood in the cranium is invariable, by adducing the absence of congestion of the cerebral vessels in persons who have died by hanging. Admitting the accuracy of such statements, I related to you the appearances in other instances of death by hanging, which fully proved that not only congestion, but extravasations of blood, were often found in the brains of those that died by hanging. I then attempted to explain the occasional absence of congestion in these cases, (1) by the imperfect compression of all the jugular veins ; (2) by the outlet afforded to the blood of the head through that beautiful plexus of sinuses which surrounds the spinal cord ; also, (3) especially by the gravitation of the fluid blood during the suspension of the body ; and, lastly, by the division of the cervical vessels before the head is opened. I also showed, by experiments, that when precautions were adopted to obviate the influence of such causes, then in death by apnœa there was intense congestion of the cerebral vessels.

Upon the present occasion I will complete my investigation of this interesting topic. And here I must remark, that those who maintain that the absolute quantity of blood in the cerebral vessels does not vary, admit a disturbance of the cerebral circulation in the following manner :—They point out the probability of a frequent alteration in the relative quantities of blood in the cerebral arteries and veins. Thus, they assert that those pathological states which have a tendency to cause influx of blood into the cerebral arteries, and accumulation in those vessels, will accomplish this change at the expense of the cerebral veins. Again, anything causing obstruction of the return of blood from the cranium will produce fulness of the sinuses and cerebral veins, but, at the same time, the quantity in the arteries will be equally diminished. They also maintain, if the quantity transmitted to the brain be lessened, the cerebral arteries will be comparatively empty; but there will be a corresponding fulness of the venous system within the cranium. These opinions of Drs. Abercrombie and Kellie are adopted by Dr. Watson, who supports them by similar reasonings. In states of anæmia, he informs us*, a diminished quantity of blood will be transmitted towards and into the cerebral arteries ; but the whole volume of blood in the brain remains the same ; therefore blood will accumulate more in the veins. " It is probably in this way that *the appearance of*

* Medical Lectures, op. cit.

congestion in the superficial veins of the brain is brought about in animals that are bled to death.'' That such venous congestion does not exist, I venture to affirm from the experiments I have performed, and the results of which have already been laid before you.

Some have gone further, and not only asserted that hæmorrhage causes venous congestion of the brain, but have also maintained the paradox, that animals bled to death die of apoplexy. True, indeed, it is that they die with symptoms analogous to those of apoplexy, and this is no new discovery, for this physiological fact was known to Hippocrates. That great man very concisely and tersely expresses the fact in one of his aphorisms, "Σπασμὸς γίνεται ἢ ὑπό πληρώσιος, ἢ κενώσιος."—Sec. vi.

Hippocrates, in this sentence, announced the remarkable pathological truth, that depletion or repletion of the vascular system produces similar symptoms of disturbance of the nervous centres.

Not only have the principles of hydrostatics and other immutable laws of physics been invoked to support the theory that the absolute quantity of blood within the cranium is invariable, or nearly so, but the symbols of algebra have been made to perform their precise evolutions to show that when any increase takes place in the quantity of blood in the arteries of the brain, there must be a corresponding decrease in the veins. If a decrease in the arteries, then an increase in the veins. Thus it is said, if the whole quantity of blood within the cranium $= C$, a constant, the quantity of blood in the arteries $= x$, the quantity of blood in the veins $= y$, then $C = x + y$ always; but let x be diminished by a quantity (a) then y must be increased by this quantity (a), otherwise the original supposition, $C = x + y = (x - a) + (y + a)$ would not be maintained.

Hence, according to the theory supported by this algebraical equation, if the carotid arteries be divided, and the quantity of blood in the cerebral arteries be thus diminished, the quantity of blood in the cerebral veins will be equally increased. But the results of experiments negative these speculations, and show that a diminution of the quantity of blood in one set of vessels is not necessarily accompanied by a state of repletion of the other system of vessels.

There must, then, be some fallacy in this part of the argument ; and the question naturally arises, where is that to be found ? I admit, with Dr. Abercrombie and others, the probability of a disturbance in the equilibrium between the quantities of blood in the arterial and venous systems within the cranium, and that such disturbance is productive of many serious cerebral symptoms.

But in such cases, I presume, there is also a change in the absolute quantity of blood within the cranium, and not a mere change in the relative quantities in the two systems of vessels.

I believe the error of this part of the argument, which I have been combating, consists in the first supposition, that the quantity of blood in the cranium is a constant quantity. On the contrary, I think that experiments and physiological considerations lead us to the conclusion that the quantity of blood within the cranium is extremely variable at different times, and under different circumstances.

The experiments which support this opinion have been already detailed.

Those who have maintained this doctrine of the constant quantity of blood within the cranium, have not, I believe, taken into due consideration that large proportion of the contents of the cranium which consists of extra-vascular serum. We know that in health the quantity which exists in the ventricles, membranes, and substance of the brain, is considerable[*]. Regarding this serum as an important element of the contents of the cranium, I admit that the whole contents of the cranium, that is, the brain, the blood, and this serum together, must be at all times nearly a constant quantity.

But variations in the quantity of serum within the cranium are quite compatible with health ; and in morbid states of the brain we know that at one time the cerebral substance, its membranes, and ventricles, will be nearly devoid of serum ; while, at another time, these parts abound with serous effusion. In accordance with the variations in the quantity of extra-vascular serum, there must be fluctuations in the quantity of intra-vascular fluid, the blood. From this consideration alone, it seems that the blood may be increased or diminished in the cranium. The increase or decrease may affect the two systems of vessels, arterial and venous, equally, or the equilibrium may be disturbed ; there may be excess in either arteries or veins, without any necessary diminution in the quantity of blood contained in the other set of vessels.

Let us now reflect how this question stands. It has been said that the brain is enclosed in a complete sphere of bone, the cranium, which removes it from the influence of atmospheric pressure, and hence no material change can take place in the absolute quantity of blood circulating in the vessels of the brain. This proposition is

[*] From the researches of M. Majendie, it would appear that in the healthy adult the cerebro-spinal serum is never under ii. oz., and often amounts to v. oz. in persons of large frame of body.

also supported by appeal to experiments, and mathematical calculation.

(1). It is maintained, that when hæmorrhage takes place from the general system, it does not affect the quantity of blood in the brain. The experiments I have performed lead me to the opposite conclusion.

(2). Posture of the body after death is said not to affect the quantity of blood within the head. My experiments show that posture has a most striking influence on the quantity of blood in the cerebral vessels.

(3). It has been attempted to prove that when individuals die of asphyxia, or apnœa, there is no excessive congestion of the cerebral vessels. Numerous observations show that in the different kinds of death by apnœa there is great congestion of the cerebral vessels, and that where it is absent it may be accounted for on anatomical and physical principles.

(4). It has also been attempted to prove, by an algebraical equation, that if the quantity of blood be diminished in one system of cerebral vessels, it will be increased in the other vessels. In reply to this, I have shown that the results of experiments negative this conclusion. The error lies in the false assumption of the elements of which the equation is formed.

But how shall we account for these variations in the quantity of blood within the head, if the cranium be a complete sphere, as it has been described by some physiologists?

Does the anatomical structure of the human cranium warrant the opinion that it is a complete sphere, capable of removing its contents from the influence of atmospheric pressure? I think not. The numerous fissures and foramina for the transmission of vessels and nerves through the bones of the cranium appear to me to do away with the idea of the cranium being a perfect sphere, like a glass globe, to which it has been compared by some writers. If there were not always an equilibrium of pressure on the parts within and without the cranium, very serious consequences would arise at the various foramina of the skull. Are, then, the contents of the cranium removed from the influence of atmospheric pressure? I think not, from other considerations. Atmospheric pressure is undoubtedly exerted on the blood in the vessels entering the cranium. This pressure, by a well-ascertained law in hydrostatics, must be transmitted in all directions through the fluid blood, and hence to the blood and other contents within the cranium. If, in the natural state of the parts, the brain is defended from atmospheric pressure, should we not expect to find the functions of that organ disturbed in some way when part of the walls of this sphere is wanting? But in children with open fontanelles, and in adults who have lost part of the bones of the cranium, we observe no peculiar disturbance of the functions of the brain from this gap in the walls of the imaginary sphere. But, lastly, the effects of gravity on the fluid contents of the cranium, and the effects of the cupping-glass, which will often draw blood from the vessels of the dura mater, causing ecchymosis there, assures us that the cranium is not a perfect sphere in the sense in which it has been supposed.

If, then, I have proved, as I believe, that the quantity of blood within the cranium, so far from being a constant, or nearly constant quantity, is, on the contrary, as variable as in other parts of the body, the pathology of many serious affections of the brain will require revision.

The principle of *pressure* is one of much importance, both in sustaining and destroying the functions of the brain.

The functions of the brain probably cannot be maintained in a healthy state without a certain amount of pressure on the cerebral substance. Any variation of pressure which we can artificially produce and estimate appears to affect the functions of this organ. Under the ordinary conditions of health, the cerebral substance is defended from the influence of all variations of external mechanical pressure, and is only subjected to causes of pressure acting within the cranium. A principal and constant cause of pressure from within is the momentum of the blood distending the arteries and veins within the skull. But some of the best writers on the pathology of the brain have maintained that this force, as a cause of pressure, is inoperative—first, because "the cerebral substance is principally composed of inelastic fluids which are incompressible"; and, secondly, "because the brain is incompressible by any such force as can be conveyed to it from the heart through the carotid and vertebral arteries."

Let us analyse these arguments. In the first "the brain is said to be incompressible, because its substance is principally composed of inelastic fluids."

The greatest confusion exists among medical writers on this part of the physiology of the brain, arising from the misapplication and misconception of the terms incompressible and inelastic. Those properties of bodies which we term incompressibility and elasticity bear no constant proportion to each other. It is well known that some of the most incompressible bodies are highly elastic, and those which are very compressible are also elastic.

Thus an ivory billiard ball is very incompressible, but highly elastic; and again, a sponge is very compressible, but also highly elastic. Hence there is neither direct nor inverse proportion subsisting between the compressiblity and elasticity of bodies. It should not therefore be affirmed, that the incompressibilty of the contents of the cranium depends on the inelasticity of the substance of which those contents are composed. In truth, the contents of the cranium, although very incompressible, are highly elastic. As long as medical writers employ the terms of the physical or exact sciences thus loosely, it will be extremely difficult to arrive at the real meaning of experimentalists.

The second part of this argument is, "that the brain is incompressible by any such force as can be conveyed to it from the heart through the carotid and vertebral arteries." The consideration of this opinion I approach with some diffidence, because it emanated from no less an authority than Dr. Abercrombie. The force which is impressed on the cerebral substance, through the carotid and vertebral arteries, is derived from the contractile power of the left ventricle of the heart, at whatever amount that power be estimated. The static force of the blood in the aorta was estimated by Hales at 50 lbs.; Poisseuille's recent experiments place this force at only 5 lbs.

It is not of great importance to my argument whether the momentum of the blood in the aorta be estimated at the greater or less amount.

I wish to show that such a force is actually operating on the cerebral substance within the cranium, and then estimate its effects, when increased or diminished. When a portion of the cranium has been removed, either by accident or artificially, and the dura mater exposed to view, phenomena are remarked which indicate pressure on the cerebral substance by a force from within the cranium, and that the force varies at different times. With every systole of the heart the surface of the dura mater rises a little, and has a tendency to transgress the level of the bones of the cranium. It again subsides with each diastole. Also during the act of expiration, while the free return of venous blood from the brain is impeded, the surface of the dura mater rises and subsides with the succeeding inspiration. Thus whatever has a tendency to distend the cerebral vessels, whether arterial or venous, appears to exert a pressure on the cerebral substance, which is manifested in the manner I have just described.

But the effects of this pressure on the cerebral substance are even more manifest after those accidents, where, with loss of a portion of the bones of the cranium, there is also a laceration of the dura mater. In such cases the distending force of the vessels, acting on the cerebral substance, is so manifest, that not only do we witness the alternate rise and fall of the exposed surface corresponding with the heart's systole and diastole, but portions of the substance of the brain are actually protruded through the aperture in the cranium. Hernia cerebri, or protrusion of the convolutions of the brain, is effected by a force from within, just as hernia of the convolutions of the intestines is produced when the walls of the abdomen are perforated.

Such phænomena more strongly assure us that considerable pressure on the cerebral substance is produced by vascular distension. If the force distending the cerebral arteries be diminished, while the foregoing phænomena are under observation, the manifestations of pressure from within are diminished in proportion.

Thus in the experiment of Dr. Kellie, when he trephined the cranium of a dog, he observed the alternate rising and subsidence of the dura mater at the opening; but having divided one of the carotid arteries of the dog, there was an evident gradual sinking of the brain from the level of the cranium, indicating a diminution of the distending force. Lastly, it has been observed that when syncope occurs, this alternating motion of the brain ceases, and again returns when the heart's action is renewed.[*]

The existence of such a force within the cranium producing outward pressure must be admitted; but Dr. Abercrombie and some others affirm that the brain is not compressible by this force. Although I cannot allow that the brain is altogether incompressible, still I admit that it is only slightly so; but although so little compressible, the cerebral substance must sustain the pressure of this force equally as if it were of the most compressible materials. On this part of the argument Dr. Alexander Monro very justly remarked, "the less compressible we suppose the substance of the brain to be, the more readily we understand how the whole of it may be affected by a plethora or increased momentum of blood in it." (Observations on Nervous System, p. 6.)

Injurious effects of this pressure on the brain would be much more often exhibited, when the quantity of the blood within the cranium is by any means increased, were it not for the peculiarity of the venous system in the cranium, which affords such ready escape for the redundant blood, and for another anatomical peculiarity of the contents of the cranium. The peculiarity which I now advert to is hardly sufficiently estimated by pathologists: it is the very large portion of the contents of the cranium, which is re-

---

* The whole of this subject of the influence of the respiration and circulation on the mass of the brain is admirably discussed by that profound and laborious writer, Albert Haller, in his Elementa Physiologiæ, vol. 4, in the sections "Refluxus sanguinis venosi, qui a respiratione pendet," and again in the section "Motus cerebri arteriosus."

movable by absorption, or by other causes. I advert to the extra-vascular fluid in the cranium; the serum in the substance, ventricles, and membranes of the brain. This fluid, very appropriately designated *cephalospinal*, varies greatly in amount at different times; and probably a portion readily changes its site from the cranium to the spinal canal, and conversely. This is not a mere hypothesis to support a theory or explain a difficulty.

Anatomy points out that the serum in the arachnoid may readily pass from the cranium to the spinal canal; also that that which is contained in the cerebral ventricles may through the fourth ventricle partly escape towards the membranes of the spinal cord. The experiments of Majendie show that this cerebro-spinal fluid may be artificially abstracted or increased.

Pathological states of the spinal column give us an opportunity of ascertaining the freedom of transmission of serum from the arachnoid of the cord to the brain. In spina bifida we remark during fits of coughing and crying the spinal tumor becomes much more tense, and by graduated pressure with the hand over the tumor it may be gradually decreased in size. With the diminution of size we may witness symptoms of pressure on the brain and cord. These considerations lead to the conclusion that this cephalo-spinal fluid may, under the influence of pressure, change its site. When arterial or venous congestion of the brain is suddenly induced, the first consequence will be increased pressure on all the contents of the cranium; the second effort will be the displacement of a portion of this extra-vascular serum into the spinal canal. When abstraction of blood from the cranium is effected, a quantity of serum occupies the vacated space. This extra-vascular serum is supplemental to the other contents of the cranium, removable by pressure or absorption, at one time giving place to the increased quantity of blood, at another making up for the deficiency of blood in the vessels. This extra-vascular serum not merely acts as supplemental to the varying quantity of blood, but also to the variable quantity of nervous matter in the brain. Thus in hypertrophy of the brain there is a more remarkable deficiency of serum in the ventricles and membranes, and ventricles are so devoid of this fluid, that they are incapable of the contrary, in atrophy of the organ the ventricles and membranes are distended with fluid.

I think it probable that this extra-vascular fluid may perform another office. Perhaps through this serum a more subtle pressure is preserved on the cerebral substance, and for the reception of the variations of pressure may be the mechanism of the arachnoid, and of these various effects of pressure.

ventricles, which dip into the central parts of the cerebral mass.[a]

The effects of increased determination of blood to the brain, or of obstructed venous circulation from it may be witnessed, even in otherwise healthy states of that organ, although those effects are probably sometimes obviated by the anatomical conditions I have just explained: but they are most strikingly displayed when there is pre-existing disease in the cranium.

When the power of the heart is inordinately increased by stimulants, general plethora, or hypertrophy of the left ventricle, we remark a train of symptoms similar to those produced by varying degrees of mechanical pressure artificially exerted on the brain.

When obstruction to the return of blood from the brain takes place, so that the blood becomes almost stagnant in the sinuses, the force of the left ventricle (which in the normal state of the cerebral circulation is expended partly in propelling the blood onward through the capillaries towards the right auricle, and partly in distending the vessels within the cranium) is under such circumstances expended upon the interior surface of the cerebral blood-vessels. This pressure is partly sustained by the resistance of the vascular tissues, and the remainder is borne by the surrounding cerebral substance.

Whatever this force may be, it becomes a source of increased pressure upon the cerebral substance; and the more so, according to the pre-existing morbid states of the encephalon. When the circulation is excited or obstructed an obvious state of congestion of the integuments of the head and face is produced, and from the experiments I have detailed, it may, I think, be inferred, that a simultaneous congestion of the internal vessels of the cranium is formed.

In previously healthy conditions of the cranium, when it contains nothing but the usual and normal quantity of serous fluid, the previous instance may read ....

brain, tumors and cysts in that organ, and in large extravasations of blood on the surface, every cause which is capable of exciting the heart's action produces an increased disturbance of the functions of the brain. The variable character of the symptoms of cerebral disturbance in these permanent lesions within the cranium are thus probably accounted for by the variable vascular pressure. Dr. Watson has offered a nearly similar explanation of the occasional recurrence of cerebral symptoms, although their supposed cause, organic disease in the cranium, is permanent. It seems to me probable that many permanent lesions within the cranium do not affect the functions of the brain by pressure, except when there is some cause in operation capable of inducing vascular congestion, or when the lesion is of a mechanical nature, or is gradually increasing.

If the force of the contractions of the heart be diminished in these morbid states of the encephalon, there is usually a corresponding relief to the cerebral symptoms; but should the same diminution in the force of the circulation be produced in healthy states of the brain, the functions of the organ are suddenly annihilated from insufficient vascular pressure: syncope is the result.

Syncope is occasioned by insufficient vascular pressure on the brain, and not from the inadequate quantity of blood supplied to the brain and its vessels, as is commonly supposed.

In the most simple form of syncope, that which arises from a strong moral emotion in a previously healthy person, we see the single effect of want of due vascular pressure on the brain. In such cases the quantity and quality of the blood in the person's body are unaltered previous to the syncope, and the suspension of the cerebral functions arises solely from the diminished energy of the heart. The blood is no longer propelled with sufficient force from the left ventricle to maintain an adequate pressure on the cerebral substance. If such a person happen to be in the erect posture, the syncope is more rapid and complete; because the enfeebled muscular tissue of the heart is unable to sustain the arterial current of blood against the force of gravity, and to preserve the proper degree of pressure on the brain. Let such a fainting person be placed in the horizontal posture, and, as is well known, consciousness quickly returns. But why? Because the enfeebled heart is equal to maintain the arterial current of blood in that favourable posture, and with it the requisite amount of vascular pressure on the brain. The same phænomena occur in syncope produced by hæmorrhage, although in this case it is not so easy to show that the suspension

of the cerebral functions is occasioned solely by want of vascular pressure on its substance. It has been forcibly pointed out by Dr. Marshall Hall, that bleeding in the erect posture is the best method of ascertaining the power of the system to sustain the loss of blood, and of the propriety of bleeding as a remedial agent. It is a matter of daily experience that a small amount of blood taken from a person in the erect posture will cause syncope; whereas double the amount of blood might have been taken from that person in the horizontal posture, without producing a similar result. Hence the posture of the individual, and not the amount of blood abstracted, is the more efficient cause of the syncope. The effects of the erect posture on the heart and brain I have just described.

In extreme states of debility, from whatever cause produced, the mere sudden assumption of the erect posture is often adequate to induce an alarming, and sometimes fatal, syncope. In this posture the feeble heart is unable to project the blood against the force of gravity in the carotid and vertebral arteries, when the brain is suddenly deprived of the vascular pressure essential to the continuance of its functions. The influence of this cause of death was not unfrequently seen in our cholera hospitals, when that disease prevailed epidemically. Patients who were in states of collapse, but still in the enjoyment of sensorial functions while reclining, upon assuming the erect posture died almost instantaneously.

There is another posture of the body which will, in some persons, induce syncope, and where the cause appears to be the sudden diminution of the momentum of the blood in the arteries of the head, and, consequently, an insufficient vascular pressure on the brain. If the arms be held extended in vertical lines above the head, this posture will quickly produce faintness in some persons. Here the heart has suddenly imposed upon it the additional labour of overcoming the effects of gravity on the blood in the arteries of the upper extremities; and the consequence is a diminution of the momentum of the blood in the arteries of the head.

It is unnecessary for me particularly to describe the remarkable disturbance of the functions of the brain which takes place in general anæmia. Does the long catalogue of nervous symptoms arise from the altered qualities of the blood in anæmia; or from an insufficient quantity of blood in the cerebral substance; or, lastly, from impaired vascular pressure on the substance of the brain? Without underrating the injurious effects of the altered qualities of the blood, in general anæmia, on the brain and all the organs of the body, still I am inclined to the opinion that some of the most remarkable symptoms arise rather from insufficient vascular pressure than from an insufficient quantity of blood in the substance of the brain.

Simple anæmia of the brain certainly does not produce that train of symptoms which is usually ascribed to a want of due supply of blood to the brain. Probably there is no condition of the brain, not even that induced by repeated hæmorrhage, in which the substance of the organ is so completely anæmic as in genuine hypertrophy of the brain. In this rare cerebral affection the membranes and substance are found dry, and devoid of blood or serum; the medullary matter is as white and firm as blanc-mange or hard-boiled white of egg. The cranium is already so completely filled by hypertrophy of the cerebral substance that the blood is unable to make its way through the vessels; and with all this bloodlessness of the organ, we witness none of the nervous symptoms of general anæmia. On the contrary, the symptoms are rather those commonly ascribed to the effects of inordinate supply of blood to the brain. In these cases of hypertrophy of the brain the force of the heart is unimpaired; the blood is propelled with its normal force into the cerebral arteries, but it cannot make its way through the capillaries; and thus the static force of the heart is expended on the surrounding cerebral substance: so that, in anæmia of the brain from this cause, there are none of the symptoms present which accompany anæmia of the organ produced by hæmorrhage, in which condition there is insufficient power of the heart to produce the amount of vascular pressure essential to the functions of the brain. Hence we infer that the simple condition of anæmia of the brain, independent of diminished vascular pressure, is insufficient to produce the peculiar train of symptoms so often observed in general anæmia.

It is in general anæmia, caused by profuse hæmorrhage, that we witness the fearful catalogue of symptoms indicating disturbance of the nervous centres in their most aggravated form. In such a condition of the body, we remark that whatever tends temporarily to assist the heart, or stimulate it to propel the blood towards the brain, alleviates the nervous symptoms; on the contrary, whatever places the heart at greater disadvantage in propelling the blood to the brain, aggravates these nervous symptoms. The loss of consciousness in syncope, the convulsions after hæmorrhage, are often immediately terminated by the horizontal posture so favourable to the momentum of the blood in the carotid arteries. The senses of sight and hearing are often impaired or lost during states of general anæmia, but posture alone will sometimes restore these functions of the brain.

Dr. Abercrombie* relates the following remarkable instance of the effects of posture on the cerebral functions. A gentleman, aged 30, came to Edinburgh for advice in regard to an obscure affection, referred chiefly to the stomach, and which had reduced him to a state of extreme weakness and emaciation. As his debility had advanced he had become considerably deaf, and this affected him in a singular manner. When standing, or sitting upright, he was very deaf; but when he lay horizontally, with his head very low, he heard perfectly. If, when standing, he stooped forward, so as to produce flushing of his face, his hearing was perfect; and upon raising himself again he continued to hear distinctly as long as the flushing continued: as this went off, the deafness returned.

In the foregoing case Dr. Abercrombie supposed there must be a want of balance in the circulation within the brain, a diminished quantity of blood and momentum of blood in the cerebral arteries, with a corresponding increase of the blood in the cerebral veins.

I think the history of this case of deafness, as recorded by Dr. Abercrombie, rather shows that the varying amount of vascular pressure was the cause both of the suspension and restoration of the cerebral functions.

For a number of curious and interesting cases illustrating the state of the nervous centres when the system is reduced to a state of general anæmia, either by loss of blood or other debilitating causes, the work of Dr. Marshall Hall "On the Loss of Blood, &c." may be consulted with advantage. In one and all of these cases of disturbed functions of the brain, an immediate, but temporary, relief to the symptoms is afforded by horizontal posture, stimulants, and other means which favour the momentum of the blood moving through the carotid and vertebral arieries.

We may remark similar effects from diminished vascular pressure on the brain in the application of that powerful, but hazardous contrivance, the horizontal revolving bed. Dr. Darwin, I believe, invented this rotatory machine for the purpose of tranquillizing the nervous system and procuring sleep†. It was subsequently employed to calm the violence of the furious maniac. Its mode of application is as follows. The patient is laid on his back, with his head close to a column or pivot, around which the bed is made to revolve in a horizontal plane with considerable velocity. A centrifugal force is thus generated, which, from the position of the patient, determines the blood from the head towards the lower

---

* Op. cit.
† Zhonomia, vol ii. p. 608.

* Op. cit.
† Zoonomia, vol ii. p. 608.

extremities. This centrifugal force, thus suddenly created, powerfully diminishes the momentum of the blood moving into the cranium : the diminished arterial pressure on the cerebral substance soon produces a sense of exhaustion or complete syncope.

I have adduced this as another illustration of the principle, that the suspension of the functions of the brain is produced by the diminished vascular pressure on its substance, rather than by an inadequate supply of blood to the organ. In this last described experiment it is clear that neither the quantity nor the quality of the blood in the vascular system is affected by the generation of this new power. Neither can we ascribe the loss of cerebral functions to an alteration in the balance of the circulation within the cranium, that is, to an alteration in the relative quantities of blood in the arteries and veins. This centrifugal force must have an equal effect upon the blood in the arteries and veins of the brain, as well as upon the removable serum. I think we can only ascribe the effects to diminished vascular pressure.

On this interesting and important principle of pressure, I have endeavoured to point out that such a force is constantly in operation upon the cerebral substance; that this pressure is produced by vascular distension; that, in health, any cause which is capable of increasing or diminishing this vascular distension has the effect of disturbing the functions of the brain; that these effects of vascular distension would be more serious and frequent if parts of the contents of the cranium were not readily removable upon increase of vascular pressure; that, in pre-existing structural diseases of the encephalon, any increase of vascular distension causes much more serious disturbance of the cerebral functions, and the symptoms so produced are analogous to those of mechanical pressure on the brain.

I have also attempted to support the opinion that variations of this vascular pressure are the causes of the intermitting character of the symptoms in cases of permanent disease within the cranium.

Lastly, I have endeavoured to explain the phenomena of syncope, however produced, on the principle of diminished momentum of blood in the arteries of the head, and consequent diminished vascular pressure on the cerebral substance, rather than on the principle that the brain is not supplied with a sufficient quantity of blood.

ON THE

CAUSES OF STRANGULATION AND DEATH IN CASES OF HERNIA,

OR THE

SIGNS OF CONSTITUTIONAL OR HUMORAL DISORDER IN SUCH CASES.

(Some Statistics: the Treatment: Dr. O'Beirne's Views, &c.)

BY T. WILKINSON KING, ESQ.

(For the London Medical Gazette.)

IN the Guy's Hospital Reports for the year 1838, I published some statistics to show that most herniæ exist for years before they become subject to violent strangulation; that the mean duration of three-fourths of the well-recorded cases had been between 15 and 25 years before danger arose.

The following were my conclusions from a considerable series of facts[*].

" First, Most herniæ being of old-standing before they become seriously strangulated, this result is not attributable to the state of the sac, but to that of the bowel; in which defective nourishment and power of vessels leads to more ready tumefaction; and all this seems attributable to the age and the organic deterioration belonging to it.

" Secondly, The common and chief danger is from a peculiar and unhealthy kind of peritonitis; the consequence, probably, of the same constitutional decay or decline of organs which induced the strangulation.

" Thirdly, The above facts lead to the conclusion, that prompt surgery, to remove the cause of inflammation, and the most cautious medicine to obviate, and not excite, inflammation, and to add nothing to the oppressed condition of the patient, are indications even more pressing than has been hitherto maintained, at least among authors and the generality of surgeons."

I am now enabled to extend the facts of my case, and, I hope, add strength to an argument which, if it has hitherto found no favour, has met no opponents, and which, if just, is important enough to claim attention, both for its own sake and for the reason

---

* See Guy's Hospital Reports, No. 7, p. 390.

effects more or less light on the
ffections of declining life.
ık it would be a consideration
; importance, if it were only
ıat the ordinary duration of
before strangulation is 15 or 16
; especially if we take into the
the fact that the age for stran-
hernia is most commonly after
ı or 40th year of life.
grand fact of my case is, that
ıalf of the cases of hernia that
with requiring immediate aid
proved to have pre-existed for
1 of 15 or 25 years, or even 40

is as undeniable as it is im-
; and it seems to me as striking
nass of surgical writers seem to
ıought it insignificant.   But it
ı cumulative argument that I
the greatest import.
:ular exertion and local con-
on are the causes of hernia : but
al or serious strangulation, at
ur times out of five, is produced
years later, when a totally dif-
state of parts and constitution
:come developed.   The acute
ılation of young persons, and its
train of comparatively healthy
ıma, may find its analogy on rare
ıns at any period of life.   It is
terised by narrow stricture and
reparative actions, and may be
of all the morbid traits of old-
ıg hernia when strangulated,
is more like what is called in-
ıted hernia, but devoid of healthy
and fraught with signs of non-
ive inflammations,—diffused ac-
ınorganized and pernicious effu-

symptoms, the course, and the
ortem appearances of the latter
re specific.
w numerical facts will, I think,
his view in a somewhat stronger
han my former tables.

In the last number of the Guy's
Hospital Reports*, 44 successive cases
are detailed. There appear to have
been—

7 cases, more or less recent ;
1   ,,   had existed for some time ;
28 ,,   ,,   stated numbers
      of years.
The mean duration of all these is 13 yrs.
2 cases had existed for some years ; and
6   ,,   ,,   several or a num-
      ber of years.

Of the same cases there were—

Submitted to operation   18
Successfully (one, æt. 9) .   .   .   9
Unsuccessfully (the gut rent in
   one, æt. 21) .   .   .   .   .   .   ,
The mean age in the 8 cases of successful operations was .   43 years
Unsuccessful 59½
22 reductions by taxis, &c. 43½
Three other cases were in the last stage,
unreduced and fatal ; one was a reduction
fatal by continued inflammation.

In the years prior to that in which
the last cases occurred, there were admitted into Guy's 55 cases of urgent
herniæ in two years, or 112 weeks : 17
between November and May, and 5
between June and October.   And by
setting the dates of these cases beside
those of the cases lately published in
our Reports, I find that of 100 cases
twice as many instances of strangulation are admitted between November
and April as between May and October ;
and that half of the whole number are
admitted between December and March
inclusive.   The increased numbers of
winter I refer, as disorganizing pneumonia, to humoral circumstances influenced by the season.
   M. Malgagne's statistics may be
made to throw some light on these
views, but, for the most part, only
indirectly. We find that of an immense number of recorded cases in
Paris, between the end of 1835 and
that of 1837—

occurred 4 times as often in males as females
  ,,   often in the first year of life†
  ,,   rarely after this, and more and more so till the 9th year.
ıbers increase after the 9th year
,   still more between 13 and 20   (in males only—exertion)
            ,,   20 and 28   (in both sexes—pregnancy.
                                     Males increased by ⅓,
                                     Females   ,,   ⅓)
            ,,   28 and 29   (and most in females)
,   stationary from   30 to 35=27½ per annum } 4 males to 1 female
,   increase   from   35 to 40=52   ,,   }
,   ,,   ,,   40 to 50=96   ,,   3 males to 1 female

* No. 1 of the New Series, April 1843.
† Chiefly umbilical and inguinal, doubtless ; and from conformation.
—XXXII.

O

Here we have a mixture of all kinds of cases—simple hernia, with instances of transitory and severer strangulation—but we may perceive that the simple cases decline in annual numbers after the 30th year, and that the largest amount of cases occur to the surgeon on all accounts (of strangulation, &c.) between the 40th and 50th years of life. From calculations of cases at Guy's Hospital, after the publication of my former paper, I find the mean ages of 26 cases fatal on various accounts to be 56¼ years, and that of 26 serious cases which recovered to be 44¼.

From my printed table I find that the mean ages of the 47 patients successfully operated on was 42$\frac{6}{7}$, or 42 years 6 weeks; and that the mean age of those 33 who were fatally operated on, was 45$\frac{11}{14}$, or 45 years 6 months. These last sets were chiefly recorded by authors as serious cases; yet I think the difference of age points to the same fact as an analysis of 70 other fatal cases now before me, in which defective reparation, unorganisable effusions, and deteriorated solid viscera, seem to be essential constitutional concomitants of old hernia becoming seriously strangulated.

Dr. Norman Chevers has lately recorded in the Guy's Hospital Reports the circumstances of a large number of unsuccessful or fatal cases of accident and operation. With disordered viscera, imperfect secretion and depurative elimination are palpable inductions in these cases,[*] and too forcible and important as arguments of humoral deterioration to be omitted or even ranked low as the causes of mischief, whether affecting cases of accidental injury, operation, or parturition, or such even as those of catarrh, pneumonia, or hæmorrhage, or epischeses.

In my former paper I thus expressed myself on this subject:—" The proneness to erysipelas or visceral inflammations, under most operations, marks them (herniæ), as well as many more who are the subject of operations at the like ages in great cities. Yet all these constitutional dispositions, as they are called, are found on inspecting the dead to be connected with very tangible and permanent alterations of the great viscera. These actual disorganizations are not incompatible with seeming health, but are highly obnoxious when reparation is in progress. If one organ is found affected after death, the change is proportionately more considerable: if several are involved, they are mostly less affected. It is to be remembered, however—though, as after all fatal operations, the changes are less severe and advanced than when the visceral affection alone seems fatal—yet they are so manifest that the wonder is that they were not alone destructive, and that much sooner: at least this has been my own reflection on many occasions."

Before the fatal period, herniæ descend almost with impunity, but at length, as in the great injuries, or rather as in cases of slight injury which have become dangerous, the reparative resources being unequal to the task, all the events till death sufficiently indicate the specific state.

It may be in a manner a test of a surgeon's principles for him to ask himself this question. Is there any fear of diffused inflammation from a circumscribed injury to the peritoneum in a healthy person? My answer is, there is no fear whatever; but I do not say, if the patient have been unduly exposed before, or during the treatment. or if subjected to violent medicines, that he is a healthy person, and doubtless there are other similar considerations. What some persons intend when they declare that certain tissues are prone of themselves to spreading inflammation, is still a problem. At one time the assertion is true of all tissues; at another it is not true of any. Of course disease is more serious in certain tissues, and also less happily repaired.

The opinion for which I contend involves of course specific rules of treatment, as I have formerly indicated. In the anticipation of fatal peritonitis, mild, speedy, and efficient remedies are the objects to be held in view. Every kind of aggravation from delay, violence, exposure to cold, or severe remedies, is to be regarded as highly dangerous. I have formerly said as much on this part of my subject as may be desirable,

---

[*] These principles have been long taught at Guy's, and the facts on which they are based run through a series of 30 or 40 large volumes of museum manuscripts which are not merely careful records of common facts. Thirteen of these volumes are, perhaps, the most valuable (no slight praise) of all the labours of Hodgkin: and I may claim an equal quantity as my own work. A tabular analysis of the whole for more than twenty years, kept up since I was a pupil, renders the examination of the whole available almost at a glance. Dr. C,'s exposition is principally based on my own autopsy-histories.

until the main principle is admitted to be a sound and essential one. I shall conclude, therefore, with some remarks on a recent theory of strangulation.

Dr. O'Beirne*, of the Richmond Hospital Dublin, some time since recommended the use of the rectum tube to facilitate the reduction of the "intestinal hernia," by giving exit to the retained gases; a simple practice, which if we were to judge from the experience recorded, cannot fail to be occasionally very useful. This distinguished surgeon's views, however, seem to me almost to demand some comments; which I have set down just in the current in which they occurred to me. If any should concur with me in recommending a trial of the practice named, they will probably see no great objection to the following brief inquiry relative to its application, the cases concerned being of so frequent occurrence and great importance, and the causes of strangulation being still subjects of useful and interesting research.

In Dr. O'Beirne's account of the causes and treatment of strangulation in hernia, he attributes the strangulation to the easy access of flatus into the incarcerated portion of bowel, and he recommends the use of the rectum tube for the relief of this air-distended portion.

It will, I think, be in conformity with the opinion of most surgical pathologists, to regard the neck of the sac in hernia as quite passive in the production of strangulation, so that we are all prepared to look for some other cause of this serious state. What commonly produces strangulation? Dr. O'Beirne says flatus does it; but of course this will not apply to the simple omental hernia; nor will it, I suppose, explain the process when only a segment of the intestinal cylinder is involved.

It is an ingenious experiment to make a perforated card represent the aperture of hernia, and then, having passed a knuckle of intestine through it, to shew the effect of rather forcibly inflating this portion of bowel; but in

connection with this, the Dr. asserts that it is not commonly the case, in strangulated hernia, that the intestinal tube is rendered impervious by the compression about the neck of the sac, and he has concluded " that no proposition in nature can be clearer than this : namely, *that as strangulation is produced by a distending force acting from within outwards, and separating the parietes of the constricted gut, and maintaining them at a greater or less distance from each other, there must be a communication.*" Now I suppose it admitted on all sides, 1st, that pressure from within the abdomen first protrudes about as much bowel as the ring will easily contain ; 2dly, that whatever may constitute the protrusion, it will generally happen that with the increase of the protrusion there will be a certain increase of calibre or mass in that part actually included in the plane of the constricting ring ; and 3dly, that with the very commencement of strangulation there begins also injection and swelling, or even additional fleshiness, of all the intestinal tunics included in the sac. I do not think that these facts warrant the assumption of a persistent " channel of communication" between the bowel in the sac and that in the abdomen, which communication Dr. O'Beirne admits must be extremely narrow. I would suggest that the *distending force* acting from within outwards may at times find a substitute in the increasing turgescence of the strangling gut*, and it cannot but be remarked that a communication between the general bowels and the strangulated portion which may transmit air, and which according to the Dr.'s experience does admit of the passage of air from the strangulated bowel, with the use of the rectum tube, certainly ought to allow of the free escape of air and fluids by the application of ordinary taxes, and still more certainly when exposed by operation. In thus adverting to what I deem erroneous, I would allow that the use of the rectum tube in hernia,

---

* Article 8th.—In the Dublin Journal of Medical and Chemical Science, for September 1838. "On the primary causes of strangulation, and on an improved mode of performing the Taxis in cases of Intestinal Hernia. By James O'Beirne, M.D. one of the Surgeons to the Richmond Surgical Hospital, &c. Dublin."

* The second part of Dr. O'Beirne's proposition above, declares the strangulated tube to be of necessity distended, and he seems to infer with air. In answer to this I would say, that the gurgling sound of air, on reduction, is often absent, and that in operations it is commonly evident that the inflation is not more remarkable than the fluid secretions in the bowel, and lastly, that the extreme thickening of its membranes is by far the most notable inherent source of difficulty in the return.

in the manner advised and illustrated by examples, may be still a valuable adjunct to surgery.

A few remarks on the deductions to be made from the cases related in corroboration of the Dr.'s views, will serve to introduce a somewhat different explanation of the result. I do not know if it is to be regretted that hitherto we have no account of the different cases in which the rectum tube is not calculated to be successful. I suppose, however, there are some; as, particularly, very small hernia, and acute cases in the young. Again, it may be quite just to conclude that the taxis, successful with the use of the tube, might in a few cases have been ultimately effectual alone. Many of the case recorded to the advantage of the tube, were for hernia in very aged patients; a circumstance involving general tympanitis almost necessarily, considering the nature of the case. Indeed, the tympanitis would appear in some measure essential to the establishment of Dr. O'Beirne's main position. With regard to the use of the tube in young hernia patients, I am tempted to infer that the result must often disappoint us, and I have to add, by way of caution, that I have known the tube (resembling that of the common stomach-pump), penetrate the rectum and peritoneum, and in very careful hands too.

A trial of the rectum tube in strangulated hernia has the advantages of requiring no delay, not interfering with other remedies, and above all it is comparatively safe; for with proper knowledge and care the thick bulbous tube of Dr. O'Beirne cannot, I think, go wrong.

It is scarcely necessary to contend for a different explanation of the use of this instrument; the cases narrated seem to prove that it has been serviceable, as far, surely, as such a number well can. My own explanation would be briefly this: that the sudden diminution of abdominal distension by evacuation per anum (as by mouth), must facilitate the taxis, and if we suppose the evacuation of flatus to be great, and the reduction attempted simultaneously, the beneficial tendency is almost certain. Of course there will often be a difficulty in determining the precise share of influence attributable to remedies when combined, and there must be some difficulty in ascertaining

well the effect of the tube with regard to the quantity of gas to which it gives exit; for I deem it important to observe that after death by strangulation of the small intestine, the whole colon is for the most part remarkably empty; as I have very often demonstrated on inspection during the last few years.

36, Bedford Square.

SOME PRACTICAL REMARKS

ON THE

EMPLOYMENT OF ARSENIC IN THE TREATMENT OF THE DISEASES OF THE SKIN.

By John E. Erichsen.

(For the London Medical Gazette.)

Among the many remedies that have been had recourse to in the treatment of the diseases of the skin, there are none about the propriety of employing which more discrepancy of opinion has been excited than about arsenic. By some, this metal has been extolled as being, in one or other of the various forms in which it is administered, an agent of the greatest value in controlling the affections in question; and by these it is resorted to, much too indiscriminately, in the treatment of every obstinate cutaneous complaint, without reference to the nature, causes, and actual condition of the disease itself, or to the habit of body and constitution of the individual in whom it occurs. By others, again, the arsenical preparations are looked upon as being frequently useless and dangerous, or, at best, as remedies of uncertain power, which are only to be had recourse to when every other available means of checking the disease for which it may be thought advisable to prescribe them has failed. This difference of opinion appears to me to have arisen from the fact, that sufficient care has not been taken by writers on the diseases of the skin to point out, not only the particular disease in which these remedies are admissible, but more especially, the particular stage of the complaint in which alone their administration may be expected to be productive of some salutary effect, as well as the kind of constitution and temperament by which only they can be borne. For it does not require a very extended observation of cutaneous affections to become aware of the fact that an arsenical preparation may be useless, if not highly injurious, in an early stage of a disease, whereas, at a later period, it may be exceedingly beneficial; and that even then it cannot be administered with safety in some constitutions, or to individuals of particular temperament. And in this, I say it with deference, lies the great defect of many of the therapeutic measures inculcated in different treatises on the diseases of the skin; that remedies of the utmost power are abundantly enumerated, but as no directions are usually given as to the precise stage of the disorder in which they should be administered, or notice taken of the circumstances that indicate or contraindicate their employment, the reader is apt to imagine that the author bases his mode of treatment rather upon the particular name that the complaint may chance to bear, than upon any circumstances connected with its stage or cause, or with the habit of body of the patient; and thus he is led to think that if he can once make out the diagnosis, and learn the name of any cutaneous affection that may fall under his observation, the proper treatment of the disease follows as a matter of course, without reference to any modifying circumstances. It is on account of the disappointment that is apt to be consequent upon such a mode of procedure that many remedies, which have been deservedly recommended to the profession as of the utmost power, have had their justly earned character depreciated, either by being administered without sufficient discrimination during improper stages of the disease, or to individuals who were, from constitution, ill able to bear them. It is my intention, then, in the remarks that I am about to make, to direct particular attention to the several circumstances, whether in the constitution or habit of body of the individual, or in the nature or stage of the particular affection under which he may be labouring, or in its complication with other diseases, that may indicate, or contra-indicate, the employment of the preparations of arsenic. For it is from a want of due consideration to these circumstances that this most powerful and valuable class of remedies has been frequently accused of having received a reputation beyond its deserts, or that, at best, it

has been allowed to be capable of curing local diseases but at the expense of more or less permanent derangement of the digestive and nervous functions.

It is to Adair and Girdlestone that we owe, at about the commencement of the present century, the introduction of the preparations of arsenic in the treatment of the diseases of the skin, and from the extraordinary effects that they were shown to possess in removing and controlling affections of this kind, even though of many years' standing, they soon came into general repute, being resorted to, almost as specifics, in those cases of cutaneous disease that had resisted other means of treatment, and even in such as would readily have yielded to less active measures.

The preparations of arsenic that are most commonly had recourse to in the treatment of cutaneous complaints are, the solution of the arsenite of potassa (Fowler's solution), the solution of the iodide of arsenic and mercury (Donovan's solution), the iodide of arsenic and arsenious acid in the form of pill. Besides these, the solution of the arseniate of soda (Pearson's solution) has been recommended by some, and that of the arseniate of ammonia by others, chiefly by Biett; but as these two last are not much employed, and as their qualities and mode of action seem in no way to differ from those of the arsenite of potassa, I shall omit all consideration of them.

The opinions of authors vary somewhat as to the dose in which we should commence the administration of the solution of the arsenite of potassa, and as to the extent to which we ought to carry it. Girdlestone recommends us to begin with the smallest doses, and never to increase the quantity taken beyond five or six drops three times a day, and only to persevere in such quantities as can be taken without inconvenience to the patient. In children, he says, the dose should not exceed two or three drops once or twice a day. The largest quantity he ever gave was twelve drops three times a day; but he soon found that half this quantity would suffice equally well. Bateman and Thomson advise us to begin with doses of four or five drops, which may be slowly increased up to eight, twice a day. Biett, who advocates the employment of arsenic more generally than any other writer, directs

us to commence with three drops of the solution every morning before breakfast, and to augment this, every fifth or sixth day, by two or three drops, until twelve or fifteen were taken daily; more than this, he says, should not be administered, and it may be expedient to interrupt the use of the medicine, in these doses, from time to time. Rayer recommends doses of from four to five drops daily, to be gradually increased until the patient takes fifteen drops in four divided doses. Thus, then, although these authorities differ somewhat as to the precise mode in which the solution of the arsenite of potassa is to be taken, they all agree that we should not carry it beyond fifteen, or at most, eighteen drops in the course of the day. I am in the habit of beginning with two minims of the solution, equal, in quantity, to 1-60th of a grain of arsenious acid, twice a-day, and to carry it up to five, six, or seven and a half minims, equal to the 1-18th of a grain of arsènious acid, three times a day; beyond which I believe it is never necessary to increase the dose, as I am convinced that the good effects of this remedy are to be obtained rather by small doses continued for a considerable time than by the exhibition of larger ones at longer intervals. But the smallest even of the quantities that have been mentioned are quite inadmissible, as will be shown in a subsequent part of this paper, in individuals of an excitable temperament.

Within the last two years another preparation of arsenic has been introduced to the notice of the profession, by Mr. Donovan, of Dublin, under the name of the " Liquor Arsenici et Hydrargyri Iodidi ;" for a full account of the chemical composition and medicinal effects of which I may refer my readers to the papers by Mr. Donovan in the Dublin Journal of Medical Science. The dose of this preparation is variously stated.   Dr. Kirby commences ·with doses of 20 minims, which he states are large enough to ensure the good effects of the remedy.   Mr. Cusack recommends from 20 to 40 minims three times a day, which may, in some cases, be pushed to a greater extent. Dr. Irvine has given as much as half a drachm three times a day, for seventy-six days, with an intermission of only two or three days on account of headache and sickness.   Dr. Graves ad-

ministered it to the extent of half a drachm four times a day for two months, with but two interruptions; and Sir Henry Marsh carried it, in the case of a boy twelve years of age, to the extent of half an ounce daily, in divided doses, which only produced very mild insalivation.   Mr. Donovan is of opinion that it is prudent to begin with Dr. Kirby's doses; but he states that, after a time, a state of tolerance is induced, and then the médicine may be gradually increased at discretion.   It has been administered to patients of all ages: thus, one of Sir H. Marsh's patients was but five years old, while both of Dr. Graves's had attained their sixtieth year, and Dr. Croker's her sixty-eighth. The composition of the liquor of the hydriodate of arsenic and mercury is, according to Mr. Donovan, as follows:—

Water, one drachm.
Arsenious acid, $\frac{1}{2}$ of a grain.
Peroxide of mercury, $\frac{1}{4}$ of a grain.
Iodine, as hydriodic acid, about $\frac{3}{4}$ of a gr.

Thus this preparation contains exactly a quarter as much arsenious acid as enters into the constitution of Fowler's solution, differing besides in other very obvious and important respects.

The iodide of arsenic, a very useful preparation of the metal, for the introduction of which into practice the profession is indebted to Dr. A. T. Thomson, is most conveniently administered in the form of pill.   The dose of this preparation should not at first exceed the twelfth of a grain twice a day; this may gradually be increased until the patient takes the sixth, or even the fourth, of a grain three times a day, although these doses are very rarely necessary.   The iodide of arsenic is most advantageously exhibited in combination with the extract of conium, which seems to sheathe its irritating qualities, and prevents it from exciting too powerfully the mucous membrane of the stomach.   By the addition of biniodide of mercury a compound pill may be formed, which resembles, in its effects, the liquor of the hydriodate of arsenic and mercury, and has been much and successfully employed by Dr. A. T. Thomson in the treatment of lupus and other diseases of the skin, and which I have found of particular service in some syphilitic eruptions, more particularly of a squamous kind. Of its use in these affections I had an interesting example last autumn, in the person of a country gentleman, the brother-in-law of a physician in this town, who had laboured under syphilitic psoriasis of the legs, the right one more particularly, for between five and six years; and who, in less than four weeks, got perfectly well under the use of a pill containing one-twelfth of a grain of the iodide of arsenic, one-sixth of a grain of the biniodide of mercury, and two grains of the extract of conium, twice a day; the iodide of arsenic being gradually increased to one-sixth of a grain, and the biniodide of mercury omitted, at the end of a fortnight, as it began to affect the gums. The diluted biniodide of mercury ointment was at the same time employed externally.

The arsenious acid, in an uncombined state, is but very seldom employed in this country, although with Biett, and some other continental physicians, it is a favourite remedy in psoriasis inveterata, and other very obstinate cutaneous affections. Its dose, in the form of the "Asiatic pill," varies from the sixteenth up to the fourth of a grain twice a day. The comparatively large quantity of arsenious acid that is required in an uncombined state to produce a beneficial action on the skin, ought, in my opinion, to militate against its employment in this form. The minimum dose of arsenious acid recommended by most writers on the diseases of the skin is one-sixteenth of a grain; now this is equal to the quantity contained in seven and a half minims, almost the maximum dose, of the solution of the arsenite of potassa, and certainly too large a quantity of this preparation for us to be justified in commencing with. This difference in effect is probably owing to the greater readiness with which the arsenious acid, when presented in solution, must be taken up by any surface, and carried into the general circulation.

Mr. Donovan lays great stress upon the small quantity of arsenic, and of the other elements, that, in his preparation, sometimes effect a cure; but in this I do not think it presents any thing peculiar, or more remarkable, than is constantly seen in Fowler's solution, and the other preparations of arsenic. I shall have occasion, in another part of this paper, to relate the particulars of a case of hereditary confluent lichen, of many years' standing,

cured by less than a drachm of the solution of the arsenite of potassa, or not quite half a grain of arsenious acid, in the course of a month; and it is by no means very uncommon to meet with cases of disease of the skin that will get well with little more than half an ounce of Fowler's solution, or two grains of the arsenious acid, if the treatment be spread over a considerable space of time, and more particularly if the effects of the arsenical be aided by appropriate topical treatment, as the iodine and citrine ointments, the nitrate of silver, and poulticing, which appear to have been had recourse to in several cases reported in the Dublin Journal.

As my experience in the use of the liquor of the hydriodate of arsenic and mercury is as yet somewhat limited, not having been extended to more than six or seven cases, I do not at present feel myself justified in giving any opinion as to the comparative merits of this and of the other preparations of arsenic in the treatment of the diseases of the skin, although I may state that it has appeared to me to be of peculiar value in the treatment of the syphilitic affections, more especially those of a squamous character, in which cases the mercury very probably exercises a greater influence than the arsenic. I may mention a case that occurred to me a few months ago, in which it not only cured the cutaneous complaint under which the patient was labouring, but also removed rheumatic neuralgic pains of twenty-four years' standing; an effect which I have not seen attributed to it, but which it is probable that it shares in common with the other preparations of arsenic.

Lawrence Keane, ætat. 46, an old sailor, of a sallow complexion, with dark hair and eyes, placed himself under my care on the 17th January last, for psoriasis of the posterior part of the neck and back, under which he had been labouring for the last four years. He states that, having been shipwrecked about twenty-four years ago, he was attacked with acute rheumatism, since which time he has never been free from pains in the limbs. I ordered him twenty minims of the solution of the hydriodate of arsenic and mercury three times a day, and a lotion of the bichloride of mercury to wash the affected parts with. On the 28th he had the dose of the solution increased to thirty minims, and on the 15th of February he was perfectly cured of the disease of the skin, the rheumatic pains, from which he said he had not been free for twenty-four years, having ceased entirely for some time past. Since this date I have several times seen him, and he continues perfectly well in every respect.

That the liquor of the hydriodate of arsenic and mercury is a most useful preparation, and one that will prove a valuable addition to our materia medica, there can be no doubt; but I think that notwithstanding the very high encomiums that have been bestowed upon it by some of the first professional authorities in Great Britain, it yet remains to be proved whether it is superior to the other arsenical preparations already in use, except, perhaps, in some cases of the syphilitic eruptions, and of lupus, in which the mercury that enters into its composition might be expected to exercise a very decidedly beneficial influence; somewhat resembling, in this respect, the pills composed of the iodide of arsenic and the biniodide of mercury. The comparative value, however, of Donovan's solution, and of the other preparations of arsenic, is too important a question to be prejudged, and is one that can only be determined by actual observation; and as the remarks that I have to make in this paper have reference chiefly to the effect of arsenicals generally upon the diseases of the skin, I shall, for the present, omit its consideration.

The *modus operandi* of the arsenical preparations, as of most other medicinal agents, is unknown to us. We are only acquainted with their secondary effects, which manifest themselves most unequivocally on the digestive, nervous, and integumentary systems; on all of which they act as excitant or stimulating tonics. When arsenic is being given in medicinal doses, one of the earliest constitutional symptoms produced by it is an acceleration of the heart's action: this, as Dr. Duffin has remarked, and as I have had occasion to observe, sometimes becomes quickened in the course of a few days after the administration of the mineral has been commenced, by ten, twenty, and even thirty beats in the minute, the pulse acquiring at the same time a hard and somewhat wiry feel. This acceleration

of the pulse is particularly observable in individuals of sanguineous or sanguineo-nervous temperament, in whom the heart's action is readily excited under the influence of physical exertion, or of mental emotion. In some cases before, but in most after this increase in the rapidity of the heart's action, evidences of some degree of irritation about the mucous membrane of the stomach will manifest themselves; there will be more or less thirst; the tongue will become coated towards the centre and root, with red sides and tip; there will be loss of appetite and a sense of weight at the epigastrium; the patient, about the same time, will complain of heaviness and pricking sensations about the eyelids, with flashes of light before the eyes when they are closed, and after a time the eyelids will become puffed and droop, giving the countenance a peculiarly melancholy and care-worn appearance; there will also be more or less headache experienced, chiefly over the eye-brows and lower part of the forehead: this pain in the head is, indeed, very frequently, one of the first symptoms indicative of the medicine disagreeing with the system. The patient will also very commonly complain of confused and horrible dreams: this is more particularly the case with children, in whom, as the nervous system is very excitable, there is a natural tendency to irritation and disturbance of it. Girdlestone has remarked that in some cases the skin assumes a uniform lobster-red colour, that erysipelas comes on, or that phlyctenæ and pustules make their appearance when the arsenic disagrees. I have very frequently had occasion to observe that the disease of the skin for which the medicine may have been administered, more particularly if it be a case of chronic eczema, has evinced a decided tendency to increased action; the patches becoming red and irritable, showing that the integuments partake in the excitement that is induced in the system generally by the employment of these preparations. If the use of the arsenic be still persevered in, which, after one or more of the symptoms which have just been detailed have manifested themselves, should never under any circumstances be the case, we shall find that great irritation will supervene about the mucous membrane of the stomach and throat; there will be nausea, vomiting, and total loss of appetite; the headache will increase in severity; the urine will become high-coloured; the countenance, which has become pale and sallow, will assume a remarkably sorrowful and anxious cast; tremors of the limbs come on, with an occasional feeling of faintness, and the foundation of incurable and permanent disease may be laid in the digestive organs or nervous system. It must not, however, be expected that all these symptoms should show themselves in every case in which the remedy has been pushed beyond its utmost limits as a medicine; far from it: in some instances the first symptom that we notice indicative of the medicine having begun to disagree, and of its employment having reached those bounds beyond which it cannot with safety be carried, is a degree of thirst, and a feeling of oppression about the epigastrium; in others, pricking sensations about the eyelids and flashes of light before the eyes; in others, again, and this very commonly, headache with disturbed dreams: and usually antecedent to, or, at all events, coincident with any one of these symptoms, will be found an acceleration in the pulse. The occurrence of any of these symptoms should be an instant warning to the practitioner to diminish the dose of the arsenic, or to intermit the use of the remedy altogether. If the patient be of a lymphatic temperament, or is somewhat advanced in years, of a languid debilitated habit of body, and the symptoms of excitement, local or general, be but trifling, it would be sufficient to diminish the dose to one half of that which is being taken, and to watch carefully the effects of the reduction before taking away the remainder. If, however, the patient be of a sanguine or sanguineo-nervous temperament, if he have been taking the arsenic for a considerable length of time, and if the symptoms of local disturbance be very unequivocal, it will be more prudent to leave off the use of the medicine for a few days, to give some saline aperient, and then, if it be thought expedient to do so, to recommence it in smaller doses. In practice it often becomes a question of considerable importance as to how far the preparations of arsenic may be carried; for this it is impossible to lay down any fixed rule as to quantity or time, as these must necessarily vary very greatly in individual cases, and our only guide in these respects must be the symptoms of local or constitutional disturbance that they may occasion. From a careful examination of many cases of cutaneous disease in which this mineral had been employed, I am enabled to state that nothing is gained by carrying it beyond a certain point, as far as the affection of the skin is concerned, and that by so doing, much mischief, perhaps of an irremediable nature, may be inflicted on the patient; that it is not a remedy that can with safety be *pushed*, to use a common phrase, but that all the good that will result from its employment can be accomplished by a careful and guarded administration of it, and by its being intermitted on the first appearance of any symptom of local or general irritation. Any marked acceleration of the pulse, or disturbance in the functions of the stomach and nervous system, should serve as a warning to us to discontinue its use. It must also be borne in mind that arsenic is a cumulative remedy, and that its deleterious effects may suddenly be manifested at a time when we least expected it to disagree. On this account patients who are taking it should be seen by their medical attendant every second, or at most every third day, and should have directions given them to omit the medicine should any of the symptoms that have already been mentioned as indicative of its disagreeing with the habit, show themselves. In illustration of the bad effects that may result from the injudicious use of the preparations of arsenic, I may mention that I have at present under my observation a young lady, of a highly nervous temperament, but otherwise perfectly healthy, and without any hereditary disposition to disease, who whilst suffering from an attack of psoriasis of the legs some years ago, was advised to take Fowler's solution, which she did in the hope of speedily getting rid of, to a delicate female, a disgusting affection, to such an extent, without the knowledge, however, of the medical attendants, that she brought on extensive derangement of the stomach, which was followed by a violent neuralgic attack, together with, at a subsequent period, a distressing train of hysterical symptoms, which have terminate.l in a state of dementia, that, having now existed for nearly four years, may almost be looked upon as incurable.

Having thus briefly passed in review the symptoms that may be produced by the arsenical preparations—their doses —and those circumstances that indicate that their use has reached that point beyond which they cannot, consistently with the patient's safety, be carried, we shall pass to an investigation of those conditions, whether of the patient himself, or of the disease under which he is labouring, that indicate or contra-indicate their employment.

[To be continued.]

SYMPTOMS LIKE CROUP COMING ON AFTER SCARLET FEVER— TRACHEOTOMY.

To the Editor of the Medical Gazette.

SIR,

RICHARD M'CLAREN, 5 years and 10 months old, came under our care as a patient of the Ardwick and Ancoats Dispensary, 15th February, 1843, in a state of most laborious orthopnœa, threatening suffocation.

Three weeks before this he had been attacked with scarlet fever and sore throat; and upon the subsidence of the swelling and soreness of the throat he was seized with dyspnœa and croupy breathing, and croupy voice, having slept the night before in the workhouse upon boards covered with a blanket only.

We found him after this long suffering worn out with fatigue, for he had not slept for many days, so painfully laborious were the efforts to inspire; and his body was wasted to the last degree. His skin was dark, rough, dry, filthy, and encrusted all over with scales of icthyosis; and the features as well as the limbs were furrowed and wrinkled, both from the effects of this cutaneous disease, and from his being emaciated almost to skin and bone. Added to these, the anxious expression of the countenance, and the painful agony of breathing, and the helpless debility of the poor boy, made him a distressing object to behold, and gave him something of an inhuman aspect.

His respirations were a continual gasping to get that breath which some obstruction about the glottis prevented from entering freely, accompanied with a croupy noise on inspiring. Some voice remained, having a different tone from that of common croup, and distinct from that which attends the formation of false membrane. The pulse was small and quick, and extremely feeble, the surface of the body cool, and the lips pale and blue.

The agonizing need for breath; the debility, and the leanness of body; the advanced period of the disease, and its supervention on scarlet fever; the probable nature of the existing lesion, and the imminent danger of suffocation, all rendered the employment of the usual remedies inapplicable, and gave no hopes of their curative action, but rather reason to fear lest they should produce hurtful effects.

The history of the case, the particular succession of the morbid events, the nature of the local disease, and its confinement to the neighbourhood of the glottis, gave us great reason to hope for aid from tracheotomy — certainly, at least, for the relief of the agony, and probably also for the cure, by a successful operation. The whole circumstances of the case were singularly favourable for the operation, and the only reasons for apprehension arose from the ill-conditioned body of the boy, and the risk attendant upon some general indisposition of the economy.

The croup was sudden in its onset, and not preceded by catarrh of the lungs; and no symptoms or signs of pulmonary disease were discoverable. There was no dulness on percussion anywhere, nor irregularity of resonance over the chest; and these circumstances, together with the absence of catarrh, and of previous indications of pneumonia, as well as the general aspect of the patient, shewed that the complications of capillary bronchitis, and lobular as well as lobate inflammation of the lungs, were happily wanting.

The sudden onset of the croup with much violence, together with its long continuance in spite of the apparent severity of the attack; the great orthopnœa, with preponderating difficulty in the act of inspiring compared to that of expiration; the persistence of the croupy sound so late in the disease, and the voice remaining when suffocation was so imminent, and the supervention of the attack upon the sore throat of scarlet fever, shewed that it was not an ordinary case of croup. The persistence of some distinctness of the voice is not commonly present at this late period of the malady, if the glottis and parts in its vicinity are clothed with false membrane.

The precedence of the sore throat of scarlet fever, under all those circumstances, afforded a strong presumption that the morbid lesion consisted in a swelling of the mucous membrane of the glottis and neighbouring structures, but complicated probably with the pigmy points of eroding ulcers, to which they are so liable in that fever. During the last mild epidemic of scarlatina we have seen some other cases in which the parts about the entrance of the windpipe were more or less affected in this manner. The inspection of the corpse of one child that died with symptoms of croup supervening on the fever, discovered no cause for death besides the extension of the swelling and ulcerous erosions from the fauces into the windpipe. Another, under the like circumstances, had some difficulty of breathing, which became suffocative whenever she cried or grew peevish; and those symptoms continued upwards of a fortnight, with complete extinction of the voice, before she manifested signs of amendment.

The two children spoken of, and the boy M'Claren, form three examples of different degrees of the same morbid state, which are worthy of notice. The one died from the utmost extension of the local disease, under circumstances in which tracheotomy would not have been proper. The other recovered without the same extension of the malady, and without absolute, but only after prospective danger, and without any need for the operation. The last was threatened with impending suffocation, when the disease had progressed too far for other treatment, and absolutely required surgical aid to restore the freedom of respiration, and to give a chance for recovery; and this was happily under circumstances, contrary to the first case, not only making tracheotomy prudent, but favourable to its success.

The scarlet fever had gone through its course, and the sore throat and tumor of the tonsils and neighbouring glands had disappeared. The swelling of the mucous membrane, probably with ulcerous erosions, which had been promoted to the parts about the glottis by taking cold whilst the throat was yet sore, now remained alone, or only with some redness of the fauces. Thus the lesion of the mucous membrane was evidently progressing fast towards recovery; being serious only by reason of its extension to the narrow opening into the windpipe, and requiring only time to heal. No feverish symptoms obtained, and the local lesion was manifestly limited to a small space. Nothing seemed to foreshow any probability of the occurrence of dropsy; but the icthyosis, perhaps, might have been a presumption to the contrary. The viscera of the belly and chest, and the functions of the brain, were proper in every respect. Lastly, the system had not been deranged by remedies.

Without a hope from medicines even for the relief of the agony, much less for saving the life of the child, we were of opinion, agreeably with our colleagues, that tracheotomy was needful and proper here, and offered the only means for the child's recovery.

Accordingly, after having obtained the consent of the mother and her friends, in the unavoidable absence of our colleague, Surgeon Harrison, on the 16th February Surgeon Dumville performed this operation in the most able manner, and with a degree of coolness and dexterity that does him great credit.

So completely had the poor boy been overcome with fatigue and sleeplessness and suffering, and so sudden was the relief obtained through the operation, that shortly after the insertion of the silver tube he fell fast asleep on the operating table, even before he was dressed or made comfortable. After the first moments of suspense, attending the relaxation of the spasm of the air-tubes, which arose from forcing the tube into the windpipe, he began to breathe with ease and freedom; and his ghastly features and his lips, which had a leaden hue before the operation, assumed their natural colour. He coughed up a little frothy mucus, mixed with blood, and quickly began to breathe with ease; and his respirations, which exceeded sixty in the minute for some hours after the operation, were only forty-eight next morning. On the evening of the third day they were thirty-four; on the fourth, thirty-two; and on the eleventh, only twenty-seven; whilst from that period they varied in frequency, sometimes above, but mostly below, thirty in the minute.

The respiratory murmur, which was inaudible before, was heard after the operation throughout the lungs without morbid accompaniment. When the freedom of respiration was restored, the feeble pulse, barely perceptible before, rallied again in strength, numbering 132 strokes in the minute that night, but only 120 next morning, which standard it seldom exceeded afterwards during convalescence, but ranged lower to 115, 108, and sometimes as low as 102.

Early on the fourth morning the child passed a good feculent stool, and afterwards he had two or three evacuations daily upon an average.

The diet was most rigid for the first few days, namely, fresh cold water as a diluent, with bits of sugar to allay appetite; but so soon as no danger was to be feared from inflammatory action, we gave him nothing but the strongest drinks of animal juices and milk, and, lastly, solid meats. We abstained carefully from administering any medicines. The boy gradually acquired strength and flesh; and as the scales of the epidermis fell off, the functions of the skin were restored, and he attained progressively his wonted vigour of body; so that he plays about as roughly as others of his age, both in the house and abroad.

The operation has proved eminently successful; and the chief features of the case seem to be, first, the sequence of the croup upon the sore throat of scarlet fever; second, the absence of pulmonary complication; and third, the limited extent of the local malady.

The tube was removed first on the morning of the fourteenth day, but it became necessary to replace it again that same evening; and since then it has been taken out and cleaned three times. When the tube was out, and the opening into the windpipe closed with a sponge, then the boy spoke audibly, but with much hoarseness; and likewise, when he stops the hole of the tube with his finger, he can pronounce some words intelligibly, and he can sound a small whistle. The respiration through the glottis is not suffi-

ciently easy to justify the final attempt at present to do without the tube; nor is it quite free from croupy sibilus.

Let no one think that this is an operation of minor importance; on the contrary, perhaps no other requires nicer care for its success, or confers greater responsibility. The successful result we attribute, next to the dexterity of the operator, mainly to the unceasing care and watchfulness which we and our colleagues were enabled to bestow upon the case, the boy never having been without medical supervision an hour for upwards of two weeks. To our colleagues, Dr. Wilkinson and Surgeon Dumville, who partook with us in the responsibility of the case, and who shared equally in the watching by night and by day, we cannot sufficiently express how much we feel indebted; but those who know what the support of a good colleague is, where so much responsibility rests, can well appreciate our feeling.

We avoid purposely making any observations on the surgical bearings of the subject, leaving them to Surgeon Dumville, to whose province they especially belong, and who will, we hope, follow up our communication with some remarks on the practical matters relating to the operation, and the management of the apparatus, as well as with his own ingenious views upon other interesting features of the case.

Your humble servant,
THOMAS HODGSON WATTS, M.D.
Physician to the Ardwick and
Ancoats Dispensary.
53, Dale Street, Manchester,
April 12, 1843.

Surgeon Dumville's remarks in continuation of the preceding case.

In the case of the boy Richard M'Claren, tracheotomy was performed in preference to laryngotomy for the following reason—that, although we had evidence in proof that the lungs were not implicated in the disease sufficiently to justify us in resorting to an operation for the relief of the dyspnœa, yet we had no proof that the disease was wholly confined to the rima glottidis. It was therefore determined to make the section as low in the trachea as we could, in the expectation of making the wound in healthy structure.

An incision was made about two inches in length over the trachea, avoiding the gland above, and not carried so far as to endanger the left subclavian vein. The edges of the sterno-thyroid muscles were carefully held apart by broad retractors. Two large thyroid veins were brought into view; and much difficulty was experienced at this point of the operation, for these veins adhered so closely to the trachea that it was no easy matter to remove them out of danger. As the thymus gland was large, and as the thyroid veins lay closely upon the trachea below, I thought it better to cut out a piece of one of the tracheal cartilages, sufficient to allow of the introduction of the large-sized canula that had been selected. I thought that there would be less risk of hæmorrhage by opening the trachea in this way than by making a longitudinal incision simply; and besides, I hoped that a more convenient aperture might be made for the introduction of the large tracheal pipe. There was, however, a little difficulty in inserting this tube, owing to the rapid manner in which the larynx rose and fell. As soon as the tube was fairly lodged, there was a free discharge of bloody mucus; the blood, I have no doubt, had been drawn in through the wound. Dr. Watts has already described the boy's appearance after the operation, and I will sum up in a few words. After the expulsion of the mucus, the respiration was performed with the greatest ease, and the contrast with the late dyspnœa was so strong that I thought the lad had ceased to breathe, when he was actually asleep.

I attribute the success of the operation mainly to the large size of the tube that was made use of, which, notwithstanding its ample calibre, required most assiduous attention to keep it pervious, and yet, after all, we were compelled four times to remove it, before we could detach the thick coating of hardened mucus which tenaciously adhered to its interior.

The experience I have had with this case convinces me not only of the necessity of employing a large pipe, but also of the propriety of disturbing it as little as possible when once inserted. However carefully it was taken out, and however adroitly it was replaced in the trachea, still the constitution suffered invariably for a time, and in every instance there was much irritation set up in the throat.

The method we adopted for cleaning the tube was, first, to moisten the mucus adhering to the interior with a small sponge attached to a flexible silver wire, and then detaching the coating by means of a scoop bent to the shape of the pipe.

One circumstance has particularly arrested my attention in the surgical treatment of this case. It is this: that every time the tube has been taken out, although the boy could talk so as to be understood, yet the voice continued croupy, and the lad was incapable of breathing through the glottis with sufficient freedom to support life. In most cases of successful tracheotomy the result has been different; a few days have often been sufficient to allow of the subsidence of the laryngeal inflammation, so that the canula could be thenceforth removed. In the case before us the success is not so complete at present; but we are sanguine in our expectation of complete recovery, inasmuch as the lad's voice becomes gradually more free from croupy resonance.

Since Dr. Cheyne's Pathology of the Larynx and Bronchi appeared before the medical world, an opinion has been very generally prevalent that croup is under any circumstances an unfit case for operation. The unfitness consists in this, that the lining of the whole bronchial tube has been found frequently involved in the inflammation. This is undoubtedly correct in many, perhaps in the majority of cases, but certainly there are some instances in which the inflammation and false membrane are confined to the larynx. Dr. Howard showed me a preparation lately taken from one of his infirmary patients, a boy about six years old, in which the inflammation and false membrane had not extended into the trachea.

I will close these observations with a sketch of a case of croup which occurred in my practice last week.

Thomas Foden, æt. 2 years and 5 months, had been exposed for a long time to cold late in the evening of April 9th, but went to bed in perfect health. Next morning he rose with a slight cough and hoarseness, and towards the evening he experienced some difficulty in breathing. On the second day he was much better. Also on the morning of the third day he appeared better; and although his hoarseness continued, still he could speak, and played about quite free from fever and having a good appetite, until about 3 o'clock P.M. when his dyspnœa and hoarseness grew rapidly worse, and he died early on the morning of the fourth day, 13th April. I only saw the little patient once.

Post-mortem.—The epiglottis was thick and inflamed; the glottis and the whole cavity of the larynx was lined with recent false membrane, and this false membrane extended but a very short way down the trachea, whilst a distinct line of demarcation distinguished the inflamed from the not inflamed structure. The trachea and bronchia contained some mucus; but the lungs were free from appearances of inflammatory disease. The preparation has been seen by many of my medical friends; and I am decidedly of opinion that bronchotomy might have been the means of saving this child's life. The freedom from fever was strong presumptive evidence that the lungs were free from inflammation.

I am, sir,
Your obedient servant,
Arthur William Dumville.

22, Higher Ardwick,
April 19, 1843.

CASE OF DIFFICULT PARTURITION.

To the Editor of the Medical Gazette.

Sir,

I take leave to transmit to you the particulars of a case, which, though it occurred several years ago, you may nevertheless deem of sufficient interest to place on record in your Medical Gazette. Time cannot deteriorate the value of facts so long as they point to practical usefulness, and a faithful relation of our own difficulties, and the mode by which they were overcome, may serve at least for some protection against the embarrassment, or difficulties, to which others are exposed.

In the night of the 13th March, 1811, Mr. Hopkinson, of Peterborough (since dead), a surgeon of acknowledged skill, and an accoucheur of great experience, being in attendance upon Mrs. —— in labour, called me to his aid. On my arrival he told me that the lady considered herself in the eighth month of utero-gestation, that the membranes had broke on the previous Sunday evening, without any pain, since which time she had not been sensible of the motion of the child, and though the head had descended into the vagina her pains had been of that distressing character which in the lying-in chamber are pronounced " wearing, yet of no avail." It may be mentioned that from the loss of her husband a few months previously, and various other afflicting circumstances, her spirits had suffered much depression, and her bodily health serious impairment. She had refused sustenance of every kind for several days; her stomach, indeed, had lost its retentive power; food even of the lightest quality, or tried in the most sparing manner, being always rejected. Her frame was naturally delicate, her person short, and the pelvis somewhat below the standard size. The face of the child presented, with the chin towards the pubes. When I was called to the patient she had no pains, and scarcely any pulse; accordingly we deemed it right, from the inert state of the uterus, as well as the exhaustion into which she had sunk, to attempt immediate delivery. Of the child's death, I may add, we had unquestionable proof, for, besides the patient's own conviction of the fact, as above hinted, the attendant fœtor was fully decisive of it: hence we were free to resolve on a mode of delivery with regard exclusively to the patient herself, and Mr. H. proposed to effect it by applying the blunt hook to the chin, and his finger to the mouth: if that method should fail it was determined to have recourse to the forceps. He succeeded at once, however, in extricating the head; but after delivering the shoulders, an obstacle, apparently unyielding and unconquerable, opposed any farther accomplishment of our object. Mr. Hopkinson gradually increased the force with which he tried to bring away the child, but to no purpose; and, after a considerable time spent in unavailing efforts, tempering force with prudence, he at length, to our dismay, extracted half the child, leaving the inferior half of the trunk, together with the extremities, in the womb. I applied my hand to the abdomen, which felt as much distended as if it contained another child, besides the remains of the mutilated one. Mr. H. next introduced his hand into the uterus and secured two feet, which, from the immense bulk of the abdomen, he suspected to belong to another child. These with some difficulty he brought beyond the external parts, and included them in a ligature : but again the same impediment presented itself. Our efforts to obtain a hold of the thighs were fruitless, and at this stage of the delivery, in attempting to draw down, I separated one of the legs of the child from its attachments above. Our next alternative was again to introduce the hand high up, which, when attempted by Mr. Hopkinson, he felt obstructed by a tense subtance or tumor, lodged at the brim of the pelvis. This he succeeded in rupturing, and an enormous discharge of fluid was the immediate result. The great obstacle being at length overcome, instead of another child, the remnant or mutilated half was instantly brought away, and the uterus, except of its placenta, emptied. Syncope immediately followed the delivery, but from this our patient rallied, and the stomach fortunately retaining the wine and nourishment we gave, I rejoice to say she progressively and permanently did well.

The tumor occupied the lower region of the back, was constituted of watery cysts, and their aggregate bulk at the time was compared to that of a full-sized adult cranium. Thus, what we considered in the first instance an evil greatly to be deplored, proved in the issue an advantage, since with such a tumor it was utterly impossible to deliver the child entire ; or, unruptured, to accomplish delivery at all.

I cannot conclude without noticing the formidable effects of pressure in this case—pressure of the gravid uterus on the subjacent or neighbouring viscera. I have already instanced the distressing sickness which the patient suffered : constipation proved another bane of equal obstinacy : despite of aperient medicines and clysters she passed the whole week antecedent to her delivery without the slightest alvine discharge : the bladder had lost its power of expulsion : moreover, the pains she suffered from the distension and weight of the uterus (pains, it may be remarked, by no means simulating those of labour), were woefully

distressing ; so urgent, indeed, as to induce Mr. H. to give a drachm of Tinctura Opii every three hours for some continuance.

This, sir, is a plain unvarnished statement of a case which, I am aware, is not of very frequent occurrence. Tumor of a child's abdomen, as well as of the back, may impede the process of delivery by its lodgment at the brim of the pelvis ; and nothing, it is manifest, in either case, but the puncture or rupture of such a tumor, will insure the life of the mother, the chief and great object of the obstetric art. In fine, my desire is to call attention not so much to that which is rare as that which is useful, and with this assurance permit me to subscribe myself, sir,

Your obedient servant,
J. WHITSED.

Wisbeach, April 28, 1843.

ON THE

DIFFERENCE OF THE BILE AS IT FLOWS FROM THE LIVER, AND THE CYSTIC BILE.

By GEORGE KEMP, M.D. Cantab.

To the Editor of the Medical Gazette.

SIR,

IN the course of my researches on the bile, it became necessary to examine the nature of the secretion as immediately given off from the liver, before its entrance into the gall-bladder. It was desirable to ascertain, in fact, whether any essential difference exists between the fluid as it flows from the liver, and the cystic bile ; and it was hoped that, by establishing the exact relation which subsists between the two, we might obtain a more accurate knowledge of the real nature of this important body.

The only written authority which has afforded me any assistance on the subject is the Physiology of Professor Müller, which contains the following sentence. " The bile which flows from the liver is of a lighter colour ; that obtained from the gall-bladder is less fluid and greener, on account of the more fluid part having been absorbed, and it is more viscid, owing to its containing mucus." Now we must infer from this that the opinion of Professor

Müller is, that the two fluids only differ from each other in the diminished quantity of water, and in the presence of mucus in the cystic bile. This is also the opinion generally received. The following results of actual experiment will I hope be considered worthy of perusal, as they differ so essentially from what we should have presumed *a priori*, and as adding one more example of the necessity of extreme caution in this interesting department of research.

The whole of the liver of an ox, with its gall-bladder attached, was obtained immediately on its removal from the animal; the gall-bladder was carefully separated, and the liver placed under a jet of water to remove the secretion from the larger hepatic ducts. The organ was then cut into small slices and placed in about a quart of distilled water for some hours, the object of this process being to obtain the fluid contained in the 'smaller branches of the ducts. Having strained the whole through cloth, a fluid was obtained strongly coloured with blood, and containing, of course, a large quantity of uncoagulated albumen. The fluid was now boiled for an hour, and again strained through cloth, and the resulting liquid submitted to examination. No reaction was produced on turmeric paper; it *was totally destitute of the peculiarly bitter taste* so characteristic of cystic bile, though highly charged with yellow colouring matter. The smell was nauseous, not unlike a solution of glue, but not in the slightest degree resembling that of the bile as usually found in the gall-bladder. After carefully evaporating the fluid to dryness, it was heated with alcohol, sp. gr. 340, by which the yellow colouring matter, and a substance (A), was dissolved. The residue (B), was very carefully washed with alcohol, and a portion burned on the platinum knife. I thought that this residue was the mucus of the hepatic ducts, and expected to obtain an ash of phosphate of lime; the result, however, was carbonate of soda. It will be remembered that the aqueous solution of this body was neutral; it is therefore an electro-negative body in combination with soda. The alcoholic solution, also neutral, was now evaporated to dryness, and a portion of the substance (A), burned on platinum; again I obtained carbonate

of soda. Each of these bodies, therefore, is principally composed of an electro-negative body in combination with soda; until, however, the ultimate analysis is made, it cannot be decided in what relation these bodies stand to the electro-negative body in the cystic bile, but I hope shortly to forward you their elementary composition.

It would seem, then, from the above, that the bile of the *ox*, at least, undergoes a remarkable change in the gall-bladder; and it seems highly probable that what has been usually denominated the *mucus* of the gall-bladder is an important agent in effecting the change. An interesting point now to be investigated is, under what condition does the bile present itself in animals which have no gall-bladder? Indeed, to make the subject at all complete, it will be necessary to commence a general research into the nature of the bile given off from the liver in animals of essentially different habits and structure.

Will you permit me, in conclusion, through the medium of your pages, to solicit the attention of the profession to one point, which has, I believe, now been clearly made out. The cystic bile, when fresh, and in a perfectly healthy state, is always neutral; at least this is the result of many more than a hundred cases which I have examined, including the ox, the human bile, the bile from several species of monkey[*], the tiger, the wolf[*], the dog, the cat, the fox, an Indian bull[*], and various kinds of fish, so that this property may fairly be presumed to be a distinctive mark of healthy bile in graminivorous, carnivorous, and omnivorous animals.

I have only met with three exceptions to this remark: the first was in the case of a child which had died from a severe burn; the second was that of an Indian bull, in which the bile was so putrid that it was unfit for particular examination; and the third was in an ox, the biliary ducts of which were completely choked up with an insect (*Distoma hepatica*).

It would be but a very trifling sacrifice of time in our large hospitals to examine the bile of every person submitted to a *post-mortem* examination

---

[*] The bile of the animals marked (*) was obtained through the kindness of Dr. Clark, Professor of Anatomy in this University.

with turmeric paper*, and I should esteem it a great favour to receive any addition to my tables on this subject by post.—I remain, sir,

Your obedient servant,
GEORGE KEMP, M.D. Cantab.

St. Peter's College, Cambridge,
May 1, 1843.

A CASE OF
STRANGULATED FEMORAL HERNIA,

IN WHICH THE SAC WAS DISTENDED WITH FLUID BLOOD.

BY J. TOYNBEE, Esq. F.R.S.

Surgeon to the St. George's and St. James's
Dispensary.

(For the Medical Gazette.)

As it is important to place on record every variety presented by so interesting a disease as hernia, I take the opportunity of publishing the following case, which displayed some peculiarities worthy of notice.

Mrs. H., æt. 50, tall and thin, and who had been losing flesh for six months, was seized with a pain in the right groin whilst exerting herself in the middle of the day of February 28th. The pain was very acute for some time, but it gradually disappeared. Towards evening the usual symptoms of strangulated hernia presented themselves, and on retiring to bed a swelling was perceived in the right groin, which was rather augmented on the following morning. During the early part of the day of February 29th, the patient walked about the house: at 2 o'clock the pain and sickness had considerably increased, and she suddenly fainted, when my attendance was requested. Upon examination I found a tumor in the right groin, of the size of a small hen's egg, produced by a femoral hernia; it was remarkably hard and incompressible, and its size was not at all diminished by the application of the taxis. An operation was therefore determined upon, which I performed the same evening, with the kind assistance of my colleague, Mr. Chapman. Nothing unusual presented itself in the steps of the operation until the hernial sac was exposed; it was of the size of

a small walnut, very tense, and perfectly black. Upon laying it open, it was found to owe a great part of its size to the presence within it of a large quantity of dark-coloured blood, of the consistence of treacle. At its upper part was a small rounded mass, also quite black, and irregular to the touch. Several coatings of firm fibrine were removed from its surface, and in its centre a very small portion of omentum was exposed, having a dark colour but possessing its natural consistence. Upon a careful examination, finding there was no oozing of blood from its surface, I divided the stricture at Poupart's ligament, and returned the protruded part into the abdominal cavity. No unfavourable symptoms supervened. The patient was quite recovered in three weeks, and has remained well to the present period. The peculiarities in this case, dependent upon the presence of thick fluid blood in the hernial sac, and of the layers of fibrine coating the omentum, are likely to afford some embarrassment to an operator who meets with them for the first time, without being aware of the probability of their existence.

12, Argyll Place, St. James's,
April 26th, 1843.

INDIAN HEMP.

To the Editor of the Medical Gazette.

SIR,

As the observations of Dr. O'Shaughnessy on the remarkable effects produced in India by the extract of *cannabis*, or common hemp, have disposed many gentlemen to make trial of its powers in this country, may I request you to give your readers the following caution.

The *apocynum cannabinum* is sold in London under the name of "Indian hemp." It is a native of Canada and Virginia, and has no resemblance to the true hemp, except in possessing a tough fibrous bark, which is applicable to the same purposes in the arts. In the U. S. Pharmacopœia it is termed "Indian Hemp." The officinal part is the root, which is powerfully emetic and cathartic. But the part which I have seen supplied as Indian hemp consists of the leaves and the follicles filled with numerous silky seeds. As the follicles are 2 to 3 inches long, and

---

* After testing the fluid it is always desirable to wash the test-paper with distilled water, as the colouring matter of the bile is otherwise apt to mislead.

P

the silky seeds are abundant, they can hardly have escaped the notice of those who may have inadvertently used this article under the idea that it was the hemp from India. The true Indian hemp, or "gunjat," is our common hemp; and consists of the flowering branches, two or three feet long, nearly destitute of leaves, and having the flowers and fruit (hemp-seed) agglutinated together by the resinous secretion. As the most powerful antispasmodic properties have been attributed to this plant, it is important that no false conclusions should be drawn in consequence of the employment of a wrong article. I am not aware that any real Indian hemp is at present in this country except the supply recently brought by Dr. O'Shaughnessy, and left with Mr. Squire, of Oxford Street. We have at present little experience of the medicinal properties of English hemp. A hotter climate, a more intense light, and a different soil, may give to it properties which are scarcely developed in this country, but as the resinous secretion is not wanting here, it appears deserving of a careful trial.

I am, sir,

Your obedient servant,

T. J. FARRE, M.D.

Curzon Street, May 1, 1843.

MEDICAL GAZETTE.

Friday, May 5, 1843.

"Licet omnibus, licet etiam mihi, dignitatem Artis Medicæ tueri; potestas modo veniendi in publicum sit, dicendi periculum non recuso."
                                        CICERO.

QUACK MEDICINES.

To suppose the extinction of quackery is almost to presuppose the arrival of the millennium; for we must either imagine disease to have disappeared from the world, or the art of medicine to have obtained such miraculous perfection that the most impatient patient could never be driven by despair to consult the quack instead of the physician. Yet it is possible to imagine that, with another century or so of education and discussion, something

short of this, yet something very good, will have been attained; and that, in four or five generations, a belief in the wonder-working powers of quack medicines will rank with a belief in witchcraft, and be found only in remote districts and among uninstructed persons. Till the arrival of this happy era, we must put our trust in reasoning, and in diffusing a knowledge of the powers of medicines and of the structure and functions of the human body; for medical dissent can no more be quelled by prosecutions and prohibitions than theological speculations can be permanently crushed by thumbscrews and Conventicle Acts.

The analogy may be carried further; for though, in every unenslaved country, freedom implies discussion, and discussion necessarily produces dissent, still overmuch dissent is a reproach to the creed of the majority: and thus a deluge of quackery implies something rotten in the profession which it supersedes. It shows that legitimate practitioners err in theory or in practice. Either they cannot explain the principles on which they act, or they cannot cure *tutò, celeriter, et jucundè*; or, perchance, they take a leaf from their adversaries' book, and copy the errors against which they declaim.

An explanation of this subject from time to time, for the benefit of the laity, must do good; and we are, therefore, pleased to find it discussed in a temperate and rational manner by Dr. T. G. Wright. His essay was lately read before the Mechanics' Institute at Wakefield, and has since appeared in the shape of a pamphlet.

A great part of it consists in a commentary on some popular errors.

Thus, it is commonly fancied that illness assumes a certain number of unalterable forms, as well defined as the provinces of a nicely-coloured map; here jaundice all yellow, and there apoplexy all red; in this corner Dropsy displaying his bloated belly, and in that one Mania shaking her iron chain. The smallest disease that takes rank in our nosologies is supposed to be distinct and immutable; he that runs may read them; and to confound one with another would argue the most culpable blindness! Moreover, it is thought by the *ignobile vulgus* of various ranks, that each skilful practitioner has a choice selection of remedies, good for particular diseases, and that doctor differs from doctor chiefly in the rare disposition of this ideal medicine-chest.

Diagnosis, in short, goes for nothing in vulgar estimation, and remedies for every thing. Hence it is supposed that one practitioner can transmit or even sell his skill to another; and hence, too, family recipes good for the gout, dropsy, or what not, are handed down from one generation to another, in sober, steady, mistaken families.

We cannot agree, however, with Dr. Wright, in confounding the doctrine of the empirics of old with medicine as practised by modern quacks or *dilettanti*. The empirics, though rejecting the theories on which medicine had been based, adopted all the refinements of treatment which had been sanctioned by experience; while the blunderers whom Dr. Wright castigates merely prescribe for a score or two of diseases, or rather of names.

We cannot allow my Lady Bountiful to suppose that she belongs to the ancient and honoured sect of empirics, though she may be an empiric in the modern sense.

The old sect consisted of educated men, to whom the registers of medicine were open, and who profited by the mistakes, as well as by the discoveries, of their predecessors; the modern one is made up of blunderers, unwilling, or unable, to be taught either by the living or the dead. Independently of this, the extremes of refinement and of coarseness make a decided practical difference between the old and the new school, and destroy the historical defence of the latter; just as a man who attempts to open a vein with an oyster-knife cannot fairly allege in his defence that it is a cutting instrument as much as a lancet.

Again, it is a popular error to attribute too much to causes inherent in the constitution of the patient, and too little to external agents. Much is said of the biliousness of his temperament, and little of the causes which have made and keep him so. In other words, Hygiene, the best and safest portion of medicine, is little regarded by the common people, and forms no part of the quack-medicine system.

Another mistake, and a very frequent one, is to confound the symptom with the disease, and to suppose that two similar aches or uncomfortable states must necessarily be relieved by the same remedy. How can they, if they arise from totally different causes? Can the headaches of Congerro, who is an alderman, and of Irus, who inhabits a Union Workhouse, require the same treatment? Assuredly not. Yet we must believe this, if we believe the advertisements of the infallible Maltese elixir. Perhaps, however, the most extravagant of all the opinions current on this subject is the belief that many or any quacks have discovered drugs good for this or that distemper. This is unquestionably the wildest of all the fictions touching nostrums with which the public is bewildered. Your cold and calculating quack may select some well-known combination of medicines, provide it with a stamp, and puff it as a panacea for every mortal ill; but as for imagining such a fellow to be among the honourable band of discoverers, one might as well imagine a caricaturist rivalling Michael Angelo.

Many of the remedies which are advertised are external applications, and it would be a good beginning, in the instruction of the laity, to teach them what can be done medicinally in the shape of salve or unguent. The surgeon can stimulate, or soothe, or simply protect an ulcerated surface; but the healing herbs of the old romances have vanished and left no successors.

A very signal triumph of nostrums over common sense, consists, no doubt, in universal specifics, in which, as Dr. Wright says, "the mighty genius of quackery delights to revel." Every Friday, it seems, the market of Wakefield is visited by a pillmonger of the comprehensive class, who cries out, "In any case whatsoever, no matter what the case may be, if you are afflicted, only take my medicine and you are *sure* to be cured!"

Now, what is the cause of all this? What is the reason that quackery is so much more prevalent in medicine than in any other art? The reason is a simple one, and though we have stated it before, it will bear telling again. The reason, then, is, that nature is to a certain extent the support of the charlatan; and while a quack or imaginary engineer could not make even a bad railway, the medical quack, or imaginary doctor, will not always prevent the disease from getting well. Nature cures fevers, but makes no tunnels. Again, although it is a sad thing to be reduced by poverty or by folly to take drugs at random, yet it is by no means the case that random shots miss every time. This is especially true of purgatives. Hence we think that Dr. Wright has overstated his case in one respect. He supposes a prescription for some common aperient pills to be taken from a physician's table, and the medicine to be administered indiscriminately to five thousand patients; and he thinks it not improbable that

three or four, or even ten or twenty, might be considerably benefited by them. Only twenty! we should have put down a thousand as much nearer the mark. Could the *Pil. Rhei C.* hit the mark only four times in a thousand? Nay, we really think that the chance of benefit to be obtained out of any respectable medicine taken by accident, from Aconitum to Zingiber, must be represented by a larger fraction than $\frac{4}{1000}$.

But boundless fame is within the reach of these same *Pil. Rhei C.*, disguised, peradventure, under the name of the Bala Hissar pills, the recipe for which was found, as the advertisement might affirm, "in the baggage of an Affghan chief!"

"It may be," says Dr. Wright, "that a not-very-clever medical man has been previously consulted, or that one of greater repute has been misled in the case; and if so, there is no end to the glory of the fortunate pills."

Hence it appears that the quacksalver has two advantages of which it would be difficult to deprive him. The one is, that he is patronized by nature, who in the cure of disease backs everything, and every body; the other is, that medicines given blindfold must sometimes do good, especially if they are purgatives. Nevertheless, the final though distant extinction of quackery is to be hoped for; it forms a fragment of that final triumph of reason and virtue which is the secret consolation of every philanthropist.

DR. LATHAM.
(For the Medical Gazette.)

LAST week we noticed the death of Dr. Latham, senior, in his 82d year. He was the father of the College of Physicians. None of his immediate contemporaries are now alive, and his juniors by ten years are almost all past away. He had himself long retired from the world, so that of the physicians now in active practice few could have known him. Yet he was eminent in his time, and enjoyed a large share of the esteem and confidence of mankind.

Half a century ago there were three physicians of St. Bartholomew's Hospital, who, each in succession and each early in life, and unaided except by their own strenuous industry and talent, ran a rapid career of success. These were, Dr. David Pitcairn, Dr. Austin, and Dr. Latham. The fortunes of all three were peculiar and instructive.

Dr. Austin, in the midst of great business and the brightest prospects, was cut off by a fever at the age of forty.

Dr. Pitcairn, between 40 and 50, had his prosperity arrested by hæmoptysis, and retired to Lisbon in search of health. He returned to a less practice but an undiminished reputation, and died about his 60th year from acute inflammation of the larynx.

Dr. Latham, at the age of 46, was worn out by the hard labour of his early success. He was believed to be consumptive, and retired into the country (it was thought) to die. But he recovered, and returned to town, and resumed the exercise of his profession. He felt, however, that, if he was to keep the health he had regained, he must never again put it to the same hazard.

Accordingly he now removed far away from the sphere of his former business. He left Bedford Row, and settled in Harley Street. And here, for twenty years, he enjoyed, with a more moderate practice, a larger share of health than he had known during the days of his greater labour and greater success.

In the year 1814, Dr. Latham was elected President of the College. In 1816, he founded the Medical Benevolent Society. He contributed several papers on practical subjects to the Medical Transactions. In 1809, he wrote a small volume entitled, " Facts and Opinions concerning Diabetes."

In 1829, having reached his 68th year, Dr. Latham finally left London. Fourteen years of life yet remained to him. For two-thirds of this period he enjoyed the comforts which are still within the reach of a vigorous old age. For the last third was reserved the sharpest of all bodily afflictions, the formation and gradual increase of stone

in the bladder. Under this he sank, and died.

The fame of physicians, except of the few in any age who have pushed forward the boundaries of physiological and pathological knowledge, does not outlive the recollection of those who knew them, or have derived benefit from their skill and care. Those who knew Dr. Latham, both his patients and his fellow physicians, speak of him with great esteem and affection. His patients remember the confidence and encouragement which accompanied his address, his sincerity, his straightforwardness, and his liberality: and there are physicians, now grey-headed, who speak of the kindness and countenance they received from him in the days of their youth.

But the highest virtues of good men are unseen by the world while they live; and are kept sacred for the solace and contemplation of their families when they die. More, therefore, need not be said of Dr. Latham, except that he was singularly temperate, when temperance was hardly yet thought to be a virtue; he was most pure in life and conversation, when to have been otherwise would have provoked no censure; and he was not ashamed to be religious, when religion had yet no recommendation or countenance from the world.

ROYAL MEDICAL & CHIRURGICAL SOCIETY.

April 25, 1843.
THE PRESIDENT IN THE CHAIR.

Cases of Strangulated Hernia reduced en masse, with observations. By J. LUKE, Esq. Surgeon to the London and St. Luke's Hospitals; and Lecturer on Surgery. [Communicated by Sir B. C. BRODIE, Bart.]

IN this paper the object of the author is to show that the reduction of a strangulated hernia *en mass*, although rare, is not so infrequent as is generally supposed; and that the occurrence should be considered as coming within the ordinary range of probabilities of surgical practice. He had seen five cases of this description, two of which had been subject to his own treatment. In these the hernial tumor had been reduced entirely, through the parietes, into the abdominal cavity, with the contents strangulated; and as no swelling was perceptible, while the usual symptoms of strangulation continued, the diagnosis was rendered extremely obscure. The author gives the details of the two cases which occurred in his own practice; and describes minutely the steps of the operation which he performed in each. In one case, owing to the deceptive nature of the symptoms, and absence of external tumor, the operation was deferred too long, and the patient died. On examination, the hernial sac was found to occupy a considerable space just within the abdominal parieties, in the vicinity of the internal ring; the fundus lay a little below its level, towards the cavity of the pelvis; while the neck, still contracted, so as obviously to have been the original seat of stricture, was between three and four inches distant from the situation of the ring, and lay in an upward direction towards the umbilicus. The whole sphacelated contents were empty, collapsed, and in a pulpy state. In the second case, the result of the operation was successful. In describing its stages, the author mentions that before the hernial sac could be reached it was necessary to lay open the inguinal canal by dividing the tendon of the external oblique muscle. Near the external ring the spermatic cord was seen lying bare, or only covered with a little fat. It was only when the finger was passed through the internal ring (the firm borders of which were distinctly perceptible), and pressed a little more deeply within the abdomen, that a round tense tumor could be felt, which was found to be the hernial sac. The internal ring was cut through, and this allowed the sac to be drawn downwards; when it was opened, the stricture divided, and the bowel returned into the abdomen. The author concludes his paper by adding observations on the propriety, in doubtful cases of strangulated hernia, of performing an exploring operation to ascertain the exact nature of the case. He points out, at considerable length, the various conditions of the parts in the inguinal canal, from which, when taken along with the history of the case, the surgeon may judge whether the hernial sac, with the bowel strangulated within it, has been forced into the abdominal cavity, and expresses his opinion that such an operation will not involve the patient in much additional danger.

FELLOWES' CLINICAL PRIZE REPORTS.

By ALFRED J. TAPSON.
University College Hospital, 1842.
[Continued from p. 104.]

CASE X.—*Splenitis (?) coming on after intermittent fever; with rheumatism and signs of incipient phthisis. The splenitis cured by leeches, blistering, and mercury, &c.*

EDWARD MORGAN, æt. 23, admitted May 6, 1842, under Dr. A. T. Thomson. A man of moderately stout conformation and sanguine temperament; complexion naturally florid, but since his illness has been much paler, and rather sallow; parents both living and both healthy, as well as eight brothers and sisters; is single, and of regular sober habits; is a sailor, and has made several voyages to India, Australia, &c. as steward.

His health was always good till December 1841, when he was returning from the East Indies; at this time he was seized with headache, feverishness, burning pains in various parts, diarrhœa, &c. and after these symptoms had lasted about three days a severe attack of quotidian ague came on; the paroxysms coming on in the evening with violent shivering, &c. and ending on the following morning with sweating. The ague lasted for eight or ten weeks altogether, but during the last three or four weeks the paroxysms were irregular in their occurrence, coming on every third or fourth day, and the intervals gradually lengthened till the paroxysms ceased to recur. In February he reached St. Helena, and was then subjected to a regular course of mercury, and severely salivated, and since that time he has never had a regular fit of ague. During the whole attack he had suffered most from pain in the left hypochondriac region; it was diminished after the salivation, but has never left him entirely; the salivation was attended with great swelling of the face, and he continued to spit a great deal for two or three weeks, after which time he gradually regained his strength and resumed his work. In the beginning of April he was much exposed to cold and wet, owing to rough weather, and he was attacked with pain in various parts of his body, especially in the knees and ankles, attended with swelling, redness, &c. and at the same time there appeared a number of dark red or purple spots on the shin-bones, and afterwards small hard swellings; the gums were swollen and bled on the least touch; the urine was very high coloured, and on three occasions it resembled blood, and his mouth now swelled again. He landed on the 29th of April, and for a few days seemed better, but on the third he walked about a great deal, and on the fourth the pain in the side became greatly increased; the legs swelled, and the rheumatic pains in the limbs returned, and he was brought to the hospital to-day (May 6th) with the following symptoms.

The surface of the body generally is warm and moist; face paler, rather sallow, and has somewhat an anxious expression; the gums are spongy, and the teeth, he says, are loose; tongue clean. He complains of a severe stabbing pain in the left hypochondriac region, extending forward to the umbilicus and backwards towards the spine, much increased by pressure and by lying on the right side; in the latter position there is a dragging sensation in addition to the sharp pain above, it is also worse after taking food; he feels most easy when lying on the back inclined to the left side; he also has pains in the knees, ankles, shins, &c.; the ankles are slightly swollen, and pit on pressure; has had a slight cough for the last two or three weeks, with expectoration of mucus; pulse 84, small, not resisting; bowels regular; urine rather pale; sp. gr. 1009; reaction acid, not albuminous.

Physical signs.—Percussion rather dull under the right clavicle and in the right supra-scapular fossa, as compared with the same parts on the left side; and in the same situations the respiration is bronchial, and bronchophony is heard. The sounds and impulse of the heart are natural, and there is no morbid sound. The dulness in the left hypochondrium, in the region of the spleen, is considerably extended, reaching from about an inch and a half below the left nipple almost down to the left groin—a distance of eight inches. It reaches forwards nearly to the umbilicus, and backwards to within about three inches of the spine.

Admoveantur Hirud. xij. parti dolenti lateris.

℞ Calomel.; Antim. Potassio-Tart.; Opii, singulorum, gr. vj. M. ft. pil. vj. Sumatur una 8vâ quâque horâ.

℞ Potass. Nitrat. gr. xv.; Mist. Camph. ℥jss. ft. haust. inter sing. dos. pilul. sumendus. Low diet.

8th.—The leeches alleviated the pain in the side almost as soon as they had been applied; it is now much easier, and there is less tenderness on pressure.

9th.—He now feels the pain at times only, and then not severe. He can lie on the right side without increasing pain. The extent of dulness in the side is much the same, except that it does not seem to extend quite so far forward. Looks and feels more comfortable. The pains in the limbs are easier, and the œdema of the ankles is almost gone; cough less; pulse natural; bowels open; urine increased in quantity; natural in colour; sp. gr. 1016; not albuminous.

10th.—No pain in the side now; has an aching pain in the epigastrium, and bowels rather confined.

℞ Haust. purgans niger q. p. sumendus. Pergat in usu pil. et Haust. Salin.

Applicetur Emplast. Cantharid. parti dolenti, et curetur pars vesicata Unguento Hydrargyri.

12th.—The size of the spleen, as ascertained by percussion, is greatly diminished; it only reaches now to about three inches below the left nipple, and its extent is di-

minished in other directions also. No pains in the limbs; feels rather weak. The mouth is sore, gums tender, some salivation, and the mercurial fœtor is perceptible. Bowels open. Urine rather scanty; sp. gr. 1012, clear, not albuminous.

Sumatur pilula nocte maneque vice ter die.

14th.—Quite free from pain; the side is quite raw from the mercurial ointment, mouth very tender, and salivation pretty considerable; urine plentiful; reaction acid; sp. gr. 1010; clear; rendered cloudy by heat and nitric acid; and on standing a precipitate of albumen falls.

Sumatur pilula omni nocte tantum.

16th.—The face is swelled considerably, especially the left side of it. The tongue is also swelled, rendering articulation indistinct. The discharge of saliva is abundant, and there is a little blood mixed with it, apparently coming from the gums; bowels open; urine very turbid, and deposits a very copious pinkish sediment of the lithates; sp. gr. 1027; reaction strongly acid, not albuminous.

Omitt. pilulæ et Ung. Hydrarg. Dress the side with water-dressing.

℞ Liq. Plumb. Diacet. ℥jss.; Aquæ, f℥viij. ft. gargarisma sæpe utend.

17th.—Swelling less on the left side of the face, and the tongue also is less swelled; it has a blackish crust on it, and some of this matter, which probably is altered blood, is mixed with the saliva.

Sumatur Haust. Salin. 6tâ qq. horâ.

℞ Liq. Plumb. Diacet. f℥j.; Sp. Vini Rectif. f℥iij.; Aquæ, f℥viij. M. ft. lotio pro ore subinde utenda.

19th.—The swelling very much less, and also the salivation: the pain and tenderness are completely gone from the left side, and he can bear firm percussion without pain being felt. The dulness is much less extensive, reaching only up to the 8th rib, so that there is a clear space of more than three inches below the nipple. In other directions also the dulness is diminished, but less so. Urine very turbid, with a pinkish sediment, soluble in ammonia or liq. potassæ, or by heat. The addition of an equal volume of nitric acid to some of the urine causes the formation of a number of crystals of nitrate of urea on cooling.

23d.—Face and tongue nearly natural in size, and salivation very trifling; gums rather pale, and tongue looks spongy, and is pitted on the margin; has no pain anywhere; can lie on either side without inconvenience; bowels regular; urine plentiful and natural.

Physical signs much the same as on the 6th instant. The expiration is loud and prolonged in the same situations as the bronchial respiration and bronchophony. The left side of the abdomen feels much softer, and more flaccid. The dulness on percussion commences a little more than three inches below the left nipple, and extends downwards about five inches, and its transverse extent is about the same.

℞ Potass. Liquoris, ♏xxiv.; Infusi Quassiæ, ℥iss. ft. haustus bis indies sumendus. Omitt. Haust. Salin. Milk diet, and a mutton chop daily.

26th.—Countenance much more natural; cheeks gaining a little red tinge; is gaining strength daily; appetite good; pulse natural; no pain anywhere; bowels regular; urine abundant and natural.

28th.—Going on very well; recovering fast. Has no pain in the side; but if firm pressure be made about three inches to the left of the umbilicus there is a little tenderness felt.

Full diet and chop daily.

30th.—Is much stronger; can walk pretty well; the dulness of the spleen reaches to the level of the umbilicus, and the lower end of it can be distinctly felt here; it is very slightly tender on its inner side, but this is scarcely worth noticing. The size seems to vary a little at different times, sometimes being rather larger than at others.

Discharged cured.

REMARKS.—Inflammation of the spleen is by no means a common disease, and, indeed, its existence is doubted by some, whilst, on the other hand, some have gone so far as to describe two varieties, one affecting the capsule, the other the proper substance of the spleen. The existence of inflammation of the capsule, independently of the substance of the spleen, may fairly be questioned, considering the multitude of processes which are given off by it, and distributed throughout the interior of the organ, and most intimately connected with the proper substance of the spleen; and even did it exist, there would be no special signs by which we could distinguish it from a local inflammation of the partial peritoneal investment of the spleen; and, indeed, it is so closely united to this membrane, that we can scarcely conceive that it could occur without exciting peritonitis. If the substance of the spleen were not affected there would be no perceptible enlargement; and as there was, in this case, we may leave this point.

In the case now under our notice the symptoms were a sharp lancinating pain in the left hypochondriac region, much increased by pressure externally—by taking food which would cause the stomach to press against the spleen, and also by lying on the right side, in which position the spleen, from its increased size and weight, produced a dragging sensation, as though there had been a weight hanging from the left side. The size of the spleen was ascertained by percussion to be very greatly enlarged, the dulness being at least twice as extensive as it is in health.

From these symptoms the existence of splenitis was assumed; but it may be argued, by those who deny this disease, that these signs may exist without there being splenitis; and therefore, as morbid anatomy has thrown very little light on diseases of the spleen, is it not better to attribute the signs to any other cause that might produce them rather than to splenitis? Thus, in this case, granting that the spleen had become enlarged during the attack of intermittent fever, would not the addition of local peritonitis account for all the other symptoms? It no doubt would account for the pain in the side, increased by pressure or by lying on the right side. The character of the pain also was such as is usual in inflammations of serous membranes, viz. sharp and lancinating; and the very fact of the greatly increased size of the spleen would tend to confirm the view, as this would act as a cause of peritonitis by stretching the peritoneum.

It seems to us most probable that the acute symptoms depended on peritonitis, produced either by the influence of fatigue and cold, on a part predisposed to inflammation from the stretching and traction resulting from the enlargement of the spleen, or else by the aggravation and extension of a chronic inflammation of the spleen, which, in the latter case, must be assumed to have been the cause of the enlargement, and of the pain which had been felt during, and ever since, the attack of intermittent fever. Hitherto it has not been shewn what is the pathological nature of these enlargements of the spleen; but it is certain, from the very rapid effects of some remedies, especially quinine, in reducing the size, that part of the increased size is due to congestion: whether there is, besides this, a chronic inflammation we cannot be certain: the influence of mercury, in the present case, in diminishing the size, as it is known to do in chronic inflammation of other organs, seems to countenance the idea that it (inflammation) did exist; but we can come to no certain conclusion on this point.

In addition to the preceding signs of disease of the spleen, there were other symptoms which would, by some persons, in accordance with their views of the functions of the spleen, be referred to the derangement of the functions consequent on its morbid condition, viz. the pale sallow complexion, the slightly yellow tinge of the conjunctivæ, the œdema of the ankles, and the symptoms of scurvy and purpura as noticed in the history; all of these clearly shewed a morbid state of the blood, but it by no means is to be deduced that this depended on the condition of the spleen; it is at least equally as philosophical to regard the condition of the spleen and that of the blood as results of a common cause, viz. malaria.

These were the chief things for which he came to the hospital; but he had besides rheumatic pains in the limbs—the remains of an attack of rheumatism a few weeks before he was admitted—and he had also some symptoms of incipient phthisis, viz. slight hacking cough, and mucous expectoration, together with the physical signs of condensation of the upper portion of the right lung: thus, there was dulness on percussion under the right clavicle, and in the right supra-scapular fossa, as compared with the left side, and in both these situations bronchial respiration, and strong bronchophony. The condensation thus indicated probably arose from tuberculous deposition; it was just in that condition in which the disease may lie dormant for many years, and it seems likely that it may do so in this case, as before he left the hospital the cough had entirely ceased, and there was not a single symptom referrible to the lungs.

Next, as regards the treatment. The symptoms of local inflammation indicated the abstraction of blood, but not to any great extent, as there was scarcely any general fever: the application of leeches to the seat of the pain was therefore deemed sufficient, and we have seen that this was followed by almost instantaneous relief. He was also ordered calomel, with opium, and tartar emetic, to be continued till the system was brought under the influence of the mercury, and nitrate of potash was added to act as a diuretic to remove the oedema and to improve the condition of the blood. Three days after this a blister was applied to the side, and the blistered surface dressed with mercurial ointment until a considerable amount of salivation was produced.

Under this treatment all the symptoms gave way, both of the affection of the spleen and of the rheumatism; his appetite returned and also his strength; the sallowness disappeared from his countenance and eyes, and the red colour began to return to his face. No other means of any importance were used; he was, for a few days before he was discharged, given a tonic mixture and extra full diet, and went out quite well on the 30th of May, a little more than three weeks from the date of his admission, during which time he had lost all symptoms of disease of the spleen, except perhaps slight enlargement and very slight tenderness at one point on firm pressure.

It is clear from the above case that mer-

cury is very useful in enlargement of the spleen with inflammation, notwithstanding that it is said by some to be injurious.

The urine underwent a considerable number of changes in the progress of the case: the only changes we shall here refer to are, the great abundance of the lithates, and the appearance of albumen in the urine for a single day (May 14th), just at the time the salivation commenced. We attribute this to the influence of the mercury, as we have seen it in several other cases under precisely similar circumstances, viz. just at the time the gums became sore, and in each case lasting only for one day. What the nature of the action of mercury in producing this may be, we cannot tell; it may be that it diminishes the cohesions of the solids, as it is stated to do by Dieterich, and thus allows the transudation of the serum of the blood through the capillaries of the kidneys, or it may produce some change in the composition of the blood; and perhaps this is the beneficial *modus operandi* of mercury in inflammation, producing a state the reverse of that produced by the disease, and thus counteracting it; but neither of these will explain why the albumen has only been found (in these cases) for a single day. The prognosis, from the age, previous good health, &c. was favourable as to the result, but so speedy a cure could hardly have been anticipated.

[We may notice that he came back to the hospital for a few minutes on 23rd June, having been in the country ever since he left the hospital: he had gained much flesh and colour, and seemed quite well.]

MEDICAL REFORM.

ANNUAL GENERAL MEETING OF THE NORTH OF ENGLAND MEDICAL ASSOCIATION.

THE members of this influential body held their anniversary meeting on Wednesday last, in the lecture-room of the Athenæum, Fawcett-street, Sunderland,—Dr. HEADLAM, President of the Association, in the chair,

Mr. C. T. Carter, of Newcastle, the Secretary of the Association, read the following REPORT:—

A period of nearly three years and a half has now elapsed since the formation of this Society; and during that period, five Reports have been submitted to general meetings. In presenting a sixth, the Council have the gratification to announce the unabated prosperity of the Association during the past year. Notwithstanding the great distance at which many of its members reside from the more immediate scene of its transactions, the little opportunity they must of necessity enjoy, from one anniversary meeting to another, of learning the nature of its proceedings,. and the difficulty (in some cases the impossibility) they must experience in attending those meetings, it is satisfactory to find that they continue to yield their support to the several objects for which it was instituted, evincing thereby a degree of zeal on behalf of their common profession well deserving of applause and imitation.

The first and foremost of these objects has ever been, to assist in procuring such a legislative reorganization of the profession as shall be adapted to the circumstances in which it is at present placed—not only in reference to its own members, but to the interests of the community at large. In the pursuit of this object, the hopes of the medical body have been alternately flattered and disappointed ; and it has been the duty of your Council to report, from time to time, the failure of every attempt which has been made, within the last few years, to legislate upon this difficult and complicated subject. Under these circumstances, it is not surprising that some gentlemen, who joined this Society in the sanguine expectation that the unsatisfactory state of medical affairs was to be rectified at once, should have become disheartened, and that, despairing of success, or doubtful at least of the utility of their individual aid, they should have deserted the ranks of the Association. But it is satisfactory to know, that if some have withdrawn themselves, there have been others ready to supply their places, and that, in spite of every discouragement, the Association has steadily kept its ground. Some who stood aloof at its formation, either from misapprehension or mistrust of its designs, have, now that time has been allowed for their development, enrolled themselves amongst its members—considering properly, that although the assistance of any one man may avail but little in the correction of evils and abuses, it should nevertheless be added to the general effort. And this, in fact, is all that is required : let the number of those who are willing to aid the cause of professional amendment, by never so little, be converted from hundreds into thousands, and that cause must, at no distant period, be crowned with abundant success. Let no one give way to despondency on account of the delay which *must* take place before the arrival of this period. Impediments and hindrances should serve but to exercise patience, and excite to renewed exertions.

Your Council deem it unnecessary to dilate on the good results which are likely to ensue from Associations such as this. It is impossible that such bodies should not exert a considerable moral influence both upon the profession and the public. Upon the former they are calculated to produce effects which cannot fail to secure the increased respect and consideration of the latter ; and

it should never be forgotten, that the interests and well-being of each are inseparably connected, and that the medical body can seek no improvement of its own condition, which would not be productive of beneficial consequences to every class and grade of the community. Members of the profession should not be disappointed if the progress of improvement be slow and almost imperceptible. The ordinary avocations of medical men are of an engrossing character, and are liable to interfere with that frequent intercourse which is requisite to the carrying out of any concerted scheme or line of action in affairs not immediately connected with the practice of their art. Your Council have to regret, that, from this circumstance, it has been found difficult to give to many topics of interest that full and careful consideration to which they are entitled ; and in resigning their functions, they would take the liberty of suggesting to their successors to consider, whether, by the appointment of Committees on individual subjects, or by some other means, this disadvantage may not in future be obviated, or at least materially diminished. The inconvenience of frequently bringing together members of this Association, scattered as they are over three extensive counties, induced the Council, some time ago, to recommend, and the Association to resolve, that, except for special and extraordinary purposes, there should be but one general meeting in the year. This arrangement was accompanied by a strong recommendation in favour of sectional subdivisions and meetings, as a means of fulfilling more particularly some of the second class of objects contemplated by the association. Such local unions might be rendered useful in a variety of ways, which will readily occur to every mind ; as in promoting harmony and community of feeling—in cherishing a due observance of professional honour and etiquette, in discussing and arranging matters of mutual interests, in affording mutual protection, and, in towns where there is no Society established for that purpose, in advancing medical literature and science.

In reference to medical legislation, the last year has been one of expectancy rather than of action. The profession has been awaiting the introduction into Parliament of the Bill announced by Sir James Graham in the early part of last session. From the peculiar nature of his office, it has been considered that on no one could the responsibility of such a measure rest with so much propriety as on Her Majesty's Secretary of State for the Home Department, and that in no hands could the carrying of a Medical Bill through Parliament be so certain of success. It has been imagined, moreover, that in undertaking a task of so much complexity, and involving so many interests, both public and professional, the Minister would feel it his duty to avail himself of all those sources of information which are peculiarly open to the Home Office ; that in deliberating on this momentous question, the *general good* would be the paramount consideration.

Your Council regret, that although two separate applications have been made for the purpose, they are unable to submit to this meeting any official outline of the anticipated Bill of Sir James Graham. From what they have been enabled to glean of its contents, they are induced to believe that its provisions are, or were, not widely different from those which, upon surmise, they ventured to criticize in their last Report ; and it is needless to say, that if such be the case, the Bill, how acceptable soever it may prove to certain parties in the profession, cannot fail, in several most important particulars, to disappoint a great numerical majority of its members. Your Council by no means wish to affirm that some parts of the Bill, as reported, would not be productive of good, nor constitute improvements on the present system. If rightly informed, it would tend to promote an incorporation of the physicians of each country, and a uniform standard of qualification for medical degrees. Upon the justice and propriety of such an arrangement the opinion of this Association has been repeatedly expressed ; and it is gratifying to know, that a growing inclination in its favour has of late years been exhibited by most of the Universities and Medical Colleges of the United Kingdom. As a natural consequence of uniformity in the conditions attached to the granting of medical degrees, the restrictions which have hitherto prevailed with regard to the right of practising in particular districts would be removed ; the power now held by the Royal College of Physicians of London to examine for its license the graduates of British Universities would be withdrawn, along with most of those questionable parts of its constitution which have entailed upon the College so much unpopularity, and occasioned so many undignified conflicts between the different classes of its members. The executive bodies of the Colleges of Physicians, it is also supposed, would be no longer self-elected, but chosen by their respective commonalties— the latter being made to comprehend all the legally recognized physicians of each country. The Colleges would thus serve as Courts of Record for Medical Degrees, and their registers would probably be the means of detecting and exposing parties who should usurp the title of M. D., or hold it merely in virtue of a purchased continental diploma.

The Bill, it has been supposed, would also

tend to promote something like uniformity in the education in the general practitioner, and would enforce a double qualification on all who should hereafter receive a license to practise as members of that branch of the profession. Such an arrangement is not only expedient but necessary. There is at present no greater evil in the profession than that arising from the unfair competition caused by the dissimilarity of qualification which prevails among general practitioners, and in consequence of which it happens, that while some parties, in order to qualify themselves for general practice, incur the labour and expense of completing the separate curricula of study, and submitting themselves to the separate examinations required for the diploma of the College of Surgeons and the license of the Society of Apothecaries, there are others, acting in a similar capacity, who have subjected themselves to the ordeal of *one only* of these Boards—an injustice which will be instantly apparent, when it is remrmbered, that the former body institutes no inquiry into the *medical* knowledge of candidates for its diploma, while the latter takes no cognizance of *surgery* in the course of study and examinations which precede the granting of its license.

It is said that the Bill of Sir James Graham would require all future English general practitioners to be examined in some departments of medical science by the College of Surgeons. The hall of the Apothecaries' Company would be no longer the scene of medical examinations. Some of its members would, however, assist in the examinations at the College of Physicians, and the license of the Company would be taken as heretofore by the general practitioner. This arrangement appears to your Council to be one of the most objectionable parts of the Bill, and would almost serve to indicate the parties by whose advice its right honourable framer would seem to have been actuated in its construction. If the general practitioner is to be no longer examined by the Company of Apothecaries, why should he continue to receive his license from that Company ? If his examination is to be conducted jointly by the Colleges of Physicians and Surgeons, under such regulations as should be approved of by a General Board or Council, why should not his license be granted by that board ?

It might have been imagined that in legislating anew for the medical profession an opportunity would have been taken to rectify the error committed by the London Colleges in the year 1815, and to atone for their supercilious disregard of that numerous and useful body of practitioners, whom they, in that year, consigned to the care and keeping of a "City Guild and Trading Company of Apothecaries."*

Your Council do not mean to assert that the Apothecaries' Company has not endeavoured faithfully to discharge the functions which, through the supineness of the Colleges, and even in opposition to its own wishes, it has been called on to fulfil. On the contrary, they willingly admit that much success has attended its exertions. The gradually increased amount of qualification now required of the general practitioner is unquestionably to be attributed to the Apothecaries' Company. Not unmindful, therefore, of its services, and with no feeling of disrespect, the Council are yet of opinion that the control of medical education, and the licensing of medical men, should never have been entrusted to this Corporation, and that, under a proper sense of duty on the part of the Colleges of Physicians and Surgeons, and a right understanding of the case by the Legislature, such an office would not have devolved upon the Society of Apothecaries. They are persuaded, that in consideration of his acquirements, and the position at present occupied by the general practitioner, both in society and the public confidence, he should cease to bear the stamp of an *apothecary;* he should no longer be identified with a functionary now all but obsolete : his authority to practise the *profession* of Medicine should no more emanate from a *trading* Company.

It is affirmed that a new order, to be entitled "*Fellows of the Royal College of Surgeons,*" is to be created, which your Council suppose will consist chiefly or entirely of that class of practitioners who may be desirous to limit their practice more particularly to the surgical branch of the healing art. The "*Fellows,*" it is believed, are intended to constitute the electoral body of the College, while the *members* or general practitioners will have no voice in the election of its officers, or in the management of collegiate affairs. From the Councils of the Colleges of Physicians and Surgeons of the three countries are to be chosen the medical members of a Central or General Medical Council, to which is to be confided the superintendence and control of the entire profession. As to the propriety of a General Council there can be no question. Its efficiency, and the respect in which it shall be held by the public and the profession, must of course depend in a great measure on the materials of which it may be composed. If the foregoing surmises be correct, the Council will be little else than an offset of the Metropolitan Colleges ; and as the mass of practitioners has been systematically dis-

* J. H. Green.

regarded hitherto, so now, according to the reputed Bill, would they be excluded from all control or influence over the medical polity of the United Kingdom. Coincident with the latter circumstance, the principle of *protection,* clearly recognized by the Apothecaries' Act, but which, from the inappropriate and defective character of the details of that measure, has been too feebly acted upon to suppress a small amount even of the unauthorized practice for which this country is notorious amongst the civilized nations of the world—this principle, it appears, would be exchanged for a species of negative restriction, or, in other words, a *discouragement* of unqualified pretenders to medical knowledge and surgical skill—a discouragement which your Council have reason to believe, and which an adequate acquaintance with the actual state of medical practice throughout the land, especially in rural districts, can hardly fail to demonstrate, would oppose but a feeble barrier to the cruel, dangerous, and fraudulent practices of ignorance, cupidity, and imposture.

Members of this association are probably aware that towards the close of the last session of Parliament Sir James Graham said it was in contemplation to propose the immediate granting of new Charters to the Colleges of Physicians and Surgeons of London, and the subsequent introduction into Parliament of a Bill for the regulation of the medical profession in general. Your Council, thinking that the granting of such Charters would prejudge the general question, petitioned both Houses of Parliament that they would not sanction such a proceeding, but withhold their support from any Charter until the whole subject of medical affairs should be brought before them. The Council took steps for insuring the presentation of similar petitions from Newcastle, Gateshead, Durham, Carlisle, Sunderland, North and South Shields, Berwick, &c., copies of petitions having been transcribed and sent for signature to those places. Members of Parliament were urged at the same time to support their prayer. After the lapse of a few days, Sir James Graham, in reply to a question put to him by Mr. D. Barclay, M.P. for Sunderland, declared that he had abandoned the idea of proposing the Charters during the session of 1842. Medical legislation having thus been once more postponed, and your Council, in reply to a recent application, having been informed that the Bill of the Home Secretary was not sufficiently matured to admit of an *outline* being submitted to their inspection, it is sincerely hoped that the interval may have been employed in framing a measure more suited to the exigencies both of the public and the profession than the *reported* Bill of 1842 could have been capable of supplying. The proper regulation of the medical profession is a matter of vital importance to society at large : its interest is not limited to medical men alone, as is too commonly supposed ; and on this account it is most earnestly to be wished that any measure having reference thereto may be carefully and attentively considered, and with a view, not to favour the designs of any particular party or institution, but to benefit the whole community. It is a question involving the safety and comfort, not of the living only, but of millions of yet unborn subjects of the British empire and its vast dependencies ; and the statesman who shall be instrumental in placing this important branch of national polity on a proper basis will have thereby earned for himself the admiration and gratitude of his country.

It would be a work of supererogation to revert, on the present occasion, to the principles of medical reform which have been advocated by this Association, seeing that they have been so frequently explained in five preceding Reports. It is a source of gratification to your Council, that those principles should have been steadily gaining ground, and that they should be identical, or nearly so, with the opinions promulgated by some of the ablest men who have directed their attention to the subject. They have been supported by the estimable Professor of Medicine in the University of Oxford (Dr. Kidd), and by the late venerated Professor of Anatomy in the University of Dublin (Dr. Macartney.) They have been urged, through a long and honourable career, by Dr. Barlow, of Bath. They have been enforced by Dr. Thomson, late Professor of Pathology in the University of Edinburgh—by Sir James Clark, Mr. Carmichael of Dublin, Dr. Marshall Hall, Dr. G. Webster, Dr. Forbes, Dr. Grant, Mr. R. D. Grainger, and many others, among whom it is but just to mention the name of one of the Vice-Presidents of this Association, Mr. Greenhow. Without wishing to make invidious distinctions where praise is due to all, your Council cannot refrain from expressing the great pleasure they have derived from a perusal of the letters addressed to Sir James Graham by Sir James Clark. To this eminent physician the thanks of the profession are justly due for his able advocacy. Occupying a foremost rank in his own department of practice, Sir James Clark has boldly stepped forward to advocate the improvement and amelioration of the *whole* professional body ; and while he maintains the expediency of divisions of medical labour (which few indeed, if any, have denied), and the persistence of the distinctions and grades already recognized in the profession, he claims for *all* practitioners a good and sufficient education, both preliminary and professional, an equal legal recognition of *all*, and the enrolment of *all* in "one great corporate institution." Sir James Clark is of opinion that there should be but one prescribed course of medical education exacted by the State ; that it should comprehend what is necessary for every medical practitioner, and should be the same throughout the empire. They who would prognosticate from such an arrangement the annihilation of prevailing divisions, distinctions, and honorary titles, may derive some alleviation of their fears from the following extract : — "Whatever department of the profession," observes Sir James, "the medical man may choose as the field of his practice, to practise that part properly he must be acquainted with the whole. When possessed of such general knowledge of his profession, the practitioner may, by devoting his attention to one department chiefly, be fairly supposed to excel, and generally will excel, the man who practises them all. Thus one man, by directing his principal attention to the investigation and treatment of diseases affecting internal organs and the general system—another, by directing his chief attention to the diseases and injuries of the external organs, and the operations and mechanical appliances required for their cure—may each attain, in their respective departments, a degree of perfection which cannot be expected of him whose attention is divided among the whole range of human infirmities and accidents. Hence there will always be physicians and surgeons, who, in addition to their individual practice, will be consulted by the general practitioner in dangerous and obscure diseases." The regulations respecting honorary degrees in medicine, the writer thinks, may be safely left to the Universities and Colleges. "Much," says he in continuation, "has been said of the necessity of requiring high literary and scientific attainments of physicians, in order to secure their high standing and character with the public. Any law for this purpose is quite unnecessary. Insist upon the general practitioner being well instructed, and you at once insure a still higher education for the physician."

Your Council beg to recommend the letters of Sir James Clark to the notice of all who are interested in the subject of medical education or medical government. They trust, moreover, that his example, and that of the other eminent individuals already named, will stimulate the profession to exert itself at the present critical moment ; and as a Bill may be possibly introduced during the present session of Parliament, no time should be lost in making known its opinions and wishes to the Legislature, through the medium of petitions. They are glad to perceive the activity which has lately been displayed by the practitioners of Surrey, Worcestershire, Liverpool, and Chichester, and would beg to suggest the propriety of meetings being convened for the purpose of petitioning both in the counties and towns of the United Kingdom. Your Council have prepared a petition, which they take the liberty to submit to this meeting; and, if approved, they trust that others of a similar kind will be forwarded from the several towns comprised within the district of this Association. They hope the profession will not rest satisfied with the mere act of petitioning, but that each of its members will feel that something more than this devolves upon him *individually*. There must be few indeed who cannot exert *some* degree of influence, both with members of the Legislature and the public; and it must never be forgotten that the progress of amendment has hitherto had to contend with no obstacle so great as the apathy and indifference of a large portion of the medical body itself.

After the length to which the preceding observations have been extended, your Council are unwilling to detain this meeting with a recapitulation of the several subjects to which, in addition to the all-absorbing one of legislative reform, their attention has been directed during the past twelvemonth. Some of these require no comment, whilst others may be said to remain *sub judice*, and might perhaps, with advantage, afford scope for inquiry by the Council which will be elected to-day. The Report on Hospital Appointments, read at the last anniversary meeting, has occasioned much discussion at different periods during the year, but nothing need be said respecting it in this place, as the Committee has of late resumed its sittings, and is prepared to submit a second Report to the meeting.

Mr. Carter, having concluded the Report, proceeded to read a statement of accounts. It was a subject of congratulation, he observed, that the Association was in a prosperous financial condition. At their former meeting in Sunderland, two years ago, they were £16 in debt. Last year, they had a balance in hand of £2. 7s. 6½d., which was increased in the present year to £30. 1s. 0½d. (applause), in addition to £40 due from members in arrear.

Dr. Brown moved that the report be received, printed, and circulated.

The motion was put and carried, and the Secretary read the following petition to parliament:—

To the Honourable the Commons of the United Kingdom of Great Britain and Ireland, in Parliament assembled.

The petition of the President, Vice-Presidents, and Members of the North of England Medical Association, in Public Meeting convened, at Sunderland, this 26th day of April, 1843,

Humbly sheweth,—That your petitioners (consisting of physicians and surgeons resident in the counties of Durham, Northumberland, and Cumberland,) have long deplored the defective and anomalous state of the medical profession in Great Britain and Ireland.

That your petitioners, having reason to believe that measures have been for some time in contemplation for reorganising and reforming the profession, beg respectfully but earnestly to impress upon your Honourable House the great importance of this question to the community at large, and its consequently strong claims to an early adjustment.

That your petitioners, having paid much attention to the subject, take the liberty of stating their persuasion, that any measure of Medical Reform, to be permanently beneficial, must provide for the union and consolidation of the whole professional body, and the proper qualification of all persons who shall hereafter be legally authorized to practise the healing art within Her Majesty's dominions. Your petitioners are further of opinion that uniformity in the qualification for a license to practise should be enforced; that honorary degrees in Medicine and Surgery should be conferred on a uniform principle; that reciprocal privileges should be enjoyed by the medical practitioners of England, Scotland, and Ireland; and that suitable measures should be adopted for protecting the public from the dangerous and fatal consequences of unauthorized medical and surgical practice.

Your petitioners therefore pray that the present state of the medical profession may receive the early attention of your Honourable House.

And your petitioners, as in duty bound, will ever pray.

Signed for and on behalf of the Meeting,

T. E. HEADLAM, M.D. President.
CHARLES T. CARTER, Secretary.

On the motion of Dr. Knott, of Newcastle, seconded by Mr. Watson, of Sunderland, it was resolved, that Mr. David Barclay be requested to present it to the House of Commons; also, that a similar petition be presented to the House of Lords, and that the Marquis of Londonderry be requested to take charge of its presentation.

After some further discussion on various points, for which we cannot make room, the thanks of the meeting were voted to Dr. Headlam for his conduct in the chair; and in the evening the members dined together at the Bridge Hotel.

NATURE AND TREATMENT OF APOPLEXY.

I PROPOSE to prove that there is no such disease as sanguineous apoplexy, and that bleeding is always prejudicial in the treatment of apoplexy. Here, I travel without a guide; no author has yet professed this doctrine; happy shall I be if, in explaining it according to my view, and as it has been revealed to me at the bedside of the patient, I succeed in eradicating a dangerous error which has been introduced into the healing art, and in enriching it with a novel truth.

Let us examine the dead bodies of patients who have died of apoplexy; and beginning with the brain, in which M. Portal believes the cause of death from apoplexy is always seated, Morgagni assures us, from his own dissections and those of Varoli, that the brain of apoplectics does not contain a larger quantity of excremental parts than that of other dead boodies.

Morgagni, who does not generally make use of repetition, repeats this assertion several times in his writings. It is strange that M. Portal should not have seen it; if he have read it, it is still more astonishing that he should have thought himself authorised to overturn a doctrine universally received, because he has found certain diseased appearances in the *brain* of one apoplectic patient.

Morgagni appears to have foreseen and condemned beforehand the system of M. Portal, when he says: " I do not agree with those who, when they find water in the cranium of an apoplectic, think immediately that it has caused the disease."

" It is the common error," says Lancisi, " of those who have no experience : when they find lymph in the cavities of the brain, they are in the habit of attributing the apoplexy to it as the cause, whilst commonly it is only the effect."

With respect to the water which is found in the cranium of apoplectics, Morgagni adds : " You are aware that authors assert that the ventricles of the brain always contain a little water, in the natural state ; besides you see very clearly that the quantity of water cannot be greater than in hydrocephalus internus ; and yet Vesalius states that he has found in a child two years old, affected with this disease, about nine pints of water ; he adds, that the child preserved its senses to the last moment ; that it had, it is true, extreme weakness in the limbs, but that they were not paralysed. Besides this," continues Morgagni, " you well know, from a number of dissections described by Bonnet, in his work, entitled *Le Cimetière anatomique*, that tumors have been found in the cranium which had not been followed by apoplexy. But I have myself seen, as I have *before* noticed in my *journal, an anormal increase* of bony sub-stance in those bones of the cranium, which presented a considerable protuberance inwards and compressed the brain, without this compression having produced either apoplexy or any other disease."

" I opened," says M. Thiéry, " fifteen bodies of persons from sixty to ninety years of age. The vessels of the head were very full; four times I found polypous concretions in the longitudinal and lateral sinuses ; in others the ventricles of the brain were filled with serum ; such are exactly the appearances I have met with, in the same proportion, in persons destroyed by apoplexy : these, however, had died without the slightest appearance of apoplexy. On the other hand, I have opened many bodies of persons who died suddenly from apoplexy, either on the third or fourth day after the attack, and have found only slight congestion of the vessels, without extravasation of any kind."

Sauvages says, that, " when water is found in the sinuses of the brain, it is not therefore to be said that this serosity has been the cause of the apoplexy. I have seen hydrocephalus to an enormous extent without apoplexy ; several authors have made the same observation."

I think it unnecessary to notice every kind of extravasation that may take place in the cranium, since the statement of Morgagni, the result of numerous dissections, embraces all the disorders which the brain presents ; and he asserts that they ought never to be considered as causes of apoplexy, whilst they are met with indifferently in patients who have died from apoplexy, and in those who have died from any other cause.

I shall observe, however, that extravasation of blood would prove the existence of sanguineous apoplexy less than extravasation of serum.

If the globules of the blood had as much tenuity, and were as fluid as the serous part, would not they escape with the latter, when it escapes ? This is self-evident. If, then, the globules remain in the vessels, whilst the serum is extravasated, they remain there only on account of their greater consistence and greater thickness ; now this consistence and thickness of the blood are allied to the state which is called *inflammatory*. Sanguineous apoplexy, which is supposed to arise from this pretended inflammatory thickening of the blood, cannot therefore present the extravasation of blood spoken of, since its density opposes it ; it is sufficient therefore to see blood extravasated in the brain, to be certain that, if that extravasation is anything else than the effect of the disease, it does not, at all events, prove the existence of sanguineous apoplexy.

* From Mr. Copeman's translation of Jean Antoine Gay's Essay on the Nature and Treatment of Apoplexy—lately published.

ON THE SIGNS OF DEATH.

Dr. Deschamps, of Melun, has presented to the French Academy of Medicine a memoir on the real sign of death. He draws the following conclusions, intended to guide public authorities in the precautions that should be taken against the danger of interring prematurely persons not really dead.

The author has observed that, in warm-blooded vertebratæ, putrefaction proceeds from the circumference towards the centre, and contrariwise in the cold-blooded; and he arrives at the following conclusions.

1. A greenish blue colour, extending uniformly over the skin of the belly, is the real and certain sign of death.

2. The period at which this sign appears varies much; but it takes place in about three days under favourable circumstances of warmth and moisture.

3. Though discolouration of various kinds, and from various causes, may occur in other parts, the characteristic mark of death is to be found only in the belly.

4. Apparent death can no longer be confounded with real death; the belly never being coloured green or blue in any case of the former.

5. This colouring of the belly, which may be artificially hastened, entirely prevents the danger of premature interment.

6. There is no danger to public health from the keeping a body until the appearance of the characteristic sign of death.—*Gazette Medicale,* April 1.

BIRMINGHAM HOSPITAL.

Mr. Jukes has resigned the office of surgeon to the Birmingham Hospital, which he long held with so much credit. He has been succeeded by Mr. Crompton, who was elected on Friday, the 29th ultimo.

COLLEGE OF PHYSICIANS.

At a Board held at the Royal College of Physicians, on Saturday the 28th ult. Sir Henry Halford, Bart., President; the following gentlemen were examined, and obtained their degrees in medicine: Mr. W. T. Ballantine, Surgeon, Royal Navy; Mr. T. Sale, Surgeon, Isle of Man; Mr. S. Newington, A.B. Oxford; Mr. G. Moor., Hastings; Mr. W. Major, Hungerford, Berks; Mr. Tomkils, Yeovil.

ROYAL COLLEGE OF SURGEONS.

LIST OF GENTLEMEN ADMITTED MEMBERS.

Friday, April 28, 1843.

J. C. Pritchard.—T. Prosser.—D. P. Evans.—D. C. Noel.—R. Tebbitt.—C. M. Smith.—J. M. Woollett.—T. Turton.—R. Worsley.—W. Hitchins.—J. M'Donogh.—S. Bowden.—J. Wheatcroft.—T. Adney.—G. H. Hopkins.

APOTHECARIES' HALL

LIST OF GENTLEMEN WHO HAVE RECEIVED CERTIFICATES.

Thursday, April 27, 1843.

W. Perkett, Petersfield, Hants.—W. Simpson, Wyken Hall, Suffolk.—J. J. Sparham, Blakeney, Norfolk.—J. B. Ashford, Plymouth.—J. Spencer, Suffolk.—J. Thompson, Whitehaven.—C. R. Francis, Bengal Army.—T. Taylor, Witney, Oxon.

A TABLE OF MORTALITY FOR THE METROPOLIS,

Shewing the number of deaths from all causes registered in the week ending Saturday, April 22, 1843.

Small Pox	6
Measles	22
Scarlatina	27
Hooping Cough	37
Croup	10
Thrush	5
Diarrhœa	4
Dysentery	2
Cholera	0
Influenza	1
Typhus	58
Erysipelas	2
Syphilis	1
Hydrophobia	0
Diseases of the Brain, Nerves, and Senses	148
Diseases of the Lungs and other Organs of Respiration	384
Diseases of the Heart and Blood-vessels	28
Diseases of the Stomach, Liver, and other Organs of Digestion	65
Diseases of the Kidneys, &c.	6
Childbed	10
Ovarian Dropsy	0
Disease of Uterus, &c.	0
Rheumatism	3
Diseases of Joints, &c.	7
Ulcer	1
Fistula	1
Diseases of Skin, &c.	0
Diseases of Uncertain Seat	113
Old Age or Natural Decay	85
Deaths by Violence, Privation, or Intemperance	28
Causes not specified	7
Deaths from all Causes	961

METEOROLOGICAL JOURNAL.

April 1843.	THERMOMETER.		BAROMETER.	
Wednesday 19	from 34 to 60		29·94 to	29·81
Thursday . 20	39	66	29 66	29·74
Friday . . 21	37	60	29·79	29·83
Saturday . 22	58	42	29·79	29·95
Sunday . . 23	28	55	29·97	30·00
Monday . . 24	28	61	29·95	29·96
Tuesday . 25	27	51	29·72	29·54
April.				
Wednesday 26	from 34 to 52		29·60 to	29·65
Thursday . 27	34	55	29·74	29·84
Friday . . 28	35	49	29 75	29·62
Saturday . 29	38	58	29·62	29·70
Sunday . . 30	44	65	29·76	29·91
May.				
Monday . 1	49	67	29 99	30·11
Tuesday . . 2	40	67	30·10	29·99

Wind variable, N.E. prevailing, except on the 25th, 26th, and 28th ult. when rain fell, generally clear.

Rain fallen, ·46 of an inch.

CHARLES HENRY ADAMS.

WILSON & OGILVY, 57, Skinner Street, London.

THE

LONDON MEDICAL GAZETTE,

BEING A

WEEKLY JOURNAL

OF

𝕸𝖊𝖉𝖎𝖈𝖎𝖓𝖊 𝖆𝖓𝖉 𝖙𝖍𝖊 𝕮𝖔𝖑𝖑𝖆𝖙𝖊𝖗𝖆𝖑 𝕾𝖈𝖎𝖊𝖓𝖈𝖊𝖘.

FRIDAY, MAY 12, 1843.

LECTURES

ON THE

THEORY AND PRACTICE OF MIDWIFERY,

Delivered in the Theatre of St. George's Hospital,

BY ROBERT LEE, M.D. F.R.S.

LECTURE XXVI.

On protracted and difficult labours from anchylosis of the coccyx and tumors within the pelvis.

Anchylosis of the coccyx.

THIS is not a common cause of protracted and difficult labour. No distinct case of tedious labour from this disease has come under my observation. Dr. F. Ramsbotham states that he has seen three cases in which the bone broke, or the anchylosed joint gave way, but there is no detailed account given by him of the duration of the labours, or of the manner in which they terminated. Dr. Haslewood, of Darlington, met with a case of severe and protracted labour, in which the forehead of the child rested on the point of the sacrum and coccyx for many hours, and the head was indented by the sharp point of the coccyx, and the skin abraded. The birth was ultimately accomplished by the forceps; as soon, indeed, as the short forceps could be effectually applied. Dr. Haslewood considered the causes of the protracted and severe labour to be smallness of the pelvis and ossification of the os coccygis, much incurvated. When pregnancy again took place, I was requested to state my opinion respecting the propriety of inducing premature labour, but before doing so, and recommending the operation, I thought it advisable to consult Dr. Merriman, whose experience on this subject was communicated to me in the following letter.

806.—XXXII.

My dear Dr. Lee,—The case you mention to me is doubtless rare, for you have never seen exactly such a one, nor have I. I recollect one patient in whom the point of the coccyx snapped in three subsequent labours and healed without difficulty; and I have known one or two others where the parts snapped in the first labours and no ill consequences followed.

One of my patients, whose case resembles most that which you refer to, had so great a *turning up*, I believe I must call it, of the coccyx, as to delay the labour for probably two hours, and I was strongly tempted to use the forceps, but they were not applied, and both mother and child did well. I attended her three or four times afterwards, and there was always some delay on account of this straitness, but not so great as at first. There was a considerable bulk of anchylosis; the mischief was produced by a fall down stairs when about 12 or 14 years old.

I agree with you in thinking that it would be right, under all the circumstances of the case, to induce labour at eight months, rather than to leave the poor woman to the chance of again losing her infant, but of course your friend will institute a careful inquiry first, as to the present condition of the parts.

Believe me, dear sir,

Very truly yours,

SAMUEL MERRIMAN.

34, Brook Street, Oct. 9, 1841.

"I find on examination," observes Dr. Haslewood, in his letter in reply, "that the last bone of the os coccygis is not ossified, but that there is the same projection as before, depending, I now think, more on malformation of the sacrum than merely on the os coccygis. I am no draughtsman, but the line above is an attempt to convey my impression of the curve; in fact, the sacrum curves forwards, so as to form an obvious obstruction, and at the end thereof the last bone of the os coccygis is moveable. My impression was that the latter bone was not

Q

moveable, but in this I believe I was mistaken, as the obstacle seems very much the same as before." Premature labour was induced, and the child was born alive without artificial assistance, but has not been reared. Pregnancy again took place, and the propriety of inducing premature labour came again to be considered. The accuracy of Dr. Haslewood's description was fully verified by the most careful examination which I could make of the pelvis, but I was induced, from the extraordinary state of mental anxiety and dread of the operation entertained by the lady, to recommend her to be allowed to go to the full period, and the delivery to be completed with the forceps as soon as it should become evident that the head could not pass without suffering from the pressure of the point of the sacrum and coccyx. The child was born by the natural efforts, and is now alive.

Tumors within the pelvis occasioning difficult parturition are not of very frequent occurrence, but when large, hard, and immoveable, they produce nearly the same consequences as distortion and exostosis of the pelvis, and require, in many respects, a similar mode of treatment. The greater number of these tumors are enlarged ovaria, which have become fixed by adhesions to the uterus and rectum. Some are fibrous tumors developed in the walls of the uterus, and others grow from the ligaments and bones of the pelvis, and are situated in the loose cellular and adipose substance lying between the bones, and the bladder, the vagina, and rectum. These latter form by far the most rare variety of pelvic tumors which obstruct the progress of the child's head during labour, and their diagnosis is extremely difficult and obscure. I shall relate the following examples of these tumors growing from the pelvic ligaments and bones, for the purpose of impressing upon you the necessity of observing the greatest caution in adopting the bold and successful plan of treatment pursued by Dr. Drew and Dr. Burns.

Difficult labour from fibrous tumors attached to the sacro-sciatic ligaments and bones of the pelvis.

In February 1803, Dr. Drew examined the body of Mrs. Shaw, æt. 37, the mother of six children, who had died from a tumor within the pelvis, which compressed the bladder and rectum. It was situated in the loose cellular and adipose substance between the viscera and bones of the pelvis, and it grew by a strong root, of a hard gristly nature, from the left sacro-sciatic ligament. Having cut through the root the tumor came away, like an almond blanched from its skin, so slightly was it attached to the parts that surrounded it. "The tumor was per-

fectly round, about 16 inches in circumference, of a fat gristly substance, without any appearance of circulation in it. No artery entering it. No vein proceeding from it. Unconnected with the arteries which run down from the internal iliacs to supply the contents of the pelvis. It seemed the production of the ligament alone. Could not an incision have been made at one side of the perineum and anus," inquires Dr. Drew, "backwards, towards the os coccygis, and the root of the tumor, proceeding from the sacro-sciatic ligament, be come at, and cut through? And as it was so easy to detach it from the contents of the pelvis, might not it have been without much difficulty removed? Should any artery in the neighbourhood of the perineum be cut, it could easily be taken up; and as the tumor itself received no branch from the internal arteries of the pelvis, the hæmorrhage, in all probability, would not be great."

Six months after this dissection the following case occurred, which is extraordinary alike for the accuracy of the diagnosis and the facility and success of the formidable operation performed. A tumor, much larger than the fist, was removed through the outlet of the pelvis, and in three days the patient "was able to suckle her child, and the wound perfectly healed."

Aug. 26, 1803, I was called on, says Dr. Drew, to Mrs. M——, of Lismore. She had been two days in labour before I saw her, and was attended by Dr. Power, Dr. Hannan, and Mr. Pack, Surgeon to the 41st Regiment of Foot. Those gentlemen were puzzled at the presentation, and so I should have been, had I not met with the preceding case. It was exactly the same. The tumor grew out of the right side, and occupied the whole cavity of the pelvis so completely as to admit of passing only one finger between it and the pubis, by which I could scarcely reach the head of the child. She said she had for some months laboured under dysuria, so that the catheter had been employed by a surgeon who attended her, and who attributed that affection to her state of pregnancy, supposing it to arise from the pressure of the gravid womb: that she had lately acquired the knack of pressing on the tumor with her finger, which enabled her to make urine without assistance. Being convinced of the nature of the case, I related that of Mrs. Shaw, and represented the possibility of removing the tumor with a prospect of success, at least with more than would attend the Cæsarean section. Embryulcia was out of the question; it could not be performed: there was no room to extract the child: and if it had been practicable, since the mother's life could be prolonged for a short time only, it involved in it a crime; and to leave our patient undelivered was cruel and unprofessional. They therefore willingly consented to the operation proposed. Having laid my patient on a table in the posture of operating for lithotomy, my assisting friends holding each a knee, and the midwife the shoulders, I made my incision by the right side of the perinæum and anus, towards the os coccygis, and with the second stroke of the scalpel brought the tumor into view. I passed my finger before and behind its root, which I easily divided with the knife, and introduced my hand, and detached it from the side of the pelvis; withdrew that hand, and introduced the other, by which I separated it with equal facility from the vagina and rectum, and, to their great pleasure and surprise, brought it away. A gush of blood now took place, and I crammed in a sponge, which instantly checked it. An artery near the perinæum spouted. This I laid my finger on, and could, if necessary, in any instant have taken it up; but all hæmorrhage completely ceased. We now turned our attention towards the support of our patient: assured her all danger was over. No fainting occurred; her pulse was sufficiently distinct and strong. We administered a little wine, but the best of cordials was the great pleasure and satisfaction she saw in the countenances of us all. A labour pain now came on, succeeded by another and another; the head descended into the cavity of the pelvis; the sponge was protruded from the wound. We retained her for an hour on the table, expecting she would soon be delivered, but finding her labour grow tedious we removed her into bed. Here we trusted to the efforts of nature for six hours. Finding the child was presenting with its face towards the os pubis, and apprehensive of her wanting strength, I applied the forceps, and delivered her of a living child, which has since continued well. The placenta came down into the vagina, and was easily removed. No hæmorrhage took place. Four stitches were passed through the lips of the wound, and a large sponge was thrust into the valves to keep the sides of the cavity which contained the tumor in contact, and all the other requisite arrangements and comforts were employed. We waited on her in the evening; found her as we could wish; drew off about half a pound of urine with the catheter, for the sponge prevented her from making it herself; left her to repose, and next morning visited her again; she slept well, and complained of little pain from the wound. We drew off her urine, and removed the sponge from the vagina, which I washed out with a syringe, and found it completely free from any injury or ulceration; replaced the sponge, and dressed the wound with a pledget and T bandage.

August 28.—An enema was administered yesterday morning without effect. Some castor oil was given in the evening, which produced rather too many evacuations; but no bad symptom took place. We removed the sponge from the vagina, and found the space which the tumor had occupied completely obliterated. But two of the stitches gave way, and left the lips in part separated. The sponge was omitted, and the lips brought together again with a strip of adhesive plaster. An anodyne was prescribed, to check the catharsis, and two scruples of bark to be taken three times in the day. Here our report ended, as no unfavourable symptom occurred: I visited her for the last time on the 29th, and found her able to suckle her child; both completely well; the wound perfectly healed, without a vestige of any ill consequence from the operation.

Mrs. M. is a slender and delicate woman, aged about 20, and married twelve months; had once before marriage some suppression of urine, but attended with no pain. The tumor measures 14 inches in circumference, weighs about 2 pounds 8 ounces, and is of the same nature and consistence with that found in Mrs. Shaw. As the above cases are very uncommon—as the operation was attended with unexpected and signal success, and the cure complete—and since many of the profession are inclined to discredit such cases, it may not be amiss to subjoin the testimony of those who were present. I have therefore obtained the signatures of Dr. Power, Dr. Hannan, and Mr. Pack.

In the histories of these very remarkable cases of tumors growing from the sacrosciatic ligaments, and situated in the cellular and adipose substance between the viscera and the pelvis, there are no symptoms described by which they could be distinguished from ovarian and uterine tumors, the removal of which in this manner no scientific surgeon would recommend. They are related in far too indefinite a manner to warrant us in drawing any conclusion from them, or proceeding to perform this operation where the diagnosis was not more clearly determined. The second case was most successful, marvellously so it is true, the patient being well in three days; but this is no test of the propriety of the operation, or proof that the case is a safe guide to us in practice. I cannot recommend you under similar circumstances to go and do likewise, as some have advised, but it is proper that your attention should be directed to the possibility of such a case occurring, and the necessity of examining in all possible ways, if such a case should present itself, so as to establish a diagnosis by which you might be prevented from being misled. I have never seen a tumor growing from the ligaments or bones of the pelvis. I have seen many ovarian and uterine tumors filling up the pelvis, but there is no symptom that I am aware of by which you can distinguish these from tumors situated between the pelvic bones and viscera.

The only case that I know of similar to the cases of Dr. Drew is the following, in which the tumor was exterior to the uterine organs, though adhering to them.

"In a dreadful case which I met with some years ago," says Dr. Burns, "the attachments were extensive, and the tumor so large as to fill the pelvis, and permit only one finger to be passed between it at the right side of the basin. It adhered from the symphysis pubis round to the sacrum, being attached to the urethra, obturator muscle, and rectum; intimately adhering to the brim of the pelvis, and even overlapping it a little towards the acetabulum. It was hard, somewhat irregular, and scarcely moveable. The patient, Mrs. Broadfoot, was in the ninth month of pregnancy. There was no choice except between the Cæsarean operation and the extirpation of the tumor. The latter was agreed on; and, with the assistance of Messrs. Cowper and Russel, I performed it on the 16th of March, a few hours after slight labour pains had come on. An incision was made on the left side of the orifice of the vagina, perineum, and anus, through the skin, cellular substance, and transversalis perinei. The levator ani being freely exposed, the tumor was then touched easily with the finger. A catheter was introduced into the urethra, and the tumor separated from its attachments to that part. It was next separated from the uterus, vagina, and rectum, partly by the scalpel, partly by the finger. I could then grasp it as a child's head, but it was quite fixed to the pelvis. An incision was made into it with a knife as near the pelvis as possible; but from the difficulty of acting safely with that instrument, the scissors, guided with the finger, were employed when I came near the back part; and instead of going quite through, I stopped when near the posterior surface, lest I should wound the rectum, or a large vessel, and completed the operation with a spatula. The tumor was then removed, and its base or attachment to the bones dissected off as closely as possible. Little blood was lost. The pains immediately became strong, and before she was laid down in bed they were pressing. In four hours she was delivered of a still-born child above the average size. Peritoneal inflammation, with considerable constitutional irritation, succeeded; but by the prompt and active use of the lancet, and purgatives, the danger was soon over, and the recovery went on well. In the month of May the wound was healed. On examining per vaginam the vagina was felt adhering as it ought to do to the pelvis, rectum, &c. The side of the pelvis was smooth, and a person ignorant of the previous history of the case, or who did not see the external cicatrix, could not have discovered that any operation had been performed. After a lapse of more than fifteen years, she still continues well, but has never been again pregnant."

Difficult labour from ovarian and uterine tumors.

Baudelocque relates a case of ovarian tumor in the pelvis, obstructing delivery, in which Lauverjat had proposed to perform the Cæsarean operation. Baudelocque turned the child, after forcing up the tumor above the brim of the pelvis, but he was obliged to extract the head with the forceps, after the body and extremities of the child had been delivered. The child was dead, and the woman died two days after. The tumor was ascertained on dissection to be an ovarian cyst filled with long hair and nine well-formed teeth. The patient had been in labour 60 hours. If there was space to admit the hand to be passed into the uterus to turn the child, there must have been sufficient space for the employment of the perforator and crotchet. Doeveren had recourse to turning in a similar case, and the mother and child both perished. Dr. Mackenzie turned the child with great difficulty in a case of large ovarian cyst, filling up the hollow of the sacrum, and pressing the os uteri forward to the pubes. The head of the child could not be extracted without long-continued and violent efforts, and the woman died the following day. Dr. Ford relates two cases of difficult labour from pelvic tumors. In the first, as the tumor was large and firm, and did not yield or diminish by the force of the pains, the head was perforated, but the patient died three weeks after. When the body was opened, the tumor was found to be an encysted dropsy of the ovarium, in which there was a considerable quantity of hair. In the latter case, which in all its circumstances resembled the former, a trocar was passed through the posterior part of the vagina directly into the tumor. A large quantity of water was immediately discharged, the tumor subsided, and a living child was born without any farther assistance. This patient recovered from the lying-in, but some time after becoming hectic, she died at the end of about six months, though from the symptoms it did not appear that the fever was occasioned either by the disease or the operation. This patient was not examined after death. "Having related these two cases," observes Dr. Denman (1795), "I have said all which I had to advance on the subject, except that I have met with more than one instance of a circumscribed tumor on one side of the pelvis which I at first suspected to be a diseased ovarium. But as these tumors have always given way to the pressure of the head of the child, the passage of which they have only retarded for a short time, I have concluded they were formed either by some soft fatty substance collecting there, or were cysts containing lymph casually effused, and forming to itself a cyst from the cellular membrane. But on making an examination after delivery, the tumors were found to have again acquired their primitive form and size."

Few if any additional facts of importance respecting tumors within the pelvis occasioning difficult parturition, were published from 1795 to 1811, when Mr. Park's paper on the subject appeared in the 2d Vol. of the Medico-Chirurgical Transactions, in which he has related clearly and precisely the following histories.

In his first case the patient had been long in labour, but the head could not enter the pelvis owing to a firm globular tumor situated between the vagina and rectum, which left very little space between this and the pubes. The head of the child was opened and extracted with much difficulty. After delivery, the tumor totally disappeared; the patient had more children afterwards, without any recurrence of the tumor. Mr. Park thought that an attempt should have been made to diminish the bulk of the tumor before having recourse to the crotchet. In his second case he found the pelvis nearly filled by a tumor similar in situation and texture to that in the former case. It was with some difficulty that the finger could be passed between the tumor and the pubis, so as to reach the os internum, till it became a good deal dilated. After a severe and protracted struggle, the delivery was accomplished by the natural efforts, and the child was born alive. After this she had four miscarriages and premature births in succession, each time of twins, from the 4th to the end of the 7th month. The seven months' children were the last of the four; and these were likewise born without any forcible measures. During these pregnancies the tumor by its pressure on the urethra frequently occasioned retention of urine so as to require the use of the catheter, although by the touch little change could be discovered in its bulk. In her next pregnancy she went to her full time of a single child, and after she had been long in labour, the head pressed constantly on the upper part of the tumor, without being able to descend into the pelvis. The lancette cachée was conducted along the finger to a part of the tumor which felt thinner than the rest, and three or four scratches were made till the parietes felt thin, and the instrument was then forced into a large cavity which was filled with a bloody serous fluid with a number of flakes of membranous substances resembling the

strippings of tripe; some of these were as large as a quarter of a sheet of common paper. The tumor was completely evacuated by the next pain, and in two or three more the child was expelled. The recovery was slow after this delivery; a very considerable offensive discharge ensued from the incision, with pains in the loins, debility, and symptomatic fever. In two months the symptoms disappeared, but the healing of the tumor and consolidation of its cavity occasioned a considerable stricture, so that the next labours were also difficult.

In the next case related by Mr. Park there was a considerable tumor, like those already described, filling up a considerable part of the pelvis, but of a less firm texture, and not so globular, being of a more irregular oblong figure. The woman had been in labour two days; her strength was not much exhausted, and the head pressed more into the pelvis than in either of the former cases. It was determined to leave the case to nature for a time, and perforate the head if requisite. The child was expelled by the natural efforts on the following day, but she died three days afterwards with vomiting and constipation. The nature of the tumor was not ascertained. In the 4th case a tumor filled the pelvis, and kept the head of the child above the brim after the labour had continued long and exhaustion had taken place. An incision was made into the tumor, but no cavity discovered. Nothing but blood was discharged. The head of the child was opened, and the patient recovered without much difficulty. In the last case an ovarian cyst filled the pelvis so completely that the os uteri could not be reached. In the evening, after slight pains had continued all day, it was reached with some difficulty above the symphysis pubis, and the head was felt presenting. The night passed over with little alteration, and the whole of the next day without much more. Strong pains then came on, and continued the whole of the following night, which dilated the os uteri to the diameter of three inches. An opening was made into the tumor after the labour had continued some time longer, and a bloody serum drained off, so as to render the head quite flaccid, and to diminish its bulk at least two-thirds. As the head descended into the pelvis, it became totally evacuated. Immediately after the puncture was made, the head began to dip into the pelvis, and to dilate the os internum more fully; but the child proving a large one, it required eight hours more of strong labour to complete the delivery, although the tumor could not oppose any further resistance. The long pressure on the head destroyed the child, but the patient recovered.

Mr. Park has given no opinion respecting the origin and nature of these tumors, most of which were probably ovarian. The practice adopted by him was certainly extremely judicious; but it did not differ from that which Dr. Ford had recourse to in his cases. In the pathology and treatment of these tumors, therefore, there is nothing absolutely new in Mr. Park's paper; but its publication was of use by directing the attention of practitioners to the subject.

In the third volume of the Medico-Chirurgical Transactions, Dr. Merriman (1812), has related a case of difficult parturition occasioned by an ovarian cyst in the pelvis, which occurred in 1804. After thirty-six hours had passed in severe and ineffectual pain, the head was perforated, and extracted with much difficulty. Soon after this child was born it was ascertained that there was another in the uterus, which, being smaller, was expelled by the natural efforts, and appeared to have been dead some hours. The patient died in a few days from peritoneal inflammation, and the right ovarium, about the size of a trap-ball, and in a state of high inflammation, was found lying between the rectum and the vagina. The brim of the pelvis was narrow. Dr. Merriman also relates a case which had occurred a short time before in one of the London lying-in hospitals, in which the labour was protracted by an ovarian tumor in the pelvis, consisting, like Baudelocque's, of fatty matter, intermixed with hair and teeth. The head of the child was perforated, and the woman was delivered, but did not long survive. "Upon the whole, therefore," he says, after alluding to all these cases, "I am disposed to believe that, where the tumor in the vagina occupies a large space, it would be a more warrantable practice to remove it by excision, if it consisted of solid substance, and certainly to puncture it if it contained a fluid, rather than to expose the child to certain death, and the mother to great hazard, by the use of the perforator." Dr. Drew's cases are quoted to sanction, in some degree, the attempt to remove solid ovarian tumors by excision during labour; although, as has been already stated, it was not an ovarian tumor which Dr. Drew removed through the outlet of the pelvis.

Other five cases, of a nature similar to the preceding, have been recorded by Dr. Merriman in the tenth volume of the same work. In the first the delivery was accomplished with the greatest difficulty after the head of the child had been opened. The tumor, which was large and elastic, occupied the back part and left side of the pelvis, which was distorted; and it was not opened, Dr. Denman and Mr. Croft not being satisfied that it contained a fluid. The patient ultimately recovered, after remaining long in extreme danger. The labour lasted ninety hours. In the second case there was a tense,

elastic, lobulated tumor, between the vagina and rectum, which was punctured with a trocar from the rectum; but the matter it contained was of the consistence of honey, and would not flow through the trocar. The patient was left twenty-four hours in labour. After this, when the tumor was somewhat diminished in volume, but the head of the child was not at all advanced, the head was perforated, and eight hours after it was extracted. The tumor had ceased to be felt before this. Eighteen months after she died hectic. The effects of chronic inflammation were apparent in the abdomen; and the ovarium, which was in its natural situation, equalled a small lemon in size, and contained sebaceous matter, and a tooth lying loose among it. The tumor in the third case was neither so large nor incompressible as in the other instances. As the head of the child was forced down at each pain, the tumor yielded or became flattened against the back of the pelvis. The hand was passed into the vagina, and the tumor pushed up above the brim; and thus room was procured for the head to pass, which in less than an hour was protruded through the os externum. The child was alive and healthy. The right shoulder presented in the fourth case, the history of which was communicated by Mr. Hardwick, of Epsom, and the tumor was not connected with the ovaria. It was situated between the cervix uteri and the rectum, forming a cushion in the hollow of the sacrum, the superior portion rising an inch or more above the projecting part of that bone. Its shape was elliptical, flattened at the anterior and posterior surfaces by the pressure it had sustained; its size was that of a large orange, or the head of a fœtus at six months. It was contained in a cyst, apparently formed of the peritoneal reflection at its superior part, and of the cellular membrane connecting the rectum and vagina. The ovaria were of their proper size and in their natural situation. The anterior part of the rectum was inseparably connected to the tumor. The whole mass was soft and compressible; and although the cyst was in most parts very thin, it had not given way by the force employed in the delivery. The contents of the tumor were regularly disposed in layers, the concave surface of one portion being exactly adapted to the convex surface of the next, and the diameter of each about the size of a sixpence. Their colour resembled tallow, and they appeared to consist of adipocerous matter. The woman was left long in labour before the operation of turning was performed. The crotchet and blunt hook were employed before the head could be extracted. Alarming symptoms took place immediately after delivery, and she died in less than half an hour, before the placenta could be extracted. She was 44 years of age, and had been delivered of six children. In her first and sixth labours the forceps were used; but no tumor existed at the time of her former labour, at least none that could be detected. The fifth case also terminated fatally. After labour had continued a great many hours, a small-sized curved trocar was passed up the rectum and pushed into the tumor, and about six ounces of a pale yellow fluid escaped. The size of the tumor was diminished so much that it was expected the child would pass by the natural efforts; but on the following day it was found necessary to deliver by opening the head.' She died in a few days, with the usual symptoms of uterine inflammation. The right ovarium was found imbedded between the vagina and the rectum: it was about the size of a sheep's bladder, and contained fatty matter, a large quantity of hair, and the rudiments of two or three teeth.

That labour was allowed to go on too long in most of these cases there can be little doubt. In cases where the tumor is large, Dr. Merriman infers, from the results, that the perforator alone cannot be trusted to, and that experience does not warrant the practice of turning and delivering by the feet. " Upon the whole," he thinks, " the evidence we at present possess is most in favour of opening the tumors; for of the nine women who recovered more or less perfectly, five appear to owe their safety to this operation; and of the three children born alive, or supposed to be so, two were preserved by the same means."

Nothing is said by Mr. Park or Dr. Merriman, in the fourth edition of his work on Difficult Parturition (1826), respecting the propriety of inducing premature labour where it is known during pregnancy that a tumor occupies the cavity of the pelvis, and is fixed within it. As early as 1815 it appears, however, from the history of the following case, No. 60, that this subject had been fully considered by Dr. Ramsbotham, Senior; and that the operation was sanctioned by other two professional accoucheurs, and would have been performed if it had been possible to reach the os uteri.

"In April 1815, I was bespoke to attend a lady near the Mansion House; and upon calling upon her, I learnt that some years ago she had passed a living child without difficulty; that about two years before she had a bad labour, in which, after its continuing for several days, the child was destroyed, and obliged to be extracted by force, and that she narrowly escaped with her life. Having now advanced beyond the fifth month of pregnancy, she suffered much uneasiness in her mind for the result of her ensuing accouchement, and wished to place herself under my care. She was tall in person and apparently well formed; but it

was evident that some malformation or disease had taken place in the pelvis between the two preceding lyings-in: I was therefore anxious to ascertain whether the same obstacle to the passage of the child still existed. An examination being allowed, I found a large tumor of considerable solidity, but of what description I am still ignorant, filling up nearly the whole cavity of the pelvis, so as scarcely to admit the free passage of two fingers to the brim. This information placed me upon the alert, and gave me some idea of the difficulties I should in future have to contend with. I extended my inquiries to the nature of the preceding labour, the degree of difficulty attending it, and the danger following it; and having made myself acquainted with these facts as far as I was able, *I proposed the induction of premature labour, as the most likely means of diminishing the patient's sufferings.* The proposition was readily acceded to. I was now desirous of a consultation, as well for a sanction to the proceeding as for determining the most proper time to put it in practice. Two celebrated professional accoucheurs met me in consultation with Mr. ——, who had been present at the preceding difficult labour. After all the inquiries we severally could make, the induction of premature labour appeared to all to be impossible, inasmuch as the tumor so far prevented the introduction of the hand that the finger could not be carried sufficiently high to reach the os uteri. In this dilemma we had no alternative but to let the woman go her full time and take her chance. Her labour commenced on the fore part of Tuesday, June 25th, and went on slowly till evening, when the pains began to quicken. About midnight I was called, and found the os uteri dilated, the liquor amnii discharged, the pains very active, the head at the brim of the pelvis, and scarcely sufficient room to admit two fingers through the pelvis. I sent to Mr. ——, who had been requested to be again present, but he was not at home. The pains rapidly increasing in power, I determined immediately upon perforating the head, with the then intention, after evacuating the brain, of leaving it a few hours for collapse before I extracted it; but this intention I did not pursue. After the perforation was made, the labour pains soon became expulsive: I was now desirous of taking advantage of their powerful efforts to assist me in the extraction of the head; I therefore introduced the crotchet, and getting a good purchase, the vagina at the same time somewhat relaxing, I got down the head by little and little, till I at length extracted it quite crushed together. The operation took up more than four hours of very great exertion on my part. The body of the child soon followed, and the placenta was naturally excluded. The tumor was still in its original situation, but the vagina felt flaccid and loose. I was apprehensive that subsequent mischief might ensue from the pressure of the head, and the degree of violent force I was obliged to exert in the extraction of the head; but none to my knowledge followed. Febrile symptoms, which took place, gradually declined, and she completely recovered.

Dr. Ramsbotham has related the history of another case, No. 61, which occurred in 1818, in which he proposed to induce premature labour in the eighth month of pregnancy, but the patient would not consent to the operation. The first volume of Guy's Hospital Reports, published in 1836, contains a paper by Dr. Ashwell, entitled, Observations on the Propriety of inducing Premature Labour in Pregnancy complicated with Tumor, in which he strongly recommends, to obviate the morbid changes in fibrous tumors resulting from pregnancy, the same operation as proposed by Dr. Ramsbotham; but in none of the six cases related in the communication was premature labour induced. In the second volume of the same work there is a case recorded by Dr. Ashwell, of cancer of the external parts with pregnancy, in which the membranes were punctured; but the woman died soon after delivery. The seventh volume of the same work contains Observations, by Dr. Lever, on Pelvic Tumors obstructing Parturition, with cases; but in none of the cases, I believe, was the operation actually performed; so that our experience upon this point is still extremely limited.

The following cases of pregnancy and difficult labour, from ovarian and uterine tumors, have come under my observation; and it will be seen that, in one of them, the induction of premature labour did not prevent fatal inflammation and suppuration of the tumor.

In the summer of 1839, I saw a patient some miles from London, whose labour was protracted by a tumor within the pelvis, probably ovarian. She had been delivered before repeatedly, and all her labours had been natural. After she became pregnant on this occasion, she thought, from feeling two distinct swellings in the abdomen, that she had twins. When I first saw her, she had been in labour nearly twenty-four hours. The head had scarcely begun to enter the brim of the pelvis, the cavity of which was occupied by a tumor the size of a cricket-ball, or larger. Whenever a pain came on, the tumor was pressed down before the head. The forceps had been applied, but the head could not be brought before the tumor, though great and long continued efforts had been made to drag it forward. I opened the head, and had much difficulty

afterwards in drawing it down with the crotchet. In 1841, the same person being in the seventh month of pregnancy, Mr. Pickering, of Hammersmith, requested me to make an internal examination, to determine the propriety of inducing premature labour. As the tumor had risen out of the pelvis, had not enlarged, and the brim was occupied with the lower part of the uterus, I thought it best not to interfere. She went to the full period, and was safely delivered of a living child.—In another case of very protracted labour, where the hollow of the sacrum was filled up with a large ovarian cyst, I delivered by craniotomy, and the patient recovered favourably.—A woman, æt. 30, in the fifth month of her first pregnancy, began to suffer from sickness, fever, and constant pain and distention of the abdomen. On examination, it was easily perceived that the gravid uterus was pressed to the left side by a hard, painful, lobulated tumor on the right. This continued rapidly to enlarge, and to become more exquisitely painful, though leeches were applied in great numbers over the tumor, and calomel, antimony, opium, and cathartics, were administered internally. The painful distension of the abdomen soon became so great that it was necessary to obtain relief by inducing premature labour. This was easily done. For a short time after delivery the symptoms were less severe, but the fever, sickness, and painful distension, soon returned, and proved fatal. A fibrous tumor, in a state of inflammation and suppuration, was found attached by a large root to the right side of the body of the uterus. The peritoneum which covered it adhered to the parietes of the abdomen, omentum, intestines, and liver. Numerous small fibrous tumors, the blood-vessels of which have been injected, were found imbedded in other parts of the parietes of the uterus. These were in a healthy state. I was called to this case by Mr. Walker, of Marylebone Street, and it occurred in the summer of 1840.—On the 6th December, 1840, Dr. Brown requested me to see a case of pregnancy complicated with an ovarian tumor. This tumor had appeared five years before conception took place, and had slowly enlarged. The patient was in the sixth month of her first gestation, and the abdomen was enormously distended, and a fluctuation was perceived on percussion. The difficulty of breathing was so urgent that it was impossible for her to remain an instant in the horizontal position. We considered it necessary to induce premature labour, but the os uteri was so high up, and directed so much backwards, that great difficulty was experienced in passing the stiletted catheter into the uterus, to perforate the membranes. The anterior lip of the os uteri could only be reached with the tip of the figer. An instrument with a sharp point and a smaller curve than that employed could not have been introduced in this case to evacuate the liquor amnii. On the 7th, labour pains commenced. Venesection and opiates were employed to promote the dilatation of the os uteri. The nates presented, and on the 9th a dead fœtus was expelled. The relief from the delivery was great, though the abdomen continued large, and the fluctuation distinct for several weeks. August 10th, 1841. The ovarian tumor has been considerably reduced in size since the repeated application of leeches and the long-continued use of the liquor potassæ. The general health is nearly in the same condition as before pregnancy. She has again been pregnant, gone to the full period, and been delivered without any artificial assistance. Inflammation of the tumor followed, but recovery has taken place.—Twelve years ago, with Dr. Merriman and Dr. John Prout, I examined the body of a woman, æt. thirty, who had died from malignant disease of the right ovarium a few days after delivery. In the 4th month she began to suffer from uneasiness in the hypogastrium, and irritability of stomach. The countenance became sallow, and the constitutional powers greatly reduced. The abdomen not long after began rapidly to enlarge, and before the end of the seventh month it had attained the size it usually acquires at the full period. An enormous cyst, which contained a dark-coloured gelatinous fluid, was found on dissection adhering to the right ovarium, and within this cyst were a number of others of different sizes and shades of colour, which, when cut open, presented the true encephaloid or hæmatoid fungous character.

I have very little to say respecting protracted labour from *cicatrices of the vagina and cancer of the os uteri*. Where it arises from the first of these causes, the pressure of the head of the child is generally sufficient to overcome the resistance, if the uterine contractions are strong. It is proper in all cases to wait, and see what the natural efforts can do, before interfering. In one case where, from the great extent and hardness of the cicatrix, it seemed impossible for the dilatation to be effected without assistance, the most striking effect was produced by a copious venesection. In another case the edge of the cicatrix was slightly cut with a scalpel. In a third, where complete exhaustion had taken place, I extracted the child alive with the forceps; but the cicatrix was extensively lacerated. To prevent women who have cancer of the os uteri from dying undelivered, if allowed to go to the full period of pregnancy, it would be justifiable to induce premature labour even before the end of the seventh month.

CLINICAL LECTURES,

Delivered at St. Thomas's Hospital,

BY SAMUEL SOLLY, Esq. F.R.S.

Assistant-Surgeon, and Lecturer on Clinical Surgery, at St. Thomas's School.

ON INJURIES OF THE HEAD.

GENTLEMEN,—One of the accidents admitted last week, permits me to direct your attention to the subject of injuries of the head. These injuries are as important in a practical as they are interesting in a physiological point of view.

For beautifully as nature has protected the brain, the case which has been contrived for this purpose cannot be interfered with, without our fearing some disturbance of the organ it contains. And we find in practice that all injuries to the skull and the membranes which cover it without or line it within, are liable to be attended with disturbance of the instrument which the mind employs in its communications with the external world. The limits of a clinical lecture necessarily forbid my entering much into either the anatomy or physiology of the subject; nevertheless I think it desirable briefly to remind you of the varied structures which are implicated in these injuries. And as in the treatment of them it is the brain which we have especially to consider, let us review them each from the surface of this organ to the external world.

This surface of the brain, from its ganglionic nature, is so vascular, that a special membrane, the pia mater, supports its vessels, and forms its first covering. Next in order is the arachnoid, a serous membrane, placed here to prevent that friction which the constant motion of the brain renders the presence of necessary.

To the physiologist the existence of this membrane affords ample proof, even if other proof were wanting, that the brain during life moves within the skull; and to the surgeon it is interesting, as it impresses him with the importance of preventing any alteration in its structure, however slight, which could interfere with this intention, or cause the friction which its healthy condition prevents.

The next is a strong fibrous elastic membrane, which lines the bony case in which the brain is placed. It is split into bands, which are stretched in different directions like the springs of a carriage, to prevent jolts and jars. The bony covering itself is not homogeneous, but constructed internally of a dense unyielding plate, which like the steel of a helmet is to protect the brain from sharp-pointed instruments; while the outer, though less dense in material, is equally well constructed for its guardian office. The very coverings of the skull itself are important in their physiology to the surgeon. The external periosteum which nourishes the bone, and with its thousand vessels inosculates at all points with those of the dura mater within; the loose and delicate cellular membrane which connects the periosteum to the firm tendon of the occipito-frontalis; and though last in our number, not the least in practical importance, the skin, which in this situation is perhaps more interesting to the surgeon in connection with its injuries and its functions, than the skin in any part of the body.

On the present occasion I shall not call your attention to the subject of scalp wounds; but I shall take the first opportunity which is afforded me by the reception of a well-marked accident illustrating this important branch of surgery. To-day we must confine our attention to fractures of the skull, their consequences, and the treatment to be employed.

The subject of the present case, John Wingrove, æt. 33, a stone sawyer, of healthy appearance, was admitted into St. Thomas's Hospital, at ¼ before 8 A.M. on April 13th, 1843, with a compound fracture of the skull. The wound was about two inches and a half in length on the right side of the head, near the posterior extremity of the vertex. The scalp was completely divided, and the bone perfectly bare. The parietal bone was fractured in a fissured form; a portion of the outer table being depressed so that the fractured edge of the skull was distinct above it. Whether the inner table was also fractured it was impossible to say positively, but my belief is that such was not the case. [A sketch was handed round the theatre, shewing the situation and extent of the injury.] Some blood flowed from the bone, but not much. A portion of the leather lining of his cap had been driven into the wound, and was nipped so closely by edges of the bone that it was not easily removed. A small artery was bleeding on the divided edge of the scalp. I saw this man at a ¼ before nine, about one hour and a quarter after it had happened. He was quite sensible; both pupils acted perfectly naturally to the light; he complained of pain in his head, but referred it principally to the forehead. There was no paralysis of any kind; pulse small, only 60 in the minute. The accident occurred at the New Royal Exchange, and was occasioned by a blow from the head of a mason's hammer which flew off from the handle, and falling about 30 feet struck him on the head and glanced off. He was completely stunned by the blow, and had no recollection of being put into the cab by which he was conveyed to the hospital, but he recovered his senses before he arrived there.

I ordered Cat. Lini. to the wound. Calomel, grs. v. 3tiâ horâ.

½ past 12 P.M.—No change.
½ past 10 P.M.—Pulse 80, but not strong; says his head is much better, but he feels very tired and cannot sleep, but this he is not surprised at, as he never can sleep well if he has not had his usual day's work.

He has taken five doses of the calomel, and the bowels have been copiously relieved; as he has no untoward symptoms, I have discontinued the calomel.

Not more than two or three ounces of blood have been lost from the wound.

14th.—Going on well in every respect; no bad symptoms; almost free from pain in his head; pulse 64; suffers a little from cough.

Linc. pro tussi.

15th.—Has had a good deal of pain in the forehead, which he attributes to the shaking of his head from his cough. His pulse 86, but not strong; loud respiration over the whole chest. No pain in the wound or neighbourhood; bowels not open to-day.

Ordered — Calomel, gr. v., 4tâ horâ; Hirud. xxx. lateri capitis dextro. Head shaved. Pil. Ipecac. c. Conio, gr. v. 6ta. horâ. Emplast. Lytt. pectori.

16th.—Much better; his cough very much relieved; free from pain in his head; bowels not open to-day; mouth tender.

Ordered—M. S. C. stat. To omit the Cal. till to-night. A poultice to the blister.

17th, 9 A.M.—Has had a bad night; head very painful in the frontal region; pulse small, 80; looks uncomfortable; wound healthy, suppurating.

Ordered—Hirud. xxx. stat.

12 P.M.—Better; very little cough.

To omit the Pil. Ipecac. c. Conio, and to rep. Hirud. h. n.

18th.—Much better as regards his head, but the cough still troublesome.

To repeat the Ipec. c. Conio, the blister on the chest not having risen well; to paint the throat and chest with tincture of iodine. Pulv. Rhei c. Cal. grs. xv. h. n.

19th.—Much better in every respect.

20th.—Free from pain in his head, and the cough nearly gone.

21st and 22d.—I did not see him.

23d.—Going on well in every respect.

Let us now direct our attention to the man's symptoms on admission, and the treatment adopted. First, here we had a fractured skull with depression of the bone. Now some 50 or 60 years ago the trephine would have been immediately applied with the view of elevating the depressed portion. This operation, however, in the present day, is not considered justifiable in the absence of symptoms of compression, or direct irritation of the brain.

In the examination of a case of this kind, then, it is extremely important · for you to enter minutely into all those signs which indicate any injury to the brain. First, the mental condition—this was perfectly normal; he was quite sensible, and his manner natural. Next, the state of the pupils—the iris is placed before that expanded surface of the optic nerve, the retina, as an intelligent curtain to guard it from injury. The vital contrivances by which it acts, and by which its action is directed, are so beautifully perfect that the extent of the opening of the curtain is indicative of the state of the nervous apparatus it is destined to protect, by preventing such an amount of light impinging upon it as would be liable to injure it. In disease of the globe of the eye, the dilated pupil indicates more or less pressure on the retina by some cause in the globe itself, such as a permanently turgid choroid, &c. But if with a healthy eye, but in connection with a blow on the head, we find a dilated pupil, then we have the sign of some pressure or injury to the nerve in its course within the skull, or the ganglia in which it terminates.

The dilated pupil, then, indicates very serious injury to the optic nerve, or the nervous centres with which it is connected, though it may happen, as in the case of very severe concussion, the injury is remediable. The contracted pupil, on the contrary, indicates an irritability of the nervous instruments, an undue excitement of their natural function, not an obliteraton of it. You will sometimes see, in the case of injury of the brain, dilatation of one pupil and contraction of the other; where this is the case you will find the most severe injury of the brain on the side opposite the dilated pupil. I have several facts to prove this assertion, which I shall relate on a future occasion.

The next point to which our attention was directed in reference to the prognosis of the case, was the state of the wound, and the blood which flowed into it. Now the blood which flowed from the depression might be from a wounded artery of the dura mater, or simply from the bone. If from the dura mater, the injury was of course very serious: this I hoped, and believed, from its extent at the time was not the case, as I stated to one of the pupils who inquired of me what I thought of it. It soon ceased, proving that this supposition was correct; which is satisfactory, as it goes far to shew that the inner table is not fractured. That the outer table may be fractured without the inner is

proved by this preparation, where you see considerable depression of the outer without any whatever of the inner table.

We will next consider our treatment of the case. I ordered him a poultice to his head of linseed meal, to be separated from the wound by a piece of thin rag. This I did in order to encourage the bleeding, at the same time giving directions to Mr. Fixot, the dresser, to carefully watch its effects. I ordered Hydr. chlorid. gr. v. 3tiâ horâ. Now, although this man was at present free from all symptoms of serious injury to the brain, notwithstanding the depression of the bone, a few hours might entirely change his condition. Reaction had scarcely taken place from the shock of the injury, and there was no indication for the abstraction of blood from the arm. The nature of the injury was, however, such as we find frequently followed by inflammation of the membranes and substance of the brain, and to avert this calamity, I ordered the calomel.

In speaking of inflammation of the membranes of the brain let me impress upon your minds that these membranes are seldom inflamed without this hemispherical ganglion either being positively inflamed itself, or directly suffering by irritation from the effects of the contiguous inflammation; and inflammation of the pia mater is in reality inflammation of the ganglion itself, which I do not think the practitioner sufficiently considers. Now as this ganglion is that portion of the brain which more immediately than any other ministers to intellect, inflammation of it causes derangement of the intellect, and of all effects of inflammatory action on the human frame, I need not say, this is most to be dreaded. You cannot, therefore, be too much on your guard to prevent its intrusion, and to distinguish it almost before it is set up; for when once set up, it is not so easy to arrest it, and when arrested it too often leaves behind consequences which are felt for the remainder of life.

The following case, the subject of which was admitted about two years ago, so well illustrates the effect of fracture of the skull in lighting up inflammation of the hemispherical ganglion, and the symptoms of that inflammation, contrasted with the natural condition of that organ after the inflammation had been arrested, that I shall briefly detail it before proceeding further to shew you what might have occurred in this case, if I had not anticipated the threatened evil by precautionary treatment.

Inflammation of the membranes of the brain, caused by fracture of the skull, arrested by antiphlogistic measures, and aconite.

Betsy Rankin, æt. 18, works at the Ropewalk, admitted April 20th, 1841, Luke's ward for Dorcas, under Mr. Travers, Mr.

Solly in attendance. Her mother stated that she had been thrown out of a swing at Greenwich fair, a week previous to admission; that she was stunned at the time, and had suffered from severe pain in the head since; but she was not considered to be seriously injured. At the time she presented herself she exhibited an unnaturally excited appearance of the eye; she complained of violent pain in the head, but her answers to questions were perfectly rational.

One of my colleagues happening to see the case immediately after she was in bed, before I came up into the ward, and finding an irregularity of the surface of skull, cut down upon it: the pain of the incision made her very violent, and disgustingly abusive in her language. The incision permitted the escape of some coagulated blood. The division of the temporal artery gave rise to a free hæmorrhage of about 8 ounces. It exposed a fracture extending horizontally through the parietal bone to the frontal bone, and another extending perpendicularly from the above.

11 P.M. same day.—Still very violent and abusive in her language when spoken to; otherwise quiet and dosing; tongue foul; pulse quick. I explained to the sister of the ward that her violent language was to be considered as a symptom of disease, and that every thing must be effected by a soothing system and by kindness. This was scarcely understood at first, but the plan was most fully carried out, and its value afterwards most thoroughly appreciated by the sister.

Ordered—M. S. C. stat. Cal. gr. iij. quâque tertia horâ.

21st.—Bowels freely opened; last evacuation about 3 o'clock was watery; her manner is still excited, but she expresses herself much relieved, adding she only wants to be quiet. On account of the diarrhœa I ordered the Cal. to be discontinued, and Hydr. c. Cretæ gr. iij. 6ta quâque, instead.

22d.—As the bowels are now quiet, ordered the calomel to be renewed; rather more rational.

23d.—Bowels relieved, but not purged; complains of pain in her head, which is unnaturally hot. Ordered 12 leeches to be applied, if the sister of the ward could persuade her to have them on, but not to use any violence.

24th. — The leeches were applied as directed without much difficulty; her head is relieved, and she is quiet, dosing nearly the whole of the day. .

I will not detain you by going through the daily reports, but refer to the most interesting.

29th.—Much better; says that she has very little pain in the head, and no heat. Ordered a little fish; her conduct and manner to-day was quiet, natural, and well-

behaved. I found her in the middle of the day sitting up in her bed knitting.

May 1st.—As she was not quite so well to-day, exhibiting some of her previous excited manner, and fearing a return of the inflammation, I ordered, as I did not think her constitution would bear any more calomel,

Aconite gr. j. ter die; Hirud. xij.; Pil. Hydr. gr. v. ter in die.

This last medicine was continued with small doses of blue pill until the 29th, when she was dismissed quite well.

Her manner now was modest and unassuming, and she expressed herself exceedingly grateful for every thing that had been done for her in the hospital.

REMARKS.—This case affords an instance of inflammation of the hemispherical ganglion caused by injury to the skull and membranes of the brain. I regarded the girl's excited manner, her disgusting violent language, and her quickness and cunning, all as true marks of inflammatory action in this portion of the brain. When I first stated to the pupils that I regarded her language as the effect of disease, and not habitual to her, it was remarked that she was not at all insane, she was quick enough, she knew what she was about as well as any girl in the ward, and that she must be a downright bad one. The correctness of my opinion was proved by the altered manner of the girl as soon as the inflammation was entirely subdued by decided but moderate antiphlogistic measures. The beneficial effect of aconite was I consider shewn by the retrogression which occurred during its accidental omission.

In the case now in the house the most practical point for our consideration is the recurrence of the pain in his head, which you will remember he complained of when first admitted, shewing that such pain, though brought back again by the cough, was but the result of the original injury, and not, as it often is, merely sympathetic with a disturbed stomach. You will naturally say how is this likely, the forehead was not the immediate seat of the injury, but the posterior portion of the skull? This is true, but it is also true that the brain as frequently suffers from the effect of the contre-coup as from the direct blow; and I have no doubt but that the force with which the anterior lobes of the brain were driven against the frontal bone by the shock of the blow was the cause of the pain in the forehead.

We may have ample proof of the fact that the brain may be actually shaken in the skull by a blow, even though the blow does not break the skull. Sometimes, indeed, the brain is actually lacerated by such concussion, but, this I believe, only occurs in old people, where the brain has partially receded from its case in consequence of senile atrophy. I am well aware that this view of the subject is directly opposed to several very good authorities, but it is not hastily or recently formed. The following cases illustrate the fact.

Laceration of the brain from a blow, without fracture of the skull.

Elizabeth Swannell, æt. 69, a cook, was admitted under the care of Mr. Green into Elizabeth's ward, St. Thomas's Hospital, on the 24th Feb. 1841, at half-past 4 P.M. having received a large contused wound, which exposed the bone over the right eye-brow; no fracture or further external injury could be detected.

Symptoms on admission.—Perfectly insensible and motionless; left pupil very much contracted and fixed; the swelling of the surrounding parts prevented the state of the right being ascertained; breathing laboured, with a stertorous noise; pulse 96, full, and not easily compressed; extremities moderately warm; fæces and urine involuntarily passed; great rigidity of the muscles, especially of the right arm and left leg; frothy saliva issuing from the mouth. No spirituous odour could be detected in the breath.

History.—Shortly after 2 o'clock, while going down stairs, she suddenly fell, and was picked up exactly in the same state in which she was brought to the hospital; was not subject to fits; nobody saw the accident.

Treatment.—A surgeon had bled her in the left arm previous to admission; soon after admission she was cupped to ℥ix. from the nape of the neck, a large blister was applied to the back part of the head, which was shaved, and hot water to her feet. Breathing slightly relieved by cupping; pulse continued full, and 92. At 9 o'clock I saw her with Mr. B. Travers, apparently exactly in the same state, except that her pulse varied in frequency from 76 to 92; it was very full, but did not indicate sufficient strength to bear further loss of blood. Her breathing was not quite so laboured. At 11 o'clock I gave her gr. iij. of calomel.

Feb. 25, 9 A.M.—No improvement in respect of sensation or motion; breathing a little impeded by mucus; much frothy saliva issuing from the mouth. She remained exactly in the same state, her pulse continuing full, and about 90, till within two or three minutes of her death, which took place at 10 minutes past 4 P.M.

Post-mortem examination.—The brain did not seem to fill the skull completely. No morbid appearance on the surface of the brain. Tentorium smeared with blood. *Interior.*—Extensive effusion of blood into the left ventricle; some into the right: this effusion appears to have resulted from laceration of the left corpus striatum and thala-

mus, also of those fibres of the great commissure which forms the anterior part of the roof of the left ventricle. The lacerated corpus striatum and thalamus were forced into the right ventricle under the fornix, and when first observed looked almost like a medullary tumor with an ulcerated surface. In this case the brain appears to have been lacerated by the contre-coup, to which it was especially exposed from its diminished size in relation to its containing cavity—the result of senile atrophy.

April 4, 1843.—Dr. Bright makes a statement, in the 2d Vol. of his Reports of Medical Cases, page 663, confirmatory of the view that I have taken of the brain not completely filling the skull in old persons. See also, p. 683.

The next case will impress upon your minds the serious effects which may be produced by contre-coup, and the necessity and advantage of combating them carefully.

Injury to the head.

William Pearson, æt. about 40, a pot-boy at a public-house, was admitted into George's ward under my care, May 16th, 1842, with a small lacerated wound on the left side of the head; he was intoxicated at the time of admission. The accident was caused by his being knocked down or run over by a cart, I could not learn which.

The case was regarded by the dresser as one of intoxication, and I did not see him until the following morning.

17th.—He now complains much of pain in his head; but, with this exception, there were no symptoms indicative of cerebral mischief, and the headache I considered more characteristic of disordered stomach than brain. There was no drowsiness, and his manner was natural; he referred the pain to his forehead, and not to the seat of injury; his pupils acted naturally.

I ordered—Pulv. Jalapæ c. Cal. ℥j. stat. M. S. C. 6ta. hor. post.

In the evening, finding that though his bowels had been relieved, the pain in the head continued, I ordered him Calomel, gr. v. 4ta. hora.

18th.—Symptoms much the same.

Ordered—Opium, gr. j. at night, and repeat the Cal. and Jalap as a purge.

19th.—Has had convulsive movements of the left side of the face of an epileptic character. Tongue drawn to the left side. Constantly spitting a large quantity of frothy saliva. Both pupils are alike, and slightly contracted, but act freely to the light. Pulse 116, weak. He is quite conscious, and answers all questions naturally, though he has not perfect power of speech. I again examined the head, and, for the first time, perceived that there was some tenderness on pressure on the right of the head, opposite the wound. Ordered—

Hirudines xx. to the right side of the head ; to be followed by a blister.

Opii Tinctura, ℈xxx. ; Spirit. Ammon. Arom. ʒss. ; Mist. Camphor. ʒj. hac nocte.

20th.—Says he found relief from the leeches, and his head is much better, though still very bad. Pulse soft.

22d.—No appearance of twitching, but tongue still drawn to the left side. Has vomited some greenish bile. Pulse soft.

Ordered—Hirudines xxx. to the right side. Port wine ʒvj. in arrow-root.

23d.—Says her head is much better, though not quite free from pain. Has only had one fit of convulsive twitching since the last report. Pulse still weak.

Ordered—Quinine, gr. ij. b. d.

24th.—Much better ; free from headache ; no twitching since yesterday ; appetite returning. Pulse weak, 80.

Quinine and a pint of porter daily, in addition to the wine.

This man perfectly recovered, and left the hospital quite well soon after the last report.

I have no doubt that the convulsive twitchings in this case were occasioned by some injury to the brain produced by the contre-coup, and the case is instructive from its showing how gradually serious symptoms will sometimes arise some days after the receipt of injury. The result of the local depletion and counter-irritation bear out this view of it, and the general tonic plan which was indicated by the previous habits of the man, and his state of constitution, is important to attend to, from the success which followed its adoption.

These two cases will, I trust, impress upon your minds the importance of attending to possible effects of the contre-coup ; and our present case shews how necessary it is to arrest as soon as possible, in all cases of injury to the head, bronchial irritation, occasioning cough. As a general rule, in all recent cases of injury to the brain you would avoid the irritation of a blister, but in the present case it was very evident that the irritation of the cough, and its influence on the brain, was more serious than the irritation of the blister was likely to be. Finally, let me warn you of considering the patient out of danger who has received so serious an injury as in the case before us, notwithstanding its present favourable progress. Its termination, whether favourable or otherwise, I shall call your attention to at our next meeting.

SOME PRACTICAL REMARKS
on the
EMPLOYMENT OF ARSENIC IN THE TREATMENT OF THE DISEASES OF THE SKIN.

By John E. Erichsen.

[Continued from p. 202.]

The circumstances that contraindicate the employment of the arsenical preparations are divisible into three classes :—

1st, Those that relate to the temperament and habit of body of the patient.

2d, The complication of the cutaneous affection with other diseases.

3d, The nature, stage, and condition of the disease of the skin itself.

1st, As regards the temperament and habit of body of the individual. It is a matter of the utmost importance in the administration of the preparation of arsenic, more so indeed than in the employment of any other remedy with which I am acquainted, to look well to the constitution and temperament of the patient to whom we are about to administer it. It will (I think, invariably) be found that arsenic, in any form, is very badly borne by individuals of a plethoric habit of body, or of a highly sanguine or sanguineo-nervous temperament ; so much so, indeed, as most commonly to be inadmissible in the treatment of cutaneous diseases occurring in such persons. This, from the stimulating properties of the metal, we should, à priori, have been led to expect. In individuals of a ruddy complexion, with blue eyes, light or fine hair, thin delicate skins, and in whom the circulating and nervous systems are naturally very excitable, whose hearts beat and cheeks flush under the influence of even slight mental emotion, it will constantly be found that the digestive organs become so irritated, and the nervous system so excited, under the use of the arsenic, that it is impossible to employ it in any such dose as can be expected to produce a beneficial effect upon the cutaneous affection. The pulse in these cases becomes rapidly accelerated, irritation and even subacute inflammation of the gastric mucous membrane supervenes, the patient complains of headache, and a sense of tension or weight in the forehead; and as the skin partakes of the general excitement into which the system is thrown, the cutaneous inflammation may very probably become aggravated rather than benefited by the exhibition of the remedy. It might, in some of these cases, be deemed advisable to prepare the system for the administration of the arsenicals by bleeding and purging; but, in the great majority of instances, such a procedure would not be advisable, as the habit of body to which I am alluding is one of irritability rather than of tone; one which, though readily excitable, will not bear depletion. The following cases may be mentioned in illustration of the effects of arsenic on individuals of this temperament:—

Miss E. B., æt. 22, came under my care on the 20th of December last, for an eczematous eruption on the neck, forehead, and scalp, under which she had laboured for four or five months. She is of moderate conformation, has blueish gray eyes, light brown hair, a very bright colour, and a quick though very irritable and weak pulse, varying from 84 to 90, and much accelerated when she is spoken to quickly, or when under the influence of any mental emotion. Has no dyspeptic symptoms of any consequence, nor does she suffer from any disease of the heart or lungs; but yet she complains of feeling weak and delicate, which she attributes to being much confined to the house, and prevented from taking due exercise. There are a number of irregular, yellowish gray, dry, laminated crusts on various parts of the scalp, with a scaly and furfuraceous condition of the forehead, ears, and neck, the skin of these parts being red, itching, and hot, with occasional exacerbations of the disease, and eruptions of the characteristic vesicles. Generally, however, the diseased parts had a dry furfuraceous aspect, and were not bedewed with moisture. The hair of the head was ordered to be cut off as closely as possible, and emollient fomentations and poultices to be used until the scabs were separated, and the irritation in the ears, neck, and forehead subdued. She was at the same time put upon the dilute nitric acid, with occasional slightly alterative and

aperient medicines; and the diet was ordered to be as mild and unstimulating as possible. She continued this plan of treatment until the 11th Jan., when, as no very decided improvement had taken place, it was determined to put her upon a course of Donovan's solution. I may mention that, during the whole of this time, the affected patches had been so irritable as to bear no application except such as were of a most emollient nature, and the oxide of zinc ointment; and even this seemed at times to irritate.

On the 11th of January, accordingly, she was ordered ten minims (the third of the usual dose) of the liquor of the hydriodate of arsenic and mercury three times a day. On the 15th the dose of the solution was increased to fifteen minims. On the 16th she complained of headache and lassitude, with some thirst; the old patches of the disease were much more irritable than they had previously been, and a fresh eruption of vesicles had taken place on them, as well as between the shoulders, and for some way down the back, where the affection had not before appeared. The solution was immediately ordered to be discontinued, some salines were given, and the irritation in the diseased surfaces was quieted by means of emollient applications. The nitric acid plan of treatment was then resumed, and persevered in for some little time, without permanent benefit.

As this was one of the first cases in which I had employed Donovan's solution, I was anxious to ascertain whether the irritation that had supervened during its use was attributable to the arsenic contained in it, or to some other cause. I therefore determined to try the effect of small doses of Fowler's solution. With this view I ordered her, on the 31st January, two minims of the solution of the arsenite of potassa, to be taken twice a day, On the 3d of February the same symptoms occurred that manifested themselves after the administration of Donovan's solution; there was some constitutional disturbance, with a decided exacerbation of the disease, so as to necessitate the discontinuance of the remedy. After this a number of different medicinal agents were employed, but none seemed to exercise any very permanent influence upon the complaint;

and the patient eventually left for Brighton, in the hope that change of air might benefit her.

Sophia Dewberry, æt. 23, a servant, a very healthy-looking girl, of small stature, florid complexion, dark grayish eyes, brown hair, with a quick excitable pulse, was placed under my care for pityriasis of the face and psoriasis of the lips, of between four and five years' standing. The pityriasis occupied both cheeks and the forehead, the skin of which part was somewhat reddened, and covered with furfuraceous scales. The psoriasis was confined to the lips, which were much fissured, and covered, in parts, with dark-coloured squamæ, the dark tinge arising from the oozing of blood from the rhagades in the lips when they were moved, as in laughing or eating. No cause could be assigned for the disease of the face. The general health was good, the tongue was clean, menstruation regular, and there were no dyspeptic symptoms of any kind.

As she had been submitted to a variety of treatment previous to my seeing her, without deriving any benefit, and as she was anxious, for obvious reasons, to get rid of the complaint under which she laboured, I determined to try the effect of the solution of the arsenite of potassa. She was accordingly ordered two minims of Fowler's solution twice a day, together with white precipitate ointment as a local application. On the third day of taking the arsenical, she began to complain of pain in the head, chiefly its fore part, of thirst, languor, and loss of appetite. On the following day I ordered her, as soon as I saw her, to discontinue the use of the mineral, and to take some saline medicine. She was then put upon a course of liquor potassa and tincture of cantharides, under the use of which remedies she soon got well.

These cases illustrate strikingly how ill able individuals of an excitable or sanguineo-nervous temperament are to bear even the most minute doses of arsenic. Both the patients whose cases have just been detailed were marked examples of the sanguineo-nervous temperament. In both the digestive organs were in a healthy condition, and in both the arsenic acted as too powerful a stimulant on the stomach

and nervous system, even when employed in so minute a dose as the forty-eighth or fiftieth of a grain twice a day.

2d, There are several diseases the co-existence of which with an affection of the skin should contra-indicate the employment of the preparations of arsenic. Amongst the most common of these is one that is very frequently met with in persons labouring under certain forms of chronic cutaneous disease, and of the non-existence of which it is always necessary to satisfy ourselves before prescribing arsenic in any form, as it would infallibly be much aggravated by the use of this mineral. The complaint in question is the irritative or inflammatory gastric dyspepsia; that form of indigestion which is characterized by slow and painful digestion— by a sensation of heat and oppression at the epigastrium, increased by food, by the pressure of the hand or of the clothes — by thirst, dryness of the mouth on waking, a sensation of heat and stiffness about the eyes — by a sharp pulse, rather high-coloured urine, unsound unrefreshing sleep, irritability of temper, more or less lassitude, and a costive state of the bowels; in short, by that train of symptoms that have been so well and accurately described by Dr. Todd, under the name of inflammatory gastric dyspepsia. It is more particularly necessary to be on our guard against the administration of the arsenical preparations to patients suffering from this form of indigestion, as the state of the stomach here described is very often accompanied by a papular and scaly condition of the skin, something between lichen and psoriasis, which might be thought to indicate these remedies in a peculiar manner, but which would certainly, in such a state of the system, not be benefited by their employment, whilst the irritation of the gastric mucous membrane would infallibly be much increased. It is, indeed, impossible for a patient labouring under inflammatory gastric dyspepsia to bear even the most moderate doses of the arsenical preparations, as these remedies have, in healthy individuals, a direct tendency to produce that very disease, the frequency of the occurrence of which, and the readiness with which it may be excited in persons of a sanguine or sanguineo-nervous temperament, explains to a certain degree, no doubt, why arsenic is so badly borne by individuals of such a habit of body.

Besides irritative gastric dyspepsia, any other local inflammatory condition of the system, or the supervention of phthisis, will contra-indicate the employment of so powerfully stimulating a tonic as arsenic.

3d, One of the most important considerations to be attended to in the employment of arsenic is the kind of diseases to which it may be administered with an expectation of success; and when this has been ascertained, the particular stage of the affection at which it should be given; for, as will immediately be shewn, it may be useless, or even injurious, at one period of a complaint, but of the utmost service at another.

In order to avoid repetition I shall here omit the consideration of the particular diseases in which the employment of arsenic is contra-indicated (the list being a long one), for as I shall have occasion, in a subsequent part of this paper, to mention those in which its administration may be useful, the others will be learnt by exclusion.

With regard to the stage of a cutaneous disease in which arsenic is admissible, it may be stated, in general terms, that it only is so when these affections have assumed somewhat of a chronic inactive character, after the irritative or inflammatory condition that characterizes the earlier stages of most of them has been removed. Diseases of the skin, with but very few exceptions, are of an essentially inflammatory nature. We find the ordinary symptoms of inflammation, as it affects other tissues, present in them, more particularly during their earlier stages; the "tumor et rubor cum calore et dolore" occur to a greater or less degree in almost all of them; and the products of inflammation also, whether consisting in the effusion of serum, pus, or lymph, or in modifications of the natural structure and functions of the skin, are observable in most. This fact is of especial value in regard to the treatment of these diseases; which, indeed, consists of nothing more than the treatment of inflammation in its active or its passive forms. As long as the inflammatory action going on in

the integuments partakes of an active character, arsenic, being a powerfully stimulating tonic, is necessarily contra-indicated; and it is not until the disease has assumed a passive or atonic condition that this mineral can be tolerated; for if it be administered in the active acute stage of an affection of the skin, more particularly of one that is connected with, or dependent upon, a phlogistic condition of the system generally, it cannot fail, from the excitant properties that it has been shown to possess, in increasing the inflammatory condition that already exists. It is from the want of due attention to this point that so much difference of opinion exists as to the real value of the preparations of arsenic, not only in cutaneous affections generally, but also in the treatment of individual diseases of the skin. A medical man finds, amongst a number of remedies, arsenic strongly recommended in a particular disease, as lepra or eczema, for example; but as there is no mention made as to the period of the affection in which it should be employed, he very probably administers it whilst the complaint is still in an active inflammatory condition: the consequence of this is, that the disease being stimulated unduly, becomes aggravated in its symptoms, and the confidence of the practitioner in a very valuable remedy is shaken; whereas, had it been employed a few weeks later, the happiest results might have attended its administration. But the question naturally arises, how is the period at which arsenic is admissible to be ascertained? It cannot certainly be a matter of time, for in one case the same disease may be in a more active inflammatory condition at the end of months, or even years, than it will in another at the expiration of but a few days or weeks. In answer to this I may state, that I think it will usually be found, with sufficiently few exceptions indeed to make it a general rule, that the administration of arsenic is contra-indicated in all those cases of cutaneous disease in which topical stimulants of a mild nature, such as the ointment of the white precipitate, or of the nitrate of mercury diluted with equal parts of the spermaceti ointment, or a solution of the sulphuret of potassium in the proportion of about a drachm to the

℞

pint, increase permanently the severity of the affection. I do not mean to imply by this that the reverse holds good, viz. that a disease in which external stimulants are employed with success should necessarily benefit by the administration of arsenicals; far from it; but I cannot recal to mind a single case that has improved under the use of this mineral that did not bear the employment of gently stimulating ointments or lotions, provided always that the disease did not occur in a person of a very highly excitable or irritable temperament, or in one labouring under irritation of the gastric mucous membrane, or other such decidedly contra-indicating affection.

In confirmation of this I may adduce as an example that very common disease eczema, which, when in its acute stage, in which it could bear no other topical applications than the most soothing poultices and fomentations, would infallibly be greatly increased in severity by the employment of arsenic even in its most minute doses, will, at a more advanced period, when it has fallen into a passive condition, improve under the use of the mineral, at the same time that it receives the most decided benefit from the application of topical excitants, such as the white precipitate or nitrate of mercury ointments, and sulphureous baths or washes. And this is nothing more than we should à priori expect; for if, as I think there can be no doubt, arsenic acts as an excitant to the integumentary system, amongst the other tissues and organs, stimulating in a peculiar way the cutaneous capillaries, we cannot suppose this stimulus to be beneficial from within, unless it also is so from without.

The circumstances, then, under which the employment of arsenic in cutaneous diseases is contra-indicated having been pointed out, we shall easily arrive at a knowledge of those cases in which its administration is likely to be attended by beneficial results. It has already been shown, that the use of the preparations of this metal is exceedingly hazardous in individuals of a sanguine or sanguineo-nervous temperament and excitable habit of body, or in those who suffer from, or are peculiarly disposed to, irritative gastric dyspepsia, or any inflammatory disor-

der. On the other hand, they are in most cases borne well by individuals of a somewhat phlegmatic, debilitated, or lax habit of body, more particularly if they are past the middle age, with a pale cachectic complexion, languid weak circulation, and a general want of tone about the system, acting upon such patients as powerful and useful tonics. In persons of this habit of body the diseases of the skin appear rather to be dependent upon a degree of debility or want of power in the cutaneous capillaries; and it is in these patients that the preparations of arsenic are of great service, in exciting, in a peculiar manner, a more healthy action in this class of vessels, thereby modifying or removing those morbid changes that are the results of an abnormal condition in their secernent and nutrient functions.

The diseases of the skin that are likely to be benefited by the employment of the arsenical preparations belong to very different orders in all classifications of these affections; but however widely they may be separated by artificial arrangement, they all agree in this one important respect, that they are characterized by the presence of scales or scurf; that even when they do not belong to the order *Squamæ*, they are usually but little benefitted until they arrive at that stage in which they assume a furfuraceous or scaly condition, in which state the boundary line between them and the real squamous diseases is, in very many cases, but very faintly marked. Thus, in the earlier stages of eczema, for example, arsenic is, in any form, decidedly useless, if not positively injurious; but when once this disease has fallen into that condition in which there is no longer any distinct evolution of vesicles, but, in their place, a serous fluid, which exudes at times, and dries rapidly into thin furfuraceous scales or laminæ, the subjacent skin being red, glazed, dry, and more or less fissured and cracked, the use of these remedies will often be productive of the most decidedly beneficial results.

[To be continued.]

———

CASE OF
SCARLATINA ANGINOSA.

By Charles Vines, Esq.
Surgeon to the Reading Dispensary.

To the Editor of the Medical Gazette.

Sir,

Should you consider the following case of sufficient interest, its early insertion in your valuable periodical will much oblige me.—I am, sir,

Your obedient servant,
Charles Vines.

5, Castle Street, Reading,
May 2, 1843.

February 26th, 1843, at 11 A.M. I was requested to visit Edwin Howel, æt. 12 years, of tolerably good constitution, and whose appearances were as follows: he was lying in bed on his left side, and perfectly insensible; complexion pale; features distorted; lips extremely livid; the head hot; eyelids closed; pupils insensible to light; the jaws closed, inside of mouth lined with a viscid mucous; breathing hurried and stertorous, carotids throbbed violently; extremities rather cold, hands clenched, scarcely any pulsation at the wrist; skin moist and clammy; on calling loudly into his ear he took no notice. His mother stated that he had been rather feverish for the last two days, and that yesterday he had a *rigor*; that she gave him an opening powder which operated freely this morning: the motions were green, offensive, and watery: he had passed a restless night. On taking a little tea early this morning he had difficulty in swallowing.

Treatment.—I first bled my patient in the arm to 8 ounces; the blood was dark and thick, and flowed slowly; mustard poultices were applied to the calves of the legs and soles of the feet, of these he took no notice; his head was then shaved and ten leeches applied to the temples and forehead; these bled freely, still the symptoms continued. My patient was then placed in a warm bath, where he remained about a quarter of an hour, cold water being applied to his head; during this time his arm commenced bleeding afresh, and he lost a few ounces more of blood; when in the bath slight reaction took place, but on being put to bed he relapsed into his former condition. His motions passed away at

this time involuntarily; at half-past seven in the evening, finding his symptoms worse, the breathing more oppressed, pulse at the wrist imperceptible, the carotids still acting violently, I ordered cupping on the crown of the head, and a cupping glass was applied immediately over the lambdoidal suture: at first he took no notice of the operation, but after 6 ounces of blood had been extracted, he raised his hand and endeavoured to pull off the glass, struggled to get away from his father who was supporting him, and evinced displeasure at the operation. On being again placed in bed consciousness was much more complete; he appeared to understand the questions asked, although he made no attempt to answer them; the pupils were more sensible to light; pulse at the wrist more distinct, and the symptoms altogether considerably relieved; the surface of the body was, however, cold and clammy. An enema consisting of 1 ounce Sp. Terebinth. and 2 drms. Tinct. Assafœtid. in a pint of gruel, was then administered: this he strongly objected to, endeavouring to force the instrument from him: about half the injection was retained. He was now able after considerable exertion to swallow a little liquid, and ten grains of calomel, mixed with a little sugar, were placed in his mouth: this, with the aid of some tea, passed into the stomach. A liniment composed of croton oil, ammonia and soap liniment, was then rubbed freely over the outside of the throat.

At half-past 9 P.M. the countenance was more calm and natural. The lips had lost their livid hue; the carotids comparatively quiet; pulse at wrist quick, but much more distinct; extremities warm, and he expressed by signs that he was better, but still swallowed with great difficulty. I ordered a tea-spoonful of gruel to be placed in his mouth occasionally, and a fourth part of the following every two or three hours.

R Liq. Ant. Pot. Tart. 3j.; Liq. Ammon. Ac. ℥ss.; Sp. Æth. Nit. 3j.; Aq. Menth. Sat. ad. ℥iij. M. ft. Mist.

27th, 9 A.M.—My patient had passed a restless night; had been delirious; bowels had not acted; head a little hotter than natural; surface of body generally warm; pulse extremely quick and small; complained much of his throat, and had a great dread of taking any thing into his mouth; the tonsils, tongue, lining membrane of mouth and fauces, very red and swollen.

To continue the mixture, and to take the following powders.

℞ Ant. Potassio-Tart. gr. ⅓; Hydrarg. Chlorid. gr. ij.; Pulv. Trag. Co. gr. iij.; M. ft. Pulvis, 4ta. q. h.

9 P.M.—Reaction more fully established, but deglutition still very difficult; bowels had been open twice.

A blister to be applied to the throat, and the medicines continued.

28th.—Had slept a little during the night; blister had drawn well; the throat slightly relieved; gums affected by the calomel; countenance calm; no pain except from the throat; pulse a little fuller.

Ordered a chloride of soda solution for the mouth. To discontinue the calomel.

March 1st.—My patient had slept much better; deglutition more easy, and consequently able to take more nourishment; pulse fuller, but soft; bowels confined.

To continue the mixture, with the addition of 2 drs. of sulphate of magnesia.

In the evening a roseolar appearance shewed itself on the hands and arms, also slightly on the face.

2d, 9 A.M.—Had slept several hours during the night; able to speak distinctly; expressed himself much better; throat almost free from pain; roseolar appearance of skin more distinct; pulse tolerably full and soft; bowels were well open during the day.

3d.—Had slept nearly all night; roseolar blush of skin had disappeared; could swallow almost as well as usual. From this period my patient gradually progressed towards recovery, and in the course of a fortnight was quite restored to health.

OBSERVATIONS.—The history of this case, in connection with others lately occurring in my practice, has suggested the few following observations. In the first place, what was the condition of the patient here described? I would answer, a state of coma or asphyxia, that kind of coma induced by unhealthy non-arterialized blood circulating in the brain. The brain had become narcotized, unfitted to perform its peculiar function. And the heart, not receiving its usual supply of nervous stimulus, nor a due share of arterial or oxygenized blood, was depressed in its action; thus vitality weakened would soon have ceased altogether. Superadded to this condition must have been that of arterial excitement, evidenced by the throbbing of the carotids, and thus, according to Dr. Kellie, the overcharged cerebral arteries, compressing their corresponding veins, would tend to impede still further the circulation within the cranium, and consequently of the vascular system generally. Hence the whole system was in a state of congestion, each vital organ participating in this depressed condition of the grand nervous centre.

To what cause, then, are we to attribute this comatose or asphyxiated condition? To an inflammatory condition of the throat, viz. effusion into the cellular membrane of the throat and fauces causing obstruction to the entrance of air into the lungs (apnœa); or to arterial excitement impeding the vascular circulation within the brain? I am inclined to suppose by a combination of the two causes. From the history of the case, the rigor which preceded the difficulty of swallowing, and the throbbing of the carotids, there can be no doubt as to the arterial excitement; and we have equal evidence that there was obstruction of the throat. Those who contend for the action of a specific poison in cases of fever might say that the symptoms were attributable to this agent exerting a depressing influence on the brain and nervous system generally; but I think that the treatment of the case disproves such a notion. Now blood-letting, in the first instance, proved to be the only efficient remedy; but a quantity of blood taken from the arm and temples produced no effect. The warm bath effected only slight reaction, followed by more decided collapse; but on the abstraction of a few ounces of blood from the vertex of the head, the brain was instantly relieved. The blood was extracted opposite the upper angle of the occipital bone, just at the junction of the sagittal and lambdoidal sutures. The longitudinal sinus traversing the upper surface of the brain in this situation communicates freely with the cranial bones, and the quick removal of blood in this situation tended to relieve the vessels immediately in the neighbourhood. A stimulating injection then served to rouse the central organs, and, by a reflex action on the nervous system, materially aided to rally the sinking powers. Reaction having been once established, no further stimulants were requisite; in fact they were contraindicated by an inflammatory tendency in the system.

It is evident, from the case in question, that the pulse afforded no criterion as to the necessity for the abstraction of blood. When the patient was first seen his pulse was scarcely perceptible. To have given stimulants, with the idea of waiting till signs of reaction manifested themselves, would have been dangerous in the highest degree, since the proximate source of the depressed circulation existed in the brain: the removal of blood, then, in order to relieve the oppressed state of the cerebral organ, afforded the patient the only chance of recovery.

Other severe cases of head affection having, as I before observed, lately occurred to me, I hope shortly to introduce them to your notice.

R E M A R K S

ON SOME

CRITICISMS ON A LATE REVIEW
IN THE BRITISH AND FOREIGN
MEDICAL REVIEW.

BY DR. GOLDING BIRD.

"Folget nun des meisters worten
Was er sagt, gilt aller orten.
Nicht die Form zeigt euch die wahrheit,
Nicht der Stoff führt euch zur klarheit,
Müsset beide gleich behandeln,
Wollt ihr nicht im Irrthum wandeln."

IN a late number of the Lancet, a letter has been published by Mr. Ancell, in which he has endeavoured to invalidate the correctness of the observations made by the author of an able review of Dr. B. Jones's work on Calculus and Gout, in the last number of the British and Foreign Medical Review. As the arguments to which Mr. Ancell particularly takes exception are the same as those which I brought forward in my lectures at Guy's Hospital, and which were published in this journal, I feel myself called upon to take some public notice of the strictures made upon them. In doing this, I shall content myself with alluding strictly to that portion of Professor Liebig's views to which Mr. Ancell has alluded; not

with a view of exciting an useless discussion, but for the purpose of shewing that he has not succeeded in proving the "futility of the objection" brought forward by the reviewer.

The opinion that urea and uric acid are formed from the destructive assimilation of effete animal tissues, advanced by Dr. Prout, and brought forward by Liebig in his late work, is now conventionally admitted. In fact, there can scarcely be a reasonable doubt on the correctness of this view. Liebig has gone further than this, and has laid it down as an axiom, that urea and uric acid are produced by oxygenation of tissues, the latter being produced when too little oxygen is present to allow the former to be generated, and hence that in reptiles slowly respiring, and consequently but little exposed to the influence of oxygen, an abundance of uric acid is excreted in the urine, which is replaced by urea, as we ascend the scale of animal life, until, in the warm-blooded carnivoræ, deposits of uric acid are unknown. I endeavoured to shew, in one of my lectures, the unsatisfactory nature of this sweeping generalization, by the case of birds, the semi-solid urine of many of which consists of a large proportion of uric acid. This objection, so far from being met by Mr. Ancell, is, in fact, avoided in defending Liebig's statement, that the ulterior conversion of animal matter into urea may take place alike at the surface of the metamorphosed tissue, and in the secreting organ,—a proposition of very little consequence, as it neither admits of proof or refutation. The winged inhabitants of the South American rocks have covered these islets with a thick layer of guano (urate and oxalate of ammonia essentially), in spite of their possessing the very conditions which Liebig assumes ought to prevent the formation of uric acid; for they possess higher temperature, more active respiration, and a greater proportionate number of blood corpuscles[*], than any other class of animals; they breathe the oxygen of the air with the aqueous vapour exhaling from the ocean surrounding their maritime resting-places; they, for any thing

---

[*] Or, in Liebig's own words, "Die Temperatur des Blutes ist im Allgemeinen bei den Vögeln höher, als bei den anderen Thierklassen, ebenso haben die Vögel die meister Blutkörperchen." HANDWORTERBUCH, B. 1. s. 202.

that is known to the contrary, drink water enough for all the conditions required by the theory, or rather hypothesis, of Liebig; and yet these sea birds, in common with many of their inland allies, pertinaciously oppose the dogma of the professor of Giessen, by dropping from their cloacæ urate of ammonia.

Mr. Ancell's criticisms are most pointedly levelled at certain deductions drawn from a table which has been quoted by the reviewer on my authority, and which was first published in my lectures as giving a view of some of M. Becquerel's clinical observations. This table, with the exception of a slight numeric error, which has been pointed out, is perfectly correct, and the numbers it contains were carefully calculated by myself. The intention with which I exhibited this table to my pupils was to demonstrate to them that the ratio between inflammatory action, or excessive oxygenation, and the disappearance of uric acid laid down by Liebig as a law, was not in accordance with recorded experience. In the cases of well-marked chlorosis, where every symptom, and even the very state of the blood, proves that oxygenation, in the view assumed by Liebig, must be most imperfect, and therefore where we ought to have excess of uric acid, we have nothing of the kind: yet no one can deny that metamorphosis of tisssue goes on in this case. Mr. Ancell ingeniously attempts to explain the difficulty by alluding to the fact that blood-corpuscules are decidedly deficient in this affection; and yet, a page further on, this gentleman uses the very same argument to explain the presence of uric deposits in inflammatory diseases. Thus the diminution of red particles (carriers of oxygen of Liebig) is used at once to explain the partial absence of uric acid in anæmia, and its excess in phlegmasiæ. I think it is not too much to denounce such ancipital arguments as utterly worthless, and destitute of any thing like a true scientific character. Let us, however, for a moment, take two cases, one of excessive pulmonary emphysema, and the other of acute hepatitis; being two of those quoted in the table. In the former, where the lung has undergone a change almost approaching to that of the turtle, and where the cold surface, the leaden lips, all attest imperfect oxygenation;

and in the latter, where the intense inflammatory fever present shows this process, according to Liebig's interpretation of the phenomena of inflammation*, to be carried on in excess. In the latter, therefore, uric acid should nearly disappear from the urine, and in the former be in excess; whilst the very reverse of this really occurs. But even if these cases did really bear out Liebig's view, how can a diminution of red particles in both cases explain such different effects?

We have an excellent illustration of the effects of extending a theory to its utmost limits, in the remarks on the urine of phthisis, which is declared to be a disease of excessive oxygenation, and therefore one in which uric acid deposits can scarcely exist. This is stated directly by Dr. Jones (p. 11), and distinctly implied by Professor Liebig (p. 137). In opposition to this, I brought forward facts which appeared to me sufficient to shew that this dogma, founded on reasoning in the laboratory, was opposed to actual experience so far as it had extended. Mr. Ancell again endeavours to explain this discrepancy between fact and theory by means of the blood-corpuscules, which, being diminished in phthisis, ought to produce an excess of uric acid. Liebig, however, states that there ought to be nothing of the kind; and thus the Professor and Mr. Ancell are opposed. In justice to the latter gentleman, however, we must not forget that he appears to be by no means satisfied with the piece of special pleading regarding the blood-discs in this disease, as explaining the existence of what Liebig denies, and in another part of his criticisms he inquires whether uric acid may not be in excess late in the disease only.

In commenting on another portion of the review, Mr. Ancell declares that the statement there made, that 100 grains of azotised solids are daily excreted by the skin, is advanced "most fallaciously." I am ignorant on what grounds this bold charge is hazarded; certainly on no facts at present before the profession. In my lecture I gave the results of the well-known experi-

---

* "In consequence of the acceleration of the circulation in the state of fever, a greater amount of arterial blood, and consequently of oxygen, is conveyed to the diseased parts as well as to all other parts."—LIEBIG, p. 256.

ments of Seguin and Anselmino, and shewed that in 24 hours the skin exhaled:—

Organic matter	107·47 grains	
Saline matter .	81·92	„
Volatile matter	15650·61	„

15840.

These 107·47 grains of organic matter are as rich in nitrogen as many other effete products of vital chemistry, and closely resemble the *extrait de viande* of Berzelius. I have in more than one instance detected distinct evidence of the presence of urea in it. Is it, then, just to denounce the statement that azotised matter is exhaled from the skin, as "most fallacious?"

Throughout the whole of his criticisms, the varying quantity of blood-corpuscules, or carriers of oxygen, in the blood, constitutes Mr. Ancell's great *cheval de bataille*. The very grounds of his defence of Liebig's hypothesis on this point are debateable; even Andral's and Lecanu's analyses, to which he refers, are not satisfactory. Their mode of determining the preparation of blood-discs is by no means free from error; in fact, we know of no means at present of doing so with any amount of accuracy; and were Mr. Ancell more practically acquainted with the difficulties surrounding quantitative analyses of blood, he would learn to be very cautious before he founded arguments of this importance upon them. The elegant and luminous researches of Dr. Rees on the anatomical and physical properties of the blood-corpuscule have thrown much light on this difficult problem in zoochemistry (Guy's Reports, April 1843).

To turn, however, more particularly to Liebig's doctrine, that blood-corpuscules are carriers of oxygen: on what proof does this rest? All the few facts he has advanced in support of this hypothesis admit of other explanations. He has, indeed, declared the iron to exist in venous blood as protoxide, and in arterial as sesquioxide: where, again, I may venture to inquire, is the proof of this statement? We look in vain for one, but find indeed the following sentence: "Let us now assume that the iron in venous blood is in the state of protoxide," p. 273. Liebig then goes on to develop his hypothesis of respiration, by grafting this, a pure

assumption, which few will feel inclined to grant, on an old and familiar theory of intra-combustion. It has not, indeed, even been proved that iron exists in blood-corpuscules as an oxide at all; there are many reasons for doubting it; if it does not exist in a metallic state, it in all probability forms a binary compound, analogous to an haloid combination. If we refer to Liebig's mode of examining the blood, every one acquainted with the structure of the corpuscule, especially since Dr. Rees' observations, must be struck with its utter unfitness to give any thing like even a distant approach to the truth. He directs dried blood, or red particles which have been separated by subsidence (cingetrocknetes Blut, oder Albumin-Blut-roth), to be mixed with strong sulphuric acid*; a paste is thus formed, which deliquesces in the air. It is unnecessary to pursue the process further, as this first step is sufficient to prevent our learning in what state the iron really exists in the blood-corpuscule, or indeed any thing else about it, as the disorganizing influence of the corrosive acid employed must be sufficient to utterly change the nature of the very body we are endeavouring to investigate. It is like attempting to study the anatomy of an animal by crushing it in a mortar before we commence its dissection. One of the most excellent chemists of the day, and one who has worked well and successfully in the path of organic chemistry under the auspices of Dumas, Professor Kane, of Dublin, differs altogether from the assumption of Liebig; he has declared that, " with the knowledge we now possess of hematosine in its pure form, we must consider the iron to be an integral part of its organic constitution, as sulphur is in albumen, or arsenic in alkarsin; and the opinion of its being oxidized, and combined with the two organic elements as a kind of salt, can no longer be supported†."

With every honest desire to do justice to the high and acknowledged talent of Professor Liebig, I feel that it must be regretted that he has left the path of pure chemistry, in which he was really a blazing luminary, to ven-

* Handwörterbuch der reinem und angwandten Chemie, b. i. § 884.
† Elements of Chemistry, 1841, p. 1147.

ture in the field of pathology unsupported by experience. In his whole work not a single case is alluded to, nor reference made to clinical experience in support of a single view. He seems to look upon the animal organism as a mere machine, in which the ordinary physical laws obtain as completely as when acting on dead and inert matter; and this has led to his making often loosely expressed statements which astonish us. I would, in illustration, refer to but two instances in which he has applied the phenomenon of exosmosis to the body, in a manner which, had any one but the professor of Giessen uttered them, had brought down on the devoted head of the writer all the gall of the critic; and yet, in all the so-called reviews of Liebig's work, they have scarcely been alluded to. He states that death often occurs by drinking "creaming" wines, containing loosely combined carbonic acid, and thus explains the cause of death. "The carbonic acid which is disengaged penetrates through the parietes of the stomach! through the diaphragm !! and through all the intervening membranes of the lungs, out of which it displaces the atmospheric air !!! The patient dies with all the symptoms of asphyxia caused by an irrespirable gas; and the surest proof of the presence of carbonic acid in the lungs is the fact that the inhalation of ammonia is recognised as the best antidote against this kind of poisoning."— p. 116. The absurdity of the first part of this explanation is sufficiently apparent: where is the proof that the carbonic acid can thus penetrate all the living tissues alluded to ? The action of ammonia affords none. A less brilliant interpreter of symptoms than Liebig would be content with a different explanation. A German toper imbibes his ill-fermented *federweisse wein*, and succumbs from the influence of his potation on the nervous system; in other words, is very drunk. The ammonia held to his nostrils exerts its well-known effect in intoxication, and gives some relief to symptoms which, from their cerebral character, might by possibility, by an unpractised eye, be mistaken for asphyxia. If Liebig's explanation were correct, ought not these cases of what he has called *asphyxia* to occur in this country among our

summer imbibers of ginger-beer, spruce-beer, or soda-water ? It is well known they do not, for the simple reason that they cannot produce intoxication, which the ill-fermented wine will readily do.

Again, in alluding to the gases exhaled from the lungs, Professor Liebig has stated that " the presence of membranes offers not the slightest obstacle to their passing directly into the cavity of the chest."—p. 117. A statement more opposed to fact can scarcely be conceived. We know that the pleura and fibrous capsule (?) of the lung completely prevent the escape of air into the chest. If this were not the case— if nature in her wisdom had not been a better physiologist than the professor—life would be in daily danger from pneumo-thorax. Where are the cases recorded in which air has escaped from the lung into the chest during life, without breach of surface ? I might point out other instances in which Liebig has allowed his brilliant imagination to outrun sober experience. I have quoted these to show that the dogmata he has laid down are not to be regarded as infallible, nor that all who venture to differ from him are to be charged with bringing forward "futile," "unfounded," or "most fallacious" statements, especially at a time when Dumas and Boussingault, in France, have severely shaken some even of his more strictly chemical inductions; and when a talented chemist of our own country, Dr. Kemp, of Cambridge, has shown that the composition of bile, and the formula he has assumed as the base of his reasoning on the products of the chemistry of life, are absolutely erroneous. It is not impossible that Liebig, high as his name must ever rank in chemistry, may one day regret that he did not apply his pathology to the test of experience, 'ere he gave it to the world.

——Heisse Magister, heisse Doctor gar,
Und ziehe schon an die zehen Jahr;
Herauf, herab und quer und krumm,
Meine schuler an der nase herum,
Und sehe, dass wir nichts wissen Kennen !
Das will mir schier das herz verbrennen.
                                        FAUST.

In conclusion, if Mr. Ancell will apply the industry and talent which so characterize him by helping those who are, and have been long working at the bedside, he will (if he will excuse the remark) confer a greater boon on the profession to which we belong, than by acting as a commentator or interpreter of dogmata which now want not a logical but an experimental criticism.

14, Myddelton Square,
May 8, 1843.

ON

NEW PERCUSSING INSTRUMENTS

FOR INVESTIGATING DISEASES OF THE CHEST.

To the Editor of the Medical Gazette.

SIR,

You were kind enough to insert in the last volume of the MEDICAL GAZETTE, page 379, an account, with an engraving, of a new percussing instrument, termed an echometer, which I invented for the purpose of producing uniform sounds. I beg now to introduce to your notice a modification of that one, involving the same principle. The present instrument, which was made by Messrs. Philp and Whicker, of St. James's Street, at my request, is much more convenient than the other, in consequence of being greatly reduced in size, and elicits louder sounds.

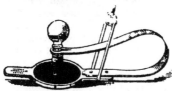

The plessimeter, surrounded by a ring, acts on a swivel. The instrument should be pressed upon the chest by the fore finger and thumb of the left hand, while the percussor, raised by the fore finger and thumb of the right hand, is propelled by a circular spring. The elevation of the percussor is regulated by a screw at the top of the regulator, which passes over the spring.

I am, sir,
Your obedient servant,
C. J. B. ALDIS, M.D.
Lecturer on Medicine at the Charlotte Street School.

13, Old Burlington Street,
May 5, 1843.

MEDICAL GAZETTE.

Friday, May 12, 1843.

"Licet omnibus, licet etiam mihi, dignitatem *Artis Medicæ* tueri; potestas modo veniendi in publicum sit, dicendi periculum non recuso."
CICERO.

LEGISLATION IN MEDICINE.

IN a late number we alluded to the fact that professional men are divided into two great natural orders; those, namely, who can afford to wait for practice, and those who cannot. We showed, also, that the time and means at the disposal of a student influenced his professional acquirements and his social position.

We should be heartily glad if every man who practises medicine or surgery in the British dominions belonged to the first division; but we fear it is scarcely possible that it should be so.

Those who have seen what the most facetious of churchmen has said of the attempt to establish a body of clergy, who, for £150 a year, should be patterns of good taste and gentlemanly bearing, as well as of all the cardinal virtues, will have no difficulty in applying the satire, *mutatis mutandis*, to the members of our own less dignified calling.

For many reasons, some obvious, others not so evident, ours is of all the professions by far the least followed by men of independent fortune. We have, as a class, no defined social position, such as is occupied by the naval and military officer, the clergyman, and the lawyer. We fill hardly any public offices, and there are no provisions for our studious youth, like those which the church has for her "poor scholars," or the honorary commissions in the two warlike services.

This undefined social position among a nation only less sensitive than their American kinsmen,—the various and almost imperceptible gradations which separate the titled physician from the obscure shopkeeper,—the disposition to cultivate professional good fellowship, struggling with the broad facts of social and educational inequality, contribute, no doubt, to produce that *géne* and want of ease so often apparent amongst our brethren. But to the same conditions is no doubt owing much of the circumspect behaviour and quiet conduct which characterize us in general, and to which, when at any time the exceptions are numerous, they are to be attributed to peculiar circumstances — such as the recent superabundance of young, ill-educated, and undisciplined members.

In speculating on the expected bill for medical reform, it will occur to some, and may prevent disappointment to remind others, that the duties, as well as the interests of the government, are totally different from those of the profession.

The minister is bound, it would appear—for we leave out the doctrine of total non-interference, the *laissez faire* system in its maturity—to insist on a minimum of qualification for those who are liable to be consulted on the bodily ailments of their fellow subjects, without the possession of which no person shall be allowed to undertake the cure of disease. He is bound to make inquiry of those best informed on the subject as to how much it is absolutely requisite to demand for this purpose; and to appoint a competent body to examine candidates and grant licenses. Having done this, his duty to the public is performed.

As a matter of detail it may be expedient to consider whether the burthen and the privilege of enforcing the law against offenders should be committed to the licensing body or to the public

prosecutor. Many think the government should undertake the punishment and the putting down of quackery. We are not of this opinion; but think that the government having obtained the proper information as to the qualifications required for a license to practise medicine, and having made it penal to practise without a license, must leave all cases of contumacy against the licensing body to be punished under the general law against such offences, all malapraxis amongst those who are licensed being punishable according to the damage done in the particular case to person or property.

This, then, or something of this kind, Sir James Graham seems disposed to do. But we do not live in a country, nor under a form of government, where a principle can be planned and laid down to have laws framed upon it and fitted to it: our materials for legislation are not so ductile. The ancient structure of our constitution is not, like an Athenian temple, formed of blocks squared and carved beforehand, but rather like the Cyclopean walls of heroic and half-fabulous ages. The huge fragments are carefully adjusted, indeed massive and permanent, but most irregular; each adopted only because found fitting, those having been rejected which were intractable. In later times, certainly, we find fragments of all sizes, shapes, and qualities, ruins of things new and old, thrown together into a soft and yielding cement. Of this cheap and tractable material, this *opus incertum*, modern utilitarianism finds it convenient to make most of its improvements.

The duty of the profession, on the other hand, seems to be to raise its own dignity and its value in the eyes of the state; to shew that it duly performs the work entrusted to its care, and deserves the privileges or the distinctions, the honours or the profits, which are considered to be its due. For this purpose it has to exact from its members much higher qualifications than those fixed by the state as a minimum; it has to create honours and rewards within its own jurisdiction, or to recommend the most deserving of its members to external patronage.

Now that the bitterness of encroachment and resistance has in great measure subsided—now that each party is conscious that much requires change, and that much must be left—now that each, sobered by time and reflection,

"Can the warmest friend reprove,
And bear to praise the fiercest foe,"

we may see, by experience of the past, how much may be left to be worked out by the moral energies of our profession, and how little need be done in aid of this by legislative interference. The Worshipful Society of Apothecaries were simply entrusted with the privilege of granting licenses to practise pharmacy to those who were not already in practice, and they have gradually raised their standard of qualification, which, before 1815, was at least as low as that of the counter-practice of the druggist, till it embraces nearly every known department of the science of medicine, and by far the greater number of its licentiates are also members of the College of Surgeons. There can be no greater proof of the disjointed state of matters than that the fact of membership with this highly educated body disqualifies for the license of the College of Physicians, and for a seat at the Council of the College of Surgeons. Wherein, however, consists the disqualification? not in the supposition that the member is unable to hold the amount of knowledge required of him as a physician, or a councilman, in addition to what he has been obliged to know as an apothecary—not, in fact, that

————"Still the wonder grew,
How one small head could carry all he knew:"

for the mere act of being disfranchised at once removes his disability. The real cause, we suspect, was a not unrighteous fear of contamination from the shop; so long as the apothecary continues a dealer in drugs, so long is he in a different category from those who abstain from such a source of profit. The surgeon with his apparatus of various kinds, his plasters, his bandages, his splints, is not a whit less mechanical in many of his details, but he has contrived totally to escape the slough in which his neighbour is fixed.

The teeth and the eyes of Englishmen are not that we know of under the especial protection of government. It is well known that dentists and oculists have flourished here for centuries, *vixere ante Agamemnona fortes*, practising without either let or license, on all who chose to submit to them. There may be some obsolete act for punishing all operators of this class; but at all events there is no college or society disposed to undertake the prosecution.

Dentistry, then, like druggistry, has grown up to its present flourishing and useful state outside the pale of all the corporations, and in spite of their laws. The art once cultivated has voluntarily sought the aid of science, scientific practice and preliminary studies have raised its professors to fortune and eminence, and it is not too much to believe that, at no very distant period, dentists who are not surgeons will be rare and despised exceptions to a general rule. But it may well be doubted whether if any even of our most eminent dentists thought it worth their while to derive a profit from some well-known shop near St. Martin's Lane, the College of Surgeons would consider them quite creditable members of their body. Much in the same way does uniting the trade of a druggist with the practice of medicine degrade the general practitioner, and we cannot but think that any arrangement amongst the members of a profession which draws a distinction between those who trust exclusively to an art or a science, and those who derive part of their gains from trade, do good service in raising and upholding the standard of professional character.

NOTICE RELATIVE TO RETURNS OF "CAUSES OF DEATH."

To the Editor of the Medical Gazette.

SIR,

I SHALL feel much obliged if you will inform the readers of the MEDICAL GAZETTE that the Registrar General has recently given the following direction to the registrars of deaths :—

" When the information given to you by the medical attendants upon deceased persons, respecting the ' cause of death,' contains also a statement of the *duration of the fatal diseases*, or is accompanied by the memorandum (*p. mortem*) denoting that the nature of the causes of death had been ascertained or verified by a *post-mortem* examination, you will not fail to enter these statements in the column of the register, headed ' Cause of Death'."

It is desirable on many accounts that the laws respecting the duration of diseases should be ascertained, and this will afford the medical profession an opportunity of entering on permanent record a sufficient number of observations for determining those laws, as well as the laws of mortality.

With regard to the registration of the " causes of death," it has been found the most convenient and satisfactory course for the medical attendant to leave a written certificate with the friends of the deceased person, to be placed in the hands of the registrar.

The registrar is directed to ask the informant whether any written statement of the cause of death has been left by the medical attendant, but the relatives, from the natural distraction of grief, or ignorant of its scientific importance, are apt to forget the medical certificate, unless the medical attendant take the trouble to state that it will be required, and place it in their hands.

If the medical profession needed any stimulus to induce them to contribute to the promotion of medical science, or to the discovery and consequent removal of the causes of untimely death, it will be found in the following considerations, to which the Registrar General has adverted in his last Report: —" I hope that the members of the medical profession, who have hitherto given their aid, will cordially assist in carrying out this national registration of the causes of death, as they alone are able to give a correct statement of the nature of the fatal diseases ; and to them, more than to the members of any other profession, must be apparent the vast importance of thus collecting accurate materials for advancing the science of vital statistics."

Copies of the " Statistical Nosology, with notes and observations for the use of those who return the causes of death," may be procured by any medical practitioner upon application (verbal or written) at the General Register Office.—I have the honour to be, sir,

Your obedient servant,

WILLIAM FARR.

CAUSES OF DEATH AFTER OPERATIONS IN THE LONDON HOSPITALS.

To the Editor of the Medical Gazette.

SIR,

IN an essay published in your journal of to-day, by Mr. T. Wilkinson King, a remark appears relative to some of my observations upon " the causes of death after operations and injuries in London hospitals," recorded in the last number of the Guy's Hospital Reports, which I cannot permit to pass unnoticed.

At page 194 of the GAZETTE, Mr. King observes, after alluding to my remarks, " These principles have been long taught at Guy's, and the facts on which they are based run through a series of thirty or forty large volumes of museum manuscripts, which are not merely records of common facts." And again, " A tabular analysis of the whole, for more than twenty years, kept up since I was a pupil, renders the whole available almost at a glance. Dr. C.'s exposition is principally based upon my own autopsy-histories." Now, sir, I must beg to observe, that Mr. King is totally in error in advancing the unfounded assumption that the principles which I have adduced are based either upon his or upon any other person's autopsy-histories. I have stated in my paper in the Reports, and I now repeat the affirmation, that the deductions which I have there drawn are wholly based upon my own observations and inquiries, pursued in the wards and dead-house of Guy's Hospital during the last eight years ; every principle which I have announced in that paper as my own is founded upon cases which I have myself seen and carefully investigated. I first gave a full exposition of the principles which form the ground-work of my last essay, in a paper (entitled, "Remarks on Asthenic Inflammations of Serous Membranes,") read before the Pupils' Physical Society of Guy's Hospital, in December 1837—a period at which, I apprehend, a very large proportion of Mr. King's autopsy-histories had not been recorded in the museum books. In that paper, as well as in the essay lately published in the Reports (note to page 91), I quoted an observation made by Dr. Hodgkin about fourteen years since, to the effect that he had observed mottling of the kidneys in patients who had sunk after operations and injuries. I had remarked the same fact before meeting with Dr. Hodgkin's observation; but I of course thought it right to append this important anticipatory remark to each of my essays. I have also expressly quoted, in my memoir in the Reports (page 97), the observation put forth by Mr. Key, in his lectures, "that he has scarcely ever seen a fatal case of lithotomy in which there was not discovered organic disease of the abdominal viscera, and more especially of the kidneys." I was first made aware of this some days after I had received the proof sheets of my paper from the printer. Beyond this I am perfectly willing to repeat, however unnecessarily, an admission which I have already made, of my obligation to the post-mortem registers for the *confirmation* of the views which I had previously committed to writing, and had advanced upon several occasions in the discussions of the societies attached to Guy's Hospital, long before I had recourse to those registers, which I looked upon merely as the most ample collection of cases to which I could refer in finally testing the correctness of my opinions before submitting them to the profession. In my essay in the Reports, I have therefore expressly stated (pp. 88, 89), that "for the purpose of confirming the observations which I had made at Guy's Hospital for several years past, I carefully examined the accounts of all the cases where death occurred from the secondary effects of operations, &c., which have been entered in the post-mortem registers of the museum during the last fifteen years." I have then given tables, in which the results of that examination are stated. I conceived it fully sufficient to mention, that these confirmatory tables were drawn from the above source, without dwelling upon the fact (often previously announced in print, and probably known to most professional readers), that these registers have been principally kept by Dr. Hodgkin and Mr. King. With respect to the "tabular analysis" of the post-mor-

tem registers by Mr. King, I must state that I did not find it very available in the above examination of those records; I certainly referred to it as an index, which it simply is, in looking over some of Dr. Hodgkin's inspections; but I preferred, in every instance, to trust to my own perusal of the cases.

I therefore beg to repeat that I am not in the slightest degree indebted to the reports or observations of Mr. King for the *basis* of any one of the results which I have advanced in my essay published in the April number of the Guy's Hospital Reports; but I freely acknowledge, as I have already done in that essay, the valuable *confirmation* which my views have received in the plain details of cadaveric inspections, by Dr. Hodgkin, Mr. King, and Mr. Roderick, contained in the museum registers of Guy's Hospital.—I have the honour to be, sir,

Your obedient servant,
NORMAN CHEVERS, M.D.

Frith Street, Soho Square,
May 5, 1843.

DIABETES.

ERROR IN TRANSLATION.

To the Editor of the Medical Gazette.

SIR,

IN the number of your valuable journal for the 21st of April ult., I observe that Dr. Percy, in his interesting case of diabetes, has called my attention to the following error in my translation of Dr. Bell's Essay on Diabetes, at page 49:—"By injecting into the vessels a solution of cane sugar, we do not find that the sugar passes into the blood or urine, but by the pulmonary transpiration. We know that cane sugar, taken into the stomach, in whatever quantity, never passes by the urine." By referring to Krimer's experiments, detailed in Horn's Archiv für Medizinish Erfahrung, 1818, the above will be found to be an exact translation of the original paragraph, at page 536, b. ii. of that work. However, the author's meaning will, I think, be rendered more intelligible by being thus stated:—"If a solution of cane sugar be injected into the veins, a very short time suffices for its complete disappearance from the blood; it does not pass into the urine, but is eliminated by the pulmonary transpiration."

If you will allow me to make this correction through the medium of your columns, you will greatly oblige me, and I am, sir,

Your obedient servant,
ALFRED MARKWICK.

North Brixton, May 5, 1843.

VIREY'S OBJECTIONS TO LIEBIG'S THEORY

OF THE USES OF RESPIRATION AND OF FOOD.

———

Liebig maintains that the chief use of the food is to supply carbon and hydrogen, which, uniting with the oxygen absorbed from the air, give rise to the generation of animal heat. He consequently holds that there is a certain fixed relation between the amount of food consumed, and the quantity of carbon and hydrogen thrown off at the lungs. M. Virey opposes this theory, as contrary to common observation, as, even though it be allowed to be applicable to mammalia, birds, and reptiles, it is by no means to those animals which respire by means of branchiæ. Thus all animals with branchiæ consume but little oxygen, comparatively speaking, and yet many of them devour very great quantities of food. Even the largest and most voracious of the reptiles, as the alligators, crocodiles, &c. which devour enormous quantities of food, under a burning climate, too, respire feebly with their vesicular lungs, and consume but little oxygen.

Fishes, whose blood is but imperfectly oxygenated by the branchial apparatus, are perhaps among the most voracious of animals, and yet, according to Liebig's theory, they ought to eat little, because they consume little oxygen.

The same holds true of the Mollusca. The cuttle-fish, *buccinum*, *strombus*, *murex*, &c. grow to a large size, but their respiration is very imperfect, and yet they are great flesh-eaters. The Crustacea, again, as the crabs, lobsters, &c. grow rapidly, because they are great eaters, but their branchial apparatus is not fitted to consume much oxygen.

In all these animals assimilation takes place very rapidly, notwithstanding their feeble respiratory powers; and they are, besides, by no means deficient in activity or muscular powers, though their flesh be but feebly azotised or animalized, and their blood is always cold.

If it be one of the characters of vitality, that the more perfect this principle is, the greater is the number of germs, or eggs, or fœtuses produced, then, quite contrary to Liebig's theory, the number of germs produced is in the inverse ratio of the perfection of the respiratory functions. Fishes and mollusca deposit their spawn or eggs by millions; but the mammalia, and even the birds, whose respiratory functions are the most perfect, are in this respect infinitely behind these. On the other hand, it is seen that the number of germs or eggs is rather proportioned to the nutrition received; for the amount of food taken is not proportioned to the respiration in the animal kingdom.

M. Virey therefore concludes, that the vital force, or central nervous energy, has more to do with the production of animal heat than the consumption of carbon at the lungs, and this for three special reasons:— 1st, Because a fecundated egg resists a freezing temperature longer than one which has not been fecundated. 2d, That a hybernating insect, reptile, or animal, or even trees during winter, by the sole influence of a vital power, resist a freezing temperature, whereas the same animals, if dead, would be instantly frozen. 3d, That many mammalia and birds keep themselves warm even in the most rigorous winters under the Pole, not in consequence of a greater amount of oxygen consumed, nor by a greater amount of muscular activity, but in consequence of a more abundant, highly azotized, or animalized nourishment. — *Journ. de Pharm.*, and *American Journal*.

———

JULES GUERIN ON STRABISMUS.

———

M. Jules Guerin has published a second Memoir on Strabismus, devoted to a rational and experimental inquiry into the distinction between the optical and the mechanical forms of the disorder; a former memoir, published in the same journal the 3d April, 1841, having treated principally of the mechanical or primitively muscular form.

Optical strabismus, the principal subject of the present paper, the author defines as a consecutive of secondarily muscular deviation of the eye, consequent on a disjunction of the axis of vision and the axis of the eye. This disjunction may be produced in three ways: 1st, from an obstacle to the passage of visual axis along the course of the ocular axis; 2dly, by a change of relation in the refracting media without alteration of their transparency, or 3dly, by an insensibility of the retina at the proper point for the reception of luminous rays. The first is characterised by the squint existing only while the patient is looking at an object. In these cases the two visual axes, though no longer concurring with the ocular axes, converge towards one point.

A squint, then, existing only during active or intentional vision, cannot depend on permanent muscular contraction. A young person, aged 19, who had a moveable clot of blood in the posterior chamber, was observed to squint from the attempt to place a transparent portion of the medium opposite to the object looked at, and thereby to avoid the inconvenience produced by the presence of the clot in different parts of the chamber. As soon as she ceased to look at an object, she ceased to squint.

A disturbance in the relation of the refracting media the author thinks is the only way of accounting for some cases of strabismus which are produced suddenly after a blow, or a jarring fall on the seat or on the feet. The first effect of displacement is double vision; and the squint, at first temporary, lasting only during attentive vision, is gradually made permanent by the repeated endeavour to escape from this fatiguing symptom.

The third form, viz. from partial paralysis of the retina, is more difficult of actual demonstration, though its presence may be inferred by induction rigorous enough for practical purposes. Amaurotic patients, when endeavouring to distinguish a light, are seen to turn the eye in different directions where they know the light does not exist; they present the various surfaces, as it were, feeling for it. Those in whom the paralysis is but partial contract a habit of subjecting to the influence of the rays the part that is most sensible.

The author believes that in no case of secondary optical strabismus will the texture of a muscle be found fibrous, and that in no case of primary mechanical muscular strabismus will such a fibrous state of the muscle be wanting. Where myotomy has been performed in cases of optical secondary strabismus, he believes that one of three things must have happened—either the case has not been watched long enough to ascertain the result, or a positive failure has followed, or the primary cause, whatever it may have been, has really been removed by the operation. The author adds a summary of the distinctive characters of the two kinds too concise to be materially abridged, but too long for our pages. The paper, which is to be continued in the next number of the journal, is well worthy of perusal.—*Gazette Médicale.*

CASES OF CLOSURE OF THE VAGINA IN INFANTS AFTER BIRTH.

By J. C. NOTT, M. D.

CASE I.—In the early part of 1837, I was requested to see the infant daughter of Mrs. P., of Mobile, aged 12 months. The mother and nurse both affirmed that the child was healthy and free from any deformity at birth, and for at least three or four months afterwards. They further stated that they had accidentally discovered, a few days before consulting me, that the vagina was closed, but were unable to say at what time this had

taken place, as there had never been any inflammation, discharge from the parts, or any circumstance to attract particular attention.

On examination, I found perfect adhesion of the labia, and closure of the vagina—the orifice of the urethra alone remaining open. The appearances were those of a congenital deformity, the parts being healthy, and the position of the os externum being marked by a superficial sulcus. The child was teething, and as I saw no good reason for immediate interference I advised that nothing should be done until this period was gone through. The parents with the child went to Scotland to spend the summer, and when they returned in the winter, I found, on examination, that the vagina had opened *spontaneously*—the parts were perfectly natural, and have remained so ever since.

CASE II.—In July last, Dr. M'Nally called on me, and asked me to see with him a child, about the same age, and under circumstances so similar in every respect, that I deem any details unimportant. I related the above facts to him, and we agreed to leave the case to nature for a few months.

We have recently examined this patient again, and find that a spontaneous opening has taken place as in the other case.

REMARKS:—These cases are not of frequent occurence, are not to be found in our common works on surgery and diseases of children, and may embarrass the inexperienced practitioner. There can be no objection to the delay of an operation, and it is always prudent to avoid cutting if possible.—*American Journal of the Medical Sciences.*

HEMIPLEGIA FROM TYING THE COMMON CAROTID ARTERY.

A MAN was wounded, on the night of the 11th April, behind the right branch of the lower jaw. A large arterial jet of blood instantly flowed, which was in vain attempted to be staunched by means of compresses. Dr. Francis cut down on the wounded artery and applied a ligature to the vessel, which arrested the hemorrhage for three days. After this it returned with double intensity, and even the tourniquet failed to arrest it completely. On the 23d of April, Professor Sedillot was called to see him, and resolved to cut down on the common trunk of the carotid artery, and throw a ligature around it, as an aneurismal tumor had formed at the site of the wound, and the parts over which the tourniquet had been applied were in a gangrenous state. A ligature was with difficulty thrown around the vessel, the diffuse phlegmonous inflammation having confused the aspect of the parts. This ligature arrested the hemorrhage, and the pulsation of the tumor disappeared. When the operation was performed the patient was in a state of extreme prostration, so that the other consequences of the ligature, other than what is stated, were not then observed. But when visited three hours afterwards, it was found that complete hemiplegia of the left side of the body and the right side of the face had taken place, and the intelligence of the patient was so far destroyed that he scarcely comprehended questions addressed to him. He died on the 2d of May.

The vessels were injected previous to opening the body, and when the skull-cap was removed and the brain examined, to ascertain, if possible, the cause of the hemiplegia, it was found that the arteries distributed to the right middle and anterior lobes of the brain were much less injected than those of the left side. These same lobes were also appreciably softer in consistence than those on the left side, but had apparently undergone no other change. No serous fluid was found in the ventricles, none on the surface of the brain. The hemiplegic symptoms, then, had apparently resulted from that side of the brain having been deprived of its due proportion of arterial blood. As the chief interest of this case depends on the hemiplegic symptom and the probable cause, it is unnecessary to detail the other morbid appearances.—*Gazette Médicale de Paris;* and *Edin. Med. and Surg. Journ.*

BIRMINGHAM SCHOOL OF MEDICINE.

We are requested to announce, that the arrangements for providing collegiately for the board, lodging, and tutelary care of the students of the Birmingham School of Medicine and Surgery, under the care of a Warden, are completed.

BOOKS RECEIVED.

Mr. Barlowe's Approved Experiments concerning the Nature and Property of the Loadstone, &c. New edition. By William Sturgeon, Lecturer to the Manchester Institute of Natural and Experimental Science, &c. &c.

Criminal Jurisprudence, considered in relation to Cerebral Organization. By M. B. Sampson. 2d edit., with additions.

ROYAL COLLEGE OF SURGEONS.

LIST OF GENTLEMEN ADMITTED MEMBERS.

Friday, May 5, 1843.

A. G. Canton.—H. Lang.—S. E. R. Jones.— F. Sopwith.—W. L. Echlin.—R. N. Rubidge.— J. Blaxland.—W. W. Wildey.—W. B. Kellock.— C. Hall.—T. B. Cowherd.

APOTHECARIES' HALL.

LIST OF GENTLEMEN WHO HAVE RECEIVED CERTIFICATES.

Thursday, May 4, 1843.

C. P. Fitzgerald, Edgar House, Sidmouth, Devon.—W. Wiblin, Southampton.—F. J. Robinson, Royal Navy.—W. M. Dowding, London.— F. Spicer, Cheltenham.—J. G. Sproston, Oldbury near Birmingham.—J. W. Barnard, Dunmow, Essex.—W. Dickson, Elvington, York.—F. R. Stradling, Bridgewater.

A TABLE OF MORTALITY FOR THE METROPOLIS,

Shewing the number of deaths from all causes registered in the week ending Saturday, April 29, 1843.

Small Pox	10
Measles	23
Scarlatina	18
Hooping Cough	50
Croup	6
Thrush	3
Diarrhœa	4
Dysentery	0
Cholera	1
Influenza	1
Typhus	62
Erysipelas	6
Syphilis	1
Hydrophobia	0
Diseases of the Brain, Nerves, and Senses	142
Diseases of the Lungs and other Organs of Respiration	262
Diseases of the Heart and Blood-vessels	24
Diseases of the Stomach, Liver, and other Organs of Digestion	66
Diseases of the Kidneys, &c.	13
Childbed	6
Ovarian Dropsy	0
Disease of Uterus, &c.	4
Rheumatism	4
Diseases of Joints, &c.	3
Ulcer	0
Fistula	0
Diseases of Skin, &c.	0
Diseases of Uncertain Seat	87
Old Age or Natural Decay	73
Deaths by Violence, Privation, or Intemperance	26
Causes not specified	13
Deaths from all Causes	896

METEOROLOGICAL JOURNAL.

Kept at EDMONTON, *Latitude* 51° 37′ 32″ N. *Longitude* 0° 3′ 51″ W. *of Greenwich.*

April 1843.	THERMOMETER.		BAROMETER.	
Wednesday 3	from 39 to 63		29·85 to	29·80
Thursday . 4	45	66	29·75	29·69
Friday . . 5	45	59	29·64	29·65
Saturday . 6	49	*44	29·36	29·55
Sunday . . 7	30	51	29·61	29·56
Monday . . 8	31	49	29·55	29·53
Tuesday . 9	40	53	29·55	29·80

Wind, S.W. and S. on the 4th and 5th; otherwise N. and N.E.

Since the 3d generally cloudy, with frequent and heavy rain.

* This temperature occurred at noon on the 6th; the extreme of the preceding night or morning was 48°.

CHARLES HENRY ADAMS.

WILSON & OGILVY, 57, Skinner Street, London.

THE

LONDON MEDICAL GAZETTE,

BEING A

WEEKLY JOURNAL

OF

Medicine and the Collateral Sciences.

FRIDAY, MAY 19, 1843.

LECTURES
ON THE
THEORY AND PRACTICE OF MIDWIFERY,

Delivered in the Theatre of St. George's Hospital,

BY ROBERT LEE, M.D. F.R.S.

LECTURE XXVII.

On the invention and use of the forceps in protracted and difficult labour.

ON the 19th August, 1670, I saw, says Mauriceau, a little woman, æt. 38, who had been eight days in labour with her first child, the liquor amnii having escaped on the first, with very slight dilatation of the uterus. Having remained in this state to the fourth day, I was called to deliver my opinion upon the case to the midwife, whom I advised to have the patient bled, and in the event of the bleeding failing to produce any good effect, to give two drachms of infusion of senna to excite uterine contractions, which was done the following day; when the uterus dilated as much as was possible. Nevertheless, the head could not pass, in consequence of the great distortion of the pelvis, and I was again called three days after, but finding, from the narrowness of the passage, that it was impossible to guide the crotchet to the head with safety, I declared to all the assistants that the delivery could not be effected, of which they being fully persuaded, urged me to draw the child from the belly by the Cæsarean operation, which I would not undertake, knowing well that it is always very certainly mortal to the mother. But after I had left this woman without being able to afford her relief, there arrived unexpectedly an English physician, named Chamberlen, who was then at Paris, and who, from father to son, practised midwifery in London, where he has since acquired the highest

807.—XXXII.

degree of reputation in this art. This physician, seeing the woman in the condition I have described, expressed his astonishment that I, whom he pronounced and affirmed to be the most dexterous accoucheur in Paris, could not deliver her, and promised that he would certainly do so in less than the half of a quarter of an hour, whatever difficulty he might encounter. He accordingly went to work, and laboured upwards of three hours without stopping to take his breath, and then being thoroughly exhausted, and seeing the poor woman almost dead, he was compelled to abandon the case, and avow that the delivery could not be effected, as I had declared. The woman died undelivered 24 hours after, and I found, on opening the body, which I did by performing the Cæsarean operation after death, that the whole uterus was torn and pierced in several places by the instruments which this physician had employed blindly, without the direction of the hand, which, being one-half larger than my hand, could not be introduced. Nevertheless, this physician had come to Paris six months before in the hope of making his fortune, having raised a report that he had a secret peculiarly applicable to labours of this kind, boasting that he could with it complete the most hopeless and desperate cases. He had even offered to communicate his pretended secret to M——, the first physician of the king, for 10,000 crowns. But the result of this unfortunate labour disgusted him so much with France, that he returned to England in a few days, seeing clearly that there were men in Paris far more skilful in the art of midwifery than he. But before setting off for London he paid me a visit to compliment me on my book, which I had published two years before, to inform me that he had never previously seen so difficult an operation as the delivery of this woman, and to praise me because I had refused to undertake it as inconsiderately as he had done. I received his congratulations as I ought, giving him to understand that he was thoroughly deceived in believing that it was as easy to deliver women in Paris as he had found it in London, to which he returned the following day, carrying with him a copy of my book, a translation of which into English he published in 1672. Since this translation appeared, he has acquired so high a reputation in the art of midwifery in London, " qu'il y a gagné plus de trente mille livres de rente, qu'il possède présentement, à ce que m'ont dit depuis peu de personnes de sa connoissance."

Dr. Hugh Chamberlen, in his preface to the translation which he published of Mauriceau's work in 1672, and which is entitled " The Diseases of Women with Child and in Child-bed, as also the best means of Helping them in Natural and Unnatural Labours, with fit Remedies for the several Indispositions of New-born Babes," &c. gives the following account of his important secret, and explanation of the reason why it was not divulged, as he obviously felt ought to have been done. " In the 17th chapter of the second book, my author justifies the fastening hooks in the head of a child that comes right, and yet, because of some difficulty or disproportion, cannot pass; which I confess has been, and is yet, the practice of the most expert artists in midwifery, not only in England but throughout Europe, and has much caused the report, that where a man comes, one or both must necessarily die; and is the reason of forbearing to send till the child is dead, or the mother dying. But I can neither approve of that practice nor those delays, because my father, brothers, and myself (though none else in Europe as I know) have by God's blessing, and our industry, attained to, and long practised, a way to deliver women in this case, without any prejudice to them or their infants, though all others (being obliged, for want of such an expedient, to use the common way) do, and must endanger, if not destroy, one or both with hooks. By this manual operation a labour may be despatched (on the least difficulty) with fewer pains, and sooner, to the great advantage, and without danger, both of woman and child. If, therefore, the use of hooks by physicians and chirurgeons be condemned (without thereto necessitated by some monstrous birth), we can much less approve of a midwife's using them, as some here in England boast they do; which rash presumption, in France, would call them in question for their lives. In the fifteenth chapter of this book my author proposes the conveying sharp instruments into the womb, to extract the head, which is a dangerous operation, and may be much better done by our fore-mentioned art, as also the inconvenience and hazard of a child dying thereby prevented, which he supposes in the twenty-seventh chapter of this second book. I will now take leave to offer an apology for not publishing the secret I mention we have to extract children without hooks where other artists use them, viz. there being my father and two brothers living that practice this art, I cannot esteem it my own to dispose of nor publish it without injury to them; and think I have not been unserviceable to my own country, although I do but inform them that the fore-mentioned three persons of our family and myself can serve them, in these extremities, with greater safety than others."

The secret which the Chamberlens possessed was the midwifery forceps, which they had invented and perfected—it has undergone no essential improvement since; and the glory of the discovery both of the forceps and vectis, notwithstanding the sordid avarice with which they were so deeply tainted, and the utter disregard to the claims of humanity which they manifested by their mysterious conduct in concealing their instruments after the acquisition of the wealth which they so eagerly coveted, must in justice be awarded to them in all future ages. A variety of forceps had been invented long before the time of the Chamberlens, but they were unquestionably the first who discovered the true principle upon which the instrument can be employed with advantage — the separate introduction and subsequent locking of the blades. But except this short notice, contained in the preface to the translation of Mauriceau's work, from which nothing can be learned respecting the construction of the forceps, the method of applying it, and the cases of labour in which it could be used with advantage, no further account was ever given by them of their secret; and the Chamberlens, father and sons, and grandsons, Hugh, Peter, and Paul, had all died, and the whole family, I believe, had become extinct (about a century and a half had passed away) before it was known with absolute certainty what instrument it was they had invented. The extraordinary manner in which this became known in 1818 has been described by Mr. Carwardine, in a short paper published in the ninth volume of the Medico-Chirurgical Transactions, which I shall read to you.

" In depositing the obstetric instruments of the Chamberlens," says Mr. Carwardine, " among the archives of the Medico-Chirurgical Society, I beg leave to offer a few facts and observations which may serve to authenticate their genuineness and their originality. The estate of Woodham, Mortimer Hall, near Maldon in Essex, was purchased by Dr. Peter Chamberlen some time previous to 1683, and continued in his family till about 1715, when it was sold by Hope Chamberlen to Mr. William

Alexander, wine-merchant, who bequeathed it to the Wine-Coopers' Company. The principal entrance to the mansion is through a porch, the masonry of which, being carried up with the building, serves as closets to its respective stories. Two or three years ago, a lady with whom I am intimately acquainted, and from whom I had the particulars, discovered in the floor of the upper closet a hinge, and tracing the line she saw another, which led to the obvious conclusion of a door; this door she soon found means to open. There was a considerable space between the floor and the ceiling below, and this space contained divers empty boxes, &c. Among those was a curious chest or cabinet, in which was deposited a collection of old coins, trinkets, gloves, fans, spectacles, &c. with many letters from Dr. Chamberlen to different members of his family, and also these obstetric instruments. Being on terms of intimacy with the family resident at Woodham, Mortimer Hall, these instruments have been presented to me, and I have now the satisfaction of depositing them with your society for the gratification of public curiosity, and to secure to Chamberlen the meed of posthumous fame due to him for his most useful discovery. With respect to these instruments, I would briefly observe that they appear to me to contain *within themselves* the most direct and conclusive evidence of originality of invention; and that even the progress of this invention may be distinctly traced in its different stages as it passed through the mind of the inventor. First we have a simple vectis, with an open fenestrum (supposed to be of much more recent invention); then we have the idea of *uniting two* of these instruments by a joint, which makes each blade serve as a fulcrum to the other, instead of making a fulcrum of the soft parts of the mother, and which also unites a power of drawing the head forward. This idea is at first accomplished by a pivot, which, being riveted, makes the instrument totally incapable of application. Then he goes to work again, and having made a hitch in each vectis for the joint, he fixes a pivot in one only, which, projecting, is to be received into a corresponding hole in the other blade after they have been applied separately. It may be observed, that although there is a worm to the projecting part of the pivot, yet there is no corresponding female screw in the hole which is to receive it. Every practical accoucheur will know that it is not easy, or always possible, to lock the joint of the forceps with such accuracy as to bring this pivot and hole into apposite contact. This Chamberlen soon discovered, and next produced a more light and manageable instrument, which instead of uniting by a pivot, he passes a tape through the two holes and winds it round the joint, which

method combines sufficient accuracy of contact, security, and mobility. From the roughness of the workmanship, I am led to conclude that Chamberlen was his own artificer: a practice, I am told, not uncommon in those days, when mystery and empiricism were not regarded as contemptible even among the enlightened professors of science."

When secretary to the Medical and Chirurgical Society ten years ago, I obtained permission from the council to have models made of all these instruments described by Mr. Carwardine, the originals of which are still preserved. These models are now before you upon the table, and if you examine them you will come to the same conclusion as he did, that they contain within themselves the most direct and satisfactory evidence of originality of invention, and that even the progress of the invention may be distinctly traced in its different stages from the vectis to the forceps as it passed through the mind of the inventor.

The two figures which follow represent a front and side view of one of the levers or vectes found among the Chamberlen instruments. The other vectis in the collection has the extremity of the handle blunt.

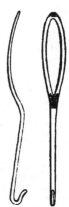

Chamberlen's lever—the front and side views. The only difference between this and the other specimen found consists in the one being blunt at the extremity of the curved handle, while this terminates in a sharp point.

If you compare the two first figures which follow, and which represent the most perfect Chamberlen forceps, with the other two figures, which represent the straight forceps of Denman, now in common use, you will perceive that they are essentially the same instruments. The wooden handles and lock of Denman's forceps were invented by Smellie, and this is the only difference which exists, and it is not an important one, between the Chamberlen forceps, and the short straight forceps of Smellie and Denman. The length and form of the blades, and the openings in them called fenestræ, are as nearly as possible the same, and undoubtedly had the same origin. It is evident from the form and construction of these forceps, and those of Chapman and Giffard, that an imperfect knowledge of the instrument employed by the Chamberlens had been obtained before 1733 by some means at present wholly unknown. I wish some evidence could be furnished to prove that this information was communicated by the authors of the discovery.

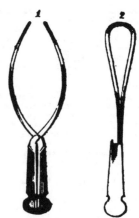

1, Denman's forceps closed.
2, a single blade.

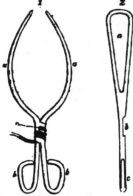

The accompanying cut is taken from a drawing of the most perfect of Chamberlen's instruments. No. 1 is the forceps locked : *a*, the blades ; *b*, the handles ; *c*, the hole in the joint, through which is passed the string to connect the blades.

No. 2, the front view of a single blade : *a*, the fenestra ; *b*, the groove in the shank, forming the lock, by which the two blades, perfectly similar in form, are adapted to each other ; *c*, the handle.

The following are the dimensions : extreme length, 11¼ inches ; length of blade, 7¼ inches : of handle, 4¼ ; greatest width between the blades, 3 inches and 3-8ths ; width between the blades at the points, 3-4ths of an inch ; greatest breadth of the blade, 1¼ inch.

It has been stated in several of the historical accounts which have been published of the forceps, that about 16 years after the occurrence of the case at Paris related by Mauriceau, Dr. Hugh Chamberlen was compelled to take refuge in Holland in consequence of espousing the cause of James II. While in Holland he sold the lever to Roonhuysen as the secret which he possessed, but there is no evidence to prove, as Alphonse Le Roy asserts, that he parted with the forceps. The vectis was afterwards sold to two Dutch accoucheurs, Bekelman and Ruysch, who afterwards, according to Osiander, made a disgraceful trade with it. It would

appear from his history of their proceedings that they not only frequently employed it for the sake of obtaining the sum which was usually paid to them for their assistance, but that they sold to others, over and over again, the same secret at an enormous price. Sometimes too they bargained for the half of what might be gained by the use of the instrument, and in the end it appears that they gave to every individual a new instrument as the true one, with the view, if any one should be inclined to betray the secret, the public might always remain in doubt which was the genuine instrument. None of the Dutch accoucheurs were so patriotic, or possessed so much humanity, as to disclose the secret of the Chamberlens. The immense gains, however, which the possessors of the secret made, rendered men of science most anxious to find out their secret. With this view Palfyn of Ghent made several journeys to Amsterdam and London for the purpose of finding out some clue to the discovery of the Chamberlens. After he had collected as much information at both these places as he was able, he had an instrument made which consisted of two steel blades like spoons, which were to be placed over the head of the child situated in the pelvis, by which with the assistance of two iron handles it might be drawn out. Palfyn went to Paris in 1723, fifty-one years after the translation of Mauriceau was published, and shewed this instrument to the members of the Royal Academy of Sciences as his own discovery. If you look at this representation of Palfyn's instrument in Mülder's plates, you will see that he had not obtained accurate information respecting either the lever or forceps of the Chamberlens. It consists of two blades without a lock, and altogether very unlike the

Chamberlen forceps, and obviously useless in practice. Palfyn's instrument underwent several changes before it acquired that form which it possessed when it received the name of Dusé's forceps, an account of which was first published by Butter in the Edinburgh Medical Essays and Observations in 1733.

"The forceps," says Butter, "for taking hold of a child's head when it is fallen so far down among the bones of the pelvis that it cannot be pushed back again into the uterus, to be extracted by the feet, and when it seems to make no advances to the birth by the throes of the mother, is scarce known in this country, though Mr. Chapman tells us it was long made use of by Dr. Chamberlen, who kept the form of it a secret, as Mr. Chapman also does. I believe, therefore, that a sight of such an instrument, which I had from M. Dusé, who practises midwifery at Paris, and who believes it to be his own invention, would not be unacceptable to you, and the publication of a picture of it may be of use to some of your readers." This figure [exhibiting it] represents this instrument of Dusé, but you see it is very widely different from the Chamberlen forceps. The handle and lock bear some resemblance to it, but the blades of Dusé's forceps are merely two deeply concave steel plates, like spoons, without fenestræ. This was, I believe however, the nearest approach to perfection in the construction of the forceps which was made on the Continent before the representation of the English midwifery forceps was given by Giffard and Chapman in 1734 and 1735. The first edition of Chapman's Treatise on the Improvement of Midwifery, which contained a description, but no representation of the forceps, appeared in 1733, or earlier; and in 1734, Giffard's Cases in Midwifery were published, with this figure [exhibiting it] of what is usually called Giffard's extractor, which, you see, is the same instrument as that delineated by Chapman in the second edition of his Treatise, published in 1735. Giffard does not lay claim to the invention of the forceps, nor is there any account of the manner in which he came to the knowledge of it; there is no intimation by him that the instrument was kept secret, and he speaks of it as well known. Chapman says, "the secret mentioned by Dr. Chamberlen, by which his father, two brothers, and himself, saved such children as presented with the head, but could not be born by natural pains, was, as is generally believed, if not past all dispute, the use of the forceps, now well known to all the principal men of the profession, both in town and country." "As to forceps," he adds, "which I think no person has yet any more than barely mentioned, it is a noble instrument, to which many now living owe

their lives, as I can assert from my own knowledge and long successful practice." He then proceeds to describe the way in which it is to be used. "This instrument, though not pointed, must yet be used with caution. You are first to pass one part thereof above, gently introducing it, and guarding and directing the bow as far as you can with all the fingers of the left hand, the instrument lying in the hollow of the hand, being careful that no fold or part of the vagina get between the instrument and the head of the child, which would at once hinder any hold of the head (and consequently foil you in the attempt), and bruise the part that intervenes. But a little care will easily prevent this. One part thus passed over the head, and under the os pubis, the other is to be passed near the os sacrum, and thus a laceration will be avoided. When those are passed, they are then to be brought close together, and if you please the screw may be put through and fastened with the button, though there is no occasion for the loss of so much time, for without doing this the hand will prove sufficient to keep them together; and thus you may extract the head, by drawing gently down. It is much better, as I have just observed, that the two parts of the forceps should not be joined or fixed by a screw, the hand being sufficient, and that for these reasons. First, because when they are screwed together, though they should not happen to be exactly opposite to each other, yet they will turn so as to take fast hold of the infant's head, and readily extract it. Secondly, in case one of the parts should slip, it is then easily returned to its proper post, without being taken wholly away; whereas, when they are screwed together, and then slip off on one side (which I have often experienced, in spite of the greatest care I could use), the instrument is to be repassed and screwed as at first. They have oftentimes slipped, and when I expected the head of the child I have been deceived, and found the handle part come close, the instrument only in my hands, and the work all to do over again. I have always found the instrument far less apt to slip since I omitted fastening the parts together; and with more ease to the patient as well as myself, and in much less time than before, have found the head of the child fairly fixed in the instrument, that is, between the two parts or bows: so that, in a few seconds of a minute, I have had the child's head with the instrument, after which little or no difficulty remains. Thus I have delivered several women since my coming to town, some of whom you will find mentioned in the cases at the end of this treatise; and Mr. Gifford, in Case xiv. and elsewhere, frequently complains that his extractor slipt, which I am fully persuaded it would not have done if the parts had been

left unjoined, as I now use them. I do in-
genuously confess that I came by this hint
and improvement by mere accident, as, I
believe, is frequently the case in discoveries
of the greatest importance. For many years
my forceps happened to be made of so soft a
metal as to bend or give way, or suffer some
alteration in their curve. They were made
as usual with the screw fixed to one part or
side of them. These I used for some years;
but they often happening to slip off sideways
(as before mentioned), my opinion of the
instrument was so much lessened, that for
many years after I used it but seldom, and
even not once in the space of ten years,
during which time, when the child could not
be turned, I employed the fillet only. This
I freely communicated to a very ingenious
practitioner, now living in the country, who
will, I doubt not, remember it upon reading
this. At length I caused another pair to be
made me, of better metal, and some other
improvements, the screw part being contrived to take out, and not fixed as in the
former. This screw I happened to lose in
the clothes at the delivery of a woman who,
with her child, is now living, and in
health, in town; and being sent for to
another presently after, and being, indeed,
forced to make the trial, found that the
instrument did its office much better without
the screw, or the two parts being fixed.
All I can say in praise of this noble instrument must necessarily fall short of what
it justly demands. Those only who have
used it to their own advantage, and the security of their offspring, can be truly sensible
of its real worth."

Chapman was aware that the forceps
could not be employed with advantage till
the greater part of the head of the child had
passed through the brim into the cavity of
the pelvis. The forceps cannot be used, he
says, "if the head does not lie very low, nor
is their use to be otherwise attempted." He
had clearly ascertained that it could not be
used with safety if the head remained above
the brim of the pelvis, and the uterus was
imperfectly dilated. "I would of all things,"
he says, "advise the operator to be particularly cautious in his inquiry whether the
infant in the womb be dead or not, if he
chooses to employ the hook, or the child
does not lie low enough for the use of the
forceps, and the parts are so streightened
that he cannot easily turn it; for there have
been many deplorable instances of infants
that have been drawn out this way as dead,
whilst they have been really living." He
admits, however, when it is past all dispute
that the child is really dead, that then the
delivery may with propriety be effected with
the crotchet. From the history of the
case of distortion of the pelvis related by
Mauriceau, it is evident that though the

Chamberlens possessed the forceps in the
most perfect form, they had not become acquainted with the cases to which it was applicable. But Chapman had discovered that
in distortion the head did not descend sufficiently low to be taken hold of by the
forceps, and that the only method of delivery
with safety to the mother was by lessening
the volume of the child's head."

"Though I have in some places of this
Treatise," he observes, "condemned the use
of the hook, and shewn that a child far advanced with its head is to be extracted
with the forceps or fillet, yet I would not
be thought to advance that it ought never to
be employed: because there are some deformed subjects, as the two last mentioned,
in whom the bones of the pelvis have so
bad a structure, and the space between the
protuberance frequently mentioned, and the
os pubis, is so very small, as to render it
altogether impossible for the head of a full-
grown child to be naturally brought away.
In these subjects the head cannot fall into
the vagina low enough to be taken hold of
by the forceps or fillet, nor can it be turned
without the greatest difficulty: and even
when it is turned, it will certainly stick
at the head. In this case it cannot be
drawn away but by the hook, which will
break into its texture, alter the form of it,
and so render it fit to pass through that
passage, which it could never do if it were
whole." It thus plainly appears that we are
not only indebted to Chapman for the first
description of the midwifery forceps, but for
the discovery of the principles which ought
invariably to guide us in its employment.

The following figures represent the forceps
of Chapman and Giffard.

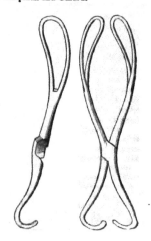

SOME PRACTICAL REMARKS

ON THE

EMPLOYMENT OF ARSENIC IN THE TREATMENT OF THE DISEASES OF THE SKIN.

BY JOHN E. ERICHSEN.

[Concluded from p. 242.]

AMONG the exanthemata there appears to be but one affection that can ever require the exhibition of arsenic; this is *urticaria tuberosa*, a rare disease, and one that I have never had an opportunity of observing. Cazenave, however, relates a case as occurring under Biett, in which it became necessary to have recourse to Fowler's solution.

The only papular disease that ever necessitates the administration of arsenic is *lichen* in its most chronic and rebellious forms. In very obstinate cases of this affection, especially in those varieties of *lichen circumscriptus* that are confined to the face or to the margin of the anus, and the genital organs, in which the skin becomes red, excoriated, chapped, and furfuraceous; or in the chronic confluent form of the eruption, when the whole of the body is covered by papulæ, capped with thin flimsy scales, having a close resemblance to pityriasis, the irritation and consequent insomnia being most distressing, it may become necessary to exhibit one or other of the preparations of this mineral. Biett was in the habit of ordering the "Asiatic Pills," one a day for a month or more. Rayer recommends either Pearson's or Fowler's solutions, due attention being paid to those circumstances that have already been spoken of as contra-indicating their employment. I would give the preference to Fowler's solution, as it is a milder preparation than the arsenious acid. It should be borne in mind, however, that these remedies are only admissible in those cases of *lichen* in which all other means of cure have failed, and in which the patients are worn out by the irritation and restlessness that are the usual consequences of this disease in its more severe and intractable forms. In proof of the value of Fowler's solution in very obstinate and chronic forms of *lichen*, I may mention the case of a girl named *Mary Ann Dockett*, nine years of age,

with delicate complexion, and dark hair and eyes, who lately came under my care for confluent lichen of the whole of the body, with the exception of the face, part of the chest, the palms of the hands, and soles of the feet. The whole of the rest of the surface was studded with an immense multitude of papulæ, somewhat resembling, but more closely set than, those which occur in the cutis anserina: these papulæ, which were particularly distinct about the outer sides of the thighs, arms, and back, were covered with exceedingly minute, flimsy, whitish scabs, giving the skin a powdery appearance. The head was very scurfy, and the hair crisp and dry. At times there was considerable irritation in the skin, which became reddened and cracked, more particularly about the bends of the arms and knees. The mother states that the child has been affected from birth, and that the disease is hereditary on the father's side. As various remedial measures had been resorted to, but without success, and as the child's health appeared to have suffered from the effects of the disease, I determined to have recourse to the solution of the arsenite of potassa. She was accordingly ordered to take one minim of the solution twice a day, to have the whole of the affected parts well anointed every night with a mixture of sweet oil and spermaceti ointment, and to take a bran bath in the morning. After having continued the treatment very little more than a month, during which time she was only obliged to discontinue the arsenic, the dose of which had not been increased, once, and that for a space of four days, the skin had recovered its natural smoothness, which has ever since been preserved by the use of the unction and warm bath.

The only disease amongst the vesiculæ that can ever necessitate the employment of arsenic is *chronic eczema*. This is more particularly the case when this affection, as has already been stated, has assumed a furfuraceous or scaly condition, closely resembling some forms of psoriasis, or pityriasis, and indeed in some instances, as Biett has shown, actually passing into these diseases; the scales becoming dry, laminated, and of a whitish, greyish, or yellowish-grey colour; the subjacent skin being red, thickened, cracked, and inflamed; the vesicular element, however, reappearing in the progress towards a cure. However obstinate this form of the disease may usually be, it becomes particularly intractable when affecting certain regions of the body, as the scrotum, labia, and inside of the thighs, and will, when of old standing in these situations, seldom yield to any remedy but arsenic. The following is a case in point:—

Mr. W. B. æt. 49, of relaxed debilitated habit of body, applied to me, in October last, for a disease of the scrotum, thighs, and breast, under which he had been labouring between four and five years. He ascribed his complaint to his having drank some porter when over-heated, soon after which act of imprudence he experienced considerable irritation about the scrotum and thighs, on which parts a vesicular eruption made its appearance: this was followed by a scaly condition of the parts, and the affection, after a time, spread to other parts of the body, as the arms and chest. He has been subjected to a variety of treatment, and has been salivated twice, but without deriving any benefit. When he applied to me, the scrotum and inner aspect of the thighs were covered by a number of thin, flimsy, yellowish-grey scabs, from under and between which an occasional exudation of a serous fluid took place; the subjacent skin was red, inflamed, and fissured, and there were several patches of a similar character upon the chest, occupying a space of about the size of the hand, as well as one on the right arm. The itching and tingling in the affected parts were severe; so much so that it was with difficulty that he could keep his hands from tearing them. When I first saw him his mouth was sore from the effects of some mercurial that had been ordered by the physician who last attended him, and by whom he was sent to me. He was, therefore, in the first instance, merely directed to take some aperient medicines, and to make use of soothing applications to the affected parts. On the 4th November he was put upon a course of Fowler's solution, beginning with two and a half minims twice a day, and increasing the quantity up to six minims three times a day : this was continued, with two intermissions on account of constitutional disturbance, up to nearly

the end of December, when the disease was entirely cured. The external applications that were had recourse to were, in the first instance, the ointment of the white precipitate, which was, as the disease became more passive in its characters, changed for that of the biniodide of mercury, diluted with four parts of spermaceti ointment.

Useful as the solution of the arsenite of potassa unquestionably is in cases similar to the preceding one, it is equally serviceable in dry chronic eczema affecting other parts of the body, as the following instance will illustrate.

Eliza Penny, æt. 16, of a lymphatico-bilious temperament, came under my care on the 17th November, 1842, for a disease of both arms under which she had laboured from the very earliest infancy (from the age of three months). The affection in question was clearly eczematous. The diseased integument appeared thicker and rougher than natural, was covered with flimsy exfoliations of the epidermis, was exceedingly irritable, itching and tingling to an intense degree when the patient got warm, and was much fissured about the bends of the elbows and wrists. There was every now and then an exacerbation of the disease with a distinct eruption of vesicles. The patient complained much of languor and lassitude, was pale, or rather sallow in complexion, and menstruated somewhat irregularly. She was ordered the diluted mineral acids internally, with the oxide of zinc ointment to the affected parts, and the pil. aloes cum myrrhâ, to regulate the bowels and menstrual functions. Under this plan of treatment the general health improved somewhat, and the irritability of the affected skin was subdued. She was then, on the 2d January, ordered to begin the solution of the arsenite of potassa in two-minim doses ; these were gradually increased to five, and subsequently to seven and a half minims, three times a day: this she continued for a space of two months and a half, until the middle of March, without being obliged to intermit its use for a single day, at the expiration of which period the arms had assumed a healthy appearance, the skin being smooth, soft, and supple, perfectly free from scales, and without any harshness; it was, however, owing probably to the very long time it had been diseased, of a yellowish or tawny colour, darker than that of the rest of the body. The only external applications used were, in the earlier stages, the ointment of the oxide of zinc, with occasional fomentations during the exacerbations of the disease; these were followed by the ointment of the white precipitate, and subsequently by a lotion of the sulphuret of potassium, in the proportions of a dram of the salt to a pint of water. The local disease was not only cured, but the general health very decidedly improved by the administration of the arsenic; the patient having gained flesh and strength, acquired a good colour, and declared herself to be in better health than she had ever enjoyed.

It is but seldom that we meet with cases of the pustular diseases that require the administration of arsenic. Biett and Rayer, however, both state that they have occasionally found it necessary to have recourse to this remedy in some very chronic and rebellious forms of impetigo. Gibert relates two cases of impetigo of the face which had existed from infancy, and which Biett cured by means of Pearson's solution, after many other plans of treatment had been employed without success. These cases are nevertheless very rare, but when they do occur it will be requisite to attend to those different circumstances that have already been mentioned as indicating, or contra-indicating, the exhibition of this metal.

Useful, however, as arsenic may be in many diseases of the skin, it is in the treatment of the squamous affections, more particularly of long-standing cases of lepra and of inveterate psoriasis, that it is incontestibly of the greatest service. For it is by no means rare to meet with cases of these diseases, which obstinately resisting, perhaps for years, milder methods of treatment, will in the course of a few weeks yield to the judicious employment of the preparations of this metal, the utility of which in this class of affections is so fully established by most dermatologists that it is almost needless to insist upon it. It was, indeed, the success that attended the employment of arsenic in the squamous diseases that first led to its introduction into practice as a most

valuable remedy in other affections of the skin. But, notwithstanding its utility in this class of diseases (the squamous), it is not admissible in every stage of their progress, nor indeed is it required in the great majority of these cases; far from it: it is only in very extensive and obstinately rebellious forms of these complaints, or when the patient is suffering some very positive inconvenience from the disease, that we should be justified in administering it, and then only in the absence of those circumstances that have already been pointed out as contra-indicating the administration of arsenic in other affections.

With regard to the stage of lepra and psoriasis in which the preparations of this metal may be administered, it should be laid down as a rule that they should not be given until the disease had assumed a decidedly chronic, inactive character. So long, indeed, as there is any inflammatory redness, heat, or irritation about the patches, they should never, under any circumstances, be employed, as the stimulus of the arsenic would almost infallibly augment the severity of the disease; besides, during the earlier periods of the complaint, we should probably be able to effect a cure by other and less heroic measures. It is only, then, in very long standing cases of an extensive and indolent squamous disease, in which all other means of treatment that are likely to benefit have been employed without success, that these remedies should be given. And even then, as Rayer justly remarks, as these diseases frequently exert no evident ill effects on the constitution, the inconvenience they occasion being but very trifling, it will be advisable to confine the treatment to a palliative one, unless the patient positively insist on some active measures being adopted, when we should not hesitate to have recourse to the employment of the arsenicals, due attention being paid to the temperament of the individual, and to the state of his digestive organs.

In the majority of cases of lepra or psoriasis, Fowler's solution will, I think, be found the most useful preparation of arsenic that we can employ. The liquor of the hydriodate of arsenic and mercury has been very successfully exhibited in cases of this description, as has also the iodide of arsenic, either alone, or, if the disease be of a syphilitic nature, in combination with the biniodide of mercury and extract of conium. Instances illustrative of the value of these preparations have been adduced in a former part of this paper. The "Asiatic pills" were strongly recommended, and, according to Cazenave and Schedel, employed by Biett with advantage, in cases of psoriasis inveterata : they are, however, open to the objection of being less manageable than the other preparations of arsenic.

When these remedies are about to exercise a beneficial influence in cases of lepra and psoriasis, it will be observed that an increased action appears to take place in the diseased cutis, which becomes red, inflamed, and irritable; the scaly patches then appear to heal up, either from the centre or the circumference, according to the nature of the affection, whether it be lepra or psoriasis, and eventually fall off, leaving the subjacent skin red, smooth, shining, and covered by thin epidermic exfoliations, which may usually be readily cleared off by stimulating topical applications, such as the ointments of tar, or of the nitrate or the biniodide of mercury; after which nothing but a red stain will be left in the site of the squamous patch. And this will soon disappear if the remedies be persevered in, which they should always be, until this blotch is entirely and effectually removed; for, until this be accomplished, the disease will be very liable to return: indeed, it is from a want of due attention to this very important circumstance, that the arsenical preparations have been so often accused of effecting merely temporary cures. We must not be content with removing the scales merely, which are secondary phenomena, but we must get rid of the primary lesion, that peculiar inflammatory or congested state of the blood-cutis, which, by giving ...ed and morbid secre-...is, is the proximate ...eases.

...y cases of squamous ...ve seen the pre-...t employed with ...ly mention one, ...r the very short ...editary affection ...ding yielded to ...owler's solution.

Sarah Partons, ætat. 20, of lymphatico-sanguine temperament, being stout, rather pale, with gray eyes and light brown hair, came under my care on the 12th January, for psoriasis of the legs, arms, knees, and elbows, of thirteen years' standing. Her father and brother (who is now under my care) labour under the same disease. There are a number of patches of psoriasis, varying from the size of a sixpence to that of a crown piece, about both legs and arms, and a few on the back. Immediately below the left knee there is one as large as the palm of the hand, and the points of both elbows, but more particularly the left one, are covered by thick scaly incrustations, extending some way down the posterior aspect of the fore-arm. The diseased patches were in a very indolent condition, there being no inflamed areola about them, and being unattended by any tingling or itching. The general health was good, and there were no dyspeptic symptoms of any kind. As the disease was of such long standing it had been subjected to a great variety of treatment, and she had been a patient at two of the metropolitan hospitals, at one for a period of eight months, without receiving any benefit. I therefore, as she was very anxious for a cure, determined to try at once the effect of arsenic, and accordingly ordered her two and a half minims of the solution of the arsenite of potassa twice a day; the biniodide of mercury ointment diluted with three parts of ung. cetacei, to be rubbed into the diseased patches night and morning. The quantity of the solution of the arsenite of potassa was gradually increased until the 27th, when she was taking seven and a half minims three times a day. By this time the diseased patches on the arms, and some of those on the legs, had been cleared of their scales; the affected skin was, however, redder than natural, and rapidly covered itself with scales of epidermis if the use of the ointment was interrupted. On the 28th some constitutional derangement, as headache, lassitude, pain in the eyes, and thirst, came on: the solution was accordingly discontinued. On the 4th February it was resumed in doses of five minims three times a day, which quantity was continued without any disturbance, either local or constitutional, until the 10th March, when, as the disease appeared to be entirely cured, with the exception of a red stain as it were, of the skin in the site of the affected patches, the dose of the solution was diminished to three minims, which quantity was continued, in order to prevent a relapse, until the end of the month. The ointment of the biniodide of mercury had been persevered in during the whole of this time, its strength having been increased to equal parts of the ointment of the Pharmacopœia and of spermaceti cerate.

It may, then, be concluded, from what has been stated in the preceding pages, that the administration of such powerfully stimulating tonics as the preparations of arsenic should be guided by the same rules that govern the exhibition of this class of remedies generally. We should avoid using them, not only in certain kinds of diseases, but in any affection so long as there is any inflammatory action of an active nature going on about it; in persons of a plethoric habit of body, or of a sanguine or sanguineo-nervous temperament; and more particularly in those in whom there exists any irritation about the gastric mucous membrane, or any other inflammatory disease; and only administer them when the cutaneous affection occurs in an individual of a relaxed, debilitated, or lymphatic habit of body, when it has fallen into an indolent, passive state; and, more particularly, if it be a squamous disease, or if it have assumed a furfuraceous aspect, and can bear, without being permanently irritated, the application of a mild topical stimulant. If the administration of arsenic be regulated with a due regard to these circumstances, the doses being slowly and gradually increased, there is no reason why its exhibition should be attended with worse consequences than that of antimony, mercury, strychnia, or of any other very active remedy which we are in the daily habit of prescribing without any fear as to the effects that it may produce upon the system. There can be no question, however, that very injurious effects have resulted from the injudicious administration of the preparations of arsenic in too large doses: but the consequences of the abuse of any medicine are not fair arguments against its careful and guarded administration; and I feel *convinced that arsenic may be exhibited with as much safety as any other powerful tonic in the Pharmacopœia,* provided due discrimination be shown in selecting the cases to which it is to be given. And it is by regarding the preparations of this metal in the light of *specifics* to be resorted to indiscriminately in the treatment of every obstinate and rebellious affection of the skin, without attention to the nature, stage, and complications of the disease, or to the habit of body and temperament of the individual in whom it occurs, that much mischief has resulted from, and opprobrium been cast upon a very valuable remedy.

MISCELLANEOUS CONTRIBUTIONS
TO
PATHOLOGY AND THERAPEUTICS.

By JAMES RICHARD SMITH, M.D.
London.

Rickets.—Pathology and treatment of the affection.—Connection with enlargement of the liver and indigestion.—Its affinity to scrofula.—Scrofula.—Its pathology and treatment.—Gastrodynia.—Sometimes cured by a dietetical remedy.—Chronic hydrocephalus.—A CEREBRAL MURMUR *symptomatic of its first stage.*

CASE I. May 27, 1839.—Wm. Kates, aged 3 years and 2 months: was born healthy and stout, and continued to be so until he was three months old, when his teeth began to appear, and he had an attack of inflammation of the lungs. About, or shortly after that time, he was transferred from his mother to her sister, to be brought up by feeding. The child's health then became much impaired, and he has been always sickly and weak since. His present condition is as follows:—skin anæmatous and pale; flesh scanty and soft; legs and thighs bowed and emaciated, and body altogether approximating to a state of marasmus; can make no effort at standing or walking, and creeps but feebly; spine curved laterally; left side of thorax enlarged and projecting laterally and posteriorly; clavicles distorted; head has always appeared larger than ordinary, and at present there is a soft fluctuating tumor situated on the left parietal bone. His mother states that previous to the appearance of this tumor the sutures of the skull were very open; that he had a fall a few days ago from a bench high, on which she pitched upon his fore the tumor appear appetite, and fall, but regular, expres rather

℞ Hydrarg. c. Cretâ, gr. iij. ; Pulv. Rhæi, gr. iv. ; Cinnam. gr. j. ft. pulvis. Mitte vj.   Sumat j. alterna nocte.

℞ Sp. Rosmar. ʒss. ; Aq. Font. ʒvss. M. ft. Lot. tumore constanter applicet.

29th.—Tumor considerably decreased ; no perceptible change otherwise.

Continuentur lotio et pulveres, et hirudo tempore iterum applicetur.

June 1st.—Tumor of head almost disappeared, and some other little improvement.

Continue the lotion and the powders, and let the child have a warm salt water bath every other night at bed-time, and let him be well rubbed with a dry cloth, both on the body and limbs, for ten minutes after coming out of the bath.

5th.—The tumor on the head has entirely disappeared, and the parietal bone on which it was situated, which was fully a line depressed below the others, has become elevated to its proper position. Head much hotter than natural ; eyes dry and glassylooking ; pupils rather dilated ; is fretful when awake, and frowns frequently in sleep, but does not start or grind the teeth ; tongue deficient in moisture, but not furred ; pulse rapid, and rather unresisting ; alvine excretions light-coloured ; is very thirsty ; hands hot. On applying the ear to the anterior fontanelle, or to the parietal bones, a murmur accompanying the cerebral circulation is very audible*.

Continue the powders, one every night, and the cold lotion to the head, and the warm bath without the salt ; let the child's diet be chiefly beef-tea, arrowroot, and milk and water.

July 1st.—Little or no alteration in any respect since last report. Head still much hotter than natural ; anterior fontanelle agitated, and cerebral murmur very loud over the entire of the head, with the exception of the os frontis ; eyes still dry and glassylooking ; no strabismus, but frequent frowning. His mother states that the child frequently complains of pain over the left ear. Otherwise as before.

Let the head be closely shaved, and kept constantly wet with the cold lotion, and let two small leeches be immediately applied to seat of pain over left ear.

℞ Hydrarg. c. Creta, Pulv. Jalapæ, as. gr. iij. ; Pulv. Ipecacuanhæ, gr. j. ; ft. pulvis mitte vi. ; Sumat j. nocte maneque. Continue the same diet.

5th.—No obvious change since last report.

Continue the cold lotion, powders, and diet, and apply two leeches again to the left parietal bone over the ear.

9th.—The leeches bled well ; the powders have been taken regularly, and the bowels have been moved thrice a day. The mother states that the child is becoming cheerful and better tempered, and more disposed to chat. Head still hot, and frequent perspiration from it and from the face during sleep ; cerebral murmur very audible even over the occipital bone ; frequent leering, but no strabismus ; abdomen hot, but arms and legs rather below the natural temperature ; appetite rather inordinate, and sleeps pretty well ; excretion of urine less frequent ; pulse frequent and resisting.

Continue the same treatment.

16th.—Has administered the treatment as prescribed faithfully. The condition of the child in all respects is much improved since last visit. He has put on flesh, and his limbs are becoming plump and firm. There is not now any frowning or leering, and the eyes are acquiring an expression of softness and animation. He has lost much of his fretfulness, and is now daily becoming more mild and more easily amused. The head is still hotter than natural, and the cerebral murmur is audible, but less intense. Renal secretion less, and appetite not so voracious. Bowels stated to be more regular, and their excretions of a more healthy character. Respiration and action of heart not disturbed.

Being struck to-day by the undiminished and still very protuberant state of the abdomen, after the use for some considerable time of aperient medicines, the thought occurred to us to examine it by percussion and pressure, when we found the liver enormously enlarged, the right lobe almost in contact with the crest of the ilium, and the left overlapping the stomach, and easily felt between two and three inches below the ensiform cartilage. The ends of the lower ribs, both on the right and left side, were considerably everted. Continue the same plan of treatment, and let us see the child again in the course of a week.

September 23d.—Had not seen the child now for more than two months. Little, if any, discernible change in its condition since last report ; but on the whole, perhaps, there is some improvement. The countenance looks better, and the child appears to have gained some more flesh ; liver somewhat reduced in size, but still much larger than natural, and very easily felt by pressure of the hand on the right side of the abdomen ; the child is not yet able to maintain the erect position, but it creeps with much more activity ; all other symptoms as before.

℞ Hydrarg. c. Cretâ, gr. ij. ; Hydrarg. Chlorid. gr. ss. ; Pulv. Rhæi, gr. iij. ; Pulv. Cinnamomi, gr. j. Ft. pulvis, mitte viij. sumat j. alterna nocte.

℞ Potassæ Bisulph. ℈ij. ; Sodæ Bicarb.

---

* Dr. Macleod, and Mr. Johnson (of Med.-Chir. Review), auscultated the head of this patient, and said they heard the murmur distinctly.

Ɔj.; Aquæ Menth. Pip. ʒix. Solve terendo, et adde Tinct. Rhæi, Tinct. Sennæ, aa. ʒiss.; Syrup Aurantii, ʒij. Ft. mistura cujus capiat cochlæaria parva tria omni mane. To have solid animal food at least once a day, and also a little beef-tea, with diluents of arrow-root or sago occasionally; to be warmly clothed, and to be as much in the open air as possible.

October 8th.—Has used the powders, mixture, and diet, and treatment otherwise, in all particulars regularly since last visit. Condition of child in all respects remarkably improved. His mother states that he sleeps well; that his appetite is not half what it was; that his disposition is quite changed, as he has lost all his peevishness; no frowning or leering, and countenance becoming full and animated; has gained considerable strength both of body and limbs, and can make some effort at standing; abdomen less protuberant, and liver further diminished in size, but still projects between two and three inches below the ribs on the right side; the ribs both on the right and left side are much less everted, and the shape of the thorax is altogether more normal; the cerebral murmur is still audible at all points of the cranium, but the forehead, and the left hemisphere of the cranium, on the parietal bone of which the tumor was situated, appears rather larger than the right. Continue the same treatment in medicine, diet, and exercise.

This patient now ceased to be under our care, and we entirely lost sight of the case; but we have every reason to suppose the little fellow continued to recover, or he would have visited us again.

CASE II. Sept. 11, 1839.—Eliz. Williams, aged two years and a half, of fair hair and fair complexion, eyes light blue, skin and subcutaneous tissue fine and soft, and the economy generally discovering a tendency to the strumous diathesis, was a very healthy child until after vaccination, which operation was performed upon her when she was about six months old, at which time, or immediately after, she commenced to cut her teeth, and a papular eruption made its appearance all over the body; and at the same time, also, the child's bowels and general health were much disordered, the alvine excretions being frequent, and showing some appearances of blood. The child has been in bad health, better or worse, ever since. Present condition as follows. Much fretfulness and irritability; sleep light and easily disturbed; countenance pale and dejected; irides decolourised; surface generally pale and chill; no emaciation, but flesh soft and flabby; no morbid curvature of the spine or of the bones of the chest, but the right leg is

very weak and bent inwards at the knee; liver considerably enlarged; it can be felt in the right hypochondrium, between two and three inches below the ribs, but it is not perceptible in the epigastrium; renal secretion stated to be natural in quantity and appearance; pulse and respiration undisturbed; no thirst, but appetite voracious. The head appears rather large, and the anterior fontanelle is still open, and on applying the ear to it or to either of the parietal bones a faint cerebral murmur is audible.

℞ Hydrarg. c. Cretâ, gr. iij.; Pulv. Jalapæ, gr. iij.; Pulv. Cinnamomi, c. gr. ij. Ft. pulvis, mitte vj. sumat j. alterna nocte.

℞ Infusi Sennæ, ʒvj.; Potassæ Bicarb. ʒss.; Mannæ Opt. ʒiss.; Tinct. Cinnamomi c. ʒj.; Aquæ Carui, ʒj. M. fiat mistura cujus capiat cochlearia parna tria omni mane. Let the child's diet be moderate in quantity, but let her have solid animal food in fair quantity once a day at least, and let her be much in the open air.

22d.—Has used the treatment prescribed regularly. Two excretions have taken place from the bowels daily of a more healthy character. The condition of the child is something improved; it is less fretful, and is more animated, and its appetite is not so voracious; little if any perceptible alteration in the size of the liver; the cheeks are still pale, but the colour appears returning to the irides; cerebral murmur and other symptomatic phenomena as before. The same treatment in all respects to be continued.

October 8th.—Has used the remedies prescribed regularly since last report; child's general condition and health altogether much improved; she is becoming lively and good-tempered, and sleeps well; countenance less exsanguineous and drooping; irides deepening in colour; appetite not voracious, but moderate; alvine excretions more regular and of a more healthy character; flesh becoming firm, and the cutaneous circulation generally more active; cerebral murmur audible now only at the anterior fontanelle, and here but faintly; abdomen much reduced in size, and softer; liver lessened considerably, but still projects below the margin of the chest.

Continue the mixture, powders, and diet, as prescribed, and let the child have a warm bath twice a week.

We saw this patient once again after some little time, when her health was all but completely restored. The countenance had acquired colour and animation, and she had become plump and active; she slept soundly, and the alvine and urinary excretions were healthy; circulation and respiration the same; the liver was further reduced in size, but still to be felt under the right hypochondrium, but not at the pit of the stomach; the cerebral murmur had ceased to be audible on auscultation of the cranium at any point.

CASE III. Aug. 17, 1838.—Wm. Rogers, æt. 19 months, of light hair, light complexion, and blue eyes; was strong and healthy till he was eight months old, when he had an attack of illness of six weeks' duration, which his medical attendant pronounced to be inflammation of the lungs. This attack consisted chiefly in feverishness with cough and much disorder of the bowels. The mother states that the alvine excretions towards the latter part of the child's illness, were unhealthy and offensive, and contained substances like pieces of flesh. He appeared to have recovered from this attack pretty well, but about a month afterwards the head was first observed to be enlarged, and it has gradually increased in size since. Present condition as follows: general health not much disturbed, but face and surface generally anæmatous and pale; no emaciation, but flesh soft; sleep unquiet; bowels generally relaxed, but their excretions and also the excretion of urine stated to be natural in character; is still at the breast, but will eat any solid food that is presented to him; appetite rather inordinate; pulse 126, and regular; head large, circumference 23 inches and a half from each meatus auditorius, over the vertex 14 inches and a quarter; no dilatation of the pupils, but considerable strabismus, and the eyes remain half open and roll a great deal during sleep; anterior fontanelle large, and of a crucial shape where the cerebral movements are perceptible to the touch, and the *cerebral murmur* very audible on application of the ear. Has not had small-pox, measles, or any other of the eruptive fevers; was successfully vaccinated.

CASE IV. Oct.16,1836.—Mrs. A.'s infant, æt. 14 months, a pretty strong and large boy for his age, has been dull and listless for the last three or four days, and has rested badly the last two nights: at present he is unusually inanimate; the skin is harsh and increased in temperature; the bowels are irregular and their excretions fluid and of a light clay-colour, without the slightest tinge of bile: the head appears rather above what is ordinary in size, and the anterior fontanelle is open, and on applying the ear to this part a *cerebral murmur* is heard very distinctly; it is also audible, but less clearly, over the parietal bones; abdomen protuberant and somewhat resisting, but no enlargement of the liver can be detected; flesh rather soft; pulse frequent. For this patient

we prescribed a powder of hepatic alterative properties, which was taken every night, and occasionally every other night, at bed-time, with a dose of a mildly aperient mixture once or twice during the day; pretty full diet with solid animal food in fair quantity at least once a day; warm clothing and exercise in the open air at all times when the weather will permit of it. This child in a short time became quite stout and well.

REMARKS.—These four cases now described present us with examples of profound chronic digestive derangement and disease in children, similar, we conceive, in their origins, causes, and natures, but in different periods of progress, and different states of development. The first case, that of the boy Kates, which will form the subject chiefly of the following observations, is manifestly a case of tabes and rickets; the cause of the tabes being, in this instance, not in the glands of the mesentery, but in a glandular structure of far greater magnitude and importance, namely, the liver. To an examination less accurate with respect to the state of the abdominal viscera, than that which was given to this case, by pressure and percussion, when, as we have seen, it had been some time under treatment, the diagnosis could scarcely have pronounced the affection other than tabes mesenterica. All the symptoms which are usually considered as peculiar to, and enunciative of, that scrofulous malady were present. There was the large protuberant abdomen, with the general and severe emaciation in contrast; the voracious appetite; the derangement of digestion, and disorder of the functions of the intestinal canal; the irregular hectic feverishness, and the diminished temperature of the extremities, with other minor symptoms. The white alvine excretions, which we find mentioned by almost all authors upon mesenteric tabes, as a pathognomonic sign of that affection, were not present. We entertain some doubts, however, on the perfect exemption from error of this diagnostic doctrine, and could give, we think, sufficient reasons for so doing. At present we will only observe, that we have seen white earthy excretions, not unlike the ashes of wood wetted, passed from the bowels, for months, by adults labouring under jaundice and organic disease of the liver. The fact, however, which deserves our first consideration, and which makes the case now under comment more particularly interesting in a pathological and practical point of view, is the immense enlargement of the liver that was present in this infantile patient. No one, we believe, however recent and imperfect his knowledge may happen to be of any disease he may be called upon to treat, but forms some notion to himself of its cause and original idea, and prescribes his remedies accordingly. The more correct, too, are his thoughts on the etiological points of the case, the more likely, it is certain, are his remedial measures of being beneficial and successful.

The question, then, of most import and utility involved in the pathology of this case, and one, undoubtedly, which it is difficult to determine, is, what place, in an analysis of its constituent phenomena, should be assigned to the hepatic enlargement; whether should it be viewed as cause, or as consequence, or as a concomitant morbid condition? Sydenham, we find, has mentioned the enlarged state of the abdominal viscera (without having particularised the liver) which is present in children affected with rickets, and he appears to have considered both the affection of rickets and the visceral disease as consequences of intermittent fever—a sort of metastatic and critical deposition of the febrile matter. "Children sometimes become hectic after both *continued* and *intermittent* autumnal fevers. The abdomen in this case swells and grows hard, a cough also and other consumptive symptoms frequently arise, which manifestly resemble the rickets." "It is worth observing, that when children have been long affected with autumnal intermittents, there are no hopes of vanquishing the disease till the abdomen (especially that part of it near the spleen) swells and grows hard; the distemper abating in the same degree as this symptom manifests itself. Nor can we, perhaps, more certainly foretel that the intermittent will go off in a short time, than by carefully attending to the swelling of the *abdomen* in children, and to that of the legs, which sometimes happens, in grown persons." "The swelling of the abdomen which happens in children after intermittents, in those years wherein the constitution of the air has a tendency to produce autumnal *intermittents epidemically*, appears to the

touch as if the viscera contained matter hardened to a scirrhus; whereas, that which comes in other years yields to the touch, as if the hypochondria were only distended by wind. Hence it is worth notice, that the true rickets rarely happen except in those years wherein autumnal intermittents prevail."— *Swan's transl. of Sydenham*, pp. 64, 65.

Baron Van Swieten, too, in his admirable Commentaries upon Boerhaave's Aphorisms, has not omitted to notice the increased bulk of the liver that accompanies the condition of rickets; but the particular part which it acts in the pathology of the disease he does not distinctly point out; he only assigns to it the place of a "concurrent cause," as he terms it, of the protuberant abdomen. "I have often, (observes Van Swieten), had children brought to me to be cured, supposed by their mothers to have been troubled with great liver, when they manifestly had the rickets." We shall hereafter see that in this disorder the liver is found of a vast size, though no other disorder can be discerned in this viscus after death. Glisson, upon examining the dead bodies of rickety children, thus testifies: "the liver, in all I have dissected, is greater than it should be; but otherwise is not of a bad colour, nor greatly indurated, or in other respects contaminated by any other remarkable vice." He excepts some dead bodies in which other diseases had been complicated with the rickets before death, as he remembered to have observed in a dropsical and extremely tabid patient. From hence the reason appears why the rickets has, in some places, been distinguished by the name of *great liver*; he found no fault in the magnitude, colour, or substance of the spleen; yet he denies not that it might happen otherwise from a complication of rickets with other diseases."—*Van Swieten's Commentaries*, vol. 17, pp. 339 and 367.

Our experience, we acknowledge, does not enable us to say to what extent enlargement of the liver, and more or less prolonged defect or vitiation of the biliary secretion in children, deranging and impairing the processes of infantile digestion and hæmatosis, may be connected with the proximate cause and early phenomena of rickets; but we could not avoid observing, during the treatment of the two first cases of the subject of this paper, in which great enlargement of the liver was present, that the return to a more healthy size of that viscus, and improvement of the general condition of each individual, and marked amendment of the rickety symptoms, were perfectly simultaneous. The great Boerhaave, it is true, has made the proximate cause of rickets to consist in "a sluggish, cold, and vapid cacochymy, together with a loose structure of the solid parts," which obviously gives to the affection a humoral origin, and places its *ens primum* in the blood; and in this respect Boerhaave is, no doubt, in a great measure correct; but the blood, it should be borne in mind, is dependent for its existence and its continuous healthy condition upon the combined and harmonious operation of a number of organs, the second in office and importance of which is the liver. The first changes wrought upon the food by the vital battery (if we may be allowed such a term) of digestion and sanguification in the abdomen, the chylopoietic viscera more usually denominated, are effected, it is almost unnecessary to observe, by the offices of the stomach; the second by that of the liver. Is it unreasonable to suppose, then, that if this latter organ should become diseased or defective in function, and continue so for any lengthened time during infancy, the period of most tender growth and conformation of the individual, it must effect in some very obvious manner the process of assimilation and healthy organic formation throughout the entire system? Look at a child the subject of slight taint, or what you might consider as the state of commencing rickets. Criticise its entire condition. Does it not bear a strong resemblance, in many points, to that of an adult whom one would suspect to be labouring under some chronic concealed affection of the liver? So has it, in fact, not unfrequently struck our observation. At all events we are firmly of opinion that the practitioner who will view the infantile affection now under consideration as one simply of hepatic disease, with more or less aggravated derangement of all the digestive functions, and so apply his remedies judiciously in accordance, will be he who is most likely to benefit, and *in all respects improve*, the condition *of his patient.* From some little atten-

tion we have occasionally paid, as opportunity offered, to the' indispositions and disorders of children, we will take upon us to observe that there is a pretty comprehensive class of chronic digestive affections, which these tender young creatures too frequently suffer from, the pathology of which is still a subject but imperfectly understood, and the treatment, as a matter of course, uncertain and unsatisfactory. In this class we place the different lesions and perversions of assimilation and nutrition as exhibited in the respective manifestations of scrofula of the vascular, muscular, and osseous structures. We coincide in opinion, it is necessary to observe, with some authors of creditable authority, who consider the malady of rickets, as regards the softness of the muscles and bones, as nothing else than a scrofulous affection of those parts. We also attribute to a taint of the same distemper the dropsical diseases of chronic hydrocephalus and spina bifida, as we are fully convinced these morbid conditions always originate in this peculiar diathesis of debility. Sir Astley Cooper, whose name we always quote with pleasure, has recommended the best measures, dietetical in particular, for the treatment of scrofula with which we are conversant. They are, we conceive, so correct and accordant with sound therapeutics, that we will venture to predict no future experience, founded on right observation, will ever find them much in error. It is the fibrine and red globules of the blood that give to it the power and means of sufficiently nourishing our organs, and of developing and supporting good health and robust strength throughout the system. Sir Astley having rightly noted that the blood of scrofulous individuals was serous and attenuated, and deficient in those important constituents, prescribed the means most likely to obviate such a state, and better its condition. To a child labouring under scrofulous debility or disease, he enjoined the use of animal food three times a day, namely, at breakfast, lunch, and dinner, and the last of these meals was to be taken at 3 o'clock P.M.; warm clothing, with frequent exercise in the open air, when wet, damp, or very cold weather did not forbid; the urging of the functions of the liver and digestive canal once a week by the administration of a solutive and alterative powder of calomel and rhubarb. This is, we truly believe, the best plan of treatment that could be devised for counteracting in childhood, or, indeed, at any period of life, scrofulous diathesis, or tendency to such a state in the economy, and for preventing the development of scrofulous abscess and ulceration locally. Many a surgical incision, sore, and cicatrice, will such therapeutics prevent from injuring the otherwise mazing beauty of many a female neck*. There is an error, in our opinion, abroad, of no little evil operation, in some instances, as regards the use of animal food. With a great many individuals, notwithstanding what the advocates of vegetable and farinaceous aliment may say to the contrary, this article of diet is unquestionably taken too sparingly, or its use is not properly timed. The presence of animal food in the stomach at an early period of the day, acts, with many persons of peculiar temperament and constitution, not only as an efficient remedy in soothing and allaying general irritability, and vascular over-action dependent thereon, but it also performs the part of an anodyne and agent of cure in various dyspeptic neuralgias and irritations. Does not the following fact, which, with some others very similar, lately came under our notice, corroborate to a considerable degree these observations? A young gentleman, who had suffered much from gastrodynia, accompanied with a feeling of cardiac distress and sense of sinking at the pit of the stomach, which generally came on between 10 and 11 A.M. (sometimes it was experienced immediately on getting up, between 7 and 8) and continued more or less severe until between 2 and 3 P.M., his usual time of dining. For the cure of this gastrodynia, by the advice of several eminent physicians, he had had recourse to a variety of medicines.

He had made trial of the extract of stramonium and extract of belladonna, of the oxide of bismuth, the oxide of iron, and of the sulphate of quinine, and some other remedial agents of less note, without having experienced any permanent benefit. When he consulted us, his countenance was pale, lean, and anxious; he was thin and somewhat irritable and nervous; his system generally had the appearance of being insufficiently supplied with blood; the pulse was rather frequent and contracted (contracted, we mean, as to the circumference of its vessel); his appetite was pretty good; the bowels were stated to be regular, and his sleep undisturbed. In the course of our inquiry into the symptoms of this case, we put the question to our patient— When do you generally observe the pain of stomach to cease? " Soon after dinner, towards the after part of the day," he replied. How often have you been in the habit of taking animal food in the day, we inquired? "Once," he replied, " at dinner." What do you breakfast upon? was our next interrogatory. " Bread-and-butter, with tea or coffee, and sometimes an egg," was the answer we received. We then prescribed a mutton-chop, with an egg, or good large slice of ham and an egg, with his usual tea and bread-and-butter, for breakfast; and the second morning after taking the mutton-chop as prescribed, the young gentleman, to his no little delight, and the gastrodynia, which had been the bane of his comfort for years, parted company, and have never since renewed acquaintance. When we last saw this patient, more than two years from the time we had prescribed for him, he still continued to take a little animal food for breakfast, and he remained free from the pain. What was the nature of this gastrodynia, then? Was it the instinct or sensation of hunger, idiosyncratic and morbid in this instance, being in the human subject, but similar to that which is naturally experienced by some of the lower carnivorous animals, the beasts of prey, and which urges them so ferociously in quest of flesh, which no other sort of food has the property to allay*. We

---

* Whatever measures it may be in the power of the physician or surgeon to suggest, that will preserve from any degree of injury and deformity the most quietly beautiful part of one of the most beautiful objects in nature, must always, we imagine, be a matter of some little interest to all. Observe that part of a beautiful woman where she is, perhaps, the most beautiful, about the neck and breasts; the smoothness, the softness, the easy and insensible swell, the variety of the surface, which is never for the smallest space the same, the deceitful maze through which the unsteady eye slides giddily, without knowing where to fix, or whither it is carried."—*Philosophical Inquiry into the Origin of our Ideas of the Sublime and Beautiful.*

---

† " In the course of this treatise we shall have frequent occasion to remark, that the *diseased* state of an organ in the human body is the physiological or *healthy* condition of the same organ in other animals.—*Andral's Pathological Anatomy*, vol. l. page 94." *Translation by Drs. Townsend & West.*

T

could adduce other instances, if necessary, equally illustrative of the good effects of a little solid animal food being presented to the stomach at the morning repast, or at a less early hour of the day, in raising the system from a state of ill health and debility, and conferring upon it the inestimable blessings of good health and strength. It is only, we will here remark, the unhealthy and infirm that ought properly to be accounted poor.

The health of the honest peasant, or labourer of any description, is his wealth, and the happiest wealth or capital, too, in all respects, which he can possess. With none other certainly does he embark so cheerfully in the business of existence, and enjoy with such fulness the fruits of his exertions, or, when they chance to come, the bounties of fortune. With none other can he contribute to the continuance of the constitution and vigour of society, in the renewal of the youth and bloom of population, by raising up around him offspring and issue ruddy with life and the light of youthful health — the *lumen purpureum juventæ* — such objects as his heart always owns and exults in, and his bosom fondly cherishes; and through which thus, by the divinity of parental affection, transmutes, it might be said, by a beautiful alchymy in the moral economy of humble life, the labourer's daily industry and toil into a daily hymn of silent happiness and content, not less acceptable and grateful to the Creator than are the most loud and lengthened orisons of the more indolent and inactive, yet dutiful and holy saint. But to return for a little to the more immediate subject of our paper.

In looking over the observations of the great surgeon, Cooper, upon the malady of rickets, we find that he places the proximate cause of that disease in the mesenteric glands, and thus identifies in a great degree *tabes mesenterica* with rickets, although the affections are unquestionably, we think, distinct both in their origins and symptoms generally. In none of the cases we have described in this paper could we detect any enlargement of the glands of the mesentery, or any tenderness on pressure of the abdomen over these vessels. *Tabes mesenterica* in the infant is more allied perhaps to the *affection of atrophy* in the adult, than *to rickets.*

Some time in the autumn of 1837,

we published a short paper in the MEDICAL GAZETTE, in which we pointed out the existence, and described the characters, of a murmur or sound accompanying the cerebral circulation in certain conditions of cerebral disease in children. We took occasion then to state that we thought such auscultic phenomenon, when present in the head, might either be received as a premonitory symptom of chronic hydrocephalus, or as a diagnostic sign of the actual existence of the disease in its most incipient state. This murmur was present, as we have seen, in various intensity, in all the four cases which form the subject of this paper, and we still rest in the opinion we took up on first observing it, that it is always concomitant with, and produced by, a morbid action of the vessels of the brain, which precedes and accompanies more or less dropsical effusion in that organ. As the phenomenon is undoubtedly one of some little interest and diagnostic novelty in the cerebral pathology of children, we would willingly direct the attention of other observers to it, in hopes that it may be found of some utility in indicating the best mode of treatment in the earliest stage of chronic hydrocephalus. Fine though it be " that nothing lives 'twixt it and silence," we take some little credit to ourselves for having been the first in this country to observe and describe this sound, and auscultic sign of disease, in the encephala of children. Shortly after the publication of our description of the phenomenon in the MEDICAL GAZETTE, one of the medical reviews* disputed our claim to originality in its observance, by the statement that we had been preceded in the matter by an American physician. We do not doubt the truth of this statement of the Review, but we have not yet seen, let us mention, a description of the phenomenon by other pen than our own. We might extend our observations here much further, but this paper has already, we perceive, grown to some considerable length.

43, Sackville Street.
    May 10th, 1843.

* The British and Foreign Medical Quarterly, we think.

CONTINUATION

OF THE

CASE OF ILEUS,

Recorded in the MED. GAZ. *for April* 28.

AND THE POST-MORTEM APPEARANCES.

———

MAY 1st.—During the past month he had slept well, and ate moderately ; the alvine evacuations two or three a day, loose, and yellow ; but the extreme emaciation had continued.

4th.—It is stated that for the last two or three days he has eaten but little, that he felt a pain yesterday on the right side. He now complains of griping pains below the umbilicus, where the abdomen is swollen and tympanitic. Pressure on the right side between the ribs and crest of the ilium gives pain. The pulse small and weak ; extremities cold ; perspiration on the face ; tongue, far back, rather coated. Sick once.

Administ. Enema Sapon. ; soon returned. R. Haust. Rhei et Mag. Carb. stat. sum.

10 P.M.—No evacuation from the bowels ; griping pain in the abdomen continues.

Adm. Enema Sap. ; returned. R. Ol. Ricini, ʒss. 3tiis. hor. sum.

5th.—No evacuation from the bowels ; nausea ; pain over the whole abdomen, which he dreads to have touched ; laborious thoracic breathing. No wish to live.

He died at 6 P.M.

Post-mortem appearances.

The contents of the bowels.—Upwards of two quarts of a brown fluid, with castor-oil, were found in the cavity of the abdomen. The convolutions of the small intestines, just below the umbilicus, were much twisted and matted together, so as sufficiently to account for the strangulation of the bowels. On the mucous surface the canal in two places was so contracted and blocked up by adhesions as scarcely to admit the passage of a probe. A portion of the jejunum was greatly distended, with a diameter of at least three inches, and lay in front of the ascending colon, which was closely contracted. In this distended portion, between the ribs and crest of the ilium, there was an opening just sufficient to admit a probe, and

taking a course of about half an inch through the coats of the bowel, which were much thickened by deposits of lymph. Near this opening on the serous surface was a conical deposit of lymph two inches from base to apex, at the base of which on the mucous surface there was a cicatrix.

———

POLYPOID TUMOR IN THE TRACHEA.

———

To the Editor of the Medical Gazette.

SIR,

SHOULD the following case be deemed sufficiently interesting to your numerous readers, you will oblige me by inserting it in your valuable journal.

I am, sir,

Your obedient servant,

J. H. STALLARD,

New Street, Leicester,   M.R.C.S.L.
May 9, 1843.

Martha Butler, æt. 40, married, was admitted into the Receiving Ward of the Leicester Workhouse, on Tuesday, April 25, 1843. She was in a most destitute and dirty state, and was labouring under symptoms of bronchitis. Her filth entirely precluded a minute examination ; but she stated that for a long time past she had been asthmatical, and had had a very bad cough, but that this cough had been much aggravated by privations and exposure. She was ordered to take the following draught every four hours :—

R Syr. Papav. Albi, Tr. Scillæ, aa. ʒss. ; Liq. Ammon. Acet. ʒiij. ; Mist. Ammoniaci, ʒj. M. ft. haust.

April 28th.—During the last few days she has been much better ; her cough is not so violent, nor her dyspnœa so urgent.

29th.—She went to bed as usual last night, but awoke about eleven o'clock, and had a violent paroxysm of coughing, which continued for upwards of an hour. She then got out of bed, and whilst sitting by the side of the bed died before any assistance could be obtained.

Sectio cadaveris 36 hours after death. — The lungs were emphysematous. The smaller bronchi were healthy, but the right and left divisions were highly congested. In the trachea was found a loose body of a polypoid nature, about the size of an almond, and having a pedicle about three-quarters of an inch long. The trachea at its lower part was much congested, and about an inch and a half below the cricoid cartilage, on the left side, the mucous membrane was considerably thickened and inflamed. About half an inch below the cricoid cartilage, at the anterior part, were the remains of the pedicle of the polypus; and above this point the trachea presented the natural appearance. The stomach was small and contracted. The liver on the whole larger than usual; it consisted of twelve or fourteen lobes, varying in size from a nut to a large orange; the larger ones, three in number, corresponding with the right and left lobes and the lobulus quadratus: in structure it appeared healthy. The kidneys and spleen were very large. The uterus was carcinomatous.

REMARKS.—When the patient was admitted, I saw no reason why a favourable prognosis should be withheld, knowing how much the comforts, cleanliness, and dietetics of the workhouse, usually accomplish in these cases. I was surprised, therefore, at the sudden termination in death, and was anxious to obtain further information as to its cause. Polypoid tumors in the trachea, so far as I have read and seen, are exceedingly rare. M. Andral states, that hypertrophy of the mucous membrane may be confined to a circumscribed spot, and produce there a tumor projecting more or less above the level of the surrounding membrane; but, he continues, they have been oftener met with in the larynx than in any other part of the air-passage. (Translated Pathology, p. 472.) I was at first inclined to doubt its origin from the tracheal mucous membrane, but the remains of the pedicle, and the thickening of that part of the membrane against which the tumor would rest, left no doubt on this point, and the separation of the tumor, produced probably by the violent coughing, was the cause of the sudden death.

MEDICAL GAZETTE.
Friday, May 18, 1843.

"Licet omnibus, licet etiam mihi, dignitatem Artis Medicae tueri; potestas modo veniendi in publicum sit, dicendi periculum non recuso."
CICERO.

LUNATIC ASYLUMS.

No department of the practice of physic can boast so great a progress within the last few years as the treatment of insanity; and it is with a particular pleasure, therefore, that we ever and anon comment on the reports of our great lunatic asylums, as they issue from the press. It is true that, as far as regards the medical part of the treatment, the improvement consists rather in the abolition of the false than in the establishment of the true. The stated bleedings and vomitings of the last generation have disappeared, like the scourgings and the hellebore of earlier times, and have left no fixed practice to succeed them. The physician prescribes for the symptoms as they arise, he gives carthartics to the constipated, and morphia to the restless, but there is no longer any specific for madness. Neither the Anticyra of the ancients, nor "the dark house and whip" of Shakspeare's age, will cure the disease; what will is a problem yet to be solved. But it is some satisfaction, at any rate, to find, in Thomas Carlyle's language, that old false formulas are trampled into destruction; the ground which they occupied, though now bare and desolate, may yet serve as a foundation for truth.

In the mechanical and moral treatment more has been effected. For, besides the abolition of chains and strait-waistcoats, which may be considered as merely negative improvements, abstaining from bad rather than introducing of good,—farm-work and manual trades, books, music, and various games, form part of the system in well-regulated mad-houses.

Perhaps some fortunate reasoner may succeed in curing the erring mind by a direct method, correcting the hallucinations of one sense by the evidence of the rest; till this happy era arrives, the physician must content himself with an indirect one. The mind of the lunatic must be withdrawn from its favourite contemplations by the allurement of other and safer objects. An asylum may be advantageously turned into a school, where the inmates are withheld from the airy nothings of their imagination; and as they advance in arithmetic, geometry, or languages, they will forget the sprites who tormented them in their ignorance. In the last annual report of the Glasgow Asylum (from which we gave an extract a few weeks ago) it appears that printing has been lately added to the previous employments of the patients. The first product of this press was a periodical, which went on vigorously for ten weeks, when it dropped, from the discharge of some of its contributors. Since then the press has been busied with other matters; and Dr. Hutcheson, the reporter, anticipates that it will not lack occupation for the remainder of the year.

The boldest proposition which he makes, and in which it is difficult, or rather impossible, to agree with him, is, that every one labouring under hallucinations must be locked up, whether mischievous or not.

"When an individual imagines himself to be a supernatural being, to be favoured with divine revelations, to be commissioned to redress grievances, to have suffered or to be threatened with injury, to be conspired against, or to be poisoned, he is *dangerous to the lieges;* and, however calm he may seem, however sane he may appear to be on other subjects, however careful and prudent, however acute he may be in business, *or skilful in the exercise of his profes-* sion, he ought not to be suffered to remain at large, but ought instantly to be placed under treatment and control."

This is a sweeping clause indeed! "If we shut up every woman who changes her mind every minute," says Dr. Smith, in the novel of 'Discipline,' "who is to make our shirts and puddings?" And if we desire to shut up all who are included in Dr. Hutcheson's comprehensive schedule, who will build asylums enough? Not the men of Glasgow, assuredly; for they are too tardy in subscribing for a single one. Whole classes of religionists, if we mistake not, imagine themselves favoured with revelations, and would demand towns metamorphosed into asylums for their reception. Authors against whom Paternoster-Row conspires, and householders constantly ill treated by their ungrateful servants, might swell the crowd, and embarrass the mad-doctors with a superfluity of employment.

The fact is, that Dr. Hutcheson has got into this scrape from an unwillingness to concede that monomaniacs are amenable to the criminal law. If we once allow that the distemperature of Macnaughten's mind, for example, rendered him an irresponsible being, and made a cell in Bethlem his extreme punishment, it will be necessary to shut up these possible criminals by the thousand. But if we admit this dangerous plea in those cases alone where the maniac is so mad that he cannot see the link between murder and the gibbet, these quiet lunatics will remain at large, and society will be satisfied to trust to the law for security. Monomaniacs, in short, will yield to social discipline, backed by Newgate and the gallows, just as they submit to asylum discipline, backed by the belt, the gloves, or a dark cell. But still some portion of danger will be left? No doubt of it. Neither law nor custom

authorises us to guard against every
possibility of danger; it is urgent and
immediate danger alone which would
justify us in imprisoning a myriad of
eccentric fellow-subjects. But the
juries must do their duty. It was said
by Burke that trial by jury was the
soul of our constitution, and that the
object of all law and government was
to bring twelve honest men into a jury-
box—on the supposition, however, we
would add, that the twelve honest men
aim at the real, and despise the
fantastic. Not a week has elapsed since
a jury acquitted the mischievous lad
who snapped a pistol at the clergyman
officiating in St. Paul's. The alleged
motive of the culprit was his indignation at hearing a usurper prayed for
instead of James Stuart; so that he
would seem not to have been in possession of his senses, and according to
different theories, might have been a
fit tenant for Newgate or Bethlem.
The former would have been the better
alternative for society; but even the
latter would have been far preferable
to the total impunity which the prisoner enjoyed by a simple verdict of
acquittal.

The influence of hereditary predisposition in producing madness is evidently considerable; and is proved not
only by common observation, but by the
records of lunatic asylums. But what
is the influence of marriages between
relations, without hereditary predisposition? The general belief is, that they
are likely to produce imbecility in the
children; but whether this belief rests
on a sufficient number of facts we
know not. It is, at any rate, probable
that repeated intermarriages between
blood relations, or breeding in and in,
as the graziers call it, will cause a
speedy degeneracy of mind and body;
and it is to be lamented that political
considerations make this practice so
general among the sovereign houses of

Europe. It certainly is not the way to
make kings *ablemen*, which, according
to Mr. Carlyle, they are etymologically,
and should be really. Of these repeated intermarriages Dr. Hutcheson
goes so far as to say, that "imbecility,
or idiocy, is the ordinary result; but
positive madness is not an unfrequent
occurrence."

He thinks that physical and moral
education might be so managed as to
be a powerful preventive of insanity;
and no doubt he is in the right. But
when he adds that this requires no
sacrifice of the passions and prejudices
of mankind, we believe that few will
agree with him. We rather side with
what he says further on, that the task
which he proposes is difficult in the
extreme, but that the issue will reward
the labour. Among the minor and
more obvious duties of him who endeavours to give a sound mind to the
children of parents who are nearly or
quite insane, will be a judicious abstinence from over-instruction. For the
first seven years of life, at least, the
hours of study should be few and far
between; and we would add, that when
the years for real study have come on,
the exact sciences should form a considerable portion of the child's education. In the records of an asylum
where poets and artists abounded, Pinel
could not find a single geometer.

Intemperance and want are frequent causes of insanity; and at
Glasgow they are unfortunately both
on the increase. Want produces despair,
and despair seeks a temporary consolation in drinking. Religious terrors are
another common source of madness;
and the intrusionist question, half
shared between religion and politics,
has of late produced a good many cases
at Glasgow.

In some cases the state of the pa
tients admitted had been made worse
by bleeding, which is still popularly

supposed to be a prime remedy in mania; and a yet more frequent error is the abuse of drastics, low diet, and tartar emetic.

This report, which is benevolent in its tone, and judicious in many of its suggestions, has confirmed us in the opinion which we offered some years since, that the more opulent inhabitants of Glasgow are so sluggish in their subscriptions, that to relieve the misery of its poor a rate should be levied on the town. The asylum now building cannot, it seems, be completed at present to contain 600 patients, but must be opened when ready to hold 350; though the sum required for the larger number would have been by no means enormous. The directors, indeed, boast of their economy, and contrast their expenditure with that incurred in building lunatic asylums in Ireland, where the cost has been greater, though the wages of labour are less.

ROYAL MEDICAL & CHIRURGICAL SOCIETY.

May 9, 1843.

THE PRESIDENT IN THE CHAIR.

Observations on the Medicinal Properties of Indian Hemp. By JOHN CLENDINNING, M.D. F.R.S.

THE author commenced his paper with general observations on the importance of narcotics, but especially of opium, in the treatment of disease. After having referred to numerous examples of the successful use of opium in acute and chronic disease, he adverted to the inconvenience occasionally attending the employment of opiates, especially to the derangement of the stomach and bowels and kidneys, and the vertiginous and other painful conditions of the nervous system they so frequently produce. He then stated that, in his experience, those inconvenient effects had occurred so frequently, and been found in many cases so difficult to obviate, without the abandonment of the use of a class of remedies of the utmost importance in a large number and variety of diseases, that he had been recently induced to make trial of the extract of hemp, recommended by Dr. O'Shaughnessy, of Calcutta, *as a substitute for opium in numerous instances. The author's object in* making this communication was to bring under the notice of the Society the results he had obtained, as in his judgment important to be made generally known with a view to further and more extended trials by other practitioners, more especially at this moment, when there was some prospect of a new edition of the London Pharmacopœia, upon which he understood a Committee of the Royal College was actually engaged.

The author then gave details of eighteen cases, from a much larger number, in which he had given trial to the new remedy with satisfactory results.

These trials included cases of acute and chronic disease, in persons of both sexes, and persons of very various ages. The number of cases detailed, although necessary to substantiate the claims advanced by the author in favour of the new narcotic, was yet such as to preclude any analysis of them in this place.

It will be sufficient to say generally, that the indications for its use in these cases appear to have been more especially to relieve neuralgic pain; to relieve irritation and spasms of chronic bronchitis, of rheumatism, &c.; and to subdue sleeplessness or disturbed rest from whatever cause, if not arising from inflammation in the head. The author found the remedy highly useful in checking cough in phthisis, and cramp and irritation in the limbs, &c. in rheumatism, without any interference with the digestive processes, or intestinal action or secretions, yet with an anodyne and hypnotic effect not less uniform than that of opium. He gave it trial also in several cases of low fever, characterized by spots, tremors, and delirious restlessness, and with very good effects; it repressed delirium and conciliated repose, and thus secured that tranquillity and refreshment the proper effects of sleep. He reported also some instances of successful use of hemp extract, as a pure anodyne to secure sleep, by suppressing pain, arising in one case from a cut, in another from a violent purgative, and in a third from rheumatic irritation of the meninges.

The author concluded his paper by a *resumé* of the objects of his trials, and the results and conclusions he had attained.

He stated that his experience had satisfied him that the hemp extract was possessed of medicinal properties sufficiently energetic and uniform to entitle it to admission into our national Pharmacopœia amongst our most useful narcotics; and that as a substitute for opium, especially in cases for which that drug was unsuited, owing to idiosyncrasy, or to the presence of active indigestion, or the nervous temperament, he had found reason to place much confidence in the extract, and to regard it as a remedy exceeding in value that of any other narcotic, or combination of narcotics, with which he was acquainted.

___

On the Removal of Blindness depending upon Palsy of the Iris. By ALEXANDER URE, Esq. [Communicated by the PRESIDENT.]

The author described the case of a female patient, who had come under his care at the Western Eye Dispensary, in consequence of having been suddenly attacked with blindness in one eye. The pupil was dilated and immoveable, and she was wholly unable to distinguish light from darkness. Judging the case to be one of idiopathic palsy of the iris, the author proceeded at once to employ the method of cauterizing the circumference of the cornea by nitrate of silver, first proposed by Serres. The result was prompt restoration of sight. He pointed attention to the importance of discriminating accurately between palsy of the iris and amaurosis; since the treatment which is so efficacious in the one would be no less improper than useless in the other.

___

On the Sugar in the Blood in Diabetes. By Dr. BENCE JONES.

The very delicate test for grape sugar which was communicated to the Academy of Sciences in Berlin, in 1841, by Professor Mitscherlich, as the discovery of Herr Trommer, was applied by him without success to the examination of diabetic blood. He found, however, that if $\frac{1}{10000}$ of grape sugar was mixed with blood, the test would indicate its presence. An opportunity occurred to the author of this paper of repeating the experiment on the blood of a diabetic patient of Dr. Nairne's, in St. George's Hospital. The disease was of about a year's standing, and the patient was in other respects in tolerable health. On the 24th of January, 1843, he was bled to twelve ounces, three hours after a dinner of bread and meat. The following morning the blood was well separated; the serum milky; the clot slightly buffed and cupped: specific gravity, ·1029,7. The serum became clear when treated with æther, and the test for grape sugar gave a negative result, as the precipitate which first formed did not redissolve, and only became much darker when heated, partly in consequence of the deep purple colour which is formed by the action of caustic potash and sulphate of copper on fibrin or albumen.

The albumen was therefore removed by evaporating the serum to dryness in a water bath. The residue was finely powdered, treated with water, filtered, and tested for grape sugar. The characteristic changes then took place. The clot of the same blood

was treated in the same way, and the test showed that grape sugar was present in it also. The urine passed between three hours before the bleeding, and nine hours after, was five pints, specific gravity, ·1031,3, and when tested by the same method the liquid first became blue, and then a very large precipitate formed, which was at first bright yellow, and after some hours became dark green.

Uric acid alone does not form the clear blue solution, although, when boiled with the potash and sulphate of copper, it will produce the same coloured precipitate as the grape sugar does.

___

BIOGRAPHICAL NOTICE OF THE LATE T. FAWDINGTON, ESQ.

(From a Correspondent.)

DIED, on the 21st ultimo, at Manchester, Thomas Fawdington, Esq. in the 48th year of his age.

The loss of this excellent surgeon and truly upright man will long be felt by those who enjoyed the privilege of his society and friendship. Possessed of an untiring zeal for the advancement of his profession, whose resources on several occasions he contributed very materially to extend, he was no less distinguished amongst his brother practitioners for the unflinching honour and integrity which ever characterized his intercourse with them and the public at large. He had been engaged in active practice for a period of about twenty years, the greater portion of which was most laboriously devoted to the cultivation of morbid anatomy, regardless alike of the sacrifice of much personal comfort, and large pecuniary expenditure involved therein. A lasting monument of these labours has resulted in the formation of a very extensive museum,—rich in almost every variety of diseased structure, but peculiarly valuable with reference to the several morbid changes of which the bones and mucous membranes are the seat. A Catalogue of all the specimens has been published, containing, in relation to very many of them, a brief but luminous sketch of the principal symptoms observed during the progress of the several diseases, of which the former are the products. The osseous preparations are most beautifully displayed, comprehending a very perfect series, from those which exhibit the anatomical structure and nutritive process of healthy bone (all very minutely injected) to the appearances observed after fracture, and the means employed by nature for its reparation. But it is to the pathological specimens that the merit of excellence pre-eminently belongs. In these is comprised almost every variety of morbid change of which the osseous structure is susceptible; and the extremely beautiful and striking manner in which they are severally preserved, affords a ready clue to their elucidation. Amongst these I may briefly allude to a preparation of malacosteon of the pelvis, the singularity of which consists in its having occurred at an advanced period of life, viz. seventy-three, the woman from whom it was removed having previously given birth to a numerous family without any difficulty or delay in the process. Amidst much that would amply merit a more detailed notice, but for its too great encroachment upon your space, it would be wrong to omit all allusion to the extensive and truly interesting series of preparations illustrative of the healthy and diseased conditions of the mucous membranes. The nature of the changes which this structure undergoes in disease was ever a favourite subject of investigation with the late Mr. Fawdington; and I have little hesitation in affirming, that, under this head, there does not exist any collection more valuable, either in point of intrinsic excellence, or in the completeness by which every link in the chain of morbid products, as applicable to the above structure, is characterised. To most of the specimens is appended a succinct history of the symptoms observed during life; and what considerably enhances their value is the circumstance of coloured drawings having been made with the utmost fidelity from the parts in a recent state, by which the otherwise evanescent characters of disease are made to stand out in prominent relief.

About seven years ago Mr. F. was elected to the important office of surgeon to the Royal Infirmary, an appointment most congenial to his wishes, and associated with many of the happiest reminiscences of his medical career. For a considerable period prior to this appointment, he had filled the chair of anatomical lecturer at the late School of Anatomy and Medicine in Marsden Street. In this capacity he was very successful in diffusing considerable interest over a subject too frequently regarded as destitute of this quality; and by those students whose privilege it was to hear him, his valuable prelections will not readily be forgotten. As a writer, Mr. F. was very favourably known to the professional public. His "Case of Melanosis," illustrated by many very accurate and beautiful drawings, published at a period when the pathology of that singular disease was but imperfectly understood, gained him no inconsiderable celebrity; and I am not aware that, up to this time, any thing very material has been added towards the more complete elucidation of the phenomena of that morbid condition. Mr. F. was likewise the author of a very valuable paper on Subcutaneous Nævus,

in which the method of treatment by the seton was vindicated, and several cases, with drawings, adduced to prove the efficacy of the plan proposed,—a mode of cure, which, though not originating with my deceased friend, was at least more clearly and definitely brought to bear upon the treatment of this affection, than had been accomplished by previous surgeons.

Mr. F. was fortunate enough to enjoy a considerable share of public patronage,—an advantage, which, although so far indicative of the estimation in which his professional services were held, was mainly prized for the opportunity thereby afforded him of extending the resources of his art, and maintaining that high sense of honour of which his whole medical career was one bright exemplification. Few practitioners, probably, have descended to the grave more sincerely lamented both by his former patients and his medical brethren, many of whom accompanied his remains to their final resting-place. By his former pupils he was universally esteemed; and the premature loss to them of his valuable counsel and friendship will long cause his memory to be " neither unwept, nor unhonoured."

T. M.

MEDICAL REFORM.

To the Editor of the Medical Gazette.

Sir,

Having thus far developed those views of Medical Reform which, in my humble opinion, seem most likely to benefit the profession, and through it the community at large, I must beg your indulgence to one more (and my last) letter on some subjects bearing upon this important question.

First, then, I would beg to draw attention to some anomalies existing under the present system, which, I conceive, would be, if not entirely removed, at least greatly diminished under the system which I have so fully endeavoured to advocate.

The College of Physicians ought to be considered the fountain-head of medical, the College of Surgeons of surgical, knowledge; and, yet, is it not strange that the diploma of the College of Surgeons should long have been considered the only requisite for army, navy, and many other public medical appointments? Although, in the army and navy, especially during periods of war, the number of important and serious surgical cases bears a much larger proportion to the whole amount of cases than occurs in civil practice, yet, taking all periods into consideration, it will be found that a vast preponderance, even of army and navy cases, falls under the strict province of the physician. Perhaps some one will say, "Yes, but then we have Army and Navy Boards, and the East India Company has a Board, to examine candidates for these appointments, as to their qualification." Surely this is no great compliment to our profession, that the person considered qualified by our Colleges should have again to submit to a test of his competency by an Army or Navy, or East India Company Board. The Bishop of London examines a candidate for deacon's orders; when he takes priest's orders, he may happen to fall under the examination of the Bishop of Worcester: having been duly passed and ordained by these bishops, it would appear to indicate some distrust in them, if, when this gentleman succeeds to a curacy or living in the diocese of the Archbishop of Canterbury, he should be compelled by a further examination to show his competency for such a post. Now, under the plan of medical reform above contemplated, the candidate for army or navy appointments would have acquired such diplomas from the two Colleges as should be thought requisite, and if this were not sufficient, an especial examination might be instituted for such purposes.

This, then, is one of those anomalies that arise out of the present confused state of our profession.

Some time since a doctor was elected physician to a London hospital who was chiefly known to the public as a skilful mechanist and operator in certain deformities. Let it it not be supposed that I for one moment doubt the fitness of this gentleman for the office; my observations are not made upon the person, but the system. A very large proportion of provincial physicians possess no kind of English or Scotch diplomas, some scarcely even nominal titles to the office and dignity of a physician. In London, vast numbers of pure surgeons, as they are called, possess no other diploma than that of the London College of Surgeons, and yet their only chance of livelihood is in the practice of medicine. Numbers of apothecaries in the country write Mr. ——, Surgeon, over their doors, who have never been inside the College of Surgeons. The genuine apothecary exists, one may almost say, in the shadow of a name,—"Stat nominis umbra." A few representatives only of this order remain in London; and what is still more curious, several persons in London, whose sole qualification is that of apothecary, are physicians in reality, if not in name, writing prescriptions, and although unwilling to soil their hands with a pill or mixture, not averse to touching the guinea.

It would be useless to adduce any further examples of the present confused state of the profession, and its inefficiency to secure to its members the rights and privileges of their respective orders.

Something has already been said upon the apothecary system, but I cannot close the subject of medical reform without again adverting to this subject. The great object of the medical profession is to confer the greatest amount of good upon the public; the duty of the government (which is the representative of the public), on the other hand, should be to foster, encourage, and protect us as a learned profession. I am well aware that in attacking the present system on which the general practitioner proceeds I may meet with many who are opposed to my views, upon high principles, and with still more who defend the system from less honourable motives; perhaps, as thinking it holds out the greatest probability of profit. I cannot, however, with propriety, withhold my views, even at the risk of opposition and personal offence, and I must again declare that my sole object is to give my opinion on a plan of reform which shall render our profession more useful, more honourable, and more respected. Let us see how the present apothecary system acts.

It is not for me to say whether more physic is poured down the throats of patients than ought to be; but it is self-evident that the present system offers a premium for such practice; and knowing human nature to be as it is, surely it were wiser to avoid temptation than to court it. Many general practitioners are no doubt above this practice; but, then, what is the result? Instead of being better paid for their honourable disinterestedness, they are not so well paid; and, what is still worse, ranked in the same class with their less scrupulous brethren.

Look, again, at the effect of this system on the scientific study of medicine. How is disease to be studied by the person engaged in making up medicines? How is that man's judgment to be considered clear and unbiassed, who, in coming to the bedside of his patient, is occupied in thinking how much medicine he can send? Indeed, I believe some persons are so sanguine on this point as almost to attribute the union of a fractured limb to an effervescing saline draught every three hours, two pills at night, with a draught in the morning, and an evaporating lotion to the limb.

Suppose a consultation between a physician and a general practitioner. By a consultation I have always felt it to be understood that two persons should consult together for the good of their patient; and, yet, often have I seen an ignorant bombastic physician meet a respectable, well-informed general practitioner, only to swagger and dictate to him as if he were a dispensing chemist, and had no share in the care and responsibility of the case. On the other hand, the general practitioner may have some pique against the physician, and send in any thing but what was agreed upon in consultation. It is to be hoped such things do not often occur, but they may, and do, happen occasionally. Under the system I have advocated they could not.

But a still more serious evil arises out of the present apothecary system, both as regards the public and profession. I allude to the contract system. Let us examine the plan by which the general practitioner contracts to supply the poor of unions and parishes with medical and surgical advice, and medicines, and see how it operates, both for the public and the profession. Driven by competition to undertake this office at the lowest possible salary, the medical man assumes this arduous and important duty, not from any hope of gain, but merely with the object of acquiring private practice, or, if he has this already, of keeping other competitors out of the field. So far the system must lead to perpetual professional bickerings and jealousy. He is necessarily obliged to economise his labour, both in visits and in the form of dispensing his medicines. How does this affect him? The clergyman or squire of the parish, or principal farmer, sees that he conducts a severe case of fever or inflammation, or a bad fracture, to a successful issue in the case of a pauper, with one half the medicine and attendance that is bestowed upon his own family in far less formidable ills. What is the result? He finds it both cheaper and pleasanter to pay a fee or two to a consulting practitioner, or even flies to a neighbouring bone-setter, or to somebody's alterative or cough pills; or he goes to a neighbouring chemist and asks for an aperient pill or draught, or a saline mixture, or "something to comfort and nourish his inside." But how does it affect the poor themselves? This is a far more serious and interesting question! Why, the medical man giving medicines and attendance for a salary that would barely pay for the former item alone, must necessarily too often use medicines defective both in quantity and quality. Let us hope that a high sense of honour and morality may lead many, nay, most parish doctors to be above such considertions; yet, the fact is evident, that human nature is human nature, and there is no check upon such conduct. Certain it is, that the more expensive remedies cannot be often, if at all, employed; and, from my own experience, I have reason to believe that the course of medical treatment so necessary after the subsidence of acute disease, is too often much neglected, and that the order for wine and mutton, though no doubt mostly *necessarily, entirely*

supplies the place of alterative medicines, tonics, and careful watching. But, supposing the profession is a body so immaculate as to be far above these errors, there yet remains one fault in the present system, even under its present modified and improved form, which is unavoidable so long as the general practitioner combines the sale of drugs with his professional character. Many parish surgeons have no assistants; consequently, many persons must be kept waiting much longer for their medicines than they ought to be. Take, for instance, a case of inflammation, in which it is proper that the abstraction of blood from the arm should be immediately followed by an opiate and the application of leeches—the delay of a few hours may render their use not only less efficacious, but absolutely hurtful. It will be said, "but the poor have the power of complaining of any neglect or mal-practice." To a certain extent they have; but when it is considered that even the richer and better educated classes of society frequently praise or blame their medical attendants upon very unjust grounds, the criticism of the poor upon any other point than the feelings, manners, and assidulity of their professional attendant, cannot be said to stand for much. Besides, they are as confiding, perhaps more so, than others, and they argue, that whatever their doctor does is right. But let the medical man undertake only the professional attendance of the poor, and let a chemist and druggist contract for supplying them with the medicines regularly prescribed by such medical attendant, and then see how much better the interests of the poor would be attended to! Here would be no self-interest to tempt him from the paths of benevolence and duty; his feelings and natural desire to obtain reputation would alike induce him to see that the orders he gave should be both promptly and properly obeyed.

The subject of remuneration for professional services is one on which much cannot be said in a letter chiefly directed to the preliminary considerations of medical reform.

Perhaps it would be well under this system that the fees of the general practitioner should be regulated by law, and constitute a legal debt, because they are most frequently called upon to attend a class of persons who would not consider themselves bound by a debt of honour; but I should be sorry to see the fees of the pure physician and surgeon made a legal debt, because this might in some degree diminish the high position which they, together with the members of the bar, at present maintain.

It would be inexpedient, even in this slight sketch of medical reform which I have ventured to attempt, entirely to omit the subject of quackery. Perhaps no part of the subject is more difficult to deal with satisfactorily than this; yet I would venture here also to cite the maxim before inculcated, that the great object of the medical profession is to bestow all the good it possibly can upon the public, and that, in its turn, it has a just and fair claim to the respect, sympathy, and protection of that public. In the course of these letters, it has been more than once hinted that the plan of medical reform therein laid down would materially lessen the necessity (if it may be so termed) for quackery, and in so doing it would probably in some measure diminish its frequency. It is hardly to be expected that any arrangements in our profession, in a free country like England, be they ever so stringent or ever so liberal, should be able entirely to put down or disarm the quack of every denomination.

First with regard to what is termed the "counter practice" of the chemist and druggist: this, if not put down by the strong arm of the law, may at least be legally discouraged, and kept within some limitations. The profession, too, being rendered more united and harmonious, would possess great power in this respect, by withholding their prescriptions from persons who were found to be infringing upon their privileges. With regard to more impudent and open quacks, perhaps a negative course would be better than a positive prohibition, the impossibility of which being carried in every case into effect would in time render it nugatory. The quack might be prohibited, under pain of punishment, from putting his name on his door or house as doctor; from advertising, &c.; and he might be rendered amenable to the law for a two-fold action for damages, both to the public whom he may have injured, and to the profession whose rights and privileges he had invaded.

But the most fearful ravages made by the quack, both upon the health and pockets of the people, is through the medium of advertisements. It is to be feared that this source of puffing and notoriety, being one of considerable profit to the government, would not be so readily put down; but let me once more remind them of the claims of a highly useful and honourable profession upon their fostering protection; let me remind them of their duty through that profession of guarding the bodily health, as well as the morals of the people, and let me tell them unflinchingly that that government cannot be altogether sound which hesitates not to derive some portion of its revenue from sanctioning the publication of the most gross and deceptious falsehoods. It is devoutly to be hoped that whenever a measure of medical reform is adopted, some measures may be taken for diminishing, if not annihilating, this at present monstrous and iniquitous system. It *would not be too much, perhaps, to aver,*

that many a quack mountebank has, aided by this system of advertising, realised a larger fortune than a Watt by the invention of the steam engine, or a Jenner by the discovery of vaccination.

A useful combination, or superior mode of preparing many remedies, has often been due to exertions of some individual practitioner, and such remedies have, in after times, been used by the profession under the names of their original discoverers; as, for instance, Dover's Powder, James's Powder, &c. &c. It might be well, in case of any one making a really useful discovery of this kind, that the matter should be laid before a medical board constituted for that purpose, and that the discoverer should receive from government a reward commensurate with the value of his discovery, which should then be made known for the benefit of the profession generally, and through it of the public.

Should this, or any other plan of medical reform, be carried out, so as to render our at present distracted and divided profession more uniform and harmonious, I have often thought that a grand scheme might be adopted of forming a quiet and united club for the benefit of the widows and orphans of medical men. In a profession like ours, in which expenses are certain, and remuneration most uncertain, in which there is no stock in trade beyond an expensive education which dies with its possessor, no salaries, and but few, very few, posts of honour and of wealth, such a scheme, if practicable, would be most desirable. My theory may be Utopian, but if it be, at least let me beg your attention to my dream. We have at present a most useful and most beneficent institution for the benefit of widows and orphans of medical men, but their charity extends only to those who are left entirely, or almost entirely, unprovided for, and that too merely to London and its immediate vicinity. Now a young man, commencing life as a married man, can ill afford to subscribe to such a society, because he says "I am possessed of a few thousand pounds, or I have insured my life for a few thousand pounds; should I die, this provision for my family, however slight and inadequate, will preclude them from the benefits of this society, and at present I cannot afford to subscribe for others' wants; I would willingly do so, but I must wait till I am richer." He goes on plodding honestly and honourably in his profession; he has reared up several children; he is just about to obtain the summit of his ambition; has means sufficient to bring out his children in the world, and to lay by a trifle for his own declining years; when, perhaps a sacrifice to the noble and honourable exercise of his calling, he is carried off, to leave a widow barely provided with decent comforts of life, and without the means to carry on that education of his family which his professional exertions had enabled him to commence. The plan I would propose is, that every person on entering the profession should be compelled to pay a fee to a society to be called, let us say, "The Society for the Widows and Orphans of Medical Men, and also for Decayed Medical Men." The entrance fee should be compulsory, and let each person afterwards use his own discretion to continue a subscriber or not, according as he likes, or at any period of life, to enter the society. The annual payments could be regulated according to age, health, &c. as in the ordinary assurance offices. The benefits of the society only to be extended to subscribers, at least their widows and orphans, and to themselves when in old age or infirm health. This benefit to be properly apportioned, and not to be given at all to persons whose other means exceed a certain income. In the present philanthropic age, no doubt such an institution would, ere long, receive liberal donations, legacies, &c. from some of our wealthier professional brethren, and no doubt also from many not of the faculty.

I have, now, sir, brought to a close my humble views on the subject of medical reform. I would willingly linger one moment longer to tell the public that we deserve their sympathy and support. From an early age we are devoted to those studies, which would repulse many a sensitive mind ; and if we are buoyed up with the expectation of some share of wealth and honour, yet are we supported by far higher and more noble views : we brave the disgust of the dissecting-room to read those pages in the history of nature that are to benefit mankind ; we lean over the sick, pestilential bed of the pauper to reap no other reward than the conscious satisfaction of doing him service, and of acquiring that knowledge of disease which is to render us useful to our fellow-men. If in after life we reap some reward of our labours we may fairly say, "Thou shalt not muzzle the mouth of the ox that treadeth out the corn ;" and this reward at the expense of how much mental as well as physical exertion is it not acquired ? As individuals we have no complaint to make, it is the fortune of many of us to be rewarded, respected, and esteemed ! It is for the medical profession as a body that I would claim the public sympathy. As a body we may be said to be almost entirely unrepresented. Our general want of wealth, our laborious professional occupations (and these, too, coming late in life), preclude us as individuals from seeking to represent our profession in the House of Commons. From the House of Lords we have been excluded. An occasional baronetcy may shed honour upon our profession, but so far from giving ease and

leisure to its possessor only requires of him increased energy and exertion to enable him to leave no empty encumbrance of honour to his heir.

Look at the present improved state of medical and surgical knowledge and practice ! Look at the mass of poor to whom our services are daily given ! Look at our army and navy medical officers, and say whether, as a body, we are not deserving of better things ? It is truly pitiful to see that one little action may place a soldier or sailor in the path of wealth and honour ; whilst very many years spent by the medical officer in the arduous and honourable prosecution of his career, exposed not only to the dangers of war, but of fever, dysentery, and plague, will barely earn him a paltry pension.

I must apologize for having trespassed at so great a length upon your columns, and
I remain, sir,
Your obedient servant,
PHILOMETHES.
April 26, 1843.

REFORM ASSOCIATION.

To the Editor of the Medical Gazette.

SIR,

ALLOW me to call your attention to the proceedings of the North of England Reform Association, at the late meeting of this body at Sunderland, as you will find them reported in the Northern Advertiser or Gateshead Observer of last week.

You will find, that while the highly-respectable president of the association, in his opening address, insists upon the necessity of grades and divisions of labour in the profession, and the propriety of supporting such grades and divisions by legislation, the report of the council expresses a somewhat unqualified approbation of the views of Sir James Clark, who would legislate only for one uniform grade, and leave the others to chance, or rather to the caprices, selfishness, and carelessness of the various University sities, British and foreign, which now undertake to give or sell degrees.

It is true that the report, and a petition also presented by the council, assert the propriety of uniformity in the qualifications on which the various honorary degrees are to be granted ; but certainly the council does not take that care to express its opinion, free from ambiguity, which is displayed by the president.

The same general proposition which is stated by the general practitioner when he wishes to be distinguished from the quack, includes the utility, nay, the necessity, of grades and distinctions in the profession ; and, in my opinion, the man who contents himself with asserting the propriety of legislating for one grade only, is no true medical reformer.

The only argument offered by those who contend against grades, which is worthy of the least consideration, is, that the various subjects of medical science are closely connected,—that it is difficult to point out the bounds which separate medicine from surgery, and so forth. We admit the utility of medical knowledge to the surgeon, and of surgical knowledge to the physician ; we likewise conceive that it is impossible to point out the distinctions or exact divisions between the animal and vegetable kingdoms, and that a general knowledge of both is highly advantageous to the man who devotes himself to the study of either ; but we are convinced that De Jussieu or Robert Brown, or Cuvier or Owen, is a proof of the utility of division of labour in a science not more vast than medicine, and where the path of the student is more discernible than in our science.

It appears to me that the branch system of medical legislation has been too little considered. The grades of druggist, general practitioner, doctor of medicine, and doctor of surgery, would realize the most appropriate scheme that can be conceived. After the degree of general practitioner had been obtained, I would allow an additional amount of time of study, passed in hospitals and at universities, or a certain time spent in private practice, to qualify for examination for the higher degrees.

Such is the general outline of the scheme of medical reform conceived by a young physician ; and after all, sir, I think you will grant that we young members of the profession are more concerned in the matter than the old practitioners.—I am, sir,

Your obedient servant,
ROBERT MORTIMER GLOVER,
M.D. Edinb.

Newcastle-on-Tyne,
May 1, 1843.

PATHOLOGY OF THE BRAIN.

To the Editor of the Medical Gazette.

SIR,

THE profession are highly indebted to Dr. Burrows for the light he has thrown on the pathology of the contents of the cranium, in his recent lectures before the College of Physicians ; for although most practitioners will, like myself, find that their practice has been in accordance not only with the facts he has brought forward, but with his deductions from them, yet it is no small satisfaction to have the results of individual experience thus agreeing with the theory of the most observant pathologists. Dr. Burrows' observations seem the more important *at the present time*, when some of your

recent correspondents have been anxious to do away with depletion in apoplexy, arguing against its use from the instances of its abuse ; and perhaps influenced by the theories of Dr. Abercrombie and others : indeed the authority of such a man as Dr. Abercrombie, if in error, cannot be unattended by injurious effects.

These remarks are, however, so obvious, that I should not have troubled you with them had it not appeared to me that neither Dr. Burrows, nor (as far as my knowledge goes) other observers, have taken sufficiently into account the probability that an *elastic* serous vapour, existing between the layers of the arachnoid, and perhaps in other parts, performs an important office in equalizing the pressure on the solid contents of the encephalon. It does not seem to me that any resiliency of the medullary mass, nor the varying quantity of extra-vascular serum, will satisfactorily account for all the phenomena, without supposing the presence of an elastic aeriform fluid : the existence of a vapour or halitus arising from the serous membranes (spoken of generally by modern anatomists) seems equally necessary, and its existence at least equally probable, in the head.

I hope that Dr. Burrows will not deem this suggestion unworthy of his notice, and that he and others who have more leisure and ability than myself, will pursue the investigation, so that our knowledge on this highly interesting and important subject may be perfected.—I am, sir,

Your obedient servant,
JOHN M. CAMPLIN.

11, Finsbury Square,
May 9, 1843.

MEDICO-LEGAL EVIDENCE IN A CASE OF SUSPECTED POISONING.

To the Editor of the Medical Gazette.

SIR,

IN allusion to Mr. Holland's letter and remarks upon the medico-legal evidence in a case of suspected poisoning, I beg to state that there are several important errors and omissions, which quite alter the view of the case, but which I decline remarking upon, as it is Mr. Dyson's intention to address you at his earliest convenience. Mr. Dyson was present at the examination solely at my request, as I knew that he was in the habit of making frequent inspections for the Coroner. There was no expectation of his evidence being required until the result of Mr. Davies' chemical examination was hinted at previous to the third sitting of the adjourned inquest, when it was thought advisable to have his opinion in conjunction with my own. As soon as it was intimated to Mr. Dyson that his presence would be required, he made notes of the principal points, which notes were produced at the inquest, but not read, as the jury desired him to give his opinion in as few words as possible, and not to enter into particulars.—I am, sir,

Your obedient servant,
JOHN GREGSON HARRISON,
Surgeon.

Manchester, 4, Piccadilly,
May 2, 1843.

CAUSES OF
DEATH AFTER OPERATIONS IN
THE LONDON HOSPITALS.

To the Editor of the Medical Gazette.

SIR,

As Dr. Chevers seems to deny that his "exposition is principally based on my autopsy-histories," I beg leave to alter the expression. Dr. C. says, "I carefully examined the accounts of all the cases where death occurred from the secondary effects of operations and mechanical injuries of every description which have been entered in the post-mortem registers of the Museum (of Guy's Hospital) during the last fifteeen years (from May, 1827)." This date is in a note, which, not observing, I concluded that fourteen years of work, instead of thirteen, out of fifteen, belonged to me and those who have done duty for me. The data which he has deduced from hence seem to be the only facts he furnishes, and as I have been employed performing the inspections, demonstrating the appearances, and recording the histories, from October 1829 till now, with some intermissions as well as with some little perseverance, I hope my hasty little note may be pardoned. Perhaps I may be allowed to say Dr. C.'s exposition is, *in some measure*, based on my autopsy-histories.

The tabular analysis of some 2000 cases may not be altogether unworthy of notice, if only for example's sake. The plan adopted is to set down : first, the disease or the injury treated ; secondly, the organs affected, in the order in which their affections seem to have been important ; and thirdly, casual appearances. For examples :

May 1835 : Wm. H——, æt. 35, fractured leg, gangrene, hæmorrhage, small kidney, brain, stomach ulcer.

Mary S—— : Femoral hernia, bloody peritonitis simulating hæmorrhage (after operation), pericarditis, dissolved œsophagus.

Nathaniel C—— : ham aneurism, ligatured, gangrene, diseased kidney.

Wm. T——, æt. 21 : amputation, pul-

monary abscesses and emphysema, meningitis, inflamed veins.

The records themselves follow the more common plan : describing, successively, changes in the head, chest, and abdomen, &c. For my own part I have generally avoided all negative statements.—I am, sir,

Your obedient servant,
T. WILKINSON KING.
26, Bedford Square, May 17, 1843.

CIRRHOSIS OF THE LUNG.

DR. STOKES exhibited to the Pathological Society of Dublin a specimen of that disease of the lung, first described by Dr. Corrigan, under the title of cirrhosis of the lung. Its general characters are, a tendency to consolidation or contraction of the pulmonic tissue, with dilatation of the bronchial tubes. Dr. Stokes' patient had been labouring for months under cough, with dyspnœa and hectic fever, and died two days after her admission into the hospital. The physical signs were dulness of sound on percussion over the upper part of both lungs, but no decided or unequivocal signs of cavities. The appearance of the lungs on dissection was very characteristic ; the left, which was the more diseased, was greatly diminished in size, and very irregular on its surface, so that when the hand was passed over it numerous small bodies could be felt, conveying to the fingers the impression of air vesicles existing on the surface of the organ ; this was produced by the presence of air vesicles. On making a longitudinal section of the trachea and primary divisions of the bronchi, the right bronchus, immediately after it branched off from the trachea, became greatly dilated, so as to exceed the latter in diameter, while the left bronchus was evidently contracted and reduced below its ordinary calibre, but dilated again a little further down.

At a subsequent meeting, Dr. Greene exhibited another specimen of pulmonary cirrhosis, with dilated bronchial tubes, closely resembling phthisical cavities, taken from a woman who had long suffered from intractable cough, and who was affected with a train of symptoms closely resembling phthisis. The physical signs were, cavernous respiration and distinct pectoriloquy in the right infra-clavicular space ; the latter sign was also found at the inferior angle of the scapula, and in the right axilla : distinct gargouillement, with bronchial respiration, could be heard in various parts of the chest. The left lung presented the signs of bronchitis. The lung, on examination after death, was found to be diminished in size and indurated ; the cavities formed by the dilatation of the tubes were of considerable size, and did not contain purulent matter ; they were largest near the surface of the lung, and towards its upper part. Their cartilaginous structure could be distinctly traced. There was not any sign of tubercular deposition in either lung. The pleura was greatly thickened, and the diaphragm was adherent to the liver.

Laennec attributed this complaint to constant cough and accumulation of mucus in the bronchial tubes. His opinion is, however, liable to objection, and his account of the causes to which the dilatation is owing is not sufficient to explain all the phenomena. According to Dr. Corrigan, the primary seat of the disease is in the web of cellular tissue which constitutes the matrix of the lung, which has a tendency to contract, so as to produce, when the disease is advanced, a very considerable obliteration of the air-cells. He thinks the diminution of the lung the first step in the disease, of which the dilatation of the bronchi is a consequence.—*Dublin Medical Journal.*

NARCOTIC EXTRACTS.

MR. BATTLEY has commenced the preparation of narcotic extracts and liquors at the Laboratory, Moorfields, and will be happy to exhibit and explain his processes to any gentleman who may be disposed to witness them prior to their publication. Mr. Battley attends at the Laboratory daily from 3 to 5.

BOOKS RECEIVED.

Practical Remarks on Gout, Rheumatic Fever, and Chronic Rheumatism of the Joints ; being the substance of the Croonian Lectures for the present year, delivered at the College of Physicians, by Robert Bentley Todd, M.D., F.R.S., &c. &c.

The Baths of Germany, considered with reference to their Remedial Efficacy in Chronic Diseases; with an Appendix on the Cold Water Cure. By Edwin Lee, Esq. Second edition, considerably improved.

ROYAL COLLEGE OF SURGEONS.

LIST OF GENTLEMEN ADMITTED MEMBERS.

Wednesday, May 10, 1843.

R. B. Yeats.—G. Gwillim.—C. L. Prince.—H. E. Brewer.—J. Pickop.—J. P. P. Chambers.—T. W. Rimell.—J. Sykes.—T. R. Wheeler.—E. Armstrong.

Friday, May 12, 1843.

D. Perkins.—F. Tinker.—F. Taylor.—R. A. Baaker.—T. Seccombe.—H. Willats.—R. H. Russell.—A. Gottreux.

Monday, May 15.

B. Pinchard.—F. R. Rose.—T. S Fletcher.—J. W. Savage.—W. Hobbs.—F. Hetley.—C. H. Brooking.—J. Eddison.—S. Fenwick.—J. Smart.—R. H. Boodle.—W. Haswell.—W. Clayton.—H. W. Watling.—J. Barrow.—J. St. J. G. Parsons.

APOTHECARIES' HALL.

LIST OF GENTLEMEN WHO HAVE RECEIVED CERTIFICATES.

Thursday, May 11, 1843.

A. Ebsworth. — W. Smith, Weyhill, Andover, Hants.—W. Haldenby, Reedness, Yorkshire.—A. N. Jones, Bristol.—L. C. Heslop, Haverfordwest.—J. P. Redruth, Cornwall. — W. Hart, North Shields, Northumberland. -J. W. Wainwright.—J. A. Carruthers.

A TABLE OF MORTALITY FOR THE METROPOLIS,

Shewing the number of deaths from all causes registered in the week ending Saturday, May 6, 1843.

Small Pox	9
Measles	23
Scarlatina	24
Hooping Cough	39
Croup	9
Thrush	5
Diarrhœa	1
Dysentery	3
Cholera	0
Influenza	1
Typhus	60
Erysipelas	7
Syphilis	0
Hydrophobia	0
Diseases of the Brain, Nerves, and Senses	124
Diseases of the Lungs and other Organs of Respiration	258
Diseases of the Heart and Blood-vessels	31
Diseases of the Stomach, Liver, and other Organs of Digestion	67
Diseases of the Kidneys, &c.	2
Childbed	12
Ovarian Dropsy	0
Disease of Uterus, &c.	0
Rheumatism	4
Diseases of Joints, &c.	8
Ulcer	0
Fistula	2
Diseases of Skin, &c.	0
Diseases of Uncertain Seat	89
Old Age or Natural Decay	63
Deaths by Violence, Privation, or Intemperance	30
Causes not specified	8
Deaths from all Causes	879

METEOROLOGICAL JOURNAL.

Kept at EDMONTON, *Latitude* 51° 37′ 32″ N. *Longitude* 0° 3′ 51″ W. *of Greenwich.*

April 1843.	THERMOMETER.		BAROMETER.	
Wednesday 10	from 43 to 57		29·94 to 30·08	
Thursday . 11	34	60	30·13	30·14
Friday . . 12	34	63	30·09	29·96
Saturday . 13	49	63	29·86	29·87
Sunday . 14	39	62	29·78	29·56
Monday . . 15	48	60	29·49	Stat.
Tuesday . 16	46	62	29·40	29·44

Wind, N.E. on the 10th and 11th; S. on the 12th; S.W. on the 13th; S. by E. on the 14th; S.W. on the 15th; E. by S., E. by N., N.E., and S.W. on the 16th.

Except the 13th, generally cloudy, with frequent rain.

CHARLES HENRY ADAMS.

WILSON & OGILVY, 57, Skinner Street, London

THE

LONDON MEDICAL GAZETTE,

BEING A

WEEKLY JOURNAL

OF

𝕸𝖊𝖉𝖎𝖈𝖎𝖓𝖊 𝖆𝖓𝖉 𝖙𝖍𝖊 𝕮𝖔𝖑𝖑𝖆𝖙𝖊𝖗𝖆𝖑 𝕾𝖈𝖎𝖊𝖓𝖈𝖊𝖘.

FRIDAY, MAY 26, 1843.

LUMLEIAN LECTURES

DELIVERED AT THE

COLLEGE OF PHYSICIANS,

MARCH 1843,

By GEORGE BURROWS, M.D.
Physician to St. Bartholomew's Hospital.

LECTURE III.

On affections of the brain and spinal cord depending on acute disease of the heart.

In my second lecture I concluded an account of the modifications which the circulation in the brain is capable of undergoing in health and disease; and particularly of the variations in the quantity of blood within the cranium, under the influence of abstraction of blood, of posture, and of obstruction to the return of blood from the brain. I then proceeded to shew that pressure was an important principle both in sustaining and destroying the functions of the brain. From physiological and pathological considerations, I supported the opinion, that a compressing force is continually exerted upon the substance of the brain, and that this pressure is produced by vascular distension. I then considered the effects of variations of this pressure on the healthy brain, suggesting the probability that the effects of increased vascular pressure are often obviated by a transference of the extra-vascular serum to the spinal canal. This led me to support the opinion of Sir Everard Home, that the serum in the cerebral ventricles was the means of diffusing equable pressure throughout the mass of the brain.

I then applied this principle of vascular pressure to explain the phenomena of those affections of the brain which are of an intermitting character, such as epilepsy, although the cerebral lesion is permanent. I also attempted to explain the phenomena of syncope as depending rather upon deficient

vascular pressure than upon insufficient supply of blood to the brain.

Lastly, I adverted to the peculiar nervous symptoms attendant on anæmia, and explained their development on the same principle of deficient vascular pressure on the nervous centres, rather than on the simple condition of anæmia of these parts.

I had proposed to have continued this argument in its application to other cerebral affections, particularly to the different forms of apoplexy; but I am unavoidably compelled to postpone these remarks to a future opportunity.

The subject of this lecture will not, however, be foreign to the principle I have been advocating, viz. the influence of the central organ of the circulation on the functions of the brain.

Upon the present occasion I shall invite your attention to a class of cases which are often misunderstood, and where all the symptoms indicate a severe affection of the nervous centres; but which, in reality, depend on disturbance of the circulation produced by active disease in the heart and its membranes.

The diagnosis of diseases of the heart has occupied so much attention during the last twenty years, that it is almost impossible to anticipate any important additions to our knowledge of this part of the history of cardiac affections. But it appears to me that the full extent of the influence of diseases of the heart upon other organs, and especially upon the brain, has not been thoroughly estimated by authors on diseases of these organs, and certainly not by the mass of the profession.

The influence of hypertrophy and valvular diseases of the heart upon the brain, has, indeed, been treated of by numerous writers in the present day, and by none more successfully, in my opinion, than by our late talented and lamented fellow, Dr. Hope. It is not, however, upon these chronic lesions of the heart, which usually afford ample opportunities to the physician to form his diagnosis, and adopt suitable treatment, that I now wish to offer a few observations : it is particularly in reference to peculiarities attending acute disease of the heart that I venture to claim your attention.

Different systematic writers on diseases of the heart have incidentally mentioned that inflammatory affections of that organ are occasionally accompanied with such severe symptoms of nervous irritation, that the primary affection of the heart is either overlooked altogether, or is so masked by the nervous disorder that it is not detected until irreparable mischief is done to a vital organ. A few cases of the same kind are to be found recorded in periodicals, and in the Transactions of medical societies, during the past twenty years. But a connected view of these remarkable and frightful cases has not, as far as I know, been hitherto presented to the medical public. Without arrogating to myself any merit for originality in the view of them which I am about to offer, I think a synopsis of them will be a suitable illustration of the great pathological principle I have been upholding in these lectures, viz. the influence of modifications of the circulation on the functions of the brain. The earliest recorded case of this kind is that detailed by Mr. Stanley*. Dr. Abercrombie, in 1821, communicated a nearly similar case to the Medico-Chirurgical Society of Edinburgh, in a paper entitled, " Contributions to the Pathology of the Heart." It is singular that this valuable essay from so distinguished a physician should have escaped the notice of (I believe) all subsequent writers on diseases of the heart. Dr. Latham was the next in the order of precedence to call attention to this deceptive form of cardiac inflammation ; and he informs us†, " that when he first related the particulars of his case to several medical friends, they looked incredulous, or rather contemptuous, of the man who would mistake an inflammation of the pericardium and heart for an inflammation of the brain." Nevertheless, I shall present to you a short account of many analogous cases, occurring in the practice of men of eminence both in Paris and in London. How many others have occurred in the practice of physicians who have been less candid in recording their mistakes, and how great a number must have happened in the practice of those who were unable, or who took no pains, to distinguish these deceptive cases, it is impossible to say. Andral‡ and Bouillaud§ have recorded cases of this kind, as well as Dr. Copland‖, Dr.

* Transactions of the Medico-Chirurgical Society of London, Vol. vii. 1817.
† Pathological Lectures on the Heart, LOND. MED. GAZ., Vol. iii.
‡ Clin. Med.
§ Traité sur les Maladies du Cœur.
‖ Dictionary.

Macleod*, Dr. F. Hawkins†, and a few others in this country. But the most interesting and valuable information upon this subject has been given to the profession by Dr. Richard Bright, in his account of " Cases of Spasmodic Disease accompanying Affections of the Pericardium." (Vol. 22, Med. Chir. Trans.)

The late Dr. Hope, in his elaborate Treatise on the Heart, remarks, that those cases of disease of that organ which simulate an affection of the brain are very rare ; and it is remarkable that with his unremitting attention to diseases of the heart, he never met with a single instance in his own experience. It has so happened that four or five such anomalous and deceptive cases have come under my observation ; and I have reason to believe that they are of more frequent occurrence than is commonly supposed.

Authors on diseases of the brain and spinal cord, have indeed, and especially of late years, pointed out the numerous extraneous sources of irritation capable of inducing symptoms of disordered functions of those nervous centres. Such symptoms have often been mistaken for the effects of morbid changes going forward in those centres ; but as far as I have been able to ascertain, these authors have scarcely ever alluded to acute diseases of the heart, as the sources of irritation to the nervous centres.

In Dr. M. Hall's recent volume, " On Diseases of the Nervous System," he devotes a chapter to the consideration of those affections which he terms " of remote origin." The effects on the nervous system from intestinal irritation, from loss of blood, chlorosis, gout, shock, and affections of the kidney, are there carefully pointed out ; but he only incidentally alludes to those remarkable disorders of the nervous centres excited by active inflammation of the heart and pericardium.

Having given this concise summary of the scattered information we possess on this interesting point in the history of diseases of the heart, I shall now direct your attention to a series of cases of inflammation of the tissues of that organ, where the disease was altogether mistaken for affections of the brain and spinal cord, or, where the prominent symptoms were referable to those nervous centres. I shall show that there is scarcely an affection of the cerebro-spinal system which may not be simulated by inflammatory diseases of the heart and its membranes.

I shall begin with citing (1) some cases which were marked with all the usual symptoms of inflammation of the brain and its membranes ; (2) cases simulating mania and dementia ; (3) cases characterised by apo-

* On Rheumatism.
† Gulstonian Lectures on Rheumatism.

plectic and epileptic symptoms; (4) cases with well-marked symptoms of tetanus and trismus, and, (5) others, still more numerous, accompained by symptoms of aggravated chorea and hysteria.

These various cases are collected from different sources, and in adapting them to the object I have in view I have necessarily been obliged to curtail the histories as they stand in the original authors.

CASE I.—*Active articular rheumatism, complicated with carditis and pericarditis, presenting the ordinary symptoms of an inflammatory affection of the brain.*

In April, 1816, one of the boys at Christ's Hospital was attacked with febrile symptoms, and pain in one thigh and knee. The pain in the limb quickly subsided, when he became restless, sleepless, and delirious. When asked if he suffered pain, he pointed to his forehead. On the third day of his illness he had a kind of convulsive fit, which soon went off. He passed another restless night with delirium, and gradually sank into fatal coma on the fourth day, never having complained of any pain in the chest throughout his illness.

It having been considered, from the general character of the symptoms, that there was inflammation going forward in the brain, all the remedies were directed to that organ; and upon examination of the body the head was first inspected. But after an attentive examination of the brain nothing further could be remarked than that the vessels were generally turgid; not more so, however, than is frequently seen when death has taken place under circumstances that led to no suspicion of affection of the brain. Upon opening the pericardium it was found to contain between four and five ounces of turbid serous fluid, with flakes of coagulable lymph floating in it. The entire free surface of the pericardium, both of the loose and reflected portions, was covered with a thin layer of lymph, exhibiting a reticulated appearance. Upon cutting through the parietes of the heart, the muscular fibres presented an exceedingly dark colour. The fibres were also very soft, and loose in their texture, easily separable, and with facility compressed between the fingers. Upon looking close'y to the cut surfaces, numerous small collections of dark-coloured pus were visible among the muscular fibres.

The internal lining, valves, and every other part of the organ, exhibited nothing worthy of remark, except a state of general turgescence of the capillary vessels, and that all the cavities of the heart were loaded with coagulated blood.

Upon this interesting case, Mr. Stanley makes the following remarks.* " We here

have presented to our consideration an instance of inflammation attacking the heart, so violent as to pass immediately into suppuration, and at the same time so destructive as to prove fatal in four days from its commencement ; and yet of the symptoms which arose, there was not one which appeared directly referable to the affected organ ; on the contrary, from their general tendency, the attention was diverted from the central organ of the circulation, the actual seat of disease, to the centre of the nervous system, where there existed no organic derangement.

CASE II.—*Idiopathic pericarditis giving rise to chorea, and symptoms of an inflammatory affection of the brain.*

A young lady, æt. 16, came under Dr. Abercrombie's care on the 8th of January 1812, complaining of acute pain at the pit of the stomach, with very short breathing : pulse generally 130, extreme restlessness, almost no sleep, with a good deal of delirium. In the third week, after antiphlogistic treatment, the pain abated, and she could take a full breath. Afterwards she fell into a state resembling chorea, with convulsive agitations of the limbs, constant motion of the head, wild rolling of the eyes and *delirium, which soon increased to such a degree, that for several days she was with difficulty kept in bed.* She no longer complained of pain ; the breathing was natural ; the pulse 120, and small. After this she gradually recovered her usual health, but on the 20th April, upon exposure to cold and fatigue, she was seized as before, but the pain was more towards the left side. It was accompanied with dyspnœa, anxiety, and restlessness. She died on April 26th, with increased dyspnœa, great anxiety, vomiting, and rapid sinking of the vital powers. Upon dissection, a thick layer of soft coagulable lymph was found interposed between the surfaces of the pericardium, which were adherent throughout. There was a deposition of the same kind upon the exterior of the pericardium, in some places nearly half an inch in thickness. The surface of the heart was dark-coloured and very vascular. The lungs were in some places indurated. The other viscera were healthy.

After detailing six other cases of pericarditis terminating fatally in the acute stage, Dr. Abercrombie observes*, " a remarkable circumstance in the history of this dangerous affection is, that it may be going on rapidly, yet insidiously, while our attention is occupied by symptoms which have no relation to it."

---

* On Carditis. Transactions of Medico-Chirurgical Society, Vol. vii.

* Contributions to the Pathology of the Heart, Transactions of Med. Chir. Soc. of Edinburgh, Vol. i. 1821.

CASES III. AND IV.—*Pericarditis, without any signs of rheumatism, giving rise to symptoms of inflammation of the brain.*

Dr. Latham has recorded* the case of a young woman, which is strongly impressed upon my recollection, who was admitted into St. Bartholomew's Hospital, in 1828, and in whom all the symptoms led to the belief that the brain was inflamed. The whole force of the treatment was therefore directed to that organ. The woman died; and upon dissection the brain and its coverings were found in a perfectly healthy and natural state, and the pericardium, towards which there was no symptom during life to induce the slightest suspicion of disease, exhibited unequivocal marks of acute inflammation.

Another woman, æt. 40, was admitted, in 1839, into St. Bartholomew's Hospital, suffering under slight delirium, fever, and other symptoms of an inflammatory affection of the brain. She was treated for this supposed affection of the brain, and did not present a single symptom referable to the heart. She sank in about four days after admission. No disease was found in the brain or elsewhere, excepting the free surfaces of the pericardium being coated with thick honeycomb lymph, which had evidently been effused within a few days previous to her death.

There appears to have been one peculiarity common to three out of the four cases I have just recited, which was, that, throughout their progress, there was no symptom present which directed attention to the organ affected. In the case recorded by Dr. Abercrombie, the patient had complained of pain in the epigastrium, and of dyspnœa, before the accession of the symptoms of affection of the brain and spinal cord; and these symptoms caused his treatment to be addressed near to the organ affected. Nevertheless, this case, as well as the other three, proved fatal.

CASE IV. — *Rheumatic pericarditis, attended with chorea and symptoms of inflammation of the brain and spinal cord.*

In April 1836, Dr. Richard Bright was summoned to attend a young man, æt. 17, who, twelve days previously, had been attacked with rheumatism. On the sixth day of the disease spasmodic symptoms appeared; and at the time of Dr. Bright's visit he was labouring under symptoms of severe chorea, the spasms being more violent than almost ever seen in that disorder. Although no particular symptom pointed out disease of the heart, still it was rather suspected. In a few days the spasms assumed the character of the most violent convulsions; his speech became indistinct, there was diffi-

culty in opening the mouth, and the mind began to wander. The *delirium* gradually increased until it was absolutely necessary to put him under personal restraint. He died at the end of three weeks. In this case lymph was found effused in abundance on the interior of the pericardium, and, to a slight extent, on the exterior of that membrane. The valves of the left side of the heart were fringed with vegetations. The brain was perfectly healthy*.

CASES VI. AND VII.—*Rheumatic pericarditis detected during life, accompanied with symptoms of inflammation of the brain, and terminating in recovery.*

In Dr. Macleod's essay " On Rheumatism, &c." published in 1842, there are two cases of rheumatic pericarditis recorded, in which symptoms of inflammation of the brain supervened, and which were both successfully treated. The first, a young woman, æt. 27, was admitted in the third week of rheumatic fever into St. George's Hospital. On the following day some incoherence was remarked, and the physical signs of pericarditis detected. On the third day constant delirium supervened, with restlessness and jactitation, so that it was necessary to put on a straight waistcoat. At the expiration of a week the delirium began to subside ; and, on examination of the heart, the friction sound had disappeared, but the sounds and impulse of the heart were feeble, distant, and intermittent. She gradually improved during the ensuing ten days, when she was twice affected with a convulsive fit of an epileptic character. From this time she progressively improved.

The treatment of this successful case consisted of bleeding, once generally, and once locally, calomel and opium, with purgatives, and blisters to the chest.

The second case related by Dr. Macleod occurred in a man of intemperate habits, æt. 39, who was admitted, September 1837, into St. George's Hospital, labouring under acute rheumatism of three weeks' duration. He was bled, purged, and took calomel and opium. On the fourth day after his admission he was observed to be incoherent, with much wildness of expression. His mouth was already affected by mercury, and he was therefore ordered a grain of opium every six hours. On the following day the delirium had increased ; so that at times he was unmanageable, and he had a fit. The physical signs of pericarditis were now detected. During the five following days the same symptoms persisted, and were treated with repeated doses of the acetate of morphia. From this period the delirium declined, and the friction sound disappeared. He gradually recovered ; and after a time the sounds of the heart became natural.

I think we can hardly attribute the success which attended the treatment of these two last-mentioned cases, as compared with the want of success in the five preceding instances, to any other circumstance than the early detection of pericarditis by its physical signs. In these two encouraging cases there does not appear to have been any symptom referable to the heart prior to the occurrence of the delirium, and the physical signs of pericarditis were not detected until after the supervention of the peculiar cerebral symptoms.

In the two following cases of rheumatic pericarditis we shall remark a still further, more serious, and permanent injury done to the brain. In both, indeed, life was preserved, the one however terminating in dementia, the second in insanity.

CASES VIII. AND IX.—*Rheumatic pericarditis, accompanied with chorea, and ending in dementia in one case, and in insanity in the other.*

A housemaid, æt. 24, was admitted into St. Bartholomew's Hospital, Aug. 23, 1838, under the care of one of my colleagues, suffering from rheumatism, affecting almost every joint of the body, and causing the most acute suffering, together with much fever. On the following day the respiration was observed to be hurried, and accompanied with pain about the præcordia. Auscultation at this time discovered no unnatural sound about the heart. She was bled from the arm; cupping-glasses were applied beneath the scapulæ; calomel and antimony administered internally, and then colchicum. At the expiration of a week her pains still continued, and as the colchicum had disturbed the stomach and bowels, it was determined to treat the case with opiates. During the ensuing week her pains declined, not uniformly, but rather remitting; her nights, however, were sleepless. On the 8th of September I was requested to see her. I found her sitting up in bed, moaning and wringing her hands, with a vacant expression of countenance. She did not appear conscious of what was passing around her, or scarcely so; she did not answer questions, or only in monosyllables, and when much urged: she occasionally put her hand to her head when questioned about pain there. During the previous night she had been wakeful, delirious, and constantly getting out of bed. I immediately suspected the nature of the case, and by a careful auscultation was able to detect a *to and fro* friction-sound over the whole præcordial region. She was again depleted twice locally, calomel and opium were administered freely, mercurial inunction commenced, and a blister applied over the cardiac region. In spite of these remedies the delirium continued during the ensuing week, the rubbing sound still being audible; she became purged and exhausted by the mercury, without affection of the gums. Milder mercurials, with opiates, leeches, and a blister to the chest, were now employed, and she was removed to a separate ward on account of her noise disturbing the other patients. Her condition remained, however, nearly the same, being delirious throughout the month of October. In the beginning of November she became more tranquil, and even took some part in the nurse's duties in the ward. She never spoke, unless to answer questions, and then very briefly. She was discharged on November 19, nearly in this condition, having had no return of rheumatism, nor at this time could any unnatural sound of the heart be heard.

On Oct. 25, 1838, a girl, æt. 16, was admitted into the same ward, suffering under rheumatism, which was not very severe. On November 2d she appeared very restless, and kept constantly moving about her arms, but not in that jerking manner commonly observed in chorea; her manner, too, appeared strange, and when addressed she did not answer the questions which were put to her, but spoke of something else, and then after some hesitation. The movements of the arms and legs became in a day or two more violent; she was continually delirious, and it was necessary to employ personal restraint. Her rheumatism disappeared, and I was informed, for I did not see her until a later period, that there was no unnatural sound of the heart.

She continued in this state until Nov. 8, when the chorea gradually subsided, but the strangeness of manner remained up to the time of her discharge, December 3, 1838. She however answered questions more readily, but was harassed by delusions, insisting that she was in Newgate, whither she had been sent for her wickedness.

It was remarkable that this and the former patient, although they never addressed any one, nor spoke to each other, were always to be found together, in whatever part of the ward they might happen to be, where they sat and looked at each other, regardless of anything else.

Although the physical signs of pericarditis were not detected in the last described case, I think that when its history is compared with other similar affections of the nervous system, coming on in the course of rheumatism, there can be little doubt as to the existence of an insidious pericarditis in this patient also.

CASE X.—*Pericarditis, attended with symptoms of apoplexy, and general paralysis.*

M. Rostan[*] relates the case of a woman

* Recherches sur Ramollissement du Cerveau.

who was admitted under his care, suffering from general uneasiness. On the second day she was suddenly seized with a complete loss of consciousness; her eyes were fixed, the eyelids open; the cheeks flushed; the pulse at the wrist, and impulse of the heart, scarcely perceptible; the limbs motionless, except when pinched. She remained in this state four days, and died.

The pericardium was found covered with false membranes, and bloody serum effused into its sac. There was no appreciable lesion in the other organs.

Case XI.—*Apoplexy occurring in the course of undetected pericarditis, not rheumatic.*

A young man, æt. 21, was admitted (March 1834) under the care of M. Bouillaud, labouring under general dropsy. Twelve days after his admission he was attacked with sudden loss of consciousness; his eyeballs were turned upwards; his breathing became stertorous; his lips covered with frothy saliva; his limbs, instead of being thrown about in convulsive movements, were completely paralysed. On the following day he had two or three similar apoplectic seizures, which however did not last many minutes. He was also observed to be occasionally slightly delirious. On the fifth day after the appearance of these cerebral symptoms the tumultuous action of the heart induced M. Bouillaud to examine the condition of that organ more carefully than he had previously done, when he distinctly ascertained the presence of the physical signs of pericarditis. On the following day the patient died.

Dissection discovered abundant effusion of lymph into the pericardium, with signs of endocarditis in the left ventricle, also recent adhesions with some serous effusion into the right pleura, with extensive consolidation and softening of the right lung. The brain presented no morbid appearances. M. Bouillaud remarks* on this case, that without the assistance of auscultation and percussion it would have been impossible to have detected the pericarditis in this man. He never complained of pain in the region of the heart, and there was no suspicion of rheumatic inflammation in any part of the body. M. Bouillaud flattered himself that this pericarditis had come on in the night previous to his detecting its presence, and that it had been brought on by exposure to cold when the man, in a state of delirium, went to the water-closet. It appears much more probable that the pericardial as well as the pneumonic inflammation had already made considerable progress at the time of the first apoplectic seizure.

Case XII.—*Undetected pericarditis, accompanied with symptoms of inflammation of the spinal cord.*

Andral details* the following case of acute pericarditis terminating fatally, where the symptoms were those of inflammation of the spinal cord, delirium and tetanic spasm being especially prominent.

A woman, æt. 26, who had recently miscarried, was brought into La Charité Hospital with so much delirium, that no account of her complaint could be obtained from herself. Her delirium was characterised by a remarkably obstinate taciturnity; her lips were observed to be drawn apart by convulsive twitches. On the following day her head was frequently drawn backwards, and her body thrown up in jerks. She appeared to understand questions, and answered, but was incoherent. On the fourth day after her admission the delirium disappeared. The muscles of the face were constantly convulsed, and her upper limbs every now and then became as rigid as in cases of tetanus. On the fifth day the delirium returned; her limbs were palsied; she fell into a state of coma, and died that evening.

On inspection of the body, the membranes and substance of the brain and spinal cord were found without the slightest morbid change; the surfaces of the pericardium were covered with soft lymph, and several ounces of turbid serum were contained in the sac. There was no disease of any other organ.

M. Andral, in recording this curious case, reconfmends it to the serious attention of his readers. It appears to him to show, that in consequence of the idiosyncrasies of individuals, the lesion of any important organ may produce, sympathetically, the most varied nervous symptoms, such as are usually the consequence of disease in the nervous centres themselves. Although M. Andral describes delirium as one of the symptoms present in the foregoing case, yet there is no evidence of delirium in the report, beyond the obstinate taciturnity, which may have arisen from the inability to command the organs of articulation.

Case XIII.—*Tetanus in its most aggravated form, occurring in a case of undetected rheumatic pericarditis, which was treated as inflammation of the spinal cord†.*

A robust lad, æt. 16, was admitted under the care of M. Bouillaud, in March, 1834. A fortnight previous to his admission he had had swelling of his hands and arms, which prevented him from working. Shortly afterwards he was seized with convulsive con-

* *Traité des Maladies du Cœur, tom i. p. 319.*

* Clin. Méd. t. i. p. 34.
† Bouillaud, op. cit. tom. i. p. 333.

tractions of his fingers, which were regarded and treated as epilepsy.

At the time of his admission his eyes were fixed and haggard, and the pupils dilated. He had the aspect of a man who apprehended some great danger; his intellect was clear, but he replied to questions with a trembling voice, his articulation being interrupted by cries and sobs, called forth by severe cramps in his limbs, and a feeling of suffocation. The fingers, hands, fore-arms, toes, and feet, were violently contracted. The muscles of the lower jaw, of the abdomen and limbs, were as hard as stone during the spasms. The mouth was opened with difficulty. The whole body, but particularly the face and chest, streamed with perspiration, which became more abundant with the return of the cramps.

During the four succeeding days he suffered from repeated attacks of spasmodic contractions of the limbs, with more urgent symptoms of trismus. Any attempt to swallow aggravated his sufferings. During the continuance of these symptoms of tetanus the circulation was frequent, the skin hot or perspiring, the bowels constipated, and some dysuria was present. The disease was regarded as inflammation of the spinal cord, and treated by venesection, and repeated local abstractions of blood along the spine. Opium was administered internally, and a warm bath every day.

The patient died on the tenth day after the first appearance of the spasms in the fingers.

Dissection detected a general increased vascularity of the pericardium, with two ounces of pure creamy greenish pus in that serous sac, and old adhesions in either pleura. The brain and spinal cord, with their membranes, were generally congested. The spinal cord was rather firm, except at the superior enlargement of the cord, where there was a circumscribed spot of softening.

In this case pericarditis was never suspected, and its physical signs were not sought after. They probably would have been more obscure than usual, on account of the absence of fibrinous exudations, and the small quantity of purulent effusion into the pericardium. It is also worthy of remark, that although this case was treated by M. Bouillaud with active depletion, and by large doses of opium, nevertheless there was no alleviation of the symptoms.

CASE XIV.—*Undetected idiopathic pericarditis, attended with symptoms of inflammation of the spinal cord.*

Dr. Macintosh* describes the case of a middle-aged man, who suffered from asthma, sleepless nights, cough, and expectoration, and at the same time from spasmodic con-

* *Practice of Physic, vol. ii. 4th edition.*

tractions of the muscles of the extremities. On examining the chest he was found to have an extraordinary curvature of the spine, and to be chicken-breasted. He was unable to inflate the lungs completely. The action of the heart was tumultuous and irregular, occasionally intermitting. On the two succeeding days he appeared to improve under the treatment adopted, the case being regarded as one of chronic disease of the lungs, with enlargement of the heart. On the third day the oppression about the chest increased; but the chief suffering arose from cramps in his extremities, and occasional spasmodic rigidity of the whole body, which was sometimes bent backwards, and supported by the occiput and heels, in complete opisthotonos. He died suddenly in the course of the following night, the spasms having been so severe that he could hardly be kept in his bed.

On dissection, the brain was found quite healthy. No trace of disease was found in the spinal cord, except one old adhesion of the membranes, and some ossific scales on the surface of the arachnoid. The pericardium was large, and contained a considerable quantity of turbid serum, with a deposition of lymph, adhering in several places to the surface of the heart. The heart itself was large; the valves were sound.

The cases of tetanus which I have now related, coming on in the course of pericarditis, should not remain mere pathological curiosities: they should suggest some useful practical rules in the treatment of that terrible nervous affection. The pathology of tetanus is confessedly obscure: numerous cases of that disease have terminated fatally in the hands of the most able practitioners, when no morbid appearances could be found in the spinal cord and membranes. We are obliged to confess our ignorance of the nature of the morbid action in such cases, and affirm that the spinal cord has suffered from irritation.

Dr. Marshall Hall has applied certain epithets to nervous affections, according as the source of irritation is situated in the brain and spinal cord, or elsewhere. When the source of irritation is within the nervous centres, he terms the affection *centric:* and when it is situated elsewhere *eccentric.* The cases I have cited upon the present occasion are examples of eccentric tetanus, the source of irritation being in the nerves of the heart and diaphragm. Considering how obscure is the pathology, and how difficult the treatment of tetanus, it behoves every one henceforth, in cases of trismus and tetanus, which are not traumatic in their origin, to scrutinize the sounds and action of the heart by auscultation, and to seek for the signs of pericarditis. It is a melancholy reflection, but, I fear, a just one, that numbers have perished from these supposed diseases of the spinal cord, when in truth the morbid action has been in the heart, although that has not been detected.

The connection of chorea with inflammation of the pericardium has already been illustrated in the narratives I have just detailed; and I therefore feel disposed to add but few observations on this part of the subject. It is, however, very fully discussed by Dr. R. Bright, in his essay "on spasmodic diseases accompanying affections of the pericardium*." No less than five cases of this complication are there recorded by Dr. Bright, who makes the following remarks on their pathology: — "The instances of the combination and alternation of rheumatism and chorea are very numerous; and though I doubt not in some cases (as supposed by Dr. Copland and others), the coverings of the cerebro-spinal mass may be, and are implicated, yet I believe that the much more frequent cause of chorea, in conjunction with rheumatism, is the inflammation of the pericardium. The irritation probably is communicated thence to the spine, just as the irritation of other parts, as of the bowels, the gums, or the uterus, is communicated, and produces the same diseases."

The series of cases which I have brought before you, I think, fully support the correctness of these opinions.

There only remains one other nervous affection, to which I alluded at the commencement of the lecture, as occasionally produced by active disease of the heart and pericardium : it is hysteria. In Dr. Bright's valuable paper is recorded a remarkable case of chronic disease of the pericardium which was accompanied with hysteria.

From this collection of cases, which I have analysed and detailed on the present occasion, we learn that all those groups of symptoms which indicate the most formidable diseases of the brain and spinal cord may arise from the irritation of the nerves of the heart, without any structural change in the nervous centres themselves.

It would thus appear, to employ the words of Andral, " qu'en raison des susceptibilités individuelles, il n'est point d'organe dont la lesion ne puisse déterminer les symptômes nerveux les plus variés, de manière à produire sympathiquement les differens états morbides dont on place le siege dans les centres nerveux et leurs dépendances†."

I may now, in conclusion, venture to offer some remarks on the pathology and treatment of these cases, as a distinct class of nervous affections.

* Op. cit.
† Clin. Méd. t. i. p. 86.

It has been supposed by some pathologists that these cases are only met with in connexion with rheumatism, and particularly where pericarditis is engrafted on rheumatism of the joints; but of the sixteen cases I have narrated, no rheumatic affection could be discovered in six of them. In two or three the pericarditis might be regarded as idiopathic; in the others, it came on in the course of chronic diseases of various kinds.

It has also been affirmed by some writers, that when peculiar nervous symptoms do appear in the course of rheumatism or pericarditis, that such nervous symptoms arise from a metastasis of the morbid action to the membranes of the brain and spinal cord. Without denying the occasional occurrence of such a phenomenon, I can only state, that in not one of the twelve fatal cases I have enumerated could a trace of disease be discovered in the brain or its membranes. In only two of the twelve did the spinal cord and its membranes present any thing remarkable. In the case of tetanus cited from the work of M. Bouillaud, the cord and its membranes were vascular, and there was also one small point in the cord softened. In the case of tetanus quoted from Dr. Macintosh, an old adhesion was discovered in the membranes of the cord, and some small ossific scales on the spinal arachnoid. I have already alluded to the opinions of Dr. Bright on the pathology of some of these spasmodic affections, and the mode in which he supposes the nervous centres to become affected. I fully coincide with the general principle of his explanation.

Dr. Bright reports, that in the cases examined by him, the inflammation was not confined to the interior of the pericardium, but existed also on that part of the external surface of the pericardium, as well as pleura, where the phrenic nerve, in its course or distribution, is to be found. Dr. Bright therefore suggests the explanation, "that the phrenic nerve is the more immediate means of communicating the irritation to the spinal cord."

In the case I have cited from Dr. Abercrombie's Essay, there was found not only a large quantity of lymph within the pericardium, but also a layer of lymph, half an inch in thickness, on the exterior of the pericardium. This additional fact gives support to the explanation offered by Dr. Bright; which also derives further confirmation from some observations of M. Bouillaud on these remarkable cases.

M. Bouillaud, in reviewing the general symptoms of pericarditis, adverts to the extraordinary disturbance of the nervous system in some cases of this disease, and proceeds to analyse the peculiarities which have distinguished them. He finds that such nervous symptoms have occurred when pericarditis has been complicated with pleurisy, and especially with extensive diaphragmatic pleurisy. This opinion he supports by reference to some of his own cases, as well as to one recorded by Corvisart, where the patient, during life, was attacked with spasms of the muscles of the face, and delirium. After death, besides the pericarditis, there was discovered extensive inflammation of the pleura covering the diaphragm. The celebrated republican, Mirabeau, also died of severe pericarditis complicated with pleurisy. The progress of his complaint was accompanied with the most distressing nervous symptoms, which caused him frequently to appeal to his philosophic friend and physician (Cabanis) to put an end to his agony by large doses of opium.

The explanation of M. Bouillaud of the pathology of these cases of pericarditis with aggravated symptoms of nervous excitement, very closely coincides with that given by Dr. R. Bright. But the details of both fatal and favourable cases of pericarditis complicated with pleurisy, recorded in the work of M. Bouillaud, shew that such cases are not necessarily attended with nervous excitement. I have known several instances of rheumatic pericarditis complicated with pleurisy, where no peculiar nervous symptoms were present; on the other hand, I have seen a few cases of pericarditis, where no pleurisy existed, and which were characterised by these strange nervous phenomena.

On this part of the pathology of the heart the late Dr. Hope made the following remarks: "There is no doubt of the fact that pleurisy, especially diaphragmatic, may produce the violent symptoms in question; it is therefore obvious, that this complication might aggravate the symptoms of pericarditis and raise them to their utmost intensity; but it does not follow that all cases of uncomplicated pericarditis should be exempt from such severe symptoms: nor are they." Dr. Hope adds, that the sardonic expression, and peculiar contortions of the features, attending the worst class of cases of pericarditis, are occasioned by the sympathy subsisting between the respiratory nerves of the face, and those of the heart. An impression is conveyed to the spinal cord through the pneumogastric nerves, and reflected to the face through the portio dura.

It would, therefore, from a more extended review of these cases, seem probable, that, although the spinal irritation may in some cases be excited through the phrenic nerves, the same amount and kind of irritation may be equally conveyed through the pneumogastric nerves. The practical value of this advance in pathology will consist in calling attention to the physical signs of the state of the heart in all obscure and intractable affections of the brain and spinal cord.

Lastly, I shall briefly allude to the subject of the treatment of these nervous affections appearing in the course of pericarditis.

In all the cases which I have adverted to, where the plan of treatment is recorded, abstraction of blood was resorted to. In some the quantity taken was considerable.

In most of the cases, in conjunction with the abstraction of blood, other remedies, usually termed antiphlogistic, were employed. In a few, in addition to abstraction of blood, opium appears to have been freely given; while in some of those where the pericarditis was detected during life, in addition to the abstraction of blood generally and locally, calomel and opium were administered freely; and mercurial inunction was likewise employed in a few: and of these various modes of treatment, the last was the only successful plan.

Of the fourteen cases I have detailed, four only escaped with their lives; and of these, three were treated on the calomel and opium plan, combined with the abstraction of blood. Of the remaining eleven, treated on the various methods I have specified, ten perished.

CLINICAL LECTURES

ON THE

THEORY & MEDICAL TREATMENT
OF INSANITY.

Delivered at St. Luke's Hospital,

May 1st, 3d, and 5th.

BY ALEXANDER JOHN SUTHERLAND.

LECTURE I.

Introduction. Different theories of the nature and seat of insanity. Reasons for considering the seat of the disease to be in the brain. Of disorders of the mental faculties. Of fatuity — incoherence — delusion. Of disorders of emotion. Hallucination — illusion — examples of each. Alterations of the sensitive nerves. Alterations of the motor nerves. General Paralysis. Foville's theory.

GENTLEMEN, — Before we go round the wards of the hospital, and before I show you particular cases illustrative of particular medical treatment, I propose to give you a brief sketch of the nature of insanity, considered not as a metaphysical subtilty, but as a disease of the body.

I am fully aware of the difficulty of the task I have undertaken, and of my inability to perform it: the end I have in view will, however, be sufficiently answered if I shall have added any thing to your previous knowledge which may hereafter be of practical use to you in your profession.

Insanity is a term which comprehends under it so many conditions of soul and body that it is quite impossible strictly to define what species and difference should constitute it 'as a genus: on the one hand we find alterations of intellect, affection, passion, and instinct; on the other those of sensation and motion.

Inasmuch as it is the brain which presides over the functions of the mind, sensation, and voluntary motion, I shall consider first how far it is probable that the disease may have its seat in that organ; secondly, the alterations in the nerves, the morbid condition of which ministers to the brain false perceptions; thirdly, the changes in the circulating fluid which either precede or follow the attack; this will lead me, lastly, to speak of alterations of function in other organs which are complicated with insanity, either as causes or effects, inasmuch as faults of secretion and excretion have an important bearing upon our subject, more especially as regards medical treatment.

The writers on the pathology of insanity may be divided into those who treat of it as an idiopathic, and those who consider it a symptomatic affection. Different physicians have often looked upon the disease in different points of view. The question—where is the seat of the disease, is a very different one from another with which it is apt to be confounded—whence did it originate. M. Esquirol, for instance, lays much stress upon the disease taking its origin in the different ganglia, and not always in the brain; but he does not say that it has its resting-place in these ganglia. So M. Guislain, although he considers the brain to be always affected in insanity, does not say that it is always primarily so affected. Again, M. Foville, who is generally placed among the advocates for insanity being an idiopathic disease, does not deny that it is both sympathetic and symptomatic. Setting aside, then, the opinions of those who take the middle, and, as I think, the safer course, there remains for us to consider two opposite theories as to the seat of insanity: the one, that it is always a primary affection of the brain, and that the other viscera are secondarily disordered; the other, that it is always a primary disease of one or other of the viscera, and that the delirium is merely a symptom.

M. Georget may be considered as one of the most active representatives of the first theory, viz. that madness is a primary affection of the brain. This theory appears to *me to be in direct contradiction to facts, inasmuch as functional and organic changes*

in the kidneys, heart, liver, and uterus, do certainly sometimes precede, and are not always the consequences of, insanity. When we find (as I often have) the kidneys marbled and granulated in our post-mortem examinations, are we to conclude that the disease of the brain produced the Bright's kidney, or rather that the diseased kidney produced those alterations in the blood which effected the first functional disturbance in the brain? If time allowed me, I could bring before you many examples of nephritis, enteritis, hypertrophy of the heart, disorders of the uterus and other viscera, which existed prior to, and which were apparently the physical cause of, the subsequent disturbance in the brain. M. Georget discards (art. Folie : Dict. de Med.), I think, rather too summarily the morbid appearances found in some of the viscera in insanity, when he says, "the heart is rarely diseased, and the kidneys are almost always healthy." Although I should agree with M. Georget, and others, in believing that madness is a disease of the brain, I cannot concur with them in thinking that the *fons et origo mali* is always to be traced to that organ.

We have next to consider the theory of Jacobi, that insanity is a symptom of disease; not a disease in itself, but secondary, depending upon disorders in other viscera. There are others of high authority who share this opinion with Jacobi; the great Pinel, for instance, considered the stomach and intestines to be the seat of the disorder, from which point he thought the evil radiated to the brain. The opinion that melancholy had its fountain-head in the colon is as old as Hippocrates; and Esquirol attributes some importance to the displacement of its transverse arch in cases of this description. Dufour places the seat of the disease in the ganglia; M. Prost in the mucous membrane of the intestines. These opinions are in some measure in accordance with those of Bichat, who endeavours to prove, from the frequent morbid appearances found in the viscera of the thorax and abdomen in cases of insanity, and from other facts, that the brain is not exclusively concerned in all psychical phenomena, but that the emotions may have their origin in other viscera. These theories are extremely plausible; and it is very difficult to answer them, because of the obscurity of the relation which exists between the viscera and the mind. Professor Müller has taught us not to confuse the mental operations with the mental principle, and here seems to lie the origin of the fallacy: the mental principle exists every where throughout the body; the mental operations are confined to the brain. He says[*], "in short it is evident that the effects of the

* Baly's Translation, 817, Vol. i.

passions upon the different organs subject to the influence of the brain in no way confirm the hypothesis of the passions, or certain mental faculties, having their seat in any other organ than the brain." If we carry our investigation farther, and appeal to comparative anatomy and physiology, as well as to morbid anatomy, it becomes a matter of high probability that the cortical structure of the brain is chiefly the instrument of mental operations. I think that no one who has had much experience in the post-mortem examinations of the insane, can fail to have been struck with the variations from healthy structure which the grey substance, generally speaking, presents. How different are the convolutions of the brain in recent mania, which are every where injected, and highly developed, and appear almost too large to be contained within the cranium, from the pale and shrunken convolutions of dementia!

Professor Owen has pointed out the importance of observing the different direction, the difference of packing, so to speak, of the convolutions in different species of animals: e. g. in herbivorous animals the median fissures which divide the folds of the hemispheres converge from the circumference to the centre; in the carnivora they are parallel, while in the human subject they diverge. When we compare the human brain with the brains of animals, we find, at a certain period of foetal existence, the total absence of convolutions, like the smooth surface of the hemispheres of the rodentia. On the other hand, in the full-developed brain of man, we have additions, not only anteriorly but posteriorly, to those folds which have their analogues in the brains of inferior animals. It would therefore seem (even though we had not the brains of idiots to strengthen the supposition) that the convolutions are mainly concerned in the operations of the higher faculties of the mind; and that if, from their deficiency in man, the soul has not the power of communicating with external nature, the reason lies not in the soul's deficiency; for it remains, notwithstanding hereditary mal-conformations, or the decay of disease, as perfect as when it first came from the hands of the Creator.

Recent physiological investigations would lead us to conjecture that the emotions and instincts have a centre of action distinct from the higher intellectual faculties; that, in fact, all psychical phenomena are not confined to the cerebrum, as was formerly supposed, but that the medulla oblongata is the chief instrument by which emotion is manifested; so that if a physiologist were called upon to draw a diagram of the principal seat of action of mind and emotion, he would represent it, not by the centre of a circle, but by the foci of an ellipse. Some doubt, however, still exists upon this subject:

some hold that the medulla oblongata, Dr. M. Hall and others that the spinal system of the nerves, is the main channel through which instinct and emotion flow.

If the brain, the organ of the mind, be diseased, it is a highly probable, though not a necessary consequence, that the mind itself should become affected. In insanity of intellect, as distinguished from that of emotion, all the faculties of the mind are liable to be disturbed in different cases—some more, some less; those, however, which most commonly suffer are attention and association, which comprise memory and imagination; for memory cannot exist without the former, and the pleasures of imagination appear chiefly to take their rise in the latter (see Diss. Encyc. Brit. i. 368). In idiotcy there is of course little or no attention; in dementia it is weakened, or almost obliterated; in mania it is distracted by a thousand ideas, furnished by sensible objects from without, and by the mind from within; in monomania it is rivetted to one predominant idea, while association, so busily at work for evil in the mind of the maniac and monomaniac, grafts its false perceptions upon those ideas most habitual to him prior to his disease.

These disorders in the faculties of the mind are usually expressed by the words fatuity, incoherence, and delusion. Fatuity expresses a state of intellect somewhat analogous to the decay of the mind in old age, which is thus very beautifully described by Locke: " Ideas often die before us, and our minds represent to us those tombs to which we are approaching, where, though the brass and marble remain, yet the inscriptions are effaced by time, and the imaginary moulders away."

Incoherence is unconnected discourse. The incoherence of mania, however, differs from that of dementia: the former is owing to a quick succession of ideas passing through the mind too rapidly for all to find utterance; the latter arises from a defect of memory; words, sometimes whole sentences, are omitted; at other times one word is substituted for another, and the whole conversation becomes disjointed and unintelligible.

Delusion is a permanent idea in the mind which is contrary to sound sense and general opinion. That the idea be contrary to sound sense is not sufficient to constitute delusion; for an uneducated man may infer many things which are contrary to sound sense, as that the sun revolves round the earth; but his opinions are not contrary to the general belief of those in the same rank of life with himself, and therefore are not, strictly speaking, delusions. Nor, on the other hand, is an idea which is contrary to general opinion necessarily a delusive one; for a philosopher before the age in which he lives, who advances theories, with sound conclusions, deduced from true premises which contradict general opinion, stands a very good chance of being considered out of his mind—instances of which must be familiar to every one. Such opinions, then, cannot properly be brought under the head of delusions.

If aberration of intellect is an important feature in cases of insanity, equally so is a diseased state of the sentiments, the affections, and the passions: a change in these is generally the first sign of the coming disorder; and when unsettled, these are commonly the last to be restored to a state of health. Cases of insanity exist in which emotion alone appears to be involved, leaving the intellect untouched: this is the moral insanity of Dr. Prichard. So common is it for that part of our nature to be changed in madness, the operation of which we recognize by the words emotion, sensibility, desire, aversion, and the like, that some men, mistaking effects for causes, have asserted that the essence of insanity consists in a wrong action of the soul, and consider all madmen to be sinners. To this theory Professor Müller answers, that "since the action of any part always induces a change in the organic structure which composes it, it necessarily follows that immoderate exertion of the mind, a continued direction of it to one object consequent on external circumstances or great mental excitement, must react on the organization of the instrument of the mental operations; the wrong direction of the thoughts is not a mental disease, but is merely one of its numerous exciting causes" (Baly's Trans. i. 820). This answer of Müller is not quite satisfactory, for it does not go far enough; because it is not sufficient that there should be a change in the organic structure of a part, for this is produced even by the healthy action of every organ; there must be such a change as to amount to disease before we can recognize it as constituting insanity. One of the most difficult questions which we have to decide is, where does passion end and insanity begin? There are many instances of passion which are unjustly attributed to insanity; and yet who is there who has yet been able to limit their shadowy confines? They approach each other so nearly that the description of the one will often pass for that of the other. Take, for example, Seneca's picture of anger, which would apply equally well to a paroxysm of furor. "Cætera vitia impellunt animos; ira præcipitat. Cæteris etiamsi resistere contra affectus suos non licet, at certe affectibus ipsis licet stare; hæc non secus quam fulmina procellæque, et si qua alia irrevocabilia sunt, quia non eunt, sed cadunt, vim suam magis ac magis tendit. *Alia vitia a ratione, hæc a sanitate dehiscit; alia accessus lenes habent, et incrementa* fallentia, in iram dejectus animorum est. Nulla itaque res urget magis attonita, et in vires suas prone, et, sive successit, superba, sive frustrata insana."

Some men quote lightly the opinion of Locke. "There is scarce any one that does not observe something that seems odd to him, and is in itself really extravagant, in the opinions, reasonings, and actions of other men," which, he says, proceeds not wholly from self-love, nor from education, but from a sort of madness. (I cannot refrain from quoting the rest of the passage, although it is somewhat long). "I shall be pardoned for calling it by so harsh a name as madness, when it is considered that opposition to reason deserves that name, and is really madness; and there is scarce a man so free from it, but that if he should always, on all occasions, argue or do as in some cases he constantly does, would not be thought fitter for Bedlam than civil conversation. I do not here mean when he is under the power of an unruly passion, but in the steady calm course of his life. That which will yet more apologize for this harsh name and ungrateful imputation on the greater part of mankind is, that inquiring a little by the bye into the nature of madness, I found it spring from the very same root, and to depend on the very same cause, we are here speaking of. This consideration of the thing itself, at a time when I thought not the least on the subject which I am now treating of, suggested it to me. And if this weakness, to which all men are so liable, if this be a taint which so universally infects mankind, the greatest care should be taken to lay it open under its due name, thereby to excite the greater care in its prevention and cure." (Ch. 33). How glad would a criminal be of such an advocate as Locke! It is easy to see how he fell into this train of thought: he had previously framed his celebrated definition, that madness consists in correct reasoning from wrong principles, without considering that some madmen reason very accurately, and others are incapable of reasoning at all; and thus, when he compared the obstinacy with which most men adhere to their opinions, with his definition, he found that either his definition must be false, or that all men must be in some measure mad; and in this dilemma he chose to conclude that the latter was correct. Locke appears to me to have been misled by a partial study of the disease: he seems mostly to have had experience of the reasonings of monomaniacs, to which his definition, and his above remarks upon madness, correctly apply, for the monomaniac is capable of reasoning accurately from false premises, and clings to his imagined sufferings and enjoyments with the greater tenacity, the more that you endeavour to convince him that he is labouring under delusion. Aware of the difficulty of drawing nice distinctions between passion and eccentricity on the one hand, and insanity on the other, our law has marked out a broad line which must be passed before a man can be recognised as insane. In order to deprive a man of his civil rights, it is not enough that he should be proved insane; he must be proved to be so far insane as not to be able to manage himself and his affairs; in order to shew that he is irresponsible for his criminal acts, it must be made evident that he was so far insane as not to be capable of distinguishing between right and wrong at the time he committed the crime. The law skilfully avoids the difficulty of measuring the capacity of men's minds; it very wisely does not attempt to determine where passion ends, and insanity begins: to define accurately the boundary between one and the other is the labour of him who would separate with distinct lines the mingling colours of the rainbow, or of Arachne's web.

In quo diversi niteant quum mille colores,
Transitus ipse tamen spectantia lumina fallit.
Usque adeo quod tangit idem est ! tamen ultima
distant.—OVID. MET. vi. 65.

Interesting as this part of our inqury is, it would be foreign to my purpose to pursue it on the present occasion; I must refer those who wish to follow out the investigation, to the works of Dr. Prichard and Dr. Conolly, and to Shelford, and Collinson, on the law of lunatics.

I must now draw your attention to those false perceptions which are furnished to the diseased mind, either by the nerves of special sense, or of nerves of sense generally: these occur in two ways; either the function of the nerves themselves is disturbed, and conveys to the mind false impressions of external objects, or the imagination conjures up the morbid perception, and acts upon the judgment through this or that nerve; it is, for instance, either the eye, or the mind's eye, which is disordered : these errors of perception are called hallucinations or illusions; words which have often been misapplied. Hallucination is a creation from within, illusion is a mistake from without: the mirage is an example of an illusion which the thirsty traveller of the desert is taught to correct. Supposed visions are examples of hallucinations; both the one and the other are compatible with perfect sanity: before they can be adduced as proofs of insanity, the condition of the understanding and of the character must be taken into consideration : e. g. our Saxon ancestors believed that they were pursued by the fauns, forest-fiends, and white women, which haunted the abodes of their fathers in the wilds of Germany : we call this superstition, not insanity. Visions of imagination also have appeared not only

to Colonel Gardner, but to Lord Herbert of Cherbury : " prophetic warnings," as the author of Distinguished Northerns says, " have occurred to young and old ; saints and sinners; to Bentley the orthodox, to Oliver Cromwell the fanatic, to Littleton the rake, to Nelson the hero, and to Alexander Stephens the buffoon." Examples analogous to these in kind, but differing in degree, are often met with in cases of aberration of intellect; the nerves of hearing and of sight are most commonly the seat of injury ; commands issuing from supernatural voices, warnings from deceased friends, persecutions from ideal enemies, visions of angels or of devils, frequently embarrass the bewildered imagination : the nerves of touch are certainly less commonly found disordered than the rest. In some cases I have seen hallucination of one sense, and illusion of another, existing at the same time. As this is a matter of some importance, I shall give you examples first of hallucinations, and afterwards of illusions.

A lady whom I occasionally visit has been blind for some years, and yet scarcely a day passes without her fancying that she sees either rays of light, bright figures, or soldiers.

J. L., æt. 45, was a patient of mine in May 1840 : he imagined that he was beset by devils, who poured all kinds of blasphemies and abuse through pipes in the ceiling of his room into his ear : at the time he was speaking to me he fancied an evil spirit was crawling over his shoulder and blowing into his left ear, while in his right ear he heard the consoling admonitions of his guardian angel, which counteracted the ill effects of the other. I ordered him some medicine, and recommended him to go into the country ; when he returned he told me that instead of having heard the abuse, swearing, and blasphemies, he had been exposed to while in London, the voices assumed the mild accents of the country people with whom he lived.

Examples of hallucinations of smell are not very uncommon, especially in the case of those who imagine they are suffering the tortures of the condemned ; these delusions also often accompany alterations of the nerve of taste. False perceptions of taste, unconnected with a foul tongue, derangement of the stomach and bowels, are rare. A patient whom I attended in February 1839, imagined she had murdered a child ; she refused her food because she thought it was the flesh of the victim she had slain, and would not drink because every thing she swallowed tasted she said like human blood. The tongue was not loaded ; the bowels were not costive : the false perception therefore must be accounted for either by supposing with M. Esquirol that it was created by the imagination, or by concluding, with M. Foville, that it was due to disease at the origin of the nerve in the brain, not to its termination in the tongue.

Hallucinations of the nerves of touch are, as I have stated, the most rarely met with : under this head the following instances may be placed.

A young officer whom I visited a year ago imagined that by touching people he had the power of magnetising and attracting them. Another patient whom I visited last week imagined that her head had been cut off, and that it was rolling about the room like a ball. The story of the turned head, so well told by the able author of the " Diary of a Physician," is not mere fiction; I have met with cases very similar to it. One man thought that his head was set on the wrong way (as the poor person who was saved from the guillotine). A patient now in the hospital fancies that all her bones are turned round.

I shall now bring before you, as briefly as I can, examples of illusions or mistakes, derived externally from morbid impressions of the nerves.

I visited Miss E. Y. on the 15th of January, 1842 : she was æt. 26, of a nervous temperament ; pulse 80, rather weak ; tongue clean ; skin cool ; head hot ; bowels costive ; urine free ; catamenia absent six months ; thorax not dull on percussion ; sounds and impulse of heart natural ; no undue action of the carotids ; abdomen not distended with flatus. She had suffered under melancholia six months. The cause of her illness was fright. Countenance anxious ; pupils and conjunctivæ natural ; complexion clear. From the cessation of the catamenia she imagined herself pregnant. She thought also that she had committed several murders, and that the robins proclaimed her guilt by their red breasts, and all the birds in the garden wore black beaks. The glass of her windows she thought was blood-red ; the flakes of snow she said were crosses and crowns of thorns ; the carts which passed the house contained the dead bodies of her murdered victims ; and she lived in continued dread of being cast into a den of wild beasts for her crimes.

℞ Infusi Quassiæ, f℥iss. ; Tincturæ Ferri Sesquichloridi, ℳ xx. bis die.

Hydrargyri Chloridi, gr. ii. ; Extracti Colocynth. Comp. gr. vilj. alt. noctibus.

February 7th.—She had been improving up to this day, when she was allowed to see one of her relations, which brought back the delusions.

Balneum calidum bis in hebdomadâ.

℞ Infusi Sennæ comp. Decocti Aloes comp. aa. f℥vi. omni mane. Omittantur pilulæ.

March 5th.—She was much the same.

Omittatur Haustus Infusi Quassiæ, &c.

℞ Decocti Aloes, comp. f℥vi. ; Tincturæ Aloes comp. f℥i. ; Tincturæ Hyoscyami, f℥ss. ; Aquæ Cinnamomi f℥ivss. omni mane. Repetatur Balneum.

18th.—She was very melancholy and desponding, and thought she was to be burnt or hung ; pulse 88, stronger ; tongue clean ; bowels open ; catamenia still absent.

Hirudines vi. regioni pubicæ.

19th.—Better.

Omittatur Haustus.

℞ Extracti Colocynth. comp. gr. x. pro re natâ. Repetatur Balneum.

April 8th.—Very much improved. She had written two letters to her friends, and seen her brother. She bore the interview well.

Perstet in usu Balnei.

14th.—The catamenia appeared on the previous evening for the first time since her illness, immediately after she came out of the bath.

20th.—She returned home cured.

I met with a curious illusion of smell in an old sportsman, for whom I prescribed the compound galbanum pill, as he was labouring under insanity with hypochondriasis : he thought from the smell of the assafœtida that I had metamorphosed him into a fox, and that he was to be turned out next morning before the hounds.

It is remarkable to listen to the misconstructions a patient places on the plainest and most harmless expressions, and sometimes the most familiar sounds. An Irishwoman who was in the hospital some little time ago stopped the clock because she thought it was calling her names.

Monsieur U. a patient of mine in 1840, became insane after reading the trial of Madame Laffarge : he fancied that every one about him intended to poison him, and was constantly searching the house, and breaking open drawers, in expectation of finding arsenic : he even imagined that the washerwoman had inserted poison into his linen, and he took his shirt to a chemist to be analysed ; the day that I visited him he had been reading the account of the arrival of Napoleon's remains at Cherbourg. He imagined at one time that the spirit of Bonaparte had been infused into his body, at another that it was all-powerful, and was about to work changes in the whole world. Napoleon's figure continually haunted him ; he saw it in the sun by day, and in the moon by night. One of his fancies was, that England was to be turned into a large British Museum, and the inhabitants placed herein as curiosities. He threatened to kill his wife because he was afraid she would be hanged into something ridiculous.

This patient very soon recovered. The treatment consisted chiefly in the use of colchicum with the sesquicarbonate of soda, which was prescribed, as well for its sedative influence, as to correct the dyspeptic symptoms bordering on gout which were present: he took also the following purgative.

R Inf. Gentianæ comp. f3vi.; Infusi Sennæ comp. f3ss.; Sp. Ammoniæ Aromat. Tinct. Hyoscyami, aa. f3i.; Magnesiæ Sulphatis, 3iij.

That which makes a strong impression on the mind sometimes serves as the nucleus of the future delusion. A gentleman who was subsequently placed under my care, and who had suffered from a coup de soleil but a short time previously, on the first evening of his arrival at Constantinople, as he walked on the terrace of a house opposite the Seraglio, mistook the rays of the moon, which played upon the waters of the Bosphorus, for a direct intimation from heaven that he was the Saviour of the world.

I need not multiply these cases; you will easily be able to supply for yourselves examples of the same kind. I pass on to false notions furnished to the mind by sensibility generally.

A young lady to whom I prescribed the potassio-tartrate of antimony to relieve the furor which accompanied her disease, had some remarkable delusions brought on by the effect of the medicine. She fancied she was on board-ship; she sang sea songs, and rolled her body about as if she were walking the deck in a heavy gale; sometimes she would imagine that she was wrecked, and when the sofa cushions were on the floor, would snatch them up, thinking she was saving her fellow-passengers from drowning.

The remedy, though it certainly caused these delusions, and made her friends anxious lest the disease might thereby be increased, yet by being steadily persevered in subdued the bodily symptoms, and was, humanly speaking, the means of her restoration to health.

Mrs. J. was a patient of mine in 1841: when æt. 18 she had an attack of erysipelas of the head with delirium. The catamenia appeared when she was 12 years old. She suffered much during the early part of her life from menorrhagia and dysmenorrhœa. She had had two attacks of puerperal mania; When I saw her she complained of "bearing down," with pain and discharge of matter from the uterus: this gave rise to the illusion that she was in the habit of committing unnatural crimes; and she imagined she brought forth monsters. She had been treated for ovarian dropsy. I found the ab-

domen resonant on percussion, when she was in a recumbent posture: it was much distended with flatus, hard, and somewhat painful on pressure: in fact she was suffering from dysentery, not from ovarian dropsy, and when I examined the evacuations I found scybala and hardened fæces, which she had mistaken for leeches and a litter of puppies. I took the precaution to measure the size of the swollen abdomen, and as the disease yielded to the remedies commonly employed in cases of dysentery, and the swelling was proved by the tape gradually to diminish, she at first began to doubt the reality of her strange fancies, and afterwards completely mastered them.

I shall make no apology for giving you so many examples of altered perceptions, because it is a matter of the utmost importance in practice: if you set them down as the mere effects of imagination, and do not stop to inquire whence they arise, and what is the probable cause of their existence, you will undoubtedly treat the disease very badly; and your attention may at last be called to the symptom when medicine is of no avail. Patients either with or without the sensation of pain about the præcordia imagine that they are possessed with devils, or have live animals in their stomach: I recommend you never to overlook such symptoms. Some madmen eat their food voraciously, and without even attempting to masticate it. A patient in St. Luke's, who was in the habit of doing this, had had a severe fall on the back of his neck: his friends said he never knew when he had had enough to eat: it is not impossible that the eighth pair of nerves might have been injured by the fall. There are those who eat their own flesh, and other matter which I need not mention here: this is always a very bad symptom. There are others who refuse food, and it has been too often the habit to order them to be fed with the stomach-pump, without taking into consideration the state of the bodily symptoms. I am confident that the majority of patients who refuse to eat do so because there is irritation of the stomach and primæ viæ: if you order an emetic or a purgative you will generally find this symptom disappear. Esquirol never saw any dangerous consequences ensue in mania from obstinate refusal of food: in monomania, however, the case is otherwise: patients who have tried every other means in vain to destroy themselves, will sometimes endeavour to starve themselves to death, and all our art is called into requisition to avoid such a catastrophe.

The capability of the insane to bear the extremities of heat and cold, and go without sleep, has, I think, been overstated. It is very true that some patients expose themselves to the rays of the sun, and go almost naked in the coldest weather, with impunity, and this is certainly due in some instances to the explanation given by Dr. Watson, viz : " that in abstraction of mind impressions which are unheeded are unfelt and inoperative :" but this in insanity is not only the result of a mental operation ; it is due also to the benumbing effect of the disease upon sensibility generally.

These patients are exactly in an opposite condition to those labouring under maniacal furor, when the least stimulus of light upon the optic nerve, the smallest sound, or the faintest smell, produce or prolong their paroxysm ; but if you think that it is of no practical importance to protect your patients against the severities of frost, or the rays of the summer's sun, you will presently find them suffering, on the one hand, from mortification of the feet, and on the other, from repeated exacerbations of furor, which too probably will end in dementia : and if you do not take proper precaution that your patient be soothed by refreshing sleep, the exhaustion subsequent to his long watchfulness will be a great hindrance to his recovery.

Alterations of motion.—The motive power of the nerves is either increased or diminished in intensity. It is increased sometimes in a surprising degree during the paroxysm of furor, and in that rare disease catalepsy ; cases of which seldom occur without disorder of intellect. To this head should be referred the inclination and power which some patients possess of taking an immoderate quantity of exercise without fatigue : it must be borne in mind, however, that this is by no means common, and that the physical power of the insane should never be overstrained. I have seen some rare cases where the patient would turn neither to the right hand nor to the left, but was impelled by an irresistible impulse to run straight on till he could go no farther, prevented either by exhaustion, or some obstacle which obstructed his course. One of these cases was a young lady, now under my care, whose insanity was manifested, in the first instance, by her getting out of bed in her night-dress, and going in a direct line over hedges, or any thing which came in her way, till she was at length with difficulty extricated from a pond. A female patient, when first admitted into St. Luke's, would get off her chair, and walk round two or three times in a circle, the left side being always turned towards the centre. These cases are interesting, when we reflect that similar results followed the removal of the corpora striata, and lesion to the medulla oblongata, in M. Majendie's experiments. M. Foville has given an account of an interesting case of a woman attacked with intermittent insanity, who, during the paroxysm, was affected with a remarkable action of the left arm.

The fore-arm, half flexed, was struck constantly against the body, while the hand remained pendant. She was seized some time afterwards with cerebral hæmorrhage, when the left arm, formerly convulsed, now became paralytic. I have a case under my care at the present time analogous to it. The patient is a gentleman who, about two years ago, received a violent blow on the side of his head while hunting, and became insane soon after. When the paroxysm comes on, he rubs the left hand violently against the right, or upon the left leg, and shudders, while the paroxysm lasts, as if struck with an electric shock. These attacks have come on more frequently lately ; in the beginning of last year they succeeded each other once a month ; they now show themselves about once in every ten days.

Whenever the motor nerves are involved in insanity it is always a bad sign. M. Esquirol has, indeed, said that the complication of insanity with lesions of motion resists all means of cure, and he holds out no hope of long life to the patient. This talented physician has also said that epilepsy complicated with mental alienation is never cured. With all deference to these opinions, still I must say that I have found that it makes an essential difference if the lesion of motion has preceded, not followed, insanity. I have seen insane patients completely recover who have been epileptic, provided the fits came on first, the madness afterwards. I attended a gentleman in 1840, who had suffered from paraplegia, which came on some time prior to the attack of insanity : this case was condemned as hopeless because of the lesion of motion, and because he had many of the wild fancies, and high ideas, which often accompany general paralysis ; yet this gentleman perfectly recovered from his insanity. This and other parallel cases have led me to think this an important distinction to draw.

Ptosis of the eyelid, and strabismus, are bad symptoms, more especially if either is permanent. Asynchronous action of the pupil, dilatation of one iris, and contraction of the other, are also bad signs ; but if the sphincters be involved the patient is not likely to recover, and if the muscles of deglutition participate in the mischief, the case is hopeless. We see from this the importance of attending to the functions of the afferent and efferent nerves in making our prognosis.

Subsequent experience has verified the opinion of Esquirol of the incurability of general paralysis ; as a proof of the justness of this opinion, patients affected with it are not admissible into either Bethlem or St. Luke's, which are hospitals for the admission of those patients only who are deemed curable. You will, perhaps, in one case in a thousand, find an exception to this rule, and you will meet with, here and there, a patient who may recover, and remain well for a short time, and then relapse. I by no means think that medicine is of no avail in these cases; I believe that some of the symptoms may be materially relieved by it. If you master this subject of general paralysis, you will gain great credit for acuteness of diagnosis. The ear once accustomed to the speech of those suffering under this form of madness is rarely deceived. The first sentence the patient utters will enable you to detect the disease. The sense of hearing is a valuable addition to our diagnosis in diseases of the lungs and heart; it is no less so in general paralysis: there is a thickness, a hesitation in speaking, which sometimes amounts to stammering; it is somewhat like what is termed "clipping the King's English," in drunkenness. Patients have a difficulty in pronouncing the letter R; if you make them say the word February they will generally fail. I have observed frequently a tremor of the upper lip when no tremor of the muscles existed in other parts of the body. The general tremor, however, of every muscle is very marked when it is present. "Tremor occupat artus" was the forcible expression of a patient of mine first seized with general paralysis, and whose case was mistaken for delirium tremens: the peculiar stammering and hesitation of speech was so marked that I did not doubt for a moment that he was paralytic, and pronounced him incurable, although he was able to repeat long passages from Virgil. My prognosis, I recollect, was considered a rash one at the time, but the patient died within a month, having passed through all the stages of the complaint in its worst form. M. Foville says with truth that it is not the power so much as the precision of the voluntary motions which is lost. If a patient, for instance, attempts to write, he will scarcely be able to hold his pen; or if he walks, there is an irregular gait, he will frequently lean over to the left side, and drag one of his legs. One very characteristic distinction between this disease and common paralysis is, that you cannot produce reflex action, because the paralysis is incomplete. The nerves of sensation are deadened, and very sluggishly conduct their oscillations to the brain. M. Foville was the first to take notice of two distinct periods in this species of paralysis. In the first, the movements, although uncertain, have still some degree of vigour, rather, he says, a kind of rigidity, which gives place to a relaxation which goes on increasing more and more. The last stage of the complaint is accompanied by sloughing sores on the sacrum, incontinence of urine and faeces, death by coma, convulsions, or epilepsy.

The delusions which accompany general paralysis are very frequently those of very great magnificence. These patients will tell you that they have millions of money; that they intend to pay off the national debt; indeed every thing they touch appears turned to gold. They also often fancy themselves happier and stronger than they ever were before. It is accurately stated that these fancies are not always found; indeed, I visited a gentleman last September who had all the bodily symptoms of this disorder, but who laboured under no delusion whatever, and his natural affections were not perverted. These unhappy patients enjoy but a short period of their elysium of happiness; a change soon takes place, the faculties of the mind fail, the imagination has no longer strength to furnish matter for delusion, and a hopeless fatuity succeeds.

Inasmuch as half the insane labour under general paralysis, it is a subject which has naturally occupied much of the attention of recent writers on the subject of insanity.

M. Esquirol, who, in 1805, first directed the attention of the profession to this subject, says that it is often a symptom of chronic inflammation of the meninges. M. Calmeil, in his work on the Paralysis of the Insane, considers that it is an affection due to disease of the cortical substance. M. Foville believes it to depend upon alteration of the fibrous structure. I find his theory generally quoted as shewing that there are adhesions of the fibres to each other; whereas he says that these adhesions are between the planes, which are easily separated in a healthy brain, but cannot be in many of those of the insane; every effort you make to do so only tears them. It is between the plane of the corpus callosum and that of the hemisphere that this morbid adhesion shews itself most frequently. In the brains of those affected with general paralysis which he had examined during the three preceding years, he had observed twice only the absence of these adhesions between the planes, and in these two exceptions the cerebral nerves, the pons and medulla oblongata, were excessively hard. Speaking of the adhesion of the fibres, he says, "It is very difficult, not to say impossible, to separate them; it appears, if we may be allowed the conjecture, that each cerebral fibre has contracted a morbid adherence to its neighbouring fibre in such a manner as to render their separation impossible." This conjecture, so seductive to the physiologist, one cannot forbear wishing to be true. I believe, however, that it will not be found to be correct, or certainly not to hold good in all cases, for I have seen, under the microscope, the primitive fibres separating from each other, and curling themselves up like the main-spring of a watch; being, in fact, quite as disunited in general paralysis as in health. If the adhesion of the fibres were the cause of the paralysis, no hope would remain of alleviating the symptoms, much less of curing the patient, whereas I have seen some cases much benefitted by treatment, and there are one or two cases on record where a permanent cure has been made. Whatever be the cause of general paralysis, it must be such as to operate on the whole body, not on any particular part. The alteration in speech is most generally the first symptom, and this would lead us to inquire particularly into the appearances which the medulla oblongata presents. A very frequent cause of the complaint is venereal excess; and this would also direct our attention to the posterior region of the same part. I recollect a case which was at first mistaken for one of general paralysis because the speech was inarticulate, and the movements of the tongue were impaired. It was, however, found on inquiry, that this patient had, a day or two previously, attempted to hang himself: he was cut down, and with difficulty saved: doubtless the medulla oblongata was injured in this case, and the nerve of the tongue paralysed. My colleague, Mr. Luke, had a patient under his care who was admitted into the London Hospital on the 25th of Dec. 1838; he had lost his speech, and never recovered it up to the time of his death, which happened on Nov. 9th, 1839. The brain was examined, and was found healthy, but at the origin of the ninth nerve was found a cyst, which pressed upon it just before it emerged from the anterior condyloid foramen : these are examples of local injury without general paralysis, and they must be carefully distinguished from it. But other examples might be adduced where the brain is first affected, and the medulla secondarily. For instance, the effects produced by alcohol and cold, which, although evanescent, are no less instructive as pointing to the part where the disease may take its rise. Professor Bouillaud has published some cases which have led him to conclude that the faculty of speech is under the guidance of the anterior lobes of each hemisphere. M. Andral says, " What our researches on this subject have led us to conclude is as follows : out of 37 cases observed by ourselves, or by others, relative to hæmorrhages, or other lesions, in which the morbid change resided in one of the anterior lobes, or in both, speech was abolished 21 times, and retained 16 times. On the other hand, we have collected 14 cases where the speech was abolished without any alteration in the anterior lobes. Of these 14 cases, 7 were connected with diseases of the middle lobes, and 7 with diseases of the posterior lobes." (Andral, Clin.) Although, therefore, we cannot conclude that the anterior lobes preside over the faculty of

speech, and although the present state of science does not allow us to point out any special part of the brain which directs it, yet from cases of apoplexy where loss of speech is the only symptom present, we should be led to expect that there are fibres expressly appropriated to its function. From the above facts it appears that embarrassment of speech may arise from local disease affecting the medulla oblongata, and from lesion of the substance of the brain.

Morbid alterations of the same parts are found in general paralysis, but they differ from the appearances found after death in paralysis from apoplexy, in that there is no disintegration of the fibres. We often find, for instance, the medulla oblongata much injected ; effusion of fluid in the subarachnoid cellular tissue and in the ventricles; the pia mater thickened ; the substance of the brain infiltrated, sometimes soft, sometimes tough and elastic, with the fibres well marked, as if the brain had been for some time steeped in alcohol. I do not think that it has been satisfactorily proved that the disease always commences in the brain and spreads itself to the spinal marrow ; I believe that it sometimes commences in the medulla oblongata and radiates to the hemispheres. A patient of my colleague, Dr. Philp, was admitted into the hospital Oct. 28th, 1842. He received a blow on the nape of the neck at the last Bath election, and became insane soon afterwards. His habits were completely changed ; he became a drunkard, having previously been a person of temperate habits. Soon afterwards his speech became thick and hesitating, and he was unconscious of the calls of nature. At 1 o'clock, P.M. Dec. 20th, he was seized with apoplexy, followed by convulsions, which occurred every ten minutes, and died at 9 P M.

In speaking of the post-mortem appearances I shall confine myself to those of the fibrous structure and medulla oblongata. The medullary structure was firm, its fibres well seen. Its cut surface presented many bleeding points. The posterior lobes of the hemispheres of the cerebrum were greatly injected ; an effusion of blood had taken place into the arachnoid from each posterior lobe ; the blood was fluid, and rested on the tentorium ; it had probably been exhaled through the membrane, and would have been converted into a false membrane had the patient lived. No ruptured vessel was discovered. The ventricles of the brain were very large, each containing an ounce of fluid. The medulla oblongata was much injected, and was small, having a pinched appearance, caused by the sliding forwards of the atlas upon the dentata. As this was exactly the place where the man received the blow, it was probably the effect of it ; and it is not impossible that the depraved desire for drink might have been caused, in the first instance, by the irritation of the pneumo-gastric nerve: however, be this as it may, the disease appears to have originated in the medulla in consequence of the blow. Again, I think that it is highly probable that the medulla oblongata may be first attacked in cases of general paralysis caused by venereal excess. Upon opening the spinal canal of a paralytic patient who died of secondary syphilis, I found the veins so loaded as completely to prevent my seeing the cord. The effect of this congestion is, we know, pressure, and its result is effusion, which will also be a cause of embarrassment to the fibres in this region.

The morbid appearances found in the brain are, however, more frequent than those in the medulla, in cases of this description, and are such as to justify us in appealing to other causes than the adhesion of the fibres, for the production of the disease. Speaking of general paralysis, M. Andral says that "he doubts not that sanguineous congestions contribute, oftener than is supposed, to produce those lesions of motion and sensation, congestions the traces of which disappear sometimes at the moment of death, but whose existence is here so much the more probable, as the entire nervous centre is the seat of greater excitation, and of a more considerable afflux of the fluids." (Clin. Med.)

Nor do I think that the effusion into the ventricles, found often in so great a quantity, is to be disregarded as a cause of the uncertain movements of these patients, since it makes its way by the calamus scriptorius to the spinal canal; and any increase to the fluid there present is, according to Majendie, attended with evil results.

Lastly, the infiltration of the medullary structure is due probably to atrophy of the fibres, just as we see atrophy of the cortical structure followed by effusion. The fibres have, indeed, retained their power of conveying the notices from the sensorium, but their excitability is more or less exhausted, and their vigour gone.

Upon the whole, I believe that there are many structural lesions, and not one only, which exist as causes of general paralysis; such lesions either directly affecting the medulla oblongata, or indirectly affecting it through the brain.

RUDIMENTARY CONSIDERATIONS
ON THE
NATURE OF IRRITATION.

By T. WILKINSON KING.

(For the London Medical Gazette.)

Definition ; rubbing; morbid, flea-bite, local achne ; secretory, catarrh ; nutrient; absorbent; nervous, pain, scald, extravasation : sympathetic pains ; worms; states of the tongue, nares, skin, and anus ; teething, epulis ; cough ; epigastric blow; shock ; cerebral irritation ; vomit ; excito-motory ; spinal, hysteric, renal, &c.

CONSIDERING the expressions of writers, and the import of many facts, irritation may, we think, be safely and advantageously defined thus :—A cause of functional disturbance, or a disturbed process, in the animal economy. So far, we shall probably find satisfactory grounds, or at least here seems a clear starting point. We shall not seek to conform to the current attempts to explain irritation, but rather endeavour to pursue a more even and less uncertain course than some distinguished writers have done.

Sir A. Cooper expressed his views thus :—" Numerous examples of sympathetic actions may be adduced ; the communication which exists between the uterus and breast is a striking instance of it." To us, the secretion of milk on the contraction of the uterus seems very little more than a physical, or rather humoral, consequence ; and all the other correlations of the generative organs, in either sex and in animals, may at least partake of humoral agencies.

Sir A. Cooper next recites examples of natural excito-motory *sympathies.* " But," he continues, " sympathetic action is also the result of injury and disease, becoming the cause of restoration, on the one hand, or of destruction on the other ; and this state of the body I call *irritation.* Irritation, gentlemen, may be defined to be an altered action excited in the system by an unnatural impression : *e.g.* the passage of an urinary calculus through the ureter occasions retraction of the testicle and pain in the thigh." It may happen that the obstructed and distended ureter acts directly on the track of the motor and sensitive nerves which are here concerned. Pain in the loins from disease of the testis seems rather like some bowel-pains referred to the wrong part through inexperience; as the toes seem pained after amputation, and there are various deep sensations that we never learn to localise accurately.

Testitis from gonorrhœa is of doubtful explanation. Continuous inflammation, or mechanical obstruction, are but common consequences. (See Sir A. Cooper's Lectures, page 10.)

We shall find that there is a great variety of irritations—simple, complex, or general; and these all may be modified by the constitution or condition of the individual subjected to any particular cause of disturbance.

Our method of reviewing these varieties will be to bring them forward in the order in which they seem to illustrate each other, rather than that of a rigorous classification, which our present knowledge will ill admit of, and which the study does not require : our plan, however, may finally facilitate a more complete and satisfactory arrangement; for we shall still endeavour to establish the basis of a natural arrangement of the phenomena of irritation.

When the back of the hand is moderately pressed or rubbed, or exposed to heat or cold, or affected by rubefacients, the result is an increase of capillary injection with reparative nutrition; and such an experiment is the basis of one definition of local simple irritation; by which we may infer here an unexplained deterioration of tissue, which is necessarily transitory in a sound body; for the consequent increased afflux of blood speedily restores the health and strength of the capillaries, and they resume their due proportions. The consequences of irritation are widely different under circumstances of disordered health, as we shall hereafter find. The above facts refer to capillary irritation in particular; and we may suppose the case to be devoid of pain, or one where no nerves are discoverable, as in the cerebrum. According to the preceding view, the simple adhesion of an incised wound, the suppuration of the same, the cicatrizing of an ulcer, sloughing, the ulcerative detachment of a slough, and the exuberance of granulations, are

very little more than so many distinct grades of capillary irritation or disturbed process, which depend first, on the kind and degree of mischief inflicted; and secondly, on the state of the materials of repair, of which the blood is the chief.

Observing a flea-bite, the puncture of a needle, or particularly the gentle wound for vaccination, a blush of redness is found to surround the injured point to a considerable extent; making its appearance soon, and gradually and shortly subsiding. This we regard as more resembling a sympathetic action than many instances commonly adduced as such. The sting of an insect produces more disorder, and the poison of the viper still more. We do not know that the more or less extensive horripilation on the application of cold to the hand is not attended with some such sympathetic capillary contraction. It is most experienced by the feebly nourished, the delicate and sensitive.

We have thought that the sudden call to micturition in such a case may be owing to the inward determination of blood causing abdominal tension. Local cold also acts on the blood and its functions universally, and we would not here exclude the idea of nervous influence.

Some regard irritation as always morbid; and this view of the subject, or rather mode of defining the term, is natural enough for those exclusively engaged in the treatment of diseases; but their position is a false one unless a physiological process of simple irritation and reparation be admitted as a basis principle.

Simple irritation, as by great heat, may be widely diffused, but it is not universal, nor even general; indeed, the idea of general or constitutional irritation is extremely complicated, and we do not propose to ourselves to do much more than explore the subject, and to show how far facts support the opinions we hold; how far we conceive the irritation to be falsely interpreted, and how we may anticipate a safer and more hopeful train of study.

Local irritation may be set up in any part of the living body. The capillaries, the nerves, the blood itself, and in short every vital organ or tissue. It is true this may be a novel mode of unfolding the matter, but we trust that a little patient attention will justify the course we take. It is to be regretted that our progress is surrounded by error as well as difficulty.

We may find a good illustration of local irritation in the circumstances of an inflamed cutaneous follicle. Inspissated secretion obstructs the orifice, or the decline of secretion allows the opening to contract, and the sudden increase of secretion from general causes produces or constitutes the irritation. A little effort re-opens the orifice, or a pustule is formed.

We shall perceive many varieties in the course and consequences of this one simple irritation (obstruction), all of which may assist to explain the state of the constitution in particular cases. Very slowly increasing distension gives rise to a large sebaceous cyst, but when inflammation is suddenly set up around, we cannot avoid the conclusion that the action is determined by the general state of the system, both as to its origin, kind, and course.

Ten or twenty pustules of achné may commence at once in consequence of exhaustion, excess, or exposure, and with a purgative, or a warm day, they may all, or nearly all, subside in twenty-four hours. Sometimes the suppurative action is rapid and confined, and the repair as speedy, or, in a similar case, we may conceive that an acute process increases the contents of the cells and their fluidity, and they are ejected without suppuration. With the renewal of the excretory aperture the inflammation disappears. This seems happier, but scarcely so natural as the mere resolutive change we have before adverted too. Occasionally the inflammation is much more chronic, often variable, and finally either suppurative or resolutive. It may be limited or diffused, attended with different degrees of hardness and tumefaction ; sometimes with sloughing or excessive suppuration, especially in the so-called strumous. The tendency to heal, to ulcerate, or form unhealthy crusts, are so many additional and distinct indications of the particular diathesis.

Let us now regard the capillaries under other circumstances of irritation or disturbance.

Secretory irritation.—All the secretory glands of the body may be supposed to act with gentleness or force according as the blood abounds little or much with the peculiar matters which they are destined to eliminate. Diuretic medicines or urinary salts may irritate the kidney ; the matters are excreted, and the organ returns to its original state of quiescence ; but habitual potations of gin, or the suppression of other excretions, as that of the skin, causes such a degree of renal irritation, that the organ, after becoming hypertrophic, becomes actually diseased.

We may assume that similar processes of irritation occasionally affect all the secretory apparatuses of the body. Thus cold and catarrh (of any mucous surface whatsoever) are in a manner justly synonymous. Probably the direct application of keen air is a cause of irritative deterioration of the conjunctiva or larynx.

In the general effects of cold to the surface of the body, we see a double cause of what is called reaction, namely, the weakness of the superficial capillaries, whose circulation has been impeded, and the stimulus of matters accumulated in the system by the suppressed secretion. And this is not all ; for it is one manifest effect of external cold to retard all functions (chemical, vegetable, or animal), and subsequently, warmth both facilitates and stimulates reaction.

Chronic catarrhs (variable or recurrent) involve hypertrophy of the secreting glands, just as the skin becomes thickened by attritions ; and in this way deafness, asthma, and prostatic stricture, may have the same cause and the same course, and may demand the same method of treatment, as constituting forms of local secernent irritation.

Nutritive irritation.—Non-secreting organs become the seat of irritation in a different way. The muscle of the arm, the heart, or the bladder, thickens by increased exertion, unless its nutrition fails ; the hand by toil ; the lung or brain, by free use, probably endures an irritation which may become excessive, and which, with deteriorated nutrition, involves absolute disease.

We have seen that hypernutrition of a gland may attend or result from secernent irritation ; yet there is still another distinct mode or kind of nutritive irritation. The growth of the parts of the body seems to be attended with a state of feebleness, or at least of great vascularity, softness, and susceptibility to disturbance and active changes; and it is likewise accompanied with a superabundance in the blood of the various nutritive materials. In another place we have dilated on the particulars of different kinds of ossific irritation;—excited nutrition, and bone deposited on bone, according to the prevalence of bone in the blood; and various irritations attended with absorption of bone, as by pressure; or defective deposition of bone from the paucity of the earth in the system. See the article Fracture, in the Cyclopædia of Surgery.)

If it be true that parts are deteriorated in proportion to the degree in which they are used or exerted, and repaired in the same ratio, that is, so long as the blood is freely formed, we may make some further inferences relating to the uses of exercise, by which blood is consumed or altered, and materials for excretion—the stimuli of the excretories—are also made abundant. Even the fluids which aid digestion seem to be more amply produced under these circumstances; and it seems that equalization and freedom of all the functions (with good nutrition) may thus lead to the exaltation of all;—assimilation, circulation, perfective or maturative assimilation, nutrition, and secretion. (See First General Laws or Fundamental Doctrines of Medicine and Surgery, by T. W. King. London, 1840.)

Nutritive irritation does not depend alone on excitement of the organ which grows or becomes hypertrophic. We must conclude that, in many cases, the mere abundance of nutritive matter in the blood is the cause of nutritive deposition; that is, of a kind of nutritive irritation.

As we know that, in the absence of sufficient nutrition, local irritation cannot cause hypertrophy, so we may understand how, nutrition abounding, secernent irritation may be attended with even great glandular hypertrophy of one kind or another.

The combination of local irritation and atrophy takes its explanation from or after these cases.

Irritation inducing absorption. — While a certain degree of local pressure or friction leads to increased nutrition, a greater amount of pressure causes absorption, as if by compressing the capillaries and arresting nutrition. *And this process, whatever its nature may be, and whatever name we give it, will often be mixed up with, though* distinct from, nutritive irritation. A tumor may cause absorption on a spot of bone, and ossification around it.

The relation between absorption from capillary compression and that from general depletion does not seem to be very uncertain.

In what has been advanced, we may see ample grounds to distinguish between several modifications of one local irritation—as a puncture. First, that connected with simple, or excessive, or deficient reparation. Secondly, that which belongs to more morbid reparative acts, according as the body may have been previously, or may become subsequently deranged; and, thirdly, that which appertains specifically to the injury inflicted as in cases of great laceration or specific poisons.

The doctrines of *nervous irritations* hitherto have been rendered unnecessarily obscure, by mingling with them a variety of false or doubtful illustrations. The most common and positive case of nervous irritation is pain in, or referred directly to, a disordered part. And what are the effects of this on the constitution? How do ordinary measures of pain affect the healthy body? We had almost said not at all! But, on the other hand, a crushed finger to a feeble person in cold weather may be followed by severe rigor, fainting, and vomiting, and the injury to a limb, without loss of blood, may perhaps be followed by a fatal collapse. We are willing that such should stand recorded as one of nervous (sentient) irritation alone, but in every such case the strength of the body, the sudden effect on the respiration, heart, capillary, and muscular systems, must be traced out; and when, after the collapse, reaction comes to be studied, even the length of time that the patient has been exposed motionless to the cold, and every collateral circumstance, must be taken into the account. The effect of an extensive scald may be compared to the preceding case, and also that of the diffusion of fæces in the peritoneum. The last two cases we deem analogous to each other, except that in the first the chief morbid agent is soon removed, while in the latter it is more persistent. In both of these cases, however, it is essential to distinguish between the local capillary irritation tending to repair, and the nervous irritation which is, as it were, one step of another process, namely, that by which the body generally may become affected. It is evident, also, that other influences tend to complicate the process. The exposure of the scalded surface, a process of depletion, and perhaps the absorption of prejudicial matters, require to be carefully appreciated.

Pain is said to be sympathetic, when, instead of being referred to the diseased organ, it seems to be seated elsewhere. Disease in the course of a sentient nerve seems to give pain where the radicles of the nerve are spread out; and this may be the explanation of many of the examples of sympathy, which are much more talked of than understood. Pain in the knee, from disease about the hip; the glans penis, from bladder disease; the inside of the thigh, from prostatic inflammation; and others may come to be thus accounted for. We have just dissected an example of sciatica dependent on medullary tumors along the right side of the loins and sacrum. We have known pains in the arm from phthisical abscess in the apex of the pleura. (See some account of pains in anginal attacks, &c. in papers on angina pectoris, by T. Wilkinson King, MED. GAZ. 1841, and of those of toothache, in the same journal, January 1842.)

Pains down the back of the leg, with disorders of the rectum, and along the inner part of the thigh with uterine diseases, seem to depend on local affections of the trunks of nerves; cramp also. There is evident reason to distinguish the various forms of pain in the head, side, back, stomach, and belly, but it is not easy to do so satisfactorily. We know almost nothing of sensibility within the pleura costalis, or in the substance of the brain, liver, spleen, and kidney. There appears to be something of definite distension in the side pains when we run after eating, and perhaps in the pains of stitch, cramp, and colic. On the whole, however, the more we know of pains, the less we know of their dangerous sympathetic effects. Pain over the shoulder has not yet been shown to depend on the liver or the stomach. Such a case as bowel irritation tickling the nose has no foundation, but such as we shall presently explain. A partial sign, and a regular sympathy, are very different things. The constitutional irritation *of worms in the bowels is at present mere hypothesis.* The delicate frame

may be infected, but myriads of the robust of all classes throughout the world are not less so, and without any sympathetic disturbance. Among the children of Jamaica, vegetable food, large bellies, multitudes of worms, and good health, did not appear to us in the slightest degree incompatible; and the same seems to hold on the continent of Europe. Our friend, Dr. Arbuckle, a very competent observer, assures us that one or two hundred lumbrici, of three or four inches in length, are sometimes voided at once, in Maranham, South America. He found tonics benefit the health of those who were put under his care under such circumstances, but that worms were too universally present for him to attribute any material or specific mischief to them. He regarded their increase as a consequence of declining health and vigour. He knows of no pathognomonic signs of worms beside the actual observation of them. It happened, though very rarely, that they were evacuated by an abscess. The people were not well supplied. Rice, vegetables, and salt fish, or salt meat, are their usual food.

It ought, we think, to appear a very difficult question with certain pathologists and doctors, that the irritation of worms may do so much harm, and harm only; while that of medicine, which is so much more evident, should be productive of so much exclusive benefit.

The *recherche* of M. Louis on Tenia presents a very good account of the symptoms of declining health, which alone are the cause of bringing the worm patient to the physician. Beyond this, his cases, we suppose, only constitute one more instance of misapplied statistics—of unequal facts, with feeble and erroneous views.

States of the tongue.—We cannot but regard the theoretical deductions commonly made from the appearance of the tongue, with reference to the rest of the system, as particularly fallacious. A natural tongue, doubtless, indicates healthy secretion; a furred tongue simply indicates undue secretion, and may very naturally accompany the increasing nutrition of the whole body. If it belongs to any kind of irritation (besides excessive secernent), it is to that of local and general hyper-nutrition. The clear and glazed tongue, said to be indicative of bowel irritation, although often no disturbance of the bowels exist, indicates only disturbed and declining secretion, with failing nutrition. The whole mouth shares the like alteration; tenderness and ulceration follow. Perhaps the larynx is similarly affected, and of course its sensitiveness betrays a different kind of irritability. Variable catarrh may be superadded. The bowels may be affected together with, or instead of, the air tube: but the glazed tongue may be attended with seemingly good digestion, as in a case of psoas abscess, or open (compound) fracture.

These remarks may tend to show that, while general deductions may be admissible with care, the true meaning of the states of the tongue is limited, and that they have no specific sympathetic connexion with those of the stomach or intestines, and their only just import (in reasoning), depends on a precise local estimation which subsequently assists to explain the general state of the body. A dry tongue almost explains itself. A simply furred tongue, then, implies a degree of secernent irritation, just as the increasing plumpness of the individual signifies a nutritive irritation. It is the decline of the secretory and nutritive actions that belongs to a red polished tongue, and if there be any peculiar irritation in the case locally, it is one of sense—imperfect nutrition and tenderness, approaching to ulceration. We shall hereafter see that the general or constitutional indications correspond to that which we deduce locally.

Itching of the nares belongs to a similar state of body to that which the morbidly clean tongue evinces; that is, a condition of deficient nutrition and secretion, with augmented or disturbed sensibility. Here varying dryness, and irritability through a sensitive nerve are mere local effects which indicate the diathesis; and just so far only as they partake of the circumstances of the entire body, they present an example of sympathy; just as the banks of a river dry and crack when its source-fountains are low: the mud sympathises with the want of clouds and rain.

The same kind of explanation seems a sufficient account of certain affections of the skin, anus, &c. The local irritation of anal worms is regulated in part by the vigour of the individual. A catarrh of the outlet, to which the feeble are liable, enables the creatures to be much more troublesome. A wasting and sensitive body is so much the more disturbed by them. Such a case of nervous irritation does, I believe, cause grinding of the teeth, by a reflex function, just as it may produce restlessness, starting, or a cry in sleep. Simple cutaneous irritation belongs to increased sensibility, to wasting, to the habit of scratching, and to the want of sound rest and full occupation.

More complicated forms of irritation of the skin may, at least in part, admit of explanation, by reference to humoral changes in the blood, as those of the spring of the year, or occurring at certain periods after exposure.

The irritation of teething must be investigated in the same cautious manner we have prescribed for other cases. Toothache is not generally supposed to excite any sympathies. Disorder of the dens sapientiæ often seems to induce a kind of earache. Active inflammation, from a cold, affecting the root of a tooth, subsides or gives rise to abscess, which will increase till its contents escape, and then it subsides. This may recur repeatedly; or a sequestrum and cloaca form, with a mass of exuberant granulation at the external opening, which mass, like that at the orifice of any granulating sinus, varies with the states of the body. With moisture and attrition the tumor may attain a larger size in the mouth than elsewhere, though never much larger than a marble. A similar tumor forms externally, in connection with salivary fistula; and, of course, with necrosis of the jaw, a fistula in the cheek with such a fungus would most probably be cured by extracting a tooth, so as to form a free opening for matter internally.

It is said that a superficial ulcer of the lip or face may be kept up by a diseased tooth irritating a nerve; and herpes of the face by teething. This requires very strong proof. The tooth may be removed, and the ulcer heal; but the one is not yet proved to be the cause of the other. Solitary and rare facts do well enough to support an imagination, but realities ought to have some more ostensible corroboration.

A state of the teeth, or rather of their connections, usually called irritable, that is, morbidly sensitive, and ready to inflame and ache, is indicative of failing nutrition, and that is premonitory of toothache, as of various general disorders which taking cold may quickly induce. The inflammation will require its specific treatment; but the cure depends on augmenting the free nutrition, and obviating the causes of inflammation both locally and generally.

Cough depends on laryngeal sensitiveness, and it may be caused by excessive secretion, with or without declining nutrition of the mucous surface, or increasing sensibility of the part. Cough from sympathy with the lungs or stomach must remain to be first proved to exist, and then we may endeavour to explain it. " Stomach-cough" implies, as we suppose, a fair digestion temporarily aggravating a bronchial catarrh. When the body begins to waste, where should we so soon look for hæmorrhage (after the gums) as to the larynx, which is so delicate and vascular, devoid of cuticle, and incessantly exposed and in motion ?

The most distinct examples of reflex function (excito-motory or other) constitute an established class of nervous irritations. It is necessary, however, to remember, that some supposed instances may be altogether erroneous assumptions on the part of those who are too exclusively wedded to a single principle.

A blow on the epigaster, causing collapse or death, is a much-vaunted instance of nervous irritation, but whether justly or not we cannot decide. We have elsewhere* suggested a different explanation. We are not sure, however, that the case is so well established as to deserve even a place among unexplained and rare phenomena. It is much more certain that men fall dead without any blow; as in cases where the openings of the coronary arteries become contracted after inflammation. Our friend, Dr. Joseph Ridge, possesses some histories of this kind, with one related by us. Those violent shocks which involve the cerebral, respiratory, and circulatory functions indiscriminately and almost universally, are not, we think, to be explained by a single word, unless by such a general term as disorganization.

Cerebral irritations, if attentively considered, seem still to require a good

* In the article on Angina, already cited.

deal of analysis. Perhaps, in strictness, we ought to consider separately all excito-motory phenomena, whether of health or disease; but these and such cases as the indirect dependence of the heart upon the brain, cannot yet be easily isolated in the study of medicine. Fear paralyses the voluntary muscles, and the blood sinks in all the veins, and fails in the cheek and head. A returning and increased current in the heart flushes the face, and even induces palpitation. These are complicated results of cerebral disturbance or irritation, but they admit of explanation in different degrees without much difficulty, and with great advantage.

Vomiting from injury of the head, or from obtuse pain or fainting, is an instance of irritation which may be called cerebral. The motions of swinging in the air, rotating the body quickly, or rocking at sea, seem analogous instances. Fear, collapse, disgust, and poisons, as antimony, whether put into the stomach or into the veins, all seem to act in a manner through the brain, in addition to excito-motor agency. Females seem more subject to sea-sickness than males, the young and aged more than the middle-aged, and invalids more than the robust. Cats, dogs, fowls, pigs, horses, and cattle, suffer, the young more than the old. We deem the affection to consist in a primary affection of the brain. Giddiness is often experienced early. Of course the only remedy for the disorder must be either to remove the cause or inure the sufferer to its effects. Perfect rest, reclining, with the head on its side, or the face upwards, decidedly assists to prevent the distress, and even to remove the feeling when it has commenced. A certain degree of repletion, and even a stimulating diet, help to maintain the powers of resistance, and obviate the tendency to debility which militates against recovery. The last attacks on a voyage may be expected before breakfast, and if the sufferer have to wait unusually for his dinner, he may find by experience, as we have done, that it may be difficult to hurry from the table to his bed in order to keep down the much-required meal; yet after an hour or two, with advancing digestion and vascular repletion, he may walk about with impunity. The wine-drinker has not to wait so long for the assimilation of his less enduring support.

We venture to class all pains under the term cerebral irritation, and also all excessive sensual and mental impressions.

The known excito-motory acts of the body may not on any account be employed to elucidate pain, or any disturbance which is not muscular, or dependent on muscle. They have nothing to do with mere sensation, and we ought to consider the philosophy which ascribes general convulsions to dental or intestinal irritation as at least very unsatisfactory — vague and undiscriminating, if not totally erroneous, since the only known cause of general convulsions is determinately in the nervous substance.

Spinal irritations may be well deserving of investigation; but we should blush to rank ourselves with some writers on this hypothetical ground. With organic lesions of the medulla and its sheaths we find here uniform signs, and there none, and so occasionally of the brain, but how different are the imaginary effects of what some call spinal irritation!

Hysteric irritation, and corresponding states in the other sex, are not simply nervous derangements; nutrient waste, and humoral deterioration and various visceral disturbances, are prominent features of the case, when the investigator is not engaged by prejudice.

Dr. Bright, in the 22d volume of the Medico-Chirurgical Transactions, has described some fatal cases of spasmodic disorder connected with pericarditis, and seems to think, with just caution however, that inflammatory or irritative action involving the phrenic nerve may have been the cause of the spasm. We have noticed such a case, in point of fact, but are far from admitting the explanation.

One prone to pericarditis is liable, though not equally it may be, to inflammation (in the same form) of any serous membrane, and when we find a more compound nerve, as the par vagum, divided by the pressure of an aneurism (as every now and then happens) without any spasm, we may not conclude, without good grounds, that slighter or even uncertain affections of a motor nerve can give rise to fatal chorea or catalepsy.

Much has been written concerning various indefinite sympathies between the kidneys and brain or spinal marrow, but we should first seek for a full explanation of all inflammations dependent on diseased kidneys; 2dly, for an account of the effects of nervous paralysis on all secretions; and, finally, the residual facts may perhaps be set down to the credit of the doctrine of nervous sympathies.

The occult part of pathology, like astrology of old, has had too great attractions for some, while simple facts and inductions require more patience than it is often agreeable to bestow on them. Paralysis of the abdominal muscles may surely have some influence on the secretory viscera; and defective digestion, secretion, and sanguineous depuration, are but a part of the intricate problem in such a case.

Constitutional irritation or general disturbance, in connexion with local or specific injury, although an extremely difficult subject, may yet admit of some analysis and elucidation upon the foregoing principles.

36, Bedford Square.

EMPHYSEMA OF THE INTERNAL ORGANS,

FOUND IN A CHILD AFTER HAVING LIVED TEN YEARS WITH GENERAL EMPHYSEMA.

By DUNCAN R. M'NAB, Esq.
Epping.

(For the London Medical Gazette.)

A BOY, æt. 10 years, labourer's child. His mother states that, at the age of four or five months, he had a severe illness, with great difficulty of breathing; that a blister was then applied to the chest; that from that time he has always been in a weak state of health, and his breathing short; that he became very puffy or full, so that, when she pressed her finger on his face, a pit would remain about two minutes; that at the age of 7 years he was brought home from school in a fainting fit, which lasted about five minutes; that from that time he used at intervals, first of four or five, latterly of one or two, months to have fainting fits, about ten in the course of two days; that after the fits he used to lose the puffiness (which she to took to be fat, but which a neighbour told her was wind-dropsy), and to become quite thin, but the fulness used gradually to come on again.

Feb. 23.—On account of the increasing frequency of the fits she brought him to me, just after the fits had left him. I did not then learn the above particulars. He took Hyd. c. Cr. gr. ij. ter die, about a fortnight, during which time he did not, as usual, become puffy, but rather thinner; the mother thought him better, and did not bring him any longer. She states that after the treatment was discontinued he gradually became again very full, till he was seized with the illness with which he died.

Nausea, pain in the head, pain in the bowels, and constipation, were at first the chief symptoms. He died in about ten days in a typhoid state, with delirium, coma, and bloody evacuations.

Post-mortem examination, 30 hours after death.

April 22. — Spleen dark coloured, large, crackling under pressure, and, on being cut into, giving out air-bubbles.

Stomach.—At the fundus two patches of air-bubbles, of the size of common shot, apparently between the mucous and serous coats: the muscles at the fundus red, and very distinct.

Gall-bladder.—Its coats very emphysematous; the contained bile very dark coloured.

Liver.—Pale; extending below the ribs and over into the left hypochondrium; on the right lobe were seen patches of minute air-bubbles, at first looked upon as a solid deposit; and on cutting into the substance of the right lobe the same were seen throughout; by pressure they might be squeezed out, and thus quite removed, or different patches might be united.

Kidneys.—The same may be said of the cortical substance as of the right lobe of the liver; there were also larger air-bubbles on the surface.

Pericardium.—A few large air-bubbles upon its outer surface.

Lungs.—Both pale and emphysematous throughout; the left with interlobular emphysema, and on its posterior surface extensive adhesions to the walls of the chest.

· The mesenteric glands generally were *much enlarged; suppuration* had taken *place* around two of them, near the ilio-cœcal valve; two inches below which, and about twelve inches above, the mucous membrane was of a dark red colour, with numerous white papillary eminences, and deep ulcerations around the larger glands. A lumbricus teres lay above the valves.

Epping, May 10, 1843.

OBSERVATIONS ON

SEMINAL AND OTHER DISCHARGES FROM THE URETHRA.

BY BENJAMIN PHILLIPS, F.R.S.

Surgeon to St. Marylebone Infirmary, and Lecturer
on Surgery at the Westminster Hospital
School of Medicine.

(For the Medical Gazette.)

IT is now many weeks since I forwarded to you two communications having reference to the subject of involuntary discharges of spermatic fluid. And as those communications have considerably enlarged my experience, and that in comparatively a very short time, so as to enable me to bring the cases more vividly to my mind than I could do on a former occasion, I have concluded that the results of my experience on the subject during the last three months might go far to shew the value of the remedy to which, on those occasions, I endeavoured to direct attention.

The number of cases which have come under my notice since that time amounts to 33; of these, 23 have been medical men—some in practice, others in *statu pupillaris.* In 24 instances it was admitted that masturbation had been practised; in some cases so frequently as twice or three times a day, but in all those cases it was stated that the habit had been abandoned. In two cases it was said that masturbation had never been practised: supposing that to be true, then the only way to account for the discharge was to assume that irritation was set up by a natural phymosis. We frequently see, even in young children, that when there is inability to uncover the glans, the secretion around the corona glandis does become acrid and troublesome. Whether in adults a similar irritation will *of itself* induce spermatic discharges, is to me very doubtful : I can readily understand that it may induce masturbation. In two cases the affec-

⸱ion was said to be the result of sexual excesses. In two cases the only apparent cause was stricture. In one case the cause seemed to be a frequent indulgence in reading lascivious books. In one instance the genital excitement resulted from study, or from the perusal of works of imagination.

Such have been the probable causes of the complaint. Its urgency was very variable; in some cases the discharge did not happen more than once in a week or ten days; in others daily; in others twice or even three times a day. The effects on the constitution were not less variable. In one case, where the discharge happened commonly three times a day, and where it had continued more or less for twelve years, the patient being at present 24, the buoyancy of his frame was very little disturbed; he could walk eight or ten miles without fatigue; whilst in other cases, where it happened once or twice a week, the physical and moral impression has been most profound. Much of this, no doubt, results from the hold the complaint obtains upon the apprehension of the patient.

In two cases the complaint coexisted with epilepsy; what direct relation the diseases bore to each other was not very evident. In two cases there was very considerable digestive disturbance; flatulence and irregularity of the bowels were much complained of. In most of them there was constipation; and unless that was carefully attended to the genital distress was increased. In five cases palpitation of the heart was complained of; in four, "swimming" sensations in the head, failing memory, inability to apply to any thing. I cannot help thinking that, in some cases, the alleged failure of memory is owing to the intense preoccupation of the mind with the complaint, and to the little impression which any other subject makes on it. Such have been the grand features in the cases to which I have referred.

With respect to treatment, the following are the results. Seven are at present under my care; five I think are doing well, two are not so satisfactory. Of the twenty-six cases which are off my hands, eighteen have been more or less completely relieved; in eight instances no sensible permanent *good was derived either from caustic or other remedies*, though there was

complete remission of the discharge for many days. In more than one of those cases I suspect the mischief has been kept up by some imprudent but concealed habit. In one case, I found the patient lay in bed till mid-day, or even later, and that the discharge generally came on once or twice between 9 and 12 o'clock. I have no doubt it was caused by conjuring up mischievous images. I requested him to get up at 9 o'clock, and the evil was, for the time, at once stayed.

With respect to the plan of treatment I employed, it depended on the circumstances of the case. In seven cases no acute pain was felt any where during the passage of the bougie; in one it occasioned a feeling as if a seminal emission was about to occur. In those seven cases I was content to try the effect of the bougie smeared with mercurial ointment, or merely oiled, and introduced twice a week; but although there was, in several cases, a considerable improvement, complete relief was obtained in only two instances. In nineteen instances I used the caustic. Of these cases ten were completely relieved by a single application; in three the amelioration was decided, though the complaint was not cured; in six there was no relief. In the nine cases in which the first application was insufficient, the remedy was again used—in three cases with complete success, in six without any evident amelioration; so that it succeeded in two-thirds of the cases in which it was applied, a result which, if confirmed by succeeding experience, would stamp it as a remedy of great value, though less certain than my previous impressions had led me to think.

On no single occasion have I known a patient to complain of the pain attendant upon the application of the caustic being severe; in many instances it did not seem to be greater than that of the inconvenience of introducing a bougie. In one single instance only did I experience any after trouble. A patient had caustic applied, without complaining of suffering; in four days afterwards he came to me with retention of urine. On the previous day he had walked far, and ate a good dinner, and it was after that he found a difficulty in passing urine. In many cases a little blood, usually a drop or two, has escaped on the next ccasion of making water after the application; but sometimes it has occurred two or three times. In no case have I known the discharge which should follow the use of the caustic extend beyond a week, and usually it is very trifling. I believe the remedy is much more effectual when it induces a pretty copious discharge.

My summary then is this: the caustic was applied in 19 cases: in 13 it succeeded, in 6 it failed; but in no case was there any aggravation of the symptoms; in no case was any complaint made of the amount of pain attendant upon the application; in only one case was any after inconvenience complained of. In several cases some drops of blood escaped with the urine; in some cases there was scarcely any appearance of discharge after it; in no case did the discharge extend beyond the seventh day.

It will be observed, then, that though the amount of good derived from the use of caustic is considerable, it is by no means a specific; but there is one class of cases in which the effect is remarkable; those in which very excited sensibility exists beyond the curvature, the disease seeming to depend upon the irritability seated in the vicinity of the opening of the ejaculatory ducts. In some cases this is so remarkable that the passage of a bougie over the part may actually induce emission. There are, however, many cases in which no such pain is discoverable, and in those cases I have not so much confidence in the efficacy of the caustic. In those cases the exciting cause of the emission is often habit. Masturbation or excesses having been long continued, the secretory action of the testicle is increased in proportion to the frequency of the calls made upon it; the vesicles are always full, the ducts are lax, and the fluid easily pressed forward. These cases improve under constant changing, occupation for the mind, and general tonic treatment. In one instance I have observed great good to result from the use of the tincture of cantharides carried to the extent of determining heat at the neck of the bladder, but in other cases I have known it fail.

I might allude to other plans of treatment, but as the present paper is merely a complement to the other, it might seem out of place.

CLOSURE OF THE VAGINA.

To the Editor of the Medical Gazette.

SIR,

ALTHOUGH I do not always approve of hasty comments on cases reported in our journals, I have been prompted to offer a few brief sentences on the cases of "Closure of the Vagina" quoted from an American journal in your number for the 12th inst.

Congenital adhesion of the labia in infants is not unfrequent: at the Royal Infirmary for Children I have had, occasionally, more than one case presented to me on the same morning, which I have not hesitated instantly to relieve.

Congenital adhesion is merely by a thin *film*, the division of which requires no *cutting*. A common probe pressed on the fissure from behind instantly relieves the labia, without any expression of pain by the child.

The epithelium is somewhat thinner in the line of the adhesion, as it usually is, indeed, when not exposed to the atmosphere. Spermaceti ointment on lint removes all irritation, if there be any, in two days.

The cases of Dr. Nott, it is stated, were adhesive *subsequent* to birth. This is, I believe, always as easily relieved without cutting, the adhesion not being the effect of plastic lymph, but a glutinous oozing probably from the follicles at the edge of the labia.

I should not have troubled you with these remarks were it not for the irritating effect often resulting from the retention of a few drops of urine, or of mucus, behind the adhesion, and the perfect simplicity and painlessness of what can scarcely be termed an operation.—I am, sir,

Your obedient servant,
WALTER C. DENDY.

May 19, 1843.

REDUCTION OF HERNIA.

To the Editor of the Medical Gazette.

SIR,

I SEND you the following case for insertion in your journal. The patient was a most unfavourable subject for an operation, and was relieved by a plan of treatment which, I understand, has been very successfully adopted in Ireland, and which, I hope, in many cases may prevent the necessity of having recourse to a painful and dangerous operation.—I remain, sir,

Your obedient servant,
CHARLES COLLAMBELL.
Canterbury Place, Lambeth,
April 19, 1843.

Mrs. Russell, æt. 51, very corpulent, ruptured herself on the right side twenty-four years since, in lifting a heavy weight, and (until within a fortnight) has not worn a truss for the last seven years, but, in consequence of its being improperly applied, has constantly had it on with the rupture down; she has not experienced much inconvenience, and has always been able to reduce it in the recumbent posture until this afternoon at three o'clock. I was requested to see her at half-past eleven P.M., April 12, and found her extremely exhausted; countenance very anxious and shrunk; constant vomiting; pulse small and thready; hands and feet cold; breathing hurried; abdomen very tender, but not tympanitic. On examination I found a protrusion of intestine through the femoral ring, larger than I could cover with my two hands, very tender, and excessively tympanitic (giving the sensation of a bladder distended with air), and no impulse on coughing. I endeavoured by very gentle manipulation, for nearly half an hour, to reduce it, without success; and as she was in a very small room, and without the possibility of having a warm-bath, I advised her removal to the hospital. This she positively refused, as she was resolved not to submit to an operation. Under these circumstances I determined to adopt the plan of treatment recommended and successfully practised by Dr. O'Beirne. I introduced the elastic tube of the stomach-pump into the rectum, and passed it on to the distance of twelve inches. I then attached the syringe, and slowly injected two quarts of warm water. When half this quantity had been thrown up a gurgling was distinctly heard in the tumor, and it gradually became less tense. Having injected all the water, I removed the syringe, and allowed the

water to run off by the tube. I then reapplied the syringe, and continued exhausting the air, when, after a few minutes, I had the gratification to find the hernia gradually subsiding; and by keeping up gentle pressure the contents were returned into the abdomen. My patient immediately pronounced herself relieved; her countenance became cheerful, and the sickness abated. She was ordered a brisk aperient of sulphate of magnesia and peppermint water, and a dose of calomel and opium. The bowels acted freely on the following morning, and she is now as well as usual.

ON THE

MECHANISM OF ABSORPTION.

To the Editor of the Medical Gazette.

SIR,

I SHALL feel much obliged by your giving insertion to the accompanying communication in an early number of your journal.—I am, sir,

Your obedient servant,
GEORGE ROBINSON, M.R.C.S.
Fellow of the Royal Medical and Chirurgical
Society.

35, Hunter Street, Brunswick Square.
May 17th, 1843.

In a memoir which was read before the Royal Medical and Chirurgical Society in February last, I attempted to prove by a series of experiments that a partial or complete obstruction to the passage of the blood through the smaller vessels of the body will cause the escape of its albuminous portion through their coats. In the present communication I wish to direct attention to the influence which the opposite condition of the circulation exercises in promoting the absorption of any fluids that may be placed in contact with the external surface of the vessels, or only separated from them by one or more membranes.

If we examine the facts brought forward to illustrate the process of absorption, we shall find that the following is perhaps the only general conclusion that can be safely drawn from them, viz. :—

That no substance can exert any influence on the whole system, unless the circulation of the blood through the vessels of the part to which it may be applied is performed with a certain degree of activity.

That the circulation of the blood must precede and accompany the act of absorption, is, among many other instances, proved by the following experiments:—

1. Magendie divided all the parts of the thigh of an animal but the femoral vessels, and then inserted poison under the integuments of the limb. While the vein was compressed no symptoms appeared, but they were immediately produced when the return of the blood was unimpeded.

2. Emmert tied the abdominal aorta, and introduced poison into a wound in the foot, but at the end of seventy hours no effects had appeared. On liberating the vessel then, the poison, prussic acid, acted within half an hour. I have repeated this experiment with precisely similar results. The aorta being compressed, a few drops of a strong solution of hydrosulphate of ammonia were introduced beneath the integuments of the thigh. At the end of seven minutes no symptoms had appeared, but on then releasing the vessel from the compression, the operation of the poison was immediately evinced, and the animal was dead in less than a minute.

A number of similar facts might be adduced in support of this assertion, but it will be sufficient to refer to those contained in all modern works on physiology: as Muller's, p. 254, &c.

This principle being established we may in the next place proceed to inquire how the circulation in favouring or rather producing absorption is to be explained.

According to the laws regulating the transmission of stagnant fluids through the membranes, exosmosis and endosmosis should be continually occurring through the coats of the vessels of the lining body; and there undoubtedly analogous processes do take place. But it appears to me highly important that we should ascertain how far these laws are modified when one or both fluids are in a state of motion.

However, Magendie, and all succeeding physiologists who adopt his opinion, suppose, that the external fluid, permeating the membrane, makes its way to the internal surface of the blood-vessel, and is then swept on by the current of the blood.

According to this hypothesis the chief part of the process of absorption is made to reside in some peculiar power possessed by the membranous walls of the vessels; the circulating fluid itself being quite a secondary agent, though, as above mentioned, its motion is necessary for the action of any poison on the system at large.

To prove the truth of his opinion, Magendie performed an experiment. He passed a stream of water through a portion of carotid artery and jugular vein, having previously applied strychnine to the exterior of the vessels. In a few minutes the water discharged had acquired the bitter taste of the poison.

Now this experiment, considered by itself, throws but little light on the mechanism of absorption; it merely proves that while a stream traverses a membranous tube, any soluble matters placed on the exterior of that tube will be absorbed. But as to the relative influence of the stream and the membrane in accomplishing that end, we are left wholly in the dark. He referred the whole of the transmitting power to the membrane; but the same experiment will, I think, prove just as much the influence of the stream in increasing that power.

It has long been known that a fluid while traversing any porous vessel will draw in a considerable quantity of air, which is liberated when the fluid is again at rest.

I now quote an experiment from Sir J. Leslie's Elements of Natural Philosophy, Vol. i. p. 364.

"If a cylinder 1 inch in diameter, and 3 inches long, be fitted into an orifice at the bottom of a cistern, and on its upper side, at the distance of half an inch from its origin, a narrow arched glass tube be inserted, having its long end carried down to a basin of water 3 feet below the insertion of the other end, when a stream traverses the cylinder with a velocity of nine feet per second it will raise the water up the glass tube to the height of two feet, and if the tube be shortened within that limit, the basin will, in a short time, be emptied of the stagnant fluid. I have now several times repeated this experiment, and, with a rapid stream, the results were always in accordance with the above statement. Having filled a wine-glass with coloured fluid, and having connected its contents (by means of a bent tube twelve inches long) with the interior of a pipe half an inch in diameter, I found that the glass was drained of the stagnant fluid in less than two minutes after the stream was turned through the pipe. I may refer to the same page for a proof of the statement that this imbibing power of the stream is proportioned to its velocity. I will, however, mention one other proof. While a cistern is full, the rate of discharge and consequent velocity of the stream through the orifice at its bottom will of course be greatest. Now if the apparatus above described be fitted into a pipe connected with this orifice, it will be found that the stagnant fluid will rapidly rise to a certain height in the glass tube; but as the depth of the column of water in the cistern diminishes, the fluid in the tube will oscillate, and fall till the stream becomes so tardy as not to exert any marked influence on the stagnant fluid. Having now proved the existence of this power, and also that it is proportioned to the velocity of the stream, the first step towards the application of the principle to the explanation of the process of absorption in the living body is to shew that the same force, whatever it may be, will act through one or more membranes.

Accordingly, the short end of the glass tube being covered with membrane, and its long end immersed in a coloured fluid, I found that within five minutes after the stream had commenced to flow, the whole of the air present in the tube (which was twelve inches long, and its bore $\frac{1}{12}$th of an inch wide) had been absorbed, and its place supplied by the coloured fluid. A continued slow ascent of the latter was still proceeding when I was compelled to stop the experiment. I repeated it again, covering the short end of the tube with two membranes instead of one, but using a tube several inches shorter than in the last case, and found that there was a very slow but steady and constant flow of the fluid towards the stream; the fluid which thus traversed the tube being opposed in its flow by gravity, and being itself of greater specific gravity than that of the water constituting the stream. By these direct experiments, and from a careful consideration of the chain of indirect evidence furnished by a number of morbid and healthy actions that

are known to occur in the bodies of animals, I am, I think, justified, even in the present incipient stage of the inquiry, in making the following statement :—

That as it has been shown that the effusion of albuminous matters through the coats of the vessels of the living body is produced, and modified in its nature, by the degree of the compression of the blood contained within them—this action being independent of, and even in opposition to, the ordinary laws of exosmosis, deduced from experiments on *stagnant* fluids —so I believe the chief part of the process of absorption in animals to arise from, and depend on, a force existing within the blood-vessels; that force being generated by, and proportioned to the velocity of, the moving mass by which, in a healthy state, they are incessantly traversed.

That something like a suction power acts in promoting or causing absorption is undoubtedly a very old opinion, and the truth of this remark is evident in the literal signification of the word itself. But so far as my present knowledge extends, all previous writers have referred that power either to the enlargement of the chest in inspiration, or to the dilatation of the ventricles. Now while readily admitting the influence of these actions in facilitating the return of venous blood, and thereby indirectly favouring absorption, I cannot think that they exercise any immediate effect in promoting the entrance of extraneous matters through the coats of the smaller vessels. But if, on the other hand, we suppose this suction power, whatever its precise nature may be, to be caused by and reside in the stream of blood, to be greatest wherever the current is most rapid, to be increased in its activity by whatever accelerates the velocity, and diminished by whatever induces a retardation of the circulation through any part, then we shall have a principle of action at once simple and efficacious, in perfect accordance with the established laws of hydraulics, and by the operation of which many morbid and healthy phenomena of the human body can be satisfactorily explained and readily understood.

In the present stage of the inquiry I shall not make many applications of this principle, but content myself with briefly alluding to some facts which seem to corroborate the doctrine herein sought to be established.

Magendie proved that a state of plethora retarded, and one of depletion promoted, absorption. These two conditions of the system are evidently attended by two opposite degrees of activity of the circulation.

For when the mass of blood is much augmented, the obstacles which naturally oppose the free passage of the blood through its vessels are materially increased, at the same time that the action of the heart is slower and more laboured than usual: consequently the proportion then existing between the moving power and the mass to be moved is unfavourable to a rapid circulation: and we may thus explain the slower action of poisons after he had injected a quantity of water into the veins.

Whereas, after bleeding or any other large depletion, the whole of the arteries contract as the quantity of blood in the system diminishes, so as to form a series of narrower tubes; and the heart being relieved of a part of its load, after the first shock is over, increases the rapidity of its contractions so much, that a more rapid circulation must necessarily result.

There are two parts of the animal economy where the process of absorption is actively carried on, and where some beautiful modifications of this principle are exemplified. I have said that compression of the blood within its vessels favours effusion: it should follow, therefore, that the compression of an external fluid against their coats, while they are traversed by a rapid stream, should promote absorption; and such doubtless is the case.

The influence of pressure in causing the absorption of effused fluids is well known, and its application is seen in daily practice. In the intestines, through which the body obtains all its nourishment, some provision for increasing the absorbing power of the vessels was required, and, accordingly, is there found. Their peristaltic action keeps up a steady continued pressure of the chyme against the vessels, thereby regulating, to a certain extent, the quantity of fluid effused from the latter, at the same time that their calibre is diminished, and the velocity of the blood traversing them consequently increased.

It has been an interesting problem in

physiology to explain how the fœtus is nourished by the maternal blood without any direct vascular communication existing. On examining the maternal vessels, it is evident from their increased diameter, great length, and tortuous arrangement, that the circulation through them must be much retarded; while, on the other hand, the shorter circuit of the fœtal blood, and the rapid contraction of the fœtal heart, render it highly probable, if they do not establish the certainty of the fact, that the velocity of the fœtal blood during its passage through the placental vessels is much greater than that of the maternal circulation.

Since, therefore, it has been shewn that the absorbing power of a stream is proportioned to its velocity, it should follow that, when two currents of blood, moving with different degrees of velocity, are in juxta-position with each other, being separated only by two thin membranes, the more rapid stream will not only draw in any fluid that the other may have already effused, but may even directly increase the quantity or rate of that effusion.

Wherever the course of the vessels is tortuous, or their coats relaxed, a retardation of, and consequent impediment to, the circulation of the blood results — effusion takes place, and absorption occurs very slowly, and *vice versâ*. We can thus understand why the surface of old ulcers should absorb more rapidly than that of more recent ones; why a ligature tied round the limb, or the application of a cupping glass, impedes the action of poisons introduced into wounds of the extremity.

In short, throughout the whole body, the two antagonistic processes of absorption and effusion are constantly in operation, the preponderance of the one or the other in any particular part being regulated by the facilities or impediments which the blood meets with in its passage through the *smaller* vessels of that part; and I believe that absorption takes place chiefly in that part of the circulating system, from the circumstance of the coats of the vessels being there thinnest, and the rapidity of the current greatest. As before stated, I consider these two processes to be, in their nature and causes, essentially different from those usually understood by the terms endosmosis and exosmosis, and to be, in a great measure, independent of the laws regulating the transmission of *stagnant* and *uncompressed* fluids through membranes.

Note.—Of course these remarks are only intended to apply to the general processes; for there is undoubtedly something more than a mere physical law in operation in all those parts where *secretion* is going on; and a certain selective influence is probably also exercised in regulating the admission of external matters within the circulation.

CASE OF

FATAL WOUND OF THE CHEST,

ACCOMPANIED WITH

DIARRHŒA AND DISTRESSING VOMITING.

To the Editor of the Medical Gazette.

SIR,

IF you think the following worthy a place in the MEDICAL GAZETTE, you will much oblige the writer by its insertion.

D. M'PHERSON,
Surgeon.

John Maitland, æt. 32, of robust constitution and temperate habits, had been standing with a pitchfork in his hand, on the top of a cart laden to the height of sixteen feet with bundles of straw. The horse in yoke, being of a restless nature, took fright at some object, and making a sudden spring forwards threw the man and the fork precipitately over the hinder end of the cart. The pitchfork had fallen first to the ground, and, while resting on its harmless end, received the man from a height of three feet upon its prongs, one of which entered the left breast about two and a half inches below the mamma, and inflicted a severe punctured wound. An old woman had administered to him a glass of gin immediately after the accident, and he was carried to bed without having sustained any considerable loss of blood. On seeing the patient three hours after, an oval wound of the size of a shilling, and resembling very much the consequence of a pistol-shot, was discovered in the situation just described; but no symptoms were then elicited which could lead to the apprehension of the *chest being entered.* Pulse full and

excited; face flushed; skin hot, and bedewed with a copious perspiration; tongue covered at the root and centre with a layer of white pasty fur, and his wife says he has had diarrhœa for the last eight days; breathing hurried and anxious. A distressing sickness had continued since the time of the accident to occasion the vomiting of a tenacious frothy mucus tinged with blood; and his strength had been so much reduced in consequence, that he begged to be let alone, and lay in a state of apparent syncope during the intervals of the retchings. No spitting of blood, or escape of air or blood from the wound. Lies easiest on his back, and does not complain of any local pain.

On examining the pitchfork, which lay still on the spot where the accident occurred, a bloody mark, extending from the point up two and a half inches of one of its toes, was distinctly discovered, and the opinion of the chest being penetrated duly confirmed.

Mitt. Sanguis ad ℥xviij. To be followed up with the succeeding mixture :—

℞ Tart. Antim. gr. ij. ; Tinct. Opii, ℨss. ; Aquæ font. ℥viij. M. fiat mist. cujus capiat. cochlear. mag. 3tiâ quâque horâ.

Wounds fomented with hot water, and dressed with adhesive plaster. On seeing patient on the afternoon of the following day, I found him almost *articulo mortis*, lying upon his back, and still making ineffectual efforts to vomit —a condition of things which, by the friends' account, had been unremitting since the period of my former visit. Respiration sonorous and abdominal ; countenance collapsed and mortally pale; coldness of the extremities and great prostration of strength ; sensibility to stimuli perceptibly impaired.

Ordered warm applications to the feet and chest, and administered at frequent intervals a little brandy diluted with water.

Went to visit another patient, and on returning a couple of hours afterwards found him still sinking. The eyes looked glassy; black sordes had encrusted his mouth and lips; and in half an hour afterwards, while in the act of changing his position in bed, he expired.

Autopsy.—The end of a gum elastic catheter passed readily down the course of the wound to a depth corresponding with the bloody encrustation upon the pitchfork. On opening the chest, I found the instrument had entered between the sixth and seventh ribs, and, running an oblique course, had severely lacerated the lung, together with the inflicting a gentle puncture upon the floor of the diaphragm. A considerable quantity (5 oz.) of effused air and blood existed in the pleuritic cavity. A high degree of inflammation surrounded the wounds in the pleura and lungs, but no morbid appearances followed upon the rasure of the diaphragm.

REMARKS.—The absence of certain pathognomonic symptoms, and the unsuspicious appearance of the external wound, would have led strongly to the conclusion that the pleura had not been injured ; but the single evidence derived from an examination of the instrument by which the wound was inflicted proved the contrary of this, and set the question satisfactorily at rest. This would seem a case in point to add to the list of injuries to the chest, the nature and extent of which are not to be determined by the information derived from the nature of existing symptoms. The presence, to be sure, of certain pathognomonic symptoms affords decisive evidence of internal mischief being done ; but their absence do not by any means assert the harmlessness of the injury. Here was a case in which there was no expectoration of frothy blood, no escape of air during expectoration, no emphysema, &c., and yet both the pleura, the diaphragm, and the lungs, were extensively and fatally wounded. The point most worthy of attention in this case was the incessant vomiting. Upon what connection between the digestive organs and the parts wounded, should the stomach be excited to such violent action as to continue its throes for a period of 24 hours in spite of medicine ; to form the most aggravated symptom of the malady, and thereby lead to the fatal consequences which ensued?

Newcastle, May 17, 1843.

MR. BRUNEL'S CASE.

To the Editor of the Medical Gazette.

SIR,

THE public sympathy and curiosity respecting Mr. Brunel were but very imperfectly gratified by gleanings from the columns of newspapers. Medical men require information of a different kind ; and now that that gentleman is happily released from his awkward predicament, they have a right to expect it from a better source. Inasmuch as their efforts to raise medicine from a conjectural art to the rank of an exact science have, in a great measure, been crowned with success, they may well be excused from reposing implicit confidence in the meagre, unsatisfactory, and unauthenticated letter upon the subject which appeared in the *Times* newspaper, and which may possibly have emanated from a non-professional person and incompetent narrator. Assuming, however, that the anonymous statement in the *Times* is substantially correct as far as it goes, it is quite clear that Mr. Brunel's case presented some features of very great interest ; and it is highly desirable that they should be fully considered and reported upon by one of the eminent surgeons who assisted him. I shall refer to one of the symptoms only to illustrate my object in thus trespassing upon your columns.

We are told that after the operation of tracheotomy the forceps could not be employed from the extreme irritation of the trachea. This is, I believe, almost a singular instance of the kind. Magendie opened the trachea of a dog, and, upon passing whalebone up into the glottis, much coughing and irritation were produced; but, upon passing it downwards through the trachea, no inconvenience ensued. A woman had a triangular portion of a sheep's vertebra impacted in the right bronchus, below the clavicle. Mr. Liston opened the trachea, and with some difficulty extracted the bone by the forceps. Not being then aware of Magendie's experiment, I was particularly struck with the very slight inconvenience felt by this patient, and subsequently by others, on the insertion of the forceps.

At a meeting of the Medico-Chirurgical Society, held about three years since, the subject of tracheotomy was introduced by Mr. Travers; and in the discussion which followed, the comparative non-susceptibility of the trachea was fully insisted upon by Sir B. Brodie, Dr. Marshall Hall, Mr. Liston, and others. An illustrative case given by Mr. Liston on that occasion is worth repeating. A man had some chronic disease about the larynx, which obstructed respiration. The trachea was opened, and the long tube, which he wore in the opening constantly, produced no uneasiness. This man habitually relieved himself from occasional attacks of dyspnœa, by passing a long feather from the tail of a turkey down into the depths of his chest, and bringing up from thence long strings of tough mucus, which he did without causing the slightest irritation or cough.

Although phthisical symptoms generally supervene if a foreign substance be long retained in the trachea, the bronchi, or air-cells, there seems to be less danger from the irritation caused by its immediate presence there than from the obstruction caused thereby to the pulmonary circulation.

Whether the excessive irritability was merely a higher order of natural susceptibility, or was morbid sensibility, or was connected with inflammatory action, or with any other cause, is one of the points which remain to be cleared up in Mr. Brunel's case, upon which, I trust, we shall shortly be provided with an efficient memoir from the pen of one of his distinguished surgeons.—I am, sir,

Your obedient servant,
REGINALD BURRIDGE, M.D.
Physician to the Taunton and Somerset Hospital.
Taunton, May 20, 1843.

ON THE

NATURE, DIAGNOSIS, AND TREAT-
MENT OF INCIPIENT
PHTHISIS.

BY CHRISTOPHER M. DURRANT, M.D.
Physician to the East Suffolk and
Ipswich Hospital.

(For the London Medical Gazette.)

SINCE the immortal discovery of auscultation by Laennec, perhaps no disease has more fully occupied the attention of pathologists than the one under consideration; and few indeed, it may be added, have advanced more progressively towards precision, or yielded more definite results.

The labourers in this extensive field have been by no means confined to a single country. England, France, Germany, America, and Italy, have alike honourably produced inquirers, who, by their zealous and successful investigations, have assuredly brought the diagnosis of phthisis, in its earlier stages, to a degree of certainty previously unknown.

The mortality caused by pulmonary consumption is estimated as producing at least one-fifth of the entire deaths in this country; which fact alone proves, with melancholy truth, the almost hopeless amount of benefit that we can expect to derive from medicine, save as a palliative in the *very advanced* stages of the malady.

That nature does occasionally, though rarely, bring the disease to a happy termination I am fully convinced; and as the views of M. Rokitansky, of Vienna, on this subject, are the most recent, I make no apology for introducing a somewhat lengthened quotation from the notice of his work on Morbid Anatomy, in the January number of the British and Foreign Medical Review for the present year.

This author has shewn that the phenomena of phthisis may proceed towards a curative termination by six different modes:—" 1st. By a callous degeneration of the tissue around the cavity, or the formation of a membrane within it, like a serous or a mucous membrane; the former being usually found when the disease is tranquil; the latter when there is much irritation. 2dly. The cavity may completely cicatrize, its walls gradually falling in and uniting, with obliteration of the bronchi and sinking in of the surface of the lung, and perhaps of the wall of the chest also. 3dly. The cavity may, after partially shrinking, be filled by chalky matter, from the metamorphosis of some remaining tubercle. 4thly. In the place of the cavity there may be produced a large callous mass of tissue, like that of cicatrices. 5thly. The tubercle may not proceed to the formation of the cavity, but being arrested in its earlier progress, may diminish in size, and may be changed into a grey or dirty white mass of chalky matter, and at last into a hard concretion. And lastly, at a still earlier stage, the tubercle being arrested in its progress, may retrograde and become *obsolete*, shrivelling into an opaque, blueish-gray, cartilaginous knot, which is indisposed to any further metamorphosis."

Such are the conclusions to which M. Rokitansky has arrived; to the correctness of some of which my own observations lead me to concur, more especially in reference to the occasional cicatrization of cavities, and the shrivelled condition of the tubercular deposit.

Nature of tubercle —This paper being professedly practical, my observations on the pathology of incipient consumption must necessarily be very brief. Without entering upon the multiform theories that have been advanced, I may state that I believe phthisis to be caused by the deposition of an unorganizable matter from the blood, presenting the form of miliary granulations, yellow caseous opaque matter, or, thirdly, as tuberculous infiltration; which latter deposit, save in the cases of acute phthisis, less frequently obtains in the early stages of the disease. This secretion forming tubercle is closely connected with the strumous diathesis, either hereditary or acquired, and, according to M. Andral, appears especially influenced by irritation, inflammation, or congestion of the blood-vessels of the part in which it is earliest deposited.

The ordinary and primary seat of tubercle, as shewn by Dr. Carswell, is principally on the free surface of mucous membranes; and at the commencement of the disease the lesser bronchi, the air-cells, and the interstitial cellular tissue, appear peculiarly obnoxious to its presence. Of the origin of the miliary tubercle, or granulations of Bayle, many different opinions are entertained. That of Laennec, who viewed them as similar in nature to the yellow crude tubercle, but existing in an incipient or nascent state, may perhaps be considered on the whole as the most satisfactory. M. Rokitansky appears to maintain a somewhat similar opinion, and believes the peculiar form of deposit to depend upon the degree of the tuberculous diathesis which exists at the time. The tubercular gra-

nulations, whether deposited singly or in clusters, appear first, according to this pathologist, in the form of miliary grains, " or, in an intense degree of the tuberculous diathesis, it may be deposited at once as the yellow tubercle."

In tubercular infiltration, the deposit appears completely diffused throughout the cellular and interstitial portion of the lungs, presenting the appearance as if the matter had been poured into the lung in a liquid form, and had subsequently become solidified.

This tuberculous infiltration is considered by M. Rokitansky as " hepatization by a tuberculous product." He maintains that the ordinary deposit of a pneumonia, when occurring in a strumous habit, instead of being absorbed or becoming purulent, is gradually metamorphosed into the yellow tuberculous matter; and farther, that the change from the fibrinous to the tuberculous secretion can be distinctly demonstrated.

This tuberculous infiltration, in which are not unfrequently detected isolated portions of caseous matter, sometimes obtains in a more fluid form; this constitutes the *infiltration tuberculeuse gélatiniforme* of Laennec, and not a deposit *sui generis*, as has been supposed by some authors.

It is now, I believe, an undisputed fact, and one which we shall hereafter find to be of great practical importance in the diagnosis, that when tuberculous deposit in the lungs takes place gradually, in almost all cases, the superior lobes will be found first affected; and of these the upper and posterior parts are most prone. Upon what circumstance this increased liability to tuberculous deposit in the upper lobes depends, I confess that I cannot decide; neither has it, I believe, hitherto been satisfactorily explained. I do, however, conceive, that the rash exposure of the upper parts of the chest in both sexes, must, by exerting a local influence on the circulation in the corresponding part of the lungs, materially increase the power of the already existing cause, whatever that may be. Another curious and valuable fact, although of less practical importance than the preceding, is this, viz. that in the earliest period of tuberculous deposit the left lung is more obnoxious to the disease than the right. As the affection, however, increases, it will be found to advance with nearly equal rapidity on both sides.

Diagnosis.—In investigating the earliest signs by which tuberculous phthisis may be detected, I may remark that it is my intention to limit my inquiry to the physical phenomena of the affection. The general symptoms are so ably and fully described by Sir James Clark, in his valuable treatise on Consumption, that to his work, especially his remarks on tuberculous cachexy, and to Dr. Todd's learned essay on strumous dyspepsia, in the Cyclopædia of Practical Medicine, I beg unhesitatingly to refer, as embracing all that can be said on the general symptoms of the disease. Notwithstanding the determined opposition and ridicule which the stethoscope long encountered in its earlier career, its value as a diagnostic agent is now, I believe, too fully admitted to require any comment.

I must, however, strenuously urge the necessity and incalculable importance of investigating the earliest and most incipient threatenings of the disease; for, as Sir James Clark graphically observes, "I do not hesitate to express my conviction, that by adopting a rigid examination on being first consulted, the greater number of cases of tuberculous phthisis would be discovered at a much earlier period of their course,—often, I am persuaded, many months, nay, occasionally years, before they now are, from the careless manner in which this class of patients is too commonly examined. In the present superficial mode of inquiry, it is too often far advanced, when the patient is said to be merely threatened with it, and tracheal or bronchial irritation are the terms employed to account for symptoms which a closer investigation would trace to a deeper source. We must not be satisfied with a few rough and slovenly thumps on the upper part of the chest, or even with the use of the ear or stethoscope for a few moments, applied as if we were afraid, rather than desirous of ascertaining the real condition of the lungs. Such superficial examination, if it deserves the name, is worse than useless : with the semblance of doing something, it really effects nothing, unless it be to deceive the patient and his friends, and bring this method of diagnosis into *unmerited disrepute.*"

Much of the apparent difficulty in stethoscopic examination may be easily removed by adopting in our investigation a more regular and methodical method; and, with this view, I may preface my observations on physical diagnosis by a few remarks on the practical application of the instrument.

In performing auscultation several rules are to be attended to, affecting both the observer and the patient. In a first examination, especially in the female sex, a nervous alarm is very commonly excited, rendering the respiratory movements irregular, abrupt, and wholly inefficient for the purpose of a correct diagnosis. This state we must endeavour quietly to overcome; we must guide, but not alarm our patient, using as little parade as possible, "Avoid" says M. Fournet, "a stern air, an abrupt address, and solemnity; these throw the patient into a state of nervousness. There is a calm, simple, benevolent mode of accosting a patient, a certain gentleness and earnestness of manner, that at once wins his confidence, and renders him composed, so that he answers correctly, does what he is desired well ; and then his features, influenced only by the morbid state, express accurately all he feels."

We must endeavour to give our entire attention to one sound at a time, avoiding with equal care any liability to distraction by surrounding noises. This faculty of concentration can, as I have personally proved, be greatly strengthened by habit, and then, like many other qualifications, it becomes more and more amenable to the will.

In examining the lungs in incipient phthisis the sitting posture is to be preferred ; the chest should be moderately rounded, and if possible uncovered; this, in the infra-clavicular regions, can generally be effected without outraging the feelings of the most delicate. The arms should be allowed to hang unconstrainedly at the sides. After glancing at the general contour of the thorax, and ascertaining the facility with which the ribs rise and fall, we should direct the patient to breathe naturally, so as in the first place to become acquainted with the normal state of the respiration.

The examination should be always conducted slowly, not trusting too much to medical tact ; at the same time it is incumbent on us to be extremely careful not to allow any preconceived judgment which we may have formed to influence us in the investigation of the true state of the lung. The stethoscope should be applied firmly, but lightly, and in close proximity to the chest; all unnecessary rustling of the clothes must be sedulously avoided. The patient should then be directed slowly to take some deep inspirations, then a *single* cough, and repeated: this latter act will frequently enable us to discover the click of incipient phthisis, when other means have failed. Both sides of the chest must be examined in a precisely similar manner : this ought never to be omitted, however clearly and indisputably the disease may be indicated. In auscultating a chest where we have reason to fear deposit, the infra-clavicular, the acromial, the supra-scapular, and the axillary regions, will obtain our especial attention. Still, however, in a doubtful case, we must never rest satisfied until the condition of the entire chest has been patiently and carefully investigated. The physical examination of the earliest local signs of phthisis may be referred to three heads. —inspection, auscultation, and percussion. To each of these I shall briefly direct attention.

Inspection. — On baring the chest, and placing the patient in a direct light, at the same time taking care that he use no muscular exertion, we are not unfrequently enabled to detect a marked difference in the form and rotundity of the upper part of the chest. This in some cases is very slight, or even unobservable, while in others it amounts to indisputable softening or flattening of the infra-clavicular region. To this is sometimes added an insufficient elevation of the three or four superior ribs on one side of the chest. The difference, if not very appreciable, may occasionally be rendered more so by the application of the expanded hands simultaneously beneath both clavicles, when we often perceive, on directing a full inspiration, that the ribs on one side rise with elasticity, as in health, while on the opposite side they remain comparatively motionless.

These signs, of minor import when isolated, yet when combined with the evidences obtained by auscultation and percussion, tend to throw considerable light on a doubtful case, and as such should never be omitted in the examination. The causes on which the above phenomena depend, are, I imagine, to be attributed to whatever obstructs the admission of air into the minute bronchial tubes. This may arise from thickening of the tubes themselves; compression by tuberculous deposit; partial atrophy of the pulmonary tissue from inactivity, often increased by adhesions; to which should be added, wasting of the thoracic muscles.

With the above phenomena may be included the occasional occurrence of diminished vocal vibration, as perceived on applying the expanded hands, upon the upper parts of the chest. This becomes more apparent in those cases in which the tuberculous matter is deposited with the greatest rapidity, and confined *en masse* to the apex of the lung.

Auscultation. — I have selected the examination of the signs deducible from auscultation, prior to those from percussion, inasmuch as I feel persuaded, that, to a practised ear, the minute changes which take place in the respiratory murmur in the earliest stages of incipient phthisis are more appreciable, and more decisive of the disease, when investigated by the auscultatory phenomena, than when too implicit reliance is placed on the minute shades of dulness as elicited by the most careful percussion. For practical purposes the physical changes affecting the normal respiratory murmur, may be advantageously divided into those pertaining to the sounds of inspiration, and those proper to expiration.

I may in this place again repeat the importance of examining and concentrating the attention on each sound separately; at the same time carefully comparing the results with the phenomena observable on the corresponding side, and in other parts of the chest.

The murmur audible during the act of inspiration may be simply decreased in duration and intensity; for instance, if fixed at 10, the nominal healthy standard of M. Fournet, it may fall to 4, or even to 2; and in cases of rapid deposit may become inaudible. The same murmur frequently undergoes great alteration in character, conveying to the ear the impression of hoarseness, roughness, or dryness; the "rude inspiration," of some authors. This depends principally upon compression of the minute bronchial tubes by tuberculous deposit, thereby causing an undue vibration in the passage of the air to the terminal cells; it arises partly, also, from a thickened state of the tubes themselves.

The occasional abrupt or jerking rhythm of the respiratory murmurs depends in part upon the same cause, and partly, also, according to Barth and Roger, upon the impediment to the free expansion of the lung, in consequence of inter-current pleuritic adhesions. This want of continuity in the act of respiration I have hitherto only met with below the clavicles. Dr. Walshe, in his valuable little work on Physical Diagnosis, just published, states that he has detected this phenomenon, at the lower parts of lungs, whose summits and upper parts presented the signs of cavities. Jerking respiration is commonly confined to the murmur of inspiration; I have, however, in a few instances, found it of a double and treble character, accompanying the expiratory sound; the inspiratory murmur, with the exception of being harsh and dry, remaining unaffected. Abrupt respiration, especially when accompanied by dulness on percussion, and flattening or insufficient expansion of the infra-clavicular region, becomes a valuable sign of incipient tubercle.

The murmur of expiration is liable to marked alteration in the earlier stages of phthisis pulmonalis, and when present is likewise a valuable indicative sign of the existence of the disease. This murmur, which, in the healthy lung, is nearly audible, (although not completely so, as stated by some), is now greatly increased both in duration and intensity. Placing with M. Fournet the ideal standard of natural respiration at 2, it may become prolonged to 20, which this author fixes as the maximum; at the same time, it passes through the different gradations of quality and intensity, to the extent in some instances of entirely masking the preceding murmur of inspiration.

Independently of the changes to which the natural respiratory sounds are liable, auscultation frequently reveals other phenomena, which, especially when coexisting with those above detailed, prove of invaluable import in *the early diagnosis of this* insidious *disease.*

Under this head are included the various rhonchi audible in the different stages of the malady: for our present purpose it will suffice to notice those only which obtain at the very commencement of the affection.

These sounds may be divided into the dry and moist: the former being almost exclusively confined to the incipient stage alone of pulmonary phthisis.

Of the dry sounds are the sensations of crackling, crumpling, &c. communicated to the ear during inspiration; these, when very marked, not unfrequently appear to blend the sounds of inspiration and those of expiration in one continuous soft rustle. I have succeeded in very closely imitating this sound by loosely enclosing a small piece of tissue paper in a large silk pocket-handkerchief; this, when gently grasped and held near the ear, at the same time using alternate compression and relaxation, yields an indistinct crumpling sound, very similar to the one in question. The mechanism of the production of this sound is somewhat obscure; as, however, it has been heard only in the first stage of tubercles, its import as a diagnostic auxiliary is very valuable. M. Fournet states that he was enabled to detect the dry crumpling sound in the wards of La Charité, in the proportion of about one case to eight of incipient phthisis. My own experience hitherto is in favour of a smaller ratio than the above.

Another sound, which I have heard more frequently, and which appears to be a mere modification of the crumpling, is an occasional plaintive whining note, audible during inspiration only, and principally at the termination of that act. This latter sound occurs only at intervals, and in general requires a forced inspiration for its development.

The only other abnormal phenomenon whose pathological signification, when confined to the apices of the lungs is strongly indicative of commencing phthisis, is the pulmonary crackling, or moist sounds above alluded to. This consists of a succession of minute cracklings, audible only during inspiration. In its commencement, it possesses the character of dryness, differing but little from the crumpling sound already described; as the disease advances, the dry crackling gradually becomes moist, and is then indicative of tuberculous softening. M. Fournet, who considers the dry crackling as distinct from the sound of crumpling, states that he recognised it in eight out of ten cases of incipient tubercular affection.

Such are the various rhonchi occasionally audible during the early stage of pulmonary consumption; and great as unquestionably is their diagnostic import, when present, still we must carefully avoid inferring from their absence (other indications obtaining) the non-existence of the disease. The only remaining physical signs revealed by auscultation are an increased resonance of the voice and cough, amounting even to modified bronchophony; together with an unusual distinctness of the sounds of the heart, below the clavicle; that viscus and the great vessels being at the same time in a healthy condition. These phenomena depend upon a condensation of the upper part of the lung, either by clusters of tubercles, by tubercular infiltration, by hepatisation, or by the three states combined, the two last being hardly distinguishable.

Percussion.—As already stated, the results afforded by this mode of investigation are not so early applicable to the diagnosis of the signs of incipient phthisis as the alterations in the character of the respiratory murmur; these latter frequently presenting, in conjunction with general symptoms, prior to the existence of any marked difference in the comparative resonance of the chest. When percussion, however, yields a dull sound, it may then, perhaps, *cæteris paribus*, be esteemed a more valuable indication of the disease than any of the foregoing signs, demonstrating as it does the positive deposition of tuberculous matter.

The amount of dulness, as elicited by careful percussion, varies greatly; in some cases a merely increased resistance to the finger is alone appreciable, while, in others, the sound resembles that obtained on percussing the thigh.

In conducting the examination, a few general rules may be advantageously borne in mind.

The position of the patient, as during auscultation, must be unconstrained, the arms being placed exactly in the same position; as the bulging out of the chest, *or irregular contraction of the pectoral muscle might materially modify the* sound, and thereby lead to error;—the chest, if possible, should be uncovered, or, if covered, the same thickness of linen should be maintained, carefully avoiding folds. Mediate percussion is preferable to immediate; while a light smart tap, frequently repeated, yields a much more delicate and accurate result than a heavy stroke. I have invariably found the index finger of the left hand the best pleximeter, and a clearer sound obtained by striking its palmar than its dorsal aspect;—the depression immediately below the clavicles yields a more accurate result than by tapping the bone itself;—in doubtful cases all the regions of the class should undergo a careful examination, as well by percussion as by auscultation; the great practical rule, however, to be followed, is to *immediately* compare the resulting sound with that elicited from a *precisely* corresponding situation on the opposite side, striking, with the same firmness, and *perpendicularly* upon the finger.

The minute shades of difference in sound may sometimes be rendered more apparent by tapping the chest during forced inspiration and forced expiration, as, by these means, tuberculous deposit may, in some cases, be discovered, even if overlapped by a portion of healthy or emphysematous lung.

In conducting the physical examination of incipient phthisis, the stethoscopist, however conversant with auscultatory phenomena, must never lose sight of the all-important principle of comparison. For example, feebleness of respiration we have seen to be a sign of commencing tuberculous deposit. True: but it is a sign also of pulmonary emphysema, bronchitis, and pleurisy with effusion; besides which, it is caused by pleurodynia, stricture of the larynx, partial obstruction of the bronchial tubes, or compression of these tubes by enlarged glands, tumors, &c.; and, lastly, the entire lungs may sometimes exhibit a naturally feeble murmur, without concomitant disease. How, then, are we to test the value of this sign as an indication of incipient phthisis? By careful comparison, not only with the corresponding sounds of the opposite side, but with those in the different regions of the same side; by investigating the other physical signs which may obtain, particularly the changes in inspiration and expiration; by percussion; and also by recollecting that phthisis almost invariably commences in, and is at first confined to, the apices of the lungs; and of these, in general, the one is affected in a greater degree, or advances more rapidly, than the other.

The same principle of comparison holds good in the differential signification of many of the other signs of incipient phthisis, and, as such, claims throughout the examination the fullest importance, as being the only mode of avoiding error, and also of arriving at a correct diagnosis.

[To be continued.]

MEDICAL GAZETTE.

Friday, May 26, 1843.

"Licet omnibus, licet etiam mihi, dignitatem Artis Medicæ tueri; potestas modo veniendi in publicum sit, dicendi periculum non recuso."
                                      CICERO.

GRATUITOUS PRACTICE.

PERHAPS in no country in the world is medical assistance given to so large an extent without fee or reward as in England; and this is not the act of government, or a matter of state policy, but due to the spontaneous exertions of individuals. The instinctive attempt to supply the deficiences of individual powers by combination has of course led us in this, as in most other things, to form societies for effecting the purposes of charity in a systematic, efficient, and economical manner; but these associations are voluntary, not compulsory; private, not public. Their magnitude and the wealth which they have gradually accumulated, has often given to them a public character, and their utility has often given them acknowledged claims to public assistance; but more often a far different effect has ensued, and the state which had no share in their foundation, has been urged to regulate their government, and administer, if not appropriate, their finances. Their wealth having become *great*, and their utility extensive, the *distribution of their benefits* profuse,

they have been first thankfully recognised as public blessings, and then looked upon as public property. The danger of spoliation, indeed, is in proportion to the degree of previous veneration; and the latter may with confidence be looked for when the former is at its height. Societies, like individuals, when they heap up riches, cannot tell who shall gather them.

Two classes of persons concur, from very different motives, in hastening this process. The one consists of men whose active benevolence and quick intelligence point out to them the vast good of which such powerful institutions seem capable, if placed under the most efficient possible management. A warm temperament, a conscientious industry, and a benevolence which has become expansive and habitual, leads such men to conceive gigantic plans of improvement, and fearlessly to undertake them. The indifference of placemen offends the best feelings of their nature, and they labour assiduously to remove, as the peculiar defects of their favourite institution, those evils which are common to the species. But the lever once applied, however tenderly and judiciously, to any part of a social edifice, is liable to be handled by the unskilful and the violent; and the force intended for raising and rectifying a part, is apt to be increased to the rending, if not the overthrow, of the whole.

The other class who conduce no less to the result above mentioned, are those who are opposed to all change, who, seeing a great deal of good effected, are unwilling to admit the propriety of attempting to do more. To them all novelty is dangerous, all projects are chimerical. An unmeaning resistance to all remonstrance however temperate, and all change however judicious, is apt to tempt disinterested reformers to alliances with those of the baser sort; similar allies are required in well-defence, good motives are gradually merged in the desire for victory, and general confusion results.

We put out of the question those low motives which by the vulgar will always be mainly attributed to the two parties, believing most firmly that a malicious desire to overthrow what is good, and a selfish intention to preserve what is bad, do not actuate the principals on either side. The perversion of noble motives and generous aims have prompted most of the actors in political dramas, whether tragedies or farces. Satan, himself a fallen angel, tempts frequently through the noblest qualities.

But the ethical view of the subject must in our pages give way to the practical. The solemn introduction to the business of Boards and Committees, which the piety of the founders has appointed in most of our hospitals, is habitually neglected by many, and apt to be forgotten by all; but for truth of description and force of satire, Crabbe's clever description of the board-room and its *habitués* is worth occasional perusal.

It is undeniably the duty of a government to provide for the medical relief of the indigent, as well as for their sustenance and shelter; and we may moreover admit that it is the duty of government to purchase that relief on the cheapest terms that are consistent with goodness of quality. There is no more reason for paying too high a price for this, than for food, clothing, or lodging. There can be no "fancy fees" in such cases.

The duty, on the other hand, of individuals is, we conceive, not only to contribute that compulsory tax which is exacted under pains and penalties, to provide for the indigent a resource against absolute starvation—that mere antiseptic which is essential to prevent the whole body politic being poisoned *by its own partial corruptions*, but also

to do the work of charity actively and voluntarily in their own neighbourhood; not only to pay a poor-rate on compulsion, but to assess themselves for the good of their neighbours; not only to provide the workhouse and the Union doctor for the sick *pauper*, lest he "prove his right of settlement by falling sick of infectious fever," but to maintain hospitals for the sick *poor*. Happily this duty is very generally recognised, though the fiercest disputes are waged as to the manner of doing it. It is the duty of the state to provide for the pauper, and of individuals to strive that there be no paupers. This seems a somewhat large exaction, and it is; yet only those who strive to comply with it are fulfilling their social duties. Like all efforts, however, made from worthy and unselfish motives, it has a rich reward—a reward reaped, it may be, by those who never recognise the connection as cause and effect between it and the duty, but which may be seen in some degree by those who look for it with the eye of wisdom.

The metropolitan hospitals, and most others which have been founded and supported by private benevolence, are served by a medical staff whose services are gratuitous, and the appointments are sought by men of the highest promise, and frequently retained after the most brilliant success. The appointment to a hospital implies the putting forward a claim to a high place in public estimation, and a willingness to wait and to work until that claim shall be recognised. The duty is done in complete publicity, under the eye of governors, pupils, and fellow-practitioners, and is submitted to the severest scrutiny of which it is capable. This publicity, which, to a Frenchman, would be an attraction, is to nearly all Englishmen a mortification of the flesh. How few of our countrymen can make a decent speech in public, how few even a decent bow; and when we find a man who can do either particularly well, we are apt to suspect that he enjoys the distinction at the expense of some more sterling qualities, or more solid acquirements. This is not mere envy; it is national instinct, often wrong, no doubt, but right in the main.

In calling appointments to public hospitals gratuitous, we have not forgotten the fees from pupils; but these are obtained under a still severer test: the dislike of his colleagues, who suffer from his unpopularity, must be a severe visitation for an incapable man. It may be remarked, that all these guarantees for efficiency, whatever they may be worth, are most secured by the elections being much influenced by the medical governors of an hospital. No doubt the medical interest, like any other, may take a selfish turn, and require wholesome correction from without; but, on the whole, the high character of medical men as a body will be best supported by the suffrages of their professional brethren; this will put them above degrading appeals to the public, where the public can only be right by accident.

Now it must be evident that a very different class of practitioners is raised up and supported by hospitals, where adult education is actively going on, from that fostered by union workhouses. This is wholly irrespective of personal respectability, and of relative efficiency, which may be possessed by individuals amongst each; the offices in our profession which are meanest to the common eye are ennobled by rectitude of purpose and of character. From hospitals gratuitously attended the easy and affluent classes are supplied with men who bring to ample opportunities of observation a long continued course *of study.* Their ambition is a proof of *earnestness; their success* of capacity;

their popularity of their being appreciated. The evils which ever attend a state of highly wrought refinement are by these men viewed *en masse;* and their palliatives (for, alas! there are but few cures which the victims will accept), are studied attentively, and applied with all the benefits of extensive experience. The rich are taught that their luxuries are the medicines of the poor, and that wisely it has been said, " It is not for kings to drink wine, nor for princes strong drink." " Give strong drink to him that is ready to perish, and wine unto those that be of heavy hearts." That physician ill performs his mission who neglects to be the exponent to the rich of the wants of the poor; his habitual contemplation of men of all ranks in a state of helplessness and selfishness should not increase his power without enlarging his charity, and deepening his responsibility.

Much has been said of the disproportion between the opportunities which hospital appointments afford for information, and the results which have been thence secured to science. Much of this is no doubt true, and is in course of improvement; but surely no reflecting or even observing man can consider what has already been obtained from hospital physicians and surgeons as small compared with that from other sources. The system of registration, indeed, now so obviously expedient, has been neglected by all parties; but it may fairly be asked, whether the naval and military services, with their advantages of centralization and discipline, have produced more men of eminence, or more works of utility, than the civil hospital appointments.

With the most sincere desire to see the general practitioner well educated, well esteemed, and well paid, we are convinced that the habit of earning same and fame, during a long period of gratuitous practice, produces some advantages which would be forfeited on a different system. It is always painful to see the payment for medical attendance made the subject of bargain and contract, still more of litigation; the latter shocks us less on account of the loss to which our brother has been exposed, than from regret that his dignity should have been compromised by the occurrence. There must have been a grievous interruption of the honourable relation which ought to subsist between a patient and his medical adviser, before matters could have reached so far; and perhaps litigation is never advisable except in the case of fraudulent executors. It is much, certainly, to have established by legal process the right of remuneration for medical attendance, without proving the delivery of medicines to the required amount; it will forward the abolition of payments by medicine, so much to be desired; but we should beware how we bring into the market the higher and more subtle implements of our art, such as knowledge, skill, and moral character. The saving of the baggage is sometimes considered as glorious as a victory; but this can only be when an engagement has been unavoidable. When the doctor gives battle for his fees, his victory seldom secures a triumph.

· No doubt gratuitous practice will recede as civilization advances. There are evils and there are virtues appertaining to barbarism; mendicancy and hospitality are of this kind. The caravanserai and the fountain on the way side bring rest and refreshment to the traveller, and call forth blessings on the pious founder; but however picturesque and welcome in the primitive East, they are gladly exchanged by *the returning* Englishman for the house cistern and the hotel, though the one exposes him to the gentle extortions of a polite waiter, and the other to arrest for arrears of water rates. While there are poor in the land, however, the philanthropist and man of science need not lack welcome opportunities of practising gratuitously; nor, it may be remarked, need the legislator be alarmed lest able men be not found willing to undertake the drudgery of attending the poor.

COMPOUND DISLOCATION OF THE FIRST UPON THE SECOND PHALANX OF THE THUMB—

REDUCTION IMPOSSIBLE—RESECTION OF THE HEAD OF THE FIRST PHALANX—CURE.

By G. W. NORRIS, M.D.
Surgeon to the Pennsylvania Hospital.

NEILL LARKIN, a stout drayman, ætat. 28, while engaged in unhitching his horse, had the end of his left thumb accidently entangled in a link of the drawing chain, when the horse starting suddenly, dragged him some distance, and produced the accident just mentioned. He was brought to the hospital late in the evening of February 17th, a couple of hours after its occurrence, when strong and well-directed efforts were unsuccessfully made to reduce it, the clove hitch being attached to the extremity, after a first failure with the hand alone. On the following morning I found the head of the first phalanx protruding considerably inwards through a wound which embraced more than one-half of the circumference of the finger; another effort at reduction was now attempted by bending the luxated phalanx and endeavouring to push its projecting head over that of the adjoining bone, but failing in this, I determined to remove the protruding extremity of the bone, which was at once done with the metacarpal saw, to the extent of three or four lines, after which the parts were easily replaced. The edges of the wound were then drawn together with strips of narrow adhesive plaster, and the part covered with dry lint, the hand and fore-arm being secured upon a splint. After the third day, the dressings were daily made, the part being only covered with simple ointment. No unpleasant symptoms followed.

March 23d.—Wound entirely closed; on the 26th he was discharged, and on the 13th of April he called at the hospital, at which time he had good use of the thumb with some motion at the point of injury.

The difficulty of reduction in cases of simple luxations of the phalangeal articulations, even when the patient is seen soon after the accident has occurred, is well known; and the same difficulty exists in reducing and retaining in place compound injuries of this class. So hard is the reduction to effect, that it is asserted upon the authority of Bromfield, that the extending force has been increased to such a degree as to tear off the second joint in efforts to reduce the first. In compound luxations of the thumb, when found irreducible upon the application of a moderate degree of force, I believe the best practice to be that which was pursued in Larkin's case, viz., to saw off the end of the projecting bone. If the wound be large, and this be not done, observation shows that, even when the part can be reduced, the dislocated end will in the majority of cases become displaced, as the inflammation necessarily following it prevents the application of a sufficient degree of force by bandages and splints, to retain it in its natural position. One case of this kind I have myself witnessed, and another instance which occurred in Guy's Hospital has recently been published, in which, although the phalanx was easily reduced immediately after the accident, so much inflammation and constitutional disturbance occurred, as to make it necessary to remove the splints and other dressings which had been applied, and resort to cataplasms; the patient being ultimately cured, after entire loss of the first, and exfoliation of the extremity of the second phalanx. Resection of the phalangeal extremity is the practice recommended by Sir A. Cooper, in compound dislocations of of these parts, when difficulty is experienced in their reduction, and has often been done with good success. Gooch states that he sawed off the head of the second bone of the thumb, and that a new joint afterwards formed. In two instances, where the head of the metacarpal bone of the thumb was dislocated towards the palm, accompanied with wound, and reduction was difficult, the protruding parts were successfully sawn off by Mr. Evans. Bobe, Wardrop, and Roux, have all been successful in like cases. The bad effects resulting from those injuries where the head of the bone is replaced, and which seem to be at least in part owing to the force necessarially made use of, and the state of tension afterwards kept up in the surrounding soft parts, by its return, has been often noticed. An instance came under my care, in which high inflammation and tetanus ensued upon *the injury* where this practice was pursued; *and Mr. S. Cooper reduced* a case at the

North London Hospital, which was followed by severe inflammation, terminating in death, a week after the accident.—*American Journal.*

ON THE PREPARATION OF MURIATIC ACID.
By Heumann.

THE preparation of pure muriatic acid is one of the easiest operations, provided that we follow Gregory,[*] and employ one atom by weight of chloride of sodium, and two of sulphuric acid. The latter must be diluted with water enough to bring down the specific gravity to 1.6, for which purpose from nine to twelve ounces of water will be required to 2½lbs. of fuming Nordhausen acid. This proportion was recommended by Dr. Wittstein[†] as the best for effecting the entire decomposition of the chloride of sodium. Moreover, the salt must be perfectly free from iron, and the sulphuric acid from arsenic.

A common glass alembic serves as the vessel for the development of the muriatic acid gas; and a glass tube, twice bent at right angles, conducts it into a receiver containing pure water, which must constantly be kept as cold as possible. By a proper management of the fire, the development and absorption of the muriatic acid gas go on easily and uninterruptedly.

The muriatic acid thus obtained varies in specific gravity according to the quantity of water employed. It is perfectly colourless, and is free from sulphuric acid, from sulphurous acid, from chlorine, iron, and arsenic.

All sulphuric acid employed in pharmacy must necessarily be tested for arsenic, as there is English sulphuric acid now in the market which abounds in this pernicious contamination. I lately examined an acid of this kind from a manufactory on the Rhine, which, when tested with sulphuretted hydrogen gas, afforded 0.7 of a grain of sulphuretted arsenic in an ounce, equal to 0.42622 of a grain of arsenic. If an acid of this kind is employed, the whole quantity of arsenic is found in the muriatic acid, not a trace of it being discoverable in the bisulphate of soda which remains.

This is the source of the arsenic so frequently found in the muriatic acid of commerce, which renders it totally unfit for pharmaceutical use. The method of detecting arsenic in muriatic acid is well known. —*Annals of Chymistry.*

---

[*] See Liebig's Annals of Pharmacy and Chymistry, vol. xli.
[†] Buchner's Repert. Band xiii.

EMPYEMA TERMINATING FAVOURABLY BY SPONTANEOUS OPENING.

THE subject of this case was a man of a stout, robust appearance, who presented the usual symptoms of acute inflammatory fever, accompanied with cough, dyspnœa, and a fixed pain near to the inferior border of the left scapula, extending across the posterior surface of the chest.

On the 3d of October, 1838, while engaged in raising a heavy piece of timber, " he felt something give a crack" in the foregoing position, which, however, did not prevent him continuing his employment during the entire day ; but on the following day, while rowing a boat, he became chilly and squeamish, and was forced to bed, when the above symptoms made their appearance.

Mr. S. saw him on the 5th of October, and took blood to syncope, and prescribed an antimonial saline mixture, some powders containing calomel and antimonial powder, and applied a sinapism to the painful part.

On the following day, there being no improvement, the blood-letting was repeated, a large blister was applied, and the medicine continued. The sputa, which now became more copious, from its rusty character, and the ordinary stethoscopic indications, enabled me to consider the inflammatory action to have extended to the substance of the lung. The usual antiphlogistic measures were continued ; blisters repeated from time to time ; and in the course of a few days, the acute febrile symptoms subsided ; but there still remained the fixed pain near the scapula, frequent cough, copious expectoration, and a total inability to lie upon the right side, any attempt at which greatly aggravated the cough and dyspnœa. Very little benefit was derived from the treatment adopted ; colliquative perspirations were superadded, to ameliorate which, mineral acid and quinine were had recourse to.

Towards the end of December debility and emaciation had advanced progressively, and a fulness was observed over the left side of the chest, although no difference in its capacity was found upon measurement ; percussion on the part elicited a dull sound ; and the respiratory murmur was very faint, although audible over the subclavian region ; and a few days after, a soft tumor appeared on the fifth intercostal space, an inch below, and to the outside of the left nipple.

The next day Mr. S. found that the surface of the tumor had ulcerated, and the patient lay bathed in purulent matter, the bed and clothes being fully saturated with it. The purulent matter continued to flow daily from the aperture, and some came afterwards by the mouth. The patient was afterwards kept comfortable by evacuating the purulent matter night and morning to the extent of a pint, which was facilitated by turning him to the left side, and requesting a full inspiration and a cough to be made, when a soft pledget with a quantity of tow and a bandage was applied.

The cough and dyspnœa were now greatly relieved ; a generous diet, with porter, together with the acid and quinine, were prescribed, under which he gradually regained so much strength as allowed him to go out of the doors by March 1839 ; and henceforward he continued still so weakly as only to be able to walk a very short distance, while the purulent matter was continued to be evacuated night and morning, in nearly the same quantities as at first, by removing the bandages, &c. until three weeks ago, when blood appeared instead of purulent matter, and the wound thereafter closed, leaving a flattened, thimble-like cavity, into which the point of the finger could be introduced ; and he has since progressed in strength.

Upon examination, the movements of both sides of the chest are equable and the respiratory murmur natural, as also the sound elicited by percussion.

The successful result of this case may, perhaps, be regarded as a support to the practice generally adopted, of gradually evacuating such collections, as it is very probable that only as much purulent matter flowed in the first instances as reduced it to the level of the aperture.—*Edinburgh Medical and Surgical Journal.*

LECTURES ON ANIMAL CHEMISTRY.

To the Editor of the Medical Gazette.

SIR,

HAVING lately heard from some members of the Apothecaries' Company that a course of lectures are being delivered by Professor Brande on Animal Chemistry, it appears to me, that if the lectures delivered to the members only were extended to the licentiates, I am sure they would gladly avail themselves of the privilege of attending ; and as the lectures delivered at the College of Physicians are open to the licentiates of its body, and the same at the College of Surgeons, I do hope that the Society of Apothecaries will confer the same boon on its licentiates. Trusting that this appeal may not have been made in vain, and as an advocate for whatever is calculated to advance professional knowledge, I am sure you will reciprocate that wish.—I remain, sir,

Your obedient servant,

AN OLD LICENTIATE.

London, May 24, 1842.

SOCIETY FOR RELIEF OF
WIDOWS AND ORPHANS OF
MEDICAL MEN IN LONDON
AND ITS VICINITY.

THE annual dinner of the above Society, which was postponed in consequence of the lamented death of the Duke of Sussex, the Patron, is now appointed to take place on Saturday, the 3d of June. H. R. H. the Duke of Cambridge has signified to the Stewards his intention to preside on the occasion.

MR. TYRRELL.

WE regret very much to record the sudden death of Mr. Tyrrell, of St. Thomas's Hospital, which took place on the 23d inst. in consequence, it is said, of disease of the heart.

BOOKS RECEIVED.

A Practical Treatise on the Diseases of the Testis, and of the Spermatic Cord and Scrotum; with Illustrations. By T. B. Curling, Lecturer on Surgery, &c.

Austria: its Literary, Scientific, and Medical Institutions, &c. &c. By W. R. Wilde, M.R.I.A. &c.

The Plea of Humanity and Common Sense against Surgical Operations for the Cure of Impediments of Speech. By James Wright, Esq.

The Educational and Subsidiary Provisions of the Birmingham Royal School of Medicine and Surgery, set forth in a Letter to the Rev. Dr. Wilson Warneford, LL.D. The whole being intended to shew the importance and practicability of applying the means actually possessed to some arrangement for providing *Collegiately* for the Board, Lodging, and Tutelary Care of its Pupils during their Residence at Birmingham for the Purposes of Study. By the Rev. Vaughan Thomas, B.D. Vicar of Stoneleigh, Warwickshire.

APOTHECARIES' HALL.

LIST OF GENTLEMEN WHO HAVE RECEIVED CERTIFICATES.

Thursday, May 18, 1843.

J. T. Pearce, Camelford, Cornwall.—C. Bond, Long Sutton, Somerset.—B. D. Adams, Nettlested, Kent.—H. M. Holman, Hurstpierpoint, Sussex.—H. S. Wharton, Brecon, South Wales.—C. Hooper, Kennington. —J. P. M'Donald, Bristol.—F. Berrington, London.—W. Folwell, London.—H. Stokes, Gibraltar.—W. M. Neale, London.—E. Russell, Bloxwich, Staffordshire.—H. Bell, Hopton, Great Yarmouth.—N. Buckley, *Rochdale Lane.* — T. E. Drinkwater, Ashford, *Derbyshire.*—E. J. L. Whitmore, Bristol.

ROYAL COLLEGE OF SURGEONS.

LIST OF GENTLEMEN ADMITTED MEMBERS.

Wednesday, May 17, 1843.
T. Lloyd.—T. Willis.—J. J. Fox.—S. S. Alford.—J. H. Browne.—R. Leach.— W. Smith. — P. Berry.—E. Labrow.—G. T. Heath.—B. R. Mudd.

Friday, May 19.
C. Girdlestone.—F. R. Manson.—W. J. Price.—W. M'Cheane.—W. M. Pinder.—J. Carter.—H. Dixon.—W. R. James.—J. S. H. Williams.—W. Davy.

A TABLE OF MORTALITY FOR THE
METROPOLIS,

Shewing the number of deaths from all causes registered in the week ending Saturday, May 6, 1843.

Small Pox	12
Measles	28
Scarlatina	10
Hooping Cough	54
Croup	10
Thrush	3
Diarrhœa	3
Dysentery	0
Cholera	0
Influenza	0
Ague	1
Typhus	58
Erysipelas	6
Syphilis	0
Hydrophobia	0
Diseases of the Brain, Nerves, and Senses	139
Diseases of the Lungs and other Organs of Respiration	273
Diseases of the Heart and Blood-vessels	25
Diseases of the Stomach, Liver, and other Organs of Digestion	64
Diseases of the Kidneys, &c.	7
Childbed	8
Ovarian Dropsy	0
Disease of Uterus, &c.	2
Rheumatism	6
Diseases of Joints, &c.	4
Carbuncle	1
Ulcer	0
Fistula	0
Diseases of Skin, &c.	0
Diseases of Uncertain Seat	104
Old Age or Natural Decay	49
Deaths by Violence, Privation, or Intemperance	14
Causes not specified	2
Deaths from all Causes	863

METEOROLOGICAL JOURNAL.

April 1843.	THERMOMETER.		BAROMETER.	
Wednesday 17	from 46 to 52		29·44 to 29·64	
Thursday . 18	41	55	29 76	29·85
Friday . . 19	44	56	29·85	29·86
Saturday . 20	46	60	29·80	29·71
Sunday . 21	48	59	29·63	29·60
Monday . . 22	40	56	29·62	29·64
Tuesday . 23	41	61	29·64	29·65

Wind variable, N.E. and S.E. prevailing. Generally cloudy, with frequent rain: thunder on the evening of the 23d.
Rain fallen, 1 inch, and ·31 of an inch.

CHARLES HENRY ADAMS.

NOTICE.—We shall be glad to have the paper on "Molecular Motion."

WILSON & OGILVY, 57, Skinner Street, London.

THE

LONDON MEDICAL GAZETTE,

BEING A

WEEKLY JOURNAL

OF

𝔐𝔢𝔡𝔦𝔠𝔦𝔫𝔢 𝔞𝔫𝔡 𝔱𝔥𝔢 ℭ𝔬𝔩𝔩𝔞𝔱𝔢𝔯𝔞𝔩 𝔖𝔠𝔦𝔢𝔫𝔠𝔢𝔰.

FRIDAY, JUNE 2, 1843.

LECTURES

ON THE

THEORY AND PRACTICE OF MIDWIFERY,

Delivered in the Theatre of St. George's Hospital,

BY ROBERT LEE, M.D. F.R.S.

LECTURE XXVIII.

On the application of the forceps.

THE midwifery forceps was invented and perfected by the Chamberlens about the middle of the 17th century, but it was first described by Chapman in 1733. " Almost every candidate for celebrity," observes Mr. Streeter, " has thought it necessary to modify the instrument; Dr. Churchill has given figures of more than fifty varieties." In the last half of the 18th century, or a few years earlier, the forceps had been altered by Mesnard, Gregoire, Rathlaw, Smellie, Levret, Bing, Burton, De Wind, Pugh, Wallis Johnson, Fried, Leake, Petit, Van De Laar, Coutouly, Pean, Sleurs, Orme, Lowder, Young, Aitken, Mayer, Starke, Saxtorph, Osborn, Denman, Hamilton, Haighton, J. Clarke, and Thynne. [Müller's plates were here exhibited, in which many of these instruments have been represented.] Dr. William Hunter appears to have been almost the only distinguished accoucheur, who lived during that period, who considered it unnecessary to modify the shape of the forceps. The instrument has undergone many changes during the present century, but that form which I prefer greatly above all others is the Chamberlen forceps, with the lock and wooden handles of Smellie—in fact, Denman's short forceps covered with leather; because it is easily applied, takes a fast hold of the head, and it may be employed with less risk to the mother, than the forceps of Drs. Hopkins, David Davis,

Naegele, Siebold, and others. But in truth I attach comparatively little importance to the shape and dimensions of the forceps you use, and think it nearly a matter of indifference whether it has a pivot lock or Smellie's lock, and whether the handles consist of wood or metal, provided the case will justify the use of the forceps where it is had recourse to, and you know the principles which ought invariably to guide you in its employment. The observations which have been made upon the forceps during the last 110 years, have proved that it is not adapted to cases of difficult labour, in which the os uteri, vagina, and other soft parts, are in a rigid, swollen, inflamed, and undilatable state; where the umbilical cord is unusually short, or is twisted once or several times around the neck and trunk of the child, where the child is hydrocephalic, or the head greatly exceeds the natural size, and where the pelvis is obstructed by tumors, or much distorted by rickets or malacosteon. It is now admitted by all practitioners in this country that the forceps ought not to be employed where a great disproportion exists between the head of the child and pelvis from any cause. It is chiefly in cases of protracted and difficult labour, from feeble, irregular, or partial uterine action, from passions of the mind, original or accidental debility in the mother, and other constitutional causes which impair the energy of the brain, and nervous system of the uterus, that the forceps is used with advantage, and where, if any disproportion exists between the fœtus and pelvis, it is only in a slight degree. The forceps is not applied because there is a great deficiency of space in the pelvis, a great want of due proportion between the head and pelvis, but because there is a want of power in the uterus to propel the child through it, the want of which power we endeavour to supply with the forceps. This is the only legitimate ground on which we can proceed in the application of the forceps, whether it be exhaustion, convulsion, hæmorrhage, or whatever the circumstance may be which renders immediate delivery necessary to preserve the life of the mother and child. It is not for our our own convenience, to spare ourselves the anxiety and fatigue of a protracted attendance upon any case of labour, to acquire skill and dexterity in the use of the forceps, that the instrument is to be applied, nor because it is in our power to do so, but in consequence of certain local and constitutional symptoms appearing in the parent, or because the child is in danger from the long-continued pressure, that we have recourse to artificial delivery. The gradual cessation of labour pains, and the descent of the head being arrested, are unquestionably the best indications we can have for the propriety of the interference of art. If the uterine contractions cease, and the head, swollen and compressed, becomes arrested or impacted in the pelvis, and there is exhaustion, fever, and disturbance of the brain, and we believe that the head of the child will not be expelled by the natural efforts, it is our duty to endeavour without delay to extract it with the forceps. To apply the instrument, when it is known with absolute certainty that the child is dead, would betray, to use the mildest expression, the highest degree of human insensibility and folly.

In a great proportion of cases they are first labours in which the forceps is required; which proves that the difficulty frequently depends on the soft parts. It is not from the duration of the process, so much as from the condition of the patient, that you are to judge of the necessity for interference. In some women, whose nervous energy is feeble, exhaustion, delirium, or some other unfavourable symptom, occurs before the labour has continued 24 hours; in others there is no unfavourable symptom witnessed, though it is greatly protracted beyond this period. In general it is a very good practical rule, and well calculated to prevent the rash and unwarrantable use of the forceps, " that the head of a child shall have rested six hours as low as the perineum, that is, in a situation which would allow of their application before the forceps are applied, though the pains should have ceased during that time." But there are exceptions to this rule, and cases occur of rapid exhaustion, or some accident takes place suddenly, in which it would be wrong to comply with it. The membranes must be ruptured, and the os uteri fully dilated, before the forceps can be safely applied. The head may not have wholly escaped from the uterus, but the greater part must have done so, to render it possible to use the forceps without great risk. *If the whole circumference of the os uteri can be felt, you must not think of the for-*

ceps, and the greatest care is required, though the posterior lip has gone up beyond the reach of the finger, if the anterior lip and cervix can be felt between the head and symphysis pubis. I have never met with a case in which the forceps was satisfactorily applied before the os uteri was fully dilated, and the head had descended so low that an ear could be felt. "Before the completion of the first stage of a labour," says Dr. Denman, " that is, before the os uteri be completely dilated and the membranes broken, the use of the forceps can never come into contemplation; because the difficulties before occurring may depend upon causes which do not require their use, or if required, they could not be applied with safety or propriety before those changes were made." In almost every case, " says Dr. Burns, " where the forceps are beneficial, the head has so far entered the pelvis as to have the ear corresponding to the inner surface of the pubes, and the cranial bones touching the perineum." " No case," observes Dr. Merriman, " is to be esteemed eligible for the application of the forceps until the ear of the child can be distinctly felt."

Smellie invented a pair of long forceps, which he sometimes used when he found the head of the child so much forward over the os pubis, by the unusual projection of the sacrum and lower lumbar vertebra, that he could not push the handles of the short forceps far enough back to include within the blades the bulky part of the head which lay over the pubes. To remedy this inconvenience he contrived a long pair, curved on one side and convex on the other; but these, he says, ought never to be used except when the head is small; for when the head is large, and the greater part of it remains above the brim, a part of the woman may be inflamed and contused by the exertion of too much force. Where the vertex presents, but only an inconsiderable part of the head, resembling the small end of a sugar-loaf, is forced down into the pelvis, after a protracted labour, we may infer that the head is either too large, or the pelvis too narrow. In these cases, indeed, a long pair of forceps may take such firm hold, that with great force and the strong purchase the head will be delivered; but such violence is commonly fatal to the woman, by causing such an inflammation, and perhaps laceration, of the parts, as is attended with mortification. In order to disable young practitioners from running such risks, and to free myself from the temptation of using too much force, I have *always used and recommended* the forceps so short in the handles that they cannot be used with such violence as will endanger the woman's life, though the purchase of them is sufficient to extract the head when one-half or two-thirds of it are equal to, or past, the upper or narrow part of the pelvis. Smellie was so fully aware of the danger of fatal contusion and laceration of the uterus and vagina necessarily incurred by the application of the long forceps, when the head of the child remained above the brim of the pelvis, that he did not venture to exhibit the instrument to the pupils of his class, from the dread that it would be misapplied; and it appears *he always used* and recommended the short forceps. Levret likewise invented a pair of long forceps, convex on one edge, and concave on the other, which have been extensively employed on the continent, especially in France and Germany, for the purpose of drawing the head of the child into the cavity of the pelvis when the brim is contracted. The common French midwifery forceps, represented in these figures, will give you some idea of the instrument recommended by Levret, though not precisely the same :—

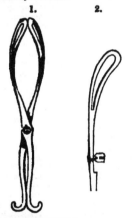

1.   2.

1. The instrument closed.
2. A partial front view of one blade, to shew the curve and peg by which it is locked.

You will meet with two very great difficulties in attempting to apply the long forceps. The first is, that the head of the child always lies transversely, or diagonally, at the brim of the pelvis; so that if the blades of the instrument are passed up along its sides, which all admit they must be, one blade will be applied over the occiput, and the other over the forehead; and you can have no hold of the head in this way upon which you can depend. If you make the experiment upon a dead child, as I shall now do before you, you will at once be satisfied that the hold which the forceps has of the head is so insecure that it would be

impossible to overcome any considerable resistance with the blades thus applied to the forehead and occiput; over the sides of the head they give you a firm hold. And in actual practice, in all the cases where I have seen an attempt made to deliver with the blades of the long forceps applied over the forehead and occiput, the instrument has soon lost its hold, and has slipped off the head, where any considerable extracting force has been applied. But if the instrument should not slip, the compression of the occiput and forehead would increase the length of the short diameter of the head, which corresponds with the contracted conjugate diameter of the brim, and the result would be an increase of the disproportion between the head and pelvis; the size of the head would be increased in the wrong direction—in fact, where it is required to be lessened. If you look at this plate of Maygrier [exhibiting it], you will be convinced of the truth of this.

But besides, before the greater part of the head has passed through the brim of the pelvis, the os uteri is never sufficiently dilated to allow of the long forceps being applied without the greatest danger. " The delivery of a female with the forceps, when the os uteri is fully dilated," observes Dr. Collins, " the soft parts relaxed, the head resting on the perineum, or nearly so, and the pelvis of sufficient size to permit the attendant to reach the ear with the finger, is so simple, that any individual with moderate experience may readily effect it. I have no hesitation in asserting, that to use it under other circumstances is not only an abuse of the instrument, but most hazardous to the patient. It is from being thoroughly convinced of these facts, by long and extensive observation, that I consider the forceps quite inapplicable when the head becomes fixed in the pelvis, and that the ear cannot be reached by the finger, except by violence, in consequence of disproportion existing between the head and pelvis, either owing to the former being unusually large, or the latter under size; in most instances measuring little more than three inches from pubes to sacrum, and in others less than this. When we consider that the blades of the smallest sized forceps used in Britain, even when completely closed, measure from 3½th inches to 3½, it is clear that were the bones of the pelvis denuded of their soft parts there would not be space to admit of their application. The French forceps measure, when closed, from blade to blade, on the upper side 2½ inches, and are about ⅜th wider on the opposite side, meeting at the point of the blades to within ⅓th of an inch. Were we even to overlook altogether the safety of the mother, where the child's head measures 13½, 14½, or 15 inches in circumference, is so compressed, as it must be when the instrument is closed, there can scarcely be a hope of life. Of course, where the pelvis is roomy, this compression of the head, so as to close the forceps, is unnecessary, and in such cases the child is uninjured. How is it possible, with the forceps, to drag a child through a pelvis where there is not space, except by force, to introduce (as is commonly said) a straw, or where the smallest flexible catheter cannot, in some instances, be passed into the bladder ? The results I have witnessed from such practice were most distressing : in some, the neck of the bladder, or urethra, either lacerated, or the injury by pressure from the forceps so great as to produce sloughing and consequent incontinence of urine ; in others, the recto-vaginal septum destroyed ; either of which renders the sufferer miserable for life ; and in two cases, where the mouth of the womb was imperfectly dilated, so much injury inflicted on this part as to terminate in death. Such melancholy consequences strongly show the necessity of having recourse to the forceps with great caution, so as to avoid the abuse of an instrument which, when judiciously applied, is occasionally most beneficial. Almost all the unfavourable results may be prevented by using the instrument only when necessary for the safety of the patient, at the same time attending to the circumstances already stated, which are dwelt upon by many of our best writers on this subject when treating of the nature of the case in which it is eligible." The accuracy of these remarks is fully confirmed by all the forceps cases which have come under my observation, and which exceed 60 in number. Four of the mothers whose cases (55) are related in the First Report of my Clinical Midwifery, died from the rash and inconsiderate use of the forceps ; seven had the perineum more or less injured ; one the recto-vaginal septum torn ; five were left with cicatrices of the vagina after sloughing ; and one with an incurable vesico-vaginal fistula. In none did any benefit result from the instrument before the greater part of the head of the child had passed through the brim of the pelvis, and the orifice of the uterus was fully dilated. In one case only was the forceps advantageous, when the blades were applied and locked with great difficulty, and great force required to extract the head of the child. Only seventeen of the children were born alive and lived. In protracted labours, when the head has made no sensible advance for hours, I repeat once more, and becomes compressed, the scalp puffy and swollen, the vagina dry, hot, and tender, the discharges offensive, and when the bladder cannot be emptied without the catheter, it is dangerous *to trust longer* to the natural efforts. If, *along with these symptoms, there is tender-*

ness of the abdomen, fever, incoherence, restlessness, and exhaustion, delaying long to deliver is invariably followed by the most injurious consequences. But if the os uteri is not fully dilated, and the greater part of the head has not passed through the brim, the forceps cannot be employed with advantage.

Most of the authors who have recommended the long forceps to be employed have been fully aware of the danger of the instrument, and the necessity for extreme caution in its use. " Sometimes it is useful," says Dr. Hamilton, " to employ a lengthened pair of forceps : but as in operating with that instrument the parts of the woman in contact with its blades must inevitably be pressed upon in a degree proportionate to the length of the instrument, the extent of its motion, or, in other words, to the force of the operator working with it, it is a very hazardous expedient in the hands of the inexperienced." When Dr. Hamilton was in London, twelve or thirteen years ago, the use of the long forceps was one of the subjects of conversation which I had with him, and I was astonished when he informed me that he had entirely for some time laid aside the short forceps. On further inquiry, however, it appeared that in no case did he ever use the long forceps until an ear could be felt ; thus admitting that he never employed the long forceps where it was not possible to deliver with the short forceps, and to derive all the advantage that could be obtained from such means with much less risk. If I recollect right, Dr. Hamilton stated on that occasion that he had used the forceps, long and short, only about forty times in the whole course of his life. In respect to the frequency with which he employed the forceps, his practice probably coincided with that of Dr. Joseph Clarke, who says, in his valuable Report of the Dublin Lying-in Hospital, " Cases of convulsion excepted, I have rarely had reason to be well pleased with the effects of extracting instruments, and not unfrequently have I had much reason to deprecate their evil consequences. Whenever labour is protracted to a dangerous length, by unusual resistance, there is nothing but mischief to be expected from their application, but when the expelling powers are impaired by debilitating diseases, the interposition of an artificial extracting power is more rational and justifiable. Let it be remembered that in the hospital such means were employed in one of 728 cases, and in private practice it is so long since I have had occasion to use, or even to think of using them, that I am persuaded a fair opportunity of applying forceps with good effect will not occur to a rational practitioner in one of 1000 cases."

Where the child is dead, where a great disproportion exists between its head and the pelvis from any cause, and the os uteri is imperfectly dilated and the parts swollen and rigid, and an ear cannot be felt, and circumstances occur demanding immediate delivery, recourse must be had to the perforator, and not to the forceps. You will never, I hope, think of applying the forceps in a secret or clandestine manner. If you were so thoughtless as to attempt to do this, you would not succeed without the attempt being discovered, and your rashness and imprudence exposed. But you might introduce the vectis or lever over the head without the patient or nurse being aware of the fact; and this is one of the many strong objections which I have to the instrument, of which the following figures are representations.

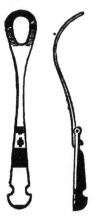

It has a joint to render it more portable, and some practitioners carry it in their pocket to every case of labour they attend, and make use of it without apprising the patient. Such conduct, I look upon, with Dr. Collins, " as unjustifiable in the extreme, and am happy to think it is the practice of those only who have little character to lose."

In all cases of protracted and difficult labour in which you consider it requisite to employ the forceps, or to perform the operation of craniotomy, or any other operation in midwifery, you will promote your own peace of mind and professional interests, and the welfare of your patients, by previously consulting another experienced practitioner, whenever it is practicable to do so. When exhausted with fatigue and watching, we are not in a condition to form a sound opinion respecting the necessity for the interference of art, and it is agreeable in all cases of difficulty and danger to have the responsibility divided by

a consultation, and mistakes in practice prevented by every means in our power. After all the circumstances of the case have been deliberately considered in consultation, and the necessity for the employment of the forceps satisfactorily proved to exist, it is right, before proceeding to apply the blades, to state to the husband and relations, and even to the patient herself, if she is in a condition to comprehend, the reasons why you have resolved to trust no longer to the efforts of nature, and even to explain to her what you are going to do. All women know well the danger they incur when delivered with instruments, and dread being cut or torn by them. This fear is often removed, and the entire consent of the patient obtained, by shewing to her one or both of the blades unlocked of the short forceps, covered with soft leather, which makes it not only in appearance but in reality a safer instrument than when the steel blades are bare.

Having obtained the patient's consent to the application of the forceps, and a promise to endure the pain with as much steadiness and resolution as possible, let her lie on the left side, with the nates close to the edge of the bed, and the knees bent and drawn up towards the abdomen. Let the nurse support the right thigh, and keep the knees separate, and let the patient take hold of the hands of a steady person before her, who can control her feelings on the occasion. Ascertain by passing the catheter that the bladder is empty before you proceed further. Then take a blade of the forceps by the handle in your left hand, and pass all your fingers of your right hand in a conical form covered with lard slowly into the orifice of the vagina, and if it is a first child, and the parts are contracted, gently dilate them, and press back the perineum. When this has been sufficiently effected, pass the four fingers of the right hand forward into the vagina deeply, as far indeed as the root of the thumb, between the head of the child and front of the pelvis. Dr. Denman says, " the forefinger of the right hand should be passed between the ossa pubis and the head of the child to the ear." I would recommend you to pass all the fingers completely over the side of the head, so as to feel the ear, and to determine positively to which side of the pelvis the occiput is directed. If you introduce only one finger, or all the fingers, in the manner represented in these plates of M. Moreau and Dr. D. Davis [exhibiting them], you cannot possibly know what the actual position of the head is before you introduce the blades, and may turn the head in the wrong direction. I believe it is possible in every case, and I consider it necessary, to ascertain exactly the position of the head before passing the first blade of the forceps. If the head is so firmly impacted that you cannot pass the fingers not only to the ear and side of the head, behind the front of the pelvis, but completely around the whole head, you will do nothing but mischief with the forceps. Pass, then, the four fingers of the right hand completely over the side of the head and ear behind the symphysis pubis, for in a vast proportion of cases an ear is felt in this situation, and not at either side of the pelvis, and when you have determined the position of the head, the point of the blade in the left hand is to be slowly and cautiously, without any force, slid up between the head and your fingers, till the blade is closely applied over the side of the head, and the lock is about an inch and a half from the fore part of the orifice of the vagina. When you begin to pass the blade, you see in the phantom that its handle is directed backward to the perineum, but as its point slides along the convex surface of the head, the handle is gradually brought forward towards the pubes. You may either have the first blade held firmly in its situation by an assistant, or you may keep it in its place with the ring and little finger of your left hand, while you are engaged in passing the second blade over the opposite side of the head, which is usually attended with greater difficulty than the first. I prefer entrusting the first blade to another person, while I am engaged in passing up the four fingers of my left hand as far as possible over the side of the head in the hollow of the sacrum, and conducting the second blade with my right hand over it. When this has been done in a satisfactory manner, the blades lock with the greatest ease—they come together almost spontaneously. But where the blades have not been properly applied to the opposite and corresponding sides of the head, but one is toward the forehead and another to the side of the occiput, the extremities of the handles are in different directions, and the blades cannot be made to lock without drawing the handles forcibly together. Where this happens, the best plan is to withdraw one or both blades, and to reintroduce them in such a manner that they shall cover exactly the opposite sides of the head.

When the blades are thus applied, take care that no part of the mother is included in the lock, before you begin to extract. When a pain comes on grasp the handles of the instrument in your right hand, place your hand over or above the handles, and bring them slowly forward towards the symphysis pubis, and after keeping them there for an instant move them backward slowly and steadily towards the perineum, exerting upon the head a slight degree of extracting force. This action must be repeated, and at the same time you should endeavour to turn the face round into the hollow of the sacrum. When the labour pain goes off, take the pressure of the blades of the forceps from the head, and merely keep the handles together to prevent the instrument from slipping, and renew the traction with the same caution, but with a little more force. Until the head is brought so low as to press upon the perineum and distend it, the extracting force should be directed backward, but when the head has advanced, and the perineum becomes very prominent, the action should be directed more forward toward the pubes. In some cases, by the exertion of very little extracting force, and in a very short time, sometimes even during a single pain, the head is brought down so as to distend the perineum, the ears are placed to the sides of the pelvis, and the face is in the hollow of the sacrum, and further advanced than is represented in the following figure.

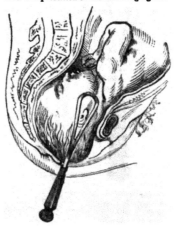

In other cases a considerable period elapses, and much force is required before the head can be brought into this situation, and occasionally we do not succeed in bringing it so low after exerting all the force we dare employ. When the head begins to advance through the os externum, and the perineum is greatly distended, you must change the direction in which you extract. Now place your hand under or below the handles of the forceps, and gently draw the head during the pains forward to the symphysis pubis away from the perineum, and move it gently from side to side. It is necessary to observe the condition of the perineum while the head is passing, and to regulate every movement with the forceps, by seeing what degree of pressure it is able to bear, and to support it with the left hand most carefully when it is rigid: imitate nature, by allowing the head to press against it for a considerable time, without exerting any considerable extracting force. The utmost circumspection is required in this part of the operation, and in some cases, where you see the perineum beginning to tear in spite of all your care, the best plan is to remove the blades of the forceps, and leave the expulsion of the head to the natural efforts.

I shall read to you Dr. Denman's account of the application and action of the forceps, which is remarkably full, plain, and easy to be understood, for the purpose of supplying any omissions or deficiencies in the previous description, and to make you more familiar with the subject.

" The first part of the operation consists in passing the fore-finger of the right hand behind the ossa pubis and the head of the child to the ear; then, taking the part of the forceps to be first introduced by the handle in the left hand, the point of the blade is to be slowly conducted between the head of the child and the finger till the instrument touches the ear: there can be no difficulty or hazard in carrying the instrument thus far, because it will be guided, and in some measure shielded, by the finger. But the further introduction must be made with a slow semi-rotatory motion, keeping the point of the blade not rigidly, yet closely, to the head of the child, by raising the handle toward the pubes. In this manner the blade must be carried gently along the head till the lock reaches the external parts near the anterior angle of the pudendum. The point of the blade, while introducing, sometimes hitches upon the ear of the child, and it then requires a little elevation. But when it has passed the ear, and is beyond the guidance of the finger, should there be any check to the introduction either of this or the other blade, it should be withdrawn a little, to give us an opportunity of discovering the cause of the obstacle, which we must never strive to overcome by violence, though we must proceed with firmness. When the first blade is properly introduced, it must be held steadily in its place by pressing the handle towards the pubes, and it will be a guide in the introduction and application of the second blade. Let the second blade be introduced in this manner. Keep the blade first introduced in its place with the two lesser fingers of the left hand, and carry the fore-finger of the same hand between the perineum and head of the child as high as you can reach. Then take the second blade of the forceps by the handle in the right hand, and, conveying the point between the finger placed within the perineum and the head of the child, conduct the instrument, with the precautions before mentioned, so far that the lock shall touch the interior part

of the perineum, or even press it a little backwards. In order to fix the two blades thus introduced, that which was placed towards the pubes must be slowly withdrawn and carried so far backwards that it can be locked with the second blade retained in its first position; and care must be taken that nothing be entangled in the lock by passing the finger round it. When the forceps are locked, it will be found convenient to tie the handles together with sufficient firmness to prevent them from sliding or changing their position when they are not held in the hand, but not in such a manner as to increase the compression upon the head of the child. Should the blades of the forceps be introduced so as not to be opposite each other, they could not be locked; or if, when applied, the handles should come close together, or be at a great distance from each other, they would probably slip, or there would be a failure of some kind in the operation, as the bulk of the head would not be included, or they would be fixed on some improper part of the head, though allowance is to be made for the difference in the size of the heads of children. But if a case be proper for the forceps, if they be well applied, and we were to act slowly with them, there would not be much risk of failure or disappointment. The difficulty of applying the forceps is most frequently occasioned by attempting to apply them too soon, or by passing them in a wrong direction, or by entangling the soft parts of the mother between the instrument and the head of the child, against all which accidents we are to be on our guard.

" When the forceps are first locked, they are placed backwards, with the lock close to, or just within, the internal surface of the perineum; and they can have no support backwards, except the little which is afforded by the soft parts. The first action with them should therefore be made by bringing the handles, grasped firmly in one or both hands, to prevent the instrument from playing upon the head of the child, slowly towards the pubes till they come to a full rest. Having waited a short interval with them in that situation, the handles must be carried back in the same slow but steady manner to the perineum, exerting, as they are carried in the different situations, a certain degree of extracting force; and after waiting another interval, they are again to be carried towards the pubes, according to the direction of the handles. Throughout the operation, especially the first part, the action of that blade of the forceps originally applied towards the pubes must be stronger and more extensive than the action with the other blade, this having no fulcrum to support it, and chiefly answering the purpose of regulating the action of the other blade. If there were any labour pains when the operation was begun, or should they come on in the course of it, the forceps should only be acted with during the continuance of the pains; the intention being not only to supply the want or insufficiency of the pains, but to follow them, and imitate also the manner in which they return. By a few repetitions of this alternate action and rest before described, we shall soon be sensible of the descent of the head; and it will be proper to examine very frequently, to know the progress made, that we may not use more force than needful, nor go on with more haste than may be expedient or safe. In every case we ought to proceed slowly and circumspectly, not forgetting that a small degree of force, continued for a long time, will in general be equivalent to a greater force hastily exerted, and with infinitely less detriment to the mother or child. But after some time, should we not perceive the head to descend, the force hitherto used must be gradually increased, till it be sufficient to overcome the obstacles to the delivery of the patient. It was before observed, as the head of the child descended, that the face would be accordingly turned towards the hollow of the sacrum, without any aim or assistance on our part. Of course the position of the handles of the forceps, and the direction in which we ought to act with them, should alter; for they becoming first more diagonal or oblique with respect to the pelvis, and then more and more lateral, every change in their position will require a differently directed action, because the handles should ever be antagonists to each other. In proportion also to the descent of the head the handles of the forceps should approach nearer to the pubes; so that, in the beginning of the operation, though we acted in the direction of the cavity of the pelvis, towards the conclusion we should act in that of the vagina. When we feel that we have the command of the head, by its being cleared of the pelvis, and the external parts begin to be distended, we ought to act yet more slowly, especially in the case of a first child, or there would be great danger of a laceration of the soft parts; and this can only be prevented by acting very deliberately in the direction of the vagina—by giving the parts time to distend—by duly supporting the perineum, which is the part chiefly in danger, with the palm of the hand—by soothing and moderating the hurry and efforts of the patient—and, in some cases, by absolutely resisting for a certain time the passage of the head through the external parts."

———

CLINICAL LECTURES,

Delivered at St. Thomas's Hospital,

BY SAMUEL SOLLY, Esq. F.R.S.

Assistant-Surgeon, and Lecturer on Clinical Surgery, at St. Thomas's School.

———

ON INJURIES OF THE HEAD.

GENTLEMEN,—The subject to which your attention was directed on the last occasion we met, shall be resumed on the present. You will, I have no doubt, remember my then warning you against considering any patient who has received a serious injury of the head as out of danger, merely because he shows no symptom of injury to the brain during the first few days. The value of such a warning has, I am sorry to say, been too truthfully illustrated in the sequence of the case I then detailed. I might well say that, in these cases, we know not what an hour may bring forth. For when we last met nothing could appear more favourable than the case related, though I have now to detail a fatal termination, from extensive cerebral lesion. I will first read to you my notes of the case to its termination, and we can then discuss the practical and physiological points of interest raised by its relation. After my lecture on the 24th, you will remember we found him apparently going on well, but as he still had pain in the head, I ordered twenty leeches, and Pil. Hydrar. gr. v. his hand.

25th.—No worse.

26th.—I received a message from the dresser saying that the man had passed a bad night, and was in a good deal of pain in his head, for which he had applied twenty leeches. I saw him at 1 P.M. His head has been relieved by the leeches, but he complains of pain at the external angle of the right orbit, which pain appears to him to rise upwards from the jaw, and to shoot over the head. He states that he is free from pain in the neighbourhood of the wound; his mouth is tender from the mercury. As the pain has so much of a neuralgic character, and possibly connected with this salivation, I ordered the mercury to be omitted, and the face to be fomented, after which an ointment containing aconitine to be rubbed into the side of the face. At 8 P.M. when I saw him again, he had been relieved by the fomentation, but had not had the ointment, as there was not any aconitine in the hospital. I ordered instead of it equal parts of the extract of belladonna and lard, to be made into an ointment and rubbed into the face.

Pulv. Jalap co. ℈j. hhe. nocte. M. & C. cras. nande.

27th, 12 A.M.—Pulse 90, soft, and rather

weak; complains of his forehead and the side of the head, but no pain in the neighbourhood of the wound. His countenance was anxious and distressed; the right pupil was dilated; the left natural. I thought at first that this might possibly arise from the application of the belladonna, but he complained of having lost the feeling in his left hand, and that he could not lay hold of things so readily with it. I need hardly say I regarded this circumstance with the greatest concern, as I feared the worst from it. He had another very serious symptom, viz. that on lying down he complained of his head throbbing violently.

I ordered the twenty leeches to be repeated, and five grains of blue pill twice a day; the head to be raised in bed. Immediately I quitted the ward I called the attention of the pupils who were with me to the serious character of his symptoms, and gave an unfavourable prognosis.

At 8 P.M. I received a message from the dresser, informing me that he had had a fit, and when I arrived I found him just recovering from a third fit. The fits were not preceded by any scream, but in every other respect they were all of a true epileptic character. As soon as he began to recover his senses he went off again, and just previous to this he became very violent, and was with difficulty retained in bed. I inquired of his wife whether he had ever been subject to epilepsy: she said no, but that she had heard from his mother that when a child he had been subject to fits. Coupling the invasion of these fits with the incipient paralysis observed in the morning, I considered it not impossible that there was some irritation from the internal surface of the fractured bone. I therefore determined to trephine. This was accomplished by making first a crucial incision of the integuments, and then, by the application of the trephine on the lower edge of the fissure in the parietal bone. After the removal of the portion cut by the trephine, I removed with the dressing forceps a small portion of bone with a sharp edge, about the size of a thumb-nail, from under the superior edge of the fissure in the internal surface, which evidently pressed on the dura mater. About eight ounces of blood were lost at the operation, but very little afterwards. I performed it just after the commencement of the fourth fit, as I found he was too excited after he recovered from one to permit any operation willingly. He had one fit shortly after it was completed, but no more during the night. The dresser, Mr. Fixot, sat up with him, and he tells me that the patient complained of a good deal of pain in his head, referring it principally to the forehead and eyebrow, but sometimes to the back part, near the wound; he dozed at intervals, and then awoke with pain;

pulse very variable, sometimes thready, and sometimes a little fuller; cough occasionally occurred, always causing violent pain in the head.

28th, 9 A.M.—He has now paralysis of the whole of the left side of the head, body, and left extremity.

He knows me: complains of pain in his head, and wishes to sit up in bed: we raised him, and then he complained of being faint. I gave him a very little weak brandy and water, and ordered some sal volatile occasionally. His pulse is weak: 100.

28th, 10 P.M.—Has had nine fits at intervals during the day, the last about half an hour before I came down; he is quite sensible between the attacks; the sister thinks that he has lost some power in the right arm. As he was now dozing I would not disturb him; pulse 80, small, but not very feeble; skin hot. In one of the fits the convulsions were very slight, and confined to the left side of the body, and he seemed scarcely to lose his consciousness. I learned from the sister that she had observed twitching of the muscles on the left side during the afternoon of yesterday.

On Saturday he continued sensible, and he did not appear to lose his consciousness even during the fits, for as soon as the convulsions ceased he would take up his handkerchief and wipe his mouth. He had fits every half hour, which began at 9 in the morning and continued till 4 in the afternoon, when twelve leeches were applied to his head, and he had no more till 11 o'clock at night, when he had a very slight one, but at 12 he had a very severe one, which continued one hour; he was perfectly conscious, and breathing natural; scarcely ever complained of his head, and then referred the pain to the right brow.

Sunday, 30th.—He had no decided fits, only twitching of the muscles; remained sensible till about 4 o'clock in the afternoon, when a great change took place; he turned very pale, and had more twitching of the muscles, and at twenty minutes after four had a fit, which lasted an hour and a half. After this he totally lost the use of his inferior extremities; all consciousness left him, and he did not have another fit, but merely twitching of the muscles, and died at twenty minutes after 3, on the 1st of May, moaning a great deal and making a great noise, but for one hour before he died he never spoke.

Post-mortem, May 1st, 1 P.M.—Head. After the cranium was sawn through, about half an ounce of yellow pus escaped, while endeavouring to detach it from the dura mater. When this was done we found the internal table of the skull fractured more extensively than the outer table, split inward from the upper edge of the fracture. A portion of this table which was thus split I had removed with the dressing forceps after using the trephine. The portion which remained could not have been removed without some force, as they were only partially separated from the surrounding bone.

At the time of the operation I did not detect this further depression, from a fear of separating the dura mater more than was absolutely necessary. But the appearance of this bone certainly teaches us that we are warranted in such cases (even in the absence of depression of the outer table, and the removal of the portions which are found at the edge of the opening made by the trephine), in searching carefully for any further portions that may have been separated.

Opposite this fracture there was a small opening in the dura mater of the size and shape of the extremity of the nail of the little finger, through which some softened brownish-coloured brain was exuding. On turning back the dura mater, we found on the same side the whole surface of the arachnoidea investiens covered with healthy yellow pus. The arachnoidea reflexa lining the dura mater was coated with a thick layer of pus, so tenacious that it almost amounted to a false membrane.

The brain, corresponding to the seat of fracture, was much discoloured. The centre of this discolouration was of a dark, dirty brownish hue, of a semi-liquid consistency, gradually becoming firmer, and shaded off to a dingy pinkish colour towards the circumference, which was spotted with deep bloody points : an horizontal section of the brain about half an inch from the surface showed this very distinctly. The disorganization extended downwards into the lateral ventricle at the commencement of the descending and posterior cornua, involving a portion of the transverse commissure, but not either the thalamus or corpus striatum. The surface of the brain, where the arachnoidea had been covered with pus, was slightly softened in many places, but most so over the inferior edge of the anterior lobes of the right hemisphere.

The hemispherical ganglion was scarcely, if at all, altered in its condition ; its colour was healthy, neither paler nor deeper than usual ; the edge, in some situations, was converted into a greyish-greenish tint, which Dr. Hodgkin attributed to a post-mortem action of sulphuretted hydrogen.

The pia mater and arachnoid on the left hemisphere were both perfectly healthy, and also on the surface of both hemispheres, where they are in contact with the falx major.

If the nature of the fracture in this case, and the injury inflicted on the brain and its membranes, as demonstrated by this post-mortem examination, could have been ascertained at the time of his admission, no one could have hesitated to use the trephine. It is, then, a question for our consideration why this condition was not detected, and how far it would be desirable to adopt a different course when a similar case comes before us.

As a post-mortem examination does not demonstrate the amount of lesion of the brain at the time of his admission, for much that we now observe is the result of subsequent inflammation and gangrene, let us endeavour, reasoning from other cases and the physiology of the subject, to establish this point.

At the time of his admission it is very clear that the internal table of the skull was more extensively fractured than the outer, and that the fractured portions were partially depressed. Notwithstanding the entire absence of all symptoms of compression, these symptoms, as almost universally agreed to by surgeons, consist of an entire loss of consciousness; the mental faculties are smothered, and they cannot be roused. Many of the functions of vegetative life are also interfered with, the breathing is laborious and stertorous, not unfrequently the sphincters are relaxed, and the excretions are evacuated involuntarily. There are sometimes other symptoms, but these are the most common.

You will naturally say, if such are the symptoms of compression, why were they entirely absent in this case, where we see that the inner table was depressed and driven in upon the brain ? I am inclined to believe that the acknowledged symptoms of compression depend upon the extent of the hemispherical ganglion which is pressed upon suddenly, and that if only a very small portion of this ganglion is pressed upon, then its functions are not naturally impaired, in this case, and many others that might be quoted : nevertheless, you must not consider it more than an hypothesis of my own, and not as an established principle. Nevertheless, I conceive this is the only truly physiological explanation of this apparent anomaly.

The splintered portion of the skull lacerated the dura mater to a very small extent, and to about the same extent, but no more, was the hemispherical ganglion originally injured. The medullary or fibrous substance beneath was so shaken that blood was effused in small points, as may sometimes be observed in cases of simple concussion without fracture. You will be surprised, on referring to treatises on injuries of the head, to find so many cases recorded in which very serious injuries to the brain have been unattended by serious symptoms of disturbed intellect, but, as far as I can judge from the loose mode in which post-mortem appearances are almost invariably detailed, they are all cases in which the injury is confined to the base of the brain, or the hemispherical ganglion has been but slightly injured in the first instance. It is a pity that surgeons who have written on this subject should have neglected to state the exact extent of the surface injured, for this fact is equally important in its physiological as it is in its pathological bearing; the ignorance of it having induced some well-meaning but foolish people to quote such uses in proof of their theory that the brain is not the organ of the mind—not distinguishing between the ganglion which is connected with the mind, and those which are not. The following case, quoted by Mr. Guthrie from Dupuytren, illustrates my view of this subject.

A young man had received a wound in the head from a knife, which healed in the usual way, leaving only a little pain which occurred occasionally round the cicatrix. Some years after he was brought to the Hôtel Dieu in a state of stupefaction, with which he had been suddenly seized. An incision having been made through the cicatrix, the point of a knife was seen sticking in the bone, the removal of which gave no relief. The trephine was then applied without any result. The paralysis continuing on the opposite side to that on which the wound had been received, it was thought right to open the dura mater, and then to plunge the knife into the brain, when a large quantity of pus escaped. The paralysis ceased that night; he recovered his speech, became sensible, and entirely, though gradually, recovered.

In this case we may conclude, from the account, that the ganglion was only injured to the extent of the breadth and thickness of the knife, and no disturbance of the mind followed until an abscess formed, which, pressing on the ganglion from within, indicated its presence by the stupefaction and paralysis that followed.

The evacuation of the matter relieved the pressure, the senses returned, and the paralysis ceased.

Whether this explanation of the fact that you do meet with cases of depression of the table of the skull without the ordinary signs of compression of the brain, be true in its physiology or not, the fact itself is a most important one for you to remember, for its practical bearings. I shall again advert to it when I criticise my treatment of the case.

On referring back to its progress, you will remember that on the 8th, 9th, and 10th days after the accident, he was almost free from untoward symptoms: so well indeed had the case gone on, that my friend Mr. Travers, who had watched it with some interest, congratulated me on the favourable result of the anticipatory treatment which I had adopted. It may be fairly considered that these antiphlogistic measures which were practised so early stayed for the time the invasion of inflammatory action, though they did not entirely arrest it. His system was brought under the influence of mercury within 24 hours of the oc-

currence of the injury, and though he was not bled from the arm, for he never had a pulse exhibiting sufficient vascular action to justify it, 148 leeches were applied to the head.

The cough was much subdued by the ipecacuanha and conium pill, a blister, and the tincture of iodine to the chest.

But still the mischief went on, and thus I believe the fibrous medulla beneath the hemispherical ganglion became softened, as indicated on the eleventh day, by slight loss of sensation in the left hand. If the medulla had been materially altered in its texture, at the time of his admission, by the blow, there must have been paralysis at that time, and the fact of its not appearing till the eleventh day shews how slowly the softening and disorganization must have proceeded. The softening increased, and then an epileptic fit takes place, quickly succeeded by another, and another, and another, until, by means of openings made with the trephine, a splinter of bone was removed.

The principal cause of irritation is removed, and one more fit occurs immediately, and then they cease for about twelve hours, when they again recur, and though occasionally stopped for a short period by local blood-letting, they return at intervals, until the patient becomes quite insensible, remaining so for twelve hours previous to his death. This loss of consciousness I attribute to the pus we found effused on the surface of the brain, for until the pus was effused there was nothing to interfere with the hemispherical ganglion, and therefore nothing to affect the intellect; and neither the quantity or quality of the pus was such as might not have been effused in the course of twelve or fifteen hours at the longest. I think the inflammatory action which caused it was occasioned *by* the epileptic fits, and not the cause of them. The cause of the fits I believe is to be found in the softening and gangrene of the fibrous or conducting substance of the brain.

Taking this view of the progress of the case, we cannot avoid the conclusion that if this patient had been trephined when he was first admitted he would have had a better chance of recovery than by postponing it; and though it is impossible to say whether the brain was or was not so much injured at first as to have been irremediable, I candidly confess that I do not believe it was; for if such had been the case there must have been some symptoms of such a lesion, and it is astonishing from what serious lesion, both primary and secondary, the brain will recover. No, gentlemen, I believe that most all the disorganization which the post-mortem examination exhibited in the right hemisphere of the brain was the result of inflammatory action, excited by the irritation of the fractured skull, and partly kept up and aggravated by the concussions occasioned by the cough. The number of cases on record in which patients have recovered whose brains have been seriously wounded, when the cause of irritation has been removed, should encourage you to make the attempt as early as possible to relieve your patient, if you can discover that any cause of irritation exists. The difficulty in the present case was to ascertain the fact of depression of the internal table.

There is no point in surgical practice regarding which there is and has been so much difference of opinion as the use of the trephine. Mr. Abernethy's Treatise on Injuries of the Head was called forth in consequence of the difference of opinion regarding the line of practice that ought to be followed in particular cases. He relates seven cases of fracture, with depression, which occurred within one twelvemonth at St. Bartholomew's, that recovered without any operation, "showing that a slight degree of pressure does not derange the functions of the brain, for a limited period at any rate, after its application." After relating other cases, he goes on to say—"Such cases ought to deter surgeons from elevating the bone in every instance of slight depression, since by the operation they must inflict a further injury upon their patients, the consequence of which it is impossible to estimate. From all, therefore, that I have learned from books, as well as from the observations I have made in practice and from reasoning upon the subject, I am disposed to join in opinion with those surgeons who are against trephining in slight depressions of the skull, or small extravasations of the dura mater."

Benjamin Bell, whose System of Surgery was published in 1801, says, "Hitherto it has been a general rule to consider the application of the trepan as necessary in every fissure, whether any symptoms of a compressed brain have occurred or not, but due attention to the real nature of the fissure, and to the effects most likely to result from perforating the skull, will show, that although fissures may be frequently combined with such symptoms as require the trepan, yet that they are not always, or necessarily so; and unless when such symptoms actually exist, that this operation, instead of affording relief, must frequently do harm; for it is by no means calculated for, or in any respect adequate to, the prevention of these symptoms, and I have already endeavoured to show that laying the brain bare is never to be considered as harmless, and therefore that it should never be advised but where it is probable that some advantage may be derived from it." In the present day these observations of Mr. Bell seem almost superfluous, *but when we find such precepts as the following inculcated by John Hunter in his*

Surgical Lectures, we need not be surprised that subsequent teachers of surgery should have felt the necessity of warning their pupils of the too free use of the trephine. "As we cannot tell for certain at the time," says Mr. Hunter, "whether the symptoms arise from concussion, compression, or from extravasation of blood, it may be more advisable to trepan, *as the operation can do no harm.*"

Mr. Lawrence relates an interesting case in a clinical lecture, published in the MEDICAL GAZETTE, vol. xxi. p. 345, of a boy who recovered without operation, in whom the skull was fractured and depressed, the brain wounded, and portions of it extravasated through a laceration of the scalp. "In this case Mr. Lawrence says, as the bone was here evidently and considerably depressed, and as it was also probably driven in upon the brain, it would, I believe, have accorded with the principles of treatment generally admitted, to have performed an operation for the purpose of elevating and removing depressed and detached portions of the bone."

"The considerations which determined me to do this were, the favourable state of the patient generally, and in particular the absence of all symptoms indicating compression of the brain; the specimens in pathological collections, of very extensive injuries of the skull repaired by a natural process; the smallness of the external wound, which brought this case nearly into the state of simple fracture; the extensive incision of the integuments, and exposure of the bone, dura mater, and brain, which an operation would have involved; and the almost invariable fatal termination of such proceedings within my own experience in hospital practice."

Dr. Hennen, in his admirable work on Military Surgery, relates many cases to show that the trephine should not be used, even when the bone is evidently depressed, in the absence of symptoms. He says, p. 288, "We have here sufficient proof that there is no absolute necessity for trepanning merely for depressed bones from gunshot, although few would be so hardy as not to remove all fragments that came easily and readily away." You will do well to read all the cases which he relates, and in the hope that most of you will do so I will only quote one short history in connection with the case before us. "A soldier was shot in the head in the Canadian campaign. A fracture was the consequence, with a depression of not less than an inch and a half; but as no untoward symptom occurred no operation was had recourse to. This man recovered, and went to the rear, where, at a distance of several weeks afterwards, he got an attack of phrenitis from excessive

drinking, and died. As the existence of
the ball in the brain was strongly suspected,
an inquiry was made after death, and on
dissection it was found lodged in the corpus
callosum."

Mr. Guthrie, in his interesting and valuable
work on Injuries of the Head, lately published,
makes some excellent remarks on the best
mode of proceeding in these obscure cases.
"The inner table, (says Mr. Guthrie) is sometimes broken in a peculiar manner, to which
I believe attention has only been drawn by
myself in my lectures, since trepanning has
ceased to be the rule in all cases of fracture.
In these cases the skull is cut rather than
broken by a sharp cutting instrument such
as an axe, sword," &c., just in fact as a piece
of wood might be, while the inner table, like
a piece of glass or brittle steel, is broken and
splintered inwards. "These cases, says
Mr. Guthrie, should be examined carefully.
The length of the wound on the top, or side,
or any part of the head which is curved and
not flat, will readily show to what depth the
sword or axe has penetrated. A blunt or
flat, ended probe should in such cases be
carefully passed into the wound, and being
gently pressed against one of the cut edges
of the bone, its thickness may be measured,
and the presence or absence of the inner
table may thus be ascertained. If it should
be separated from the diploe, the continued
but careful insertion of the probe will detect
it deeper in the wound ; a further careful
investigation will show the extent in length
of this separation, although not in width,
and will, in all probability, satisfy the surgeon
that those portions of bone which have thus
been broken and driven in are sticking in
or irritating the brain. In many such cases
there has not been more than a momentary
stunning felt by the patient ; he says he is
free from symptoms, that he is not much
hurt, and is satisfied he shall be well in a few
days."

"An officer was struck on the head in
Halifax, Nova Scotia, by a drunken woman
with a tomahawk or small Indian hatchet,
which made a perpendicular cut into his
left parietal bone and knocked him down.
As he soon recovered from the blow, and
suffered nothing but the ordinary symptoms
of a common wound of the head with fracture, it was considered to be a favourable
case, and was treated simply, although with
sufficient precaution. He sat up and shaved
himself until the fourteenth day, when he
observed that the corner of his mouth on
the opposite side to that on which he had
been wounded was fixed, and the other
drawn aside, and that he had not the free
use of the right arm, so as to enable him to
shave. He was bled largely, but the symptoms increased until he lost the use of the
right side, became comatose, and died. On

examination the inner table was found
broken, separated from the diploe, and
driven into the brain, which was at that part
soft, yellow, and in a state of suppuration."
After relating several other instructive cases
bearing on this point, he says, " the principle
being laid down that it is right and proper to
examine all such wounds with a blunt flat
probe, in order to ascertain if possible
whether the inner table is depressed or
broken, the question necessarily arises, what
is to be done when such depression and
breaking down of the inner table is ascertained to have taken place ? There can be no
hesitation in answering that in all such cases
the trephine should be applied, although no
symptoms should exist, with the view of an-
ticipating them."

" The old doctrine, it may be said, in regard
to fractures generally, is revived in these
cases, but on a principle with which our predecessors were not sufficiently acquainted.
A patient very often survives a mere depression of the skull ; he may, and occasionally does, survive a greater depression of the
inner than the outer table ; but I do not
believe that he ever does survive and remain
in tolerable health, after a depression with
fracture of the inner table, when portions of
it have been driven into the dura mater. If
cases could be advanced of complete recovery
after such injuries, I should not consider
them as superseding the practice recommended, unless they were so numerous as to
establish the fact that wounds of the dura
mater and brain are not extremely dangerous.
I have referred purposely to many cases in
which a cure was effected after a lapse of
time by the bone being removed; but they
rather support than invalidate the principle
I have inculcated. There are great objections, I admit, to the trephine being applied
in ordinary cases of fracture, which are not
attended by symptoms of further mischief ;
but the nature of the cases which I have
particularly referred to having been ascertained, I maintain that the practice should be
prompt and decisive in every instance in
which the surgeon is satisfied that there is
not merely a slight depression or separation
of the inner table, but that several points of
it are driven into the dura mater."

I have thought it incumbent on me to
dwell very fully on the justifiableness of the
use of the trephine in such fractures of the
skull where there is an absence of cerebral
symptoms, lest I should have practically
misled you by attaching too much importance to this circumstance in my former
lecture. Nevertheless, I cannot recommend
the use of the trephine in any case, unless
you have very decided evidence of a wounded
dura mater from splintered portions of the
inner table. " If there be any doubt," says
the same authority, " on the mind of the

surgeon whether there are, or are not, any portions depressed and irritating the brain or its membranes, he should wait; and in this it is that the real difference between modern surgery and that of the olden time exists, with respect to adults.

The nature of the fracture in this case rendered it almost impossible to ascertain the fact of fracture of the inner table by means of the probe, as recommended by Mr. Guthrie.

You will perceive, gentlemen, from these few quotations, that there is still considerable difference of opinion as to any general rule for the use of the trephine in fracture of the skull. It must, indeed, be admitted that no general rule can be laid down, but that every surgeon must be guided by the peculiar circumstances of each particular case, bearing in mind that there are cases of injury of the brain in which the trephine may be required, though all the symptoms of *compression* are absent. Such cases, it is true, are rare, and their diagnosis difficult, but it is only by the remembrance of their occasional existence that you will ever detect them.

And, on the other hand, scarcely any extent of wound of the skull, the brain, and its membranes, accompanied with unequivocal depression of bone, should discourage you from the operation, if the functions of vegetative life are not so seriously interfered with as to make a fatal result inevitable; for the records of surgery teem with cases showing from what serious injury of the brain some patients will recover.

The following case, which some of you may remember, will come under this head, and also illustrate the usual symptoms of compression, and the first effect of such an operation.

James White, æt. 49, was admitted into St. Thomas's Hospital at half-past 9, A.M. of the 13th of July, 1842. When I visited him at 12, I found him with an incised wound of the scalp, with a corresponding fissured fracture of the skull on the left side, extending from the occipital bone across the parietal bone and coronal suture into the frontal bone. The brain was oozing out at the posterior portion of the fissure, and it was reported that he had lost a large quantity of blood. The wound was inflicted with a large bill-hook as he lay asleep (by a man who intended robbing him.) When admitted he was quite sensible, and answered all questions rationally, but when I saw him about two hours subsequently it was difficult to rouse him, and his answers were not clear. The muscles of his face were paralysed both as regards sensation and motion, for he was *quite unconscious of my touching him, even when I pinched him sharply. On examination of the wound I found a portion of* depressed bone driven under the edge of the upper portion of the parietal bone, and as it was evident that it could not be removed without a larger opening in the skull, I determined, with the advice of Mr. Green, to trephine the cranium, and remove it. The operation was performed without difficulty, and with scarcely any expression of pain on the part of the patient.

Three pieces were removed, two about the size of a square inch, one the size of a finger-nail, besides the portion removed by the trephine. A smaller, but very sharp, portion was driven through the dura mater and wounded the brain. The immediate effect of the removal of the bone was very striking. The patient at once complained of pain, and articulated quite distinctly, which he could not do before the operation. The sensibility of the skin of the thigh was also restored, as he felt my fingers when I touched him, though not so distinctly as in the perfect state. The arterial blood flowed very freely, but the bleeding did not last long after the removal of the bone.

Ordered him Hyd. Chlorid. gr. v. 4tâ. quâque horâ s., and cold water to the wound.

11 P.M.—Much the same as when I left him; has been dozing.

14th, 1 P.M.—Not quite so sensible as yesterday; skin hot; very thirsty; pulse 120; has taken six doses of calomel; mouth slightly affected; mercurial fœtor; bowels open once pretty freely.

Cal. gr. j. 6tâ horâ s.; Hirud. x. capitis lateri sinistro et.

9 P.M.—Has been dozing all the afternoon; complains of his head when roused; cannot speak distinctly, but his answers are rational; skin very hot; pulse 140, sharp and small; very thirsty.

Ordered—V.S. ad ℥xvj. Enema Communis.

Expressed himself, in answer to my inquiry, relieved by the bleeding.

15th.—Much the same; still sensible, and complains of pains in his head; mouth scarcely so tender.

Hirud. xxx. capiti.

16th.—Scarcely any difference in his condition; says his head is not so painful; wound gaping; no fungus cerebri. Mr. Green advised my not pushing the mercury further, and to apply a poultice instead of the lint, considering it of great importance to establish suppuration.

Ordered—Cataplasma Panis. To omit the mercury.

19th, 10 A.M.—Much the same; pulse 120; skin very hot; complains of pain in the head.

Ordered Hirud. xxx.

10 P.M.—Sinking; quite rational, but very low, can scarcely answer; pulse too quick to count; gave him two ounces of brandy; had very little effect upon his pulse. Ordered it to be renewed in the night if he lived.

20th.—9 A.M.—Sensible, but more depressed than last night; has taken some more stimulus during the night: sank gradually, and died about 11 o'clock.

Post-mortem.—Fracture extending from the centre of the frontal bone across the left parietal bone into the lambdoidal suture, which was separated slightly, so as to admit blood enough to make its course for about an inch in extent. The dura mater was divided for about four inches. The surface of the brain opposite the wound was softened, red, and pulpy. The disorganization extended downwards for about an inch and a half in its deepest part. Surrounding this softened portion for about half an inch, the brain was dotted with red points, and a little beyond it was in spots rather yellow. The surface of the brain on the left side was coated by a very thin yellow tawnish layer of ill-formed pus. The right side normal; the corpora striata, thalami nervorum opticorum, and the rest of the brain, healthy.

This case is interesting in many points of view.

First, the intellect remaining so perfect, notwithstanding the extent of the brain that was injured. This circumstance confirms the theory stated elsewhere, that incised wounds of the hemispherical ganglion do not, in the first instance, affect the intellect so much as a compressing force; because the extent of surface which is injured is less in the former than the latter injury in the first instance; though as soon as blood is extravasated, and softening of the ganglion follows, then the senses are oppressed and subsequently obliterated.

Secondly, that the removal of the bone should have almost perfectly restored the functions of the nerves of sensation, which had been obliterated by its pressure, while it had no effect upon the motor tract.

Thirdly, the proof it affords that both motion and sensation may be interfered with, without the corpora striata and thalami nervorum opticorum being injured. In a practical point of view, I had some doubt as to whether I had pushed the depletion too far, as the man seemed exhausted; but the membranes exhibited quite sufficient indication of inflammatory action to justify the treatment most fully, and shewed how high it would have run if it had not been checked.

To return to Wingrove's case: the next practical point which the consideration of it suggests is, whether you are justified in opening the dura mater when it has been exposed by the trephine, in those cases in which there are symptoms of pus beneath its surface.

The dura mater, when exposed by the removal of a portion of the skull, will be seen to rise and fall with the pulsations of the brain, if it is not separated from the dura mater by anything else than the other investing membranes. It is true that in a tranquil state, and with a small opening, the motion is very slight. The absence of this motion is stated by Mr. Guthrie as diagnostic of fluid beneath. "I have seen," says this author, "on the removal of a portion of bone, the dura mater rapidly rise up into the opening, so as to attain nearly the level of the surface of the skull, totally devoid however of that pulsatory motion which usually marks its healthy state; and an opening into it under these circumstances has allowed a quantity of purulent matter to escape, proving that the unnatural elevation of the dura mater was caused by the resiliency of the brain, when the opposing pressure of the cranium was removed. I consider this tense elevation, and the absence of pulsation, to be positive signs of there being a fluid beneath requiring an incision into the dura mater for its evacuation. It is a point scarcely, if at all, noticed in English surgery, although much insisted on in France. It was not in the slightest degree understood till the commencement of the war in the Peninsula, and was one of those points which particularly attracted my attention."

In Wingrove's case no such phenomena were exhibited at the time of the operation, nor did I perceive it when I examined the wound at my daily visits, which would rather confirm the opinion that the pus was not effused until about twelve or fifteen hours before death.

If I had observed this sign of the presence of matter under the dura mater, I confess that I should have punctured it, though I cannot believe, from the post-mortem examination, that the operation would have altered the result, as nothing could have changed the gangrenous condition of the brain. There are many other points of interest connected with injuries of the skull, and the use of the trephine, which do not bear upon the present case, but which I shall take the first opportunity of bringing before your notice.

I cannot conclude these remarks without expressing the hope that the study of this case will impress you with the importance of making a very careful diagnosis and prognosis in all injuries of the skull; and that while you value the trephine and elevator as most useful instruments for the relief of a compressed and irritated brain, that you will never be tempted by the prospect of performing (what, if successful, is certainly a brilliant operation, but blamefully mischievous if the condition of the parts should not absolutely require it,) without having first a well-grounded conviction that their use can alone save the life of your patient; remembering that in all such injuries the great danger to be apprehended is inflammation of the brain and its membranes, and that nothing is so likely to produce it as their exposure to their air, and the forcible removal of their natural protectors.

REMARKS
ON
THE INJURIOUS EFFECTS OF MESMERISM.

By GEORGE SOUTHAM,
Surgeon to the Salford and Pendleton Royal Dispensary, Manchester.

(For the Medical Gazette.)

IN November 1841, Monsieur La Fontaine visited Manchester to exhibit the phenomena of animal magnesism; and having succeeded in producing its influence on a few individuals of known respectability, it soon acquired great popularity. It became the subject of conversation and experiment among almost all classes of society, and several persons were found more or less susceptible to its effects. Somnolency and catalepsy were produced in some; others were seized with various anomalous symptoms bearing the strongest affinity to those of hysteria; and, in a few instances, convulsions of a tetanic or epileptic character were excited. Such surprising effects soon made converts amongst the lovers of the wonderful and marvellous, but the profession generally received them with caution. Accordingly, with a few exceptions, the practice of the art continued in the hands of the charlatan, who, always ready to take advantage of the credulity of his fellow creatures, seeks every means which folly and imposition can invent to seek temporary fame and wealth. Besides the thumbing and staring, as practised by La Fontaine, other methods are stated to be capable of producing its phenomena; and, either from ignorance of the known physiological truths, or more probably from a desire to delude, new theories, so framed as to excite the curiosity of the ignorant, *have* been continually vaunted *forth to explain effects* which, in many instances, are merely those of monotony and an excited imagination. With the cool effrontery peculiar to such people, they have pretended to restore sight to the blind, hearing to the deaf, and speech to the dumb. The bedridden and paralytic have been said to walk at their pleasure, and women to have had no longer occasion to fear the pains of labour.

It is unnecessary, in a medical journal, to prove the futility of such extravagant pretensions. If animal magnetism has any claim on our notice, it is not on account of any remedial power it possesses, but from the mischievous consequences it produces by exciting dangerous diseases of the nervous system.

Its advocates regard it as a peculiar agent existing within the living body under the direction of the will, which may be transmitted from one person to another, producing effects in the recipient which are not possessed by the individual communicating the impression. Doubtless such an agent is necessary to explain those anomalous symptoms presented by the O'Keys, and numerous other individuals, whose cases have operated so wonderfully on the credulity of its partisans; but to those whose minds are accustomed to more cautious reflection and observation, the proofs adduced in support of such a doctrine are too ambiguous and contradictory to enable them to admit the existence of such an agent. Besides, we are sufficiently familiar with the laws of the nervous system to explain many of the phenomena produced by mesmerism, provided we separate the real effects which it occasions from those merely the result of imposition and collusion.

The following case appears to illustrate its nature, and is a good example of the dangerous consequences arising from its application. A young man, aged 18, was mesmerised by one of his companions in December 1841, in the following manner. They pressed their thumbs together, and looked steadfastly at each other in the face, the operator at the same time gently moving his fingers over the palms of the patient's hand.

In about twenty minutes from the commencement of the experiment, his fingers, which had previously been half bent, gradually extended themselves; the arms became similarly affected; afterwards, the muscles at the back of the neck, and those over the whole body. A feeling of coldness came over him, and a sense of tightness across his head, as if it had been bound firmly with a bandage. After remaining motionless and stiff a few minutes, he was seized with slight convulsive movements in the face; shortly the whole body was violently agitated, and he fell from the chair on which he had been sitting. These convulsions continued about 15 minutes, and in three quarters of an hour from the commencement he had perfectly recovered. He had allowed the experiment to be repeated several times before I saw the effects. This was a week after the first experiment. I mesmerised him in the manner described, and in less than five minutes the whole of his body was in a state of tetanic rigidity. This was quickly followed by contractions of the muscles on the right side of the face, afterwards of the whole body. The vessels of the head and neck became distended with blood, and the countenance bloated. The eye was turned upwards, or rolled about in the socket, the pupil sometimes dilated, and insensible to light; at other times it was contracted to a pin-point. The action of the heart was much increased, and the pulsations of the carotid distinctly seen. He frothed at the mouth, and his face at times was violently distorted. In about ten minutes the convulsions began to subside, and he fell into a deep sleep, from which he awoke in a quarter of an hour, suffering no other inconvenience than a slight but transient headache, and feeling of lassitude. During the paroxysm the power of feeling was destroyed, but consciousness remained. He states that at the onset he has sufficient control over the symptoms to cut short the paroxysm; but when the convulsions have set in, all power is lost, and he feels as if he had the will to rouse himself, but has not the power to do so—a sensation similar to that experienced on awaking suddenly from a profound sleep. Six weeks afterwards I witnessed a second attack in company with Mr. Jordan. Here it was produced by looking at an image, at the same time keeping the mind abstracted from all other subjects. In less than five minutes the patient fell backwards in my arms, and before I could place him on the floor his body was in a complete state of tetanic rigidity. To this succeeded convul-

sions and their attendant symptoms, which continued longer, and were more violent, than on the previous occasion. On recovering, he mentioned some conversation that passed between Mr. J. and myself, proving that consciousness remained; but, as on the former occasion, pinching and pricking gave him no pain. Some weeks afterwards I found that his system had become so susceptible from repeated impressions that he could excite a paroxysm in a few minutes by a mere effort of the will. With respect to his previous history, it may be stated that he is of an excitable and nervous temperament, but has always enjoyed good health. There appears to be an hereditary tendency to nervous affections in his family; for similar symptoms have been produced by mesmerism in his sister, who is about 14 years of age. His maternal grandfather is paralytic, his mother had an attack of the same disease in her 36th year, and two of her uncles died from apoplexy. The case presents several remarkable circumstances. It at once points out the dangerous consequences of mesmerism, and satisfactorily shews the means through which it exerts its influence. The symptoms certainly differ from those generally produced, and it may be stated that they are not the result of mesmerism. But the same objection would apply to those met with in the O'Keys, and in Mons. La Fontaine's two travelling patients. Further, those on whom it produces any influence are generally characterised by a similar condition of the nervous system, and the actions of the body in such persons being more under the control of the imagination than the will, they are very susceptible to external impressions, whose effects are in proportion to the individual's susceptibility. Precisely as the same feeling which excites pleasure in one produces a degree of ecstacy in another, and may be so exalted in a third as to occasion death, so likewise mesmerism may cause any of the various forms of nervous affections, from hysteria to catalepsy and epilepsy. The first application may require to be long continued before any effects follow; but when once excited they may be reproduced from the same impression more slightly applied; and thus by frequent repetition the system may be rendered so susceptible from a superinduced

2 A

habit as to act without any perceptible influence of the will.

Hence we may easily conceive how mesmerism exhibits its numerous phenomena, when we consider that it combines several means, all of which are powerful excitants of the nervous system. Externally the sense of touch and the sensibility of external parts are acted upon, by pressing the thumbs and gently moving the fingers over the palm of the hand; and vision is powerfully stimulated by the continual staring.

Internally it operates through the mind by mental emotion and the influence of attention, which enables us to transfer the sensorial power from one part of the body to another, giving rise to torpidity in the one, and an exalted condition in the other. The mesmeric power, therefore, is but a combination of exciting causes of disease, which are merely the " sparks that set fire to the train," their power of doing mischief depending on the degree of susceptibility of the constitution.

In the case described, besides an excitable temperament, there was an hereditary tendency to disease; two conditions extremely favourable for the production of a highly susceptible constitution. On stimulating the organs of vision and touch, with the co-operation of mental emotion, symptoms were excited closely allied to those of epilepsy; and from frequent repetitions the system became so extremely susceptible that a paroxysm might be produced by stimulating either of the senses; and ultimately the susceptibility had reached such a high degree, that, through the stimulus of the will alone, he could excite a paroxysm in a few minutes. A similar explanation may be given of the real effects produced in the O'Keys. One of these girls was subject to epilepsy, the other to hysteria, for the cure of which they were admitted into the University College Hospital. Dr. Elliotson states that one was said to have fits at such distant intervals that he could not tell whether she had any thing the matter with her. (See his Elements of Physiology.) By the aid of mesmerism he reproduced the disease, which has continued from time to time, with the addition of a variety of phenomena which can only be classed with the mysteries of witchcraft.

In the same way we may account for the catalepsy and cataleptic ecstacy sometimes produced by mesmerism; and their comparative frequency amongst its phenomena may be regarded as a strong proof that the mind is chiefly concerned in their production, for when these diseases have occurred naturally they have generally been induced by inordinate excitement of the affections and passions, especially from contemplating some religious topics, in individuals with a highly excitable nervous system. The Estatica of Caldaro, and the Adolorata of Capriana, were probably instances of the real form of these diseases; by repeated attacks their systems have become so susceptible that they can produce a paroxysm voluntarily. The history of these remarkable deceivers proves that their diseases were excited by religious fanaticism. In addition to the cataleptic ecstacy they are said to possess marks of the stigmata and crown of thorns of Christ. The latter Lord Shrewsbury describes as being regularly and distinctly marked across the forehead by a number of small punctures, as if they had been pricked with a large pin, which was very probably the case: from the wounds he states that blood flows on certain occasions, generally on Saint days. Such effects being quite inexplicable by any of the known laws of nature, are attributed by their believers to the direct interference of God; consequently the girls have been named the Holy Virgins of the Tyrol. Religion is frequently used as a cloak for deception, and phenomena have been referred to Divine Agency by individuals who are as ignorant of the true principles of religion as they are of the laws of nature.

[To be continued.]

ON THE

NATURE, DIAGNOSIS, AND TREATMENT OF INCIPIENT PHTHISIS.

By CHRISTOPHER M. DURRANT, M.D.
Physician to the East Suffolk and Ipswich Hospital.

(For the London Medical Gazette.)

(Concluded from page 330.)

Recapitulation. — Having now examined in detail the various physical signs which obtain in the earliest stages of phthisis pulmonalis, it may be ad-

prior to considering the treatment; briefly to recapitulate these phenomena, in the order in which they already stand.—We have, then—

1. Alterations in the form of the two sides of the chest, amounting, in some cases, to complete sinking in of the supra and infra clavicular spaces.

2. Insufficient expansion in the upper parts of the corresponding sides of the chest.

3. Decreased vocal and tussive fremitus, as felt below the clavicles.

4. Comparative diminution of the duration and intensity of the inspiratory murmur.

5. Augmentation of the intensity and duration of the expiratory sound.

6. Alterations in the character and quality of both murmurs, becoming rough, harsh, dry, &c.

7. The various rhonchi; the crackling or crumpling sound, dry at first, becoming afterwards moist; the plaintive, whining, or cooing note; and other occasional abnormal sounds, all indicative of the commencement of the disease.

8. Increased resonance, both of voice and cough, becoming more or less bronchophonic.

9. Undue transmission of the sounds of the heart through the tuberculated part of the lung.

10. Comparative dulness on percussion, with alterations in the quality of the sound elicited.

It will seldom occur, indeed it is scarcely possible, for all the above signs to exist at the same time in any one case of incipient consumption, although we are not unfrequently enabled to detect their successive appearance as the disease advances. The greater number that can be combined in any particular case, the more marked their character, and especially if conjoined with general symptoms, the more accurate will our conclusion be, and the more decidedly may we pronounce on the positive existence of the disease.

Treatment.—Recent pathological investigations tend to prove that phthisis is not so invariably fatal as is generally supposed; "that it is not, like cancer, a disease of itself incurable, but that its extreme danger chiefly depends on the ordinary seat, extension, and relapses of the malady." Such are the conclusions arrived at by M. Boudet, *and recently communicated by him to* the Academy of Sciences at Paris. This author's investigations lead him to believe that recovery is possible at any period of pulmonary consumption; but that nature, independently of remedies, works the entire cure. That such will be the case in the occasional terminations of the advanced stages I am ready to admit; but that in the commencement of the deposit, very much towards a cure, or at least a suspension of the disease, may often be effected by treatment, I am fully prepared to affirm; and, as such, shall now consider the remedies which have, from time to time, proved decidedly beneficial, dwelling especially on those which my own experience has found of most value.

Blood-letting.—Among the various remedial measures had recourse to in the treatment of incipient phthisis pulmonalis, perhaps none has canvassed the opinions of the profession more than bleeding. Among its advocates are included many authors of the last as well as the present century, some of whom, acting under the impression of various preconceived theories, carried the practice to a very great extent. Like many other remedies, however, which have been proposed in this affection, the abuse, rather than the adoption of depletion, has, from the earliest period, given rise to the most conflicting opinions.

Viewing phthisis not as inflammatory in itself, but as peculiarly liable to excite that condition in the surrounding tissues, I am disposed to limit the use of general blood-letting (and then only in small quantity and seldom repeated), to such cases as clearly indicate signs of plethora, pulmonary congestion inflammation, or hæmorrhage.

Laennec, speaking of bleeding in phthisis, says, "it ought never to be employed, except to remove inflammation, or active determination of blood, with which the disease may be complicated; beyond this, its operation can only tend to a useless loss of strength." In a note by Dr. Forbes (to whom the profession is much indebted for first pointing out the importance of investigating the earliest changes in the respiration in phthisis, with a view to treatment), we read : "I have seen blood-letting much employed, and have myself used it much in this disease. I have seen great benefit derived from it, but chiefly in relieving the inflammatory complications of phthisis. With our present knowledge of its pathology, it can hardly be expected to benefit the tuberculous affection, and my experience leads me to condemn its use in every case of pure phthisis."

Having, however, subdued pulmonary congestion, &c. by small general blood-lettings, the adoption of local depletion, by leeches or cupping, ought then to be substituted, especially in those cases in which co-existing bronchitis, hæmoptysis, or pneumonic consolidation, resulting from tuberculous deposit, still remain. At this period I strongly advise the application of six or eight leeches below one or both clavicles, or the withdrawal of four or five ounces of blood from between the scapulæ, by cupping. The former method is preferable, and should be repeated according to the exigency of the case, once a week or fortnight. This practice, by unloading the apices of the lungs, I have found to afford marked and permanent relief in the majority of cases, more especially by removing the sensation of tightness, pain, and general uneasiness, often so distressingly felt at the upper part of the chest.

It is in those cases of incipient phthisis accompanied by hæmoptysis, or complicated with bronchitis, that small, general, or repeated local depletions, so frequently prove of such decided benefit; in the purely chronic form even topical bleeding is less called for, save to remove accidental complications.

Counter-irritation.—Many have been the forms proposed, and great has been the testimony in favour of the adoption of this important remedy; important both as a palliative and also as a frequent preventive against the farther extension of the tuberculous deposit.

The use of counter-irritation in the treatment of phthisis appears to claim considerable antiquity. Both Celsus and Galen, whose attention however was only directed to the advanced stages of the malady, recommended the free application of revulsive plasters, and even the actual cautery, to the chests of their patients in this disease.

From a tolerably extended observation and experience of the comparative amount of benefit derived from the use of different counter-irritants, I am disposed to place the greatest reliance on the timely application of blisters, and the use of a liniment of turpentine and acetic acid. If, however, much febrile excitement attend the disease, it will be advisable, in all cases, to postpone the application of blisters until after its removal by appropriate, general, or local depletory measures; otherwise they not unfrequently increase the evil they are intended to remove.

Small blisters, about an inch and a half in width, placed below the entire length of the clavicles, operate very favourably. Should, however, dyspnœa prove urgent, a large blister over the sternum seldom fails in affording marked relief. With a view to excite and keep up a moderate degree of counter-irritation, and, at the same time, to render the skin less easily affected by atmospheric changes and external impressions, I have hitherto found no application so useful and so manageable as a liniment of turpentine and acetic acid, first proposed by Dr. Stokes, and since advocated by Dr. Hughes. The latter author adopts a formula, which, for extemporaneous prescription, amply fulfils the intention: viz. one ounce of strong acetic acid and two ounces of the oil of turpentine, simply shaken together. I have, however, in a few cases of delicate skins, found it necessary to reduce the proportion of the acid.

The original formula employed by Dr. Stokes is the following:—

℞. Olei Terebinth. ʒiij.; Acidi Acet. ʒss.; Vitelli ovi. j.; Aq. Rosar. ʒijss.; Olei Limon. ʒj. M. fiat Linimentum.

After applying this remedy freely to the chest night and morning for a few days, patients have often expressed themselves in almost enthusiastic terms of the relief afforded. The various lotions containing vinegar, alcohol, ammonia, mustard, &c., from time to time recommended, are all much inferior to the above. Tartar emetic, either in the form of ointment or solution, proves a useful, though, in chronic cases, by no means so decidedly effectual a remedy as the turpentine and acetic acid liniment. Croton oil has been held in considerable repute, and certainly fulfils the intention, especially as an application to the larynx and trachea.

Issues, setons, moxa, and even the actual cautery, have severally found their advocates; of the latter, from their painful application, and the great irritation which they inevitably pro-

 once, no further mention is necessary. The insertion of setons or issues is to a certain extent open to similar objections; nevertheless, an issue introduced alternately in each arm, and allowed to heal, will be a prudent course, especially at the age of puberty, in all cases whenever from hereditary or acquired predisposition an attack of phthisis is apprehended.

Emetics.—Since the publication of Sir James Clark's valuable work on Consumption, the practice of treating incipient phthisis by frequently repeated emetics has lately been revived, with a prospect, if persevered in, of beneficial results. The testimony of the numerous authors of the last century in favour of this measure, valuable as is their authority, must not be received without due limitation. The uncertain knowledge that then existed in detecting incipient phthisis, and the imperfect manner in which the pathology of mucous membrane and its secretions was at that time understood, renders it exceedingly probable that the majority of cases reported as relieved, or even cured, were not phthisis, but chronic bronchitis. One fact, however, is unquestionably proved, viz. that emetics may be administered for months, not only without injury, but with positive advantage; the appetite improving, the complexion becoming clear, and the patient gaining both flesh and strength under their continued use.

I have now had an opportunity of watching and treating very many well-marked cases of incipient phthisis, and the large amount of benefit which, in the great majority of instances, I have seen derived from a persevering use of emetics, makes me the more anxious to add the feeble weight of my own testimony and experience to that of others, in favour of the adoption of this remedy, both as a palliative and curative measure, in the treatment of the commencement of this too frequent disease.

The visible effects of the emetic treatment are, in general, the great alleviation, and frequently the entire removal, of the cough and dyspnœa, together with the pain and oppressive uneasiness in the chest, so frequently complained of in this affection. The changes in the expectoration under the *use of emetics are very various*; in *some it is increased, in others di-*

minished, or altogether checked. The complexion clears, and the appetite, if previously defective, I have generally found to improve; at the same time the secretions flowing more freely, and the bowels acting with greater regularity. The physical signs of the disease also frequently undergo a corresponding and equally favourable change; the expiratory sound becoming less loud and of shorter duration; the rhonchi cease; and nothing frequently remains but a slight roughness, audible only on a deep inspiration. The emetic which I have found to answer best, causing vomiting to occur twice or thrice, has been twelve to fifteen grains of powdered ipecacuanha, taken in warm water an hour before breakfast, and repeated daily, or less frequently, according to the peculiar exigencies of the case. A wine-glassful of cold camomile infusion, taken immediately the vomiting has ceased, imparts tone to the stomach, and prevents the distressing nausea which sometimes succeeds its operation.

The *modus operandi* of this remedy is, I imagine, two-fold—partly local, by dislodging the recently deposited tuberculous matter, and at the same time preventing its increase, and partly general, by giving a shock to the whole system, thereby improving the secretions, and restoring the due balance in the circulation.

In the selection of proper cases for the exhibition of emetics, some care and circumspection are necessary. If the tuberculous matter be deposited to a considerable extent, very little advantage can be expected from the use of emetics; indeed, the propriety of adopting them at this period becomes very questionable. The incipient stage alone is the period in which we clearly derive benefit from this practice; and, as a general rule, the more chronic the character of the malady, the more decidedly and sanguinely may we employ the remedy.

In those instances in which bronchitis or hæmoptysis co-exist, these should first be removed by appropriate treatment, and then the emetic plan may be safely adopted.

The existence of gastric irritation, as evinced by a dry, red, shining tongue, with prominent papillæ, thirst, a congested and swollen state of the fauces, and upper part of the pharynx, with or without epigastric tenderness, strongly contra-indicates the use of emetics.

The only objection of which I am aware, that has been advanced against this practice, is the opposition with which the remedy would be met by the patients themselves. Hitherto, I confess, I have found very little difficulty in ensuring its regular adoption, and am disposed to attribute the non-compliance of the patient more to the want of decision and firmness on the part of the physician in enforcing the measure, than to the disagreeable nature of the remedy prescribed. One great recommendation of this practice is, that it need not, and indeed ought not, to interfere with any other treatment, which, according to the existing symptoms, may be considered most suitable to the peculiar condition of the case.

Iodine.—From the palpable effects which this substance exerts in the removal of enlarged glands, and scrofulous deposits in various parts of the body, which latter, in their intimate nature, do not apparently differ from the tuberculous, and from the very favourable testimony of several authors, founded on extensive trials of the remedy, the use of iodine and its preparations, in the treatment of incipient phthisis, unquestionably lays claim to the fairest considerations. The operation of this medicine is very slow, but acting, as it does, on the hepatic, renal, and uterine functions, the general health of the majority of patients rarely fails to improve under its use; and if the morbid deposit in the lungs be limited, the probability in many cases, of its absorption, is by no means chimerical.

The iodide of potassium, in doses of two or three grains three times a day, with a few grains of the sesquicarbonate of soda in any light infusion, is the form in which I have found the remedy to agree best. In leucophlegmatic habits, and where a more tonic effect is required, the iodide of iron may be advantageously substituted.

Sedatives.—The employment of sedatives, however valuable as a palliative measure in the more advanced stages of the malady, I have seldom found to be of much service in the very commencement of the disease, save in diminishing the irritation of the cough, *and occasionally in procuring rest.* The *hydrocyanic acid does not appear to have*

sustained the reputation in the treatment of phthisis which its advocates at first raised in its favour: nevertheless, in combination with morphia or conium, it is sometimes exceedingly useful in quieting the paroxysmal cough, which often, even at the commencement of the disease, proves so harassing and wearing to the sufferer. Hyoscyamus, in the form of tincture, is a valuable addition to the mixture of iodide of potassium and soda, above alluded to.

Digitalis may be advantageously prescribed in those cases of phthisis co-existing with cardiac affection, and especially if the habit be phlegmatic. The effects, however, of this remedy must be carefully watched, since by deranging the gastric and alvine functions, and permanently reducing the force of the circulation, the constitution will be thereby injured, and the disposition to deposit tuberculous matter in consequence increased. Perhaps, on the whole, the salts of morphia, commencing with very small doses, may be esteemed the most useful. In the inflammatory complications of the complaint, the tartrate of antimony, in combination with a sedative, will operate beneficially; but, from its liability to disorder the stomach and bowels, its use should be discontinued immediately the inflammatory symptoms have been subdued.

Mercury.—The exhibition of mercury in phthisis, save as an alterative, or in combination as a mild aperient, has been considered by the greater number of authors as decidedly injurious. More recently, however, the attention of the profession has been ably directed to the subject by Sir Henry Marsh, Dr. Graves, and Dr. William Stokes, of Dublin; and still more lately, in an interesting paper on the treatment of incipient phthisis by mercury, by Dr. Munk, published in the MEDICAL GAZETTE for Oct. 1840.

From the high talent and undoubted testimony of the authors above mentioned, and from the numerous well-marked cases which they have detailed, little question can exist but that in some cases of incipient consumption the production of ptyalism is attended with the happiest result; in reference to the adoption of this treatment, however, the precaution of Dr. Stokes should never be lost sight of: viz. "that the remedy is a two-edged sword, and its exhibition must not be lightly attempted."

The form of the disease best adapted for the mercurial treatment is that in which the symptoms present more or less of an inflammatory character. In these cases, by the judicious use of mercury, the irritation of the pulmonary mucous membrane and parenchyma may be removed, the deposition of tuberculous matter probably arrested; and thus, by the suspension of local action, time is gained for the adoption of other remedies, and the improvement of the general health.

In my own practice I have tried the mercurial treatment of incipient phthisis in a very limited number of cases; where I have done so, however, the result has been more or less favourable.

Inhalation.—Of the utility of inhalation as a remedy in the early stage of consumption, I have at present had very little experience. Like the majority of curative measures, it has its advocates and its opponents; and on weighing the testimony of each, it is extremely probable that by judicious management, where there exists but little disposition to inflammatory action, it will prove a useful adjunct to the therapeutics of pulmonary disorders. Sir Charles Scudamore strongly recommends a mixture of iodine with conium, inhaled from a glass apparatus with large tubes, by which treatment, combined with general measures, he reports that he has effected several cures. Dr. Corrigan prefers impregnating the air of the patient's room with iodine. Perhaps the most ingenious and economical method of introducing this substance into the system by inhalation, is that proposed by Dr. Leigh, of Jersey, who directs the patient to apply a sufficient quantity of iodine ointment on the ribs, under both axillæ, and then, by covering the head with the bed-clothes, to inhale the iodine that is volatilized by the heat of the patient's body. This practice may be advantageously adopted in hospitals, and as the ointment produces counter-irritation, I would suggest its simultaneous application below the clavicles.

Tonics.—After the removal of local, especially gastric irritation, and the more prominent symptoms caused by the presence of tubercles, the free exhibition of tonic remedies (with a view *to improve the general health,* by altering the condition of the fluids and solids of the body, upon the depraved state of which the secretion of tuberculous matter undoubtedly in a great measure depends) may be most advantageously had recourse to: of these, iodine, the preparations of iron and zinc, the sulphate of quinine, and the mineral acids, are to be preferred. The sulphates of iron and quinine, with an excess of acid, I have repeatedly found, in conjunction with the exhibition of emetics, to act most favourably in this disease; indeed, the salts of iron, by improving the condition of the blood, have, and still most deservedly enjoy, a high reputation in the treatment of the early stages of pulmonary consumption.

Among the best tonics in incipient phthisis may be included—early hours, both in reference to rising and going to bed; at the same time, carefully avoiding excitement of any kind that may at all interfere with a quiet and unbroken slumber; a diet at once nutritious, unstimulating, and easy of digestion. Thus, for breakfast, I would recommend a lightly-boiled egg, with dry buttered toast, or bread a day old, and tea or cocoa, with a large proportion of milk; coffee, with an equal quantity of milk, may be taken if it agree, but in general I have found it too stimulating. For dinner (which should be an early hour, viz. 1 or 2), meat, principally mutton, beef, and game: veal, pork, and salted meats, are objectionable: fried fish and salmon must be rejected from the dietary of the phthisical patient; boiled sole, whiting, and haddock, however, are nutritious and digestible, and may therefore be allowed; a moderate proportion of well-dressed vegetables may be taken with the meat, with a small quantity of mild home-brewed beer; this is far preferable to porter or wine, which are too stimulating. The tea and supper should be combined, and consist principally of milk, or thin arrow-root, with toast or bread and butter; the last meal ought to be taken at least one hour before bed-time. In addition to the above, I would strongly recommend a tumbler of asses' milk to be taken twice a day, viz. on rising in the morning, and again immediately before retiring to rest.

Another admirable tonic is a residence where the air is mild and dry, to the invigorating influence of which the patient should expose himself as much as possible, carefully avoiding easterly and northerly winds. He should live much in the open air, taking gentle exercise, the best of which by far, when attainable, is that derived from horse exercise. Sailing on the sea, when moderately agitated, if it do not excite too great nausea, is another valuable remedy in the early stage of the complaint; and, at this period, seldom fails in affording marked relief; cruising round the coast, at repeated short intervals, by avoiding the inevitable *ennui* consequent on a protracted sea expedition, is preferable. Travelling (provided the circumstances of the patient admit of the comforts of home, combined with the strictest regard to the improvement of the general health), by varying the air and scene, and at the same time tranquillizing the mind, proves, in many cases, a valuable auxiliary to the tonic treatment.

The shower-bath, if possible, should never be neglected by those in whom there exists the slightest predisposition to the tuberculous habit. It is astonishing the amount of benefit derived from this remedy as a tonic; it enables the invalid to bear with impunity the vicissitudes of climate, braces the system, gives tone to the digestive organs, and, by diminishing the susceptibility to the impressions of cold, prevents, in many cases, the first assumption of the disease. It should be taken every morning throughout the year on rising, and its use followed by brisk friction with the coarsest towels. If, in delicate individuals, the shock of the bath cannot be borne, or reaction does not immediately follow, rapid sponging of the entire surface of the body, succeeded by friction, must be substituted. In commencing either practice, it will be advisable to use the water slightly warm; the temperature, however, must be daily reduced, until it becomes cold, at which point it must be steadily kept and persevered in. Flannel ought always to be worn next the skin; and, during the winter months, I would strongly advise a chamois leather waistcoat being worn over thin flannel during the day, by all those who, from whatever cause, are more or less prone to the disease.

Having brought to a conclusion the consideration of those remedies which have proved, both in my own practice as well as in that of others, of unquestionable benefit in the treatment of the early stage of pulmonary phthisis, it now only remains for me, in a few words, to notice the especial treatment of those forms in which the disease commonly obtains at its commencement, more particularly in reference to its complication with inflammation and hæmorrhage.

When bronchitis or pneumonia coexist with tuberculous deposit, the proper remedies will be depletion, saline aperients, antimony, low diet, and the cautious exhibition of mercury to the extent of *slightly* affecting the system. Having, by one or more of these measures, subdued the inflammatory condition, the period then arrives for emetics, counter-irritation, and mild tonics; at the same time, by way of precaution, frequently repeating the topical bleeding by leeches below the clavicles.

When hæmoptysis is a prominent symptom in the early stage of phthisis, small and repeated general bloodlettings are advisable; saline aperients; nauseating doses of antimony or ipecacuanha; the mineral acids, with opium; the acetate of lead, with opium and acetic acid; or creosote, with opium; or lastly, in the event of all these remedies failing to arrest the bleeding, we may try what is now believed to be the active ingredient of Ruspini's styptic, viz. gallic acid, in doses of half a grain, three or four times a day.

Having, by the above practice, succeeded in stopping the bleeding, we may then, with advantage, commence the exhibition of emetics; the application of blisters to the chest; the use of tonics, especially iron and the mineral acids; with the other general measures already fully detailed.

If the disease be uncomplicated either by hæmoptysis or inflammation, which in the majority of instances is the case, we should at once commence the practice of emetics, counter-irritation, and iodine, with strict attention to the rules for diet and regimen above prescribed.

To ensure the beneficial effects of the foregoing treatment, it must be commenced *early, boldly*, and *continued perseveringly ;* and although, in so fatal an affection as phthisis pulmonalis, and one the tendency of which to a progressive and fatal termination is so great, many cases will inevitably occur in which apparently little benefit is derived from any mode of treatment; yet, on the other hand, I do conscientiously affirm, that by the timely and judicious exhibition of remedies, the disease, if not cured, may often be indefinitely suspended; and the lives of hundreds, in whom it now too frequently runs unchecked to its close, may be long preserved in a state of happiness and comfort.

CASE OF ARTIFICIAL ANUS,

SUCCESSFULLY TREATED BY INCISION OF ITS DIVIDED EDGES.

To the Editor of the Medical Gazette.

SIR,

IF the following should be thought worthy of the pages of the MEDICAL GAZETTE, an early insertion will much oblige the writer.—I am, sir,

Your obedient servant,
D. MALCOLM, M.C.

Boston, May 20th, 1845.

John Barclay, æt. 47, farm labourer, for the last two years has been troubled with periodical prolapses of a reducible inguinal hernia, attaining sometimes the size of a hen's egg, and occupying an elevated position in the left groin. Previous to the last two months it has occasioned him but inconsiderable pain, and very little inconvenience, save that of assuming the horizontal position and reducing the tumor with his own hand. Never wore a truss, and says the rupture has frequently continued down for spaces of thirty-six and forty-eight hours without the occurrence of any unpleasant symptoms. About eight weeks ago, however, after a hard day's work, an unusual pain began to be felt in the seat of the tumor, which had now become exquisitely painful to the touch and defied all his attempts at reduction. The pain increased rapidly with the continuance of the rupture, and in seven hours afterwards all the symptoms of strangulation had supervened. A surgeon had been immediately called in, who, failing in all his attempts to effect reduction, and perceiving the alarming advance made by the symptoms, intimated to the patient the danger of his condition, and held out an operation as the only available means

of affording him relief. An operation accordingly was consented to, and in a few hours afterwards was carried into execution. The consequences were, that the bowel was reduced, and the urgency of the symptoms abated; but in lieu of the danger of the former tumor, there succeeded the loathsomeness and inconveniences of an artificial anus. Up to the present time the patient had been discharging his fæces partly by the rectum, but in greater quantity from the opening in the groin; and had thereby, by the acrimony of the discharge, incurred extensive excoriation round about and in the neighbourhood of the latter situation. The wound occupied the middle third of the sulcus which divides the thigh from the abdomen, was two inches long, irregular in its edges, but capable of complete closure by the semi-bent position of the thigh upon the belly. Patient felt exhausted, and complained of great pain and tenderness in the back and sacrum, occasioned by the continued pressure of the mattrass on which he lay on these parts. On dilating the edges of the wound, which were much inverted, and covered with spongy-looking skin, a quantity of wind and liquid fæces made their escape, and obscured the internal orifice for a time, but which, by sponging and drying, was afterwards determined to be of the size of a shilling. As the patient was much reduced in strength, and on the point of being threatened with bed sores; and, moreover, as there were no marks of incarnation in the bottom of the wound, and no external evidence of a disposition to heal, it was proposed to the patient, as a means of increasing his present comfort and adding greater certainty to his recovery, to submit himself to the chances of a second operation. The proposal was readily acceded to; and on the following day, with an instrument prepared for the purpose, I proceeded to incise the edges of the wound, and afterwards to keep them in close contact, with the object in view of producing adhesion of their surfaces, and effecting a favourable termination to the disease. The instruments I employed for the purpose were a piece of iron wire bent into a parallelogram of the length and depth of the wound, and a common scalpel. By inserting the former perpendicularly into the wound, and pressing first on one side and next upon the other, so as to make the respective walls of the wound to protrude through the opening, the necessary slice to be removed was thus conveniently brought within reach of the scalpel, and the operation was done without pain or loss of blood. The results fully realized my expectations : union took place by the first intention ; and the man, grateful for his recovery, was able to resume his usual occupations in thirteen days.

EXTRACTION OF A NEEDLE FROM THE LEG,

SUPPOSED TO HAVE BEEN PREVIOUSLY SWALLOWED.

To the Editor of the Medical Gazette.

SIR,

MANY cases are on record, and some in the early numbers of your journal, of needles which, after being swallowed, have subsequently escaped from the surface of the body. Such results are usually described as attended with more or less unfavourable symptoms, local or general irritation, abscess, &c. I forward you a case, thinking it may be worthy of remark, in which a needle passed from the leg of a female, without giving rise to any thing but the most trifling degree of irritation.

A young woman, æt. 24, consulted me about eight weeks back respecting a small swelling about the size of a walnut, situated on the outer side of the calf of the leg. It was hard and very moveable, did not implicate the adjacent skin, and gave no pain unless roughly handled. When pressed with some force it gave a distinct sensation of crackling, and altogether disappeared, at the same time causing the patient to complain of a " pricking pain," which lasted until the tumor re-formed, which took place in a few hours. This was repeated several times. The inconvenience caused by the swelling was so slight, that no active remedies were called for. A light bandage and cold lotions afforded all the relief required.

At the expiration of eight weeks the swelling was not changed ; but I was *summoned* to see her, and found the *point of a needle* projecting a line or *two through the skin*, directly in the centre of the tumor. I easily extracted about two-thirds of an ordinary-sized sewing-needle, which had its surface completely oxidized, and the edges, where it had been broken, rounded and perfectly smooth. No pain, redness of the surface, or even the most trifling bleeding, followed its removal. A small quantity of thin colourless serum only escaped. The tumor almost immediately disappeared. The patient could not remember having swallowed such a body ; but there can be little doubt of it, as I know her to be above deceit, and the fact of the point being the first to escape disproves any other notion.

I infer that this needle was surrounded by cysts : the crackling and subsequent temporary disappearance of the tumor upon pressure would justify such a conclusion.

This case may be of service to any who are consulted by persons rendered anxious on account of having swallowed a similar body.—I am, sir,

Your obedient servant,
C.

London, May 11, 1843.

MEDICAL GAZETTE.

Friday, June 2, 1843.

" Licet omnibus, licet etiam mihi, dignitatem *Artis Medicæ* tueri ; potestas modo veniendi in publicum sit, dicendi periculum non recuso."
CICERO.

THE REVENUE IN JEOPARDY FROM SPURIOUS CHEMISTRY.

IT was well said by Boerhaave that chemistry, though an excellent handmaid to medicine, was a bad mistress ; and we may add that all the ordinary affairs of life admit with advantage her oc-casional interference, though they would be damaged by her constant direction.

. Several instances have lately oc-curred where the revenue has been pro-tected by skilful analysis from frauds which might have appeared at first too difficult even for modern chemistry to detect. Dr. Ure, whose analytic dex-terity has conferred this benefit upon the country, has given the history of his success in a pamphlet, of which we have placed the title at the head of this article.

It appears that in September 1842, a cargo of eighteen casks was entered at the Custom-house of Liverpool by Messrs. Tennants, Clow, and Co., under the title of *naphtha*, at a valuation in the whole of £50. It was suspected that the cargo was not really naphtha, and after the matter had been referred to the Board of Customs in London, a sample bottle was forwarded for analysis to Dr. Ure. In his report he stated that the liquor was not naphtha, but pyroligneous acid mixed with alcohol; or rather, as it should seem, spirits masked by a slight admixture of pyroligneous acid. One hundred parts of the fluid in the bottle contained ninety-one of proof spirits. "*The sprits thus distilled may be rendered quite palateable by rectification with potash, so as to be fit for making English gin.*"

In consequence of this report, the Commissioners ordered the goods to be detained for having been entered under a false denomination. The importing merchants now procured a contrary certificate from the Apothecaries' Hall at Liverpool, as well as one from Professor Graham, of the London University College. The Professor stated that the liquor was not convertible into gin by potash or by any other process; that it was not alcohol; that the small proportion of alcohol, if any, which it contained, was not separable from it; and that it contained no pyroligneous acid.

A memorial embodying these points having been presented to the Board of Trade, the matter was referred to the Board of Customs for re-consideration. Mr. Ross, the surveyor-general, was accordingly instructed to invite Dr. Ure to a consultation in his office. This took place on the 5th of January, when the *certificates of Professor Graham*,

and of Mr. Waldie, practical chemist t[o] the Liverpool Apothecaries' Company, were laid before Dr. Ure. Mr. Graham's certificate, which appears to be the one already quoted, affirms that a small quantity of spirit in naphtha is exceedingly difficult of detection, owing to the impossibility of separating them when once mixed. He is unable, therefore, to say whether the naphtha contains a small quantity of alcohol or not; but he affirms that the alcohol could not be separated, nor used in making English gin by distillation from potash, or any other process whatever.

David Waldie, again, certifies that the naphtha gave no evidence of the presence of alcoholic spirit; but that it was merely pyroxylic spirit, or wood-naphtha, with less impurities than usual, on which account its flavour was more agreeable than ordinary: nor could it, in his opinion, be made a drinkable liquid by any chemical process.

Dr. Ure, having reserved the greater portion of the original sample bottle, performed a series of fresh experiments with it, and furnished the Surveyor-General's office with the result on the 7th of January.

He allows that alcohol and naphtha, being equally volatile, cannot be completely separated by distillation, or by any direct method: yet the thing can be done indirectly. In the present instance, however, it was easy to ascertain the presence of a large proportion of alcohol, without effecting this separation. The method was as follows:—When alcohol, fifty or sixty per cent. above proof, is mixed with its own weight of sulphuric acid, and distilled, it affords sulphuric ether; but when wood-spirit, or wood-naphtha, is treated in the same way, it affords, not a liquid, but an acriform product. Moreover, in the former case, if the distillation is continued too long, the residuum in the retort becomes black, thick, and froths up with such impetuosity as to be projected out of the vessel, though fifty times as large as the liquid required before its intumescence; in the latter, the mixture neither thickens nor froths up. Now, after rectifying the imaginary naphtha by repeated distillations, Dr. Ure treated it with sulphuric acid, when it yielded a fine, fragrant, *liquid* sulphuric ether, and almost as much as the same quantity of alcohol would have done. A very little ligneous or methylic ethereal gas also appeared. In due time the residuum became black, frothed up, and was projected out of the vessel with great violence. "Thus by the product of fine liquid ether, and the intumescence in the retort, two infallible proofs of abundance of alcohol in the said naphtha are obtained—proofs which will be recognised in every chemical court in Christendom." Dr. Ure found, too, that four fluid ounces of the pyroligneous acid residuum saturated as much carbonate of potash as two fluid ounces of ordinary vinegar.

He naturally thought that the matter was now settled; but on the 18th of February he was again summoned to the Custom-House to consider two certificates signed by Mr. Brande, both denying the presence of alcohol in the supposed naphtha. Some little doubt, however, overshades the denial, and Mr. Brande suggests the propriety of submitting the question to some third chemical authority.

Dr. Ure now requested to have a sample from each of the casks at Liverpool, and he accordingly received 18 bottles full of the naphtha, with the corks sealed with the Custom-House arms. The liquor was like the former sample. It had a sour empyreumatic smell, an acidulous taste, reddened litmus, effervesced with carbonate of soda, and had a specific gravity of 0·942.

Dr. Ure and Mr. Scanlan were occu-

pied for three weeks in experiments with this liquid, which fully confirmed the former ones, and showed that the "naphtha" was merely alcohol disguised with a little pyroligneous acid.

In the first place, Dr. Ure and his friend took half a gallon of the liquid from five of the bottles indiscriminately, and having distilled by the heat of a water-bath, obtained a spirit of sp. gr. 0·901, while an acidulous residuum, as before, was left in the still. A part of the alcohol thus obtained was then rectified, and afterwards afforded a fine ether of specific gravity 0·752. A gallon of the Liverpool naphtha was then distilled with a rectifying apparatus of Dr. Ure's own invention; and a portion of the alcohol obtained from it was made into twenty ounces of ether, of sp. gr. 0·742. This is lighter, and therefore finer, than the standard ether of the Pharmacopœia.

Dr. Ure finds that when ten parts of wood-naphtha are mixed with ninety of alcohol, and the mixture is treated with sulphuric acid, it does not afford ether, but a pungent and offensive fluid, thus showing that the Liverpool mixture contained little or no real naphtha, but owed its peculiar taste and flavour to the pyroligneous oil of the wood-vinegar.

Dr. Ure and Mr. Scanlan were equally successful in making sweet spirit of nitre, and gin, with the rectified Liverpool liquor.

They afterwards ascertained that the pretended naphtha consisted of seventy parts of alcohol, 14·3 above proof, and thirty of pyroligneous acid.

They then tried a variety of experiments with genuine naphtha from the manufactory of Messrs. Hill, of Deptford, and proved, if more proof were needed, how different was the reality from the Liverpool fiction. Among other differences, Hill's naphtha of sp. gr. 0·870 boils at 144° Fah., while alcohol of the same specific gravity boils at 180°°.

Besides these chemical proofs to shew that the casks at Liverpool did not contain naphtha, Dr. Ure gives a commercial one, which is worth mentioning. The casks were imported from New York. Now naphtha is made only from pyroligneous acid; and where there are no great calico-printing establishments (as there are none in the United States) little or none of this acid is prepared. But the casks in question contained about 2000 gallons of " naphtha," equivalent to about 200,000 of pyroligneous acid, " a quantity certainly far greater than has been made there since the days of Elizabeth.' The simple fact is, that coarse ardent spirit is excessively cheap in the United States, and pyroligneous acid can easily be procured to give it a flavour.

It appears, moreover, that this same introduction of alcohol, under its masquerade name of naphtha, has become very frequent of late; sometimes it comes from abroad, and at other times it is of native growth.

A sample of some "naphtha" imported from Havre in the " James Watt" was analysed by Dr. Ure, and found to contain at least 95 per cent. of alcohol of sp. gr. 0·842, or about 53.7 over proof!

Ten more samples of sham naphtha were sent to Dr. Ure for analysis, by the fiscal authorities, within one fortnight. Two came from the Customs, and eight from the Excise. The first of the former was an approach to the genuine stuff, and, as Dr. Ure pleasantly

* During these and other researches, Dr. Ure had the good fortune to discover the solution of the following problem: as he does not give the solution, we enunciate the difficulty, for the diversion of chemical experimentalists:—" Given a mixture of wood-naphtha and alcohol, each of the same specific gravity, or otherwise, and which suffer no change of density by admixture; to determine, in the course of twenty minutes, the proportion of each."
The problem is solved without the aid of heat.

supposes, was intended as a puzzle for our professors of chemistry; for it consisted of sixty parts of real wood-spirit and forty of alcohol. The eight samples seized by the Excise were nothing but alcohol impregnated " with the dead coal oil of the coal-tar distillers."

It would be unjust to conclude without mentioning that Mr. Brande made the amende honorable in the handsomest manner, and allowed that he had committed an error, in the tone that befits a gentleman.

We have assumed that Dr. Ure is in the right; but should arguments or facts appear to show that he is in the wrong, we shall not let them drop without notice. The only fault we have to find with him at present is that he treats his opponents with a leetle too much asperity. It is obvious, however, that his discovery is of high importance : were the nation served by many men as zealous and as skilful as Dr. Ure, the income tax would have been unnecessary.

EXAMINATION OF THE BODY OF THE LATE MR. TYRRELL.

56 HOURS AFTER DEATH.

Chest.—The pleura closely adherent throughout the whole of the right side of the chest, by old adhesive bands. On the left by a few only.

The right lung hepatised, or consolidated, nearly throughout its whole extent; there being only a very small portion that was crepitant on pressure. The mucous membrane of the lower portion of the trachea and right bronchus thickened, and of a dark brick-dust hue. Left lung engorged with blood, but crepitating tolerably on pressure.

The pericardium considerably distended, and containing from an ounce and a half to two ounces of dark fluid blood. On the posterior aspect of the right auricle the investing pericardium, to a considerable extent, had a rough, depressed, and by the aid of a lens, an ulcerated appearance; while the opposite surface of the loose pericardium, to the same extent, had a granular or tuberculated appearance, very similar to the tuberculous accretions which we find occasionally on the peritoneum; there were two or three adhesive bands connecting these two surfaces.

The heart itself was twice the natural size; the muscular fibre pale, flaccid and flabby, and collapsing; the cavities of both ventricles much dilated, but without hypertrophy of the walls; the left ventricle more especially dilated; in the right ventricle were two or three delicate filaments of lymph of considerable strength, stretching between the carneæ columnæ and chordæ tendineæ, and across the cavity, the evident result of former endocarditis. All the valves of the heart and aorta were perfectly natural.

The liver was enlarged, very much indurated, especially at the superior portion of the right lobe, and granular throughout.

Signed, { H. S. ROOTS, M.D.
C. ASTON KEY.
GEORGE BEAMAN.
JAMES DIXON.
WILLIAM TREW.

NOTE.—The fluid blood in the pericardium was most probably exuded from the depressed and apparently ulcerated surface of the pericardium before stated.

ROYAL MEDICAL & CHIRURGICAL SOCIETY.

May 23, 1843.

THE PRESIDENT IN THE CHAIR.

A few Observations on Encysted Hydrocele. By ROBERT LISTON, F.R.S. Surgeon to the North London Hospital.

THE author commenced by referring to the excellent manner in which the subject had been treated of by former writers, both ancient and modern, and stating, as an apology for introducing it, that he had recently made an observation which induced him to believe that some collections in the scrotum are more intimately connected with the testicle, or its seminiferous tubes, than has been generally supposed. When swellings of this kind have attained a large size, it is difficult, if not impossible, to distinguish between the encysted and the common hydrocele; so that it is only when we have the opportunity of examining them at an early stage of their formation, that we can ascertain their nature correctly. He adverted to the description given by several authors of

eminence, of cysts formed in immediate proximity to the testis or epididymis; and pointed out some of the principal characters by which encysted hydrocele is distinguished from collections in the tunica vaginalis. One peculiarity of the former is, that the fluid contained in it is clear and limpid, and exhibits no traces of albumen; and another is, that in the operations for radical cure its walls are not so prone to take on inflammatory action as those in common hydrocele. One object of the author's communication was to give a rational explanation of this circumstance.

About nine or ten months since he was consulted by a gentleman beyond the middle period of life, on account of tumor of the scrotum. There was plainly fluid on both sides. The largest cyst was punctured, and gave exit to some eight or nine ounces of thin fluid, resembling distilled water with a little soap diffused through it. The other side was punctured a few months afterwards, and five or six ounces of ordinary serum discharged. A short time since the patient returned, to have the first cyst again emptied. The fluid had the same appearance as before; it contained scarcely a trace of albumen. On the second day after it had been drawn off a small quantity was examined with the microscope, when it was found quite full of spermatozoa. It contained also some of the primitive cells in which the spermatozoa are developed, and mucous globules. Had the fluid been examined sooner, probably the animalcules might have been found in motion.

The preceding observation was lately confirmed by the examination of the fluid withdrawn from a small cyst in the scrotum of a man æt. 53, who had applied to be treated for bad stricture. It was nearly transparent, and colourless; and was found to contain numerous spermatozoa, some of which continued to move actively for a considerable time after the fluid had been drawn from the cyst.

The author referred next to several preparations of cysts connected with the body of the testis and epididymis, which he had attentively examined, with the view of ascertaining if possible the nature of the connection between these collections of fluid and the glandular structure of the testis. He concluded with proposing the three following questions for investigation:—

1st, Does the limpid fluid drawn from cysts of the scrotum, or inguinal region, uniformly, or often, contain spermatozoa?

2d, What connection subsists between the seminiferous tubes and these cysts?

3d, Whether dilatation of parts of the epididymis or vas deferens, from obstruction or otherwise, may not in some instances give rise to these collections?

If it be established that these cavities are always lined by mucous membrane, we should have an easy solution of the difficulty regarding a radical cure not following injection, as in the serous cyst.

Some account of an Epidemic which prevailed at Teheran in the months of January and February 1842. By C. W. BELL, M.D. attached to H. B. M.'s Mission at the Court of Persia, in a letter to his Brother, Dr. G. J. BELL, Travelling Fellow of Oxford.

The disease described by the writer occurred nearly simultaneously with an anomalous complaint, presenting symptoms like those of angina pectoris, which broke out as an epidemic at Baghdad, and carried off many persons suddenly. The disease which the author witnessed was attended with a nervous excited action of the heart and arteries, periodical, but neither preceded by chill, nor succeeded by perspiration. Many of the patients were seized with fits, which in some instances resembled epilepsy, and in others were like apoplexy, with palsy of one or other of the extremities; in some cases the patients suffered only from numbness and sleeping of the hands and feet, and they had always more or less palpitation of the heart at the same time, sometimes amounting to pain. The attacks of spasm and loss of power in the extremities returned periodically in some instances, but passed off as single attacks in others. The author was induced at first to employ antiphlogistic measures; but these he soon abandoned, and had recourse to quinine. This last medicine he did not find so effectual as a combination of iron and manfactida, which he gave on first accession of the disease, and commonly with speedy success. Numerous cases are related to illustrate the disease and its treatment.

ON ELECTRO-PUNCTURE IN THE TREATMENT OF DEAFNESS,

DEPENDING ON A PARALYSIS OF THE ACOUSTIC NERVE.

BY M. JOBERT.

THE paralysis of the acoustic nerve may be produced by exposure to a current of air, to too great a shock of the head, to waves of sound too violent, to affections of the teeth or of the gums. Electro-puncture has been already employed in these cases, but it had fallen into disrepute. The author believes that he uses it in a manner more direct and more rational; here is his proceeding:— Stard's sound, he says, is introduced through the nasal fossa into the eustachian tube, and in this sound a long thin acupuncture needle is inserted, so as to fix itself in a point of the parietes of the eustachian tube, while the other end projects from the end of the sound; another acupuncture needle is implanted in the membrane of the tympanum. This being done, one of the conducting wires of a galvanic battery, of which the trough is filled with water and muriatic acid, is passed through the eye of one of the needles, and the end of the other conducting wire is made to touch the opposite needle. I have used, in the beginning, eight pairs of the battery, then I got to ten, to twelve pairs; finally I have been as high as eighteen, and at present I have patients who have undergone several sittings, and on whom I have acted with the entire pile, the trough of which contains forty metallic pairs. At the moment that the two poles are put in contact, there is a very painful shock in the ear and in the head, with convulsive motions; but this shock and this pain cease immediately. In a single patient the impression was felt during eight days, but it never extended beyond a slight pain, which ceased of itself. It must be added, that the patients who were submitted to electricity in this manner, were, during some moments, as if stunned, and preserved some time after the experiment a bewildered look. The sitting was usually confined to a single shock when the patients were irritable; I have given two and even three shocks in people whose sensibility was obtuse, and who have been already submitted to electro-puncture. In general I allow eight days to pass between each trial. The author then relates four cases of well marked deafness, and in which the cure was complete; in the first after a single shock, in the second after two shocks, and in the third after two sittings, each composed of three galvanic shocks. — *L'Examinateur Medicale;* and *Dublin Journal.*

LUXATION OF CERVICAL VERTEBRÆ.

PROF. HORNER presented to the class an example of recent occurrence of this rare and commonly fatal accident. A boy, Thomas Brierly, aged ten years, in clambering about an unfinished house, towards the latter part of November, missed his footing on the second floor and fell through the stairway to the cellar, head foremost, a distance of twenty feet. He was stunned by the fall, and was found, as stated by the friends, with his head bent under his body. He was conveyed senseless and motionless to his home. He gradually regained his perceptions, but in an incoherent and perplexed manner: his head was much bruised by the fall, his neck was stiff and distorted, forming a large serpentine bulge on the left side, and a deep concavity to the right: his face was inclined downwards to the right side. Circumduction of the head was arrested and the neck motionless. The practitioner, Dr. Henry, who attended him in this stage of the injury, applied leeches to the part, emollients and frictions in succession.

In two days after the accident his common and accurate perceptions returned, but he was affected for some time with tingling and numbness in the left upper extremity.

At the period of his exhibition to the class the deformity of the neck is still obvious, but much reduced ; the rotatory motions of the neck can now be executed to some extent, but are much more to the right than to the left side. On tracing the line of the transverse processes of the vertebræ, the upper ones starting from the fourth are about half an inch forward of the lower, indicating clearly the advance of the vertebra on that side, and consequently proving that the left lower oblique process of the fourth vertebra had been luxated in advance of the upper oblique of the fifth, and was there fixed.

We may presume from this state of the accident, that the intervertebral substance there had been partially or wholly ruptured, and that the two vertebræ were held together by the other ligamentous attachments and by the muscles. An attempt at the replacing of such a luxation is viewed with great apprehension by surgeons. Desault, in a case analogous, absolutely declined making the effort, for fear of its fatal issue ; and it is related by M. Petit Radel, (Boyer, Malad. Chir. vol. 4, p. 118,) that a young patient at La Charité expired in the hands of the surgeons, upon such an attempt a few days after the accident. This result is very intelligible when we reflect that to disengage an oblique process thus placed, it is necessary to begin by increasing the inflection forwards, or in other words, by augmenting the displacement, which must in all probability tear up more of the natural fastenings of the bones, and thus subject the spinal marrow to compression or even laceration. Under these circumstances Brierly was dismissed with some general directions for his treatment, and the expectation that his youth would insure a still further erection of that part of the spine. At the period of his exhibition, say about six weeks after the accident, his general health was good, he enjoyed the use of all his faculties, and was going to school.—*American Medical Examiner,* Jan. 21, 1843.

ROYAL COLLEGE OF SURGEONS.

LIST OF GENTLEMEN ADMITTED MEMBERS.

Friday, May 26.

W. C. Small.—D. Grantham.—E. Wright.— W. W. Kershaw.—S. Wilson.—W. G. Carter.— A. T. Thomson.—P. P. M'Donogh.—F. Kelly.— C. T. Male.

WIDOWS AND ORPHANS OF MEDICAL MEN.

WE beg leave again to draw attention to the dinner of this Society, advertised to take place to-morrow, and especially to the request of the Stewards, that those who intend to be present will give notice of their intention.

A TABLE OF MORTALITY FOR THE METROPOLIS,

Shewing the number of deaths from all causes registered in the week' ending Saturday, May 20, 1843.

Small Pox	5
Measles	33
Scarlatina	21
Hooping Cough	56
Croup	7
Thrush	4
Diarrhœa	4
Dysentery	1
Cholera	1
Influenza	2
Ague	0
Typhus	39
Erysipelas	2
Syphilis	1
Hydrophobia	0
Diseases of the Brain, Nerves, and Senses	147
Diseases of the Lungs and other Organs of Respiration	271
Diseases of the Heart and Blood-vessels	17
Diseases of the Stomach, Liver, and other Organs of Digestion	70
Diseases of the Kidneys, &c.	5
Childbed	10
Ovarian Dropsy	1
Disease of Uterus, &c.	0
Rheumatism	1
Diseases of Joints, &c.	2
Carbuncle	0
Ulcer	0
Fistula	1
Diseases of Skin, &c.	0
Diseases of Uncertain Seat	39
Old Age or Natural Decay	64
Deaths by Violence, Privation, or Intemperance	12
Causes not specified	4
Deaths from all Causes	**871**

METEOROLOGICAL JOURNAL.

Kept at EDMONTON, *Latitude* 51° 37' 32" N. *Longitude* 0° 3' 51" W. *of Greenwich.*

April 1843.	THERMOMETER.	BAROMETER.
Wednesday 24	from 50 to 62	29·48 to 29·54
Thursday . 25	45 62	29·55 29·66
Friday . . 26	42 60	29·66 29·92
Saturday . 27	44 61	29·52 29·42
Sunday . . 28	42 63	29·48 29·73
Monday . . 29	41 53	29·83 29·95
Tuesday . 30	32 60	30·00 29·96

Wind variable, S. and S.W. prevailing. Except the 25th and 30th, generally cloudy, with frequent rain. Rain fallen, 1 inch, and ·225 of an inch.

CHARLES HENRY ADAMS.

NOTICE.—The note of Dr. C. appears to us wholly unnecessary, on which account we have omitted it.

THE

LONDON MEDICAL GAZETTE,

BEING A

WEEKLY JOURNAL

OF

Medicine and the Collateral Sciences.

FRIDAY, JUNE 9, 1843.

LECTURE XXIX.

On the operation of craniotomy, the induction of premature labour, and the Cæsarean section.

WHERE the child is dead, where a great disproportion exists between its head and the pelvis from any cause, and the os uteri is imperfectly dilated, and the parts swollen and rigid, and an ear cannot be felt, and circumstances occur demanding immediate delivery, recourse must be had to the perforator, and not to the forceps. It is in difficult labour from distortion of the pelvis that we are most frequently compelled to open and extract the head; and where this exists in a high degree, and the brim is so contracted that the head cannot enter it, the operation of craniotomy often requires the employment of strong extracting force for several hours; and fatal contusion and laceration of the uterus, vagina, bladder, and rectum, can only be prevented by the greatest caution and dexterity, and a perfect knowledge of the structure of all the parts. It unfortunately happens that, in some cases, before the operation is performed, the soft parts have already been injured by the long-continued pressure they have sustained,—the same thing happens here which takes place in strangulated hernia, where the operation has been delayed too long,—and sloughing follows. In cases of slight disproportion between the head and pelvis, or *where there is none, but delivery becomes necessary in consequence of convulsions,*

810.—XXXII.

hæmorrhage, or exhaustion, the operation is attended with little difficulty and danger; much less than the application of the forceps. The position of the patient ought to be the same—the left side, near the edge of the bed—whether you are going to use the forceps, perforate the head, induce premature labour, deliver by turning the child, or remove a retained placenta. The difficulty of all these operations will be greatly increased if you allow patients to lie upon the back, as they do during labour on the Continent, or on the left side at a distance from the edge of the bed. No practitioner, whatever the extent of his experience may be, ought, in my opinion, to open the head of a child, without the most urgent necessity, unless he is absolutely certain that the child is dead, before consulting another accoucheur. Where the bladder is distended with urine, and the urethra is much pressed upon by the head of the child, you will introduce the catheter more easily and safely after the head has been lessened than before perforation.

If the head is in the cavity of the pelvis, or the greater part of it has passed through the brim, and it is not impacted, and the os uteri is fully dilated, no difficulty can be experienced in perforating and extracting the head. With the fore-finger of the right hand carefully examine the situation of the head; and if you can feel a suture or fontanelle, let the point of the perforator pass into it; but if the head is much swollen, and you cannot distinguish either of these, resolve to open the head in the most depending part; and if the instrument is of sufficient strength, it will pass without much difficulty, even through the centre of either of the parietal bones. Having with the fore-finger of the right hand determined the point where the perforator is to enter, slide up the fore and middle fingers of the left hand, before withdrawing the fore-finger of the right, to this point; and in the groove formed between these fingers of the left hand, slowly and carefully introduce the perforator, previously warmed ; and when it has reached the head, press it firmly forward, during a labour pain, through the integuments and bones, as far as the rests will permit it to go, by a boring or semi-rotatory motion.   Where a great effusion is formed under the scalp, if the instrument is not driven forward with sufficient force, you will open the tumor of the scalp without opening the skull, as I have seen happen more than once, to the annoyance of practitioners.   When the perforator has been introduced, in the manner represented in the following figure, withdraw the fingers of the left hand, while with the right you keep the

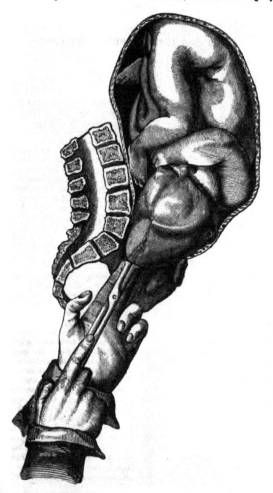

instrument from receding.   If you remove the pressure with the right hand from the *handles at this time, the point will escape from the head, and the skull, if perforated at all, will not be so to a sufficient extent to enable you afterwards to use the crotchet.* Having by firm pressure prevented this accident, take hold of one of the rings of the handles of the perforator with your left hand, and the other with the right, and draw the handles widely asunder, and at the same time press the handles forward, that

the points may not slide back from the head. Having made a large lacerated opening in the integuments and bones, close the handles, and with the fore-finger of the left hand ascertain that the points are still within the head as far as the rests, and then turn the handles round about a quarter of a circle, and open them slowly, with the same precautions, and to a similar extent. Having made a large crucial incision, pass the perforator within the skull, and turn it freely around in every direction until the brain is completely disorganized, and a considerable portion of it has escaped. It is right to do this effectually, and to allow an interval of a quarter of an hour or longer to elapse, that more of the brain may escape, and the bones collapse, before attempting to extract the head with the crotchet. All syringes and instruments for scooping out the brain are quite unnecessary. Then, in your right hand, take the handle of the common crotchet, which should neither be very sharp nor very blunt in the point, and with the fore and middle fingers of the left hand introduce it through the opening in the head, and still more completely destroy the texture of the brain, and draw out as much of it as you can through the opening. Then fix the point of the crotchet on the inside of the head behind—I mean on the part which corresponds with the hollow of the sacrum, at as great a distance as possible from the opening in it made with the perforator, and pass up the fore and middle fingers of your left hand between the posterior wall of the vagina and the head, till their extremities are exactly opposite to the part where the point of the instrument is fixed within. When a pain comes on press the point of the crotchet against the bone, laying firm hold of its handle with your right hand, while you press firmly the points of the fingers of the left hand on the outside of the head, and at the same time turn the ring and little fingers of this hand around the handle, or rather shank, of the crotchet, close to the orifice of the vagina. In this manner you form a double crotchet, far more safe and powerful than that which was invented by Smellie [exhibiting it], which has fallen into complete disuse, because it tore the bones and integuments to pieces, but did not extract the head. With the crotchet fixed on the inside of the bones of the head behind on the part lying in the hollow of the sacrum, and the fore and middle fingers of the left hand on the outside, and with the other two grasping the shank of the crotchet, you can exert a great degree of extracting force, and you will often succeed in completing the delivery in a short period if the perineum is not rigid. The head should always be drawn backward till

the perineum is put upon the stretch, and to prevent the bones from being torn, and the hold with the crotchet lost, the traction should be made slowly and steadily, and during the pains, and time given for the parts to dilate. But if there is any considerable obstruction to the head, however carefully the extracting force may be applied, the point of the crotchet will tear away the bone upon which it is fixed, and it must be placed upon another part of the bones of the head; or you may lay aside the crotchet altogether, and employ the craniotomy forceps, which undoubtedly does in some cases possess advantages over the crotchet. If you know how to form the double crotchet which I have described, and which is one of the most safe and powerful weapons in midwifery, and most frequently sufficient to complete the delivery without any other means, the mother is exposed to no danger from laceration of the bones of the head and slipping of the crotchet, for the point of the instrument is constantly covered with the extremities of the fingers, and the two hands never act but in concert. But where the bones are readily torn, and you are compelled repeatedly to seek a fresh hold, and perhaps meet with some difficulty in fixing the instrument again, I would recommend you to lay aside the crotchet, and try the craniotomy forceps, which is represented in the following figure, the blades of which resemble somewhat the jaws of a crocodile, and which I have employed satisfactorily in many cases of difficult labour from distortion of the pelvis and other causes. The lock is the same as the lock of the common forceps, and the blades are likewise introduced separately and then brought together and fixed. One

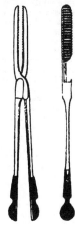

blade is introduced within the head, and the other on the outside, with the same caution as the second blade of the common midwifery forceps. The ragged edges of the bones should be covered with the integuments before you begin to extract, and in operating with the crotchet it is of great importance frequently to pass the finger around the opening in the head, to ascertain if there is not some sharp and uncovered portion of bone pressing against the vagina. When the craniotomy forceps is applied so as to include a large portion of the integuments and bones of the head, the hold you obtain with it is very secure, and you may not only exert a much greater degree of force than you could employ with the crotchet, but you can accommodate the head much better to the axis of the outlet of the pelvis, and protect the perineum, which is exposed to great danger from laceration in all cases of craniotomy. When the head is drawn entirely forward out of the vagina with the crotchet, the perineum must, as you require both hands to wield the instrument, be supported by an assistant, who cannot know the degree of force which you are exerting at any time. If the craniotomy forceps be employed, you can support the perineum with your left hand, while you are operating with the right and drawing the head forward toward the pubes. With the forceps the perineum is certainly exposed to less risk than with the crotchet, but I admit that it may be seriously injured with the forceps if it be a first child, and the bones of the head, compressed into a shape like a wedge, are drawn hastily forward.

In cases of great distortion, where the head cannot enter the brim of the pelvis to any extent, and the os uteri is imperfectly dilated, there is no instrument after perforation so efficient—none to be compared with the crotchet. I have tried all varieties of craniotomy forceps in such cases, and can assure you that they are totally inapplicable unless the os uteri is widely dilated and the head has made considerable progress through the brim into the cavity of the pelvis. M. Baudelocque has invented a huge instrument, weighing four pounds, for crushing the head in these cases, called céphalotribe [exhibiting a figure of it], but it cannot be applied to the head above the brim of the pelvis, and if the os uteri is undilated. In M. Baudelocque's cases the effects of injurious pressure were striking, and they would probably have been much slighter had the perforator and crotchet been employed. Great care must be taken in perforating the head in cases of extreme distortion, that the os uteri *is* not wounded with the sharp edges of the *instrument*. *To obviate this*, if the outlet *is not so much contracted as* to prevent the

hand from being introduced, the fore and middle fingers of the left hand, or all the fingers, should be passed up within the os uteri to the most depending part of the head, and the opening made in the same manner as already described, while the orifice is protected by the fingers expanded. The undilated state of the uterus adds greatly to the difficulty. In extracting the head with the crotchet, it not unfrequently happens that the bones of the cranium are all torn to pieces, and removed, before the base of the skull has entered the brim of the pelvis. It is impossible, under such circumstances, to fix the point of the crotchet in the foramen magnum, as some recommend; and the best mode of proceeding is to pass the fingers of the left hand over the head as far as possible, and to slide up the crotchet between the fingers and the outside of the head, and fix its point in one of the orbits, about the angles of the lower jaw, or wherever a secure hold can be obtained. In this manner, as recommended by Smellie, I have sometimes succeeded in extracting the head in a short time, where I had begun to despair of ever doing so by fixing the crotchet on the inner surface of the base of the cranium, or by any other means. Indeed, in cases of this description you must be prepared to encounter very great difficulties; but when you look at this distorted pelvis from malacosteon, which measures only 1¾ inches from the last lumbar vertebra to the symphysis pubis, and know that two children, at the full period, were drawn through it without destroying the mother, you may conclude that few cases of distortion can possibly occur where you will not ultimately succeed in effecting the delivery with the crotchet. What the degree of distortion is which renders the operation of craniotomy impossible I am unable to state; what is impossible to one may not be so to another practitioner possessed of greater power, dexterity, and patience.

In this table (see pp. 375-8) the results are contained of 127 cases of difficult labour in which it was necessary to deliver by opening the head. After carefully examining all the details of these cases, I feel satisfied that in none was the interference premature, and that in several had the delivery been sooner effected the fatal consequences which ensued would have been prevented. I do not believe there is one of these cases in which the operation was resorted to without a consultation, and the necessity and propriety of the measure fully admitted.

On the Induction of Premature Labour.

The history of this operation, which is the greatest improvement in midwifery since the invention of the forceps, was first given by Dr. Denman about 1795. "We have before alluded," he says, "to this operation as a method of preserving the lives of children, without adding to the danger of women ; if in any case the pelvis were so much distorted, or so small, as absolutely to prevent the passage of the head of a full-grown child, and yet not so far reduced in its dimensions as to prevent the head of a child of a much less size from passing through it. Melancholy are the reflections, where a woman has a very much distorted pelvis (and such women have usually wonderful aptitude to conceive) that there should be little, if any, chance of preserving the lives of their children ; and yet, in the course of practice, I have in several instances been called to the same woman in five or six successive labours, merely to give a sanction to an operation by which the children were to be destroyed. It is to the credit of the profession that every method by which the lives of parents and children might be preserved has been devised and tried : and though frequent occasions for using some of these methods cannot possibly occur in any one person's practice, it is right that all should be acquainted with what has been proposed and done in every case, with or without success.

"The first account of the method of bringing on premature labour was given to me by Dr. C. Kelly. He informed me, that about the year 1756 there was a consultation of the most eminent men in London at that time, to consider of the moral rectitude of, and advantages which might be expected from, the practice, which met with their general approbation. The first case in which it was deemed necessary and proper fell under the care of the late Dr. Macaulay, and it terminated successfully. (The patient was the wife of a linen-draper in the Strand.) Dr. Kelly informed me that he himself had practised it, and, among other instances, mentioned that the operation had been performed three times upon the same woman, and twice the children had been born living. The thing has often been the subject of conversation, and proposed by writers, but some have doubted the morality of the practice ; and the circumstances which may render the operation needful and proper have not been stated with any degree of precision."

The morality, perfect safety, and the utility of the operation, have been fully established, not only in cases of distorted pelvis, but in some of the dangerous diseases of pregnancy, by the experience of all the most eminent practitioners in Great Britain during the last 87 years, and I do not know that it has often, if ever, been employed for criminal purposes in this country. In cases of slighter distortion recourse should not be had to this operation until it has been proved by one or more labours that a child at the full period would not pass without lessening the head. Labour should not be brought on until the $7\frac{1}{2}$ month of gestation, or a little later, where it is known that the pelvis is very little contracted. In cases of very great distortion of the pelvis, the induction of premature labour at an early period, even of the first pregnancy, (as has already been stated, before the sixth month,) is likewise known to be a safe operation, and to render craniotomy and the Cæsarean section wholly unnecessary. The only effectual method of bringing on premature labour is to puncture the fœtal membranes and discharge the liquor amnii. I have repeatedly detached the membranes with a catheter from the lower part of the uterus, but labour has not followed. I have strong objections to the exhibition of ergot for the purpose of inducing premature labour, without taking the uncertainty of its effects into account. I have successfully employed this probe-pointed catheter (represented in the figure above), with a stilette in many cases to puncture the membranes, when I could not do so with instruments less curved and having sharp points.

When you are about to induce premature labour, pass up the fore-finger of the right hand to the os uteri, and when you have ascertained its precise situation slide up along this finger the fore and middle fingers of the left hand to the posterior lip ; the points of the fingers should if possible touch the posterior lip ; then withdraw the fore-finger of the other hand, and take the handle of the instrument with it, and pass up the point in the groove formed between the fingers of the left hand to the os uteri, and gently press it forward along the cervix into the cavity of the uterus, about $1\frac{1}{2}$ or 2 inches, when the membranes will generally be felt offering a slight degree of resistance. The stilette should then be pressed forward with the thumb, and a second puncture made through the membranes before withdrawing the instrument. The blunt point of this catheter enables us to pass it into the uterus with safety, where the os uteri is so high up that the finger cannot even reach the anterior lip. When the liquor amnii has escaped, labour follows, and if the presentation is natural no peculiar treatment is required.

I have been informed that some accoucheurs on the continent induce premature labour by forcing a piece of sponge into the os uteri, which I consider very objectionable. Uterine contractions might be excited, it was stated to me last year by a German physician, without forcing the sponge into the os uteri—by simply pressing it into the upper part of the vagina. I have lately had an opportunity of putting this plan to the test, and it completely failed.

On the Cæsarean section.

Having already defined, as clearly as I possibly can, the cases of difficult labour in which it is justifiable to employ this method of delivery, I have nothing further to say on the subject. I have never seen the operation performed on the living body. On the dead body it is not a difficult matter, for the gravid uterus is at once brought into view by a long incision through the abdominal parietes in the direction of the linea alba. But the child soon dies after respiration has ceased in the mother.

When Dr. Hull, of Manchester, performed this operation on a woman with distorted pelvis, he made a transverse incision nearly six inches in length, and higher than the umbilicus, in the right side of the abdomen, to which part the fundus uteri was inclined, through the integuments, muscles, and peritoneum. He then made an incision of the same length and in the same direction through the parietes of the uterus, and with great ease and expedition extracted a child which had been dead for some days. The placenta was extracted at the wound without any difficulty. The intestines now began to protrude at the wound, and it was not without a great deal of attention and trouble that they were reduced and retained in the cavity of the abdomen, whilst he stitched the external incision by means of the uninterrupted suture, carefully avoiding the peritoneum. The quantity of blood lost during the operation did not exceed 3 or 4 ounces, and no artery was divided that required a ligature, or any application made to it for the purpose of restraining hæmorrhage. The patient died.

Graefe performed the operation at least once successfully. The time of operation, he says, should if possible be that of natural labour; the place of the incision the linea alba: but if the uterus does not lie in the middle of the abdomen, and cannot be brought there, the incision must be carried in a line over the fœtus. To prevent protrusion of the intestines they must be carefully removed from the face of the uterus, and fixed with three warm sponges, each a foot long and six inches wide, so as to leave a free space 8 inches long and four broad for an incision of 9 French inches in length through the abdomen, and of 4½ through the uterus. In dressing the wound three sutures and circular plasters should be used.

Mr. Knowles has related a successful case of Cæsarean section in the fourth volume of the Provincial Medical and Surgical Association. The woman was 36 years of age, and had been delivered of several living children. During a pregnancy in 1829 she had pains in the hips and loins, with loss of power in the lower extremities. She miscarried after this several times. In her ninth pregnancy Mr. Knowles was called to see her on the 15th May, 1835, labour having commenced about 4 P.M. of the 14th. The sacrum, with the lower lumbar vertebra, projected, and at the same time descended far into the cavity of the pelvis, and occupied a large portion of it, and resembled the child's head. The ossa pubis were bent inwards so much that they approached very near to the distorted vertebræ. The presentation could not be ascertained. The space left by the deformity did not exceed two inches in length by less than one in breadth. The head could not be felt, and therefore could not be opened. The Cæsarean operation was performed by Mr. Knowles 30 hours after the commencement of the labour; the external incision, about ten inches in length, was made through the linea alba immediately on the left side of the umbilicus. A portion of intestine immediately protruded. The incision into the uterus was commenced near its fundus by passing the scalpel carefully through its parietes, which were about an inch in thickness, so as to allow the admission of two fingers: using the fingers as a director, the opening was rapidly enlarged, by which the placenta was exposed and a brisk hæmorrhage produced. Passing my hand by the side of the placenta, says Mr. Knowles, I ruptured the membranes, and without difficulty took out the child, which was living. The placenta was then detached, some coagula were removed, the uterus contracted, and the hæmorrhage, which probably did not exceed ʒxvi., was arrested. The external integuments were brought together by stitches, which were inserted at somewhat more than an inch apart. Adhesive straps were applied in the intervals, and the whole was secured by a compress and bandage. Tympanites and several alarming symptoms followed the operation. The wound did not heal by the first intention, so that the serous and purulent fluids readily escaped. Had the condition of this woman been known during pregnancy, which probably was not the case, as it is not alluded to in the history, the necessity for the operation would have been obviated altogether by puncturing the ovum in the early months.

A TABULAR VIEW OF ONE HUNDRED AND TWENTY-SEVEN CASES OF DIFFICULT LABOUR

in which Delivery was effected by the Operation of Craniotomy.

No.	Date.	Cases of Difficulty.	Hours in Labour.	Result.
1	June 28, 1823	1st labour—Impaction of head; small pelvis; swelling of soft parts: long forceps	72	Recovered—Vesico-vaginal fistula.
2	July 12, 1823	1st labour—Rigidity, ...tion, ...missions: long forceps	50	Recovered—Uterine inflammation.
3	July 28, 1824	1st labour—Pelvis and extremities distorted by rickets	67	Recovered—Uterine inflammation.
4	August 1, 1824	Face ...tion	58	Recovered.
5	October 29, 1827	9th labour—Uterine ...morrhage from detachment of placenta	12	Died—Inflammation of uterus.
6	Nov. 2, 1827	1st labour—Distortion of pelvis; head and arm presenting; child dead	72	Recovered—Uterine inflammation.
7	Dec. 3, 1827	Distorted pelvis; arm ...sion with head; turning; head impacted	90	Recovered—Severe inflammation.
8	Feb. 29, 1828	1st labour—Head impacted many hours; ...sion of urine; great exhaustion	36	Recovered.
9	March 2, 1828	3d labour—Head fixed in brim; great ...sion; extraction difficult	40	Recovered.
10	March 12, 1828	Hydrocephalus of foetus; dropsy of amnion; sixteen pints liquor amnii	30	Died—Uterine inflammation.
11	April 3, 1828	1st labour—Distorted pelvis; prolapsus of cord; swollen and tender ...gina	84	Recovered.
12	May 9, 1828	1st labour—Convulsions; rigidity [brim; cord prolapsed	—	Recovered—Severe inflammation.
13	July 3, 1828	1st l ...—r...rtion of ...ight a and ...teal parts; head and foot impacted in	24	Recovered.
14	August 6, 1828	Enormous œdema of ...ighs and ...teal parts; a large exomphalos	24	Recovered.
15	Sept. 19, 1828	Swelling of scalp; head impacted; pains feeble	48	Recovered.
16	Nov. 5, 1828	Uterine hemorrhage from detachment of placenta	21	Died—Hæmorrhage.
17	Nov. 18, 1828	Distortion of pelvis; regular labour pains	48	Recovered—Uterine inflammation.
18	Dec. 16, 1828	Impaction of head; retention of urine; abdomen tense and painful; delirium	48	Recovered.
19	Feb. 4, 1829	2d labour—Head swollen, and impacted in brim of pelvis	48	Recovered—Uterine inflammation.
20	March 27, 1829	1st labour—Rigidity; impaction; exhaustion; delirium; lacerated perineum	72	Died—Sloughing.
21	April 29, 1829	1st labour—Cessation of uterine contractions; head fixed in brim; bladder distended	144	Recovered.
22	July 14, 1829	Hydrocephalus of foetus; dropsy of amnion	60	Died—Phlebitis; gangrene of lung.
23	August 18, 1829	Exhaustion; child dead two days	20	Recovered—Recto-vesical fistula.
24	Autumn, 1829	1st labour—Impaction of head; feeble uterine contraction; exhaustion	48	Recovered.
25	September, 1829	1st stage protracted; labia immensely swollen	74	Died—Gangrene of vagina.
26	October, 1829	Induction of labour at 7½ months; distorted pelvis	48	Recovered.
27	Nov. 8, 1829	Distorted pelvis; arm presentation; swollen vagina	20	Died—Laceration of os and cervix uteri.
28	Nov. 18, 1829	Accidental uterine hæmorrhage; rigid os uteri; vomiting; exhaustion	4	Died two hours after delivery.

No.	Date.	Causes of Difficulty.	Hours in Labour.	Result.
29	Dec. 5, 1829	1st labour—Distorted pelvis from rickets	40	Recovered—Uterine inflammation.
30	Dec. 27, 1829	Head impacted in brim; exhaustion	48	Recovered.
31	Jan. 17, 1830	Great distortion of pelvis; exhaustion; os uteri half dilated	50	Recovered.
32	October 30, 1830	Distortion of pelvis; labour induced at 7½ months; arm presentation; turning performed with difficulty; head perforated behind the ear	—	Recovered.
33	Dec. 6, 1830	Head compressed in brim; feeble uterine action; vagina swollen and painful	72	Recovered—Vesico-vaginal fistula.
34	Feb. 17, 1831	Slight distortion; impaction of head; delirium; labour-pains gone	Many	Recovered.
35	March 6, 1831	Tumefaction of labia and vagina; cessation of uterine action	72	Recovered—Sloughing of vagina.
36	March 27, 1831	Exhaustion; inflammation and tumefaction of vagina	72	Recovered—Sloughing and cicatrix.
37	March, 1831	Impaction of head twelve hours; abdomen tender; despondency; restlessness	48	Recovered.
38	April 16, 1831	Impaction of head in brim; exhaustion; perforation in a previous labour	24	Recovered.
39	Dec. 1831	Severe fits; cessation of pains; head above brim	—	Recovered.
40	October, 1831	Deformed pelvis; nates presentation; head impacted	—	Recovered.
41	March 15, 1832	1st labour—Exhaustion; distorted pelvis	50	Recovered.
42	April, 1832	Os uteri rigid; head impacted in brim; distortion; ergot given	60	Recovered.
43	May 9, 1832	Convulsions and unconsciousness for several hours	48	Recovered.
44	July 11, 1832	Distorted pelvis, in the highest degree, from malacosteon	30	Recovered.
45	Sept. 18, 1832	Distortion from rickets in infancy; rigidity; pulse rapid	36	Recovered.
46	Sept. 13, 1832	1st labour—Great distortion of pelvis; extraction difficult	36	Recovered.
47	Sept. 14, 1832	Valvular disease of heart; dyspnea increased by labour; danger of immediate asphyxia [sentation	—	Recovered.
48	October 5, 1832	Highly distorted pelvis; induction of premature labour at 7½ months; nates presentation	—	Recovered.
49	—— 1832	Head wedged in brim; bladder enormously distended; vagina hot and swollen	72	Died—Uterine phlebitis.
50	April 11, 1833	Impaction of head	30	Died—Inflammation of bladder.
51	March 30, 1843	Head, left arm, and funis without pulsation	12	Recovered.
52	July, 1833	Distortion of pelvis; shoulders jammed in brim; head nearly separated from trunk	48	Recovered.
53	July 5, 1833	1st labour—Head above brim; great prostration; incoherence	64	Recovered.
54	July 5, 1833	1st labour—No progress for twenty-four hours; delirium	—	Recovered.
55	July 5, 1833	1st labour—Delirium; convulsions	24	Recovered.
56	Nov. 10, 1833	Exhaustion from being allowed to remain too long in labour; abdomen painful; vagina swollen	72	Recovered.
57	Nov. 11, 1833	1st labour—Small pelvis; child large; rigidity	46	Recovered.
58	Dec. 1833	1st labour—Violent convulsions; exhaustion	16	Recovered.
59	Dec. 31, 1833	Incoherence; cessation of pains; swelling of soft parts	72	Recovered.

	Date	Description		Result
60	——1833	2d labour—Spontaneous rupture of uterus; vomiting; distortion	15	Died.
61	May 23, 1834	Pelvis small; head impacted; convulsions	12 or 15	Recovered.
62	August, 1834	Impaction of head; vomiting; exhaustion; distended bladder	—	Died.
63	Dec. 27, 1834	Nates presentation; difficulty in extracting head	60	Recovered.
64	——1834	1st labour—Hydrocephalus of foetus	6 or 8	Died—Uterine inflammation.
65	March 3, 1835	Convulsions at eighth month	—	Recovered.
66	April 14, 1835	Great distortion of pelvis in a dwarf at Chelsea	50	Recovered.
67	May 10, 1835	1st labour—Head and soft parts swollen; cessation of pains	48	Recovered.
68	June 23, 1835	Impaction of head; retention of urine; swelling of vagina	60	Recovered.
69	July 8, 1835	1st labour—Distorted pelvis from rickets	30	Recovered.
70	Dec. 6, 1835	2d labour—Head and arm impacted in pelvis; cicatrix of vagina	144	Died—Ruptured uterus
71	Jan. 19, 1836	Distortion of pelvis; induction of premature labour; nates presentation	—	Recovered.
72	Aug. 30, 1836	Great distortion of pelvis from rickets	46	Recovered.
73	Sept. 21, 1836	Impaction of head	120	Recovered.
74	Dec. 3, 1836	Impaction of head; delirium; abdomen tender	—	Recovered.
75	Feb. 8, 1837	Severe convulsions in eighth month of pregnancy	24	Recovered.
76	May 8, 1837	Partial placental presentation; hæmorrhage; prolapsus of cord	—	Recovered.
77	Aug. 15, 1837	Puerperal convulsions	—	Recovered.
78	Aug. 15, 1837	Face presentation; much swelling; pains feeble	21	Recovered—Ruptured perineum.
79	Aug. 24, 1837	1st labour—Threatened rupture of uterus; great exhaustion	—	Recovered.
80	October 1, 1837	Distortion of pelvis from rickets	—	Recovered.
81	Jan. 19, 1838	1st labour—Distortion of pelvis from rickets; induction of premature labour at seventh month	48	Recovered.
82	March 9, 1838	1st labour—Exhaustion and vomiting	144	Recovered.
83	April 20, 1838	1st labour—Exhaustion	—	Recovered.
84	June 2, 1838	1st labour—Head impacted; pains feeble	81	Recovered.
85	August 11, 1838	1st labour—Impaction of head	53	Recovered.
86	Dec. 13, 1838	Nates presentation; head arrested in brim	—	Recovered.
87	Feb. 16, 1839	1st labour—Puerperal convulsions	—	Died in convulsions.
88	June 22, 1839	Hæmorrhage from detachment of placenta	—	Died.
89	July 8, 1839	1st labour—Complete exhaustion; os uteri thick and rigid	50	Recovered. [of urine.
90	July 9, 1839	1st labour—Impaction of head; exhaustion	36	Recovered—Inflammation and retention
91	July 26, 1839	Distorted pelvis; cicatrix of vagina	24	Recovered.
92	July 22, 1839	Exhaustion	50	Recovered.
93	Summer, 1839	Large tumor in pelvis, pressed down before the presenting part; forceps	36	Recovered.
94	Sept. 2, 1839	Arm presentation; rigid os uteri; head left in uterus	48	Died.
95	October 23, 1839	1st labour—Head swollen, and firmly impacted in brim of pelvis	72	Recovered—Vesico-vaginal fistula.

No.	Date.	Causes of Difficulty.	Hours in Labour.	Result.
96	Jan. 13, 1840	Slight distortion of pelvis; face presentation; head impacted in brim; right labium immensely distended, burst, and great haemorrhage	Many	Recovered.
97	Feb. 1, 1840	1st labour—Exhaustion; fever	52	Recovered.
98	April 14, 1840	1st labour—Head compressed in brim; rigid os uteri; exhaustion; fever	72	Recovered.
99	May 1, 1840	Malignant disease of os and cervix uteri	24	Died—Ruptured uterus.
100	July 7, 1840	Head firmly fixed in pelvis; exhaustion	48	Recovered.
101	Dec. 31, 1840	1st labour—Exhaustion	40	Recovered.
102	Jan. 12, 1841	Head impacted in brim of pelvis; vagina swelled, and an offensive discharge from it	94	Recovered.
103	Feb. 11, 1841	1st labour—Head impacted; great tumor of scalp; exhaustion	38	Recovered.
104	April 1, 1841	Head, hand, and funis presentation; delirium [lirium	48	Recovered.
105	May 3, 1841	1st labour—Impaction of head; peculiar nervous irritability; exhaustion and de-	34	Recovered.
106	June 13, 1841	Head and right arm presenting; would not allow child to be turned	—	Recovered.
107	Sept. 14, 1841	Head swollen and fixed in brim of pelvis; delirium	72	Recovered.
108	Oct. 14, 1841	Distorted pelvis; incoherence	92	Died.
109	Oct. 30, 1841	Head impacted in brim of pelvis; exhaustion	35	Recovered.
110	Dec. 12, 1841	1st labour—Brim and outlet of pelvis distorted; threatened rupture of uterus	48	Recovered.
111	Jan. 8, 1842	Rigidity; nates presentation; head impacted; child dead	—	Recovered.
112	Feb. 12, 1842	1st labour—Distortion of pelvis from rickets	72	Recovered.
113	June 4, 1842	Exhaustion; thickening of vagina	96	Recovered.
114	June 18, 1842	Hydrocephalus of foetus; rupture of uterus	72	Died.
115	June 20, 1842	Hydrocephalus of foetus; rupture of uterus	22	Died.
116	July 15, 1842	1st labour—Impaction of head; swelling of scalp; exhaustion	60	Recovered.
117	1838	Distorted brim of pelvis; impacted head; swollen vagina; forceps used	48	Died.
118	1830	1st labour—Pelvis small; head impacted in brim; parts rigid	48	Recovered.
119	1836	Violent puerperal convulsions; not relieved by venesection	—	Recovered—Sloughing of vagina.
120	1839	Head impacted in brim; soft parts enormously swollen; delirium	—	Died.
121	Feb. 4, 1843	Impaction; great exhaustion	24	Recovered.
122	Feb. 13, 1843	Uterine action suspended through terror; delirium; V.S.; os uteri undilated	24	Recovered.
123	April 12, 1843	Great distortion of pelvis; 2d labour; 1st child delivered by craniotomy	70	Recovered.
124	May 6, 1843	Great distortion; nates presentation; head perforated behind	30	Recovered.
125	May 31, 1843	Small pelvis; impaction; retention of urine	60	Recovering.
126	May, 1843	Impaction; child dead; vagina swollen and inflamed	60	Recovered.
127	June 1, 1843	Great distortion; has had four dead children, and very protracted labours	24	Recovered.

CLINICAL LECTURES

ON THE

THEORY & MEDICAL TREATMENT
OF INSANITY,

Delivered at St. Luke's Hospital,

May 1st, 3d, and 5th.

BY ALEXANDER JOHN SUTHERLAND.

LECTURE II.

Alterations in the blood; pulse; diagnosis between phrenitis and insanity; signs of acute inflammation seldom met with in insanity; congestion, whether active, passive, or mechanical, generally accompanies the disease; hyperæmia; anæmia; alterations in the quality of the blood; M. Couerbe's theory, refuted by M. Frémy; post-mortem examinations; alterations found in the scalp, bone, dura mater, in the cavity and cellular tissue of the arachnoid, in the pia mater; acute and chronic alterations of the cortical structure, those of the fibrous structure, spinal marrow, nerves; morbid appearances found in the viscera of the thorax and abdomen.

IN my last lecture, gentlemen, I endeavoured to lay before you examples of insanity with lesions of innervation; it is my intention in my present lecture to speak of the disorders met with in the circulating fluid. When a nerve has become exhausted, two things are necessary to restore it to a healthy state: rest from its particular function, and contact with good arterial blood. The state of the circulation, then, the quantity and quality of the blood, are very material points for our consideration. Some practical writers have said that the pulse is not affected in insanity; this does not accord with my experience, as the following table will show, in which the number of pulsations per minute are given, the state of the pulse on admission into the hospital and upon the discharge of the patient, the form of the disease, and the result of the treatment.

The cases are placed in the order in which they come in my note-book, and are not selected.

MEN.

		Pulse on admission.		When discharged.	
Initials	Form of disease.	Pulse.		Result.	Pulse.
1. P.	Melancholia	80		uncured	64
2. F.	Mania	100		cured	96
3. M.	Melancholia	64		cured	120
4. M.	Mania	100, very weak		paralytic	84 weak
5. B.	Melancholia, Intermittent	100		on trial	88
6. P.	Melancholia	120, weak		cured	100, stronger
7. F.	Mania	60		on trial	64
8. G.	Mania	68		cured	100
9. W.	Mania, Intermitting	120		uncured	88
10. H.	Mania	120		uncured	80
11. S.	Catalepsy	100		cured	84
12. T.	Mania	100 full, intermittent, and regular		cured	88, not full, intermittent
13. E.	Melancholia	100		cured	80
14. H.	Melancholia	100, weak		uncured	84
15. S.	Melancholia	100		cured	100
16. G.	Mania	100, weak		cured	100, stronger
17. O.	Acute Dementia	100, weak		cured	88, of good strength
18. H.	General Paralysis	100		paralytic	108
19. B.	General Paralysis	96		paralytic	88
20. W.	Melancholia	120, weak		cured	100, stronger
21. P.	Mania	104		cured	80, intermitting
22. S.	Mania	100, weak		cured	88, of good strength
23. S.	Melancholia	64		cured	80, strong
24. O.	Acute Dementia	92, full		cured	100
25. H.	Mania	112		cured	104

WOMEN.

1. W.	Mania	80, strong		uncured	120, weak
2. O.	Melancholia	100, full		uncured	96, full
3. R.	Mania	110, weak		cured	100, weak
4. E.	Melancholia	120		uncured	88, weak
5. C.	Melancholia	120		cured	88

Initials	Form of disease.	Pulse on admission. Pulse.		When discharged. Result.	Pulse.
6. G.	Melancholia	80		cured	100
7. P.	Mania	100, weak		cured	100, strong
8. W.	Melancholia	120		cured	112
9. B.	Mania	100, weak		cured	100, weak
10. H.	Melancholia	120, weak		cured	100, weak
11. W.	Melancholia	64, weak		cured	88
12. M.	Melancholia	120, very weak		cured	100, of good strength
13. P.	Acute Dementia	180		uncured	114
14. S.	Mania	100		uncured	76
15. M.	Mania	100, very weak		cured	52, of good strength
16. R.	Mania	100, weak		cured	100, weak
17. M.	Mania	100, weak		uncured	84
18. C.	Melancholia	90, very weak		cured	80, much stronger
19. P.	Mania	84		cured	80
20. S.	Melancholia	80, very weak.		cured	128, weak
21. H.	Melancholia	120, weak		cured	88, weak
22. F.	Melancholia	100		cured	140
23. L.	Mania	84		cured	84
24. H.	Monomania	96		cured	96
25. S.	Melancholia	108, very weak		cured	112, very weak

The most superficial glance at the above figures will serve to show, that in cases of fact,—

insanity the pulse is accelerated; it was, in

		On admission.		On discharge.
		from 40 to 50	. .	in 1 case.
In 5 cases	. .	from 60 to 70	. .	in 2 cases.
		from 70 to 80	. .	in 1 case.
In 6 cases	. .	from 80 to 90	. .	in 21 cases.
In 4 cases	. .	from 90 to 100	. .	in 3 cases.
In 34 cases	. .	from 100 to 120	. .	in 20 cases.
In 1 case	. .	above 120	. .	in 2 cases.

The pulse was slower than on admission when the patient left the hospital in 31 cases, quicker in 12 cases, equal in 7 cases.

M. Foville's table very nearly corresponds with the above. In 62 cases, indiscriminately selected from men and women,

In 5 cases the pulse was, in the minute, from					60 to 70.
In 18	"	"	"	"	from 70 to 80.
In 23	"	"	"	"	from 80 to 90.
In 6	"	"	"	"	from 90 to 100.
In 10	"	"	"	"	from 100 to 120.

Disease of the heart is not uncommon in cases of insanity, but I have not met with it so frequently as M. Foville; he says that at least five-sixths of the patients at his hospital had diseased heart. Hypertrophy is more frequently found than disease of the valves; and this is what we should be led to expect, when we take into consideration the obstacles to the circulation which the heart has to surmount in mental diseases. In recent cases throbbing of the carotid and temporal arteries is frequently observed, and this should draw our attention to the quantity of blood circulating in the body, for undue pulsation of these arteries is not found only in hyperæmia, but it is observed when animals are bled to death. In considering the state of the blood and of the blood-vessels in insanity, we have been too apt, I think, to attribute everything to inflammation, without considering how many different states of the capillary vessels that term im-

plies. We have also overlooked almost entirely that the same functional disturbances are produced not only in the brain, but in other organs, by a minus quantity as well as by a plus quantity. That a state of anæmia can be produced in the vessels of the brain by depletion has been proved by Dr. G. Burrows, in the Lumleian Lectures delivered this year at the College of Physicians. It very seldom happens that we find in insanity acute inflammation — what would serve to distinguish the disease from phrenitis, if symptoms of acute inflammation were present: if there were fever, great intolerance of light and of sound, contracted pupil, and hard pulse. The ancients, and indeed the moderns, have, in their definitions of insanity, always referred to the absence of fever. It is nevertheless sometimes present, and this will guide you in your diagnosis. The fever precedes the delirium in phrenitis, but follows it in mania.

In delirium the mind is occupied solely with the past, in madness with the past and present also. In phrenitis the blood presents the buffy coat, in mania it does so very seldom. In the early part of the present century it was the fashion to bleed insane patients every spring and fall, as it was called, a custom by the way long practised in the veterinary art. Crowther, on one of these occasions, bled 150 patients at a time: the blood in every case, without exception, was free from inflamed appearance.

Dr. Haslam also says, that in more than 200 patients, male and female, who were bled, in six only was the blood sizy.

In post-mortem examinations of the insane we meet with the results of congestion and chronic inflammation, but seldom or ever those of acute inflammation. This is a subject highly deserving of your attention in a practical point of view ; for if you are called in to see a patient in a paroxysm of mania, and have read that the disease owes its origin to inflammation, you would be doing very wrong if you were to bleed him freely. I believe that every variety of congestion exists in insanity, whether active, passive, or mechanical. The blood is either in excess, or deficient in quantity, and the circulating fluid acts sometimes as a poison to the brain. The reason why we find variations, I had almost said contradictions, in the mode of treating the same case of insanity, is, because one thinks only of inflammation, and bleeds, another considers the symptoms due to irritation, and employs opiates or stimulants. The same differences long prevailed with regard to the treatment of diseases of the eye, which bear a striking analogy to those of the brain : we have now pretty sure signs to guide us in applying soothing lotions to the eye, or stimulating collyria. In the treatment of a hidden organ like the brain we can never hope to be guided as infallibly ; still, I trust that at some future day we shall know more fully how much to attribute to undue susceptibility, how much to passive turgescence, or how much to active congestion.

Few, I think, will be inclined to deny that there is active congestion of the capillary vessels in some cases of insanity, particularly in those of recent mania, attended with paroxysms of furor. The full pulse, the throbbing of the carotids and temporal arteries, the ferretty eye, the burning forehead, and the cold extremities, are all proofs of local plethora. But the opposite state, anæmia, has not been sufficiently considered ; indeed, many, from a close resemblance of some of the symptoms, would be inclined to deny its existence, yet we know that vertigo is produced by the latter as well as by the former; and sometimes the only way we have of distinguishing the one from the other

is by making the patient stoop, and then judging whether the symptoms are aggravated or not by the gravitation of the fluid : this means of diagnosis I frequently find occasion to employ in insanity, and it serves as a useful guide in the employment of remedies.

I attended a young gentleman in 1840, who, shortly before his illness, had received several severe blows upon his face when boxing, and had lost much blood from the nose in consequence : there were also other causes which produced a drain upon the constitution, and great prostration of strength. When the first excitement of the mania had passed off, and the symptoms had somewhat abated, upon one occasion when I visited him I found the pulse reduced from 100, as it was in the first instance to 64 : he was lying on a sofa, and talked to me for about ten minutes rationally : he got up to get a book which was lying on the table, and the mere change from the horizontal position brought back the delusions : he became confused and giddy, and said that he was Robert the Bruce. I have seen two cases of insanity, in one of which the disease followed a copious bloodletting ; in the other it came on after frequently repeated small bleedings and violent purging. Sir B. Brodie, in a clinical lecture delivered at St. George's Hospital, Feb. 19, 1839, mentioned the case of a gentleman whom he attended who had been thrown from a high phæton, and injured his head ; symptoms soon occurred which rendered venesection necessary ; at the end of a week, however, he became maniacal : his ravings were like those of deliri im traumaticum. One of the medical men with whom he acted recommended the blood-letting to be repeated ; to this Sir Benjamin reluctantly consented. The blood drawn had scarcely any colouring matter : it hardly stained the linen on which it dropped. The mania became infinitely worse, and wine was then ordered to be administered, upon which plan of treatment he gradually became quite well.

I need hardly call your attention to the importance of this case as shewing the necessity of drawing a correct diagnosis between the delirium from an injury to the head, and maniacal furor, and the opposite manner in which mania, with anæmia and delirium, are treated. I do not, of course, mean that tonics and stimulants are to be given in every case of insanity with poverty of blood, for in this very state of the circulating fluid local plethora is frequent, and it will be necessary to subdue it before recourse is had to tonics and stimulants ; I have seen much harm done by a too speedy application of these remedies. Prostration of strength, with poverty of blood, is very commonly present when the acute stage of mania has subsided. Patients are then in a very similar condition to those in the convalescing stage of fever, and the same remedies are found beneficial in both. Passive congestions, when the blood appears to stagnate in the capillaries, not unfrequently occurs in cases of insanity.

Patients in this condition are generally weak and sluggish in their movements; little animal heat is evolved; the skin loses much of its sensibility; the pulse is so weak as scarcely to be felt. Mechanical congestion frequently accompanies this form of congestion; the extremities become livid, and effusion takes place into the cellular membrane. If you press upon the capillaries, and empty them of their contents, they are sluggishly refilled. We find also in post-mortem examinations proofs of mechanical congestion. The sinuses are found loaded with blood, and the large veins flowing into them are often very turgid. This species of congestion is also well marked during life; and it is not surprising that it should occur, considering the impediments in this disease which prevent the free return of blood to the heart. You will sometimes observe venous blood circulating in the small arteries. The lips of the patient are often blue; and if you make him bend downwards, and thus increase the impetus with which the blood is sent to the head, the lips immediately resume their natural colour. I have a gentleman under my care at the present time who labours under mechanical obstruction to the circulation, which is shewn only in the winter. There are other variations in the symptoms during hot and cold weather. In the summer he is very lively, takes a great deal of exercise, talks incessantly and incoherently; his pulse is generally between 80 and 84, of good strength; the skin is of a proper temperature, and its colour natural; his appetite is good, and he gets up of his own accord and dresses himself. In the winter all is changed; he frequently has attacks of catalepsy; he is torpid; if he walks it is in a circle; he never speaks; his pulse was 100 and very weak, the thermometer being 26° Fah.; his hands become livid; his appetite fails; he is unconscious of the calls of nature, and the attendant has great difficulty in inducing him to get out of bed.

Cold weather is always prejudicial in head affections. The statistical tables of London, Paris, Holland, and Turin, shew that cerebral congestions are most frequent in winter; and this corresponds with Dr. Heberden's opinion. We shall not therefore be surprised at finding that a severe winter increases the symptoms of those suffering under general paralysis. It is an interesting fact connected with this circumstance, that those who have been long exposed to

severe cold have a thickness of speech, and stagger as if they were drunk. M. Larrey informs us that many of the soldiers who died in their retreat from Moscow were seized with dizziness and vertigo, to which a state of somnolence and profound coma succeeded.

The insane are liable to sudden attacks of congestion, which frequently end in apoplexy. These attacks, however, are not invariably followed by disturbance either of sensation or motion. A woman who was admitted into the hospital on the 14th May, 1841, and who was labouring under puerperal mania, was on the 16th of August following seized with one of these attacks of congestion, accompanied with nausea and vomiting. She complained previously of pain in the right side of her head, and she told me that she was conscious during the whole of the time that the fit lasted, and that she felt numbness of the left side. The symptoms very soon abated, and she went out cured on the 30th August of the same year. A man, æt. 57, fell down in a fit, Oct. 22, 1841: he remained insensible only for five minutes. This case also did well. It is, nevertheless, always an alarming symptom, and one never to be treated lightly.

Congestion of the liver, not uncommon in cases of insanity, is another cause of mechanical obstruction to the circulation; the vena portæ becomes loaded, and dropsy sometimes follows: it is, however, rare, as we shall see afterwards, to meet with organic disease of this organ.

There is no symptom so common in the early period of insanity as sleeplessness. Dr. Bright attributes the frequent attacks which epileptics have in the night to slight congestion, which he says always accompanies sleep. This is the reason that the insane so often do not enjoy this temporary release from care. Unless there be some bodily disease, as fever, present, a patient should never be allowed to remain in bed during the day, as the recumbent position will of course favour the congestion.

There remains for us to consider the quality of the blood in cases of mental alienation: so intimate is the connection between the capillaries and the ultimate filaments of the nerves, both at the periphery and at the centre, that what affects the one is likely ere long to affect the other. Not only do we perceive this in the blush of shame and the paleness of anger, and in the effect which the passions have upon the action of the heart, but we see also that injury to the nerves produces stagnation in the capillary tubes, thereby of course greatly interfering with nutrition and secretion. The division of the par vagum, we learn from the experiments of Dr. Reid, is followed by disturbance of the latter, arising from paralysis of the nerves of the stomach, and not, as stated by Dr. W. Philip, from want of secretion of the gastric juice, such secretion being in nowise impeded. It is not material whether the alteration in the quality of the blood is the cause or consequence of the disease. The alteration of the blood is the cause of the disease when it is deprived of the qualities necessary for supplying proper nourishment to the brain, and also when, owing to the skin, the uterus, the liver, or the kidney, not performing their proper functions, it is not properly elaborated. On the other hand the alteration is the consequence of the disease; for though nutrition and secretion are not dependent upon the nerves, yet they are materially influenced by them; and in this and other disorders of the nervous system the circulating fluid must undoubtedly suffer.

Familiar instances of the influence of poisoned blood upon the brain are to be found in the effects of alcohol and opium. · No less striking are the consequences which follow when the elements of the blood are not repaired by proper nutrition. "In the progress of starvation," says Liebig, "it is not only the fat which disappears, but also, by degrees, all such solids as are capable of being dissolved. In the wasted bodies of those who have suffered starvation, the muscles are shrunk, and unnaturally soft, and have lost their contractility; all those parts of the body which were capable of entering into the state of motion have served to protect the remainder of the frame from the destructive influence of the atmosphere. Towards the end, the particles of the brain begin to undergo the process of oxidation, and delirium, mania, and death, close the scene; that is to say, all resistance to the oxidising power of the atmospheric oxygen ceases, and the chemical process of eremacausis, or decay, commences, in which every part of the body, the bones excepted, enters into combination with oxygen." Chemical analysis has not aided us at present in detecting any characteristic peculiarity in the brains of the insane. The brain of man is chiefly composed of albumen, a large proportion of water, and a peculiar fatty matter. The latter presents us with results of most interest: it was in this that phosphorus was detected by M. Vauquelin. M. Couerbe, following up these experiments, thought he could appreciate distinct variations in the quantity of phosphorus in the brains of the sane and insane. In the former he asserts that it is present to the amount of from 2 to 2½ per cent.; in the brains of violent maniacs to that of 3, 4, and 4½ per cent.; while in those of idiots he says that it is deficient in quantity, being not more than from 1 to 1½ per cent. The value of these

experiments has been rigorously tested by M. Frémy, in a very interesting paper published in the 3d series of the Annales de Chimie et de Physique. "All my efforts," says he, "have been employed in studying the fatty matter which can be obtained by digesting the brain in alcohol or ether. It was after evaporation with ether that M. Couerbe discovered cholesterine, the white substance containing phosphorus, which he calls cérébrote, and moreover three fatty substances which he considers neutral, and which he calls céphalote, stearoconote, and éléencephole; (see Annales de Chimie, tom. lvi. p. 164.) The results which I have obtained differ in every point from those just quoted, for I have not seen in the substances of M. Couerbe anything but an acid fatty agglomeration in combination with a saponaceous compound. Setting aside the fatty substances which are found common to other animal matter, we find that the brain is characterized by the presence of cholesterine, and by two peculiar fatty acids. This composition is much more simple than M. Couerbe has been inclined to admit. M. Frémy goes on to state that, in fresh brains, the oleophosphoric acid is found, but that it soon becomes decomposed, and in a brain which has not been examined for some days you find phosphoric acid in a free state, and oleine." M. Vauquelin found the same alteration in ramollissement of the brain, which he considers to be exactly analogous to what takes place in putrefaction. It is interesting in connection with this subject to know that M. Chevreul has found in the blood the fatty matter of the brain, and M. Boudet cholesterine. M. Vauquelin has, also, in some cases, found the peculiar fatty matter of the brain in the liver, which is certainly a discovery of much importance: it may, perhaps, throw some light upon the subject of sympathy between the brain and the liver. We must rest contented for the present with the theory of sympathy to explain the mutual action and reaction of the central organs of the nervous system with each other, and with the nerves themselves. Esquirol lays much stress upon this subject, and draws our attention to the connection existing between the ganglia of organic life and the brain, as leading us to trace the source of the disease to the ganglia. The central parts of the nervous system do, as we know, sympathize with the functional and organic disturbance of all organs of the body. The opinion, therefore, that insanity is sometimes a sympathetic disease, is not so very improbable as some have supposed; but, whether sympathetic or idiopathic, it becomes a matter of great importance in practice to consider the diseases with which insanity may be complicated, and to relieve the symptoms not only which take their origin from the disease of the brain, but those also which are due to the disease existing at the same time in any other organ, as the mental disease will undoubtedly be much aggravated if attention is not paid to the latter. As there is no disease in the body with which insanity may not become involved, so there is no medicine in the Pharmacopœia which you may not have at some time or other to prescribe in treating mental affections. The search after specifics for the cure of madness does, therefore, appear to me to be as vain as the labours of the alchymist to discover the philosopher's stone. Although there is no disease with which insanity may not be complicated, yet there are some more commonly met with, in conjunction with it, than others; e. g. scrofula, phthisis, inflammation of the lungs, disease of the heart, congestion of the liver, diseased kidneys, inflammation of the mucous lining membrane of the intestines, diarrhœa, erysipelas, epilepsy, apoplexy. Sometimes an attack of diarrhœa, of phthisis, or of fever, will put a stop to the attack of insanity; sometimes the attack will be merely suspended. The approach of the catamenia is always a critical period with our female patients; the disease is then often aggravated, and paroxysms of furor occur; the return of the monthly period sometimes gives an intermitting character to the disorder, and the hopes of the friends and of the physician are alternately raised and depressed. It is not uncommon to meet with insanity manifesting itself in one member of a family, while nervous disorders akin to it develope themselves in the rest. This takes place, also, occasionally, with respect to other diseases, which are not of a nervous type, e. g. scrofula and phthisis. A patient under my care, who died of general paralysis, was the only one of ten children who did not die of phthisis.

[To be continued.]

ON A NEW TEST FOR CORROSIVE SUBLIMATE.

To the Editor of the Medical Gazette.

SIR,

ALLOW me, through the columns of your journal, to call the attention of those interested in the science of toxicology to a method of detecting corrosive sublimate, which I am not aware to have been previously brought before the public.

It is now upwards of two years since, *reflecting on the strong affinity of metallic silver both for metallic mercury* and for chlorine, I triturated a grain of corrosive sublimate with several grains of pure metallic silver in powder, as it is procured by precipitation with copper from a solution of the nitrate, and in a dry state; and I was soon encouraged by the blackened appearance of the mixture to believe that decomposition of the bichloride had taken place in some degree at least; and that this decomposition was complete became evident when, upon placing the powder in the bulb of a small tube (such as is used in reducing arsenic), I obtained a distinct ring of metallic mercurial globules in the neck of the tube. Since that time, in obtaining metallic mercury from corrosive sublimate, I have always used silver, which I have not known to fail in producing its reduction, and have found much more convenient and manageable than the potassa fusa, commonly employed; this last not being easily pulverised, and attracting moisture to an inconvenient extent very rapidly. This objection, however, scarcely applies to the use of the bicarbonate of soda or potass.

I have subsequently endeavoured to ascertain whether metallic silver possessed the same power, and to what extent, over corrosive sublimate in solution; and in successive trials I have been able to obtain distinct, nay abundant, metallic globules from the amalgam formed by boiling metallic silver in a solution containing one grain of corrosive sublimate in four ounces of distilled water, and even in a solution of half that strength, i. e. of one grain to eight ounces. My time does not allow me to make numerous comparative experiments, but I am disposed to believe that silver acts slowly, or not at all, on solutions of corrosive sublimate at the ordinary temperature.

I next tried this method of experimenting on organic mixtures; and having added one grain of corrosive sublimate to four ounces of tea, made with sugar and milk, I boiled the liquor with the powdered silver, and after allowing time for subsidence, the fluid was poured off. Liquor potassæ was boiled for some time upon the metal, to dissolve organic matter, and liquor ammoniæ afterwards added to the sediment, in order to dissolve the chloride of silver. This was also poured off, and the sediment having been washed and thoroughly dried, was placed in a tube as before, and metallic mercury obtained in abundance.

Two other experiments have also given very satisfactory results, in one of which one grain of corrosive sublimate, dissolved in a little distilled water, was mixed with a gelatinous fluid, made by diffusing ʒj. by weight of the patent gelatine of the shops in 4 oz. of New River water. In the other, one grain of the same substance in powder was added to 5 oz. of a sanguineous fluid, which had been obtained five days previously, by tapping, from the head of a hydrocephalous infant. The only modification in these cases was, that the mixture was acidulated with hydrochloric acid before adding the silver; this proceeding having been suggested by M. Reinsch's plan of testing for arsenic. It is necessary to moisten the silver by agitating it with a little distilled water in a tube, before adding to the suspected mixture; but, in the cases detailed, the metallic sediment has been very easily obtained, subsiding rapidly, and the results have been very satisfactory.

No actual case of poisoning has occurred to me since I have tried this method, and my professional engagements leave me little time for pursuing the investigation of its powers; but I submit it your readers not without a hope that in other and more skilful hands it may be productive of important results.

I have the honour to be, sir,
Your obedient servant,
ALGERNON FRAMPTON, M.D.
Assistant Physician to, and Lecturer on Toxicology at, the London Hospital.
29, New Broad Street,
May 31, 1843.

ON THE PRODUCTION OF UREA AND URIC ACID.

To the Editor of the Medical Gazette.

SIR,

IN Dr. Golding Bird's "remarks" published in your journal of May 12th, I have been misinterpreted on the subject of Liebig's doctrines. I shall feel obliged by your insertion of this note of explanation.

Dr. Bird appears to understand that, in my observations upon a recent review, I attempt to explain the fact of a diminished proportion of uric acid having occurred in certain cases of chlorosis by 810.—XXXII.

the existence in that affection of a decided deficiency of blood-corpuscles. This is an error. On turning to my paper in the Lancet of April 15th, it will be found that I refer the fact to a diminished nutrition and change of matter in the tissues, and a more perfect oxygenation of the effete particles than would happen if the usual quantity of matter had been changed in the vital process. At the same time, I admitted that the reasoning is hypothetical, and that the case furnishes an apparent exception to Liebig's views. Dr. Bird employs his own misrepresentation of my statement for the purpose of rendering one part of the subject inconsistent with another part.

Dr. Bird leads his readers to the inference that I "denounced" the statement, that 107 grains of organic matter are daily excreted by the skin, as most fallacious. This, again, is an error. I admitted the fact, being fully aware of the source from which it was derived. The writer of the review in question resorted to it for the purpose of showing that the function of the skin is of great importance in the removal of azotised compounds from the body, and I stated my belief that the fact was thus employed most fallaciously. Until it be proved that urea is a general, and not merely an occasional constituent of the cutaneous secretions, or, as respects the particular animal substance which the skin is said to secrete, until a description is given, more accurate than a vague resemblance to an undefined compound and, in particular, until the amount of azote which that substance contains is determined, I am likely to remain of the same opinion. Allowing for the nitrogen contained in the cast-off epithelium scales, I am aware of nothing which justifies the conclusion that the elimination of azotised compounds by the skin is an important part of its function.

For the purpose of invalidating Liebig's theory of the uric acid of the urine being one step in that series of metamorphoses by which the azotised compounds cast off by the living structures become more and more highly oxidised, until they finally disperse in the atmosphere in the forms of carbonic acid gas and ammonia, Dr. Golding Bird asserts that he has advanced a fact. Birds, we are informed, void a large quantity of uric acid, which

2 C

ought not to be the case. The Doctor complains that I have omitted to notice this objection of his to the Professor's theory.

I do not think we have as yet sufficient data to enable us with accuracy to apply the principles of Liebig's physiology to all classes of animals. This is the case with some graminivorous animals, and still less do we know of the carnivorous birds, on which the objection is founded. Among the few facts published regarding the metamorphoses occurring in the latter, there is one which Berzelius states on the authority of Coindet. " The urine of carnivorous birds contains *urea*, but it is wanting in the urine of those birds which live on vegetable food, notwithstanding this consists of acid urate of ammonia." This fact is derived from a foreign source; perhaps, therefore, Dr. Bird regards it as one which should be deemed valueless. The above objection as well as others advanced by Dr. Bird, is founded on a partial application of Liebig's theories to states of life in which some only of the data are as yet known.

With regard to the state of the iron in the blood, I believe Dr. Kane has not as yet given us any facts. If Dr Bird will draw a different conclusion from the experiments of Gmelin and Liebig than they themselves—if he will also come to a different conclusion as to whether Dumas is to be considered more trustworthy than Mulder, Liebig, and Scherer, in analysing fibrin—and Dr. Kemp is equal in analysis, and as good an authority on the bile, as Berzelius—I hope we shall be allowed the exercise of our judgment in receiving those conclusions.

Dr. Bird, finally, misinterprets me with regard to personality towards himself or others in my observations. My object is only to forward the truth, and not even to reply to those personalities in which Dr. Bird indulges. I feel, accordingly, that I am precluded from entering further than is necessary with him into these deeply interesting topics.

I am, sir,
Your obedient servant,
HENRY ANCELL.

3, Norfolk Crescent, Oxford Square,
May 20th, 1843.

———

ON PSEUDO-ERUCTATION.

By G. C. CHILD, M.D.

Physician to the Westminster General Dispensary.

(For the London Medical Gazette.)

IT is well known that there is no more frequent attendant upon hysteria than flatulence. This is easily accounted for by the fact, that hysterical affections are usually associated with more or less of indigestion and irregularity in the evacuation of the bowels. In many cases, however, the production of air in the intestines is so enormous and so sudden that dyspepsia of the ordinary kind has been deemed inadequate to account for it, and it has accordingly been attributed to a special effect of the hysteria upon the secreting vessels of the intestinal mucous membrane.

No sign of hysteria is better known than this excessive flatulence. The abdomen sometimes becomes tympanitic even during the short period of the patient's examination : the eructation is loud, well-marked, and distressing. Anti-flatulent medicines are indicated, and produce the best effects.

But there are hysterical disorders, common enough in practice, where the flatulence is only *apparent*, and belongs to the class of mimoses. This fact is, I have no doubt, familiar to those who have seen much of the disease; but I infer that it is perhaps not so generally known as it ought to be, because I have had patients under my charge whose most troublesome symptom was, as they imagined, flatulence, for which they had been perseveringly treated with stimulants and carminatives, but of course without the least benefit.

I never saw this species of mimosis displayed better than in a patient who is at present under my care. This woman, about the middle period of life, is a pew-opener, exceedingly nervous and hysterical. During the last seven or eight years she has received a good deal of medical advice for headache, indigestion, palpitation, and pains in the abdomen; for the last of these complaints she has been frequently bled and cupped, and, I fear, too actively treated. At present she complains of fluttering at the heart, faintness, with occasional sharp pains, and anomalous sensations in various parts of the body. One of the symptoms from which, she says, her greatest suffering proceeds is "wind." According to her account she sometimes belches up enormous quantities of it for hours together. The abdomen is swollen, and resonant on percussion.

In the course of treatment I have had several opportunities of observing these "attacks of wind," and what I am now about to remark is gathered from this and from similar cases.

When the face of a person affected with this pseudo-flatulence is watched steadily for a minute or two, a characteristic expression may be observed, although it is difficult to describe it; I shall only say that it is quite different from that of a person who is actually bringing up wind. The face is kept averted from the practitioner, and the quantity of air which passes out seems very little when compared with the efforts made for its expulsion. It will be remarked that the mouth is kept shut, so that the air passes from the nose only, and sometimes the mouth is held firmly by the hand, or even the nostrils are partially closed by it. This act has of course a tendency to impede rather than to favour the exit of the air: but the reason for it will immediately appear.

As in the paroxysms of hysterical cough or convulsions, so also in this complaint, there is much irregular and tumultuous action about the upper part of the throat, the muscles of the tongue, pharynx, and the levators and depressors of the larynx, being chiefly involved. A loud rumbling or forcible movement of air may be perceived in the same situation, but there is seldom any distinct flatulent "rapport." Under the heart, and over the abdomen generally, there is no movement of flatus to be detected; occasionally there is a short quick contraction of the diaphragm, as in hiccup.

The fit can be instantly stopped by simply causing the patient to keep her mouth open. This is the diagnostic mark between true and pseudo-flatulence. It is obvious that keeping the mouth open cannot impede the passage of air from the stomach, but it deprives the patient of the power to emit those sounds which simulate eructation. To produce these sounds the mouth must be shut and the posterior nares closed. The various muscles of deglutition are then thrown into *strong and irregular action*, and by this means the compressed air is forcibly made to circulate about the different parts of the mouth and pharynx. During these efforts air is often pressed into the gullet, whence it either returns into the mouth again, or is swallowed into the stomach. Of this fact I am very sure, that in many cases of hysterical flatulence there is more air swallowed into the stomach than expelled from it.

If any one will try to imitate the act above described, he will, I think, be able to produce sounds more or less resembling eructation. I know some who can mimic it perfectly, but on causing them to open their mouth the air is no longer enclosed in a shut cavity, and the power to produce the pseudo-eructation is lost. In making the trial one will generally be conscious of swallowing air involuntarily.

In a patient who fancied that her complaint was a "windy dropsy," it was found that pressing or rubbing the arms or legs immediately brought on a paroxysm of this pseudo-flatulence. I could not help remarking how similar this case was to those mentioned by Morgagni (De Sed. et Causis Morb. Epist. 43): the first reflects credit on the practical tact of Santorini:—

"I was at Venice when a woman sent for surgeons and physicians, and among them Santorini, in order to ascertain the nature of the tumor, which was prominent in one of her groins, as she feared lest it should be a bubonocele; for this reason, that it appeared suddenly, as she was straining to discharge the hardened excrements from the intestines. All signs of a hernia were absent, except that immediately upon applying their hands to that part, the woman discharged wind by eructation. Santorini, observing the physicians to be in doubt merely on this account, smiled, and said to them, 'Whatever part of my body you touch, you will have eructations come on.' They instantly made the experiments, and found it to be as he had said. When Santorini related these things to me, and to some more friends, others wondered at it as an unheard of circumstance; but I (Morgagni) said it is extraordinary indeed, yet not unheard of. In Bartholin you will really find the observation of a man 'who from a slight friction of any part of the body, immediately fell into so enormous an eructation, that he did not cease to eructate before the friction ceased*."

The above sentence, marked with inverted commas, applied exactly to the woman with " windy dropsy," to whom I have alluded. I have no doubt they were all examples of pseudo-eructation. On reading the quotation just made, I am inclined to suspect that Santorini knew the trick, and was quizzing his brother practitioners : but it does not appear that Morgagni was aware that it was simply a deception, otherwise his surprise and wonderment would scarcely have been so great.

MEDICAL GAZETTE.

Friday, June 9, 1843.

"Licet omnibus, licet etiam mihi, dignitatem Artis Medicæ tueri; potestas modo veniendi in publicum sit, dicendi periculum non recuso."
                                        CICERO.

SOCIETY FOR RELIEF OF
WIDOWS AND ORPHANS OF
MEDICAL MEN.

We publish this day a notice of the annual dinner of the " Society for Relief of Widows and Orphans of Medical Men in London and its Vicinity." This inconveniently long name it seems has been borne by the institution ever since the year 1788, and is somewhat remarkable in these days of rapid movement, and of successful search after ease and material comfort. It reads almost as laboriously as the titles of some old books, where the author appears hardly to have been restrained from putting the whole table of contents into his title-page.

This peculiarity, by the way, though generally abandoned, is still found in some controversial tracts, and seems to be a natural result of people earnestly putting forth what they have to say, and being more anxious for the success of their cause than for the elegance of

* Translation of Morgagni by Dr. Alexander, 1769.

their style. Towards the close of a controversy, when zeal has cooled, when the less informed, but not less earnest, have made room for the stronger or more skilful disputants, those in whose hands the contest is left shew more skill in their weapons and more judgment in their selection, knowing how much depends on their length, their weight, their balance. " See that my staves be sound and not too heavy," is one of the Duke of Gloster's commands on the eve of Bosworth Field. " Last night it more fatigued my arm than foes," is the Corsair's complaint of his scimitar.

Homer makes a burly hero do much execution with a huge stone; but this great poet,—or to avoid controversy this " able editor" of all the hero-poetry of his day,—the blind Ionian balladsinger,—would never have put such a weapon into the hands of Achilles or of Ulysses. Long, awkward, and laborious names, then, are apt to be faithful exponents of real facts, while shorter and more concise ones are often mere theories and professions of things which ought to be, but are not.

The title, however, of this society has at least this virtue, that it does not mislead the reader, but faithfully sets forth its purpose, and an inspection of the annual statement of its affairs will convince those who take the trouble to inquire that it is doing, with no small success, what it professess.

This society seems to have been originally a club formed by certain London practitioners of eminence for the purpose of making a fund the proceeds of which should be divided amongst the widows and children of members, or rather amongst such of them as should be left in a state of indigence.

From the high professional standing of the first founders, it is evident that their intentions were principally benevolent, and that their contributions were destined for the families of their less opulent neighbours, rather than for their own; but the encouragement held out soon induced many to subscribe from motives of prudence, and the gradual increase in the proportion of those whose families became claimants for relief proved the expediency of contributing to the fund, and brought into full relief its value as a provision against the contingencies of early death and inadequate savings.

The union of provident and benevolent objects which this society accomplishes, while it is calculated to attract two very different classes of subscribers, must nevertheless tend also to deter many of each class; and the very small number of members, which has never exceeded 350, is a sufficient proof that many of each class fear that their own personal objects may not be the most effectually attained by its means. Unlike an insurance office, the investment in this fund can never be profitable, except in case of a degree of destitution which few are willing to believe will be the probable lot of their own families, and many defer the securing an income for their surviving dependents until they can afford to provide one which shall do more than place them above the reach of want. By some, indeed, who have contributed largely to the support of this institution as the best hitherto formed, strong objections are entertained to the principle on which it acts. They consider it as a temptation to neglect adequate and liberal provision for a family, and to be content with a state but one remove above pauperism, which may be dangerous to industry and burdensome to society. But it is urged on the other hand that life insurance even to a moderate amount is very expensive, even if commenced early in life, and if long deferred often becomes impossible. It is difficult,

too, to believe that those who in early life have, by joining a society like this, insured their families against absolute privation, will be on that account less likely, with the increase of their ability, to make further provision by ordinary modes of insurance.

It is also contended that this society is deficient in not having a purely benevolent fund, the benefits of which might be extended beyond the families of its own members. Such an addition would be very desirable, but as many of the subscriptions are obtained from members who ought not in common prudence to indulge largely in the luxury of alms-giving, it is perhaps more desirable that a separate institution should be formed which should accomplish this object, and the contributions to which should be left more to the discretion of the benevolent according to their respective means.

Another very forcible objection to this society is, that those who do require its assistance are obliged to solicit that assistance, as a favour, which they should have a claim to as a right: many men dislike their families being exposed to this humiliation: but if the original object of the society, and the mutual good will which suggested and sustains it, be duly kept in view, and if proper kindness and delicacy be preserved in the *manner* of affording relief, this objection will lose all its force.

When trades and crafts first emerging from mere feudal vassalage protected themselves by corporate alliances, the admission of each member into a trading company was subjected to certain restrictions. These kept the numbers of those who were admitted within convenient bounds, and gave to each, when once admitted, a sort of family interest in the whole body of which he became a member; the trades of each town even had their respective powers of excluding from the local exercise of their calling all who had not contributed by servitude or compensatory payments, or both ; in return for which the member obtained a claim for protection in his calling, and for support in old age and destitution. But as monopolies and exclusive privileges became obnoxious, and were gradually diminished or abolished, the protection which they afforded was withdrawn at the same time, and their place has been gradually supplied by voluntary associations for the relief of the decayed and the destitute, for the widow and the orphan ; so that, at the present time, there is hardly a trade or a profession which has not a fund raised for these purposes. But it is obviously much easier to keep up by stringent regulations the levy of customs or dues on entering a profession, than to awaken and keep in action that prudence and forethought in individuals which are required to supply their place, when those customs are disused, and perhaps the efforts of clear-sighted and earnest philanthropists cannot be more beneficially exerted than in pressing home on the indolent and the indifferent the urgent necessity that exists for individual forethought and self-denial. Compassion and alms-giving will never cease to be estimable, but the more extensively the need for them can be diminished, by a sound and healthy self-dependence, the better for a nation and for society. The parliamentary evidence elicited by the contemplated Poor-law for Ireland shows how grievous are the effects of shameless mendicancy and reckless almsgiving, though the one be called contentment, and the other charity. Perhaps at no time did members of the medical profession stand more in need of mutual support and co-operation than at the present. The claims of

our art to public estimation are trenched upon by quackery ; the most obvious truths and established axioms denied by those who have neither sufficient information for argument nor docility for belief ; and the advantages of our recent discoveries are neutralized by undue contempt of former theories : the honest refusal to assert for itself that infallibility which is impudently claimed by quackery, all concur to diminish the aggregate of our gains, while the numbers who are to share these gains are far beyond what can be supported—all these things concur to render the preservation of individual and general independence more than ever difficult. Yet on this independence must we rely for the power of sustaining our present difficulties, and of amending our future condition.

The constitution of this society appears to be purely democratic; the members elect by ballot their own officers, and surrender the entire management of affairs into their hands, the acts of the Court of Directors being finally subject to the veto of the General Court. The ordinary Courts of Directors are held four times a year : perhaps, considering the amount of business to be done, and how desirable it is to keep up a spirit of activity in promoting the accession of new members, this is too seldom. The General Courts are held half yearly.

The Medical Benevolent Society was established in the year 1816, and is intended for assisting such of its members as may, by illness, or other causes, be incapable of supporting themselves. It has a wider range of operation, but, though established 27 years ago, contains but 150 members, yet it has afforded much very effectual and seasonable relief, and has received the gratitude and the pecuniary support of some who had accepted its assistance. The constitution and government are almost exactly similar to those of the "Widows and Orphans'" Society, to which most of its members are also contributors.

Public dinners, and public advertisements, are no doubt highly useful for promoting harmony and good feeling amongst the members of a society, and can hardly be dispensed with in this country, but the speeches which follow are not calculated to promote a deliberate consideration of its claims to support, nor do public advertisements appeal with sufficient distinctness to individuals. Surely a statement of the nature, objects, and efficiency of these two most laudable institutions should be addressed to every member of the profession, and the deliberate opinion of each should be taken as to the propriety of giving them his support. The corporate bodies especially should be appealed to, that each member of the profession might have the subject pressed upon his attention immediately on admission. These bodies might take a useful hint from the Medical Association, which has established a fund for the relief of destitution, the benefits not being confined to its own members. We cordially agree with the wish expressed by Dr. Wilson, "that the Councils of this Society" (for the Relief of Widows and Orphans of Medical Men, &c.) "instead of being held at a coffee-house in Holborn, should transact their business in the hall of a Royal College; and that its limits should be extended till they included every member of the profession in the United Kingdom, or even in the British possessions." The Army and Navy have each a fund for medical officers; it is, we believe, obligatory on all to subscribe to it, and its operations are very much of the nature of an insurance.

Perhaps not one of our readers has escaped an appeal for relief from a medical man, or his family, in complete destitution: such appeals he has been unwilling either to reject or to encourage on insufficient grounds: he may have given without hope of conferring real benefit, or refused without feeling justified in withholding. Joining a society such as we have described, he may, by his recommendation and his example, encourage sound prudence, and confer effectual relief.

THE DINNER.

THE annual dinner of the society above alluded to took place last Saturday, at the Freemasons' Tavern, Great Queen Street, and was attended by about 70 of the members and their friends. H. R. H. the Duke of Cambridge presided. *Non nobis Domine* having been sung, and the usual loyal and patriotic toasts given, his Royal Highness called attention to the objects of the society, which were to provide a fund for relief of the families of deceased members, who might have failed in struggling against the difficulties of their profession, or been worn out in its practice, and died without having realized a sufficient maintenance for their surviving relatives. His Royal Highness felt assured that such an institution was exceedingly necessary, from the very great difficulties with which medical men had to struggle, and the casualties to which they were liable; and he was most happy to find how much this society had done to relieve those who had been obliged to make claims on its funds. His Royal Highness read part of the annual statement laid upon the table, from which it appeared that the society had relieved, within the past year, 31 widows and 20 children, distributing for that purpose nearly £1300, in half-yearly payments; and that £385 had been added to the capital stock, which now amounted to nearly £41,000.

His Royal Highness expressed a hope that the society would not only continue to afford the same amount of relief, but to increase it when necessary, and that many would prove by their contributions that evening that they felt, as he himself did, warmly interested in its prosperity. His Royal Highness subsequently added, on his own health being proposed, that it gave him great pleasure to express thus publicly his best wishes towards the society; and that as it had been intimated that he could serve its interests by becoming the Patron, he had much pleasure in accepting that office, and hoped that he should at all times be found able and willing to promote the society's welfare. This gracious announcement was of course received with hearty cheering.

Mr. Bacot, the acting treasurer, announced that the investment of the capital with the Commissioners for the Reduction of the National Debt had already produced a considerable increase in the half-yearly income, and stated the present condition of the society to be certainly flourishing; but that it must be borne in mind, that according to calculations made long ago, and which had hitherto proved correct, the number of claimants, though actually smaller this year than the last, would *increase for the next twenty years.* To meet this demand, therefore, and to secure permanent efficiency and stability, would require the most careful management on the part of the directors, and the utmost exertions of friends and supporters. The recent investment with the Commissioners was owing, he said, to the suggestions of three members, viz. Dr. Mann Burrows, Mr. Dover, and Mr. Maclure.

The usual toasts were given in succession, and duly responded to; and we are happy to add that 308*l.* 15*s.* were collected on the occasion.

FELLOWES' CLINICAL PRIZE REPORTS.

By Alfred J. Tapson.
University College Hospital, 1842.

[Continued from p. 217.]

CASE XI.—*Melancholia coming on during pregnancy, without much, if any, derangement of the general health; considerably relieved by aperients, morphia, and tonics.*

ANNE HUNTER, æt. 31, admitted July 6, 1842, under Dr. A. T. Thomson. A woman of rather slender conformation; melancholic temperament; dark complexion; naturally rather florid, but now sallow; black hair, &c. Is married, and had four children, two of which only are living, and the younger is only five weeks old. Her father died some years since: about two years before his death he was deranged for four months, owing to disappointment in business and loss of property; he however recovered from this perfectly, and died sane, but was hemiplegic. No other member of her father's family was ever deranged. Her mother is living, and well; she has two cousins on her mother's side now in lunatic asylums.

She has been a map-colourer ever since she was quite a child, and has had consequently much confinement, and sometimes works as many as eighteen hours in the twenty-four. Her health has always been good, and habits regular. She used to be very nervous about ten years ago, but this she got the better of.

The present attack, she states, came on

about six months since, when she got into a very violent passion with another woman, without any definite cause, and since then she has always felt distracted, never having a moment's peace of mind, and constantly so much discomposed, that she has been able to do nothing, neither to read nor think, nor follow her employment; is worse sometimes than at others, but not at any particular times, nor worse in one posture than another, but generally a little better towards evening.

It is not easy to describe correctly the state of her mind: she does not brood over any particular point or event, but feels a great desire to die, so great indeed that she says she would destroy herself if she had the means in her power; her feelings are so horrible that she says she cannot live; she seems to be persuaded that she is destined to eternal misery, do what she may; she says it is only running against providence to think differently: as a proof of her lost condition, she declares that she now hates her elder child, whereas she used to love him very much.

This state of mind came on quite suddenly, without any other apparent cause than that already mentioned; she was on good terms with her husband, never had any fits, &c.: she thinks her recent confinement had very little effect on her mind in any way, and thus disappointed her, as she had hoped to have got well then.

From the commencement the most prominent symptom had been sleeplessness, and this caused her to apply to a surgeon soon after it began. He gave her some "sleeping powders," and ever since she has been obliged to take opium, in order to obtain any sleep, though before the present attack she used to sleep very well. She has been in the habit of taking enough hard opium to make a good-sized pill every night, and sometimes another during the day, but never more. The effect of each dose she has always found to be to cause her skin to tingle and perspire, and to render her more composed and tranquil; her mouth and throat are dry in the morning, and indigestion and constipation have been produced, rendering aperients necessary. Her appetite does not appear to have been impaired, but it was never very good. Also, since she has taken the opium, her complexion and skin in general has become very yellow, and this was never the case before, except when she had a bilious attack, to which she was rather subject, and this temporary derangement of the secreting function of the liver was always increased by the opium. She has also got thinner and weaker. Latterly the opium seems to have lost its specific quieting effect, and her only hope of obtaining rest being thus annihilated, she was reduced to despair.

July 8th.—The surface of the body generally is warm and comfortable, except the feet, which, she says, are always cold, even after taking the opium; the complexion has a very dingy sallow tinge; the eyes are surrounded by a very dark circle; the expression of the countenance is very much depressed, and she frequently sighs deeply; the tongue is coated with a thick white fur; the appetite moderate; thirst normal; pulse 74, regular, moderately full and soft. During the two nights she has been in the hospital she has slept much better, though she has taken no opium; bowels costive; evacuations not particularly pale; urine free. The heart's sounds are natural, and the breath sounds quite healthy.

Habeat Haust. Purg. Statim.

9th.—The bowels have been freely opened.

℞ Morphiæ Acetatis, gr. ij.; Micæ Panis, gr. xij. M. f. pil. viij. Sumatur una quinque quáque horá.

℞ Tinct. Gent. Comp. f3j.; Infusi Gentianæ, f3xj. M. f. haustus. Inter sing. dos. pilul. sumendus.

11th.—Slept very well last night, except being much alarmed by a dream; did not feel so oppressed when she awoke this morning as she commonly does, and now feels much less irritable, and is in better spirits, and looks considerably more cheerful; pulse 84, tolerably full and firm; pupils natural.

12th.—Talks with more freedom about herself, and now, though still very indifferent about living, yet she seems to have no desire to destroy herself. Dr. Thomson recommended her some active employment.

14th.—Improving steadily; sleeps soundly all through the night, without dreaming, also sleeps in the day-time after taking the morphia; expression of countenance much more animated; eyes brighter; pupils natural; no headache; says she will live now if she can; appetite increased, though it has never been very bad; bowels keep regular without the aid of medicine.

16th.—Has unpleasant feelings at times, but not very frequently; the tongue has a milky villous appearance on the surface, but there is a purplish tinge beneath this, and some of the papillæ are enlarged.

Adde Haust. Quinæ Disulph. gr.j.; et Acidi Sulph. Dil. ♏viij.

20th.—Continues to improve; complexion becoming clearer, and is less dark round the eyes; the feet are never cold now as they used to be, indeed they generally feel quite warm; she feels that she is gaining strength, and is active and cheerful; the head feels clear, and she can command her thoughts sufficiently to read a little at a time. The morphia produces just the same effects as it did at first, she sleeps as long after each dose, and the skin tingles a good deal after it.

23d.—Does not seem to have made much progress during the last few days, but on the whole she is very much better than she was.

26th.—She was allowed to leave the hospital yesterday for an hour, but did not return till this afternoon, and says she feels much worse for not having slept last night.

28th.—Improved again considerably; slept well; spirits improved; appetite much better than it has been for a long time.

Cont. Pilul. Omitt. Haust.

℞ Quinæ Disulph. gr.j.; Infusi Gentianæ, f3x.; Sp. Æther. Nitrici, f3ss.; Acidi Nitrici diluti, ♏viij. M. f. haustus ter die sumendus.

August 1st.—Discharged at her own request.

REMARKS.—In the preceding history we have a description of the state of mind in a well-marked case of melancholia; or if it were desirable to give it another name, it might almost be termed "suicidal monomania," her leading desire being to die, either by her own hand, or by some other means.

The reasoning faculties of her mind did not appear to be much, if at all, perverted, except when she thought of her destination, as she believed, to eternal misery. She seemed to fancy that she was possessed of some evil spirit, over which no being, either human or divine, could exercise any authority. Even on this point, however, she was able in a limited degree to reason correctly; for after stating that her only wish was to die, and that had she the means of death in her power she would use them instantly, she added, "It's a dreadful thing to hurry into eternal misery, which I know I must do if I destroy myself."

Thus it was evident that her mind was much perverted on this subject. No motive urged seemed to have sufficient influence to rouse her to voluntary and cheerful exertion: so great was the mental dejection, that all hope seemed to be extinguished, and a settled despondency held undisputed possession of her mind; so that whilst to outward appearance the mind seemed to be in a state of tranquillity, "it was," as Dr. Prichard remarks, "a deceitful calm, concealing profound grief and misery."

Almost the only bodily symptom accompanying this state of mind was sleeplessness; and this may reasonably be attributed to the state of the mind: indeed, all her organs seemed to be perfectly healthy. This freedom from bodily disease forms one of the means of diagnosis from hypochondriasis, in which disease there are almost always dyspeptic symptoms, on which the patient continually dwells, and which he delights to magnify. It was also distinguished from this by the suicidal disposition that was evinced; for in hypochondriasis, notwithstanding that they fancy they shall soon die, they take extremely good care not to injure themselves. Again, in this latter disease there is a disposition to dwell with tedious minuteness on all their sufferings, real and imaginary; whereas here there was a marked disinclination to talk at all: all the patient's desires might be summed up in that one word—rest. We shall say nothing more respecting the diagnosis, as it was so well marked, and there is no other disease besides hypochondriasis with which there is any chance of confounding melancholia; and by attending to the preceding points there can be no difficulty in that respect. The patient, when brought into the hospital, was said to be labouring under puerperal mania; but besides wanting the characters of that, it had existed long before delivery, and that process, we have already stated, had no marked influence on the mind either one way or the other.

Several causes probably co-operated in producing it. As predisposing causes we may mention, 1st, that her father was deranged, though not till many years after the patient's birth; and in his case the madness appears to have been produced by disappointment in business; also the patient had two cousins on her mother's side in lunatic asylums at the time of her admission: therefore we may fairly assume that there was an hereditary predisposition to some form of mental derangement. 2d. Her temperament was decidedly melancholic; and this is stated by Dr. Prichard to be a very powerful predisposing cause to melancholic madness. 3d. Her employment was sedentary in the extreme, and had often been very severe: this would, of course, tend to weaken the body, and thus to unnerve the mind. 4th. Her age was that at which this species of mania usually shews itself.

The only exciting cause appears to have been of a moral nature; at least she attributed the attack to her getting into a very violent passion about six months before her admission: from that time she has never felt as she did before. At the same time, she scarcely seems to believe that this could have been a sufficient cause, for she said that had she done anything very bad she should not have thought so much about it; but she knows no other cause. The attack was not preceded by pain any where, nor fits of any kind. No symptoms of disease of the brain or of any other organ.

In noticing the treatment, we shall first consider that which had been used previous to her admission into the hospital. It is stated that she had been in the habit of taking an opium pill once, and sometimes *twice a day, almost ever since the commencement of the attack; it used to compose her mind, but was beginning to lose its*

effects. As a natural consequence of this habit, her digestion became deranged, her bowels were costive and aperient medicines necessary, and her complexion became sallow. The last is a well-known consequence of a habit of taking opium; and here there seemed to be a particular reason why it should do so, for it appears that she had been subject to bilious attacks, at which times her skin used to become yellow, and opium would be sure to increase it by diminishing the secretion of bile.

At the time of her admission, the principal indications of treatment were—1st, to quiet the nervous system, and to procure sleep; 2d, to attend to the secretions generally, especially of the bowels and liver; and 3d, to give tone to the system in general, so that it might not be necessary to continue indefinitely the use of the means for fulfilling the first indication. The treatment was commenced with a purgative draught, to open the bowels freely; and this was ordered to be repeated afterwards as often as it might be necessary. To fulfil the first indication she was ordered a quarter of a grain of morphia every five hours; and to fulfil the third, a draught containing gentian, &c.

The effects of this treatment were soon apparent. We find that in two days she slept well, but was alarmed by dreams, and very soon slept soundly without dreaming; and her desire for dying left her, and that natural desire for the prolongation of life returned. Her appetite increased, and with it her strength and spirits; and her complexion became clearer. Her improvement was gradual and steady, except at the time when she remained out of the hospital for a night: she soon recovered this, and was not long after discharged at her own request.

MEDICAL REFORM.

To the Editor of the Medical Gazette.

Sir,

The subject of medical reform having received fresh interest from the great probability that something definite is soon to be brought forward in parliament, I request a small space in your journal for a few remarks upon a subject connected with that question; and knowing how valuable that space is, I will endeavour to be as brief as possible.

Without therefore entering into the point of the necessity for this reformation, I shall at once take it for granted that the measure is to be carried; but at the same time I shall conclude that even if the general practitioner is to be in future a bachelor of medicine*, his position with the public, and the public

* Vide Sir James Clark on Medical Reform.

demand for the general practitioner will remain much in the same state as at present; that is, there will always be, 1st the consulting practitioner or physician; 2d, the general practitioner, or the practitioner who sends his own medicine and gives a lengthened credit, and there will be also the prescribing chemist, who sells at a cheaper rate behind the counter. The public must have the family attendant; that attendant must supply all medicines and give a lengthened credit; in other words he must be in one respect in exactly the same position as the tradesman. This has been the case from time immemorial, and as long as the public demand exists there will always exist a sufficient number of medical men to supply that demand. It is on the preliminary education of the medical practitioner, be he called what he may in the forthcoming measure, that I wish to make a remark. This education has heretofore commenced by a term of apprenticeship, and I think I am justified in declaring that there exists a decided feeling throughout the profession against the system; but I wish to invite a calm consideration of this old-established institution before it is too late, before reform shall have swept it away as useless and unnecessary. I admit that its utility has much diminished, and that in too many instances it has been made a vehicle for oppression, and its duties converted into drudgery. It was instituted when the medicine of the apothecary was an art and mystery, and consisted in pure empiricism; it took its origin before lectures were generally delivered in London; and therefore a period of eight years in the apothecaries' shop was well spent, and was the only means of obtaining medical knowledge. The student's channel for the prosecution of medicine in the country is not only diverted, but his duties have, from the more perfect division of labour throughout the profession, been confined to one monotonous duty, that of dispensing. This office, too, in many instances has precluded the possibility of reading, which is now essential, and these idle habits have been engendered at a most important period of life. These are some of the evils, it must be allowed, which have too often acted prejudicially, not only to the student himself, but have done much to disgrace the whole system of apprenticeship. The evil appears to be, that while every other part of the profession has advanced, this useful institution has remained all but stationary; or, if it has altered at all, it has become more monotonous and tedious.

I would first show in what I consider its usefulness chiefly to consist, and therefore that it should be preserved, in at least a modified form, in any future measure affecting medical education.

I have concluded, I think justly, that the demand for the practitioner practising pharmacy, or rather sending his own medicines, will continue of necessity, allowing that all scientific knowledge is now obtained at the hospital and medical schools. I maintain that there is much essential though not scientific knowledge which cannot be taught there, nor in any other place than in the surgery of the general practitioner; the species of knowledge to which I allude is not easily described, but consists in an infinity of small matters relating to the proper management of the surgery, the method of book-keeping generally adopted, the proper economy of time, including all the more commercial part, down to the proper receiving and attending messages at the door. But this is not all; a student can obtain but a very limited knowledge of the materia medica, the cost of drugs, the best mode of buying them, preserving them, and their state of purity, by merely attending lectures on the subject, and examining the specimens in rotation. It is by having them constantly before him, weighing them, dividing and subdividing them, that a more thorough and intimate knowledge can be obtained of them. I will allow that physicians obtain a knowledge of materia medica without this dispensing, but the general practitioner has something more to attend to.

He has to purchase them, and is himself always responsible for the quality; he ought therefore to know more than merely their medical properties.

I would here state, however, that though I think that the total abolition of apprenticeship would be inexpedient, I would allow that the period of it might be shortened to three years; and it must be allowed that the above duties, to be obtained in the surgery only, and which require but very little mental exertion, might be taught in much less time than three years, and that three years' exclusive attention to them would be great waste of time; yet they require a lengthened practice rather than any close application.

But there is another reason for the continuance of medical apprenticeship, and that is, the youth, at the age at which he enters on his medical studies, requires to be properly overlooked, which he could not be at any hospital or collegiate establishment in London, or in the provinces; for even in Oxford and Cambridge, where the whole town is under the authority of the Universities, there is difficulty in exercising proper control over the student. How could this, then, be done in the heart of London, or in any other large city?

I conceive, therefore, that there is a necessity that the youth entering the profession should be placed under the eye and surveillance of a medical practitioner; for if

consider the following are only
... on the proper instruction of ... edu-
... prentices; and if six apprentices could
... ceived at the same time, they could be
... ed, though to one or two pupils they
... ld be impossible. In the first place,
... ly every drug, and every preparation in
... London Pharmacopœia, should be kept
... the surgery, and, as far as possible,
... should be prescribed occasionally. A proper
laboratory for the preparation of the chemi-
...als, and for the pursuit of practical chemistry, should be established, and it should
be furnished with all necessary philosophical
apparatus for elementary instruction in
chemistry and general physics. An her-
barium, illustrating at least all the natural
and artificial orders of plants; the skeleton,
and a good collection of separate boxes for
the study of osteology; a library, consisting
of anatomical botanical plates, and most of
the elementary works on medicine. I consider that with six or eight pupils, and the
usual rate of remuneration given to clergymen who take pupils, that is, at least £100
to £120 per annum, all the above advantages could be given—a sum, by the way,
which is frequently denied to the medical
man, but which is freely given to the lawyer,
clergyman, architect, engineer, or farmer.
The depreciation, however, is as much, it is
feared, to be attributed to the profession,
because they have consented to take less,
than to the public. The outlay would be at
first considerable, but it would never have
to be repeated, and the pleasure and gratification of having efficient apparatus and
ample opportunities for scientific pursuits,
and inducements for keeping pace with every
discovery and improvement of the day,
which is often next to impossible with the
routine of a private practitioner, would fully
compensate many for the first expense.

As I have too far trespassed on your space,
I will reserve what I had to say on the manner in which this plan could be developed,
and at present subscribe myself

Your obedient servant,
W. H. O. SANKEY.

Margate, May 29, 1843.

ANEURISM CURED BY PRESSURE.

*Case of Popliteal Aneurism cured by Com-
pression of the Femoral Artery.* By ED-
WARD HUTTON, M.D. Surgeon to the
Richmond Hospital.

MICHAEL DUNCAN, æt. 30, a labourer of
rather healthy appearance, but of intemperate
habits, was admitted into the Richmond
Hospital on the 3d of October, 1842. He
stated, that ten days previously, while suffering from cramp in the right leg, to which
he had been subject for the last year, he, for

[illegible]

Nov. [illegible] being informed [illegible] Mr. [illegible] of which [illegible] Having [illegible] for the suppression of secondary hemorrhage after ligature of the femoral artery I applied it in this case. It was so constructed as to admit of pressure being made by a screw and pad upon the course of the femoral artery, and the counter-pressure upon the opposite surface of the limb without interfering with the collateral circulation.

In the first instance the compression was made upon the femoral artery in the middle third of the thigh, and although it was effectual in compressing this vessel it produced so much uneasiness that it could not be sustained, and after a few applications the apparatus was removed and adapted to the upper part of the limb.

12th.—The femoral artery was compressed as it passes from the pelvis under Poupart's ligament, and the pressure maintained for more than four hours.

14th.—The tumor feels rather more solid; the purring thrill, before felt on the re-entrance of the blood into the sac, is no longer sensible; the pulsation as before.

18th.—No change in the tumor.

19th.—The circumference of the limb at the seat *of the tumor is a quarter* of an inch *less than at the last measurement.*

[illegible]

		Aneur.	Sound limb
Dec.	12th.—Temperature	[illegible]	[illegible]
"	[illegible]	[illegible]	[illegible]
"	[illegible]	[illegible]	[illegible]

On the 21st of December the tumor was reduced to the size of a small walnut, and felt very hard. He was this day discharged, at his own request.

[illegible] the hospital at my request. The tumor was then of the size of a nutmeg and solid. He has been at his usual employment.

Remarks.—Since this case occurred Dr. Cusack has treated with success by similar means a case of popliteal aneurism in Dr. Steevens' Hospital, and Dr. Bellingham another in St. Vincent's Hospital. It would appear that this plan of treatment has been too hastily abandoned by the profession, probably from the compression employed being so excessive as to render it quite insupportable to the patient. The least possible pressure which may be sufficient to close the vessel should be used, and when this cannot be sustained, it will prove of use to partially compress the artery so as to lessen the impulse of the circulation. In cases where the aneurism [illegible] exists, this treatment would [illegible] before recourse should [illegible]

We are happy to be able to add Mr. Cusack's case.

Case of Popliteal Aneurism cured by Pressure. By Mr. CUSACK.

JOHN LYNCH, æt. 55, a tanner, of short stout build, admitted into Stevens' Hospital, No. 4 Ward, January 17, 1843, under Mr. Cusack. Last autumn he had a bad fever, from which he recovered slowly; about five weeks since he began to experience burning pains running from the knee down to the ankle, particularly along the outer and anterior part of the leg; these continued until seven days before admission, when, as he was walking in the street, he suddenly felt a very acute pain in the ham, running to the ankle, and compelling him to sit down; he put his hand to the part, and, for the first time, felt a lump there the size of his fist; he got home with some difficulty, but the pain gradually decreased, and next day he went about his business as usual; during the following days the lump became much smaller, so that, on admission, it was not more than half its original size.

He has been in the habit of carrying heavy burdens up a ladder; has had cough and palpitation of the heart since the fever; used to drink freely, but has lived temperately for the last twenty years; never used mercury.

On examination, there is a tumor in the lower angle of the left ham in the course of the popliteal artery, about the size of a hen's egg; it is elastic, and pulsates synchronously with, but more powerfully than, the heart; the pulsations are as evident laterally as on the superficial surface; moderate pressure on the femoral artery stops them, and empties the tumor, so that it can scarcely be felt; the skin is not discoloured, nor is the tumor tender on pressure, except at a point on each side the size of the top of the finger; it is smooth and even on the surface, and a distinct bruit can be heard when the ear is applied to it; the anterior and posterior tibial arteries cannot be felt in either feet; what vessels can be felt appear to be large, and to have thin coats; no morbid sound can be detected in the heart, but its impulse is weak, and the pulsations very intermittent and irregular; the pulse at present is 70, small and irregular, but it varies from 60 to 90, without any apparent cause; the left lung is emphysematous; the superficial veins of his cheeks are much enlarged, giving a dusky red appearance; temperature of both limbs the same.

22d.—A roller was applied lightly from the toes up to the groin.

Habeat tinct. Digitalis gtts. v. ter in die.

Feb. 4th.—No apparent difference; if the *bandage is not very carefully applied, it gives him severe pain in the instep* after ten or twelve hours; to-day a compress was laid over the tumor, and the bandage put on as before.

Tinct. Digitalis gtts. x. ter in die.

22d.—No change in the tumor. Mr. Hutton came to-day and applied his instrument; the pad being screwed down on the femoral artery at as high a point as possible, and with a force sufficient to stop completely the pulsations in the tumor; a compress was then laid over the aneurism, and secured by a flannel bandage, beginning at the toes: he soon began to feel uneasy, but when it had been on for one hour and a half, his face became pale, his pulse weak and slow, and he complained of faintness, with a feeling of weight in the situation of the pad, running up to his heart, and the sensation of a rush of blood to the head, accompanied by profuse perspiration on the forehead and vertex; the instrument was now loosened, and he soon rallied; when quite recovered, the pad was again screwed down, but he could not bear it for more than half an hour at a time.

Cont. tinct. Digitalis gtts. x. t. d.

24th.—He bears the instrument as long as he can, and then loosens it, screwing it down as soon as he is free from pain; he complains most of the rush to his head; the pad slips off the artery very easily; he says he can tell by a peculiar sensation of something running up from the situation of the pad, when the pulsations in the tumor are stopped, but he often gives an erroneous opinion; to-day the instrument was put on loosely, so as only to lessen the force of the pulsations.

Cont. tinct. Digitalis gtts. x. t. d.

27th.—He has been very patient and quiet, but no effect has been produced on the aneurism. Mr. Hutton's instrument was left off, and a bandage applied. Temperature of both legs the same throughout.

Cont. tinct. Digitalis gtts. x. t. d.

March 4th.—Same as at last report.

Tinct. Digitalis gtts. xv. ter die.

16th.—Sir P. Crampton's instrument, modified by Mr. Daly, was put on, so as merely to lessen the impulse in the aneurism; no compress or bandage was put on the tumor. Pulse 63, very intermittent: it soon rose to 90.

Cont. tinct. Digitalis, gtts. xv. ter die.

18th.—He bears this instrument much better than the other; has none of that unpleasant rush to the head; complains chiefly of soreness produced by the pressure of the pad; this is relieved by dusting the part with flour. No change in the tumor.

Omitte tinct. Digitalis.

22d.—The tumor is decidedly harder and smaller, the impulse being greatly lessened; at times there is only a thrill in the aneurism; sometimes there is no motion whatever in the tumor, even when the pressure is removed, but it returns on the slightest movement of the body; he observes that the two spots before mentioned have lost all tenderness on pressure. Complains of cough. Pulse 67, very irregular.

Mist. expect. c. tinct. opii camph.

23d.—Pulsation has totally ceased; the tumor is very hard, and about the size of a large walnut; a large artery can be felt running down superficially to the aneurism, over which it can be easily rolled with the finger; it then divides into two branches: the articular vessels do not appear to be enlarged.

On the 19th he had some œdema of the leg, for which a bandage was put on the limb; for the last two nights he has had a most intolerable itching in the thigh, but there is no redness or mark of any kind.

25th.—Instrument was removed to-day. The femoral artery can be distinctly traced as far as the opening in the tendons of the triceps and vastus int.

Mist. expect. c. Aq. lauro cerasi.

April 1st.—The tumor is decreasing; the enlarged artery above mentioned is much smaller than at last report; the relative temperature of the limbs, as ascertained by thermometer, has not varied.

7th.—Tumor continues to decrease; the entire artery can be traced until it enters the aneurism, but in the lower third of the thigh and in the ham the pulsation is so weak that it can only be felt on a careful examination.

Cont. Mist. expect.

April 14th.—Tumor can now be grasped with facility; the enlarged artery has become very small, while the popliteal of the affected limb now pulsates as strongly as that of the sound one; a number of hard cords can be felt passing over the tumor. The palpitations of the heart still continue. Pulse 68, intermittent.—*Dub. Journ. of Med. Science.*

ON THE

REMOVAL OF CALCULI FROM THE BLADDER OF THE HORSE.

By Mr. Mogford, V. S.

My attention has been arrested by an article in your number for January on lithotomy; a few observations on which, as they are the result of my own experience, will not, I am sure, give offence to that justly respected operator, Mr. Field. I cannot forbear from again expressing my surprise that, in operations of this kind, veterinary surgeons do not make use of the means so peculiar accessible to them, viz. inverting the bladder through the rectum. Mr. Percivall has very kindly noticed my mode of operation in the third volume of his Lectures and the second of his Pathology.

I first extracted a stone from the bladder in this way in the year 1820, and the case was published by Mr. White in 1824. No operation could be more simple or less exposed to dangerous consequences. There was no inflammatory symptom whatever, and the horse was soon after hunted. In fact, all that is required is a scapula and a probe-pointed bistoury, for the arteries are easily avoided without any guide.

In proof of my assertion I may state that I have more than once introduced a stone into the bladder, and extracted it in the same way.

About two years ago I introduced, by way of experiment, an egg into the bladder of a mare, and extracted it again, whilst she was in a standing position. As this was done in a private manner, I thought it advisable to have witnesses. I, therefore, introduced the egg into the bladder again, and left it there until the following morning, when I found that the bladder was full to bursting, as the mare was afraid to stale.

At my request, three medical gentlemen of this island kindly accompanied me the next morning to witness the operation; but being puzzled by the fulness of the bladder, and having no catheter at hand, I introduced, as a substitute, the nose of a bellows, which answered the purpose pretty well, although the large quantity of water in the bladder retarded the operation. Notwithstanding this, however, the operation was performed within a minute, and without breaking the egg, although the shell had been considerably softened by the action of the acid of the urine. In order to put the whole matter beyond a doubt to the spectators, I again introduced the egg. The mare was then killed, the bladder taken out, and shewn to them with the egg in it.

There is some degree of tact required in the operation, the want of which has probably, on many occasions, prevented its adoption. When the arm is first introduced into the rectum, the animal forces against it, in order to expel it; the arm must remain quiet, until these struggles have ceased, when the operator may proceed without difficulty. If the finger should not be sufficiently long to reach the neck of the bladder from the opening, the latter may be pushed towards the finger from the rectum.—*Veterinarian.*

HEMIPLEGIA FROM TYING THE COMMON CAROTID ARTERY.

M. SEDILLOT applied a ligature to the common carotid to arrest hæmorrhage, in a man who was wounded behind the right branch of the lower jaw. Complete hemiplegia of the left side of the body, and of the right side of the face, followed, and the patient lost his intelligence so far that he could scarcely comprehend questions put to him. He died nine days after the appplication of the ligature, and the post-mortem examination showed that the hemiplegic symptoms had resulted from the right side of the brain having been deprived of its due proportion of arterial blood.—*Gazette Médicale;* and *American Journal of the Medical Sciences.*

BOOKS RECEIVED FOR REVIEW.

Medico-Legal Reflections on the Trial of Daniel M'Naughten for the Murder of Mr. Drummond ; with Remarks on the different forms of Insanity, and the irresponsibility of of the Insane. By James George Davey, M.D. &c. &c. &c. With an Appendix.

Practical Treatise on the Diseases peculiar to Women, illustrated by Cases derived from Hospital and Private Practice. By Samuel Ashwell, M.D. &c. &c. Part 2— Organic Diseases.

The Transactions of the Provincial Medical and Surgical Association, Vol. XI.

Mental Hygiene, or an Examination of the Intellect and Passions, designed to illustrate their Influence on Health and the Duration of Life. By William Sweetser, M.D., late Professor of the Theory and Practice of Physic, and Fellow of the American Academy of Arts and Sciences.

Clinical Remarks on Certain Diseases of the Eye, and on Miscellaneous Subjects, Medical and Surgical, including Gout, Rheumatism, Fistula, Cancer, Hernia, Indigestion, &c. &c. By John Charles Hall, M.D. &c.

Essays on Partial Derangement of the Mind in supposed connexion with Religion. By the late John Cheyne, M.D. F.R.S.E. M.R.I.A. Physician General to His Majesty's Forces in Ireland, &c. &c.

ROYAL COLLEGE OF SURGEONS.

LIST OF GENTLEMEN ADMITTED MEMBERS.

Friday, June 2, 1843.

E. B. Clayton.—J. A. W. Thomson.—W. Gompertz.—T. B. Stone.—C. H. F.. Routh.— J. T. Pearce.—J. Cross.—J. W. Wainwright.— R. Field.—M. F. Bush.—T. Berryman.—F. H. Hewitt.—J. C. Foulkes.

Monday, June 5, 1843.

G. Lister.—J. H. Blount.—J. Duigan.—A. B. Semple.—T. Dawson.—W. Smith.—W. W. Clarke. —W. C. Northey.

APOTHECARIES' HALL.

LIST OF GENTLEMEN WHO HAVE RECEIVED CERTIFICATES.

Thursday, May 25, 1843.

Josiah Blomfield, London. — William John Preston, Great Yarmouth. — Sidney Rudge Robinson.—John Moore Woollett, Monmouth.— John James Bunch, Wolverhampton.—Thomas Mallabar Clewley, Ashby-de-la-Zouch.—George Frederick Giles.—John Howells Thornhill, Darlaston.—John Gray Henry, London.

Thursday, June 1, 1843.

C. Withington, Pendleton.—S. T. Frost, Bradistone, Norwich.—A. Markwick.—C. Meeres, Herts.—A. C. Ayres, Ramsgate.—E. H. Ambler, Churchstoke, Montgomeryshire.—T. M. Gunn, Chard, Somersetshire.—R. Cammack, Berrington, Boston.—R. B. Penny.—C. W. Blashfield, Abergavenny.—J. H. Coveny, Stilton.—P. Chawner, Burton-on-Trent.

A TABLE OF MORTALITY FOR THE METROPOLIS,

Shewing the number of deaths from all causes registered in the week ending Saturday, May 27, 1843.

Small Pox	10
Measles	34
Scarlatina	27
Hooping Cough	35
Croup	5
Thrush	2
Diarrhœa	3
Dysentery	1
Cholera	2
Influenza	0
Ague	0
Typhus	59
Erysipelas	4
Syphilis	1
Hydrophobia	0
Diseases of the Brain, Nerves, and Senses	129
Diseases of the Lungs and other Organs of Respiration	256
Diseases of the Heart and Blood-vessels	23
Diseases of the Stomach, Liver, and other Organs of Digestion	68
Diseases of the Kidneys, &c.	7
Childbed	9
Ovarian Dropsy	0
Disease of Uterus, &c.	3
Rheumatism	0
Diseases of Joints, &c.	8
Carbuncle	0
Ulcer	0
Fistula	0
Diseases of Skin, &c.	0
Diseases of Uncertain Seat	88
Old Age or Natural Decay	65
Deaths by Violence, Privation, or Intemperance	17
Causes not specified	3
Deaths from all Causes	859

NOTICE.

We regret that we cannot give insertion to the paper of Mr. T.

WILSON & OGILVY, 57, Skinner Street, London.

THE

LONDON MEDICAL GAZETTE,

BEING A

WEEKLY JOURNAL

OF

Medicine and the Collateral Sciences.

FRIDAY, JUNE 16, 1843.

LECTURES

ON THE

THEORY AND PRACTICE OF MIDWIFERY,

Delivered in the Theatre of St. George's Hospital,

BY ROBERT LEE, M.D. F.R.S.

LECTURE XXX.

On the causes, symptoms, and treatment of preternatural labours.

IN preternatural labours, which form the third class of Smellie and Denman, the head of the child does not present as in natural labours, but the nates and inferior extremities, or one of the shoulders and arms. Cases of prolapsus of the umbilical cord, and twins, may be included in the same class. It is very difficult, or impossible, to explain why the head of the child does not invariably present in labour, or assign a cause for the same women having preternatural presentations in several successive labours, the head of the child being rarely if ever in them the presenting part. Violence inflicted on the mother during pregnancy will not explain their occurrence once or oftener in the same individuals, for they take place where there has been no shock sustained during gestation, and they are seldom met with after the most severe accidents experienced during pregnancy. That they are not the result of accident is proved by the fact that in some women the same shoulder and superior extremity has presented in different labours, and the children have certainly been placed transversely in the uterus before the commencement of labour.

On July 31st, 1836, I attended a lady in labour, in whom the left superior extremity of the child presented, and the operation of turning was required: I was informed that in both her previous labours the left superior extremity had presented at the beginning of the labour; the situation of the child was the same, and it was alive in all the three labours at the commencement; yet she had been exposed to no shock or accident of any kind during pregnancy. Another patient had eight preternatural labours in succession. The arm presented in the first four or five, and the nates and inferior extremities in all the others. A woman was delivered twice at the British Lying-in Hospital in three years, and in both labours the right shoulder and arm presented. In a woman with distorted pelvis the inferior extremities presented in the first and third labours, and an arm in the fourth. Another, who has been delivered five times, had presentations of the nates and inferior extremities in four labours, the first only being natural. It is highly probable that some cases of preternatural presentation may arise from twisting of the umbilical cord around the neck, trunk, or extremities of the fœtus. Of the sixty cases of arm presentation related in these Clinical Reports, there was prolapsus of the funis in fifteen. The death of the fœtus in utero is, I believe, a more common cause of preternatural labours than twisting of the cord around the child. Of thirty cases of arm presentation related by Dr. Denman, in which spontaneous evolution took place, or the children were expelled double, only one was born alive, and the greater number were premature, and probably dead before the labour commenced. "One hundred and twenty-seven cases of presentation of the feet occurred in the Dublin Lying-in Hospital during the mastership of Dr. Collins, not including those met with in twins. Sixty-two of the 127 children were still-born; forty of which were *putrid*. Thirty-six of the 127 were premature, viz. four at the fifth month; seven at the eighth month; twenty-eight of the premature children were *putrid*; four were dead, but not putrid, and four were born living."

Mauriceau states that when the fœtus is dead the labour is almost always protracted and difficult, and the reason he assigns for this is probably correct: "à cause que son corps n'ayant plus de soutien, et étant devenu tout mollasse, ses parties s'affoissent tout en un tas les unes sur les autres : ce qui fait qu'il vient aussi pour l'ordinaire en mauvaise situation, ou quoiqu'il se présente par la tête en figure naturelle : les douleurs de la femme sont si foible and si lentes en cette occasion, qu'elles ne le peuvent pas faire expulsion." But there are other and more obscure causes of preternatural presentations than the death of the fœtus and twisting of the cord around the trunk and extremities, of which we at present know as little as Dr. Denman did when he wrote the following passage in 1795. " It seems doubtful, therefore, whether we ought not to exclude accidents as the common causes of these presentations, and search for the real cause from some more intricate circumstance; such as the manner after which the ovum may pass out of the ovarium into the uterus ; some peculiarity in the form of the cavity of the uterus or abdomen; in the quantity of the waters of the ovum at some certain time of pregnancy ; or, perhaps, in the insertion of the funis into the abdomen of the child, which is not in all cases confined to one precise part, but admits of considerable variety."

Women often suspect during the latter months of pregnancy that the child is not in the natural position, and that when labour comes on it will be a cross birth, when their fears are unfounded. But they are not always mistaken, for some who have before had natural labours have been firmly persuaded, from something unusual in the form of the abdomen, that the child was unfavourably situated, and their suspicions have been confirmed by the result of the labour. In the greater number, however, it is only after the labour has commenced and made some progress that we ascertain that some other part than the head presents. In preternatural presentations, particularly when the extremities present, the membranes are either ruptured at the commencement of labour or soon after, or they have a peculiar conical pointed shape, not the ordinary globular form, and protrude far into the vagina. Sometimes, before the os uteri is much dilated, the membranes, filled with liquor amnii, pass into the upper part of the vagina, and form a considerable sac with a narrow neck. The presenting part either cannot be felt, or it is lighter, and when touched gives less resistance, than the head usually does, and is less smooth, hard, and regular. A hand, or a foot, or the umbilical cord, may sometimes be distinctly felt *through the membranes, but more frequently* the membranes burst as soon as the dilation of the os uteri commences, and the first thing we touch on making an examination is an extremity in the vagina, or perhaps protruding through the external parts. The spontaneous and premature rupture of the membranes, or something peculiar in their shape —the presenting part lying so high up within the os uteri, after it is considerably dilated, that it cannot be felt by an ordinary examination —the presenting part, if felt, being more moveable, less smooth, and globular, and resisting, than the head, are the chief circumstances which should induce you to suspect that the presentation is preternatural, and make you, by all means in your power, preserve the membranes entire, and prevent the escape of the liquor amnii until the uterus is so much dilated, or is so dilatable, that the operation of turning, if necessary, may be performed. As soon as we are certain that the head does not present, it is right to state the fact to the nurse, if not to the relatives of the patient.

Before the membranes are ruptured, it is difficult in some cases to determine positively whether the head presents, or the nates; and it is not unusual for those who have been some years in practice, and who are not afraid of committing mistakes, to make a hasty examination, and to believe and state that it is a natural labour, but afterwards discover, to their mortification, that the nates present. If you touch one of the nates through the membranes, you will feel that it is round, like the head, but much softer, and that there is no suture nor margin of the parietal bones to be felt, however carefully you endeavour to make out the presentation. After the most careful investigation, if you remain in doubt about the nature of the case, whether the head presents or the nates—if you are certain that it is not the shoulder—there is no ground for anxiety; the only circumstances requiring attention are, that the membranes should not be ruptured artificially, and that you should not state to the nurse and patient that all is going on favourably before you are positively certain of the fact. After the membranes give way, you will readily ascertain that the nates present by the cleft between the buttocks, the anus and external parts of generation, and the escape of the meconium. The shoulder is much more pointed than one of the nates, and if you can pass the finger carefully around all the parts within your reach, where a shoulder presents you will not fail to distinguish it by feeling the ribs and the scapula. The parietes of the thorax communicate a peculiar sensation which you cannot fail to recognise. The hand is much flatter and broader than the foot, the fingers are much longer than the toes, and they differ from one mother in length much more than the toes do, and are more separated from each other; their extremities are uneven. The middle finger is the longest and the thumb the shortest part, and it is at a distance from the fingers. The foot is thicker and heavier than the hand, the great toe is the most prominent part, and near to the other toes; the toes are shorter than the fingers, their ends form nearly an even line, descending from the great toe. But the heel projects in a remarkable manner, and it is by feeling this heel that you will never fail to distinguish the foot from the hand in the uterus: you may forget all these distinctions between the fingers and toes during the operation of turning; but if you will take the trouble once to examine attentively the heel of a new-born child, you will never bring down an arm

into the vagina instead of a leg, as I have seen done.

Treatment of presentations of the nates and inferior extremities.

If the nates present to the centre of the brim of the pelvis, the abdomen of the child may correspond with the spine or abdomen of the mother; it may be directed backward or forward, or the back of the child may be directed to either side of the mother. Some of these positions are more favourable than others; that which is most so is represented in the following figure from Smellie's plates, in which the fore-parts of the child are to the posterior part of the uterus; and the funis, with a knot upon it, surrounds the neck, arm, and body. "I have sometimes felt," he says, "in these cases, when labour

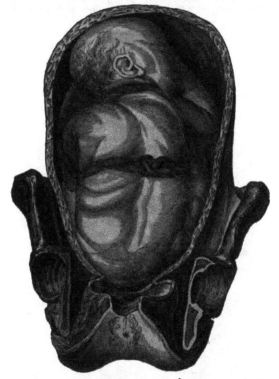

was begun, and before the breech was advanced into the pelvis, one hip at the sacrum, the other resting above the os pubis, and the private parts to one side; but before they would advance lower, the nates were

turned to the sides and wide part of the brim of the pelvis, with the private parts to the sacrum, as in this table; though sometimes to the sacrum, as in the following table. As soon as the breech advances to the lower part of the basin, the hips again return to their former position, viz. one hip turned out below the os pubis, and the other at the back parts of the os externum.

In this case the child, if not very large, or the pelvis narrow, may be often delivered alive by the labour-pains; but if detained long at the inferior part of the pelvis, the long pressure of the funis may obstruct the circulation. In most cases, adds Smellie, where the breech presents, the effect of the labour pains ought to be waited for till at least they have fully dilated the os internum and vagina, if the same have not been stretched before with the waters and membranes. In the meantime, whilst the breech advances, the os externum may be dilated gently during every pain, to allow room for introducing a finger or two of each hand to the outside of each groin of the fœtus, in order to assist the delivery when the nates are advanced to the lower part of the vagina.

But if the fœtus is larger than usual, or the pelvis narrow, and, after a long time and many repeated pains, the breech is not forced down into the pelvis, the patient's strength at the same time failing, the operator must, having introduced a finger into the vagina, raise or push up the breech of the fœtus, and bring down the legs and thighs. If the uterus is so strongly contracted that the legs cannot be got down, the largest end of the blunt hook is to be introduced, and cautiously drawn down with it. As soon as the breech or legs are brought down, the body and head are to be delivered, as described in the next table, only there is no necessity here to alter the position of the child's body.

This figure, also from Smellie's plates, shows, as he states, in the same view as the former figure, the breech of the fœtus presenting: with this difference, however, that the fore parts of the child are to the fore

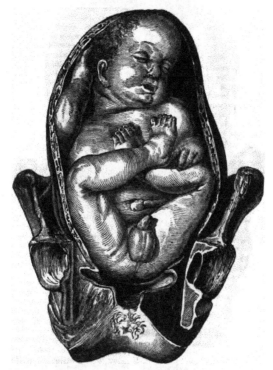

part of the uterus. In this case, when the *breech, coming down double as it presents, is brought down to the hams, the legs must be extracted,* a cloth wrapped round them,

and the fore parts of the child turned to the back part of the woman. If a pain should in the meantime force down the body of the child, it ought to be pushed up again in turning, as it turns easier when the belly is in the pelvis than when the breast and shoulders are engaged; and as sometimes the face and forehead are rather towards one of the groins, a quarter turn more brings these parts to the side of the pelvis and a little backwards, after which the body is to be brought If the child is not large the arms need be brought down, and the head may vered by pressing back the shoulders,wn, body of the child to the perineum, and that the chin and face are within the vagina, to bring the occiput out from below the pubes, according to Daventer's method. Or the operator may introduce a finger or two into the mouth, or on each side of the nose, and, supporting the body on the same arm, fix two fingers on the other hand over the shoulders, on each side of the child's neck; and in this manner raise the body over the pubes, and bring the face and forehead out with a semicircular turn upwards from the under part of the os externum. All this may be easily done when the woman lies on her side; but if the child is large and the pelvis narrow, it is better to turn the patient on her back, and after the legs and body are extracted as far as the shoulders, the arms are to be cautiously brought down, and the head delivered. If the woman has strong pains, and when, by the felt pulsation of the vessels of the funis umbilicalis, or the struggling motion of the fœtus, it is certain that the child is still alive, wait with patience for the assistance of the labour; but, if that and the hand are insufficient, and the pulsation of the funis turns weaker, and if the child cannot be brought double, the breech must be pushed up; and if the resistance of the uterus is so great as to prevent the extraction of the legs, the patient ought to be turned on her knees and elbows. When the legs are thus brought down, the woman, if needful, is to be again turned to her back, to allow more freedom to deliver the body and head, as before described. If the head, after several trials, cannot be delivered without endangering the child, from overstraining the neck, the long curved forceps ought to be applied. If these fail, and the patient is not in danger, some time may be allowed for the effect of the labour pains; which likewise proving insufficient, the crotchet may be used, when it is certain that the child is dead, or that there is no possibility of saving it."

The treatment adopted in cases of nates presentation by Dr. Burton, a contemporary of Smellie, was still more artificial and objectionable; for as soon as he discovered that the nates presented, he was accustomed to thrust up against the buttocks with all his strength, *and to endeavour to turn the child with its belly towards the os uteri*,

and then search for the feet. "Were this rough and barbarous recommendation of Burton generally followed," observes Dr. Merriman, "the most lamentable consequences, both to mother and child, could not fail of being often experienced. Smellie was too fond of this pushing up; indeed it was the doctrine of the day; and Dr. Hunter, in the early part of his practice, used to follow the same plan in breech presentations; but, from a conviction of its impropriety, he afterwards discontinued it." "At this time I lost the child in almost all the breech cases," says Dr. Hunter, "but since I have left these cases to nature, I always succeed." Portal, who first described the best method of treating face presentations, was probably also the first who discovered that cases of nates presentation might often be left to the natural efforts, and that they did not require the operation of turning upon the head, or that attempts should be made to bring down the feet. "In such a case as this," he says, "you must not be impatient, for though the labour proceeds very slowly, yet it is not much more difficult than a natural birth; whence it is that our midwives say, by way of proverb, that where the buttocks can pass, the head will follow of course. The position of the child in this case is doubled, with his thighs upon the belly, and the passage being once open for the buttocks by the reiterated pains, the head follows without much trouble."

Having ascertained that the nates present, whatever the position of the fœtus may be, whether the abdomen look backward or forward, we cannot alter it with safety, and no change can be required to be made till the nates and lower extremities are expelled. The os uteri dilates slowly in most cases of nates presentation, but we cannot employ any means with advantage to accelerate the delivery, and in most cases, if we do not interfere, but wait patiently, they are gradually pressed lower and lower into the pelvis, and at last escape from the vagina without any assistance. If the os uteri and vagina are imperfectly dilated, and the nates are drawn down or pass rapidly through the pelvis, the child is often lost. The membranes should not be ruptured, and the expulsion of the nates should be left entirely to the natural efforts, unless the labour is protracted and exhaustion takes place. Except supporting the perineum, nothing is required in a great proportion of these cases before the nates and lower extremities have been expelled, when it becomes necessary to ascertain precisely the relative position of the child to the pelvis, to rectify this if it is unfavourable, and artificially extract the superior extremities and head, to prevent the fatal compression of the umbilical cord. If we find, after the expulsion of the nates and lower extremities, that the toes are directed forward, or that the child is in the position represented in the second figure, with its abdomen applied to the anterior part of the uterus, and that its back lies along the spine of the mother, we should wrap the nates and sides in a soft napkin, and turn the child very gently round during a pain, observing to which side the feet are inclined to turn, till its abdomen is to the spine of the mother, and the toes are directed backward to the hollow of the sacrum, or to the side of the pelvis. In many cases, the nates turn round in the passage spontaneously, so that it is not required artificially to alter the position. It is necessary always to recollect that it is possible to turn the body of the child round without turning the face round into the hollow of the sacrum, and that the chin may be over the symphysis pubis when the front of the chest and abdomen are turned backward. After the lower extremities and body of the child have been expelled, and placed in the most favourable position for the extraction of the superior extremities and head, it is necessary to proceed without loss of time to draw these through the pelvis, that the child may not be destroyed by compression of the umbilical cord. As pressure upon the cord for a very short time will in some cases kill the child, it is proper to watch closely the pulsations of its arteries. Draw the body of the child forward as far as the arm-pits, and place it in this manner [exhibiting it upon the phantom] over the palm of your right hand and forearm, and gently draw the body towards the left thigh of the mother; then pass the fore and middle fingers of your left hand along the back part of the left arm of the child to the elbow-joint, and press down the arm with your fingers along the thorax of the child, and extract it. Then transfer the body of the child and left arm to your left hand and fore-arm for support, and with the fore and middle fingers of your right hand disengage and bring down, in the same way, the right arm of the child; then pass the fore and middle fingers of your left hand into the mouth of the child, or rather over the lower and upper jaw, and at the same time place the fore and middle fingers of your right hand over the back part of the neck and occiput, and with the fingers of the two hands thus applied extract the head, in the line of the axis of the pelvis. The perineum is very rigid in some cases of nates presentation, where it is the first child, and it will be torn if the head is extracted hastily, and not drawn forward to the symphysis pubis. When you feel the pulsations of the cord beginning to cease, you may be tempted to employ greater extracting force than the neck of the child and perineum can bear, and both may be destroyed. The only me-

thod of obviating this is to press back the edge of the perineum, that the air may gain admission into the mouth of the child, and the respiration go on, when the circulation in the cord has been arrested, until the perineum is sufficiently dilated to slide back over the face, and allow the head to pass. I have seen from twenty minutes to half an hour elapse in some cases after the cord had ceased to pulsate, before the perineum would allow the head to escape, during which time the respiration was regularly performed. This is not a new practice: it has been alluded to by some of the older accoucheurs, and some others; and the advantages to be derived from it were fully pointed out some years ago by Dr. Bigelow, in a paper published in the American Journal of the Medical Sciences, "On the Means of affording Respiration to Children in Reversed Presentations." The object of Dr. Bigelow in this paper is to show that in many cases the life of the child may be saved by forming a communication between the mouth and atmosphere previous to the delivery of the head. If the head be low down, the fingers alone can give the necessary assistance; but if it is high in the pelvis, and is reached with difficulty, the assistance of a tube may be necessary. He recommends a flat tube, which is to be guarded, and kept within the fingers of the inserted hand.

Where the pelvis of the mother is small or distorted, and the child large and unfavourably situated, the efforts of nature may be insufficient to expel the child, either alive or dead. The nates may become so firmly impacted in the pelvis, that they cannot advance without artificial assistance. A finger should be passed up to one of the groins, and when a pain comes on a considerable extracting force may be exerted with it, without injuring the child; or a soft handkerchief may be passed between the thigh and abdomen, and the nates drawn down; but this cannot be done unless they have descended low into the cavity of the pelvis. Where these means fail, and it is impossible to extract the child alive, the blunt hook or crotchet must be employed. In cases of nates presentation, where the pelvis is distorted, after the extraction of the trunk and extremities, it is necessary to perforate the back part of the head, and complete the delivery with the crotchet. In presentations of the feet and knees, the treatment does not essentially differ from that required in presentations of the nates.

CLINICAL LECTURES

ON THE

THEORY & MEDICAL TREATMENT
OF INSANITY,

Delivered at St. Luke's Hospital,

May 1st, 3d, and 5th.

BY ALEXANDER JOHN SUTHERLAND.

———

LECTURE II.—concluded.

Post-mortem examinations.

I HAVE now to draw your attention to the morbid appearances found after death in the brain and viscera of the thorax and abdomen. It must not be expected that the exact nature and seat of the alterations in the encephalon can be pointed out as manifesting the disease; I have never found any thing in the brain of the madman which could be said to be characteristic of his disorder; although there are very few cases which have not presented some morbid appearance either of the brain or its membranes. I think that medical men generally expect too much when they are called upon to examine the encephalon in a case of insanity. The brain is sliced to the centrum ovale, and the examination ends in disappointment. It was not thus that Foville examined the brain; every minute alteration in the cortical and medullary structure was carefully noted by him, and a healthy brain was compared with the madman's brain as often as circumstances would permit.

In laying the results of my post-mortem examinations before you, I shall commence with the scalp, and describe the morbid appearances according to the order in which the structure presents itself. The integument of the cranium is sometimes remarkably thin, and loosely attached to the parts beneath, and I have occasionally observed beneath the scalp a round circumscribed swelling containing fluid.

The shape of the cranium does not appear to have any connection either with the production or species of the disease. Many of our uncured patients have very well-formed heads; some, on the contrary, with badly-formed heads have got well. Georget says, one encounters, among madmen, the same formation of the head as among those of sound mind. Foville asserts that this is not strictly correct; there were more than 50 malformations of the cranium in the 300 patients then in the hospital. I conclude that this remark applies to the madmen only, and not to the idiots under his care. The *receding of the forehead is the most striking alteration of the bone, and therefore, perhaps,* most frequently observed in insanity. I have seen a patient the shape of whose head corresponded exactly with the description of that of Thersites, φοξος την κεφαλην. The bones of the cranium differ very much in appearance in different madmen. Sometimes they are so thin as to be translucent, at other times they are preternaturally thickened; the thickness is also sometimes unequal. In some, the diploë has entirely disappeared, and the bone is hard and brittle; in others it is more than usually developed, and the external table is comparatively soft and yielding. Rough deposits of bone and spiculæ are found in various parts of the inner surface. The eburnated cranium which is sometimes found was supposed by Gall to have been accompanied by a disposition to commit suicide: this has been proved not to be correct.

Alterations of the membranes.—As in all cases of chronic inflammation, so in insanity, the dura mater adheres firmly to the inner table; so firm has been the adhesion sometimes that I have been obliged to remove the divided membrane with the skull-cap. In one case only I have observed extravasation of blood between the bone and the dura mater. The patient died of epilepsy. The first fit came on Dec. 6th, 1838, from which day to the 10th she had about fifty (they came on in such rapid succession that it was difficult to remember the exact number); coma followed, which terminated in death on the 13th. The dura mater was found much injected; separating this membrane from the inner table was an extravasation of blood the size of a half-crown; corresponding with this was an extravasation of blood beneath the scalp. In injuries to the head I need not say that such appearances are often found, and there is little doubt that the patient must have had a severe fall during one of the fits. There was, however, in this case, an appearance more rarely met with, there was no falx cerebri; the hemispheres were joined together by cellular membrane, which adhered to either side of the longitudinal fissure. The vessels and sinuses of the dura mater are sometimes gorged with blood. The arteria meningea media is frequently injected to its most minute ramifications. The membrane itself is sometimes also much thicker than natural; small deposits of bone are also occasionally found, particularly on the falx. Dr. M. Hall has directed our attention to the influence of irritation of the membranes of the brain in inducing spasmodic affections (Med. Chir. Trans. xxiv. 122). He removed the cranium of a dog; every kind of irritation, puncture, laceration, &c. of the cerebrum and cerebellum was entirely inoperative: when the brain was cut away, leaving the medulla oblongata, to his surprise he found that laceration or pinching of the dura mater induced peculiar spasmodic movements of the eye-ball, the eye-lids, the head, &c. These effects are probably induced through branches of the trifacial nerve, which, as in the recurrent of Arnold, is well known to impart branches to the dura mater, and which may do so to other membranes within the cranium. This experiment of Dr. M. Hall's is extremely interesting, but I think we should not too hastily conclude from it that irritation of the membranes, as by deposition of bone on the dura mater, or inflammation of the arachnoid, will always produce spasm; for we must remember that the dog's brain was removed, and the spinal marrow, having lost its controlling influence, was in a state most favourable to the production of reflex phenomena.

The glandulæ pacchioni are not more numerous in insanity than in other diseases. I cannot think, with M. Andral and others, that these are the result of disease because they are so universally found; but if they are not they must have some use. Can it be that, imbedded deeply in the inner table as we sometimes find them, they afford additional support to the brain, and prevent more effectually the interference of the hemispheres with each other when we lie on one side? They may be so far the effect of disease (or rather, I should say, of a provision of nature to counteract its effects), if it be necessary that they should be multiplied to ensure a firmer adhesion of the dura mater to the bone, when the weight of one hemisphere, from the presence, for instance, of a tumor, is likely to interfere with the functions of the other. I considered this supposition to be probable from observing in a patient who died of organic disease of the brain a greater number of these so-called glands than I had previously observed.

The arachnoid membrane is very commonly found opaque and thickened: I have seen this in a patient whose insanity was only of five weeks' duration; it depends, however, more upon the intensity than the duration of the disease. The opacity is sometimes general, sometimes partial. It is more frequently met with on the surface of the hemispheres than at the base of the brain: and this accords with the lesions found in acute inflammation of the meninges. M. Foville considers the opacity and thickening of the arachnoid, and its adhesions with the pia mater, not to be the simple effects of inflammation, but of a deposit of albuminous layers.

I have, in some few cases, met with false membranes in the cavity of the arachnoid. Some have believed these membranes to be deposited between the dura mater and the arachnoid. M. Boudet (Mém. sur l'Hemorrhagie des Meninges), and others have, I believe, satisfactorily made out that the false membrane is in the shut sac of the arachnoid. The blood which forms this false membrane is not effused from a ruptured vessel, but exhaled by little and little through the arachnoid; it expands itself gradually in its cavity till it exactly represents a true serous membrane. If its adhering portion be peeled off, the arachnoid will be found beneath; somewhat rough and tarnished, however, from its contact with the pseudo-membrane. After the effusion of blood has taken place the serum is gradually absorbed, and the clot of blood left. If death occurs soon after the effusion, liquid blood is found; if at a more advanced period, a fibrous sheath is seen enveloping the blood; at a still later period, black clots, which become paler and paler till they lose at last their colouring matter (see Boudet).

Mr. A. had an epileptic fit about two months previous to his coming under my care in Sept. 1839, at which time he laboured under dementia. In December of that year he had a second fit, after which there was thickness and hesitation in his speech, with impaired motion of the limbs, particularly of the left leg.

The fits became more and more severe, and terminated in death on May 23d at 10 A.M.

Post-mortem examination, May 25, 3 P.M.

There was much emaciation of the body. The skull-cap being removed presented great inequality in its thickness. The parietal bones were thin and translucent, and had no diploë. The occipital and frontal bones were natural. The dura mater adhered very firmly to the bone, and was much injected with blood. The arachnoid membrane was much thicker and tougher than natural, and here and there over its surface opaque milky spots were observed. In its cellular tissue, on the upper surface of both hemispheres, but more on the right than left side, there was a great quantity of serum effused, which raised it about a line above the pia mater. In the cavity of the arachnoid was a false membrane, exactly resembling it in appearance, between the layers of which was an effusion of dark red blood, spreading on either side in parallel lines from the crysta galli to the squamous portion of the temporal bones. The layers were thick and tough, but not so shining as the arachnoid. The upper layer was so closely connected with the arachnoid that at their point of junction the one could not be distinguished from the other. This pseudo-membrane extended from each side of the falx to the tempero-occipital sutures, and from before backwards over the whole of the superior surface of the hemispheres. The parallel lines of dark blood appeared at first like small arteries, but under the microscope the blood-globules could be distinctly seen, not confined within vessels, but running in the folds of the false membrane. The pia mater separated very readily from the brain. The convolutions were atrophied; externally they were paler than natural; when sliced, there was very little depth of cortical structure. The cut surface of the brain presented numerous bleeding punctæ. The substance was soft and very wet; when taken up in the hand it felt like a spongeful of water. The ventricles of the brain were larger than natural. Five ounces of sero-sanguineous fluid were collected, which had filtered from the brain and ventricle. The cerebellum was natural. On raising the spinous processes of the vertebræ the vessels of the dura mater were enormously turgid. The spinal cord itself was both externally and internally highly injected, and uniformly so from the occiput to the lumbar vertebræ.

In another patient who was admitted into the hospital, November 3d, 1838, and who died of apoplexy, May 18th, 1839, there was not only found a similar membrane to the one above described, but a layer of lymph of a red colour, and resembling a honeycomb, was spread over the whole surface of the pericardium, which was filled with bloody serum.

I have only two other cases of pseudo-membranes in my note-book; they are very similar to the one I have already detailed. The one died of epilepsy, the other of apoplexy.

The arachnoid is sometimes perfectly dry, its surfaces are not lubricated by the smallest quantity of serum. In general, however, there is much effusion of clear transparent fluid into its cellular tissue; it is not often that this fluid is coloured. This appearance must not be taken as an unequivocal proof of inflammation of the arachnoid; for it may be caused by congestion of the veins, or be the result of poverty of blood. Dr. Kellie, of Leith, in his experiments upon animals bled to death, found effusion of serum in the brains of all.

I think that this effusion is often the consequence of atrophy of the convolutions; for I have observed in some cases where the atrophy has been very limited in extent that serum is collected here under the arachnoid, which has shewn no signs of inflammation: upon one or two occasions this effusion of fluid has been so circumscribed by the membrane that I at first mistook it for a transparent cyst.

The most extensive disease of the arachnoid membrane which I have met with in insanity was in the case of a gentleman who died of epilepsy on February 22d, 1838. The *duration of his illness was five years and a half. The evidences of his insanity were,*

that all his friends were dead, that the whole population of London had been swept off by disease; that our ships were rotten, our banks had stopped, our trade had failed: he latterly sank into a state of complete fatuity.

In the early part of 1839 symptoms of amaurosis shewed themselves; in September he became totally blind. He never had any illusion of hearing, nor was he at any time deaf. There were deposits of the triple phosphates in the urine, but it was not albuminous. He was subject to attacks of vertigo, when he would fancy that he was being run away with in a cart; he would call out to those about him to stop the horse, and would lay hold of a chair to prevent him, as he said, from being jolted out.

Physical symptoms preceding death.— Epileptic fits, followed by fever; twitching of the muscles more on right side than left; no paralysis of arms or legs; difficulty of swallowing two days before death. No reflex action when the finger was drawn across the eyelids.

Post-mortem examination, February 23d, 13½ *hours after death.*

The body was not emaciated; there was injection of the capillaries in the depending parts; the scalp was natural; the cranium very thick.

The dura mater adhered firmly to the inner table, and was removed with the skullcap. It was much injected. The veins were loaded with blood.

The arachnoid membrane on the upper surface was universally thickened and opaque, and studded all over with white spots the size of a millet-seed; in the situation of the anterior lobes of the cerebrum it was so thick that I could with difficulty cut it with the scalpel; it was as firm and elastic as fibro-cartilage; at the anterior and centre part of each lobe, there was on this membrane a deposit of bone with sharp spiculæ, the diameter of which was half an inch on the left, an inch on the right side, the spiculæ on the latter being more prominent. The colour of the arachnoid in this part was of a dirty yellow for the space of three inches; it was universally adherent to the pia mater on the anterior lobes; there was much effusion into the subarachnoid cellular tissue, which being collected with the sero-sanguineous fluid from the base of the cranium, amounted to half a pint by measure. The pia mater was much injected. The convolutions externally were pinched and atrophied, the sulci between them were wide, and the vacant space left by the absorption of the cortical structure was filled with the thickened pia mater and serum. The colour of the convolutions was pale externally; their cut surface shewed scarcely any definite line between the cortical and the fibrous structure. They were paler at their circumference than their base, and in some parts not more than a line in breadth : when a sponge was placed on the surface of the brain it was so soft that a portion of the convolutions came off with it : the white bands which separate the cortical structure into three parts were no where seen. Dark purple points were seen on the cut surface of the fibrous structure, and not the bright red points so commonly found. The substance of the brain was every where softened, and when taken from the skull did not in the least degree preserve its elasticity. The whole of the anterior lobe of the cerebrum of the right side, except the convolutions of the lower surface, was converted into a pulpy mass of ramollissement, the softening being greatest beneath the points of bone of the arachnoid. The lateral ventricles were twice their natural size, and gaped open without elasticity : on the arachnoid membrane lining all the ventricles were deposited innumerable small pellucid shining tubercles, varying in size from a pin's head to a pin's point; these were thickly studded over the optic thalami and corpora striata, and were traced down the iter a tertio ad quartum ventriculum, where they also existed in great number, particularly in the situation of the calamus scriptorius. The anterior cornua of the ventricles were as large as the ventricles themselves. The posterior cornua were also enlarged. The left hippocampus major of the posterior cornua was converted into a cyst containing a limpid fluid with no lining membrane. The optic nerves were one-third their natural size, flattened, yellowish, without any pearly lustre : all the other nerves of the cerebrum were softened. The thalami were extremely soft; the corpora quadragemina were natural ; the cerebellum was very soft ; the pons varolii and upper part of the spinal cord were much injected. The basilar and internal carotids, to their remotest ramifications, were studded with atheromatous deposits; some of the smaller arteries were quite plugged up by them.

Thorax healthy; heart flabby and contained a firm yellow coagulum; there were atheromatous deposits on the inner lining membrane of the aorta.

Abdomen, stomach, pancreas, spleen, healthy; liver congested. There was a gall-stone in the gall-bladder the size of a marble. The veins of the intestines were congested ; their mucous lining membrane was healthy. The kidneys were of a leaden colour and marbled.

The pellucid tubercles of the arachnoid, seen under the microscope, appeared like transparent eggs surrounded by small *granules*. They were very hard, and with *difficulty broken up*. *The tubules of the fibrous structure easily*

took on the varicose appearance, became granular when the smallest pressure was made, and had no elasticity whatever.

In parts of the anterior lobe (under a one-eighth eye-piece), were seen small round pellucid bodies corresponding exactly with the tubercles on the arachnoid : nearly the whole pulpy mass was composed of these bodies, mixed here and there with debris of arteries, and granular structure without any trace of fibrous structure. These small tubercles were composed of many other tubercles, and appeared like a bunch of grapes.

Adhesions of the pia mater are found with the arachnoid on the one side, and with the convolutions on the other. It is sometimes much thickened, and in recent cases generally injected. If we wanted other proofs of the variation of the quantity of blood, and of the state of the capillary vessels, in insanity, we should find them here. I have seen the colour of the plexus choroides in some cases a bright red, in others of a dirty white, or quite blanched. Sometimes arterial, sometimes venous congestion is found : I have seen this plexus loaded with varicose veins.

I have now to mention the alterations in the cortical structure. In acute mania the convolutions have a tendency to hypertrophy, in chronic mania to atrophy. In acute cases their external surface is round, and their colour intensely red. In chronic cases it is flattened and pale. As there is so much difference between the appearance of the one and the other, it will be more convenient if I first describe the morbid alterations found in the acute stage of the disease, and afterwards those found in the chronic.

In acute cases the pia mater is seldom found adhering to the surface of the hemispheres; the convolutions are well developed ; when cut there is as well defined a separation between the cineritious and fibrous structure as in a healthy brain; the white bands may be traced in every part running parallel to the external and internal surface ; but the cortical structure is much injected, and what is called the marbled appearance by French writers is very generally seen. Foville has frequently observed small red points in the marbled lines, which appear to him very small effusions of blood, afterwards converted, he thinks, into cysts filled with serosity.

The chronic alterations of the cortical structure are more marked than those of the acute. The pia mater frequently adheres to its surface; and a layer of softened grey matter is sometimes separated in the attempt to peel it off. The diminution of bulk takes place both on the surface and in the centre of the convolutions ; so that wide sulci are left between the folds, and a very thin layer is spread over the fibrous structure ; the white bands have either disappeared, or the colour of the ganglion globules is so faded that they cannot be distinguished. The external layer of the cortical structure is sometimes firm, while the internal layer is soft. It then assumes the appearance seen in Dr. Bright's Work, Plate 1, fig. 6. Medical Reports, Vol. ii.

Softening of the substance of the convolutions is either partial or general; it is sometimes confined to one or two folds; sometimes to one, at other times to both hemispheres.

The two following cases of acute and chronic insanity may serve to exemplify what I have said of the difference of appearance of the brains of each after death.

A woman, æt. 39, who had suffered under mania with violent paroxysms of furor, was brought to the hospital, October 28th, 1842, in a dying state. She died October 29th, at 6½ A.M. of exhaustion. The duration of the insanity was 10 days. Her occupation was a dress-maker. The cause of her illness was disappointment in her affections.

Post-mortem examination, October 29th, *13 hours after death.*

The body was bloodless and emaciated. The skull-cap thin : in the centre on the right side was an indentation which nearly pierced through the parietal bone; it corresponded with a swelling the size of a small marble, where the arachnoid had collected some effused serum. The vessels of the dura mater were turgid ; the arachnoid membrane was every where transparent ; fluid was effused into its cellular tissue. The pia mater separated with some difficulty from the convolutions, but did not tear them : its veins were much injected. The cortical structure was both externally and internally of its natural colour and consistence ; the white median bands were well seen. The convolutions were sharply cut, and in high relief. The arteries were distended with blood. The cut substance of the brain presented a deep blush of red throughout the cerebrum, cerebellum, pons and medulla oblongata, but more especially in the region of the posterior lobes, where there was also more serum effused. The lateral ventricles were rather large, and contained more fluid than natural. The substance of the brain was firm. An ounce and a half of sero-sanguineous fluid was left in the base of the cranium.

Thorax.—Some firm adhesions of the pleuræ on the left side ; lungs, heart, liver, gall-bladder, spleen, pancreas, and stomach, healthy. Left kidney healthy ; right slightly marbled ; both of the natural size. Mucous membrane of the ileum very slightly injected. No ulceration present.

A *woman,* æt. 51, who had been a boarder *or uncured patient in St. Luke's,* since January 1833, died January 7th, 1843, of phthisis.

The duration of her insanity had been 16 years.

Evidences of her madness.—Incoherent ; imbecile.

Physical symptoms prior to death.— Dulness of percussion over the whole of the right side of the thorax ; no respiratory murmur heard here. There was scarcely any expectoration. Anasarca of the left leg.

Port-mortem examination, January 7th, 8 P.M.

The frontal bone receded very slightly from before backwards. The body emaciated and bloodless. After the skull-cap had been removed, the diploe were found to have disappeared, except in a small portion of the frontal and occipital bones. There was a small depression in the centre of the inner table of the occipital bone, which was translucent ; there was another in the frontal bone.

The *dura mater,* externally, was much injected with red blood. The arteria meningea media was large ; the membrane adhered firmly to the bone. The arachnoid was dotted all over with minute opaque spots ; into its cellular tissue yellowish transparent serum was effused throughout its whole extent.

The *pia mater* was rather more injected than usual ; it separated from the convolutions without tearing them. Under the hollow of the occipital bone, above described, the convolutions were flattened and atrophied for three lines in extent on either side of the longitudinal sinus ; the arachnoid had here formed a circumscribed cyst. The cortical structure externally was pale. Its outer layer was soft, and separated readily from the external white band, under which the substance was firm and of a reddish hue in the frontal region. Serum was infiltrated into the substance of the brain, and about three ounces of fluid were left in the basis of the brain. There were numerous bleeding punctæ on the cut surface of the cerebrum and cerebellum ; the pons and medulla were also injected. Their substance was firm. The ventricles were rather larger than natural ; the hippocampi not altered. The basilar artery was joined by two internal carotids ; one pair of which was much constricted and of the size of a pin, and most atheromatous deposits were upon it. There were small dots of extravasated blood of a dark red colour, the size of a pin's point, in the right lobe of the cerebellum.

Thorax.—Slight adhesions of the pleuræ on the left side—the lung healthy ; universal adhesions of the pleuræ on the right side—the lung was with difficulty taken out ; it was studded all over with miliary tubercles ; there was a dark vomica near its apex and posterior part. Heart healthy, small, a firm dark coagulum in the left ventricle; stomach, spleen, pancreas, healthy; liver pale, of a dirty white colour, and of a fatty consistence; kidneys small, and very slightly marbled; their capsules were with difficulty separated. Intestines—there was a small portion of the ilium constricted to the size of the little finger, extending about a foot; the mucous lining membrane was here injected.

Alterations of the fibrous structure.— Upon slicing the substance of the brain numerous bleeding punctæ from the gaping mouths of the vessels are frequently seen, giving it the appearance of being sprinkled with sand — the *aspect sablé* of French writers. This varies in intensity from the few specks seen in healthy brains to patches of extravasated blood, a deep blush, or marbling and mottling over the whole surface [Bright's plate]. We have a salutary warning from Dr. Seymour not to lay too much stress upon this appearance. "There is, perhaps," he says, "no appearance to which more importance has been attached than to congestion of the vessels of the head; the mechanical physician having his scruples satisfied by a very slight injection of the vessels of the brain, while the morbid anatomist must have observed almost every variety of intensity of this appearance often unattended by corresponding symptoms of excitement, or disturbance of the brain, during life." As a proof that these remarks of Dr. Seymour's are just, I may state that I have met with some brains in madmen marked by the entire absence of bleeding points.

In speaking of the hardness or softness of the brain of lunatics I shall not refer to cases of a questionable nature, as every one must have seen much variety of density in this organ, depending upon the time of making the examination after death, and the season of the year. There are some brains of lunatics which are remarkably tough and elastic; when they are taken from the cranium they preserve their shape perfectly, and when you attempt to cut them you will think your scalpel is blunt, however sharp it may really be: these brains appear like hard albumen. On the other hand, the brain of the lunatic is found remarkably soft; and when taken in the hand feels like a wet sponge. Ramollissement is not very uncommonly met with. I have found the greatest degree of softening correspond with a spicula of bone either adhering to the cranium, dura mater, or arachnoid. I have, however, likewise found it accompanied with atheromatous deposits on the arteries; and, on the *other* hand, I have found a spicula of bone *pressing on the convolutions* without any *sensible alterations in the part pressed upon.*

Tubercles are not often met with in the substance of the brain; their slow growth rarely interferes with the functions of motion or sensation; if, towards the close of the disease, there is aberration of intellect, it partakes more of the nature of delirium than insanity.

The ventricles are frequently distended with fluid; their walls are also found gaping and inelastic. I have sometimes seen vesicles on the choroid plexus, and once I found sabulous matter deposited in it when it was absent in the pineal gland. This gland I have seen converted into a transparent cyst, a morbid appearance which would have been highly prized by a disciple of Descartes.

The pons varolii is occasionally found injected. Upon one occasion I found one half highly vascular, the other half natural; upon another occasion I found a lesion in an interesting case, which I will detail to you. A young woman was admitted into the hospital March 19th, 1841. She was a nurse, and was seized with mania on March 14th. The cause of her illness was stated to be anxiety in having to leave the children of whom she had the care, as she was about to be married. The evidences of her insanity were incoherence, excitement; she fancied she was nursing a child, would sing, and rock herself backwards and forwards, &c.

Physical symptoms. — Very weak and emaciated; when she attempted to walk she staggered from side to side as if she was drunk. March 27th she was attacked with fever; violent convulsions soon after showed themselves, which succeeded one another very rapidly. She died April 2d, 1841.

Post-mortem examination, April 2, half-past 9 P.M.

Body emaciated. Dura mater more injected than natural. Arachnoid and pia mater healthy, except that the vessels of the latter were turgid. Convolutions and cortical structure natural. Substance of the brain firm. On slicing it to the centrum ovale, a remarkable difference between the anterior and posterior half presented itself, the former being of a natural colour, the latter of a deep red; the division between the white and red colour was so defined that a line drawn from ear to ear separated the one from the other. Fluid blood was effused over the surface also of both posterior lobes; there was more than an ounce of blood left in the basis cranii. On cutting into the pons varolii an apoplectic cyst was seen, the blood contained in it being changed and mixed with the broken-down substance of the pons. *Thorax.*—The lungs did not collapse on opening the chest; they felt solid, but a piece placed in water floated. The bronchi were gorged with frothy mucus, and were deeply injected. Heart.—The auriculo-ventricular ostium on the left side was so small that it hardly admitted the point of the little finger to pass through, as the mitral valve was nearly obliterated, not by disease, for it was perfectly smooth, but by a malformation. The parietes of the left ventricle were thinner than natural ; those of the auricle thickened and dilated. The uterus of a dusky brown colour, from engorgements of the vessels. Spleen, liver, kidneys, ovaries, intestines, healthy.

It now only remains for us to consider the morbid appearances of the nerves. The evidence upon this part of our subject is not so satisfactory as one could wish ; we cannot, however, be surprised at this, considering how difficult it is to detect disease of the nerves even in those cases where there has been great functional disturbance existing in them during life. Disease may spread along a sensitive nerve, gradually affecting it till the spinal marrow becomes involved ; and it is probable that the same may take place with regard to the brain.

In January 1839, I attended a gentleman who laboured under general paralysis occasioned by taking large quantities of morphia to relieve the pain of tic douloureux, for which the supra-orbital nerve of the right side had been divided previously. He died on the 22d Feb. 1840. At the post-mortem examination I found three sharp spiculæ of bone on the ridge of the petrous portion of the temporal bone under the fifth and seventh nerves. In tracing the auditory nerve to its origin in the fourth ventricle, the iter a tertio ad quartum ventriculum was found inflamed, and the floor of the fourth ventricle presented a deep blush of red, and was somewhat softened, the transverse white bands being involved. In this case hearing was perfect. "In the museum at Berlin," according to Müller, " there is the brain of a young female who, in consequence of a fall upon the neck and occiput, was gradually attacked by paralysis of the whole body ; and here, upon the floor of the fourth ventricle, and upon these transverse white fibres, an effusion of lymph had taken place, although the sense of hearing had not suffered. We must, then, agree with him that these bands have by no means the important influence on the sense of hearing which is often attributed to them."—Baly's Trans. 828.

Disease at the origin of the nerves, although the most careful anatomist may fail to detect it, is doubtless frequently the source to which the subsequent delusion may be traced.

A patient under the care of my father in 1813, imagined that snakes were crawling about his arms, and frequently asked for a knife to cut them out. At the post-mortem examination, on opening the spinal canal, something having the appearance which

effused blood assumes after it has been deposited a considerable time, was discovered lying between the processes of the vertebræ and the membrane ; this substance was nearly two inches and a half in length, half an inch in breadth, and one-sixth of an inch in thickness ; it extended from the 3d to the 5th cervical vertebra, and adhered firmly to the bone.

In a patient who died of epilepsy combined with general paralysis, and who fancied that wild beasts were tearing the flesh off his back, I found the membranes of the spinal marrow injected, and the minute vessels of the cord much inflamed in the cervical region : its cut surface, from the situation of the 1st to that of the 7th vertebra, presented a deep blush of red.

It will be needless that I should take up your time in detailing minutely the morbid appearances which I have found in the viscera of the thorax and the abdomen. I shall merely state them in a general manner.

In 50 cases, which I select from my case-book, where the thorax and abdomen were examined the lungs, were diseased in 31.

Adhesion of the pleuræ . . . in	25
Effusion into ,, . . .	11
Pneumonia.	13
Bronchitis	5
Tubercles and Vomicæ	8
Emphysema	3
Gangrene	2
The heart was diseased in . . .	25
Hypertrophy	12
Diseased valves	10
Hypertrophy with dilatation . .	2
Atrophy with dilatation. . . .	3
Fluid in pericardium.	4
Flabby	6
Alterations in the liver were observed in	12
Congested in	3
Gall-bladder contracted without bile	2
Gall-stones.	5
False membrane on surface. . .	1
Fatty degeneration	1
Granular	1
Disease of the kidneys	19
Disease of the uterus and ovaries .	7

I must say, in justice to M. Pinel's theory, that in the majority of the cases the intestines were only partially examined, as I often had to work single-handed, and had not completed my labours when the friends came for the corpse.

The intestines were found diseased in	12
Mucous lining membrane injected in .	6
Ulceration in	1
Stricture in	3
Arch of the colon displaced in	2

In concluding the observations I have

make on the examination of the brain of insanity, I have to draw your attention—1st, To the many different morbid appearances which accompany the disease; 2dly, To the many similar appearances which give rise to its different species, and are found where insanity does not exist; the best proof of which is, that I have been able to illustrate many of the post-mortem alterations by the plates of Dr. Bright and Dr. Carswell.

Now although we may look to the cortical substance as giving us the most conclusive evidence of variations from healthy structure, yet we are far from being able to say in what the first departure from such healthy structure consists. Do we call it congestion? This is the mere effect of something which has caused previous irritation: we know well how different in their nature the causes are which produce congestion—whether passion, over-exertion of intellect, diseases of the heart and lungs, stomach and intestines, narcotic poisons, &c. It would appear, then, that beyond what morbid anatomy teaches us, there is some change in the brain which, influenced by individual susceptibility, is the primary cause of the various phenomena which we recognise in madness. In this, as in every other disease, morbid anatomy alone cannot guide us in establishing just views of pathology. It is the better, perhaps, that such is the case, as it makes us attend more particularly to the symptoms during life, the relief of which is of far greater importance than a correct knowledge of the primary source of the disease.

OBSERVATIONS

ON

CERTAIN SOURCES OF FALLACY IN THERAPEUTICS:

THEIR CAUSES, CONSEQUENCES, AND THE MEANS OF PREVENTING THEM.

By ROBERT VENABLES, M.B. &c. &c.

(For the London Medical Gazette.)

THERE are fallacies in anatomy; fallacies in physiology and pathology; and, what is of still greater moment, fallacies in medicine. Hence it is that virtues are frequently ascribed to particular remedies, which subsequent experience or more ample and careful observations refuse to confirm. This is much to be lamented; because, from a first disappointment, really valuable remedies are often consigned to unmerited neglect. In illustration it will only perhaps be necessary to state the

following facts, and to show that careful and cautious examination into all the circumstances is essential to guard against over hasty and unfounded conclusions.

A bottle of urine, containing about half a pint, was presented to me, with a request to examine it, and report the result. I was informed "that, on examination previously, it was found highly *alkaline*, and strongly effervesced on the addition of an acid." The urine when presented to me had been standing at rest for some days, was clear and transparent, of the natural colour, devoid of smell, unctuous to the touch, deepened the natural blue of litmus paper, but strongly affected turmeric, turning it to a reddish brown. To the bottom of the vessel had subsided a layer of a whitish-looking powder, somewhat coloured apparently by the colouring matter of the urine. This powder, on subsequent examination, proved to be the triple phosphate, with a small proportion of the earthy carbonates*. Thus, it dissolved with slight effervescence in diluted hydrochloric acid, and fused into a globule before the blowpipe. The specific gravity of the urine was found to be between 1·033 and 1·034. Such were the more immediate phenomena in this case.

This being considered a case of highly alkaline urine, and presenting a fair opportunity of testing the efficacy of benzoic acid in restoring alkaline urine to its natural acidulous condition, as urged by Mr. Ure†, ten grains of this acid were given as a dose, and repeated three times, the patient taking thirty grains in all between this and the subsequent visit. The urine examined on this occasion was found to possess its natural acidulous reaction upon litmus paper, did not effervesce with the strong acids, threw down no sediment, and presented the ordinary sensible properties.

The inferences about to be drawn from the phenomena and facts above stated were—

1. That the urine, when passed from the bladder, was in a highly *alkaline* condition.

2. That three doses, or thirty grains, of benzoic acid—in conformity with the views of Mr. Ure, that this acid

* I have since ascertained that such would be the result of those re-actions, which must have occurred in the present instance.
† See MED. GAZ. Feb. 10th.

undergoes decomposition *in transitû,* and appears in the urine as *hippuric acid*—had sufficed to restore to this strongly alkaline urine its normal acidulous reaction. Several of the phenomena, however, above described, appeared to me wholly irreconcileable with any of the observed and known morbid states of urine, and even in themselves quite incompatible. The urine is very seldom alkaline when first voided. Even in the phosphatic diathesis it is either neutral for the most part, or even acidulous*, becoming alkaline—in a time greater or less, in proportion to the severity of the diathesis—after being passed †. The only marked exception is when the mucous lining of the bladder, in a diseased state, throws off a large quantity of vitiated mucus, the fixed alkali of which reacting on the urea converts this principle into carbonate of ammonia in the bladder, and the urine then has an alkaline reaction even when first passed. In such cases, too, the urine, if not actually putrescent when voided, speedily putrefies, and exhales a strong ammoniacal odour. Such were the facts in the case detailed by Mr. Ure.

But the case under consideration presented no such phenomena, and, although strongly alkaline, yet, after having stood for four or five days, presented no turbidness, no alkaline odour, nor any mucous subsidence. The specific gravity, too, 1·033, greatly exceeded any compatible with the sensible conditions or properties presented, and could only, pathologically considered, result from either the presence of sugar, or an excess of urea. The presence of sugar was negatived by the sensible properties—the large deposition of the triple phosphate, the strongly alkaline state, and the capability of effervescence. Neither the nitric nor the oxalic acid, after four hours, separated any urea, and consequently this principle ‡ could not have been the cause of the high specific gravity. The usual reagents, also, shewed that the urine was completely freed from its earthy principles, as neither caustic potass, nor even oxalate

of ammonia, precipitated a single particle of earthy matter.

The anomalous characters and irreconcileable phenomena presented by the urine in this case inclined me to suspect one or other of the fixed alkalies in a carbonated state as their source, and I determined, in the first instance, to examine for potass, as admitting of more positive identification. For this purpose, a portion of the urine was diluted with rather more than an equal volume of water in a test-tube, and to it a concentrated solution of tartaric acid was added in considerable excess; violent effervescence took place, and a large quantity of the crystals of bitartrate of potass speedily subsided, and which, when completely deposited, exceeded in bulk the volume of urine employed by about one-half. A volume of the urine undiluted, treated in the same manner, instantly became a solid mass of crystals of cream of tartar. On adding to a portion of the same urine a solution of chloride of calcium, a large quantity of chalk, or carbonate of lime, separated and speedily subsided. Thus the presence of potass, and of carbonic acid, in large proportion, were unequivocally proved.

The facts above stated leave no doubt but that the anomalies furnished by this case arose entirely from the artificial impregnation of the urine with carbonate of potass, and that this impregnation had been effected after the urine had been voided from the bladder. The presence of carbonate of potass does not form the principal feature in the anomaly, as it is well known that the citrate, tartrate, acetate, &c., are converted *in transitû,* and appear as carbonate of potass in the urine, and may be detected and identified by the appropriate methods. But no bladder, however hardy or callous, could tolerate, even for the shortest period, urine so highly loaded with carbonate of potass; nor could it endure even the injection of water so strongly alkaline. The urine in this case was capable of dissolving, or at least of disorganising, the cuticle, as was manifested by the unctuosity of feel which it communicated. I found that it takes nearly half an ounce of carbonate of potass to raise the ordinary specific gravity of half a pint of urine to that of the specimen in question.

A question here naturally presents; how was the impurity in this instance

* The term acidulous is to be understood as referring to the reaction on litmus paper.
† See Guide to the Urinary Cabinet, &c.
‡ Subsequent observation shewed this principle to be, if not actually deficient, at least in no excess.

effected? was the adulteration intentional, with a view to imposition; or was it the result of accident rather than design? Although I think we may generally attribute such contaminations to design, yet I have been informed that in this instance there was no assignable motive; on the contrary, that many circumstances concur to lead to a diametrically opposite conclusion. But although these circumstances may acquit the individual of any attempt at intentional deception, still they will not alter the absolute facts. The alkaline impregnation might have been the result of accident, from not carefully examining the vessel into which the urine had been just passed, or into which it was subsequently transferred*. Be this as it may, still the history presents matter by no means uninteresting in several points of view : first, it shews how careful and diligent we should be in the examination and analysis of morbid phenomena, especially if intended as the basis of either pathological or therapeutical inductions. It proves the necessity of great caution and circumspection before we admit the natural existence of such phenomena, more especially if of an anomalous or incompatible nature; and that we do not reason upon nor draw conclusions from equivocal facts. Secondly, how much more rigidly and strictly we should analyse the various phenomena, and examine their compatibility, when we intend them as the foundations for special therapeutical axioms.

To apply these principles in the present instance, it is evident that a blind confidence in the obvious phenomena, and an over anxiety too hastily to corroborate new theories or modern discoveries, might have led to serious errors, not only as regards pathology, but also therapeutics. The three doses or thirty grains of benzoic acid might have been supposed capable of rendering even the most strongly alkaline urine acidulous, as the urine passed on the first visit after taking benzoic acid, but in the presence of the practitioner, was found, so far from possessing any alkaline property, to be naturally and unequivocally acidulous. A therapeutical fact, especially if new and previously unobserved, commands attention, and interests in a degree proportionate to

its value in pathology, or the benefits which it is likely to confer upon practical medicine; hence it must be evident that a rigid examination of the premises is as essential to correctness as that of the conclusion. The conclusion may be legitimate, but still, if the premises be unfounded or erroneous, evidently the conclusion must be false.

There is no department of medicine more subject to fallacies of this sort than that of urinary diseases. This, perhaps, is owing to various causes : first, to the little attention given by earlier observers to the subject in question; secondly, the ease with which superficial observers may be imposed upon, either through accident or design. But it is to be hoped that the greater assiduity, and the greater degree of importance attached to this particular subject by more modern inquirers, will greatly limit both such fallacies and their ordinary causes.

Since the above, two cases of alkaline urine have presented to me, in which the urine was alkaline, or at least neutral, even when passed from the bladder; and the general details, perhaps, may form a useful contrast to the above. They both occurred within a few days of each other.

April 29th, I visited Mr. G——, who came to London from the country in consequence of the state of his health. He complained of pain in his loins, and pain in the urethra, especially near the orifice, on passing water. Had frequent desire to pass water, and was obliged to get up frequently in the course of the night to pass it. The urine on being voided was muddy, alkaline, or perhaps rather neutral, not rendering turmeric brown, although litmus reddened by a very weak acid was after a minute or two turned blue again; the specific gravity, 1·022, never getting lower than 1·020 during the four weeks that I have been attending, at least twice in every week. Heated, the urine coagulated; and this took place by nitric acid. On being allowed to remain at rest it did not become clear, but deposited a quantity of purulent-looking matter, intermixed with blood, the red particles distinctly shewing themselves. There was no excess of urea; on the contrary, this principle might be considered, if anything, deficient. A strong acid caused slight effervescence, but

* This specimen was brought to, not passed in the presence of, the medical practitioner.

nothing like what occurred in the former case. It seemed to depend upon the presence of carbonate of ammonia. The earthy bases were not in excess.

May 2d, I was requested to visit Capt. E——, whose symptoms were very similar to those above stated. The urine, passed frequently in my presence, was turbid on being passed; it was occasionally alkaline, not sensibly so to turmeric, but when tested by litmus reddened by a very weak acid largely diluted; occasionally neutral; on remaining at rest for a time — 24 or 30 hours — deposited a muco-purulent deposit, often intermixed with blood. Specific gravity varying from 1·019 to 1·022, but never becoming clear. No urea in excess, but if anything deficient. Earthy bases not superabundant. Exercise, such as walking rather fast, or an unusual distance, causes the voiding of a considerable quantity of blood, which falls to the bottom as a clot, while a portion of the red particles remain uniformly diffused through the urine; and a specimen passed on the 16th instant, and left at rest ever since, now the 28th, exhibits precisely the same appearance, viz. a portion of the red particles still uniformly diffused.

I examined the effects of a saturated solution of tartaric acid in excess in these cases. An effervescence took place; the urine, though clear, became cloudy, and gradually deposited a muddy-looking precipitate, but which evidently had not the crystalline appearance of bitartrate of potass, neither did it form or separate as this salt invariably does when suddenly and artificially precipitated. The precipitate collected, washed, dried, and heated over the spirit-lamp, became black, and deposited charcoal evidently from the decomposition of the tartaric acid. The ash, tested by an acid, feebly effervesced; on being urged by a stronger heat—the blow-pipe in a platinum spoon—it diminished in bulk, and ultimately became white. This white ash, applied to moistened turmeric paper, turned it of a reddish brown. Another portion, dissolved in acetic acid, but feebly diluted with water, without effervescence, and the solution yielded a precipitate when treated with oxalate of ammonia; nor was this precipitate dissolved by even concentrated acetic acid, however considerable the quantity. In a word, all the evidence

tended to shew that the tartaric acid had precipitated the earthy tartrates, principally tartrate of lime, and that the proportion of the earthy bases was by no means great. The alkaline bases in these instances, if we except ammonia, seem to have been deficient. The ammonia, too, will perhaps account for the deficiency of urea, as it was probably derived from the conversion of this principle into carbonate of ammonia. It is evident, however, that there is a marked difference in both the sensible and chemical properties of the two specimens of urine in contrast with each other.

In these two cases I endeavoured to render the urine acidulous, by means, first, of hydrochloric acid, and, failing, I conjoined the phosphoric. After, as I conceived, a sufficient trial, and the urine still remaining neutral, I gave the benzoic acid in doses of fifteen grains three times a day. In the case of Capt. E. the urine was rendered acidulous on the third day, and continued so although left exposed for several days; and the benzoic gradually was reduced in dose, and he now feels tolerably well.

In the case of Mr. G., the same effect did not occur for two or three days longer, when I found the urine immediately on being voided acidulous, but becoming neutral in a time varying from 20 to 30 hours. However, the last time I examined this gentleman's urine I found it much improved, although still frequently intermixed with blood in very small proportions, but the intermixture of mucus much greater than natural, although now greatly reduced from what it had been.

From the circumstances just now detailed, I think we have every reason to infer that benzoic acid exerts a greater acidulating agency upon neutral or alkaline urine, than the acids upon which we have hitherto relied for this purpose. Thus the hydrochloric, and the phosphoric, though tried sufficiently, had not the desired effect; but in a comparatively short space of time after the benzoic acid had been administered, the urine in both these cases became acidulous; and exhibited this one of its natural characters the last time I had an opportunity of investigating the matter, and which was on the 23d instant. It is true that as hydrochloric and phosphoric acids had been given in the first instance, and continued at the same time with the benzoic, it may be a matter of question, and indeed one difficult to determine, whether any, and how much, of the acidulation can be justly attributed to each agent.

From the foregoing it is evident that the first case has no value whatever in a therapeutical point of view, but is highly instructive as shewing how easily we might be betrayed into errors, and of serious character. The two latter are of importance, and tend much to corroborate, or rather to confirm, the therapeutical principles laid down by Mr. Ure No doubt they will excite to farther investigation, while the first will serve as a beacon to guard us against incautious induction, and satisfy us of the true mode of giving a real value to our researches, whether intended as philosophical investigations, or therapeutical facts and observations.

5, St. Vincent Place, City Road,
May 29, 1843.

ILLUSTRATIONS

OF THE

ALLEGED FALLACIES OF
AUSCULTATION, &c.

By H. M. HUGHES, M.D.

(For the London Medical Gazette.)

THERE are, perhaps, few, if any, members of the medical profession who would, at the present day, think it proper to assert that the practice of auscultation and percussion had not materially contributed to accuracy of diagnosis in thoracic, and in some forms of abdominal, disease. Facts almost innumerable would be adduced to confute such an opinion. But there are not a few who, while they concede to the stethoscope and plessimeter a limited praise, appear disposed to magnify their occasional failures, and relate, with a measure of exultation, the comparatively rare mistakes of those who take a higher estimate of their importance. Such persons are generally, either not in the habit of employing auscultation in their investigations, or, from physical defects or want of practice, are incapable of fully appreciating its advantages. They may, I think, be divided into those who are too old, or consider themselves too

experienced, to learn, and who, therefore, will not hear;—those who are incapable of distinguishing minute differences of sound and tone, and really cannot hear;—those who never tried to learn, and, consequently, do not expect to hear;—and those who, partly from want of education, and partly from deficiency of tact, combined with some obtuseness of auditory perception, hear imperfectly.

"Ah! Dr. Hughes," said an old and really experienced practitioner to me, while examining the chest of a medical gentleman in a distant part of Sussex, "I am sorry I have not learned to use this new means of examination; I ought to have done so before, but I cannot do so now." I gave a very decided opinion that our patient was suffering from acute tuberculous disease of the apex of the right lung, and prognosticated a not very distant fatal termination to his complaint. This opinion was received with kind deference, though opposed to one previously entertained. My senior friend subsequently told me in private that, as our patient had already been in confinement, he feared disease of the brain more than of the lungs. In about two months he died from rapid consumption.

"I really cannot hear it," said a gentleman whose attention was directed to a particularly well-marked pleuritic rubbing, which was clearly audible by a number of pupils who immediately afterwards examined the patient. This gentleman, however, acknowledged that his ear is far from being delicate in reference to other, and especially as to musical, sounds.

"As to your pericardial sounds," said another, "I don't believe a word about them." "Have you ever heard the rubbing noise which is supposed to have its seat in that membrane?" "No, I never tried." A case was pointed out to him in which the sound was especially harsh and superficial. He acknowledged it was *strange*, and different from any thing he had heard before. This patient recovered, and, when adhesion had taken place and the sound had disappeared, was again examined by the same individual. Another patient, however, in the wards nearly at the same time, with exactly the same physical signs, died, and was examined after death. The pericardium, covered with rough solid deposit, was shown to him, and he was convinced, not only of the reality of the sound, but also of the correctness of the usual explanation of its origin. He believed in the existence of a pericardial rubbing; no longer thought it *strange*.

A fellow pupil, now dead, having very considerable talent, but comparatively little experience as an auscultator, and not possessing the advantage of a fine ear, was accustomed, publicly, to dispute the reality of the sound last referred to, which had then been only recently discovered, but which has since proved such an invaluable aid to the diagnosis of pericarditis. But the principal or only reason he was accustomed to assign for his incredulity was that *he* could not distinguish it from the bellows murmur or other sounds arising from diseases of the valves. I am not aware whether his opinions upon this subject were in any respect changed or modified before his death.

The preceding are genuine, and may, perhaps, be regarded as fair examples of persons who, though not actual objectors to, or detractors from, the merits of "physical diagnosis," believe that its importance has been too highly extolled, and its advantages exaggerated.

That opinions founded upon the practice of auscultation and percussion, as upon every other mode of investigation, are liable to error, is of course readily conceded; that mistakes sometimes occur to the most experienced is undeniable; but they are frequently, perhaps generally, attributable either to want of experience or the too hasty conclusions of the auscultator.

To employ these *aids to diagnosis* with advantage, they should be used constantly and for a long period: a protracted education is required: in them, as in other arts, practice is necessary for perfection, and repeated examinations are often indispensable to correctness. Yet the mistakes of the inexperienced are sometimes referred to as the fallacies of the art itself, and opinions, unwillingly given after a single explanation, are advanced as proofs of its imperfections.

Though it may not be correct to say that in all cases, and under all circumstances, the auscultatory or other physical signs should be regarded as the mere handmaids of the general symp-

toms, as many cases might be adduced in which a correct diagnosis has been founded upon the former independently of the latter, yet is it incumbent upon the practical auscultator diligently to weigh every feature, and each attendant circumstance, of the complaint under investigation, and in all cases to exercise his judgment as well as his hands and his ears. The stethoscope and plessimeter should in most cases be regarded as very important adjuvants to the other means of arriving at a correct conclusion as to the nature of a malady, rather than as instruments for their exclusion. Mistakes have perhaps sometimes arisen from neglect of these considerations: the physical indications have been too implicitly trusted, and the history and general symptoms have been too lightly esteemed. Fallacies also sometimes arise from a disregard of the fact, which should ever be borne in mind, and which has been recently forcibly stated by a lecturer on clinical medicine, that physical signs, with very few exceptions indeed, are indicative not of particular diseases, but of physical conditions. Thus metallic tinkling indicates the presence of an admixture of gas and fluid in a circumscribed space, and may exist in pneumo-thorax, a large vomica, or a distended stomach.

Fallacies are also not unfrequently attributed to auscultation, in consequence of changes taking place in the diseased organ subsequently to the examination, and to the expressed opinion of the physician. After death fluid is found in the pleura, or consolidation of the lung, or a cavity is discovered, the presence of which had not been ascertained, for the simple reason that it did not exist at the time of examination. Rapid changes occurring a short time before death are far from uncommon, and unfounded charges of the fallacies of auscultation in consequence are, I am convinced, not unfrequent.

I shall now relate some cases occurring under my own notice, in which, with due consideration of the history, general symptoms, and physical signs conjoined, fallacies, apparent or real, might have existed, without affecting in the remotest degree the credit of the auscultator.

CASE I.—*Disease of the lung; history, symptoms, and some of the physical signs, those of empyema and pneumothorax.*

E. G., aged 32, a small woman of light complexion, married, and the mother of several children, was admitted into Guy's Hospital, Oct. 5, 1842. Two years before she had been a patient of the Surrey Dispensary, under my care, suffering from what was believed to be empyema, or at least chronic pleuritic effusion. She had some weeks before I saw her been attacked with pain of the side, which was then enlarged and bulging, quite dull on percussion, and inferiorly afforded no traces of natural respiration. She continued under my care for about a fortnight only, during which she certainly improved considerably by the use of blisters, slight mercurials, and tonics. She then went into the country for two weeks, and continued to improve for two months subsequently. She became pregnant, and during her pregnancy, which terminated in the birth of a living and healthy child, she suddenly expectorated a large quantity of fœtid yellow matter. Expectoration of the same kind of matter had continued, and had caused gradually increasing debility up to the date of her admission into the hospital. She was then considerably emaciated; her face was pale, her features contracted, and the expression of her countenance somewhat anxious. She lay upon the back, with considerable inclination to the right side; her cough was not frequent except upon motion, but was constantly induced by turning towards the left side, and was accompanied by an abundant expectoration, which streamed from her mouth almost without effort, and which consisted of a sero-purulent fluid, yellowish, homogeneous, frothless, fœtid, and of the consistence and tenacity of thin gruel. She had no pain, and appeared in tolerable spirits, and of a quiet contented disposition. She had never suffered from hæmoptysis, but was occasionally troubled with diarrhœa, and was liable to hectic flushes, especially of the left cheek, and in the afternoon. She perspired considerably at night; and though she continually felt drowsy (perhaps from medicine administered), *she slept but little.*

Physical signs.—The entire left side of the chest, both before and behind, afforded very good, perhaps greater than the natural, resonance on percussion; and throughout its whole extent the respiratory murmur, a little increased in intensity, but quite free from rattles or other morbid sounds, was distinctly audible. The right side was considerably altered in form, was flattened below the clavicle, and raised very imperfectly during inspiration. The resonance upon percussion anteriorly was generally less than natural, but in no part could extreme dulness be discovered, while in the inferior lateral region there occasionally, but only occasionally, existed tympanitic resonance. Posteriorly this side was scarcely dull, but not so resonant as the left. Throughout the whole of the upper part of the right side, both before and behind, was distinctly heard a loud and shrill gurgling, possessing at some parts, particularly below the inferior angle of the scapula, a tolerably pure metallic character; while in the lower parts was heard a loud, shrill, and loose mucous rattle. The voice also was loud, shrill, and ringing, throughout the whole of this side, but especially at the upper part. The patient was too feeble to attempt succussion. The sounds of the heart were natural, and were audible in the præcordial region, but were most distinct between the cartilages of the second and third ribs of the right side, where alone the impulse could be felt, and where the apex of the organ appeared constantly to strike the thoracic parietes. She was ordered ten grains of compound chalk powder, with opium, in a draught containing ammonia and gentian, every six hours. A mutton-chop, two eggs, and six ounces of wine daily, and subsequently an opiate enema at night, as the diarrhœa was not effectually checked by the medicine previously prescribed. She obviously improved under this treatment, and appeared to gain flesh; but as she continued to sleep badly at night, half a grain of opium, with ten grains of compound chalk powder, was ordered to be given at bed-time, in addition to her other medicines.

On November 6th Mr. Stocker was called to her on account of a severe pain of the left side, and ordered a mustard poultice to be applied, and a pill containing antimony, opium, and a grain of calomel, to be given directly, and to be repeated every four hours if the pain continued. The next day the pain was relieved; and as she had no fever, and no increase of cough, but was still troubled with diarrhœa, and too low for physical examination, she was ordered ammonia and decoction of bark, with twelve grains of confection of opium, every six hours, and half a grain of opium if the pain returned. She now became more depressed; she had no cough; her skin was generally moist; and she died rather suddenly during the night of November 10th.

Inspection eleven hours after death. —The head was not opened. Thorax: On raising the sternum the heart was found to occupy nearly its natural situation. The left pleura was slightly adherent inferiorly by tender false membrane, evidently the result of recent pleuritis. The left lung was large, and about its inferior half was of a palish red colour, fleshy and œdematous, from recent pneumonia. The upper half was tolerably healthy, and, as well as the inferior, was free from tubercular deposit. On the right side the lung was so firmly adherent to the costal pleura, except over a small space inferiorly, where there existed only a few old bridles, as not to be detached without tearing away that membrane. The right lung was much contracted; the upper third was of a dark iron-grey colour, dense, and without air, except in that contained in some enlarged bronchial tubes. One or two small cavities existed therein, filled with dirty yellow pus, around which the lung was soft, friable, and uneven. The inferior two-thirds of the lung contained a number of cavities of different sizes, in the midst of a dirty gray-coloured consolidated pulmonary tissue, quite devoid of air. Among these cavities, as they appeared upon an incision being made into the organ, were some evidently produced by the section of greatly dilated bronchial tubes; others, varying in size from a pea to a pullet's egg, communicated freely and by large openings with the bronchial tubes, but were lined with a soft, loose, flocculent, but not decidedly membranous substance, which alone separated *them from the pulmonary tissue. These were generally of a* rounded or oval form. One, however' appeared to differ from all the rest: it was situated about the centre of the organ, rather posteriorly; it was of the superficial extent of the palm of the hand, very shallow, and so close to the surface as to be covered only by the thickened pleura, or at most by an exceedingly thin layer of the tissue of the lung, *if indeed any could be proved to exist.* Its internal surface was smooth and polished, crossed by thick bands, and was continuous with the lining of the bronchial tubes, several of which communicated with it by large openings. The whole of these cavities *were quite empty*, excepting those in the upper lobe, which appeared not yet to have opened into the bronchi. Abdomen: The liver was pale, and the right acute edge elongated, coarse, and tumid. The kidneys were firm, and slightly granular; the ovaries hard, wasted, and rugous; and the other organs examined natural.

Upon a review of all the circumstances connected with this rare and very interesting case, it will be observed that almost every thing tended to support the notion that the disease was empyema with pneumothorax. The history and general symptoms in particular appeared alone sufficient to mark the origin and nature of the complaint. The pain of the side, the bulging and immobility of the part affected, the subsequent sudden and copious expectoration of matter, and the excretion of the same for many months, seemed especially to attest the probability of that disorder. The physical signs, though imperfect in some respects, might be supposed not unnaturally to confirm, or certainly not to oppose, the diagnosis derived from the general symptoms. The mis-shapen and contracted parietes, the partial dislocation of the heart, the loud and ringing voice, the shrill metallic gurgling, the occasional tympanitic resonance, were in its favour. It is true that the extended, marked, and continued tympanitic resonance upon percussion, often supposed to be an invariable and almost a necessary sign of pneumothorax, did not exist. But independently of those related by others, I have myself seen, and have notes of, a well-marked case of pneumothorax, in which at no period while the patient remained

under my observation was there even
the natural amount of resonance upon
percussion. It is also true that the
phenomena produced by succussion
were not ascertained to exist. These,
however, might have been present,
though a feeling of humanity towards
the suffering and debilitated patient
would not permit her attendants to
make an attempt to produce them.
Upon examination after death, no empyema, no pneumothorax, was discovered; and though the physical signs
were admirably and beautifully explained by the physical conditions that
were found to exist, and though the
history and general symptoms might
properly cause under ordinary circumstances those physical signs to be attributed to empyema and pneumothorax,
yet might the case be adduced as an
illustration of the fallacies of auscultation. In respect to the true morbid
anatomy of the disease, as well as to its
pathology, different opinions existed.
Some believed that all the cavities, of
whatever shape and size, were in truth
dilated bronchial tubes, and others
that they originated in the softening of a diseased lung. My own
belief is, that neither opinion was
exclusively correct—that both conditions clearly existed; that in fact the
case had been one of pleuro-peripneu-
mony, and that it was a genuine example of chronic pneumonia, with softening and dilated bronchial tubes, without a trace of tubercle; and that it is
even highly probable that the large superficial cavity, with scarcely any covering but the pleura, and perhaps with
that of the costal pleura alone, had
been an empyema which had communicated with the bronchial tubes, the
air from which had not extended into
the general cavity of the pleura, in consequence of the old and firm adhesion
of that membrane. It is, however,
sufficient for my present purpose to
show that the physical state was exactly
indicated by the physical signs, that
there existed a large cavity containing air, freely communicating with
a large bronchial tube immediately
under the costal pleura, and that this
was clearly indicated by auscultation.
Two other circumstances are worthy of
notice before closing the remarks upon
this interesting case. All the cavities
in the lung that opened into tubes, and
all the tubes themselves, were found

empty after death, though the expectoration during life had been profuse.
The heart, which had been distinctly
and constantly felt pulsating between
the second and third ribs upon the
right of the sternum, drawn over by
the contraction of the diseased side,
assisted probably by the increased action and development of the left lung,
was found after death, and when that
lung had collapsed by the admission of
air upon the thorax, in its normal
position.

[To be continued.]

CASE OF MENINGITIS.
BY CHARLES VINES, ESQ.
Surgeon to the Reading Dispensary.
(For the London Medical Gazette.)

THE following case, in which depletion
to an unusual extent was necessary,
affords also a few other points of interest.

Elizabeth Joseph, æt. 19, a servant,
of plethoric habit and nervous temperament, who had enjoyed a good state of
health up to June 7th, 1842; was
seized at 10 in the morning with rigors,
and shortly afterwards with headache
and fever. She was visited for the first
time at 8 in the evening, and presented
the following symptoms. She was in
bed lying on her back, and complained
of severe lancinating pains in the forehead and back part of the head; the
face and neck flushed; slight protrusion
and wildness of eyes; pupils dilated and
insensible to light; head very hot;
carotids and temporal arteries throbbed
violently; tongue rather coated, but
moist; skin hot and dry; respiration
hurried, unusual quickness of hearing
and speech; nausea; pulse 130, sharp,
contracted, and intermittent; bowels
had been open during the day.

Treatment.—Bleeding from the arm
in the upright posture. After the removal of 36 ounces of blood faintness
was induced, and the symptoms were
much relieved. The head to be shaved
and an evaporating lotion to be continually applied. To take the following
powder directly:—

℞ Hydr. Chlorid. gr. vi.; Pulv. Jalap.
gr. xv. M. ft. pulv.

After the powder had operated, the
pills and mixture as follows:—

R Hydr. Chlorid. ; Pulv. Antim. aa. gr.
xij.; Conf. q. s. ft. pil vj. Cap. unam
4tà quàque horà.

R Liq. Ant. Potas. Tart. ʒvj. ; Magn.
Sulph. ʒij. ; Aq. Men. sat. ad ʒvj.
M. ft. mist. Cap. coch. ij. mag. 2dà
quàque horà, post sing. pil.

The diet to consist of gruel, tea and toast,
and water.

8th, 9 A.M.—Had passed a sleepless
night, had been restless and incoherent;
all the symptoms as yesterday; bowels
had been open; no sickness produced
by the antimonial mixture; blood taken
yesterday highly buffed and cupped.
So long as the faintness induced by the
bleeding continued, the symptoms were
relieved; but on reaction taking place,
they again recurred.

Ordered another full bleeding, and 30
ounces were taken. To continue the
medicines.

9 P.M.—The bleeding relieved the
head, as before, about four hours, when
the pain returned; and this evening all
the symptoms were aggravated. The
pulse had become rapid and thready;
pain in the head excessive; the blood
taken in the morning was cupped, and
exhibited the buffy coat. The vein
of the arm was again opened, and 16
ounces of blood removed, which relieved the head slightly. Cupping
at the back of the neck was then
resorted to, and 16 ounces were
taken. This last abstraction of blood
had a most decided effect over all the
symptoms. The pupils immediately
acted freely; the pulse became soft and
fell to 90; the pain in the head was
quite relieved.

To continue the calomel and antimonial
mixture, and a blister to be applied to
the crown of the head.

9th, 9 A.M.—Had slept well at intervals during the night; had been
quite free from pain; complained of
lightness and giddiness of the head;
pulse 100, fuller, but rather sharp; respiration less hurried; pupils natural;
bowels open; tongue clean; skin moist;
expressed herself much better.

To continue the medicines.

9 P.M.—The former symptoms had
again returned, viz. the quick thready
pulse, with pain in the head. Took 12
ounces of blood from the arm.

10th. - Has had no sleep; been very
restless; vomiting several times; suspect improper food was taken yesterday; pupils dilated and sluggish; pulse
100 and thready; spasmodic twitchings
of the arms; pain at the back part of the
head; pain in bowels with tenesmus.

To discontinue the calomel and antimony.
Took 12 ounces of blood from the arm;
directed a mustard poultice to be applied
to the bowels, and ordered the following
mixture :—

R Potas. Bicarb. Ɖij. ; Pulv. Tragac. Co.
ʒj. ; Sp. Ether Nitr. aa. ʒj. ; Aq. Men.
sat. ʒvj. M. ft. mist. Cap. coch. ij.
mag. 4tà. q. h.

11th.—Has had no sleep; bowels
open twice during the night; pupils
act better; pulse 90 and soft; catamenia made its appearance, being a
fortnight before the proper period;
pain in head and bowels relieved; symptoms altogether better.

12th.—Slept five hours during the
night; general condition of the patient
improving.

13th.—Slept well; the bowels confined. Ordered the following mixture :—

R Magnes. Carbon. ʒj. ; Magnes. Sulph.
ʒiij. ; Sp. Ether. Nitr. ʒj. ; Aq. Men.
sat. ad ʒvj. M. ft. mist. Cap. coch. ij.
mag. 4tà. q. h.

14th.—Passed a good night; bowels
had been open twice; going on well.

15th.—Going on favourably.

17th.—Passed a sleepless night; complained of pain in the head and right
side; head hot; pupils again dilated;
pulse 100, and thready; appeared strange
and incoherent in manner; countenance vacant; answered slowly to
questions; skin hot and dry; bowels
confined.

Bled to 16 ounces. To repeat the calomel
and antimony. A blister to be applied to
the nape of the neck, an evaporating
lotion to the head.

18th.—has had no sleep; symptoms
nearly the same as yesterday.

Ordered a blister to be applied to the
whole crown of the head.

19th.—Passed a better night; symptoms generally relieved. From this
period a gradual restoration to health
took place, and in two months the
patient was enabled to resume her
former situation. In the course of her recovery, occasional blisters were applied

to the temples and behind the ears, and a due caution observed with regard to diet and the regulation of the bowels.

OBSERVATIONS. — A peculiarity of some importance in the symptoms of this patient was, the occurrence of dilated pupil and insensibility to light at so early a stage of the disease. It cannot be supposed that this amaurotic condition of the eye was produced by effusion, or other more general symptoms of coma would have been present ; but we must, I think, infer that it arose from a plethoric or congested condition of the vessels immediately supplying the ophthalmic apparatus exerting an undue pressure on the retina and optic nerve; the origin of this cause being arterial excitement, just as in the first stage of cerebral inflammation, we may have in one case extreme acuteness of the auditory nerve, in another extreme dulness, admitting, I believe, of explanation on similar principles.

Another symptom worthy of notice, was the peculiarly rapid pulse, as though receding from beneath the finger. The abstraction of blood from the nape of the neck appeared to afford much more decided relief than general blood-letting, and would have been repeated but for the strong objection of the patient ; and here I refer with great pleasure to the excellent lectures lately delivered by Dr. Burrows before the College of Physicians, in which he has demonstrated that the brain does actually contain more blood at one period than at another, and consequently that local depletion, when properly applied, must have the effect of diminishing vascular plethora, and, as a necessary consequence, vascular pressure within the cranium. In accordance with these views, I would suggest that in severe cases of cerebral congestion, or inflammation, where it is desirable to produce a most decided and speedy effect on the vascular condition of the brain, and where a general blood-letting has failed to effect this important object, that the abstraction of blood by cupping on the vertex of the head, or nape of the neck, is a preferable plan to the application of leeches, or the opening of the temporal artery, the cupping-glass being applied in all cases where practicable to the crown of the head, at the junction of the lambdoidal and sagittal sutures. *It will be remarked in the* preceding history, that two or three relapses occurred, attributable, I believe, to improper diet ; so complete is the sympathy between the head and stomach. The close contiguity of the brain to its investing membrane renders it probable that those cases are rare in which inflammation exists in one tissue without the adjacent one being, to a certain extent, implicated. The hitherto imperfect state of our knowledge in this branch of pathology ought to stimulate us to increased exertion and most attentive observation, in every case that may occur to us. The experienced Dr. Abercrombie, to whom we are so much indebted for our present knowledge of these diseases, confesses that we are often at a loss to distinguish the true origin of the symptoms.

ANALYSES AND NOTICES OF BOOKS.

" L'Auteur se tue à allonger ce que le lecteur se tue à abréger."—D'ALEMBERT.

Practical Remarks on Gout, Rheumatic Fever, and Chronic Rheumatism of of the Joints, &c. By R. B. TODD, M.D. &c. London, 1843. 12mo. pp. 216.

THIS sensible and judicious work is the substance of the Croonian Lectures delivered this year at the College of Physicians. Dr. Todd's object is to show that rheumatic fever and gout are diseases of the blood ; his book, however, is by no means limited to the proof of this proposition, but is full of practical hints.

We are much pleased with the author for insisting on the importance of studying the natural history of disease; without which we cannot assign their due shares to nature and to medicine in its cure.

Some of the points in the following extract are far from universally known.

"The sebaceous glands are not so numerous [as the sudoriferous ones] ; they are most abundant in the vicinity of hairs. Their form is that of small vesicular bags, which open by minute orifices into a hair follicle, or quite close to one. When sebaceous matter is suffered to accumulate in these glands, a peculiar disease of the skin is induced, called *acne*, which often shows itself on the face, nose, or forehead, and very frequently on the back.

In a simple form the accumulations are denoted by numerous black points, produced by particles of dust being entangled in the sebaceous matter, which chokes the orifices of the glands. The skin around them will often inflame, and angry pustules result.

Nothing favours the excretion of this sebaceous matter so much as cleanliness and friction. If any additional arguments were wanting to enforce the propriety of adopting means for these purposes, it is derived from the curious, and in some measure humiliating, fact lately discovered by Dr Simon of Berlin, that these glands are the habitat of a parasitic insect, which has been called the *entozoon folliculorum*. This creature is of considerable size, and may exist alone, or in clusters of several, in a single gland. In the perfectly healthy state they are few in number; but when sebaceous matter, their proper food, is suffered to accumulate, they abound. Through the kindness of my friend, Mr. Erasmus Wilson, who has lately read a paper to the Royal Society on their structure and habits, I have been enabled to see the insect alive and had a favourable opportunity of watching its movements, as well as carefully observing its form and structure. Cleanliness and friction remove sebaceous matter, and, therefore, oppose the accumulation of those insects; and the local application of a solution of corrosive sublimate is often very beneficial in removing the points of acne which result from the retention of the sebaceous secretion."—p. 84-5.

Austria: its Literary, Scientific, and Medical Institutions. With Notes upon the present State of Science, and a Guide to the Hospitals and Sanatory Establishments of Vienna. By W. R. WILDE, M.R.I.A. &c. Dublin, London, and Edinburgh, 1843. 8vo. pp. 325.

AMONG the subjects treated of by Mr. Wilde, are the present state of science in Vienna; the great General Hospital; public clinical instruction; the young school of Vienna; auscultation, and pathological anatomy; syphilis; the lunatic asylum; midwifery and the lying-in hospital; the foundling hospital; the veterinary institution, and Josephinum Academy; homœopathy, poor laws, and minor hospitals of Vienna; and the general and medical statistics of the Austrian empire.

The general hospital contains 2,214 beds, and receives from 18,000 to 20,000 patients annually.

The lying-in hospital forms part of the general one, and the mortality in it is quite frightful. Of 4453 women admitted in 1838, no less than 179 died—ought we not to say were put to death? This is a mortality of 1 in 25; in this country 1 in 80 or 100 is the common proportion; but even this is so much greater than occurs in dispensary practice, that it is questionable how far lying-in hospitals can be considered charities. The great size of the one at Vienna, and the fact of its forming part of the colossal general hospital, must tell strongly against the recovery of the patients. Women in child-bed require pure air above all things; and as puerperal fever is, unfortunately, an infectious disease, the only wholesome hospital for their care would be a series of cottages, as was suggested some years ago by Dr. Ferguson.

The tables exhibiting the result of 25,906 deliveries, which Mr. Wilde gives at p. 223, *et seq.*, he supposes to be the most extensive "in British print;" but we think he will find more comprehensive ones at the end of Dr. Merriman's Treatise on Difficult Parturition.

Mr. Wilde's work will be consulted not only by the student who intends to proceed to Vienna, but by the accomplished practitioner who desires to improve the institutions of his own country by culling the best regulations of foreign states.

The British Quarterly Journal of Dental Surgery. Edited by J. ROBINSON, Esq. No. 1. London, March 1843. 8vo. pp. 64. With a Lithograph and Woodcuts.

AMONG the articles in this number we may mention—A review of dental surgery; Successful treatment of irregularity of the central and lateral incisores in an adult, by the editor; Report to the *Académie des Sciences*, Paris, on a memoir by A. Nasmyth, Esq.; Artificial Teeth; On the necessity of a faculty of surgeon-dentists, by J. L. Levison, Esq.; Scale of charges in America; Osseous union of deciduous teeth; A case of complicated double congenital hare-lip, with an excessive

formation and projection of an inter-
maxillary bone, by John Martin, Esq.;
The process of development of the
epithelium; Association of dental surgeons; Mania from decayed teeth;
&c.

Mr. Robinson's bold attempt (the
first of the kind, we believe, in this
country) deserves every encouragement; and, by securing the services of
numerous and skilful *collaborateurs*,
he will be certain to attain success.

MEDICAL GAZETTE.

Friday, June 16, 1843.

---

*" Licet omnibus, licet etiam mihi, dignitatem
Artis Medicæ tueri; potestas modo veniendi in
publicum sit, dicendi periculum non recuso."*
CICERO.

THE COLLEGIATE SYSTEM.

ALL who have read the Pickwick
papers—that is to say, every one—
must have been struck with the say-
ings and doings of certain medical
students immortalized in the pages of
the great novelist. Unrivalled as he
is in his delineations of the more unfavourable phases of London life, he
has surpassed himself in the painful
fidelity of these medical sketches.
After making a slight allowance for
the colouring with which the artist
enriches the sombre tints of dull reality, what is left is enough to surprise
the indifferent reader, and to urge the
philanthropist to the mitigation of
the evils so picturesquely described.
Meantime, while the benevolent sa-
tirist attacks the present system—the
system of neglect—like a light-armed
horseman, the heavy cannon of grave
remonstrance and entreaty have been
brought against it by other writers.
It is satisfactory to think that the combined efforts of these allies have produced some effect, and that the collegiate system will probably be commenced in London this very year. We

have been favoured with some of the
details of the new plan, and lose no
time in laying them before our readers.

Six houses have been appropriated
by the Governors of St. Bartholomew's
Hospital, for the purpose of carrying
out the Collegiate system. They are
all situated in Duke Street, within the
hospital walls, and will be finished for
the accommodation of twenty-four students, each of whom will have his separate sitting and bed-room. The sets
of rooms will be furnished alike, but
the rent, of course, will vary in proportion to the distance from the ground.
Its precise amount is not yet settled,
but it will be less than students
usually pay. Now, it has been stated
that the average cost of a lodging to a
medical pupil in a metropolitan or
great provincial town, is about fourteen
shillings a week. Assuming this to be
pretty near the mark, we should conjecture that the rents for apartments in
Duke Street would vary from ten to
twenty shillings a week. Moderate as
these rents are, they will no doubt,
afford a fair return for the outlay: so
that the Governors would be justified in
thus employing the property of the
hospital, even were we to look upon
the design merely in the narrow light
of a commercial speculation; but
when we consider, on the one hand,
the noble object which is to be fulfilled,
and, on the other, scan the overflowing
coffers of St. Bartholomew's Hospital,
it would almost be a crime to neglect
such an opportunity of benefiting the
common weal.

Moreover, a dining-hall, with a
kitchen and other offices, will be built
in a middle space between the six
houses, thus affording a comfortable
spot for dining to resident as well as
non-resident students; while it is obvious that for the same money it will
be easy to give a far better repast than
at the chop-houses commonly resorted

to. The bill of fare will probably contain, besides the established dishes, some extra luxuries, like the commons and sizings of a Cambridge dinner. We do not know whether it is intended that each student shall dine separately, after the fashion of a chop-house, or together in the style of a *table-d'-hôte;* the latter, if feasible, should be preferred; for the gloomy practice of solitary repasts is one of the most uncomfortable points about English manners. The expenses of lodging and attendance have been carefully computed from the known expenditure of many students living, as they ordinarily do, in lodgings; and both the rent and cost of dinner being brought within those limits, it is pretty clear that the sum total of the comfortable will be less than that of the uncomfortable mode.

Much care will be taken to prevent the frauds so common in lodging-houses,—frauds which, petty though they be, are provoking in themselves, and inconvenient to the purse of the young beginner. The rooms will be attended by laundresses or their analogues, persons of unimpeachable honesty, (and, of course, *anti-Hebes*); and by them breakfast, tea, and small meals, will be served to each man in his own room. As much as is possible, the items of food, drink, coals, candles, &c. will be supplied by persons empowered by the managers of the College; and their accounts, so far as concerns the prices charged, will be watched by the same authorities.

But it is time to quit these household details, and turn to the weightier matters of discipline and superintendence, where more difference of opinion must arise.

Divine service will be performed every morning at eight in the Hospital Church, which is within twenty paces of the College rooms; and the students will be particularly invited, but not compelled to attend it.

No arrangement has yet been made for the immediate superintendence of the College, nor is the amount of discipline to be exercised yet determined upon. The general opinion is, that there must be a resident tutor, one who by his standing and knowledge should exercise authority, even when silent. Some have suggested that a senior student would be fit for this office; but such a man would soon become either a spy or an accomplice in the frays which he should have checked; and if he did not join with his juniors, they would certainly hate and probably annoy him.

Whatever he is, the Warden (as he will be called) must have educational authority. From the very first he must guide the studies of the resident pupils, and examine them in the progress they have made. He will naturally succeed to the lectureships in the school, or it may, probably, be deemed necessary that he should already hold one as a qualification for the office of Warden.

These matters are still open for discussion, and, indeed, are being discussed at this very time. Had we a vote in the divan, we should certainly hold up hand against the appointment of a senior student as Warden; for this officer should unquestionably be a man who has held a diploma for several years, and who is visibly older than the oldest pupil committed to his charge.

The more difficult question remains, how tight should the reins of discipline be drawn, to observe the happy mean between the irritatingly severe and the uselessly feeble. We may imagine some objector startled at the very name of discipline, and exclaiming—" What! are our sons never to see real life? Is mamma's apron-string to be indefinitely prolonged into an iron chain of constant discipline? Instead of fine-spirited men, are we to turn out the prim and bitter progeny of restraint, like so many victims of a dissenting academy?" By no means, Sir Critic; nothing of the kind is contemplated;

Est inter Tanaim quiddam, socerumque Vitelli;

There are many resting-places between the Sawyer of the novelist, and the unfavourable specimens of the favoured Caucasean race whom you hint at in your queries. We should anticipate that the discipline at St. Bartholomew's would incline to the side of the agreeable; and though the rigid might call it lax, the lenient would not term it severe. Even if, in the course of years, it should be raised to the pitch of our two antique Universities, this could not be called unreasonably strait-laced, nor one calculated to form harsh puritans, instead of philanthropic citizens of the world.

All these arrangements will be brought into full play, it is hoped, by next October, and there can be no doubt that all which is possible to make the system work well, will be done. A chief mover for this excellent purpose among the hospital authorities is the treasurer, a man of strong common sense, and thoroughly devoted to the hospital and school; a man, in short, of genuine English energy.

" Nil actum reputans, si quid superesset agendum ;"

He is cordially seconded by the chaplain, and by all the influential governors; so that we may consider the approaching good to be not merely in posse, but almost in esse.

CHANGES IN THE HOSPITALS AND SCHOOLS.

Mr. STANLEY having resigned his lectureship on anatomy and physiology, it has been determined to adopt the same division of lectures as at King's and University Colleges. There will be no course of demonstrations, but a course of lectures on descriptive and surgical anatomy; and one on general and morbid anatomy and physiology. Mr. Skey has been appointed lecturer on the former, and Mr. James Paget on the latter subject.

Dr. Bright has resigned his office at Guy's Hospital, and Dr. Golding Bird has in consequence become assistant-physician.

Mr. Guthrie has retired from the Westminster, and the death of Mr. Tyrrell occasioned a vacancy at St. Thomas's Hospital, which was filled by the election of Mr. Macmurdo on the 14th.

MEDICAL REFORM.

To the Editor of the Medical Gazette.

Sir,

I conceive, as stated in my last letter, that it is only by six or eight apprentices being received into the surgery of a general practitioner, that proper advantages could be afforded to them, or proper time devoted to their studies and superintendance. I proceed to detail the plan by which I consider their instruction could be conducted.

If the practitioner's private practice be extensive, an assistant should be kept, though I do not think it any advantage that the practice should exceed 1000, or 1500 cases yearly, if the surgery is carried on methodically; and perhaps it might be in some measure considered the perquisite of the junior practitioner to receive pupils; and it must be confessed in many instances he would be the most competent instructor in the scientific department.

Supposing, therefore, eight pupils were taken, they might be divided into two classes; one class taking the duties of the surgery, the other confined exclusively to the study. In the surgery, again, the four might alternate morning and afternoon in their duties of dispensing and bookkeeping. Again, the dispensing admits of subdivision into extemporaneous prescriptions, or the putting up of medicines for the patients, and the preparations and prescriptions kept always ready, as the preparations of all tinctures, masses of pills, &c. The bookkeeping might be also divided into the posting of the ledger and day-book, and into the proper keeping of the drug-book, registers, &c. &c., and several other small accounts, the detail of which would occupy too much space here. The spare time of the students in the surgery could be occupied in studies of several subjects, that would not suffer by an occasional interruption, as translations of Latin, German, French, or Greek; the practice of drawing, and readings in the materia medica, as in Drs. Pereira's or Thomson's works; and their reading, as well as all prescriptions and entries, should be overlooked by the assistant or master. This division or class of students, on the following week should change places with the other class, and take their place in the study.

The subjects to be prosecuted in the study are such as require the whole and uninterrupted attention, as anatomy and the first principles of medicine; and this species of application could be diversified by a regular time in the laboratory in practising chemical manipulation, taking, perhaps, the 25th section of Faraday for their direction; and in the preparations of all the chemical formulæ in the London Pharmacopœia; while their hours of relaxation, which should not be stinted, might be taxed, if in the country, in the cultivation of the many medical plants, and in the collection of herbs.

The students should be called upon at an early hour every morning, and also every evening, to attend a lecture on a subject connected with their studies, especially on natural philosophy and chemistry, by which the practitioner's time would not be too much interfered with; and early rising, and occupation in the evening, would be useful in a moral view. I consider that instruction by lectures is also essential, because students unused to this method at first cannot learn much by it; and therefore the first lectures in town are often wasted and lost to the pupil. The master would often have opportunities of encouraging the proper employment of the hours of relaxation, by fostering any desire they might evince for any of the collateral sciences, as in the collection of various objects of natural history, geology, and mineralogy, &c., and also by allowing time and procuring masters for other branches, as in drawing, modelling, casting, &c.

I would undertake that by this method, the outline of which is here sketched, and the details of which would be filled out best by each person for himself, that any pupil in three years might be sent to the hospital, having a sound elementary knowledge on the following subjects:—

Elementary and practical chemistry.

Botany—and in this subject considerable progress might be made by the aid of botanical excursions.

Pharmacy—by the actual preparation of all the chemicals, and also by preparing all the extracts, &c. contained in the Pharmacopœia.

Anatomy. — The students could obtain, by the aid of plates and the skeleton, a thorough knowledge of human osteology,

and a good general idea of the situation of all the muscles.

Physiology—the rudiments.

Medicine—the theory, especially as treated in the Conspectus of Gregory. As to the practice, though generally considered so essential a part of apprenticeship by nonprofessional persons, most medical men will agree, that until further advance is made in physiology and the theory of medicines, it would not be of much service. If, however, any one should consider it advisable, a dispensary can be supported for a very small annual cost; and many charitable persons would be induced to lend such establishment their help, when started for legitimate purposes.

Toxicology—the chemical portion practically.

Natural philosophy—the outlines.

I need not add how essential it would be that the master's treatment and conduct towards his pupil should be strictly in accordance with the rules of gentlemanly bearing. Such things having been heard of, it is almost painful to acknowledge it, as a difference made to the apprentice at the table, than which nothing can be more detrimental.

The advantages of a sound scientific instruction of the apprentice would act beneficially, both mentally and morally.

Mentally—because it would begin early to instil industrious and studious habits, and because the pupil would go to town, not only with a sound elementary knowledge, but with a *method of study*; and, to use the exact words of the Apothecaries' Company, the "neglect of regular and systematic study will usually be found to terminate in failure and disappointment;" and it would also, of course, greatly facilitate the labour while at the hospital, and therefore give the greater opportunity of obtaining a better insight into more important matters: and, morally, because it would be no difficult matter to show that the dissipation of medical students on their arrival in London, depends upon the idle habits engendered during servitude, and from the sudden escape from a most rigid confinement to absolute and ungoverned liberty: besides, the previous instruction would give them an immediate interest in all the lectures they are now called upon to attend, and from the first it would place the profession of their own choice in the most pleasing and fascinating light, and it would therefore strengthen their predilection for it, and increase their ardour in its study.

But another point remains, and in the natural order of things should have been first discussed, which is—how is the practitioner at the present day to obtain the six pupils.

It is beyond a doubt that the number of

young persons entering the profession has very considerably diminished during the last few years; and I am sure that in my own neighbourhood there is scarcely one pupil to a dozen practitioners. The current seems to have turned, and is now directed to the professions chiefly of engineers, barristers, solicitors, all which require either no examination, or a very slight one. There is little doubt but the difficulties imposed have acted materially, at least on the young men themselves; I imagine, therefore, by somewhat dignifying the apprentices from the mere dispenser of medicines, to the private pupil, would have some effect in increasing the supply. Nevertheless, I do not doubt there would be some difficulty at first in forming such an establishment, especially with parents who naturally view innovation with suspicion.

I consider, however, that the Apothecaries' Company especially, by whose law it is that apprentices exist, have a right to demand a matriculation. Every member of the profession will cordially join in acknowledgment of the services which they have rendered the profession by their attention to the studies of the licentiates; but the Company have hitherto confined their bye-laws to that period of those studies that commenced after the student's arrival at the hospital; and happy as have been the results already, there cannot be the least doubt an equally beneficial effect would be produced, if the same superintendence was extended to that period of apprenticeship prior to the student's attendance at the hospital. They might test the student's progress by a matriculative examination of a very elementary character, and allow the present curriculum of studies to date from such matriculation. Indeed, when the student is compelled to pass at least two years and a half in the profession before he arrives in town, it is only common justice to ascertain that proper advantages and instruction have been afforded him, and it would be by no means an ill-spent bounty, if some substantial reward could be given to the pupil acquitting himself in the best manner at such examination.

There will be few to deny that education to the extent that I have described would be highly desirable. I trust I have also shown strong reasons why that education should be combined with the sort of knowledge to be obtained only in the surgery of the general practitioner; and that from the pupil's age, and from other grounds, the continuance of medical apprenticeship is expedient. I have also endeavoured to point out how an improved education could be effected, and I leave the method to the *consideration of any whom it may concern, whether to the legislature or to the present*

authorities, with whose regulations it is perfectly compatible; or, lastly, to any general practitioner who may think well ·of it, who might adopt it without any alteration whatever even in the present curricula taking place.—I am, sir,

Your obedient servant,
W. H. O. SANKEY.

Margate, June 2, 1843.

DEATH FROM A LARGE DOSE OF SULPHATE OF QUININE.

A MAN 26 years of age, No. 11 Saint Madeline's ward, was affected with acute articular rheumatism; he had been shortly before treated in the Hôtel Dieu for small-pox, and having probably left the hospital too soon was exposed to cold, and contracted acute rheumatism, in consequence of which he was admitted under the care of M. Recamier on the 27th of November; he then laboured under general fever without any complication; the heart, lungs, and head were not implicated; there was derangement of intelligence; no headache; both wrists were very painful and swollen, but the skin was not red; the knees were also painful, but in a less degree; no pain in the hips. The diagnosis was thus stated. *Acute rheumatism of the joints, with fever of medium intensity;* as to the prognosis it was stated that they would probably be of tolerably long duration; that complications were to be expected, such as inflammation of the serous membranes of the ²thorax, through nothing of the kind yet existed.

M. Recamier having just witnessed an admirable cure affected in an analogous case, by the administration of sulphate of quinine, to a lady, in private practice, resolved to employ the same treatment in this case. He prescribed the first day three grammes (36½ grains) in twelve papers, one to be taken every hour. No bad effect resulted.

The next day the pains were diminished in the lower extremities, but were more severe in the wrists. On a careful examination of the heart, no bruit de soufflet could be detected, but its pulsations were not quite so distinctly clear as natural.

The second day five grammes (77 grs.) of sulphate of quinine were prescribed; to be taken in the same manner as the first day. The patient had only taken 3½ grammes when he was suddenly attacked with extreme agitation, followed by furious delirium, and death occurred in a few hours.

On dissection the signs of a general and most intense meningitis were discovered; considerable sanguineous effusion of the meninges; penetrated vascularity of the surface of the brain, of which some points, more intensely inflamed, presented a commencement of softening; the quantity of serum in the ventricles was natural.

While the foregoing case was in progress, a similar but less disastrous one occurred under the care of M. Husson, in the person of a patient affected with symptoms of rheumatism, closely resembling the above mentioned. Six grammes of sulphate of quinine were administered; after the ingestion of the last dose, the patient fell into a state of prostration, rapidly followed by extreme agitation and delirium, to which soon succeeded excessive debility and complete immobility. The pains, however, had disappeared.—*Gaz. des Hopiteux*, Dec. 8, 1842.

LIGATURE OF THE COMMON ILIAC ARTERY.

Dr. Peace, one of the Surgeons of the Pennsylvania Hospital, has recently tied the common iliac artery with success. The operation is stated by the author to have been "a modification of that of Sir A. Cooper, but retaining the great advantage —that of the greater facility of separating safely the peritoneum." He thus describes his operation:—

The patient having had his groin shaved, and placed upon a table of a convenient height, on the morning of the 29th of August, before the medical class, assisted by my colleagues, Drs. Randolph and Norris, and the experience of Dr. J. Rhea Barton, I proceeded to make an incision seven inches in length through the integuments, commencing at a point, on a level with the umbilicus, two inches within and three inches above the anterior superior spinous process of the ilium, and approaching to within an inch of Poupart's ligament, and terminating one half an inch above the external ring; this divided the arteria ad cutem, which was twisted by the artery forceps; no ligature was required; next the superficial fascia was divided, then the tendon of the external oblique was exposed, nicked, and with the aid of a director was cut the whole length of the first incision as far inwards as the spermatic cord. There was considerable difficulty in raising up the lower edge of the tendon of the internal oblique and transversalis, owing to the thickening and induration of the surrounding tissues from the pressure of the tumor: this was finally accomplished by means of the handle of the knife, and a careful division of the layers as they presented themselves, until we arrived at the peritoneum, having cut some of the fleshy fibres of the transversalis; the peritoneum was then carefully and with some difficulty detached from

the tumor, which was found to involve a great portion of the external iliac artery; we continued raising the peritoneum till we came to a part of the artery which appeared to be healthy; this was about one-half an inch above the bifurcation of the common iliac. The artery was separated from the vein by the finger nail, and a silk ligature was passed underneath from within outwards, by means of the admirable aneurismal needle of Professor Gibson. Notwithstanding the precautions that we had taken to have the bowels well evacuated, and the length of our first incision, it was some time before we were able to get a view of the curve of the needle still held under the artery, on account of the projection of the tumor and the protrusion of the abdominal contents. Finally, by means of broad, curved steel spatulas, and drawing forward the artery by means of the aneurismal needle that was underneath, we managed to get a view of the common iliac artery, and the iliac vein underneath, on the side of the sacro-vertebral promontory, with the ureter crossing the artery, and attached to the raised peritoneum. The ligature was without the slightest difficulty passed out of the wound by the watch-spring of the needle, and was tied by the tips of the fingers with a simple double knot; both ends of the ligature were allowed to remain hanging together from the wound. Immediately the pulsation of the tumor ceased, and its volume sensibly diminished. The edges of the wound were brought together by three interrupted sutures and adhesive plaster, and dressed with lint spread with cerate, and retained by two adhesive strips. The patient was removed to his bed, placed on his back, his leg slightly raised by a pillow under the knee, his shoulders raised, his body flexed and inclined towards the affected side. The needle was placed under the artery in seventeen minutes, but thirty minutes more were required before the patient was removed to his bed. The ligature came away on the 35th day.—*American Journal.*

WENZEL THE OCULIST.

This tradition is current in Vienna:—A lady attached to the court of the empress, becoming blind, was pronounced amaurotic by the medical man called in; her malady continuing to increase, the Baron Wenzel was sent for, and he at once declared it to be cataract, and operated on it with success. So amazed was Maria Theresa at this display of Austrian surgery, that she forthwith established a special lectureship of ophthalmology, and Barth was the first that filled this chair in 1773; and in 1776 he was appointed oculist to Joseph II. He was a most expert extractor, and there are still several who have witnessed his operations—the invention and use of Beer's knife (that now so generally adopted) is in a great measure due to him, for although his was longer in the blade, and somewhat broader towards the handle, yet it was upon an enlarged scale the same. The objections urged against it, of pricking the nose from the great length of its point, and not cutting itself out (as it is termed) with facility, is now obviated in that introduced by his pupil, Beer. His mode of operating was remarkable; he did not require an assistant, (and was, perhaps, the first oculist who did not), but placing the patient standing in the corner of the room near a window, he opened the lids, and fixing the eye with one hand, he passed his knife through the cornea with the other, as is now so dexterously performed by Mr. Alexander; but, different from that very distinguished oculist, he stood before his patient. It is needless to add that he was ambidexter. He died in 1818; his portrait bespeaks him a man of noble and prepossessing appearance, and his ad captandum, but engaging manner and address, added to his acknowledged talents, procured him many admirers.—*Wilde's Austria.*

CASE OF
RHEUMATICO-CATARRHAL FEVER
WITH METASTASIS TO THE TOES.

By Dr. Leopold Beer, of Brünn.

The patient was tall, and eighteen years of age; the prominent symptoms of his protracted fever were weakness, attenuation, sleeplessness, and increasing pain in the legs. In the fourth week of his illness, these pains extended to the soles of the feet, which were sensitive to the touch; their skin, too, was somewhat reddened, hot, and as it were, detached. In the 5th week of his illness, the nails, all of which projected far beyond the toes, degenerated, and were unbearably painful, when pressed towards their roots, sensations which extended as far as the knees. Gradually, and with considerable difficulty, the horn-like points of the nails were pulled off; and first of all dry, and afterwards fluid pus was found under each one. A few days after this operation the pains disappeared, and the patient recovered perfectly.—*Osterr. med. Wochenschr.* and *Schmidt's Jahrb.*

ROYAL COLLEGE OF SURGEONS.
LIST OF GENTLEMEN ADMITTED MEMBERS.
Friday, June 9, 1843.

E. Phillips.—J. Lyddon.—P. O. Brien.—J. S. S. Lang.—H. Gimlett.—F. G. Jackson.—J. W. Willows.—C. Rogerson.—G. E. Aldred.—G. R. Elliott.

APOTHECARIES' HALL.
LIST OF GENTLEMEN WHO HAVE RECEIVED CERTIFICATES.
Thursday, June 8, 1843.

R. W. Watkins, Towcester, Northamptonshire.—William Fisher, Kendal, Westmoreland.—L. Roberts, Exeter, Devon.—R. P. Roberts, Denbigh.—F. J. Genet, London.—S. Wilson, Gateshead on Tyne.—J. Pestell, Bedford.—J. W. Tripe, London.—B. Bird, Rusherline.—J. Eastwood, Meltham, Yorkshire.
Omitted May 11—James Phillips, Redruth, Cornwall.

A TABLE OF MORTALITY FOR THE METROPOLIS,

Shewing the number of deaths from all causes registered in the week ending Saturday, June 3, 1843.

Small Pox	6
Measles	33
Scarlatina	29
Hooping Cough	39
Croup	9
Thrush	4
Diarrhœa	3
Dysentery	2
Cholera	1
Influenza	0
Ague	1
Typhus	73
Erysipelas	6
Syphilis	1
Hydrophobia	0
Diseases of the Brain, Nerves, and Senses	134
Diseases of the Lungs and other Organs of Respiration	243
Diseases of the Heart and Blood-vessels	35
Diseases of the Stomach, Liver, and other Organs of Digestion	63
Diseases of the Kidneys, &c.	2
Childbed	11
Ovarian Dropsy	0
Disease of Uterus, &c.	0
Rheumatism	3
Diseases of Joints, &c.	9
Carbuncle	0
Ulcer	0
Fistula	1
Diseases of Skin, &c.	1
Diseases of Uncertain Seat	77
Old Age or Natural Decay	54
Deaths by Violence, Privation, or Intemperance	23
Causes not specified	10
Deaths from all Causes	875

METEOROLOGICAL JOURNAL.

Kept at Edmonton, *Latitude* 51° 37' 32" N. *Longitude* 0° 3' 51" W. *of Greenwich.*

June 1843.	THERMOMETER.		BAROMETER.	
Wednesday 7	from 42 to 57		29·84 to	29·70
Thursday . 8	48	62	29·41	29·39
Friday . . . 9	50	61	29·37	29·36
Saturday . 10	49	64	29·69	29·86
Sunday . . 11	48	64	29·97	Stat.
Monday . . 12	47	57	29·95	29·92
Tuesday . 13	47	55	29·80	29·75

Wind S. and S.W. till the 10th; since N.W. and North.
Generally cloudy, with frequent rain.
Rain fallen, ·785 of an inch.

CHARLES HENRY ADAMS.

WILSON & OGILVY, 57, Skinner Street, London.

THE

LONDON MEDICAL GAZETTE,

BEING A

WEEKLY JOURNAL

OF

Medicine and the Collateral Sciences.

FRIDAY, JUNE 23, 1843.

LECTURES

ON THE

THEORY AND PRACTICE OF MIDWIFERY,

Delivered in the Theatre of St. George's Hospital,

BY ROBERT LEE, M.D. F.R.S.

LECTURE XXXI.

On Preternatural Labours. Presentations of the shoulders and superior extremities.

ALL the varieties of preternatural labours have usually been divided into two orders; the first comprehending presentations of the nates and inferior extremities, and the second those in which the shoulder and superior extremities present. Cases in which the back, abdomen, or sides of the fœtus present, are so rare, that some practitioners believe it to be almost impossible for them ever to happen at the full period.

In 20,517 cases, delivered in the Maternity of Paris, Madame Boivin states, that no instance of such presentation occurred at the full term of gestation. The representations which have been given by her in the 117th and 118th Plates of her Memorial de l'Art des Accouchmens, of presentations of the abdomen and back, were therefore not made from nature; and I can hardly believe that a fœtus ever lay within the uterus with his heels and occiput in contact, as you see delineated in the last of these figures. Smellie's 33d table, which exhibits the fœtus compressed into a round form, the belly or umbilical region presenting at the os internum, and the funis hanging out of the vagina, is probably also to a great degree an imaginary representation. In the extensive practice of Dr. Merriman and his uncle, amounting together to nearly 20,000 labours, no instance occurred of either of these presentations, except in one or two cases where

the mother had not completed her seventh month of utero gestation; and in these the children passed double through the pelvis. Dr. Hunter says in his MS. Lectures, 1765, " I have read much in authors where the navel is said to present, or, on the contrary, where, on introducing the finger, you feel the middle of the spine. I do not believe there is the possibility of such a thing in nature: the shape of the uterus, pelvis, &c. all deny it." Dr. Denman says, " I do not mention the marks by which the back, belly, or sides might be distinguished, because these, properly speaking, never constitute the presenting part : that is, though they may sometimes be felt, they never advance foremost into the pelvis, in the commencement at least of a labour."

Presentations of the shoulder and superior extremities.—In these difficult and dangerous cases of preternatural labour, usually called cross births, the fœtus lies transversely in the uterus, the nates and lower extremities being directed to one ilium, and the head to the other, and the abdomen backward to the spine of the mother, or downward to the os uteri. The thirty-first table of Smellie represents, in a front view of the pelvis, the fœtus compressed by the contraction of the uterus into a round form, the fore parts of the former being towards the inferior part of the latter, and one foot and hand fallen down into the vagina. (Exhibiting it.)

The thirty-second table represents, in the same view with the former, the fœtus in the contrary position : the breech and fore parts being towards the fundus uteri, the left arm in the vagina, and forearm without the os externum, the shoulder being likewise forced into the os uteri. (See next page.)

The thirty-fourth table shows, in a lateral view of the pelvis, one of the most difficult preternatural cases, the left shoulder, breast, and neck of the fœtus presenting, the head reflected over the pubes to the right shoulder and back, and the feet and breech stretched up to the fundus, the uterus contracted at

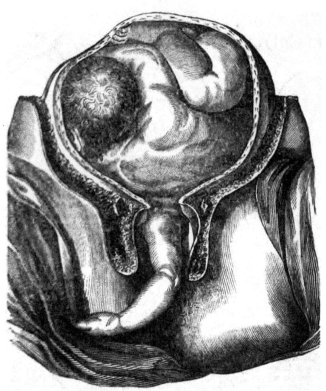

the same time, in form of a long sheath round the body of the fœtus. (See next page.)

In some favourable cases of shoulder and arm presentation, the uterus is widely dilated before the membranes are ruptured and the liquor amnii discharged; and no difficulty is experienced in passing the hand into the uterus, laying hold of the feet, and extracting the child by the operation of turning. If the uterus is not contracting strongly and at short intervals, little resistance is offered to the introduction of the hand, and the delivery may be speedily accomplished with safety both to the mother and child. But if the membranes have burst, the liquor amnii escaped, and the uterus has been contracting firmly upon the child many hours before the operation of turning is attempted, the child is often destroyed by the pressure, and the coats of the uterus exposed to great danger from contusion and laceration in passing up the hand and bringing down the feet. The shoulder and thorax become so strongly impacted in the pelvis, that great force is required to introduce the hand into the uterus to grasp the feet, and much exertion necessary before the position of the child can be changed.

In other cases of shoulder and arm presentation, the membranes burst and the liquor amnii escapes at the commencement of labour, and the os uteri is rigid and undilated, so that the hand cannot be passed into the uterus after the labour has continued many hours. The difficulty and danger of these cases are greatly increased when theu terus is contracting with violence, and the pelvis is distorted, or a disproportion exists between the child and pelvis from any other cause. The greater number of women, if abandoned to the efforts of nature under these circumstances—the uterus having no power to alter the position of the fœtus, would ultimately die undelivered from exhaustion or rupture of the uterus and vagina. Where the pelvis is large, the fœtus premature and dead, and the uterine action strong, the child, it is true, has sometimes, where no artificial assistance is afforded, been expelled double or what has been called by Dr. Denman spontaneous evolution of the

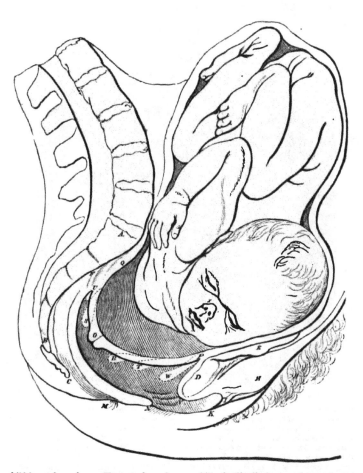

child has taken place. The arm here descends, and the shoulder and thorax are forced lower and lower into the pelvis, and gradually advance by the pains till they escape through the outlet, and the head and other parts soon follow. This expulsion of the fœtus double was observed by Puzos, and the proper treatment recommended where it was about to take place. He says, " Si l'enfant plié en deux se précipite dans l'orifice et qu'il s'engage aussitôt les eaux percées, les douleurs continuant de porter en bas, il vaut mieux laisser venir l'enfant dans cette situation, que de faire violence à la matrice pour aller chercher les pieds, l'enfant ne périt pas pour vénir de cette façon : il n'ouvre pas non plus une femme

au-delà de l'ordinaire : puisque souvent après les fesses sorties avec les cuisses repliées sur le ventre, la tête a encore peine à franchie ce detroit : quand l'enfant plié en deux à les fesses au passage, il faut le tournée alors le ventre en dessous, mettant les doigts de châque main dans ses aines, ce qui s'exécute fort aisément, et le degazement de ses pieds ne donne pas plus de peine." Dr. Denman observed a considerable number of cases of shoulder and arm presentation in which the child was expelled double, and he gave the following account of the process. " As to the manner in which this evolution takes place, I presume that after the long-continued action of the uterus the body of the child is brought into such a

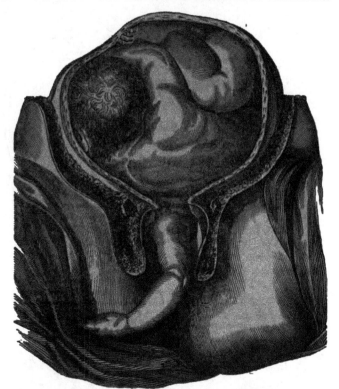

the same time, in form of a long sheath round the body of the fœtus. (See next page.)

In some favourable cases of shoulder and arm presentation, the uterus is widely dilated before the membranes are ruptured and the liquor amnii discharged ; and no difficulty is experienced in passing the hand into the uterus, laying hold of the feet, and extracting the child by the operation of turning. If the uterus is not contracting strongly and at short intervals, little resistance is offered to the introduction of the hand, and the delivery may be speedily accomplished with safety both to the mother and child. But if the membranes have burst, the liquor amnii escaped, and the uterus has been contracting firmly upon the child many hours before the operation of turning is attempted, the child is often destroyed by the pressure, and the coats of the uterus exposed to great danger from contusion and laceration in passing up the hand and bringing down the feet. The shoulder and thorax become so strongly impacted in the pelvis, that great force is required to introduce the hand into the uterus to grasp the feet, and much exertion necessary before the position of the child can be changed.

In other cases of shoulder and arm presentation, the membranes burst and the liquor amnii escapes at the commencement of labour, and the os uteri is rigid and undilated, so that the hand cannot be passed into the uterus after the labour has continued many hours. The difficulty and danger of these cases are greatly increased when the uterus is contracting with violence, and the pelvis is distorted, or a disproportion exists between the child and pelvis from any other cause. The greater number of women, if abandoned to the efforts of nature under these circumstances—the uterus having no power to alter the position of the fœtus, would ultimately die undelivered from exhaustion or rupture of the uterus and vagina. Where the pelvis is large, the fœtus premature and dead, and the uterine action strong, the child, it is true, has sometimes, where no artificial assistance is afforded, been expelled double, or what has been called by Dr. Denman spontaneous evolution of the

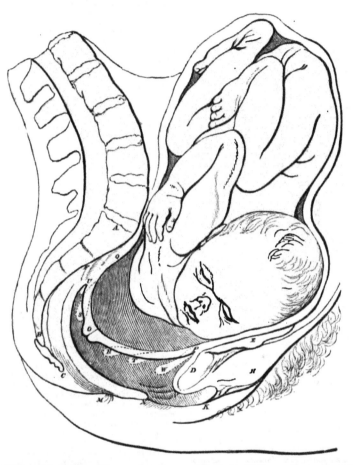

child has taken place. The arm here descends, and the shoulder and thorax are
forced lower and lower into the pelvis, and
gradually advance by the pains till they
escape through the outlet, and the head and
other parts soon follow. This expulsion of
the fœtus double was observed by Puzos,
and the proper treatment recommended
where it was about to take place. He says,
" Si l'enfant plié en deux se précipité dans
l'orifice et qu'il s'engage aussitôt les eaux
percées, les douleurs continuant de porter
en bas, il vaut mieux laisser venir l'enfant
dans cette situation, que de faire violence à
la matrice pour aller chercher les pieds,
l'enfant ne périt pas pour venir de cette
façon : il n'ouvre pas non plus une femme

au-délà de l'ordinaire : puisque souvent
après les fesses sorties avec les cuisses repliées sur le ventre, la tête a encore peine
à franchie ce detroit : quand l'enfant plié
en deux à les fesses au passage, il faut le
tournée alors le ventre en dessous, mettant les
doigts de châque main dans ses aines, ce qui
s'exécute fort aisément, et le degazement de
ses pieds ne donne pas plus de peine."
Dr. Denman observed a considerable number of cases of shoulder and arm presentation in which the child was expelled double,
and he gave the following account of the
process. " As to the manner in which this
evolution takes place, I presume that after
the long-continued action of the uterus the
body of the child is brought into such a

compacted state as to receive the full force of every returning action. The body, in its doubled state, being too large to pass through the pelvis, and the uterus, pressing upon its inferior extremities, which are the only parts capable of being moved, they are forced gradually lower, till the body turning as it were upon its own axis, the breech of the child is expelled, as in an original presentation of that part."

Since the publication of Dr. Douglas's essay in 1811, entitled, An Explanation of the real Process of the "Spontaneous Evolution of the Fœtus," it has been almost universally admitted that, in these cases, the arm and shoulder do not recede; that the child does not turn upon its axis; and that the nates are not expelled as in an original presentation of that part. The arm, shoulder, and thorax, are first expelled, and the nates and head afterwards. As the term spontaneous evolution is still in common use, and is calculated to convey an erroneous idea of what does actually take place in these cases of preternatural labour, I shall read to you what Dr. Douglas, who first gave a correct explanation of the fact, states on the subject :—" So far as the foregoing detail my observations coincide with those of Dr. Denman and others; but I cannot comprehend how successive repetitions of the same propelling power which forced the child into this situation, should subsequently, at any period, produce a counter effect, causing the shoulder to retreat into the uterus. The fact, however, is, that the shoulder and thorax, thus low and impacted, instead of receding into the uterus, are at each successive pain forced still lower, until the ribs of that side corresponding with the protruded arm press on the perineum, and cause it to assume the same form as it would by the pressure of the forehead in a natural labour. At this period not only the entire of the arm, but the shoulder, can be perceived externally, with the clavicle, lying under the arch of the pubis. By further uterine contractions the ribs are forced more forward, appearing at the os externum as the vertex would in a natural labour; the clavicle having been, by degrees, forced round on the anterior part of the pubis, with the acromion looking towards the mons veneris. But in order to render as clear as possible the successive movements in this astonishing effort of nature, I will endeavour to describe still more precisely the situation of the fœtus immediately prior to its expulsion. The entire of it somewhat resembles the larger segment of a circle; the head rests on the pubis internally; the clavicle presses against the pubis externally, with the acromion stretching towards the mons veneris; the arm and shoulder are entirely protruded, with one side of the thorax not only appearing at the

os externum, but partly without it: the lower part of the same side of the trunk presses on the perineum, with the breech either in the hollow of the sacrum, or at the brim of the pelvis, ready to descend into it: and by a few further uterine efforts, the remainder of the trunk with the lower extremities is expelled. And to be still more minutely explanatory in this ultimate stage of the process, I have to state that the breech is not expelled exactly sideways, as the upper part of the trunk had previously been; for during the presence of that pain by which the evolution is completed, there is a twist made, about the centre of the curve, at the lumbar vertebræ, when both buttocks, instead of the side of one of them, are thrown against the perineum, distending it very much: and immediately after the breech, with the lower extremities, issues forth; the upper and back part of it appearing first, as if the back of the child had originally formed the convex, and its front the concave side of the curve."

There is now a premature acephalous fœtus upon the table before you, the left arm and shoulder of which presented in labour a few days ago, and the body passed through the pelvis double, in the manner here described; or spontaneous evolution took place. I have repeatedly witnessed the same occurrence where the fœtus was premature, and flaccid from putrefaction; and on the 14th August, 1831, I saw a child at the full period expelled in this manner, in a woman who obstinately refused to allow the operation of turning to be performed. The right shoulder and arm presented in that case; and after the labour had continued three days and nights, the child was at last forced through the pelvis doubled up, in a putrid state, the head being flattened, and the viscera of the abdomen pressed through the parietes. It is only in a few rare cases, however, that the delivery is completed in this manner—where an unusual combination of circumstances exists; and it would be improper to calculate upon the occurrence of spontaneous evolution, or allow the possibility of its taking place, to influence the treatment we adopt in cases of arm presentation. It does not occur in cases where the operation of turning is performed with difficulty, and it is not a resource to which, in practice, we ought ever to trust—it ought never to be considered as a substitute for turning. It is now a general rule, established in all countries where midwifery is understood, that in cases of preternatural labour, where the shoulder and superior extremities of the child present, the operation of turning ought to be performed. But the hand must not be forced into the uterus if the orifice is rigid and undilatable; it should be dilated nearly to the size of half a crown piece or more, or the margin ought to be very thin, soft, and yielding, if it is expanded to a smaller extent than this when turning is attempted. If the os uteri will not admit the extremities of the fingers and thumb in a conical form to be introduced without much force; if it is thick, hard, and unyielding, some delay is necessary that the parts may relax, death being almost always the consequence of thrusting the hand with violence through the orifice of the uterus in a rigid and undilatable condition, whether the membranes be ruptured or not. But as soon as it will admit of the safe introduction of the hand, where you have ascertained that an arm presents, no time should be lost in completing the delivery, otherwise the membranes may give way, the liquor amnii be evacuated, and a case of little difficulty and danger be suddenly converted into one equally hazardous to the mother and child. In all cases of labour, where the first stage is far advanced without the nature of the presentation being positively determined, or a superior extremity is felt through the membranes, the patient should be kept in the horizontal position, that they may not be ruptured; and you should remain in constant attendance upon the patient, and be prepared to interfere the instant the necessity arises.

When the operation of turning is required before the membranes are ruptured, and when the orifice of the uterus is widely dilated, and there are long intervals between the pains, it is accompanied with little difficulty and danger. Having explained to the patient and her relatives the nature of the case, let her lie on the left side near the edge of the bed, with the knees drawn up to the abdomen. Sit down by the side of the bed and quietly take off your coat; lay bare your right arm by turning up the shirt above the elbow, and cover the back of the hand and the whole fore-arm with cold cream, lard, or a solution of soap. Introduce one finger after another into the vagina, and slowly and effectually dilate its orifice. The hand in a conical form, and in a state of half supination, must then be pressed steadily forward with a semi-rotatory motion against the perineum and sides of the passage, till it clears the orifice of the vagina. This should always be done very slowly and gently, as it is accompanied with great pain. Let the hand remain some time in the orifice of the vagina, that it may be fully dilated, and offer no resistance in the subsequent steps of the operation of turning. When the hand has dilated the vagina sufficiently, in the absence of pain gently insinuate the points of the fingers and thumb into the os uteri in a conical form; and if it is not sufficiently open to allow the hand to pass, you must proceed *next to use* artificial dilatation *here also, very gently* and slowly, always *stopping as soon as* a pain comes on, but not

withdrawing the fingers altogether at the time from the os uteri. Having succeeded in dilating the part without rupturing the membranes, slide the hand up between the membranes and the anterior part of the uterus into the cavity, and grasp the feet when the membranes give way. Most frequently the membranes burst as the hand is entering the uterus, before it reaches the feet, and the liquor amnii rushes out and is lost, if it is not prevented by pressing the hand forward firmly into the orifice. Never be contented with one foot when it is possible to grasp both; and this can always be done when the liquor amnii has not escaped, and the uterus is not closely contracted around the body of the child. Seize both feet and legs, and when there is no pain, draw them down into the vagina; and as the nates descend through the os uteri, the shoulder and arm will gradually recede or be retracted, and will offer no obstacle to the remaining part of the operation, which should be completed as if the nates and inferior extremities had orginally presented, and which has already been very fully described. In actual practice, except in twin cases, the membranes have been ruptured and the liquor amnii is gone, in a great proportion of cases—in about ten to one—long before we are called upon to deliver by turning, and the operation is then a much more serious affair. Sometimes when the os uteri is half dilated, there is an interval of freedom from pain for several hours after the rupture of the membranes, and partial escape of the liquor amnii. Here it is advisable to turn without delay; and the hand can be passed up into the uterus and the feet brought down with little more difficulty than if the membranes had not been ruptured.

The shoulder and arm may present, and the operation of turning be required where the membranes have burst at the commencement of the labour, the liquor amnii has escaped, and the os uteri is rigid, and is not dilated in a sufficient degree to allow the hand to pass. You can learn from experience alone, when there is a probability in such cases of artificially dilating the os uteri without the employment of too much force; it is best to wait patiently, in such a state of the os uteri, till relaxation takes place, before attempting to overcome the resistance, and to obviate the danger of spontaneous laceration of the uterus by venesection and opiates.

A much more difficult case of turning than any of those already described, is that in which the liquor amnii has long been evacuated, the uterus has contracted strongly around the body of the child, and the arm, shoulder, and a part of the thorax, have become firmly impacted in the pelvis. No attempt in such a case should ever be made to force back the presenting part into the uterus, but the hand should be cautiously c ducted to the feet along the arm of the child, and the shoulder pressed aside. It is impossible in all cases to determine positively the position of the child and the side of the

hand ought, however, invariably to be passed up between the front of the pelvis and the presenting part of the child, however the trunk and extremities may be situated; and as both hands are frequently required in these cases to turn, it is of no importance whether you employ the right or left first. I believe the two most important rules which you ought to remember in the treatment of these cases are, first, to pass up the hand between the anterior and shallow part of the pelvis, and the presenting part of the child; and secondly, when one hand is rendered powerless by the pressure from the contractions of the uterus, to withdraw this hand and replace it by the other By the observance of these rules there are few cases, I believe, of arm presentation, in which the operation of turning may not be safely accomplished. It is in rigid and irritable states of the uterus that we encounter the greatest resistance to the introduction of the hand and where these exist in a high degree, recourse should be had to a copious venesection and a large opiate, before the operation is again attempted. Where these means have been vigorously employed, it will rarely be necessary to remove the arm of the child at the shoulder joint, perforate the thorax, and draw it through the pelvis with the crotchet doubled up as in spontaneous evolution.

Sixty-six cases of shoulder and arm presentation have come under my observation since 1823. In a great proportion of these the operation of turning was undertaken in the most unfavourable circumstances, both for the mothers and their children, after the liquor amnii had entirely escaped, and the uterus had not only been contracting for many hours around the child, but repeated unsuccessful efforts had been made to deliver. Seven women died from rupture of the uterus, and three from inflammation of the uterus. Laceration and inflammation of the uterus are therefore the consequences of turning chiefly to be dreaded. Four of these cases of rupture occurred in the practice of other accoucheurs, and three in patients under my own care, and where no great difficulty was experienced, or force employed in turning. The most perplexing cases were those in which there was distortion of the pelvis, with arm presentation; and the most easy and successful, those twin cases in which the superior extremity of the second child presented, and the operation of turning was promptly performed. Edmund Johnson, Esq. has had the kindness to make the following tabular view of the histories of these cases, sixty of which have been recorded *in my Clinical Midwifery.*

A TABULAR VIEW OF SIXTY-SIX CASES OF SHOULDER AND ARM PRESENTATIONS.

	Date	History	Result
	October 10, 1823	Arm in vagina; uterus firmly contracting around the child; repeated attempts to turn; uterus ruptured on left side, either from or before operation; foetus escaped through rent, afterwards extracted; none of the ordinary symptoms of ruptured uterus present	Died seven days after delivery; adhesions by lymph around rupture, which, when peeled off, exposed the rent; peritonitis.
	August 1, 1824	Right arm with funis low in the vagina; shoulder and thorax squeezed in brim; liquor amnii escaped; operation of turning performed with difficulty	Died forty-eight hours after from peritonitis.
3	October 15, 1824	Right arm, swollen and livid, protruded through the os externum; pelvis distorted; shoulder and thorax wedged in brim; uterus firmly contracted; membranes ruptured four hours; repeated efforts to turn, without success; thorax perforated; arm separated at shoulder; child dragged through the pelvis, doubled up	Recovered.
4	Feb. 12, 1827	Triplets; arm of first and second child presented; turned without difficulty; presentation of third natural; all still born	Recovered.

No.	Date	Particulars	Result
5	April 9, 1827	Arm presentation; liquor amnii discharged; uterus firmly contracting; turning difficult; child dead	Died from uterine hæmorrhage.
6	May 1, 1827	Left arm presenting, with cord twisted around it; not pulsating; uterus firmly contracted; frequent attempts to turn, without success; thorax perforated, and child extracted	Recovered.
7	May 14, 1827	Presentation of left arm; shoulder and thorax fixed low in pelvis; umbilical cord prolapsed, without pulsation; uterine contractions strong and violent when turning was attempted; thorax perforated and child extracted	Recovered.
8	Dec. 3, 1827	Presentation of arm with head; turning attempted; one foot brought down, and left in vagina a day and a night; distorted pelvis; labour completed by craniotomy; extraction difficult.	Recovered, after severe inflammation of uterus.
9	Dec. 18, 1827	Presentation of arm and funis; os uteri partially dilated, and high up; membranes ruptured three hours; cord pulsating; turning difficult	Recovered.
10	March 25, 1828	Right arm with funis; liquor amnii escaped four hours; slight uterine contraction; operation of turning performed without difficulty; in extracting head the chin hitched over pubis; child dead	Recovered.
11	April 20, 1828	Twins; arm of second child; pains not strong; turning easily performed; one hour between the birth of first and second child; both children alive	Recovered.
12	April 26, 1828	Right arm with funis hanging out of external parts; no pulsation; turning easily performed; placenta retained; rupture of uterus discovered, when placenta was extracted	Died, with delirium and vomiting.
13	June 15, 1828	Left arm with funis; no pulsation; liquor amnii evacuated; strong and violent uterine contractions; tinct. opii employed; turning easily performed	Recovered.
14	August 19, 1828	Right arm; liquor amnii evacuated; no uterine contractions; turning accomplished with great ease; child alive	Recovered; severe inflammation.
15	Sept. 18, 1828	Twins; arm and shoulde of second child protruded through external parts; operation of turning difficult	Recovered.
16	Dec. 15, 1828	Left arm and thorax pressed deeply in pelvis; liquor amnii discharged; strong uterine contractions; V.S. and opiate used with advantage; turning at last performed with ease; child dead	Recovered.
17	Jan. 3, 1829	Presentation of arm; rigid os uteri; pains strong and frequent; thorax perforated; arm divided from trunk; delivery completed with crotchet	Recovered.
18	Jan. 9, 1829	Right arm protruded through os externum; pains slight; turning difficult; child dead	Recovered.
19	May 29, 1829	Presentation of left arm, much swollen; os uteri firmly contracted around shoulder; liquor amnii evacuated; V.S. employed with benefit; turning accomplished with ease; rigors and feeble pulse after operation	Recovered.
20	June 3, 1829	Twins; second child, arm presentation; pains strong; operation of turning not accomplished; arm and shoulder drawn through the outlet of the pelvis, and child delivered doubled up	Recovered.

No.	Date		Result
21	July 28, 1829	Presentation of right arm; membranes ruptured; os uteri dilated; pains few and feeble; operation of turning performed with ease	Recovered.
22	Autumn, 1829	Arm with umbilical cord in vagina three days; would not allow the operation of turning to be tried; complete exhaustion; turning at last effected	Recovered.
23	Nov. 8, 1829	Distorted pelvis; presentation of arm; arm removed by another practitioner, and turning repeatedly attempted; thorax impacted in pelvis; foot grasped with craniotomy forceps, and turning at last effected; head unable to pass through brim; perforated behind ear; delivery completed with crotchet	Died; rupture of orifice and neck of uterus.
24	May 22, 1830	Presentation of left arm; membranes ruptured seven days; irregular uterine contractions; shoulder and part of thorax jammed in brim; turning unable to be performed; arm removed at shoulder; thorax perforated; delivery accomplished with crotchet	Recovered.
25	August 29, 1830	Twins; second child, presentation of arm; membranes entire; uterus in state of rest; first child born four hours previously; turning easily performed; both children alive	Recovered.
26	October 24, 1830	Left arm descended low in vagina; pains very strong, but intervals long; liquor amnii evacuated; turning easily effected; child alive	Recovered.
27	Dec. 4, 1830	Arm low down in vagina; membranes ruptured; great difficulty experienced in turning	Died; rupture of muscular and mucous coats of uterus.
28	June 1831	Twins; arm presentation of second child; membranes entire; turning easily performed; child alive	Recovered.
29	August 14, 1831	Presentation of right arm; would not allow turning to be performed; three days and nights in labour; child putrid, and forced through pelvis doubled up; head flattened; contents of abdomen pressed through parietes	Recovered.
30	Nov. 3, 1831	Presentation of arm; membranes long ruptured; liquor amnii discharged; uterus firmly contracted around child; great difficulty in turning; child dead	Recovered.
31	Dec. 1831	Twins; presentation of arm of second child; membranes entire; no time lost in bringing down the feet; child alive	Recovered.
32	Feb. 1, 1833	Twins; presentation of arm of second child; pelvis large; child small; expelled doubled up; child dead	Recovered.
33	Feb. 13, 1833	Presentation of right arm; membranes ruptured some hours; uterine action suspended; turning easily accomplished; head arrested in brim; delivery completed by crotchet.	Recovered.
34	August 18, 1833	Presentation of arm; useless efforts had been long used to push back arm, and allow head to descend; turning accomplished; child dead	Recovered.
35	October 23, 1833	Twins; arm of second child presented; turning easily effected; child dead; delivery followed by dangerous hemorrhage	Recovered.

36	Jan. 2, 1834	Presentation of right arm; membranes just ruptured; shoulder and arm low down; turning performed with difficulty; child dead	Recovered.
37	July 14, 1834	Distorted pelvis; premature labour induced; presentation of left arm; turning performed; child dead	Recovered.
38	March 2, 1836	Presentation of left arm and funis, without pulsation; pains feeble; os uteri half dilated; but not rigid; turning easily performed	Recovered.
39	July 31, 1836	Presentation of shoulder; os uteri high up; membranes entire; operation of turning performed with ease; child dead	Recovered.
40	August 2, 1836	Presentation of left arm and large portion of funis; liquor amnii gone; os uteri dilated; pains feeble	Recovered.
41	August 4, 1836	Presentation of left arm; liquor amnii discharged many hours; uterus firmly contracting; child expelled putrid and doubled up	Died; uterine phlebitis and peritonitis
42	Nov. 3, 1836	Presentation of left arm with funis; turning ineffectually attempted; V.S. employed; pains increased; trunk pressed down into brim; turning at last completed with safety; child dead.	Recovered.
43	Nov. 14, 1836	Sudden rupture of membranes; left arm hanging out of external parts, and right arm in upper part of vagina; foot grasped with great difficulty	Recovered.
44	May 24, 1837	Right arm with umbilical cord, not pulsating, hanging out of external parts; many ineffectual efforts had been employed to turn; the operation at last performed	Recovered.
45	Dec. 23, 1837	Presentation of left arm; uterus firmly contracted; operation of turning tried, but failed; opiates used; arm removed from shoulder; uterus contracted on trunk, and caused it to recede, rendering application of crotchet difficult; trunk separated from head; head extracted without much difficulty	Died; laceration of uterus
46	Jan. 18, 1838	Twins; presentation of left arm of second child; liquor amnii evacuated; arm and shoulder thrust to outlet; right arm also descended; turning accomplished with great difficulty; child dead	Recovered.
47	Nov. 6, 1838	First labour; left arm hanging out of vagina; shoulder strongly impacted in brim; os uteri dilated; liquor amnii evacuated; turning completed with difficulty.	Recovered.
48	March 15, 1839	Presentation of right arm and funis, without pulsation; os uteri widely dilated; pains feeble; great difficulty in turning, on account of violent uterine contractions	Recovered.
49	May 24, 1839	Twins; presentation of head and foot of first child; foot brought down with ease; second child natural	Recovered.
50	Sept. 22, 1839	Presentation of right arm and funis; membranes ruptured; os uteri rigid; turning attempted; V.S. and opiates administered; turning again attempted; V.S. repeated, but turning again ineffectual; arm removed at shoulder-joint; child eviscerated; head left in cavity of uterus; head delivered with difficulty by crotchet, on account of rigidity	Died.

No.	Date	Description	Result
21	July 28, 1829	Presentation of right arm; membranes ruptured; os uteri dilated; pains few and feeble; operation of turning performed with ease	Recovered.
22	Autumn, 1829	Arm with umbilical cord in vagina three days; would not allow the operation of turning to be tried; complete exhaustion; turning at last effected	Recovered.
23	Nov. 8, 1829	Distorted pelvis; presentation of arm; arm removed by another practitioner, and turning repeatedly attempted; thorax impacted in pelvis; foot grasped with craniotomy forceps, and turning at last effected; head unable to pass through brim; perforated behind ear; delivery completed with crotchet	Died; rupture of orifice and neck of uterus.
24	May 22, 1830	Presentation of left arm; membranes ruptured seven days; irregular uterine contractions; shoulder and part of thorax jammed in brim; turning unable to be performed; arm removed at shoulder; thorax perforated; delivery accomplished with crotchet	Recovered.
25	August 29, 1830	Twins; second child, presentation of arm; membranes entire; uterus in state of rest; first child born four hours previously; turning easily performed; both children alive	Recovered.
26	October 24, 1830	Left arm descended low in vagina; pains very strong, but intervals long; liquor amnii evacuated; turning easily effected; child alive	Recovered.
27	Dec. 4, 1830	Arm low down in vagina; membranes ruptured; great difficulty experienced in turning	Died; rupture of muscular and mucous coats of uterus.
28	June 1831	Twins; arm presentation of second child; membranes entire; turning easily performed; child alive	Recovered.
29	August 14, 1831	Presentation of right arm; would not allow turning to be performed; three days and nights in labour; child putrid, and forced through pelvis doubled up; head flattened; contents of abdomen pressed through parietes	Recovered.
30	Nov. 3, 1831	Presentation of arm; membranes long ruptured; liquor amnii discharged; uterus firmly contracted around child; great difficulty in turning; child dead	Recovered.
31	Dec. 1831	Twins; presentation of arm of second child; arm lost in bringing	Recovered.
32	Feb.		

36	Jan. 2, 1834	Presentation of right arm; membranes just ruptured; shoulder and arm low down; turning performed with difficulty; child dead	Recovered.
37	July 14, 1834	Distorted pelvis, premature labour induced; presentation of left arm; turning performed; child dead	Recovered.
38	March 2, 1836	Presentation of left arm and funis, without pulsation; pains feeble; os uteri half dilated; but not rigid; turning easily performed	Recovered.
39	July 31, 1836	Presentation of (...Mr; os uteri high up; membranes entire; operation of turning performed with ease; ...ild dead	...dor red.
40	August 2, 1836	Presentation of left arm and large portion of funis; liquor amnii gone; os uteri dilated; pains feeble	Recovered.
41	August 4, 1836	Presentation of left arm; liquor amnii ...gd many hours; uterus firmly contracting; child expelled putrid and died up	Died, uterine phlebiti and peritonitis
42	Nov. 3, 1836	Presentation of left arm with funis; turning ineffectually attempted; V.S. employed; pains increased; trunk pressed down into brim; turning at last completed with safety; child dead.	Rec...d.
43	Nov. 14, 1836	Sudden rupture of membranes; left arm hanging out of external parts, and right arm in up...er part of vagina; o...t grasped with great difficulty	Recovered.
44	May 24, 1837	Right arm with umbilical cord, nt pl ...tg, hanging out of external parts; my ineffectual efforts ...d ...d to turn; the operation at ...t performed	Recovered.
45	Dec. 23, 1837	Presentation of left arm; uterus firmly ...t; ...on of turning tried, but failed; ...us contracted on trunk, and caused it to ...s ...d; arm 1 ...d from shoulder; ...het difficult; trunk separated from head; ...d ex...; ...ring application of ...het ... ...ted without ...mb difficulty	Died; laceration of uterus
46	Jan. 18, 1838	Twins; presentation of left arm of ...d child; liquor amnii evacuated; arm and shoulder thrust to outlet; right arm also descended; turning a ...complished with great difficulty; child dead	...led.
47	Nov. 6, 1838	First ...thr; left arm hanging ...ut of ...gtc; ...lr strongly ...pacted in brim; os uteri ...d; liquor ...d; turning ...ud, ...pl ted with ...lity.	Rec...d.
48	March 15, 1839	Presentation of right arm and funis, ...ng, on account of ...tc; ...t pl ...; os ...tri widely dilated; p ...s feeble; great difficulty in ...ng, on account of ...tt ...tne ...tractus	Rec...d.
49	May 24, 1839	...ms; presentation of ...ead and ...t of first child; ...t ...ght down with ease; ...nd ...ild natural	Recovered.
50	Sept. 22, 1839	Presentation of right arm ...l funis; membranes ...pd; os uteri rigid; turning ...ped; V.S. ...d ...ss ...ld; turning again ...d; V.S. ...d, ...t turning ...gn ineffectual; arm removed at shoulder-joint; ...ild eviscerated; ...ad left in ...ity ...rus; head delivered with difficulty by ...het, on account of rigidity	Died.

No.	Date	Case	Result
51	Nov. 8, 1839	Presentation of left arm; membranes ruptured; os uteri fully dilated; turning favourably performed	Recovered.
52	Dec. 18, 1839	Left arm hanging out of vagina; uterus firmly contracted around child; turning accomplished with difficulty, on account of uterine contractions; great assistance derived from a tape fixed around ankle in his and several other cases	Recovered.
53	Oct. 14, 1840	Presentation of hand with head; hand pushed back into uterus; head descended, and case terminated naturally	Recovered.
54	April 1841	Presentation of right arm; membranes thro; turning easily performed	Recovered; uterine inflammation.
55	Aug. 16, 1841	Right arm in vagina; membranes long ... and uterus contracting ten hours, but not strongly; turning performed without ...; hand passed between child and part of pelvis, fore finger in hm; child dead	Recovered.
56	Nov. 24, 1841	Presentation of right arm; membranes ruptured; uterus acting forcibly around child; turning	Recovered.
57	Jan. 19, 1842	Left arm ... in brim; os uteri partially dilated; uterus firmly contracting; ... ruptured ... days; turning safely completed; adhesion of placenta; seized soon after with ...	Died; hæmorrhage from the lungs.
58	June 20, 1842	Twins; presentation of arm of second; turned ... ease; two hours elapsed since birth of first ...; child alive	Recovered.
59	August 2, 1842	Presentation of arm, foot, and part of funis; great ... in turning	Recovered.
60	Sept. 8, 1842	Presentation of ... arm ..., without pulsation; liquor ... evacuated forty-eight ...; ... contracted firmly on ...; ... difficulty in turning,	Recovered.
61	Sept. 16, 1842	... discharged twenty-four hours; an ... in ... vagina; ... oly a few hours; both feet brought down into ...; ... not be ... ted till	Recovered.
62	October 25, 1842	Twins; arm of ...; ... turning easily ... completed;	Recovered.
63	Nov. 19, 1842	Left arm in vagina; ... great ... forcibly, ... hold; the def ... arose ... on the fore ... to change the hands; part of the pelvis;	Recovered.
64	Feb. 16, 1833	... arm presenting; a foot brought down into the vagina, but the version could not be completed; on putting a ... child dead, arm, and funis, without ... in ... extraction with the crotchet	Recovered.
65	April 31, 1843	Child premature; turned and extracted without ...	Recovered.
66	April 9, 1843		Recovered.

CLINICAL LECTURES

ON THE

THEORY & MEDICAL TREATMENT OF INSANITY,

Delivered at St. Luke's Hospital,

May 1st, 3d, and 5th.

BY ALEXANDER JOHN SUTHERLAND.

LECTURE III.

The medical treatment.—The faculty of attention a good test of the amount of insanity.—Caution necessary in estimating the value of a medicine in the treatment of madness.—Of purgatives.—Hellebore.—Opinions of Alex. Trallianus and Oribasius.—The preparations of mercury.—Taraxacum, croton oil, &c. —Emetics: potassio-tartrate of antimony.

IN speaking of the medical treatment of insanity, gentlemen, I feel that I stand the chance either, on the one hand, of dealing too much in generalities; or, on the other hand, of wearying you with details. To avoid this dilemma as far as possible I shall in the present lecture give you only a brief outline of the treatment of the disease, leaving the remainder to be filled up by the cases which I shall hereafter bring under your notice. I have one warning, however, to give you before you draw any conclusion as to the effect of medicine in particular cases; viz. that the patients here are of course under moral as well as medical treatment—I mean the separation from friends; the regular hours and exercise to which they are subject in the hospital; the withdrawal from those heart-rending scenes of privation and misery which have harassed too many before their admission.

The utility of establishing some receptacle for the insane was long ago felt. We find that so early as the sixth century a lunatic asylum (the first which was built) was erected at Jerusalem, for the poor monks whose distempered fanaticism had deprived of reason: here, too probably, the severities of "the Laura," and the stern authority of the abbot, followed them; and the chains under which they sank, and the collars, bracelets, gauntlets, and greaves of massive iron, which confined their emaciated limbs, might possibly have been converted from a means of penance into one of restraint.

In confining my present observations to the medical treatment of insanity, I wish neither to overrate its effects, nor to undervalue the moral treatment, as the one and the other must go hand in hand in order to insure success. My reason for now speaking only of the former, is, because it is a subject which has from various causes been much neglected.

In the treatment of insanity we must constantly revert to first principles—to those general laws which are our guide in the treatment of other diseases: experience alone teaches us how these laws are to be modified in each particular case, according to the species or stage of the disease, the difference of age and of individual temperament. You must of course bring with you a knowledge of disease learnt at the bedside of the sane patient before you will be able to detect it when it becomes masked by insanity. If you cannot treat symptoms when a sane patient describes them, much less will you be able to treat them in the case of a madman, who either cannot or will not describe them to you. We cannot take too much trouble in endeavouring to separate the real from the imagined pains of the lunatic. Active disease may all at once shew itself; and if the pain which it causes be, without investigation, set down as the effect of imagination, the patient is soon in a condition in which no medicine is of any avail. Our old patients sometimes sink without any apparent cause: they have no cough, no expectoration, no fever, no pain in the chest; they often cannot tell whether they have night-perspiration. When they are examined by percussion, dulness is found over almost every part of the thorax. It is seldom possible in these cases to hear pectoriloquy, as the patient is too weak, or too much lost, to speak; but the respiration is almost inaudible, and they cannot expand the thorax. I need scarcely say that, at the post-mortem examination of such patients, we find the lungs filled with tubercles and vomicæ. The numerous questions asked of the friends of patients who apply for admission at the Hospital of Siegburg, prove how much trouble is taken in each case; and not without reason. The previous diseases, the habits, even the occupation of the patient, may tend to throw some light upon the method of treatment. Esquirol has well said, " From the gestures, movements, looks, expression, discourse, from shades of difference inappreciable to any one else, the physician often derives the first hint of the treatment which is suitable to each case consigned to his care." Our chief endeavour must be, in the first instance, to ascertain as far as we can the cause of the disease, whether it be moral or physical; we have then to consider what consequences to the general health have ensued. As in the treatment of epilepsy we try to discover whether the disease depends on irritation of the stomach, bowels, uterus, &c., so, in insanity, we must see whether, prior to the attack, there has not been suppression of the catamenia, of the discharge of an old ulcer, or whether an eruption has not suddenly disappeared—whether the patient has at any time been attacked with fever, delirium tremens, gout, and the like.

I advise a systematic arrangement in each case. Observe the state of the pulse and the skin; feel the head; see whether it is hot all over, or in one part only; whether the extremities are cold; whether the tongue is loaded and dry; whether the bowels are open, the urine free, and, if the patient be a female, whether the catamenia are regular. Next observe the breathing, and the action of the heart; pass your hand over the right hypochondrium, and feel whether the liver is enlarged, or whether the abdomen is distended with flatus; and whether there be tenderness about the præcordia. Examine also the beating of the carotids and temporal arteries. When the patient has his head back, and his neckcloth unfastened, you may perhaps see a scar on the throat, which will let you into a secret. The expression of countenance, the complexion, the colour of the conjunctivæ, and the action of the iris, must all be carefully noted. When you are observing the eye, ask the patient whether he sees moats floating before him; and this may lead him to speak of his illusions or hallucinations. When you have exhausted these, ask about his sense of smelling; you may discover, perhaps, that he smells brimstone, and imagines himself lost to all eternity. Now inquire whether his taste is altered; if it be, he may fancy that his friends have conspired to poison him. Then pay attention to the sense of hearing; and lastly, to that of touch. You will now be prepared to draw him into conversation, in order to ascertain whether his emotions are changed, or whether one or more of the faculties of the mind be disordered.

The faculty of attention often serves as a useful test of the amount of insanity. In the commencement of mania the patient will tell you that he cannot read or write, because he cannot apply his mind to any given subject, particularly if the subject be a new one. As the disease progresses the ideas become more and more distracted; he cannot fix his attention for an instant upon the subject matter before him; he is incapable of conversation; he becomes incoherent. On the other hand, the monomaniac, when the disease first appears, is now and then only absorbed in the day-dream of his imagination. As it advances it swallows up, like Aaron's serpent, all the other ideas of his mind, and he is inattentive to every thing else, even to the common decencies of life. As both mania and monomania sink

into dementia, attention becomes more and more weakened, till it is destroyed by a state of complete unconsciousness. Dr. Holland, in his Medical Notes and Reflections, p. 239, 1st edition, says, "No principle of practice in mental disorders can probably be successful, which does not recognise their relation to the phenomena of mind in its healthy state;" and he states that some of the more remarkable cases which he has known, "where physical causes of the infirmity did not exist, have been effected really, if not professedly, by a discreet application of this method." It must be confessed that we sometimes meet with cases where there are no physical symptoms to guide us in the employment of remedies, and we are obliged either to trust solely to the moral treatment, or to have recourse to empiricism. If such be based upon rational principles, I see no reason for not adopting it; nor do I understand how we are to advance our art of prescribing in these cases, unless, when all else fails us, we call in this to our aid. Our two rules in applying remedies are, first, to do good; secondly, not to do harm. The scales may hang even between doing nothing and trying a new remedy: indolence always throws her weight in on the side of the former. Some remedies have borne a high reputation in the treatment of insanity, from their success in individual cases; but experience upon a large scale has either proved them to be worthless, or useful only in removing symptoms. No one can be surprised at the reputation which a medicine sometimes acquires as a specific, when he knows the effect which confidence in the prescriber inspires in weak minds. Many of us, I fear, are prone to attribute too much importance to the last prescribed remedy: in the treatment of insanity we cannot be too careful to guard against such an error. In testing the value of a medicine in any disease, more especially in a mental disease, we should never leave out of our consideration the element of time. "Time," as Locke says, "cures some diseases in the mind which reason cannot;" and some too, I may add, which medicine cannot.

It is not the medicine which has produced some effect in this or that case that we are to regard as useful in all cases, but it is that which has produced effects by relieving parallel symptoms in the great majority of cases, that we may expect to derive benefit from, when similar indications present themselves.

Purgatives.—The first class of medicines which claims our attention, as having been used in the treatment of insanity in all ages, are cathartics. The great remedy for insanity among the Greeks was hellebore; its healing power over this disease had passed into a proverb as early as the time of Aristophanes. It is, however, a mistake to suppose that the ancients employed no other means of cure. Alex. Trallianus employed the bath, warm drinks, bitters; and says that the Armenian stone is better and safer than the hellebore. We have a prescription of his preserved:—

℞. Pieræ, ʒss.; Scammonii, ʒj.; Agarici, ℈iv.; Lapidi Armeniaci, ℈iv.; Caryophillorum, gr. xx. M. ft. massa.

a certain portion of which was to be taken. This celebrated physician seems also to have had recourse to stratagem when he could not succeed by other means. He gives us the case of a woman who was cured of melancholy in the following manner. The case seems to have been one of monomania (which you have all heard so much of lately). She imagined that she had swallowed a serpent. An emetic was administered, and a little worm was skilfully inserted into what came off her stomach, and she immediately recovered. Nor was moral treatment neglected by him; for he says, "Know that I have cured many by an appeal to ethics rather than pharmacy."

Oribasius gives us minute details as to the manner of preparing and prescribing the hellebore; but he confesses that it should not be given in every case to the infirm and old, and those of a timid disposition. He says, moreover, that a very unpleasant hiccough followed the administration of this remedy.

Anticyra, as every one knows, was the place most famous for the growth of this plant; so that " naviget Anticyram" became a proverb. When Livius Drusus was seized with madness, he was sent by his physician to Anticyra, where he recovered by means of this ancient specific. One would be inclined to suspect that the sea voyage, and change of air and of scene, did more towards the recovery of the patient than the boasted effects of the hellebore. This drug has, indeed, lost all its popularity. Dr. Cullen and Dr. Perfect speak strongly against the propriety of employing it. I believe that most practitioners are now agreed upon its inefficacy, because we possess much safer and better remedies. Many have been the revolutions which fashion has caused in the treatment of insanity; but the popularity of cathartics has always more or less prevailed, if we may except the latter part of the last, and the beginning of the present century—an age apparently not very famous in its treatment of mental diseases; for we find the following remarks in Dr. Crowther's work:—" Those who superintend the management of mad patients cannot be too attentive to the state of their bowels. In my practice," he says, " I have witnessed very criminal neglect as to this point. In one case the intestines were so distended that the transverse arch of the colon gave way." These remarks would have been unnecessary, had not some at least of the practitioners of that period neglected the advice of the father of physic, who recommends us to have recourse to purgatives for the cure of melancholy.

It is of no small importance that we should be careful in our selection of our cathartics; it may be that it is necessary to employ merely a laxative; or the case may require stronger measures, sometimes even a hydragogue cathartic.

The importance of making use of these medicines is obvious, from the frequency of constipation as a symptom in insanity and all other head affections, and from the fact of some cases having recovered after a severe diarrhœa. At the time when there were so many rivals for the honour of winning the hand of the Queen, I asked a patient of mine how his suit prospered. He said, " Oh! I have given up the idea of marrying the Queen." I asked him how that happened, and he said that his bowels had been well purged in the morning, and that his ambitious hopes had vanished. Cathartics should be prescribed in insanity for the purpose of emptying the bowels of their vitiated contents, of correcting depraved secretions, of favouring the peristaltic movements of the muscular fibres of the intestines, of calling into aid the sluggish action of the neighbouring viscera, especially the liver, in order that the circulation of the portal system may be relieved; and, above all, to create a copious serous discharge from the exhalant vessels, by which means we create an artificial point of irritation, and thus, as it is usually called, derive from the head.

The preparations of mercury are of the utmost importance in the treatment of insanity, and are perhaps more generally used in this country than those of any other medicine. They are not only useful for their purgative effects, for stimulating the liver and relieving it of the congestion so often found in recent cases, but they are of great service in equalizing the circulation in the capillaries; thus in those cases where, from the heat of head, the injected conjunctivæ, and other symptoms, we have to fear congestion of the cerebral vessels, their use is manifestly indicated. In those cases also where we have reason to suspect incipient paralysis, or even where the disease has begun to develop itself, I have derived much service from the liquor hydrargyri bichloridi, given in ʒss. to ʒij. doses two or three times daily, with occasional purges. The importance of continuing this medicine for a

compacted state as to receive the full force of every returning action. The body, in its doubled state, being too large to pass through the pelvis, and the uterus, pressing upon its inferior extremities, which are the only parts capable of being moved, they are forced gradually lower, till the body turning as it were upon its own axis, the breech of the child is expelled, as in an original presentation of that part."

Since the publication of Dr. Douglas's essay in 1811, entitled, An Explanation of the real Process of the "Spontaneous Evolution of the Fœtus," it has been almost universally admitted that, in these cases, the arm and shoulder do not recede; that the child does not turn upon its axis; and that the nates are not expelled as in an original presentation of that part. The arm, shoulder, and thorax, are first expelled, and the nates and head afterwards. As the term spontaneous evolution is still in common use, and is calculated to convey an erroneous idea of what does actually take place in these cases of preternatural labour, I shall read to you what Dr. Douglas, who first gave a correct explanation of the fact, states on the subject :—" So far as the foregoing detail my observations coincide with those of Dr. Denman and others; but I cannot comprehend how successive repetitions of the same propelling power which forced the child into this situation, should subsequently, at any period, produce a counter effect, causing the shoulder to retreat into the uterus. The fact, however, is, that the shoulder and thorax, thus low and impacted, instead of receding into the uterus, are at each successive pain forced still lower, until the ribs of that side corresponding with the protruded arm press on the perineum, and cause it to assume the same form as it would by the pressure of the forehead in a natural labour. At this period not only the entire of the arm, but the shoulder, can be perceived externally, with the clavicle, lying under the arch of the pubis. By further uterine contractions the ribs are forced more forward, appearing at the os externum as the vertex would in a natural labour ; the clavicle having been, by degrees, forced round on the anterior part of the pubis, with the acromion looking towards the mons veneris. But in order to render as clear as possible the successive movements in this astonishing effort of nature, I will endeavour to describe still more precisely the situation of the fœtus immediately prior to its expulsion. The entire of it somewhat resembles the larger segment of a circle ; the head rests on the pubis internally ; the clavicle presses against the pubis externally, with the acromion stretching *towards the mons veneris*; the arm and *shoulder are entirely protruded*, with one *side of the thorax not only appearing at the*

os externum, but partly without it ; the lower part of the same side of the trunk presses on the perineum, with the breech either in the hollow of the sacrum, or at the brim of the pelvis, ready to descend into it ; and by a few further uterine efforts, the remainder of the trunk with the lower extremities is expelled. And to be still more minutely explanatory in this ultimate stage of the process, I have to state that the breech is not expelled exactly sideways, as the upper part of the trunk had previously been ; for during the presence of that pain by which the evolution is completed, there is a twist made, about the centre of the curve, at the lumbar vertebræ, when both buttocks, instead of the side of one of them, are thrown against the perineum, distending it very much ; and immediately after the breech, with the lower extremities, issues forth ; the upper and back part of it appearing first, as if the back of the child had originally formed the convex, and its front the concave side of the curve."

There is now a premature acephalous fœtus upon the table before you, the left arm and shoulder of which presented in labour a few days ago, and the body passed through the pelvis double, in the manner here described; or spontaneous evolution took place. I have repeatedly witnessed the same occurrence where the fœtus was premature, and flaccid from putrefaction ; and on the 14th August, 1831, I saw a child at the full period expelled in this manner, in a woman who obstinately refused to allow the operation of turning to be performed. The right shoulder and arm presented in that case ; and after the labour had continued three days and nights, the child was at last forced through the pelvis doubled up, in a putrid state, the head being flattened, and the viscera of the abdomen pressed through the parietes. It is only in a few rare cases, however, that the delivery is completed in this manner—where an unusual combination of circumstances exists ; and it would be improper to calculate upon the occurrence of spontaneous evolution, or allow the possibility of its taking place, to influence the treatment we adopt in cases of arm presentation. It does not occur in cases where the operation of turning is performed with difficulty, and it is not a resource to which, in practice, we ought ever to trust— it ought never to be considered as a substitute for turning. It is now a general rule, established in all countries where midwifery is understood, that in cases of preternatural labour, where the shoulder and superior extremities of the child present, the operation of turning ought to be performed. But the hand must not be forced into the uterus if the orifice is rigid and undilatable ; it should be dilated nearly to the size of half a crown piece or more, or the margin ought to be very thin, soft, and yielding, if it is expanded to a smaller extent than this when turning is attempted. If the os uteri will not admit the extremities of the fingers and thumb in a conical form to be introduced without much force; if it is thick, hard, and unyielding, some delay is necessary that the parts may relax, death being almost always the consequence of thrusting the hand with violence through the orifice of the uterus in a rigid and undilatable condition, whether the membranes be ruptured or not. But as soon as it will admit of the safe introduction of the hand, where you have ascertained that an arm presents, no time should be lost in completing the delivery, otherwise the membranes may give way, the liquor amnii be evacuated, and a case of little difficulty and danger be suddenly converted into one equally hazardous to the mother and child. In all cases of labour, where the first stage is far advanced without the nature of the presentation being positively determined, or a superior extremity is felt through the membranes, the patient should be kept in the horizontal position, that they may not be ruptured; and you should remain in constant attendance upon the patient, and be prepared to interfere the instant the necessity arises.

When the operation of turning is required before the membranes are ruptured, and when the orifice of the uterus is widely dilated, and there are long intervals between the pains, it is accompanied with little difficulty and danger. Having explained to the patient and her relatives the nature of the case, let her lie on the left side near the edge of the bed, with the knees drawn up to the abdomen. Sit down by the side of the bed and quietly take off your coat; lay bare your right arm by turning up the shirt above the elbow, and cover the back of the hand and the whole fore-arm with cold cream, lard, or a solution of soap. Introduce one finger after another into the vagina, and slowly and effectually dilate its orifice. The hand in a conical form, and in a state of half supination, must then be pressed steadily forward with a semi-rotatory motion against the perineum and sides of the passage, till it clears the orifice of the vagina. This should always be done very slowly and gently, as it is accompanied with great pain. Let the hand remain some time in the orifice of the vagina, that it may be fully dilated, and offer no resistance in the subsequent steps of the operation of turning. When the hand has dilated the vagina sufficiently, in the absence of pain gently insinuate the points of the fingers and thumb into the os uteri in a conical form; and if it is not sufficiently open to allow the hand to pass, you must proceed next to use artificial dilatation here also, very gently and slowly, always stopping as soon as a pain comes on, but not

withdrawing the fingers altogether at the time from the os uteri. Having succeeded in dilating the part without rupturing the membranes, slide the hand up between the membranes and the anterior part of the uterus into the cavity, and grasp the feet when the membranes give way. Most frequently the membranes burst as the hand is entering the uterus, before it reaches the feet, and the liquor amnii rushes out and is lost, if it is not prevented by pressing the hand forward firmly into the orifice. Never be contented with one foot when it is possible to grasp both; and this can always be done when the liquor amnii has not escaped, and the uterus is not closely contracted around the body of the child. Seize both feet and legs, and when there is no pain, draw them down into the vagina; and as the nates descend through the os uteri, the shoulder and arm will gradually recede or be retracted, and will offer no obstacle to the remaining part of the operation, which should be completed as if the nates and inferior extremities had orginally presented, and which has already been very fully described. In actual practice, except in twin cases, the membranes have been ruptured and the liquor amnii is gone, in a great proportion of cases—in about ten to one—long before we are called upon to deliver by turning, and the operation is then a much more serious affair. Sometimes when the os uteri is half dilated, there is an interval of freedom from pain for several hours after the rupture of the membranes, and partial escape of the liquor amnii. Here it is advisable to turn without delay; and the hand can be passed up into the uterus and the feet brought down with little more difficulty than if the membranes had not been ruptured.

The shoulder and arm may present, and the operation of turning be required where the membranes have burst at the commencement of the labour, the liquor amnii has escaped, and the os uteri is rigid, and is not dilated in a sufficient degree to allow the hand to pass. You can learn from experience alone, when there is a probability in such cases of artificially dilating the os uteri without the employment of too much force; it is best to wait patiently, in such a state of the os uteri, till relaxation takes place, before attempting to overcome the resistance, and to obviate the danger of spontaneous laceration of the uterus by venesection and opiates.

A much more difficult case of turning than any of those already described, is that in which the liquor amnii has long been evacuated, the uterus has contracted strongly around the body of the child, and the arm, shoulder, and a part of the thorax, have become firmly impacted in the pelvis. No attempt in such a case should ever be made to force back the presenting part into uterus, but the hand should be cautiously ducted to the feet along the arm of the child, and the shoulder pressed aside. It is impossible in all cases to determine positively the position of the child and the side of the uterus to which the feet are directed the hand ought, however, invariably to be passed up between the front of the pelvis and the presenting part of the child, however the trunk and extremities may be situated; and as both hands are frequently required in these cases to turn, it is of no importance whether you employ the right or left first. I believe the two most important rules which you ought to remember in the treatment of these cases are, first, to pass up the hand between the anterior and shallow part of the pelvis, and the presenting part of the child; and secondly, when one hand is rendered powerless by the pressure from the contractions of the uterus, to withdraw this hand and replace it by the other By the observance of these rules there are few cases, I believe, of arm presentation, in which the operation of turning may not be safely accomplished. It is in rigid and irritable states of the uterus that we encounter the greatest resistance to the introduction of the hand and where these exist in a high degree, recourse should be had to a copious venesection and a large opiate, before the operation is again attempted. Where these means have been vigorously employed, it will rarely be necessary to remove the arm of the child at the shoulder joint, perforate the thorax, and draw it through the pelvis with the crotchet doubled up as in spontaneous evolution.

Sixty-six cases of shoulder and arm presentation have come under my observation since 1823. In a great proportion of these the operation of turning was undertaken in the most unfavourable circumstances, both for the mothers and their children, after the liquor amnii had entirely escaped, and the uterus had not only been contracting for many hours around the child, but repeated unsuccessful efforts had been made to deliver. Seven women died from rupture of the uterus, and three from inflammation of the uterus. Laceration and inflammation of the uterus are therefore the consequences of turning chiefly to be dreaded. Four of these cases of rupture occurred in the practice of other accoucheurs, and three in patients under my own care, and where no great difficulty was experienced, or force employed in turning. The most perplexing cases were those in which there was distortion of the pelvis, with arm presentation; and the most easy and successful, those twin cases in which the superior extremity of the second child presented, and the operation of turning was promptly performed. Edmund Johnson, Esq. has had the kindness to make the following tabular view of the histories of these cases, sixty of which have been recorded in my Clinical Midwifery.

A TABULAR VIEW OF SIXTY-SIX CASES OF SHOULDER AND ARM PRESENTATIONS.

1	October 10, 1823	Arm in vagina; uterus firmly contracting around the child; repeated attempts to turn; uterus ruptured on left side, either from or before operation; foetus escaped through rent, afterwards extracted; none of the ordinary symptoms of ruptured uterus present	Died seven days after delivery; adhesions by lymph around rupture, which, when peeled off, exposed the rent; peritonitis.
2	August 1, 1824	Right arm with funis low in the vagina; shoulder and thorax squeezed in brim; liquor amnii escaped; operation of turning performed with difficulty	Died forty-eight hours after from peritonitis.
3	October 15, 1824	Right arm, swollen and livid, protruded through the os externum; pelvis distorted; shoulder and thorax wedged in brim; uterus firmly contracted; membrane ruptured four hours; repeated efforts to turn, without success; thorax perforated; arm separated at shoulder; child dragged through the pelvis, doubled up	Recovered.
4	Feb. 12, 1827	Triplets; arm of first and second child presented; turned without difficulty; presentation of third natural; all still born	Recovered.

5	April 9, 1827	Arm presentation; liquor amnii discharged; uterus firmly contracting; turning difficult; child dead	Died from uterine hæmorrhage.
6	May 1, 1827	Left arm presenting, with cord twisted around it; not pulsating; uterus firmly contracted; frequent attempts to turn, without success; thorax perforated, and child extracted	Recovered.
7	May 14, 1827	Presentation of left arm; shoulder and thorax fixed low in pelvis; umbilical cord prolapsed, without pulsation; uterine contractions strong and violent when turning was attempted; thorax perforated and child extracted	Recovered.
8	Dec. 3, 1827	Presentation of arm with head; turning attempted; one foot brought down, and left in vagina a day and a night; distorted pelvis; labour completed by craniotomy; extraction difficult.	Recovered, after severe inflammation of uterus.
9	Dec. 18, 1827	Presentation of arm and funis; os uteri partially dilated, and high up; membranes ruptured three hours; cord pulsating; turning difficult	Recovered.
10	March 25, 1828	Right arm with funis; liquor amnii escaped four hours; slight uterine contraction; operation of turning performed without difficulty; in extracting head the chin hitched over pubis; child dead	Recovered.
11	April 20, 1828	Twins; arm of second child; pains not strong; turning easily performed; one hour between the birth of first and second child; both children alive	Recovered.
12	April 26, 1828	Right arm with funis hanging out of external parts; no pulsation; turning easily performed; placenta retained; rupture of uterus discovered, when placenta was extracted	Died, with delirium and vomiting.
13	June 15, 1828	Left arm with funis; no pulsation; liquor amnii evacuated; strong and violent uterine contractions; tinct. opii employed; turning easily performed	Recovered.
14	August 19, 1828	Right arm; liquor amnii evacuated; no uterine contractions; turning accomplished with great ease; child alive	Recovered; severe inflammation.
15	Sept. 18, 1828	Twins; arm and shoulde of second child protruded through external parts; operation of turning difficult	Recovered.
16	Dec. 15, 1828	Left arm and thorax pressed deeply in pelvis; liquor amnii discharged; strong uterine contractions; V.S. and opiate used with advantage; turning at last performed with ease; child dead	Recovered.
17	Jan. 3, 1829	Presentation of arm; rigid os uteri; pains strong and frequent; thorax perforated; arm divided from trunk; delivery completed with crotchet	Recovered.
18	Jan. 9, 1829	Right arm protruded through os externum; pains slight; turning difficult; child dead	Recovered.
19	May 29, 1829	Presentation of left arm, much swollen; os uteri firmly contracted around shoulder; liquor amnii evacuated; V.S. employed with benefit; turning accomplished with ease; rigors and feeble pulse after operation	Recovered.
20	June 3, 1829	Twins; second child, arm presentation; pains strong; operation of turning not accomplished; arm and shoulder drawn through the outlet of the pelvis, and child delivered doubled up	Recovered.

No.	Date		Result
21	July 28, 1829	Presentation of right arm; membranes ruptured; os uteri dilated; pains few and feeble; operation of turning performed with ease	Recovered.
22	Autumn, 1829	With umbilical cord in vagina three days; would not allow the operation of turning to be tried; ... ex ...; turning at last effected	Recovered.
23	Nov. 8, 1829	... pelvis; presentation of arm, arm ... by ... practitioner, and turning repeatedly ...; thorax ... sted in ...; foot grasped with craniotomy forceps, and turning at last effected; head unable to pass through brim; perforated behind ear; delivery ... with ...	Died; rupture of orifice and neck of uterus.
24	May 22, 1830	Presentation of left arm; membranes ruptured even days; irregular uterine contractions; shoulder and ... art of thorax ... ed in brim; turning ... ... to be performed; arm re-moved at ... ...er; thorax perforated; ... ery accomplished with crotchet	Recovered.
25	August 29, 1830	...; ...ond child, presentation of arm; membranes ...re; uterus in state of rest; first ... born four hours	Recovered.
26	...ber 24, 1830	Left arm descended low in vagina; pains very ...g, but intervals long; ligor amnii ...; ...; child ...	Recovered.
27	Dec. 4, 1830	Arm low down in vagina; ...es ruptured; great difficulty ...ed in turning	Died; rupture of muscular and mucous coats of uterus.
28	June 1831	Twins; arm presentation of second child; membranes entire; turning easily performed; child alive	Recovered.
29	August 14, 1831	Presentation of right arm; would not ...w turning to be performed; the days and nights in labour; child putrid, and ...ed through ...is ...led up; head fixed; ...ts of abdomen pressed through parietes	Recovered.
30	Nov. 3, 1831	Presentation of arm; membranes long ruptured; liquor amnii discharged; uterus firmly con-tracted around child; great ...lty in turning; child dead	...ld.
31	Dec. 1831	Twins; presentation of arm of second child; membranes entire; no time lost in bringing down the feet; child alive	...d.
32	Feb. 1, 1833	Twins; presentation of arm of ...ond child; pelvis large; ...ild small; expelled doubled up; child dead	Recovered.
33	Feb. 13, 1833	Presentation of right arm; membranes ruptured some hours; uterine action suspended; turning easily accomplished; head arrested in brim; delivery completed by crotchet.	Recovered.
34	August 18, 1833	Presentation of arm; useless efforts had been long used to push back arm, and allow head to descend; turning accomplished; child dead	Recovered.
35	...ber 23, 1833	Twins; arm of second child presented; turning easily effected; child dead; delivery followed by dangerous haemorrhage	Re...ed.

36	Jan. 2, 1834	Presentation of right arm; membranes just ruptured; shoulder and arm low down; turning performed with difficulty; child dead	Recovered.
37	July 14, 1834	Distorted pelvis; premature labour induced; presentation of left arm; turning performed; child dead	Recovered.
38	March 2, 1836	Presentation of left arm and funis, without pulsation; pains feeble; os uteri half dilated; but not rigid; turning easily performed	Recovered.
39	July 31, 1836	Presentation of shoulder; os uteri high up; membranes entire; operation of turning performed with ease; child dead	Recovered.
40	August 2, 1836	Presentation of left arm and large portion of funis; liquor amnii gone; os uteri dilated; pains feeble	Recovered.
41	August 4, 1836	Presentation of left arm; liquor amnii discharged many hours; uterus firmly contracting; child expelled putrid and doubled up	Died; uterine phlebiti and peritonitis
42	Nov. 3, 1836	Presentation of left arm with funis; turning ineffectually attempted; V.S. employed; pains increased; trunk pressed down into brim; turning at last completed with safety; child dead.	Recovered.
43	Nov. 14, 1836	Sudden rupture of membranes; left arm hanging out of external parts, and right arm in upper part of vagina; foot grasped with great difficulty	Recovered.
44	May 24, 1837	Right arm with umbilical cord, not pulsating, hanging out of external parts; many ineffectual efforts had been employed to turn; the operation at last performed	Recovered.
45	Dec. 23, 1837	Presentation of left arm; uterus firmly contracted; operation of turning tried, but failed; opiates used; arm removed from shoulder; uterus contracted on trunk, and caused it to recede, rendering application of crotchet difficult; trunk separated from head; head extracted without much difficulty	Died; laceration of uterus
46	Jan. 18, 1838	Twins; presentation of left arm of second child; liquor amnii evacuated; arm and shoulder thrust to outlet; right arm also descended; turning accomplished with great difficulty; child dead	Recovered.
47	Nov. 6, 1838	First labour; left arm hanging out of vagina; shoulder strongly impacted in brim; os uteri dilated; liquor amnii evacuated; turning completed with difficulty.	Recovered.
48	March 15, 1839	Presentation of right arm and funis, without pulsation; os uteri widely dilated; pains feeble; great difficulty in turning, on account of violent uterine contractions	Recovered.
49	May 24, 1839	Twins; presentation of head and foot of first child; foot brought down with ease; second child natural	Recovered.
50	Sept. 22, 1839	Presentation of right arm and funis; membranes ruptured; os uteri rigid; turning attempted; V.S. and opiates administered; turning again attempted; V.S. repeated, but turning again ineffectual; arm removed at shoulder-joint; child eviscerated; head left in cavity of uterus; head delivered with difficulty by crotchet, on account of rigidity	Died.

found adherent; there was not a drop of fluid to be found therein. And another instance might be hereby added to the so-called fallacies of auscultation. But considerable effusion was predicted, and considerable effusion was found to exist. The general symptoms, as well as the physical signs, might naturally induce the belief that this effusion was partly fluid—it was found solid.

CASE III.—*Pneumonia, with tubercles; rapid and extensive consolidation a few days before death.*

I was, on the 3d of January, 1843, requested to visit a gentleman by Mr. Collambell, of Lambeth, from whom I received the following account of his history and ailments. He was 23 years of age, married, the father of two children; by occupation an engraver on wood, of some celebrity and considerable merit. His mother died of phthisis. Some weeks before, he had been attended by Mr. Collambell for a rather severe attack of hæmoptysis, accompanied by marked dulness of the right side of the chest, and principally affecting, if not wholly confined to, the middle lobe of the lung. The hæmoptysis yielded to treatment; the dulness on percussion, and other signs of pulmonary apoplexy, disappeared almost entirely, and he was prudently advised to go into the country to re-establish his health. While there, according to his own statement, he was again attacked with hæmoptysis, and was treated by nauseants. The after symptoms rendered it probable that the medicine was antimony administered for the cure of pneumonia, the rusty sputa of which had by himself been supposed to prove that he was again suffering from "spitting of blood." After some days he came to town, and again placed himself under the care of Mr. Collambell. I saw him the day after his return. His complexion was fair; his hair long, and black; his breathing was frequent and difficult, rendering it necessary that he should be supported in bed by pillows; his cough was not very frequent; his expectoration frothy, mucous, viscid, generally white, but intermixed with portions of a reddish brown colour; the skin was hot and dry; the tongue moist and not much loaded; the pulse small, feeble, and frequent.

The physical signs were as follows:— The entire right side and the upper part of the left sounded well on percussion, and afforded pure respiratory murmur, only a little increased in its intensity of sound. The whole of the left side was imperfectly raised during inspiration, and the inferior part anteriorly, and all below the scapula posteriorly, were dull upon percussion; affording well marked, but not very fine crepitating rattle at the end of each inspiration, and, below the scapula, decided bronchophony approaching the tone of Punch upon speaking. The patient was considerably depressed in spirits, and very anxious, especially in reference to the probable existence of tubercles in the lungs. After minute examination I felt justified in stating that, whatever might be the probability of their presence arising from other symptoms, I was unable to detect any *physical indication* of their existence.

He was ordered the tartrate of antimony in small but frequently repeated doses, and, as depletion appeared from his debility to be contra-indicated, a succession of blisters to the affected side.

January 9th.—He was represented to have been much lower this morning; but at my visit in the afternoon had considerably improved. The dulness upon percussion had almost disappeared; the bronchophony was no longer audible; the cough had considerably decreased; the affected part of the lung was clearly much more permeable, and the inspiration therein was accompanied with a general muco-crepitating rattle. Just below the heart alone was there a space about as large as the palm of the hand, under which, from the dulness on percussion and the absence of respiratory murmur, or morbid rattles, it appeared probable that the lung was still consolidated. The infra-clavicular, acromial, and scapular regions, were again examined attentively, but afforded no evidence of disease or obstruction. He was still very anxious, weak, and pale; but the skin was still rather hot and dry, and he was ordered to repeat the medicine less frequently, and to persist in the use of the blisters.

I saw him about ten days after this, but discovered little difference in his general or local symptoms. He was now recommended to take a milder tonic, and to continue the blisters.

February 12th.—He had considerably increased difficulty of breathing, and was rather weaker. He had in no respect improved. The muco-crepitating rattle of the left side inferiorly, the dulness and absence of respiration in a small defined portion of the lung, and the absence of the indications of disease in the upper part of both lungs, remained as before. But the tongue was red, and he had some diarrhœa; the pulse as usual was small, frequent, and feeble.

Ordered—Small doses of Hydr. c. Creta and Pulv. Ipec. C. at bed-time, and a mixture containing Compound Chalk powder, Mucilage, and Infusion of Cusparia, during the day.

19th.—No improvement; aphthæ had appeared on the tongue and cheeks, which were red and tender; the diarrhœa continued frequently to trouble him, and though occasionally checked by medicine, materially contributed to exhaust his little remaining strength. His chest was again examined as carefully as his debility would permit. The portion formerly affected therewith presented the same muco crepitating rattle as before. The part below the heart was still dull, but was now supposed to be breaking down. This at least appeared to be indicated by a peculiarly shrill and resonant mucous rattle being distinctly heard over it. The upper parts of the chest were again carefully examined, and again found to be freely expansible on inspiration, perfectly resonant upon percussion, and free from all morbid sounds, excepting a slight increase of the natural respiratory murmur approaching to puerile respiration. In the lower part of the right lung there was now, however, heard some muco-crepitating rattle.

Ordered—To use a croton oil liniment as a counter-irritant, as the blisters caused considerable inconvenience by stranguary. To take Infusion of Catechu, and aromatic confection with other astringents, and if the diarrhœa should be checked, to replace it with Tr. Ferri Sesquichlorid. and Infusion of Quassia, or some other preparation of iron, should that be found not to agree.

23d.—The diarrhœa continued unchecked; the dyspnœa had considerably increased. The lower parts of the chest presented the same physical signs as before: the upper, in consequence of the distress caused by the exploration, were not upon this occasion examined. His pulse was now exceedingly small and feeble, and his debility very great. The expectoration, as throughout the complaint, was frothy, mucous, and small in quantity. Sulphate of copper and opium were now recommended to be given in addition to the catechu and aromatic confection, previously ordered by Mr. Collambell, but they were ineffectual in checking the relaxation of the bowels; his dyspnœa gradually increased, and latterly became most distressing, and he expired during the evening of February 27th.

Inspection 84 hours after death, by Mr. Collambell and myself.—Externally considerable emaciation was evident, but there existed no appearance of decomposition. The chest alone was permitted by the friends to be examined. The pericardium contained a few drachms of clear serum. The heart was moderately distended with very dark and nearly fluid blood. It was rather loose, pale and soft in structure, but free from any other marks of disease.

Left side.—The two folds of the pleura were connected by adhesions of different sizes and various characters; some were close and membranous; others soft and opaque; while small portions of semi-transparent lymph were found on other parts of the membrane. The inferior two-thirds of this lung, or thereabouts, were soft, dark, friable, and congested from the receding pneumonia, but were thinly sprinkled throughout with small transparent tubercles. A small portion, about an inch and a half square, at the anterior and inferior part, just below the heart, exactly in the situation indicated by dulness and absence of respiration during life, was consolidated, of a dirty white or fawn-colour, from the infiltration of pus, and contained small cavities partly filled with the same sort of fluid, and communicating with the bronchial tubes. The upper third of this lung was generally very solid, and quite destitute of air, of an iron grey colour, friable, and opaque, but containing a few transparent tubercles interspersed through it, and also many small depôts of well-formed healthy pus, varying in size from a large shot to a small bean. These collections of matter were lodged in cavities which were of a rounded form, were lined with a fine layer of opaque lymph, were quite filled with the fluid, and appeared to have no communication with the external air. Quite at the apex of the lung was an irregularly shaped cavity, which was broken by the efforts used in tearing away the strong adhesions by which it was connected to the parietes. It appeared to be nearly as large as a pullet's egg, to have walls which were loose, flocculent, and dark-coloured, and to have been multilocular.

Right side.—The upper third of this lung adhered firmly to the ribs, and was in other respects precisely in the same condition as that of the left, excepting that there was no cavity in the apex, but a small one, about the size of an almond, with a smooth lining of semipurulent lymph, and nearly empty, at the posterior part. The middle lobe contained several defined. portions as large as nuts or almonds, of a dirty pale pink colour, firm, friable, dry and airless, probably the remains of the preceding pulmonary apoplexy. With these were commingled masses of grey consolidation of the lung from pneumonia, approaching in character that existing in the apices, but without any purulent depôts. Irregularly distributed between these two specimens of diseased structure were portions of lung perfectly healthy. The inferior lobe of the right side was the least diseased of any part of the lungs. Posteriorly it was dark-coloured from gravitation, but anteriorly was light coloured, dry, soft and crepitant, and contained only a very few transparent tubercles thinly scattered through it.

In the preceding case is presented an example of consolidation of the upper parts of both lungs so extensive and complete as to render a considerable portion of the organs almost perfectly impermeable by air. This consolidation, nevertheless, was not discovered during life. It offers also a very remarkable illustration of some of the supposed fallacies of auscultation. Nothing could be more striking. Those parts of the lungs which afforded during life natural resonance and almost pure respiratory murmur, and were pronounced to be comparatively free from disease, were found after death not only more diseased, with one trifling exception, than any other part, but impermeable, solid, and suppurating.

The explanation is evident. This disease was not *discovered*, simply because it did not *exist* at the time the exploration of the chest was made. Ten days intervened between the examination of the chest and the death of the individual. During this period his general distress had much increased, his debility from diarrhœa had considerably advanced, and his dyspnœa especially had become gradually but greatly aggravated. During this period, then, this new disease had been set up and had run its course. It did not exist—it may, indeed, be asserted to be physically impossible that it could have existed—at the time of the preceding examination. Even if this, however, were not true, it would appear incredible that a portion of the lung not so large as the palm of the hand, in a more difficult position for examination and detection, should be constantly pronounced to be consolidated, till it was stated, only a few days before death, to be breaking down and forming cavities, and should be afterwards found exactly in the situation, and precisely in the condition that had been predicted, and yet that this far more extensive and obvious disease should have remained undiscovered. The case, then, was an instance of rapid consolidation of the lung, with purulent deposits, occurring in a scrofulous subject a short time before death. Such rapid changes are, I am convinced, especially in persons of bad constitution, by no means unfrequent. Thus a person, not many weeks since, was admitted into the hospital, the duration of whose entire illness was not more than eleven days, but upon the examination of whose body after death the middle lobe of the right lung was found not only perfectly consolidated, but softened, and of a dirty fawn colour, from the infiltration of pus, the consequence of an active but low form of pneumonia. Thus also it arises that cavities are sometimes found where none had been predicted; that large caverns are exposed to view, where small abscesses were supposed to exist; and that consolidations and effusions are discovered after death which had not been prognosticated during the life of the patient.

———

REFLECTIONS
ON THE
INFLUENCES OF COLD UPON THE LIVING BODY.

BY T. WILKINSON KING.

Admitted effects; chemical; vital — Safety valve—Heat depends on many functions — Five effects of cold — States of Nerves—Congestion—Delay of functions; reaction; irregular— Diathesis; fever; wasting; irritation.

AT a time when cold and cold water are becoming so much reputed among the ignorant and the careless, it may not be unacceptable to many to find an attempt made towards determining the medical value of these agents. We hope to be able, in a small degree, to correct the received doctrines relative to the subject of cold, but it is not so much our intention to treat of it systematically as to prepare the way for other considerations.

We cannot but observe that the compiled notices concerning cold appear to us to comprise much that is erroneous and unsatisfactory, especially in the way of theory.

There does not appear to be any cause of disease so well appreciated or so generally admitted as cold. We do not mean that its agency is understood, but merely that authors and observers of all kinds, and in all places, attribute the rise and modification of the greatest variety of affections to the influence of cold, and to us it seems almost impossible, medically, to attach too much importance to the study of the agent in question.

" The theories of sympathy and of associated motions are hardly adequate to an explanation of the phenomena of torpor from cold. There must here, as in other cases, be a regular series of events, a succession of antecedents and consequents in the relation of cause and effect, from the first to the last event, which it is the business of philosophy to discover and enumerate. The narration is still incomplete, from

* In respect of principles, these thoughts are, in part, a repetition of what has been elsewhere advanced. In respect of illustration, they are left somewhat deficient, to avoid repeating more. We may refer generally to former papers in this journal, and in the Guy's Hospital Reports, and particularly to one in the latter, On Variable Disorders.

defective facts and limited observation. Some links of the chain, however, are perhaps within our reach. The terminations of the sanguiniferous system on the surface of the body have their action immediately diminished by the local abstraction of caloric*." Thus wrote a highly intelligent physician, Dr. G. Kellie, of Leith, near forty years since. It is little to his reproach that the existing knowledge and doctrines did not enable him to extend his reflections with much greater success. With reference to severe cold, he argued farther thus:—" The whole series of changes, from the first torpor of the skin and lungs to the complete suspension of the voluntary powers, may be connected and illustrated by the theory (of pulmonic sympathy and influence); if, as there is some reason to conjecture, *the blood suffer changes at the cutaneous surface* similar to those it undergoes in the lungs—if there be a co-operation of the functions of these two organs in freeing the blood from carbon, hydrocarbonate, or carbonic acid."

The words in italics have our concurrence, but, as will be seen, we do not accompany the physiologist to the conclusion. Dr. K. quotes a particularly happy apology from the Essay on the Sublime and Beautiful :—" A theory founded on experiment, and not assumed, is always good for so much as it explains. Our inability to push it indefinitely is no argument at all against it. This inability may be owing to our ignorance of some necessary mediums—to a want of proper application—to many other causes besides a defect in the principles we employ."

When we see how much chemical reactions are influenced by temperature, and observe that the functions of vegetable life are similarly controlled, we may well conclude that there is no more important subject in medicine than that of the influence of temperature on the animal body. Temperature or heat must be a main element in every process of health and disease, and in the operation of every remedy.

Chemistry shows us very clearly that water is at least a triple compound of oxygen, hydrogen, and matter of heat : thus it is, we must remember, that heat

* See the Edinburgh Medical and Surgical Journal, vol. i. p. 308. 1805.

is one of the essential elements of the blood and animal tissues. The degree and variations of temperature of a living part are necessary consequences of its nutrient functions, and when we have considered the heat which is indispensable to the integrity of the part, our next great concern probably should be with the temperature which disturbs the function of the part, and finally the functions of the body generally. In all this, however, the caloric evolved may be considered chiefly as an index of the more material changes by which it is eliminated.

With reference to the influence of cold, we should not neglect to consider what is best known with regard to the temperature of our bodies.

Thus it is highly important to remember that all parts have their own natural and pretty definite proportions of heat. The following is probably a well-observed instance:—In the month of July, the left ventricle itself was about 103° Fah., its blood a little less, and so successively less and less, the right ventricle and its blood, and then the mouth and rectum, the hands, the groin and axillæ, the cheeks, the feet, and the surface of the hypochondria exposed, on which the thermometer stood at 95°.

In the main, the *heat of the body decreases towards the surface;* there is a difference of three or four degrees between the layers half an inch deep on the chest, legs, and arms, and the muscles an inch and a half deeper. Other circumstances modify this statement.

Parts are warm in proportion to their depth, central situation, vascular supply, and immediate vascular activity.

When the artery of a limb is compressed, the heat of the whole limb begins immediately, though slowly, to decline, and on removing the obstruction, so soon the temperature begins to rise*.

On the approach of summer, or the like, while the thermometer is rising from 60° to 80°, the heat of our bodies is rising from 90° to 100°, and so that of birds from 100° to 110°.

Again, we find it a general law, *that*

to raise or lower the temperature of any one part is to do the same by the rest. Put one hand in water at 110°, and in a short time it and all the remotest parts will gain 1° of heat. With one hand in iced water, the opposite one will pretty speedily lose 9° or 10°. These are facts of the utmost importance, and of the most constant use in our reflections on health and disease, prophylactics and remedies*.

It is a remarkable fact that the temperature of warm-blooded animals follows very closely in inverse proportion to the degree of safety-valve-function attributed to each; that is, in direct proportion to the force and precision of the general circulation†. The temperature of the body seems in most cases to be in proportion to the frequency of the pulse.

Harvey put a ligature on the arm until the veins were distended, and then cooled the limb down considerably, and he found that suddenly relaxing the ligature produced a deep sense of cold in the thorax. This may seem a rude experiment, yet it cannot but have its fellow in every-day life, and the most valuable corollaries depend on it. It is in vain to impute all delay of secretions and the like to mere obstructions of nervous influence; cooling the blood is a certain means of retarding all capillary functions. Subsequent reactions are the necessary result of such retardations. If the reaction be general and equal, it is salutary, but if it be only partial, it can scarcely fail to be excessive and mischievous. It has been very commonly advanced that the respiratory function is that which especially and almost exclusively regulates the heat of the body, but we should not forget that the supplies of digestion are equally essential. We make this remark, however, chiefly for the sake of a more general observation, that the condition of the blood and its function are dependent on many organs, and that we must be careful not to impute an undue share of uses to any particular organ, however essential it may be in some one respect.

The function of respiration is no

---

* See an explanation of the changes after tying arteries, in a paper "On the Open State of the *Ductus Arteriosus* after Birth," by T. W. King, *London and Edinburgh Monthly Journal of Medical Science, July 1842.*

* See the article Animal Heat, in the Cyclopædia of Anatomy and Physiology.
† Vide Accounts of the Safety Valve-function in the Heart of Man and Warm-blooded Animals, by T. W. King, Guy's Hospital Reports, Nos. 4 and 11.

doubt essential to the processes of circulation, nutrition, and evolution of heat, but the full development of many functions (as to a series of animals) is scarcely less indispensable than that of respiration. We have nothing which serves to prove that the highest grade of respiratory function could of itself be equal to any useful end.

Medically, the influence of cold seems to demand a threefold consideration. We have to seek for the explanation of its morbid agency, of its curative actions, and of its peculiar influence in regulating the functions of the body, as we observe them changing with the advance of winter, or a visit to colder climates. Thus, we find a physiological, a pathological, and a therapeutic series of views, which require distinct investigation, but it may for the present suffice, if we are enabled, by reference to these various points indiscriminately, to establish more accurate notions of the influence of cold generally.

It is desirable to consider, but not easy to decide, how far cold may operate locally. It does not seem to affect the feet, or the neck and arms; yet a disordered tooth, or perhaps a chronic laryngitis, are directly disturbed by it. We do not imagine that if half a dozen square inches of the subclavicular space were alone exposed to cold air, that this would particularly affect the lung; but in the case of a skin disease, or an ophthalmia, the case seems different.

Cold directly applied may affect any organ, and especially if it be already weak. Remote cold, as at the feet, may affect any organ, but especially the weak one; as the lung, or the eye, as in the case of rheumatism or headache. Some nodes seem to be the effect of direct cold; chilblains, also, and the cutaneous irritation of the winter's evening.

Cold extremities are to be considered as general indications both of the influence of external things and of the internal dispositions. They are the first marked indications; but we do not think it wise to impute disorder to this local affection, without admitting that the surface as well as the system has been at the same time much more generally affected. The patient may complain of having had cold feet; but the physician *must* conclude that the cold has operated almost over the whole surface.

The first great effect of the application of cold to the surface of the body is, to diminish the vitality, or rather nutrition of the part. The consequences of this result will be various, according to the degree, extent, and the duration of the cold, and according to the powers of resistance which the individual may possess. Five different changes at least demand attention,—

   1st, as affecting the state of the surface;

   2dly, with regard to superficial local reaction;

   3dly, the simple determination of blood to the interior;

   4thly, the depression of functions generally; and

   5thly, the determination of active functions generally, or in particular parts, by reaction.

Dr. Copland, the focus of authorities, observes (Dictionary, p. 355), "The *primary effects* of the abstraction of heat from a part, to the extent of producing a decided sensation of cold, appear to be exerted upon the *nervous system*, whose sensibility and vital manifestations it lowers, and, when excessive, entirely annihilates." Now we do not deny this statement, yet we believe that the partial view it affords is a great and prevalent error. The concomitant effects on the blood and capillaries, as independent organs (suppose frost-bite superadded to old paralysis), are much more essential local changes; and there is reason to suppose that the effects of cold on the mass of the blood are of the first consequence, independently of all the nervous functions. Some may infer with Mr. Travers that the blood-globule has its own peculiar nervous organization, which is susceptible of disturbance or irritation; but even this is an insufficient evasion, for it is a much more certain and not less important fact, that the chemical or material organization of the blood is the subject of disorder, and a cause of diseases.

Cold applied to a part in some intensity operates very much as a slow or steady pressure; the nutrition of the capillaries, &c. is suspended or disturbed, and subsequently they yield more than adjacent vessels to the distending blood. By this their reparation is effected, and their strength restored, so that they resume their natural calibre; and in this manner, so far as the local changes are independent, we see merely decline of capillary function, reaction, and restoration, occurring as natural and simple sequents and consequences.

The application of cold in syncope is possibly a simple transfer of blood; or is there here nervous agency in addition?

The salutary effects of cold belong to the study of therapeutics; and amongst medical authors the use of cold has had strong advocates. I shall but briefly reflect on its mode of operation. Topical cold reduces inflammation, and seems often admissible; but the more the inflammation is healthful, the less it needs to be cut short; while the more it is morbid, the less it is safe to subdue it. Applied to the head in cases of brain affection, cold is generally sanctioned; in erysipelas of the scalp it is mostly prohibited. Certainly the most frequent known explanation of metastasis is by the action of cold. Sponging the surface of the chest is only equal to any equally free ablution; it may be harmless, refreshing, or fatal.

The *cold bath* is said to be in many cases invigorating; and it may be pretty evident that the glow which it induces must tend to the freer nutrition of the skin, if it be not rather an absolute index of the augmented nutritive process. The general ease of body, sense of health, "feeling light," as it is called, are indications of the internal functions being at least free from oppression. But what is to be inferred from all this? May we conclude more than this, that a well nourished skin, able to resist casual impressions of cold, may thus sometimes be obtained? whilst the means often fail or prove pernicious; and the desired object is not less surely promoted by the warm or tepid bath, frictions, or common exercise. Cold, frictions, and even heat, applied generally, with judgment, are all calculated to produce a free nutrition of the surface, which may be regarded as equally salutary in itself, however produced. It is in vain, however, to promote this state at the expense of other organs; and, of course, it is still more in vain to expect such a result while general wasting is in progress. Nutrition of

the skin can only be promoted while the proper materials prevail in the blood. If it be an object to be desired, it would appear that friction offers the simplest means of insuring cutaneous nourishment. The use of warmth, while it excites superficial actions, is more calculated, according to experience, to facilitate many functions, both nutrient and secretory, or even to induce wasting. The application of cold, however judicious, may not be free from danger; its advantages seem to depend on moderating (retarding and perhaps equalizing) the internal functions. So far it would seem to resemble the medicines which retard excretion, and add force to the circulation.

A gentleman informed us that he was in the habit of accelerating his circulation to a considerable degree before taking his seat on or in a coach, and he believed that thus he was better and longer able to resist the cold while inactive. In this we conceive he may have judged rightly, and especially, supposing as a contrast the case of one taking his place after a long period of rest. The general action of the system, free distribution of the blood, and evolution of heat, would take time to subside. Our approval is not to be understood of a state of perspiration, by which, with evaporation, the body is rapidly cooled down, nor will it apply to that exercise which may produce any material waste of the circulatory fluids, for under such circumstances protracted exposure would find the body too rapidly becoming exhausted of its nutrient and calorific materials. If cold could be made to effect the simple purposes of abating perspirations and cutaneous loss, we might easily understand the advantage. This object, however, in delicate persons, is at least of doubtful security. Long-continued cold is out of the question. The most transitory cold may be tried with but little risk. The safest mode of cooling the surface is by exercise in the air with light clothing; for, while the first equalizes the functions of the body, the latter tends to moderate them; but even this attempt, in our own experience, requires much caution. It is sometimes scarcely necessary that more than a small part of the frame be partially clothed to produce more effect than is healthful or safe. With respect to exercise it should be remembered likewise that it not only tends to regulate all functions, but first favours the nutrition of a great part of the body, and so prepares matters for excretion (to stimulate excretories), and even induce freer digestion.

Cold applied generally to the surface to a limited degree, when the body is sufficiently vigorous, scarcely seems to produce a decrease of activity. It may be that the sudden impediment leads at once to a commensurate reaction of the capillaries of the skin. Hence the glow after immersions, &c. But these pleasing effects are not constant, and the man who has enjoyed a bath in the morning may take severe mischief by cold in the evening. This indicates conclusively the grand point on which all our medical reflections must turn; namely, the constitution or state of the individual concerned. One takes cold, another does not. One and the same exposure shall produce, in so many different persons, catarrh, pleuritis, and rheumatism,—strumous, fibrinous, serous, and purulent effusions. It is little to say, that age, sex, and habits, help to decide these results. Relapse and metastasis will often find their explanation in a similar way.

The simple determination of blood to the interior of the body, which is so commonly adverted to as a mischievous effect of external cold, does not seem in itself competent to disturb any organ in particular, nor is it in fact equal to any thing beyond that of simple repletion. If all the other causes of diarrhœa, local and general, exist, external cold may readily induce it, or reproduce it when it has just subsided; but, under ordinary healthy circumstances, the so-called inward congestion from sudden cold is only adequate to the common effects of repletion, such as a fuller and more active heart, deeper respiration, and more free secretion and nutrition of the deeper organs generally. That some even tender frames may endure exposure and inactivity with impunity, is possibly true, yet not without many limitations. The appearance of tender health may depend on exposures; both it and the impunity may be deceitful, or only temporary; and, at the best, it would seem that the powers of resisting and of maintaining a general equipoise of the animal functions, under great dif-

ficulties, is the ultimate limit of health and safety.

That the material diminution of the superficial functions of nutrition or secretion, &c. will leave more to be disposed of by other actions, we need not stay to explain; yet we should recollect that the pathological irregularities of this compensatory process deserve much attention. One organ is already more prone to excitement perhaps; the individual more prone to concoct the stimulus of one particular secreting organ, or even to determine specific deposits, as tubercle or pus. It is not only certain that cold may arrest the functions of the skin, but, by diminishing the temperature of the whole mass of the circulating fluids, we cannot but conclude that all the nutritive and depurative functions are, in a definite measure, impeded, and perhaps still farther perverted; and hence it follows that difficulty must be expected, both generally and locally, in various degrees, according to the quantity of heat abstracted, and to the sufferer's natural powers. The fatal sleep from cold is not mere narcotism, but rather to be compared to hybernation. It is an increasing retardation of all functions, beginning at the surface. Dr. Marshall Hall concluded from experiment that hybernants presented but insensible degrees between ordinary sleep and the deepest hybernation. The torpor of tropic reptiles, and of fish in mud, seems analogous: one animal may be frozen, and another dried up, and still be capable of renewed life. In what other ways cold may affect the system must remain to be seen elsewhere.

It may illustrate our reflections, to consider how, by degrees, all the organs may adapt themselves to a low diet, stimuli, or excesses; and thus it is with regard to the depression of functions which a cold climate may induce. All nature shews a rapid and full development of life in warm regions, and tardy evolutions in cold climates. Excessive heat brings on premature decay, and a cool region tends to moderate actions and longevity; but still much depends on the peculiar disposition of individuals.

It cannot be denied that many persons in health suffer nothing from exposure of very severe kinds; and perhaps it is true that a very transitory, though severe, application of cold is mostly harmless even to the delicate; but to these last the effect of any continued cold, though at the time unperceived, is very generally pernicious: hence one great advantage of warm climates to persons in delicate health.

Dr. James Blundell and others have recommended the free use of cold in cases of dangerous uterine hæmorrhage; and it must be admitted that facts are brought forward which seem both to justify and uphold this practice in various analogous cases. We offer no decided opinion on the merits of such a plan of treatment, but we hold that some reserve is imperatively called for. Oozing of blood from a mucous surface, the open veins of a relaxed uterus, or tangible perforation of an artery, surely demand different methods. The constitution, and also the instant condition of the patient, involve particular considerations. We cannot question the fact, that cold may arrest the catamenia, or any other secretion, and the administration of warmth may restore the function. The spontaneous arrest of epistaxis is so constant, that cold is hardly proved to have any decided effect. The circumstances of inflammatory hæmorrhage, as from the bowels, would seem strictly to contra-indicate the use of cold.

The case of bleeding from the most minute vessels is probably that in which the sudden stoppage of blood by remote cold is most likely to be effected.

Some attribute almost as much harm pathologically to warmth as to cold, but we think not justly. External warmth promotes much superficial capillary activity and secretion; and thus it frees the internal functions, and perhaps even enervates. A person with catarrhal affection of the chest, well clothed or active, goes into the cold air in the upright posture with comfort; and this even increases for hours, especially if perhaps there is some excretory diminution of the circulating fluids, and not an increase, as by renewed meals. Subsequently he returns to his warm room and comfortable meal, and he sits or reclines inertly; upon which a general increase of vascular fulness and activity, and local obstruction and secretion, commences and pro-

ceeds, until the general secretions have disburthened the circulation, and he is again at ease by a partial restoration of the balance. This exposition applies in a manner to a great variety of chronic disorders, such as discharges, rheumatism, strictures, and skin disorders. With us capillary distension comprises the chief mystery of *spasmodic* stricture, the proper name for which we conceive to be transitory, or transitory aggravation of, stricture.

A great variety of pains, catarrhs, inflammations, and fevers, are said to arise from cold, and doubtless, where the vigour is wanting to resist, external cold greatly disturbs the balance of the circulation, and obstructs both the superficial secretions and deeper functions. A person affected with any variable chronic discharge, which is excited by every little cause of disturbance to which the body is exposed, seems in a great measure exempt from fevers and phlegmasiæ; but the case is widely different if the habitual discharge becomes arrested.

We think we have often sufficiently noticed, that chronic disorder, repeatedly aggravated by cold or the like, is often attended by a short train of febrile symptoms, which the local excitement seems to carry off.

Now we may suppose that one in strong health may throw off the effects of severe exposure by a simple and general reaction, yet not without loss or waste; and may we not still farther suppose, that such causes of decline, and similar but less complete restorative eliminations, often repeated, may be among the substantial causes of febrile and inflammatory attacks? These are not always to be attributed to "a cold," without previous disorder. How universal and just is the idea of an accumulating morbific cause; and is not temperature as much an imaginable cause of deteriorations as a suppositious state of the air?

All men readily draw inferences from the appearance of emaciation; but we do not know of any reflections which pretend to give a rational account of the wasting body, and of its connection with different morbid states. We may endeavour to clear up the approaches of this important topic; and it is perhaps some recommendation of our attempt to say, that our observations have been corroborated by personal experience, as well as by some experimental attention to the subject of declining health in former periods.

It is not necessary to dwell on the effects of deficient food, or simply impeded nutrition, nor on the palpable results of wasting discharges, yet it is desirable to state here that the considerations which remain are calculated to define and limit the application of the above mentioned causes. Asthma imposing abstinence, the functional or organic impediments to digestion, excesses or anxiety, are more or less intelligible causes of marasmus. The influences of cold are occasionally evident also.

A delicate patient is heard to say, "It is a matter of surprise to my friends every year, that, while others grow thinner and feebler during the hottest weather, I invariably grow larger and stronger." And the medical observer will hardly fail to call to mind cases of wasting which have recurred almost as regularly as the winter season. We know that susceptible infants, convalescents, and the aged, waste with cold, and fatten with warmth. This, as a general remark, is amply corroborated in different climates. The mortality among infants in France is great in proportion as the season or the "department" is cold. The deaths in foundling hospitals, where scarcely one in 19, 27, and 37 are reared, we attribute greatly to the want of warmth and comfort. If any thing like 5 out of 6 of our poor infants are cut off (see Underwood), has cold no share in the result? It is notorious that young infants flourish in the tropics, and also many delicate and aged. To such person each successive exposure, though only to moderate cold, and for a short time, without ample care, clothing, and activity, is speedily followed by languors, and perhaps pains, catarrhs, cutaneous itching, and, unless suppressed, often perspiration; and also by irregular digestion, turbid urine, some falling off of the hair, &c. These, all or in part, may occur without any consciousness of the cause, and pass off in twenty-four hours, and be renewed still more rapidly. Half a family only eat more heartily after sitting in a cold church; the rest become weary and restless, complain of

aching legs and feet, and fall asleep. Repeated relapses of this kind, however little the effects are manifested, and however little the causes are suspected, are a common source of wasting and decline.

We do not dispute that cold, proportioned to the powers of endurance, may often invigorate, as there are doubtless instances in which high temperatures accelerate the functions of secretion to the wasting of the body; but those who, setting aside the natural prejudices of a vigorous body, carefully look into the progress of declining health, with or without the presence of chronic disease, will, we are assured, find reason to accuse cold as a morbid cause alike of declines, relapses, and aggravations, and also of those new and fatal seizures which cut short many obstinate diseases.

These reflections are offered to the reader as rational though feeble suggestions on a difficult and neglected subject. Many points have been passed over to render them brief; and some conclusions to which these views tend are for the present omitted, to avoid offence. Our object has been to regard the effects of cold as a form of irritation or disturbance, both local and general. We hope to strengthen and extend these remarks, by examining the subject of heat in a somewhat similar manner.

36, Bedford Square.

REMARKS ON MESMERISM.

By George Southam,

Surgeon to the Salford and Pendleton Royal Dispensary, Manchester.

(For the Medical Gazette.)

[Concluded from p. 354.]

Sleep appears to be one of the most frequent effects of mesmerism. It has been produced in different degrees, from slight drowsiness to profound stupor; in some instances accompanied with an exalted state, or partial suspension of sensation, thought, and voluntary motion, giving rise to somnambulism or ecstacy in those of ardent imagination. Such effects are similar to the various conditions of natural sleep, which, when perfect, is characterised by the senses ceasing to perceive external impressions, the ideas and emotions being suspended, and the will no longer controlling the voluntary movement; when imperfect dreaming and somnambulism arise, from the conception of ideas by the mind not entirely ceasing, one portion of the mental faculties remaining awake when the rest are asleep : with this addition in somnambulism, that the voluntary muscles, and generally one or more of the senses, are called into activity. In ordinary cases, sleep is induced by mental and corporeal fatigue, but it is not necessary that all the functions of the body and mind should be equally exposed to exhaustion; for such is the power of association and habit, that when one organ or faculty experiences fatigue, the others participate in the same condition; thus the body becomes drowsy from study, and the mind by corporeal exertion*. When sleep is partial (which is frequently the case if produced artificially), this association of the functions of the body and mind does not take place, and some of the senses, or particular sets of the muscles, are awake while the rest are asleep. For instance, if we look steadily at an object for a length of time, the whole field of vision becomes darkened; and if the object is placed in such a position that the action of the levator† muscles of the eyelids are powerfully excited, closure of them is induced‡. Temporary blindness will be the only consequence, if the faculties of the mind and the voluntary actions have not participated in the drowsiness; but generally a tendency to sleep arises in some of them, from having been indirectly influenced in the operation, or from having sustained a degree of exhaustion in consequence of their share of the nervous energy being contributed to the support of the organ which has been the object of attention. This experiment, regarded as a striking proof of the mesmeric power, depends on the concentration of the sensorial energy on the organ of vision, and its gradual exhaustion by constantly directing the attention to the part; on the same principle as the blind and the dumb acquire occasionally such an extraordinary acuteness of touch, that it is apt to be mistaken for the faculties of hearing and seeing. The withdrawal of this energy, under the influence of mental motion, from the external senses, produces insensibility to pain and outward impressions, just as intense reverie on abstract subjects renders the individual almost dead to every thing around him—as in the well-known examples of Archimedes and Sir Isaac Newton.

Every practitioner of experience knows with what activity similar influences operate in persons of excitable dispositions, especially where the balance and harmony of the functions of life have been weakened from previous disease. Some forms of dyspepsia, affections of the respiratory and circulating organs, are frequently aggravated by the continual direction of the mind towards them, which ultimately proves the most troublesome part of the complaint. The same powers are still more active in those nervous diseases which more peculiarly belong to females, who, as Hunter observes, " being less acquainted with the real properties of natural things, are more apt to imagine preternatural ones ; and their reasoning powers not being so strong, they indulge the actions of the mind more, and allow it to take possession of the body*." Thus hysterical attacks are frequently brought on by the mere expectation of them, in addition to the morbid state of the system, which originally caused the disorder. In fact, as Müller remarks, " any state of the body which is conceived to be approaching, and which is expected with perfect confidence and certainty of its occurrence, will be very prone to ensue as the mere result of that idea, if it do not lie without the bounds of possibility†." In illustration of such phenomena, he mentions a case detailed by Pictet in the German translation of Sir H. Davy's Researches on Nitrous Oxide. " A young lady wished to inspire this intoxicating gas, but in order to test the power of the imagination, common atmospheric air was given to her, instead of the nitrous oxide.

---

* Mason Good's Study of Medicine, vol. iii.
† Dr. M. Hall " believes the levator palpebræ, and perhaps the four recti muscles of the eye, to be, of all the muscles of the animal frame, the most purely cerebral, or voluntary, and unendowed with fibres from the excito-motory system. When awake volition raises the eyelid. During sleep, the excito-motory property induces constant contraction of the orbicularis, as it does of the other sphincters."—*Diseases and Derangements of the Nervous System,* 1841.
‡ The success of this experiment is much facilitated by the remarkable association which exists between the actions of the eyelids and the iris.

* Works edited by Palmer, vol. i. p. 360.
† Elements of Physiology, vol. ii.

She had scarcely taken two or three inspirations of it, when she fell into a state of syncope, which she had never suffered previously." Few examples, however, are more conclusive than those observed in some mesmeric patients, which frequently border on the marvellous. Elizabeth O'Key, obedient to every wish of her master, was told by him that nickel was capable of retaining and transmitting the magnetic fluid in an extraordinary degree, but that lead possessed no such virtues: accordingly when nickel was produced, and a few passes made, she was thrown into one of her fits of ecstatic delirium. It need scarcely be remarked that these alleged magnetic properties of nickel have been very satisfactorily refuted[*]. Kluge says, that such is the wonderful sympathy between the magnetiser and the patient, that he has known the latter to vomit and be purged in consequence of medicine which the former had taken. Whenever he put pepper on his tongue, or drank wine, the patient could taste these things distinctly on her palate; and I have seen a person suffering from deafness, who, whilst in the mesmeric sleep, imagined she heard the tick of a watch, which was found afterwards not to have been going.

The idea that a structural defect will certainly be removed by a particular remedy, has sometimes increased the organic actions of the part to such a degree as to remove the disease[†]; hence the miraculous cures said to have been performed by our kings laying their hands upon persons afflicted with scrofula, and other wonderful effects worked by the numerous empirical remedies which have been in vogue at different periods; but the ingenious and simple experiments of Dr. Haygarth[‡] on the tractors, have satisfactorily explained the virtues of such agents, and proved that their success depends chiefly on the power of transferring the nervous energy from one part of the body to another, under the influence of an excited imagination.

The epidemic nature of certain forms of insanity, and of those remarkable convulsive diseases formerly so prevalent in Scotland, America, and the continent, may be accounted for on the same principles; and the facility with which the latter appear to have been propagated amongst a crowd, shows that much of the success of Mesmer and his followers is owing to the public exhibitions, and the other imposing means they have adopted.

On this subject, the French commissioners[*], after observing how inconsiderable the effects were which isolated patients exhibited, stated that even in the public process, the crises do not commence in less than the space of two hours. They further remark, that the impressions are communicated from one to another, and reinforced in the same manner as the impressions which are made by theatrical representations. " The applause by which the emotions of individuals at the banquet are announced, occasions a general emotion, which every one partakes in the degree in which he is susceptible. The same observation has been made in armies upon a day of battle, where the enthusiasm of courage, as well as the impressions of terror, are propagated with so amazing rapidity. The drum, the sound of the military musical instruments, the noise of the cannon, the musketry, the shouts of the army, and the general disorder, impress the organs and exalt the imagination in the same degree. In this equilibrium of inebriation, the external manifestion of a single sensation immediately becomes universal: it hurries the soldiers to the charge, or it determines them to fly. In a numerous assembly, individuals are more subjected than on other occasions to their senses and imaginations, and less capable of consulting and obeying the dictates of reason. Hence the origin of that religious frenzy which formerly affected so powerfully both the minds and bodies of the enthusiasts of the *Cevennes*; and hence the acts of insanity into which public bodies are apt to be hurried in times of political revolution.

Magnetism, then, or rather the operations of the imagination, are equally discoverable at the theatre, in the camp, and in all numerous assemblies, as at the banquet; acting, indeed, by different means, but producing similar effects[†]."

---

* Lancet, 1837-8.
† Müller's Physiology, by Baly, vol. ii.
‡ On the Imagination as a Cause and as a Cure of Disorders of the Body. London, 1800.

* Report of the Experiments on Animal Magnetism by a Committee of the French Royal Academy of Science, 1831.
† Dugald Stewart, Elements of Mental Philosophy.

These observations lead me to notice phreno-mesmerism.

The influence of the will over the train of thought being suspended in sleep, we ascribe to the objects of imagination a real and present existence, similar to those of perception when awake. In dreaming, then, some of the faculties, as the will, perception, and judgment, being in a state of torpidity, whilst the memory and imagination are active, the mind becomes crowded with ideas, which, in the absence of the governing powers, are in most instances subject to the laws of association, and occur with more or less irregularity according to the cause which gives rise to them. Generally, dreams consist of the simplest forms of ideas and emotions; but when they are caused by any train of thought or reasoning which has had a certain persistency in the mind whilst awake, they are produced with greater regularity and vividness.

Further, particular ideas may be associated with certain bodily sensations: a person feeling himself in an uneasy position in bed fancies he is tied down, or that he is falling from a precipice: another, having a bottle of hot water applied to his feet, dreamt that he was making a journey to the top of Mount Etna, and found that the heat of the ground was almost insupportable. Dr. Reid relates of himself, that the dressing applied after a blister on his head having become ruffled so as to produce considerable uneasiness, he dreamt of falling into the hands of savages, and being scalped by them; and every one who is in the habit of dreaming will remember similar instances in his own person.

Moreover, dreaming and somnambulism can be produced in some persons by whispering into their ears when they are asleep. An interesting case of this description is alluded to by Dr. Abercrombie, on the authority of Dr. Gregory. "The subject of it was an officer in the expedition to Louisburg, in 1758, who had this peculiarity in so remarkable a degree, that his companions in the transport were in the constant habit of amusing themselves at his expense. They could produce in him any kind of dream by whispering into his ear, especially if this was done by a friend with whose voice he was familiar. At one time they conducted him through the whole progress of a quarrel, which ended in a duel; and when the parties were supposed to be met, a pistol was put into his hand, which he fired, and was awakened by the report. On another occasion, they found him asleep on the top of a locker, or bunker, in the cabin, when they made him believe that he had fallen overboard, and exhorted him to save himself by swimming. He immediately imitated all the motions of swimming. They then told him that a shark was pursuing him, and entreated him to dive for his life. He instantly did so with such force as to throw himself entirely from the locker upon the cabin floor, by which he was much bruised and awakened, of course. After the landing of the army at Louisburgh, his friends found him one day asleep in his tent, and evidently much annoyed by the cannonading. They then made him believe that he was engaged, when he expressed great fear, and showed an evident disposition to run away. Against this they remonstrated, but, at the same time, they increased his fears by imitating the groans of the wounded and the dying; and when he asked, as he often did, who was down, they named his particular friends. At last, they told him that the man next himself in the line had fallen, when he instantly sprung from his bed, rushed out of the tent, and was roused from his danger and his dream together by falling over the tent-ropes. A remarkable circumstance in this case was, that after these experiments, he had no distinct recollection of his dreams, but only a confused feeling of oppression or fatigue; and he used to tell his friends that he was sure they had been playing some trick upon him[*]."

Similar cases have been related by Smellie in his Natural History, and by Beattie in his Moral and Critical Dissertations.

It is evident, therefore, that there are some individuals, accustomed to dreaming, in whom the slightest suggestion, or bodily impression, is sufficient to call into action a certain train of ideas; and those who have watched the experiments of the phreno-mesmerists cannot but admit that they

---

[*] Inquiries concerning the Intellectual Powers, page 262, Edin. Rev.

depend on similar principles; with this addition, that by associating a particular set of ideas with a certain bodily impression, they may be renewed on other occasions by the mere repetition of the impression. Accordingly, they have associated the different faculties and propensities with impressions on the corresponding phrenological organs; and the remarkable facility and precision with which they appear to be renewed, when once formed, have led the "men of skulls" to regard these phenomena as indisputable facts in favour of phrenology. Unfortunately, their experiments were confined to the phrenological organs: had they extended their inquiries, they would have discovered that benevolence, veneration, self-esteem, &c. might have been as easily associated with corresponding places on the foot, or any other part of the body, as on the head.

Malebranche said, "that to become a philosopher we must see clearly; but to be endued with faith, we must believe blindly:" and certainly, from the recent acts of the phrenologists, it would appear that having discovered their inability to bring their general views into accordance with known facts, they have wandered into the paths of mysticism, and brought to the aid of their science "some dim and disfigured images of truth," which have been ascribed to supernatural powers.

With regard to the reputed advantages of mesmerism, it has been asserted that such a degree of insensibility can be produced under its influence that individuals have undergone severe operations without feeling pain.

Ordinary sensation, it is well known, is frequently suspended from mental emotion, and from disease. We have no means of ascertaining the limit beyond which absence of feeling does not extend; but when such a condition occurs in an extreme degree, it generally arises from some morbid state of the nervous system; and as we have seen that several of these formidable affections are produced by mesmerism, we may infer that any remarkable insensibility to pain can only exist as a symptom of disease.

There is little probability of it possessing any salutary effects (although we are told that it is an infallible cure for most intractable complaints); for a power so energetic in exciting disease can scarcely be expected to have any remedial virtues. If its application could be limited to the production of sleep, or to regulating the supply of nervous energy, it might, under the influence of faith, be successful in the cure of those affections arising from, or modified by, imaginary causes.

CONTRIBUTIONS
TO
ANATOMY AND PHYSIOLOGY.

By ROBERT KNOX, M.D. F.R.S.E.

Lecturer on Anatomy and Physiology, and Corresponding Member of the French Academy of Medicine.

Some Remarks on the Structure and Arrangement of the Spinal Arachnoid.

A FEW years ago I published in the MEDICAL GAZETTE a translation of a memoir, by Arnold, on the Membranes of the Brain and Spinal Marrow; to the translation I added a commentary. My chief object was to point out to anatomists the existence and the peculiarities of a tissue subjacent to the arachnoid (sub-arachnoid tissue), connecting that membrane to the pia mater as well cerebral as spinal. 2. To explain my reasons for differing with M. Magendie in respect to those "communications" he supposes to exist between the fourth ventricle (cerebellar) and the general sub-arachnoid space. And, 3. To describe the true nature of that membrane which invests the cerebral and cerebellar ventricles (ventricular membrane) and the surfaces of the convolutions of the brain where they oppose each other. These observations I now make from memory, not having the memoir before me, but I believe that these were the points at which I chiefly aimed.

Since then, some additional observations on the arrangement and structure of the spinal sub-arachnoid tissue have been made by an anatomical writer who, though evidently young and but recently in the field, has already, by the remarkable clearness of his descriptions, earned for himself a reputation which must be lasting. The observations to which I allude are contained in a foot-note to the admirable descriptive work of Mr. Viner Ellis. They are not put forward as his own, but described as having been furnished him by an old and much esteemed friend of mine, Dr. Sharpey; they refer to an anatomical structure to which, for many years, I had occasionally given a good deal of attention, and bestowed on its examination a good deal of labour. Surprised at the discrepancy between us, I repeated with, if possible, still greater care, my previous observations. To avoid every chance of error, I requested my assistants to repeat the dissections. I next made them, in presence of large classes of students. After reading to them the various passages alluded to as occurring in Mr. Ellis's work, and finding that hitherto I have met with nothing to alter my previous description of this membranous structure, which, by the by, simply accords with the usual descriptions of others, I now venture to submit the matter in dispute to my brother anatomists and physiologists: the ultimate structure of these important membranes can scarcely be too frequently examined*.

Mr. Ellis's text is as follows :—" Dissection of the Spinal Cord." " A small portion of the cord is to be cut off, and the dura mater, having been laid open both before and behind, placed in water, with the dura mater pinned out on a piece of board, and with the posterior surface uppermost. If air be gently blown beneath the visceral layer of the arachnoid, the sub-arachnoid space is perceived, and it is found to be divided into a right and left portion by a septum extending along it."—P. 150.

As a lecturer on anatomy for nearly twenty years, and the conductor of large practical classes, I have been much in the habit of laying open the spinal column with the view of demonstrating the structures to classes and to individuals. Now, what I have observed having a reference to the passage just quoted is simply this, confining my remarks as strictly as I can to the *dorsal* aspect (posterior of Mr. Ellis) of the spinal marrow and its membranes. I am quite within bounds when I say that I have opened and examined the spinal marrow and its membranes, or caused it to be opened and examined in my presence, at least a hundred times.

On laying open the spinal column in the usual way, by removing the arches of all the vertebræ from the atlas to the last sacral, and incising cautiously the dura mater, the visceral layer of the arachnoid presents itself. This generally adheres by a few points here and there to the parietal layer, an arrangement which I once thought might have some remote connexion with the speculations of Goethe, Frank, Oken, Dumeril, and De Blainville, but which were supported neither by comparative dissections nor by abnormal structures. If the visceral layer of the arachnoid be now punctured, and a blow-pipe introduced into the sub-arachnoid space, air may be blown in with the greatest ease, so as to fill large portions of this space, of some inches in length, and extending quite across the medulla, or, in other words, from side to side : the examination of the same aspect of the membrane under water gives precisely the same result. Thus the septum has no existence as a complete septum ; its existence as an incomplete one I think extremely doubtful. It is worthy of remark, that neither M. Cruveilhier*, nor the learned authors of the Encyclopédie Anatomique, now in the course of publication, make the slightest mention of this septum on the dorsal aspect of the spinal arachnoid, nor, indeed, on any other. This is negative evidence, it is true, but of an important kind in a matter of this sort. M. Magendie's opinions must be known to these anatomists. To their works I shall afterwards return; in the meantime, I may remark, that although varieties in the connexions of the visceral layer of the arachnoid (on its dorsal aspect) with the proper membrane of the medulla are occasionally met with, they amount to nothing more than the adhesion of the two membranes to each other at more numerous points by a fine filamentous and sometimes fibrous-looking tissue. Mr. Ellis continues—

" The sub-arachnoid space is much larger in the lower than in the upper part of the cord ; it contains the sub-arachnoid fluid, and is divided, as Magendie has shown, by a partition along the middle line, and it communicates with the interior of the brain by the aperture in the fourth ventricle, as proved by Magendie. Dr. Sharpey

---

* When I commenced these observations I was in hopes of putting my hand on the "Translation of Arnold, with a Commentary," already referred to; it was published, so far as I can recollect, in the GAZETTE (perhaps in the Lancet) some four or five years ago, but I have failed in putting my hand on the volume, so that I am compelled reluctantly to quote it from memory.

considers this space to be lined by a thin membrane, that (which?) he describes as a loose serous sac; this is reflected around the cord by its visceral layer, and on the arachnoid by its parietal; it is separable from the arachnoid, and it may be raised with care, as a thin membrane, from the cord, roots of the nerves, and ligamentum dentatum. He suggests, also, that the portion extending along the posterior part of the space is formed by a reflection of this thin membrane inwards to the cord; that the sub-arachnoid fluid is secreted by this, and contained in it; and that it is continued into the ventricles of the brain, which it lines, by the aperture of the fourth ventricle into the posterior sub-arachnoid space of the brain,"—pages 150 and 151. Again, at page 14 of the same volume, "This space (the posterior sub-arachnoid space) situated between the medulla oblongata and the hemispheres of the cerebellum, is wider before than behind, and communicates in front with the anterior space by the side of the medulla and pons; on the sides and behind with the under surface of the cerebellum, and below with the large sub-arachnoid space of the spinal canal. When this space is opened, the aperture of the fourth ventricle is exposed. By this aperture the cavities of the interior of the brain communicate with the sub-arachnoid spaces both of the brain and of the medulla; and Dr. Sharpey thinks it probable that the membrane which he considers to line the interior of the sub-arachnoid space of the medulla is continued into the cavities of the brain by this opening."

In a foot-note is added—" We might conceive this membrane (the internal arachnoid), to be prolonged from the external arachnoid by the canal of Bichat into the interior of the ventricles, after lining them to be continued through the opening of the fourth ventricle into the so-called sub-arachnoid space, which it lines, being applied to the surface of the spinal cord, the nerves, and the ligimentum dentatum on the one hand, and on the other to the surface of the external sac of the arachnoid; the two by their mutual adhesion forming the loose arachnoid."

Now if it be meant by the above passage that the arachnoid membrane transmits into the interior of the brain by the great cerebral fissure, a mem-

branous sac lining the ventricles, then it will be quite unnecessary for me to say one word in refutation of an opinion already proved false in all our elementary works; a statement involving in fact a physical impossibility : but the passage no doubt admits of another meaning, namely, that a serous sac lining the ventricles passes through the fissure of Bichat to communicate with the sub-arachnoid space there, and through the fourth ventricle, to communicate at the anterior spinal sub-arachnoid space. Now this assertion equally involves a physical impossibility, or nearly so.

Before venturing to offer any critical remarks on the passages now quoted, I shall first beg the reader to remember what I said regarding the disposition of the spinal arachnoid, as high at least as the lower extremity of the medulla oblongata observed on its *dorsal aspect ;* secondly, I shall state the result of several dissections of that portion of the arachnoid extending from the point until fairly traced over the cerebellum ; thirdly, the dissection of the arachnoid and its space on the anterior or ventral aspect of the spinal marrow ; fourthly, the distribution of the arachnoid with reference to the cerebral anfractuosities, and the great posterior cerebral fissure, so called, of Bichat, so well described by Veselius and Galen; and lastly, I shall compare these dissections with the passages just quoted from Mr. Ellis's work.

1st. We have seen that in the vast majority of dissections air may be blown into the posterior sub-arachnoid spinal space freely; that there exists no septum here; that the points of adhesion between the visceral layer of the arachnoid and the proper covering of the medulla spinalis are extremely few. Now trace the arachnoid upwards towards the medulla oblongata and cerebellum, and it will be found that the parietal layer of the arachnoid generally adheres with sufficient firmness towards the lower end of the medulla oblongata as to prevent the passage of air upwards into that large sub-arachnoid space formed by the sudden passage of the arachnoid across to the cerebellum, leaving thus a large space immediately behind the fourth ventricle. If the arachnoid be very cautiously opened where it forms the posterior wall of this space, another membrane will be found either close to

2 H

it, or separated by a considerable quantity of filamentous tissue : this membrane I believe to be a layer of the pia mater, or proper membrane of the medulla spinalis and oblongata, which quits the medulla along a line more or less distant from the margins of the calamus to reach the cerebellum by a nearer point : it varies in its position, and often seems to be merged in that deeper layer of the spinal neurilema which, approaching the aortic margins of the calamus, passes from these to the vermiform process, and aided by the valves of Tarin completely shuts in the fourth ventricle behind, cutting off all communication between the fourth ventricle and the posterior sub-arachnoid space. The "opening," then, of Magendie must be generally artificial. I say generally, because that a deficiency should occasionally exist in the pia mater as it shuts in the ventricle is neither impossible nor improbable. But if any additional serous sac exists exterior to the arachnoid in this space, communicating at this point with the interior of the ventricles, it can only do so by forcing its way through a real barrier which the pia mater presents against the escape of the ventricular fluid into the posterior sub-arachnoid space. This fact I have verified over and over again, and I find it constantly proved by every case of chronic hydrocephalus internus.

No mention is made of any septum in the posterior sub-arachnoid space ; the internal arachnoid, as it is called, seems to commence in the interior of the ventricles whose walls it lines, communicating with the sub-arachnoid spaces chiefly at two points : 1st, at the great cerebral fissure ; 2d, at the pretended foramen of Magendie. Now at the great cerebral fissure there exists a physical obstacle to such a communication, which is this : the cerebral pia mater as it passes from one edge of the fissure to the other, shuts it closely in ; it adheres, in fact, (as it does to the edges of the convolutions) to each edge firmly, passing from one to the other, and in passing transmits into the interior of the brain two distinct processes, namely, the excessively delicate ventricular lining, and secondly, the tela choridea and choroid plexuses. These structural arrangements were pointed out in my Commentary on Arnold. Thus it is physically impossible that any serous

sac can pass across the brain by the wall of the ventricles, as described in Mr. Ellis's work. The ventricular lining is in fact a layer of the pia mater, and the ventricular cavities are excluded from all communication with the sub-arachnoid space by the firm adhesions of the same membrane at the margins of the great openings into the interior of the brain, viz. the great cerebral fissure, and the fourth ventricle : the prolongation of the vascular layer of the same membrane, under the name of choroid plexuses, contributes to shut up the openings.

I promised to return, thirdly, to the dissection of the arachnoid membrane, and sub-arachnoid space on the ventral aspect of the cord ; and, unquestionably here, great varieties exist.

A very common arrangement is a loose adhesion of the visceral layer of the arachnoid to the pia mater, so that on blowing up the space by introducing the blow-pipe, the arrangement was found to be very similar to that on the dorsal aspect. Sometimes, on the contrary, the space is crowded with filamentous tissue to such an extent, and at the same time so short and dense, as to prevent the passage of the air amongst its meshes for any great distance at least, although considerable force be used. Now between these extremes every variety exists, and it has not unfrequently happened that four or five specimens examined in succession with a view to determine this very question, have presented each of them structures quite dissimilar to the others. To look for a serous sac here was quite out of the question ; supposing it to exist in some cases (which is not impossible). Mr. Ellis has omitted mentioning how it terminates upwards.

I find that I had promised to compare these dissections with the statement in Mr. Ellis's text ; but perhaps the reader had better do this for himself. Much, no doubt, remains still to be inquired into with respect to these membranes ; I shall be happy to repeat the dissections with any anatomist situated within a convenient distance. It were easy for me to extend these notes, by pointing out several contradictory passages in the generally very clear and eminently descriptive work of M. Cruveilhier ; but this is unnecessary. The work was published in 1835, and in a new edition they may not be found. My object is not criticism; merely truth.

In conclusion, it only remains that I should notice, with surprise, the extremely meagre and imperfect account of these structures which has just appeared in the " Encyclopedie Anatomique," a work leading necessarily to great expectations, as well from the celebrity of its translator, M. Jordan, as from the host of distinguished and original contributors to the work, and more especially from the celebrity of that high name, Valentin, attached especially to the volume containing the " Neurologie."

ON THE

CIRCULATION IN ACARDIAC FŒTUSES.

To the Editor of the Medical Gazette.

SIR,

IN the last number of Dr. Cormack's Monthly Journal of Medical Science is an article by Dr. Marshall Hall, on the circulation in *acardiac* fœtuses ; from which article it appears that Dr. Hall is of opinion, that the propulsion of the blood through the hepatic and general systems of an acardiac fœtus is effected by the heart of the perfect fœtus, by which the acardiac one is usually, if not invariably, accompanied. Now, before we give credence to so extraordinary a doctrine as this—that the heart of one fœtus can propel the blood through the two distinct systems which compose the circulation of another and acardiac one—Dr. Hall should prove to us that the heart of a perfect fœtus is capable of propelling the blood through *both its own systems ;* that is, through the hepatic system as well as the general. By *hepatic system* I mean the *roots* of the umbilical vein in the placenta (and of which roots the placenta chiefly and essentially consists), the *trunk* of the umbilical vein, the *branches* of the umbilical vein in the liver, the *portal plexuses,* and the *hepatic veins.* By the term *general system,* I mean the heart and all the other vessels, arteries, and veins, except the *spleno-hepatic* vein. There is no *pulmonary system* before birth ; for owing to the communication, first, between the two auricles by means of the foramen ovale, and secondly, between the

pulmonary artery and aorta by the ductus arteriosus, the pulmonary vessels are only a part of the general system.

I confess, sir, I should much like to see what sort of facts and arguments Dr. Marshall Hall could adduce in support of the present all but universal opinion, that it is the heart which propels the blood through the liver both before birth and after. It may seem somewhat heretical, and indeed presumptuous, in me, to call in question the truth of so venerable a doctrine ; but it so happens that I am acquainted with a simple fact, which, in my mind, clearly proves it to be erroneous. That fact is, that more blood enters the heart by the hepatic veins *before* birth than is propelled through the umbilical arteries ; and, *after* birth, than is propelled through the cœliac and mesenteric arteries. Now for the left ventricle to be able to propel the blood through the liver after birth, it would be necessary for it to be able, by propelling a certain quantity, say one ounce, through the cœliac and mesenteric arteries, to displace and drive out of the portal vein, and propel through the portal plexuses and hepatic veins, a *greater* quantity, say ten drachms ; and again, for the fœtal ventricles to propel the blood from the placenta through the umbilical vein and fœtal liver into the fœtal auricles, it would be necessary for them to be able, by propelling a certain quantity through the long and tortuous umbilical arteries, also to effect the propulsion of a *greater* quantity through the vessels of the hepatic system ; that is, through the roots, trunk, and branches of the umbilical vein, the portal plexuses, and hepatic veins. If this be *possible,* if the heart *can* propel the blood through the liver either before birth or after (much more the heart of one fœtus propel the blood through the hepatic and general systems of another fœtus!) · it is not true that a power cannot overcome a resistance greater than itself; for the heart must do so—must always be performing a physical impossibility from the very moment of its formation.

It is evident that more blood *does* pass through the umbilical vein than through the umbilical arteries ; for if as much was continually being returned from the fœtus to the placenta, by the umbilical arteri~ ~~ passes from the placenta to the fœtus by the umbilical vein, it is clear nothing could be *deposited* in the fœtus; and, as *ex nihilo nihil fit*, how could the development of the fœtus then be effected? That more blood passes through the hepatic veins into the heart after birth than is propelled through the cœliac and mesenteric arteries, is indubitably true, because all the fluids taken into the stomach pass through the gastric and duodenal veins into the splenic vein, and so *through* the liver into the heart; and not, as most of us have been taught, through the thoracic duct and *behind* the liver, through the chest, into the neck! I have no doubt in my own mind that even the nutrient juices derived from the solids pass from the digestive tube through the hepatic system into the pulmonary, and not through the trunk of what are called the absorbents. I must state, however, that I ask no one else to believe this. I am by no means desirous of undermining the present physiological creed as to the office of the *thoracic duct.* Nevertheless, I am prepared to defend my own opinion against any one who may feel disposed to advocate the aforesaid creed, either in your pages or elsewhere.

But, to return to Dr. Hall and the acardiac fœtuses. Will that physiologist deny the truth of the fact which I have adduced—that more blood does pass through the liver before birth than is propelled through the umbilical arteries, and after birth than is propelled through the cœliac and mesenteric arteries? And if he will not deny its truth, and I think he cannot, will he oblige me by endeavouring, in his next paper concerning acardiac fœtuses, to reconcile that particular fact with his present views concerning the circulation?

In conclusion I may state, that I entirely concur with Dr. Hall in the opinion that the capillaries have nothing whatever to do with the propulsion of the blood through the veins. I cannot conceive any thing to be more evident and certain, than that they must necessarily retard its motion, and that such retardation is proportionate to their length and minuteness. I am very far, however, from agreeing with Dr. Hall and others in the belief that the heart is the sole agent in the propulsion of the blood. I admit the

right ventricle propels the blood through the lungs, and the left through all other parts and organs except the liver; but with the propulsion of the blood through that organ, I hold the heart has nothing whatever to do, either before birth or after. The hepatic system is always a distinct, perfect, and independent system; and the two veins, of which the spleen and placenta are essentially only the roots, perform in that system, the one before birth, and the other after, the triple function of recipient cavity or auricle, propulsive agent or ventricle, and afferent vessel or artery. Of each of those two veins it may be said, " tria conjuncta in uno;" for each is an auricle, a ventricle, and an artery, although a vein.—I am, sir,

> Your obedient servant,
> JOHN JACKSON.

June 10, 1843.

ON THE

TISSUE UPON WHICH THE RE-MOTE* ACTION OF POISONS IS EXERTED.

BY W. WATES, M.D.

(For the London Medical Gazette.)

OUR ignorance regarding the *modus operandi* of the agents we daily use in the treatment of disease has ever been the fertile source of false theories; has given rise to the bitter, because hitherto unanswered taunt of the empiric and sceptic; has proved a stumbling-block to the pharmacologist at the outset of his task, and is the acknowledged opprobrium of our whole profession. To endeavour to do away with this is the object with which the following remarks are made.

---

* In order that no misconception may arise regarding the position in the chain of sequence which the phenomena induced by poisons, acting on the organised frame, occupy, to which the term remote applies, I copy from Dr. Copland's Dictionary of Medicine, page 558, par. 8, the meaning that word is understood by nosologists to convey; in which it is used throughout the following remarks.

" The division, however, which has been most generally adopted is into remote and proximate or immediate, according to their relation to the disease occasioned by them : the remote being the first in the chain of causation, the proximate or immediate those early changes which they effect in the economy, and which constitute the primary condition of the disease, or, in other words, the pathological states arising directly from the operation of the remote agents."

It has been observed, that we never can know how our medicines act, and, therefore, that it is almost vain to attempt the research: but this, I apprehend, is nothing more than pleading ignorance as a plea for idleness. Whilst the laws which regulate all the various constituents of the universe amongst themselves are gradually being discriminated and fixed, is there any just reason why those by which the effects of agents upon the human frame are produced should remain undefined? I believe not: nor would they so long have been misunderstood, if the same strict rules had been applied in the reasonings based upon the observations made upon the latter, as have been upon those made upon the former. Medical writers have been too apt to permit the opinions springing from a few imperfect observations to colour the results of their investigations, which have been made, though perhaps not intentionally, to prove certain hypotheses, instead simply of defining the strict relations of cause and effect between certain phenomena.

In order that my mind might be as little swayed as possible by any particular theory, I determined, whilst making the investigation into the modus operandi of medical agents and poisons, not to make any experiments myself, but to take those executed by men of acknowledged skill and observation; and by collating them, to endeavour to deduce the various points in which they agree; hoping that thus I might be enabled to lay down some of the laws which they obey in such a way as that they might become fixed data in our reasonings, and prove sure starting-points for fresh research.

Perhaps no little confusion upon this subject has arisen from the mind of the student not fully comprehending what is included under the expression "the action of poisons." In it are necessarily implied the capability, 1st, in the agent to produce an impression upon the organ to which it is applied: 2d, of that organ for receiving that particular impression: and 3d, of the organ impressed to manifest its being acted upon by the impression created by the agent.

The first of these relates to the individual properties of each poison, and as they are universally conceded I shall not stop here to notice them, but

pass on to the consideration of the second and third divisions of the subject. In discussing the former of these two propositions, the question to be first determined is, "upon what tissue are the remote actions of poisons exerted."

No point has been more debated than this, and each succeeding writer seems to have enveloped the matter in greater mystery than he found it, and none more so than Messrs. Morgan and Addison, whose "Essay on Poisons" is written in such an obscure style, that it is almost impossible clearly to understand the meaning they wish it to convey.

Much, if not all, the difficulty met with in determining this most essential part of the inquiry, has arisen from the remote effects of the poison being entirely overlooked, and from the proximate effects, or pathological states, the consequence of the remote action, having been mistaken for them. For instance, some poisons are said to exert their remote action upon the brain, and others upon the heart, the spine, and lungs respectively, because the organs present symptoms of derangement of their functions when a poison is introduced into the system. Yet it will be seen that those very poisons still produce their full effects upon the system, when the particular organ it is supposed to have its remote action confined to, either is removed from the body, or when the chain of communication between the part poisoned and it is destroyed. Yet that organ, when present, is indisputably affected, and the question arises, does the poison act remotely on it, or are they the proximate effects of the poison which it exhibits? This we will now proceed to examine.

What, then, is the tissue remotely acted upon by poisons?

It is admitted on all hands that poisons have the power of affecting the system in two ways. One, in which the impression is not transmitted beyond the part to which it is primarily applied, and in which the general powers of life manifest no symptoms of partaking in any, or to a very slight degree, in the effect of the agent; the other, in which the proximate effects of the remote action of the poison are such as shew that the whole system is affected. The former is the local, the latter the general action of poisons; each consequent upon the remote action.

Several organs are said, by various authors, to be the seat of the remote action; as the brain, the spinal cord, the heart, the lungs, the liver, the stomach; and the blood itself is classed along with them.

Dr. Christison, in his work on Poisons[*], says, "poisons are commonly, but I conceive erroneously, said to affect remotely the general system. A few of them, such as arsenic and mercury, do, indeed, appear to affect a great number of the organs of the body. But by much the larger proportion seem, on the contrary, to act on one or more organs only, not on the general system."

The brain is supposed by many to be the organ remotely acted upon by certain poisons, and among those that hold this opinion may be enumerated Christison, Brodie, and Magendie. I imagine Messrs. Morgan and Addison entertain the same opinion, but am not certain, although I have carefully perused their " Essay" three or four times, and have collated the various passages. I shall therefore give them the benefit of the doubt.

Under the head " remote action," at page 19 of his most valuable work, Dr. Christison writes : " A great number of the poisons now under consideration act upon the brain. The most decided proof of such an action is the nature of the symptoms, which are, convulsions, giddiness, delirium, palsy, coma. All narcotic poisons act on the brain, and most narcotico-acrids too ; but very frequently other organs are acted on at the same time, in particular the spine, and heart."

Sir B. Brodie, as quoted by Morgan and Addison, at pages 21 and 31 of their Essay, infers from his experiments that the brain was affected when death was produced by hydrocyanic acid, and by ticunas. Magendie, also, is represented by the same writers (at page 40) as supposing that the brain is the organ remotely impressed by the action of poisons.

As it will avoid repetition, I shall here introduce the opinions of those who contend for a remote action upon the spinal cord, either in connection with, or independent of, a similar action upon the brain, and also those which advocate the remote action upon the heart, lungs, and blood, and then consider the evidence which affects them.

" It has been maintained by some, that all poisons which have a remote action exert it through the medium of the brain ; but it does not apply well to those which act on remote organs, such as the heart or spine, without causing any sensible symptom referrible to the head. The infusion of tobacco paralyses the heart, and nux vomica irritates the spine, without causing any disorder of the mind : which could scarcely happen through the medium of the brain[*]."

" Few poisons act specifically upon the spinal cord. The only species, indeed, which are known to possess such an action, are nux vomica, the other species of plants which, like it, contain strychnia, and the false angustura bark. Their action on the spine is quite independent of any action on the brain, if indeed such action exist at all, for when the spinal cord is separated from the brain by dividing the medulla oblongata, the effects on the muscles supplied by the spinal cord are produced as usual. Many poisons which act on the brain also act on the spinal cord."[†]

" Some very interesting experiments were made by Emmert with this poison (false angustura bark), to show that it acts upon the spine directly, and not on that organ through the medium of the brain."[‡]

Of the remote action upon the heart. —" Of the poisons which act remotely through a sympathy of distant parts with an organic injury of the textures directly acted on, many appear to act sympathetically on the heart alone."[∥]

"Some poisons of this kind act chiefly if not solely on the heart. The best examples are infusions of tobacco, and upas antiar."[§]

Dr. Christison also places the active principle found in hemlock by Geiger, on his authority, in the list of poisons which act remotely upon the heart, either alone or in conjunction with other organs : together with arsenic, and oxalic acid, on the authority of Dr. Campbell, Dr. Coindet, and himself.[*]

The remote action on the lungs.— Regarding the lungs being the seat of the remote action of poisons little is

---

[*] 3d edition, p. 17.

[*] Christison on Poisons, p. 19.
[†] Ibid. p. 19.
[‡] Ibid. p. 807.
[∥] Ibid. p. 17.
[§] Ibid. p. 17-18.
[*] Ibid. p. 18.

known. Dr. Christison writing on it says, "other poisons act upon the lungs: but we are not acquainted with any which act on them alone."* Magendie found that in poisoning with tartar emetic, the lungs are commonly inflamed, and sometimes hepatised. Mr. Smith, and M. Orfila, both remarked similar signs of pulmonary inflammation in animals poisoned with corrosive sublimate. But these poisons produce important effects on the organs likewise.

These remarks, like the others, are included under the head of "remote action" of poisons, in Dr. Christison's work.

Before I enter upon the consideration of each of the above remote actions, I will make an observation regarding the capability of organs in general to receive and to transmit impressions caused by external agents, of whatever nature they may be.

It is a general law throughout nature that particular functions have each a structure specially constructed for its performance, and that function is alone capable of being produced by its own particular organ: further, each portion of the frame is capable of receiving such impressions only as are calculated to act upon its peculiar structure. In conformity with this law, the brain is constituted for reasoning upon impressions created by external agents acting upon the extremities of, and transmitted by, the cerebro-spinal nerves, and has for its sole function the formation of ideas of external objects from the impressions thus transmitted, and is in nowise necessarily connected with the control or regulation of the functions of organic life. The same remark applies to the spinal cord; its function is to receive impressions created by external objects, and to react upon those organs, whose function is to be in relation with, and to be exercised upon, the external objects creating the impression. Therefore, the cords of communication between the object impressing, and the brain, or spinal cord remotely impressed, are constituted for appreciating and transmitting external forms and properties alone.

As poisons do not differ essentially in their external qualities from other substances which are perfectly inno-

cuous, it will not surprise us to find that these organs (the brain and spinal cord), having functions in connection with the nature of external objects only, are not in any way necessarily connected with the remote reception of the impressions created by substances whose capability of action is quite independent of their external properties.

I shall now proceed to shew that, in conformity with this law—

1st. Poisons do not act when applied to the cut surface of the brain, spinal cord, or to the cut extremities of cerebro-spinal nerves.

2d. Poisons do act when the nervous connexion between the brain and the part inoculated is destroyed by division of the spinal-cord.

3d. Poisons do not act when the inoculated part is connected with the trunk cerebro-spinal nerves alone.

4th. Poisons continue to act though the cerebro-spinal nerves supplying the inoculated part be divided.

1st. Poisons do not act when applied directly to the cut surface of the brain, spinal cord, or cerebro-spinal nerves.

Dr. Copland, speaking on this subject, says, "for when the poison has been applied to the cerebro-spinal nerves, it has been found by Orfila, Fontana, and others, to have no further operation, or even less than when applied to other tissues*." Again: "The celebrated and accurate experiments made by Fontana on the venom of the viper, and ticunas, can be justly estimated only in accordance with this view, for when those substances were applied to the cerebro-spinal nerves, no more rapid effect was produced than when applied upon any other tissue; but when injected into the veins, the result was almost instantaneous." In another work[+] he says :—" It may be concluded from this that the opinion of many physiologists, that poisons act mortally when they are applied to these parts of the nervous system" (i. e. the brain, spinal marrow, and cerebro-spinal nerves), "are not well founded, and are devoid of direct proofs."

On the same point Dr. Christison writes[‡]—"The experiments of Emmert,

---

* Christison on Poisons, p. 18.

* Dictionary of Practical Medicine, vol. 1, page 194, par. 141.
† Appendix to Richerand's Physiology, 3d edition, p. 599, par. 14.
‡ On Poisons, 3d edition, p. 697.

Coullon, and Krimur, shew that it (dilute hydrocyanic acid), has no effect when applied to the trunks or cut extremities of the nerves, or to a fissure made in the brain or spinal marrow; and that its action is not prevented by previously dividing the nerves;" and again,[*] " as to the nervous tissue, it is a singular fact, and well worthy of mention, that the poisons which appear to act on the sentient extremities of the nerves, on the brain and spine, do not act at all on the cut surface of the brain or nerves, or upon any part of the course of the latter. This has been proved with respect to hydrocyanic acid, opium, strychnia, and all active narcotics."

Messrs. Morgan and Addison made the following experiment, to shew the same thing[†]. " The brain of another rabbit of the same age and condition" (as one previously poisoned), " was then laid bare, and a small portion of the cerebrum sliced off horizontally; in the surface thus exposed a portion of woorara, of the same size as that used in the experiment on the first rabbit, was inserted, the greatest care being taken to prevent its contact with any part except the brain itself. After an interval of three quarters of an hour had elapsed from the time of the inoculation, the animal was, from motives of humanity, destroyed ; but during the whole of that time not the slightest symptoms of the effect of the poison upon the system was observed; the animal under excitement leaping about the room as usual."

Dr. Christison[‡] remarks that " some poisons retain their action although the brain be removed," though he does not give the experiment, or the authority upon which the statement is based.

2d. Poisons do act when the nervous connection between the brain and the part inoculated is destroyed by division of the cord.

Widemeyer relates the following experiment. " In a dog the spinal cord was divided at the top of the loins, so that no movements took place when the hind legs were pricked; hydrocyanic acid being then introduced into a wound in the left hind leg, symptoms of poisoning commenced in one minute, and

the hind legs were affected with convulsions as well as the fore legs."[*]

" In a second frog we divided the spinal marrow below the origin of the tracheal plexus, and applied strychnine as before. The anterior extremities became tetanic first, after an interval of twenty minutes, and the posterior extremities became tetanic after an interval of fifty minutes."[†]

" Emmert found that poisoning took place in an animal in whose hind leg the extract of false angustura bark had been inserted, and in whom the spinal cord had been severed in the loins; and in others, where the medulla oblongata was cut across, and artificial respiration kept up, the usual symptoms were produced over the whole body by the administration of it internally or externally."[‡]

" The spinal marrow of a half-grown rabbit was divided; the leg was inoculated with strong prussic acid ; the animal died in three minutes after the introduction of the poison, this being the usual period of time in which that poison was found to operate upon these animals under common circumstances, when introduced into the same part.[§]"

3d. Poisons do not act, when the inoculated part is connected with the trunk by cerebro-spinal nerves alone.

" A fact somewhat analogous has been established by the same experimentalist (Emmert) in regard to the woorara; he found that it does not act when introduced into the limb of any animal connected to the body by nerves alone."[||]

Mr. Brodie " tied a tape half an inch wide round the thigh of a rabbit, excluding the sciatic nerve, and although the leg was wounded, and poisoned with ticunas, yet no sensible effect was produced at the end of an hour from the operation ; after this interval of time had elapsed, the ligature was removed, and in twenty minutes the rabbit was found motionless and insensible[¶]."

" A. Herr observed the same results in a corresponding experiment made with hydrocyanic acid and strychnine on frogs: the thigh of a frog was divided

* On Poisons, p. 25.
† Essay on Poisons, p. 76.
‡ On Poisons, p. 19.

* Ibid. p. 628.
† Gulstonian Lectures for 1842, by Dr. Hall, p. 69.
‡ Christison on Poisons, p. 807.
§ Morgan and Addison's Essay, p. 25.
|| Christison on Poisons, p. 9.
¶ Morgan and Addison's Essay, p. 29.

except the nerves, and the artery was tied; then ticunas poison was applied to the foot, without any effect on the system following.*"

" In another rabbit of the same age a ligature was tied round the leg to the careful exclusion of the sciatic nerve; six drops of prussic acid were then applied to a wound in the foot of the strangulated limb, and without producing the slightest possible effect,"† though a rabbit had just previously been killed with four drops of the same acid.

These four experiments, and all similar ones, are open to some objection, which I shall not notice here, but when I come to consider the circumstances which modify the action of poisons I shall advert to them.

‹ 4th. Poisons continue to act though the cerebro-spinal nerves supplying the inoculated part be divided.

To shew this the following experiment by Sir B. Brodie is quoted from Morgan and Addison.

" The axillary plexus of a rabbit is next divided, and the same poison" (woorara), " is inserted into the limb which produced death in the usual period of time‡."

" Next, many poisons act with unimpaired rapidity when the nerves supplying the part to which they have been applied have been previously divided, or even when the part is attached to the body by arteries and veins only. Dr. Monro *secundus* proved this with regard to opium; the same fact has been extended by Mr. Brodie and Professor Emmert to woorara; by Magendie to nux vomica; by Coullon to hydrocyanic acid; by Charret to opium; and by Coindet and myself to dilute oxalic acid."§

[To be continued.]

MEDICAL GAZETTE.

Friday, June 23, 1843.

" Licet omnibus, licet etiam mihi, dignitatem *Artis Medicæ* tueri; potestas modo veniendi in publicum sit, dicendi periculum non recuso."
                                    CICERO.

PROFESSIONAL SUCCESS.

CLOSELY related to the subject of provision for families by different modes of mutual assurance, as suggested in our last number but one, and strongly recommended by us to the members of our hard-working and ill-paid profession, is the consideration of the qualities, the conduct, and the circumstances which wisdom suggests, or experience proves, conduce to success or failure, to honour or discredit, in a professional career.

We need not do more than advert to those general principles of morality, beyond the limits of which all praise however flattering, all wealth however abounding, falls lamentably short of true success. These principles, if they have not been firmly inculcated during early youth, while the mind is receiving that imperceptible direction in favour of good which sound early education can alone afford, must be taught in the more exciting and violent methods which it is the office of the preacher to use: for to his office is often reserved the arresting that tendency to evil, which seems natural to man, and the bringing, by all the energies at his command, the distorted mind and perverted faculties to an upright and becoming direction. Setting aside these general principles, we would consider our subject within the more special limits of professional ethics, and examine some of the circumstances which seem most frequently to have caused success or failure.

The following advice has been given to a candidate for success at the bar :—
" Spend your patrimony, the larger the better, as elegantly, indeed, but as completely as you can. Marry an heiress, and spend her fortune also; and when your necessities shall have made you industrious, your knowledge of mankind will enable you to make a profitable use of the connections you have formed." This counsel, which has much of the brilliant profligacy of Lord Chesterfield, or the broad satire of Dean Swift, has of course this capital disadvantage, that if deliberately

† Herr's Theorie der Arzneiwirkung. Freibourg, 1836.
    ‡ Morgan and Addison's Essay, p. 31.
    ‖ Ibid. p. 29.
    § Christison on Poisons, p. 9.

acted on it would make a man a scoundrel, and if found by experience to be true, it would be needless. At forty, every man is a fool or a physician, well acquainted with his own mental as well as bodily infirmities; but to this degree, "in nature's good old college," there is no admission *ad eundem.* All the terms must be rigorously kept; the diploma cannot be obtained, like some recently advertised, " for fifty pounds without absence from practice, or thirty-five pounds with two months' residence abroad, including travel through the most delightful part of Europe,"—in company, of course, with the intelligent advertiser. The graduate in self-knowledge—the most difficult of arts—will often have to say with Crabbe—

> " We've trod the maze of error round,
> Long wandering in each devious glade;
> And when the torch of truth is found,
> It only shows us where we strayed.
> Light for ourselves, what is it worth
> When we no more our way can chuse?
> To others when we hold it forth,
> They in their turn the boon refuse."

But the advice above given is brilliant—

> "Se non è vero, è ben trovato,"

and not a few have acted and will act on it. But it scarcely is good for our profession, whatever it may be for the law. Seriousness, not occasional but habitual; earnestness, not affected but real, are useful in securing the confidence of the sick, and indispensable in the studies which prepare us for practice: and if the unvarying liveliness of a mercurial temperament, seems, in some instances, to have been a prime element of professional success, we may rely on it that such unwearied cheerfulness has only lightened the labours of conscientious activity; that it has been kept up by a consciousness of duties performed, not used as a substitute for duties neglected. Of those who can set the table in a roar, how many can leave it at the calls of duty ?

Those who are dissatisfied with their position and success are too apt to throw the whole blame on outward circumstances, when the fault has been mainly in their own conduct. This would be a mere harmless vent for their wrath or repinings, did it not too often tempt them to seek in a change of place or of circumstances that success which can only be fairly expected from a change of conduct. Now of all defects in education, that is the greatest which omits instruction in the art of bearing and suffering. Man's burden of work and trouble is to be borne steadily up the hill of life, and those who are perpetually stopping to shift it, or perpetually seeking less wearisome roads than the direct one, will find themselves, towards the close of the day, hardly less wearied, though far less advanced, than steadier travellers, whom they will have the mortification to see resting while they continue toiling. We certainly do see some of our fellow travellers carry burdens of needless bulk, and in a very awkward manner, which makes us long to give them a hint or a hand for diminishing the weight, or for its better adjustment; but such sturdy fellows do get along surprisingly, and we cease to wonder at their contempt of advice and interference when we see the progress they have made. The old apprenticeship system, and the old school drudgery, had some useful qualities, and produced some useful results, which we may be very thankful if we find secured by the "reading-made-easy" plans so largely tried of late years. The whole advantage of skilled labour, which makes a man and his work so valuable in the eyes of the Benthamec political economist (and not of him only), is forfeited by perpetually shifting from one pursuit or one place to another. The fact of having aimed, and missed an object, is a good reason for aiming again and again, till we hit it, and making their dinners depend upon their success—as is sometimes practised towards young savages, who are to live by their bow and arrow—may furnish a useful hint for more civilized education. The encroaching sea of Holland—the lagoons of Venice—the frost and the thaw, the swamp and the torrent, at St. Petersburgh—all the physical disadvantages which great nations have overcome, have not caused a mere worthless expenditure of toil and treasure; they have been occasions of discipline,—they are crabbed passages in the national grammar, invented seemingly for the mere vexation of pupils, but which once diligently mastered, enable nations not only to correct their early mistakes — their " nonsense verses"—but to write for themselves on the pages of history those great world epics which will, for ever be remembered and quoted, however dimly or traditionally.

Diligent labour, patient application, repeated trials after repeated failures, must be, sooner or later, the portion of all who would win success in any department of life: the object makes no difference in the means required, though it may make a fearful one in the reward earned. The applause of the posture-master, or the blessings which follow the philanthropist, can be won in no other way, though circumstances, talents, taste, or even education, may determine our lot, or direct our choice.

It is often complained that a devotion to science is ill rewarded; this may be true in appearance, but is false in fact. Pure science does not contend for the same objects, nor seek the same rewards, as art or skill. It must be fed and clothed, indeed, but of material outward gains it can receive but little more. Its market value is often not found out till after the death of the inventor, when, with the aid of art, it has been wrought into forms and patterns which men admire, wish for, and find useful or pleasant; but has science, therefore, no rewards? ask the earnest cultivator of physiology, of comparative anatomy, of mechanics, mathematics, or others, for his cash estimate of his labour of love. When he requires to use some art as a bread-winner, he will be all the better workman for being a scientific one, and his science may thus procure him better wages, but he will live by his art, and for skill in this he must labour like other arts men, and will receive the arts-man's reward, and no other. Men agree to deal at certain or uncertain prices, for law, physic, and divinity, for they want justice, health, and piety; but these, the several professors do not pretend to sell.

ROYAL MEDICAL & CHIRURGICAL SOCIETY.
June 13, 1843.
THE PRESIDENT IN THE CHAIR.

On the Characters and Structural Peculiarities of a group of Morbid Growths in which cancerous affections are included. By DR. HODGKIN.

THIS paper was in continuation of a subject which had already been brought before the society on a former occasion by the same writer.

After describing the different appearances revealed by the improved microscopes of the present day, the author endeavoured to connect the nucleated cells, which Müller has shewn to exist in these structures, with the production of those compound cysts which were described in the former paper, and pointed out as affording the type of the adventitious structures referred to.

The following are the conclusions which the author is desirous of drawing from the observations contained in the paper :—

1st. The unrestricted confirmation of the views contained in the former paper as to the existence of the type of compound serous cysts in the adventitious structures referred to. The author had not only found it in man, but in several of the inferior species of mammalia, and in birds. Several able observers had, on examination, coincided with his views, and he mentioned the late Professor Delpech, and the present Professor Rokitanski, having personally informed him of their having, independently, been induced to adopt his views.

2d. That the microscopic examination of these tissues, though extremely interesting, does not furnish perfectly conclusive tests of any particular form of adventitious structure to which a specimen may belong, but that it demonstrates the application of the nucleated cell theory, whilst it is fatal to that of cancerous matter being formed in the blood and eliminated at the spots at which the tumors become manifest. It therefore furnishes an important argument in favour of operation, though other practical considerations require to be attended to before operation is decided on.

3rd. That to have a complete view of the mode of production of these structures, we must combine the cell theory of Schwann and Müller, the coagulation principle which the author had previously suggested, and the process of organization investigated by Mr. Kiernan — three stages of development which appear to occur in the order just enumerated; and that none of the phenomena, taken singly, is an adequate test of malignancy, which, as stated in his first paper, must be regarded as the sum of several characters.

4th. That chemical analysis, though extremely important and interesting, affords an imperfect and inadequate criterion, as the principles concerned may vary or be changed in the progress of development.

5th. That, in operating for the removal of a tumor of this class, it is extremely important to leave behind none of those minute cysts which often form granules in the surrounding cellular membrane, though it may appear in other respects perfectly healthy. This appears to be a mode of extension of the disease independent of inflammation.

6th. That experience teaches us that the infiltrated form of these diseases occurs in the structures in the neighbourhood of the purely adventitious growth, when these structures have been the seat of inflammation, and that the chances of success from operation are consequently infinitely diminished when such surrounding inflammation has taken place. The presence of the peculiar matter of the disease in the interior of vessels appears to be one of the modes in which infiltration, the result of inflammation, exhibits itself, and is, therefore, not a valid argument in favour of the pre-existence of such matter in the circulating blood.

On the Nature of the Ossification of Encysted Tumors. By JOHN DALRYMPLE, Esq. Assistant-Surgeon to the London Ophthalmic Hospital.

The author removed from the upper eyelid of a patient an encysted tumor, about the size of a pea, which was found to consist of concentric layers of hard earthy material. Upon examining the structure by the microscope, he found that the layers were composed of epithelium scales closely agglutinated together; but instead of the usual transparent and thin lamina, with its central nucleus, they were thickened and hard, and

contained granular earthy molecules, which could be removed by immersion in weak muriatic acid. No amorphous earthy deposit existed around or among the scales, which were opaque, of a light brown colour, with a clear and large central nucleus. Having added some observations on the microscopic appearances of other encysted tumors, the author concluded by noticing shortly the difference between the origin of proper ossific growths and that of the tumor described by him. Accompanying the paper was a drawing which exhibited the epithelium scales of which the tumor consisted, with the granular earthy material disseminated through them.

On the Varieties, Causes, Pathology, and Treatment, of the Inflammatory Affections of the Retina. By EDWARD OCTAVIUS HOCKEN, M.D.

After some general remarks on the frequency of retinitis occurring as a secondary affection consequent on other diseased conditions of the eye, the author drew attention to three tables, which shewed the relative numbers of cases of idiopathic inflammation of the retina, met with in three large Eye Infirmaries during several years. According to the records of the West of England Eye Infirmary, there were 20 cases of retinitis in 3,926 patients admitted for various ophthalmic diseases during four years. Of these, 6 were acute, 9 chronic, and 5 not specified. Combining with these the results of the Glasgow Eye Infirmary, and the London Ophthalmic Hospital tables, the author found that acute retinitis only occurred once in every 1755 cases of other diseases of the eye; and this corresponded with his own experience: that the proportion of sub-acute cases was 1 in every 500; and that of chronic cases 1 in 330. He then proceeded, in accordance with the title of his paper, to make observations on the pathology and treatment of the different forms of retinitis, and illustrated his views with the details of some cases.

On the Presence of Spermatozoa in the fluid of Common Hydrocele. By E. A. LLOYD, Esq. Assistant-Surgeon to St. Bartholomew's Hospital, and Surgeon to Christ's Hospital. [In a letter to the President.]

The object of the author was to announce the fact, that in two cases of common hydrocele, in which he examined the fluid withdrawn by tapping, by the microscope, he found numerous spermatozoa. The first case occurred in the early part of last winter. Subsequently to that, in the course of a few weeks, he examined the fluid in four other cases, but without finding any animalcules in them. Three months ago, the second case occurred. The patient was 63 years of age, and had been operated on previously for hydrocele, about fifteen times. Sixteen ounces of a greenish yellow fluid, so albuminous as to be quite adhesive, were drawn off. The author counted forty of these microscopical beings in one drop of this fluid. Some of the animalcules were observed to retain their power of motion for three hours after the fluid had been withdrawn. Blood-globules, transparent cysts, and small granular bodies, also portions of epithelium, or what much resembled it, were likewise found in the fluid. The author concluded by mentioning that since the last case he has examined the fluid of many hydroceles, but had not met with spermatoza in any of them.

The next and last meeting of the season will be held on Tuesday, the 27th inst.

FELLOWES' CLINICAL PRIZE REPORTS.

By ALFRED J. TAPSON.
University College Hospital, 1842.
[Continued from p. 394.]

CASE XII.—*Measles in an adult; the characteristic eruption abundant; coryza; slight sore-throat; bronchitis, and a copious peculiar expectoration, much like that of phthisis, &c. Treated by mercury, saline draughts, tartar emetic, &c.*

SUSAN HENRY, æt. 29, admitted May 16, 1842, under Dr. Taylor. Conformation moderate; black hair, and rather dark complexion. Has been married twice, and had two children, and is now in the fourth month of pregnancy. Her habits have been regular. During the last few months she has not been able to get sufficient food. Lives in Sussex Street, in a dry, but confined, situation. Her mother died seven years ago of consumption; her father is living and well.

She has been subject to a cough in the winter, and slight expectoration, for the last six years; also has occasionally suffered from mild attacks of rheumatism, and has usually had an attack of colic about twice a year for five years. Has never had measles, and is not aware that she has been exposed to it now; has not seen any one with it.

The *present attack* commenced on the 10th inst. with chills alternating with flushes of heat, pain in the back and in the limbs, headache, sickness, and vomiting, faintness, and general weakness. On the 12th, these symptoms had increased, and she noticed a few red spots on the back of the right hand. On the 13th, there were more of the spots

on both hands and on the feet. At this time she felt so ill that she kept her bed; her throat was sore, and she had a cough; the eyes and nose were also sore, and discharged a thin fluid; she fainted once or twice, and was very feverish. On the 14th, the eruption appeared on the knees and elbows, and then on the thighs: on the 15th, on the abdomen, and she believes also on the face at this time. She has been very sick, and vomited repeatedly almost from the commencement; and the soreness of the throat, and running of the eyes and nose, sneezing, &c. have increased. She has had no medical advice, nor has she taken any medicine.

The *present symptoms* are as follows:—The skin feels rather hot and dry; there is an abundant eruption on the face, hands, feet, elbows, and knees, and some, also, on the chest and arms, but it is most abundant on the joints; she says it has been worse on the feet and knees than it is at present. The eruption consists of slightly elevated papulæ, which are confluent in those parts where they are most numerous, and the patches are chiefly semicircular or crescentic; the colour is dull, red, not at all vivid, and disappears on pressure. The face is rather swelled; the tongue is tremulous when protruded, and is covered with an uniform dirty-white fur; the throat feels sore, she says, and the mucous membrane of the fauces, uvula, and back part of the pharynx, is rather redder than natural, but not much swollen. She is very thirsty; has headache and running from the nose and eyes; the conjunctivæ are not inflamed, and the pulse is 108, moderate in volume and force; the breathing is very quick (54 respirations in a minute), but probably is quickened by temporary excitement. She has a hacking cough, which troubles her very much during the night, and is attended with a good deal of thick, frothy, mucous expectoration, similar to that of acute bronchitis. The bowels are rather relaxed, being open three or four times a day, and the evacuations watery; she has had slight pain in the bowels at times, and there is some tenderness on pressure, limited to the right iliac region. The urine is rather scanty, natural in colour, acid reaction, and contains a flocculent deposit of the phosphates; it is not albuminous.

Physical signs.—There is no morbid sound heard with the respiration; the vesicular murmur is somewhat rougher than natural, and there is a slight murmur heard with the first sound of the heart at the apex.

℞ Pulv. Hydrarg. c. Cretâ. gr. v., ter sumend. Low diet. To be kept cool and quiet.

May 17th.—Has not slept during the

night; the skin still feels hot (it is 104° F. in the bend of the elbow), and she complains of itching very much. The eruption is increased on the chest and back, but is somewhat faded on the face, hands, and arms; the redness here is of a more purplish tinge, and more diffused; the crescentic patches are still distinct. The running at the eyes and nose is not diminished, but the eyes are suffused and too sensitive of the light; headache and soreness of the throat less. Breathing much less rapid, only 28 respirations in a minute; she, however, feels more oppressed. The respiratory murmur is too rough, and there is a little sonorous rhonchus; the cough is troublesome; the expectoration contains some thick opaque masses; pulse 112, full, and rather firm. The lips are dry and cracked; the tongue congested and indented at the edges; the papillæ much enlarged; the fur on it is rather brownish along the middle; thirst considerable. Bowels open seven or eight times since yesterday, and the abdomen feels tender on pressure, especially in the hypogastric region; the urine rather scanty and dark coloured, and contains a cloud of mucus.

℞ Acidi Tartarici, ʒij.; Sodæ Sesquicarb. ʒij.; Aquæ, f ʒviij. M. f. Mist.; Sum. cochl. tria magna. 2da. vel. 3tiâ qq. horâ.

18th.—Did not sleep well, in consequence of her breathing being oppressed, but now feels much easier. The skin is warm and rather moist; the eruption is almost gone from the hands, arms, and face, and also is faded somewhat on the chest, but is pretty red on the lower parts of the body and the legs; very little itching to-day; no coryza or sneezing. The cough is rather less troublesome, and the expectoration freer and more abundant; it is a mixture of mucus and of opaque separate masses of a yellowish green colour; it is of a loose character, and altogether very like the expectoration of phthisis. When first expectorated it is of a pale yellowish white colour, homogeneous, and almost gelatinous in consistence, but after standing a little while it separates into a thin nearly transparent mucus, and the masses above mentioned, which sink to the bottom of the vessel. The gums are a little tender to the touch. Has no pain anywhere, but there is some tenderness on pressure in the epigastric and umbilical regions, and during the night she had several sharp pains in the abdomen, which were relieved by vomiting; pulse 96, moderately full; bowels open; urine increased in quantity, reaction acid, sp. grav. 1027; it contains a copious pale brown sediment of the phosphates, and when heated and nitric acid added, a flaky precipitate of albumen is produced.

Cont. Med.
Milk, half a pint daily.

19th.—Slept much better; breathing easier; the rash nearly gone from the whole body except the legs and back. The gums feel more tender and the teeth rather loose; tongue pale; pulse 82, not so full as it was; she feels rather weaker.

Omittantur pulveres.

20th.—The rash quite gone, except from the lower part of the back; no soreness of the throat, and the cough has been very troublesome during the night; the expectoration rather less in quantity, but the appearance is much the same as on the 18th. The respiratory murmur is rough both anteriorly and posteriorly; not otherwise morbid; the sound on percussion is the same on both sides—tolerably clear; pulse 80; bowels open; urine neutral in reaction, not albuminous.

℞ Antim. Potassio Tart. gr. ¼. Mist. Camph. f ʒiss. f. haust. 6tis horis sum.

21st.—The cough, she says, is harder and more frequent, and the expectoration less; there has been considerable running from the nose during the night, and she has perspired very much; has no pain in the chest; tongue covered with a white fur; pulse 78, soft, but moderately full. The medicine griped and purged her two or three times, and also made her vomit three times.

23d.—The eruption is completely gone, and there is a slight exfoliation of the cuticle over the arms and face, but it does not appear to be general over the body. The cough is not at all better; the expectoration is about the same in quantity and in appearance; the fluid part of it is almost transparent, like mucus; the respiratory murmur is still rough, and is accompanied with a sonorous rhonchus. The medicine has not made her sick since the 21st.

Emplast. Canth. pectori applic.
℞ Antim. Potassio Tart. gr. ⅓; Tinct. Camph. Co. ♏xx.; Mist. Camph. f ʒj. ft. haust. 4tâ. qq. horâ sum.
Milk, a pint daily.

25th.—The blister relieved the chest and cough considerably; there is still a good deal of expectoration, and it is mixed with frothy mucus.

Bread, a pound daily.

27th.—The breathing is more free and cough less troublesome; she still expectorates the same mixed kind of matter, and to-day it is slightly tinged with florid blood; the respiratory murmur is less rough, and no sonorous rhonchus can be heard.

30th.—Cough is now quite gone; she feels rather weak, but in every other respect is quite well.

. Discharged cured.

REMARKS.—The above account of the mode of attack, and of the symptoms on the patient's admission, readily leads to a correct diagnosis as to-the nature of the disease. It commenced on the 10th instant, with the usual symptoms of fever, which were followed on the 12th by the appearance of an eruption, coming out successively on the hands, feet, arms, legs, abdomen, face, back, &c., and continuing to come out on the back till the 17th, at which time it was commencing to fade on the parts where it had appeared first. By the 21st it had disappeared entirely from the whole body; so that it lasted in each part about four or five days, and terminated in partial desquamation of the cuticle on the arms and face.

It was clearly, therefore, an eruptive fever; and the only doubt that could exist was, whether it was rubeola or scarlatina. The eruption appeared on the third day of the fever; but this would not help in the diagnosis between these two diseases, as it usually appears on the second in scarlatina, and fourth in rubeola. Again, there was some soreness of the throat, but it was inconsiderable in amount, and was conjoined with a catarrhal affection of the mucous membrane of the eyes, nose, and bronchi, which almost always occurs in rubeola, and not often in scarlatina. But leaving these comparatively unimportant points, the dull or purplish red colour of the eruption appeared at first sight quite characteristic of rubeola; the eruption was in small slightly elevated spots, which manifested a great tendency to arrange themselves in small crescentic or semilunar patches, leaving the intermediate skin of the natural colour.

There are some points in the case deserving a rather particular notice: thus—1st. There was an almost universal affection of the mucous membranes: that of the eyes, nose, and bronchial tubes, discharged a great quantity of mucous secretion; that of the mouth was also probably affected in some way, causing the tumid flabby appearance of the tongue, &c.; that of the alimentary canal was also affected, giving rise to the diarrhœa that existed almost from the first, and most likely also to the pain and tenderness of the abdomen, and lastly, very probably a few of the changes in the urine were due to some affection of the mucous lining of the urinary passages. Of these mucous membranes, that which lines the nasal passages, &c. is especially apt to be affected in the early stages of the disease; whereas the bronchial and alimentary mucous membranes are more likely to be affected at the decline of the eruption, at which time inflammatory complications are most common.

2d. The expectoration presented a very remarkable appearance: at first it was little else than simple frothy mucus, as in bronchitis, but it very soon acquired the peculiar appearance described in the report of the 18th inst., at which time it bore so striking a resemblance to the expectoration of phthisis, that in itself it would create in most persons' mind a very strong suspicion of the existence of that disease. Dr. Taylor, however, stated at the time in the ward, and also subsequently in his clinical lecture on the case, that Chomel had noticed this resemblance between the expectoration of measles in adults and that of phthisis, and said they could only be distinguished by the fluid portion being of a whitish colour in measles, and not in phthisis: in this case, though the expectoration had at first a decidedly whitish colour, yet the fluid portion which separated on standing was not white (vide report). We presume that Chomel in the above statement does not include the microscopical characters, for these, surely, must be different in the two cases.

3d. The urine underwent several changes at different periods of the disease; it contained a good deal of mucus on several occasions: in the earlier part of the disease there was an excess of the phosphates, and shortly after this a considerable excess of the lithates, and also a small quantity of albumen. This has been mentioned by Becquerel as a common occurrence in fevers generally, and is attributed by him to the congestive state of the kidneys produced by the fever; and in such a case as measles, where the functions of the skin must be materially interfered with, we can easily believe that congestion would be likely to arise in these organs: but at the same time we are much inclined to attribute the presence of the albumen in this case to the influence of the mercury on the system, rather than to the fever. How mercury causes it we do not know, whether by its operation on the solids, or, what is more probable, by altering the constitution of the blood; but that it does cause it we have seen instances where it was given in rheumatism, and in all the albumen appeared in the urine just at the time the influence of the mercury on the system was evidenced by the tenderness of the gums, and in these cases, as here, the presence of the albumen could not be detected more than one or two days. Further, we have not found albumen in those cases of rheumatism where mercury has not been given, so that we can hardly ascribe it to the rheumatism itself.

The cause of the disease was, no doubt, contagion, though the patient believed she had not been exposed to it in any way; and she was predisposed to any contagious disease in consequence of being in a weak state from poor living; and besides, she had never had the measles, which, in itself, is almost a predisposing cause, considering how few, comparatively, escape measles altogether.

The treatment of measles is generally very simple, but little being required beyond watching for any complications that may arise, so as to be able to attack them at their very onset. This patient was given small doses of the Pulv. Hydrarg. c. Cretà so as slightly to affect the gums; she was also ordered low diet, and to be kept quiet and cool, and some saline draughts. Under this treatment the fever and eruption passed off in about the usual time without any serious complication having arisen. There was a tendency to bronchitis from the first, and it increased after the decline of the eruption, but was soon removed by a blister and antimonial draughts, and the cough and expectoration had quite ceased before she left the hospital.

HOW TO MAKE LEECHES BITE.

THE leech which it is intended to apply is to be thrown into a saucer containing fresh beer, and is to be left there till it begins to be quite lively. When it has moved about in the vessel for a few moments, it is to be quickly taken out and applied. This method will rarely disappoint expectation, and even dull leeches, and those which have been used not long before, will do their duty. It will be seen with astonishment how quickly they bite. — *Weitenweber's Beitr.*, and *Schmidt's Jahrb.*

CAT'S MINT.

The *Nepeta cataria* of Linnæus is recommended by Dr. Guastamacchia as a sovereign remedy for tooth-ache, whether it proceeds from catching cold, or from caries. The leaves of the plant are placed between the affected tooth and the opposite one; this causes a copious flow of saliva, and in two or three minutes the most violent pains are relieved. If the patients cannot keep the leaves in contact with the diseased tooth, they must chew them, and the object is equally attained by the flow of saliva thus excited.—*Filiatre Sebezio,* and *Schmidt's Jahrb.*

APOTHECARIES' HALL.

LIST OF GENTLEMEN WHO HAVE RECEIVED CERTIFICATES.

Thursday, June 15, 1843.

T. Hawksley.—H. Chambers, Donington, Lincolnshire. — J. Wade, London. — W. Clayton, Hull.—E. Lawford, Leighton Buzzard.—H. Hill, Worcester.—F. Forwood, London.—R. E. Lutley, Wiveliscombe, Somersetshire, — J. Bosdell, Tiverton, Devonshire,

ROYAL COLLEGE OF SURGEONS.

LIST OF GENTLEMEN ADMITTED MEMBERS.

Friday, June 16, 1843.

J. B. Langley.—R. Bullock.—J. Hooper.—P. M'Intyre. — H. Nathan.—S. M. Marshall. — G. Royde.—T. L. Henley.—J. Warwick.—J. Duke. —A. Kidd.

A TABLE OF MORTALITY FOR THE METROPOLIS,

Shewing the number of deaths from all causes registered in the week ending Saturday, June 10, 1843.

Small Pox	10
Measles	29
Scarlatina	33
Hooping Cough	56
Croup	4
Thrush	3
Diarrhœa	4
Dysentery	1
Cholera	0
Influenza	1
Ague	1
Typhus	48
Erysipelas	7
Syphilis	2
Hydrophobia	0
Diseases of the Brain, Nerves, and Senses	130
Diseases of the Lungs and other Organs of Respiration	294
Diseases of the Heart and Blood-vessels	22
Diseases of the Stomach, Liver, and other Organs of Digestion	67
Diseases of the Kidneys, &c	9
Childbed	2
Ovarian Dropsy	1
Disease of Uterus, &c.	3
Rheumatism	2
Diseases of Joints, &c.	8
Carbuncle	0
Ulcer	0
Fistula	0
Diseases of Skin, &c.	0
Old Age or Natural Decay	58
Dropsy, Cancer, and other Diseases of Uncertain Seat	92
Deaths by Violence, Privation, or Intemperance	17
Causes not specified	3
Deaths from all Causes	848

METEOROLOGICAL JOURNAL.

Kept at EDMONTON, *Latitude* 51° 37′ 32″ *N. Longitude* 0° 3′ 51″ *W. of Greenwich.*

June 1843.	THERMOMETER.		BAROMETER.	
Wednesday 14	from 53 to 64		29·92 to	29·85
Thursday . 15	55	69	29·94	29·93
Friday . . . 16	48	69	29·90	Stat.
Saturday . 17	46	72	29·96	29·95
Sunday . . 18	50	72	29·90	29·83
Monday . . 19	50	56	29·89	29·80
Tuesday . 20	49	55	30·00	30·10

Wind, N. and N.E. Cloudy with frequent showers till the 15th; since generally fine. Rain fallen, 9 of an inch.

CHARLES HENRY ADAMS.

NOTICE.

We regret that we cannot make room for the communication of Mr. B.

WILSON & OGILVY, 57, Skinner Street, London.

THE

LONDON MEDICAL GAZETTE,

BEING A

WEEKLY JOURNAL

OF

Medicine and the Collateral Sciences.

FRIDAY, JUNE 30, 1843.

LECTURES

ON THE

THEORY AND PRACTICE OF MIDWIFERY,

Delivered in the Theatre of St. George's Hospital,

BY ROBERT LEE, M.D. F.R.S.

LECTURE XXXII.

On Presentations of the Umbilical Cord, and Labours with two or more Children.

THE umbilical cord may present along with the head, nates, or extremities of the child. Dr. Saxtorph has collected together, from various authors, 292 cases of prolapsus of the cord, in 212 of which the head presented; in 41, the head and extremities; in 5, the nates; in 20, the feet; and in 12, the arm or shoulder. Of 116,277 labours, the funis presented 480 times, being about 1 in 242. Dr. Churchill states, from nearly the same sources, that prolapsus of the cord, in Britain, occurred 226 times in 47,377 cases, or about 1 in 209½: in France, 82 times in 36,621 cases, or about 1 in 446½: in Germany, 93 times in 14,514 cases, or about 1 in 156. Putting the whole of these together, we have 98,512 cases of labour, and 401 examples of prolapsed cord, or about 1 in 245½. Of 355 of these cases, 220 children were born dead, and there is no difficulty in explaining the cause of this great mortality. The cord is sometimes felt through the membranes, pulsating in the progress of the first stage of labour, but when they burst, and the liquor amnii flows out, a portion of the cord passes through the os uteri into the vagina, or out of the external parts, and is exposed to more or less pressure from the head of the child as the labour advances. The vessels of the cord continue to beat for some time, but their pulsations gradually become more and more feeble, and at last entirely cease, if the compression is great and long continued. The circulation of the fœtal blood through the placenta is interrupted—the necessary changes in it are not effected by the maternal blood—and the consequence is the death of the child before its expulsion, by a process similar in all respects to asphyxia after birth. In the operation of turning, the child is not unfrequently destroyed by unavoidable compression of the cord with the hand, when it has not escaped from the uterus, and been exposed to the cold air; and the same occasionally takes place in the vagina, from the pressure of the nates or head interrupting the circulation in its vessels. It is generally believed that the child is exposed to much greater danger when the cord descends in the anterior than in the posterior part of the pelvis. Some children appear to perish much more quickly than others, from prolapsus of the funis. In the last case of this kind which has come under my observation, the membranes were ruptured, and a great part of the liquor amnii discharged at the commencement of the labour, and a long coil of the cord immediately after passed into the vagina; but though the labour continued for eight or ten hours, and the vessels must have been subjected to great pressure from the head in the pelvis, yet the child was born alive by the natural efforts. It seemed more advisable to trust to these, than to any of the means hereafter described. If the circulation in the cord be arrested for a few seconds only in some children, they cannot be made to breathe after birth, while in others, even when the blood has almost entirely for some time ceased to flow through the vessels—at least, has been so feeble that it could scarcely be felt—respiration has been established readily on exposure to the air.

Prolapsus of the cord has been observed, like other preternatural presentations, to occur repeatedly in the same persons in

successive pregnancies, and where no satisfactory cause could be assigned for the
occurrence. Sudden rupture of the membranes, and escape of a great quantity of
liquor amnii ; unusual length of the cord ;
attachment of the placenta to the inferior
part of the uterus, and the cord terminating
in its lower margin ; irregular shape, or
irregular action of the uterus ; unfavourable
position of the trunk and extremities of the
child ; the death of the child and distortion
of the pelvis, have all been considered causes
of presentation of the umbilical cord, and
probably may, in certain cases, assist in
producing the accident.

I regret being obliged unreservedly to
acknowledge that no generally successful plan
of treatment has yet been discovered for
prolapsus of the cord. If it does not pulsate,
the child is dead, and the case should be
treated as if the cord had not descended before
the child : the condition of the mother alone
is then to be considered.

If a shoulder or arm presentation is complicated with prolapsus of the cord, the
operation of turning should be performed as
soon as the circumstances of the case will
permit, and compression of the cord be avoided
as much as possible. Should the cord pass
down before the nates or lower extremities,
the rules which have been already pointed
out for the treatment of cases referred to this
order of preternatural labours should be
strictly observed, and the condition of the
umbilical arteries closely watched. If we
could by any means contrive to effect a
reduction of the portion of prolapsed cord,
or push it back into the uterus above the
head, and retain it there till the head had
passed through the os uteri, or completely
distended it, or if we could by any means
hasten the delivery, the danger to which the
child is exposed would evidently be averted.
The whole hand must be introduced into the
vagina, and not the fingers merely, if you
would succeed in reducing the cord. This
I have found to be the case in actual practice,
and I am persuaded there is no other method
upon which any dependence can be placed.
" It has been proposed," says Dr. Merriman,
" to carry the cord upon the points of the
fingers, or upon a forked piece of cane or
whalebone, through the os uteri and above
the head of the child, so as to prevent the
funis being pressed upon as the head descends through the pelvis. But this expedient has been often found to fail, for upon
withdrawing the fingers, or the forked stick,
the funis usually sinks again into the vagina."
Dr. Aitkin says, " that a grooved piece of
ivory tied on the edge of the point of the
lever, to retain and carry the cord, returns it
with certainty." But many of Aitkin's
recommendations are very fanciful. Dr.

Mackenzie informed Dr. Denman of another
method which he had tried. " Instead of
attempting to replace the descended funis in
the common way, he brought down as much
more of it as would come with ease, and then
enclosed the whole mass in a small bag made
of soft leather, gently drawn together with a
string, like the mouth of a purse. The
whole of the descended funis, enclosed in this
way, was conveniently returned, and remained beyond the head of the child till this
was expelled ; and the bag containing the
funis having escaped compression, the child
was born living." But he very ingenously
told me, that he had afterwards made several
other trials in the same manner without success. Dr. Denman does not, however, state
whether a pitchfork, or the fingers, or what
other means, were employed on these occasions to push up into the uterus the piece of
cord tied in the soft leather bag. " Many
years ago," says Dr. Denman, " Mr. Croft
also informed me of a method which he had
successfully used in these cases. When he
had in vain attempted to replace the funis
in the common way, he carried up the descended part beyond the head till he met
with the limb of the child—suppose the leg
or arm. On this he suspended the funis,
and then withdrawing his hand, suffered the
labour to proceed in the natural way." Mr.
Croft met with other cases in which he had
been equally successful in suspending the
funis over the limbs of the child. " There
may be much of accident in the success of
these different methods," observes Dr. Denman, who had sagacity enough to know their
real value, " but I should believe, whenever
it may have been thought necessary to introduce the hand into the uterus, that it would
be found more expedient to complete the
business by turning the child and delivering
by the feet." " Dr. Davis recommends an
instrument," says Dr. Merriman, " consisting of a thin plate of flat elastic steel, gently
curved, and fixed into a wooden handle.
Near the point are two or three small apertures ; through these apertures it is proposed to pass, by means of a needle, sufficiently strong threads, and to connect by
these threads the prolapsed funis to the
instrument, and *then to remove the funis
out of the way of confusion* by carrying the
point of the instrument above the head of
the child." Dr. Merriman does not inform
us of the number of cases in which Dr. D.
Davis succeeded by this instrument *in
removing the funis out of the way of confusion*, but merely observes, that " any of
the foregoing methods which appear practicable in particular cases may be attempted,
but there is reason to fear they will frequently fail."

In 1835, Dr. Michaelis, of Kiel, published

some Observations, in a German journal, on the Reposition of the Umbilical Cord, and recommended the hand, or an elastic catheter with a silk ligature, to be employed for this purpose. The following is the account of Dr. Michaelis's method of treatment, contained in the 1st Vol. of the British and Foreign Medical Review. " From what has been stated, reposition of the cord consists in carrying it above that circular portion of the uterus which is contracted over the presenting part. The reposition of the cord may be effected by the hand, or by means of an elastic catheter and ligature. In replacing the cord by the means of the hand alone, Dr. Michaelis remarks that we shall effect this more readily by merely insinuating the hand between the head and the uterus, and gradually passing it further round the head, pushing the cord before it; in this manner we do not require to rupture the membranes where we have felt the cord before the liquor amnii has escaped—a point of considerable importance. The reposition by means of the catheter is effected by passing a silk ligature, doubled, along a stout elastic catheter from 12 to 16 inches in length, so that the loop comes out at the upper extremity; the catheter is introduced into the vagina, and the ligature is passed through the coil of umbilical cord, and again brought down to the os externum. A stilet, with a wooden handle, is introduced, and its point passed out at its upper orifice, and the loop of the ligature hung upon it; it is then drawn back into the catheter, and pushed up to the end. The operator has now only to pull down the ends of the ligature, passing the catheter up to the cord, which now becomes securely fixed to its extremity. When the reposition has been effected, he has merely to withdraw the stilet; the cord is instantly disengaged. To prevent any injury, &c. the ligature should be brought away first, and then the catheter."

" Dr. Michaelis has recorded eleven cases of prolapsus of the cord where it has been returned by the above means, in nine of which the child was born alive. In three cases the arm presented also, which was replaced, and the head brought down; in two of these the child was born alive." This is the first time I ever read or heard of the reposition of the cord being attempted before the rupture of the membranes and escape of the liquor amnii. Nothing but mischief could possibly result from "insinuating the hand between the head and the uterus, and gradually passing it further round the head, pushing the cord before it," before the rupture of the membranes. The most important part of the treatment in cases of funis presentations is to preserve the membranes entire as long as possible. Let me entreat you, therefore, to avoid all inter-

ference at this period, for the cord is never exposed to dangerous compression before the membranes are ruptured and the liquor amnii is discharged. I should have thought the catheter and ligature, and stilet with wooden handle, as here recommended to be employed in the reposition of the cord, would be the best means you could possibly adopt for putting the cord into " the way of confusion." But not on'y is the cord here stated to have been replaced by this awkward contrivance, and nine out of eleven children saved, but in three cases of arm-presentation *the arm is replaced, and the head brought down*, and in two of these the child was born alive.

In the Dublin Lying-'n Hospital, the practice which Dr. Collins found of most benefit in cases of presentation of the umbilical cord was keeping it up with great diligence with the fingers, assisted often by a piece of sponge. " It is quite impossible, however," he says, " in the majority of cases, to succeed in this way in protecting the funis from pressure, as it is no sooner returned, than we find it forced down in another direction. We tried in a few instances to return the funis completely into the uterus, by passing a piece of soft twine through a long gum elastic catheter, so as to retain the funis exactly at its extremity, and when thus fixed a strong copper wire was introduced into the catheter in order to render it sufficiently firm to carry up the cord; when elevated as far as practicable by these means, the wire was withdrawn, and the catheter retained in its position during the subsequent expulsion of the child. With this contrivance there was not a sufficient number of trials, as it was but a short time previous to my retiring from the hospital that this expedient was had recourse to." " The total number of cases of prolapsus of the umbilical cord, met with by Dr. Collins, was 97; of these, 24 children were born alive; none of the mothers sustained any injury in the delivery. 12 of the 97 occurred in twin cases; and in 7 of the 12 it was the cord of the second child. Nine occurred where the feet presented (not including two met with in twin children), which was in the proportion of one in every 14 of such presentations; two only, where the breech presented, which was in the proportion of 1 in every 121 of such presentations—this approaches nearly the proportional average in all deliveries, which is one in 171½; four occurred where the shoulder or arm presented—this is in the proportion of 1 in 9 of such presentations. Seven occurred where the hand came down with the head. Seven of the 97 children were born putrid; three of the 97 were premature births, viz. two at the 7th, and one at the 8th month."

Without attempting to press up the prolapsed portion of cord above the head, it has been recommended to place the cord towards one of the sacro-iliac synchondroses, with the view of diminishing the danger of compression. As there is no angle in the gravid uterus corresponding with either sacro-iliac synchondrosis in the dried pelvis, little good would probably be effected by any such attempt to remove the funis out of the way of compression.

Where the head has descended into the pelvis sufficiently low for the application of the short forceps, and the pulsations of the cord are becoming weak and indistinct, there can be no doubt about the propriety of delivering as expeditiously as possible with the forceps; the misfortune is, however, in the greater number of cases of this description, that the child has been destroyed by the pressure before the head is within reach of the instrument, and it can seldom be applied till the child is dead. In two cases Dr. Merriman succeeded by means of the forceps in bringing the children alive.

The operation of turning has been had recourse to in many cases of presentation of the umbilical cord, and in some instances with success, the child's life having been preserved, and the mother having escaped all injury. Guillemeau, Portal, Mauriceau, Giffard, Chapman, and Smellie, and the most eminent practitioners of all countries, before the commencement of the present century, delivered by turning the child in most of these cases, and sometimes they did so when they knew that the child was dead, and when it would have been better practice to have perforated the head and extracted it with the crotchet. In some cases there can be no doubt that the child's life has been saved by the operation of turning, and that the mother has not been injured, but in the reports of the greater number of such cases there is little or nothing stated respecting the mothers' recovery. In 33 cases of prolapsus of the funis recorded by Mauriceau, who was more successful in the treatment of these cases than any other practitioner, he delivered by turning 19 times, and all the children were born alive except one, and most of the women were uninjured. Of 21 cases related by Giffard, in a great proportion of which, if not in all, the operation of turning was performed, or his extractor employed, 17 of the children were born dead; and how many of the women recovered it is impossible to tell, as he does not state. Had Giffard's cases been all left to nature, the probability is a much greater number of the children would have been born alive, and the women would have escaped the danger to which they were exposed by the operation of turning. The following passage proves, I think, that Giffard must have left some cases of prolapsus to nature. " If you cannot return

the navel-string, and there retain it, you ought as soon as possible to turn the child, although it presents with the head, and bring it by the feet, unless it is sunk very low into the vagina, and that a few pains will protrude it." " If the navel-string comes down" says Smellie, " by the child's head, and the pulsation is felt in the arteries, there is a necessity for turning without loss of time; for unless the head advances fast, and the delivery is quick, the circulation in the vessels will be entirely obstructed, and the child consequently perish. If the head is low in the pelvis, the forceps may be successfully used: no doubt, if the pelvis is very narrow, or the head too large, it would be wrong to turn; in that case we ought to try if we can possibly raise the head so as to reduce the funis above it, and after that let the labour go on: but if the waters are all gone, and a large portion of the funis falls down, it is impossible to raise it, so as to keep it up, even although we could easily raise the head; because as one part of the funis is pushed up with the fingers, another part falls down and evades the reduction: and to raise it up to the side and not above the head, will be to no purpose: when a little only jets down at the side, of the head, our endeavours will be for the most part be unsuccessful." In the ninth case, related at p. 255, vol. 3, the head and funis presented, and the membranes were ruptured: he tried to pass the cord above the head, but finding as he pushed up the different folds of the funis they again descended, he turned. " When the head is not uncommonly large," he observes upon this case, " nor the pelvis narrow, this method of delivery seems most advisable to save the life of the child, for unless a very small part of the funis is come down, it seldom can be slipped up so high as to prevent the pressure of the head, and obstruction of the circulating fluids in the vessels of the cord."

Where you have reason to anticipate any difficulty in turning, and even in cases where the uterus is dilated, the membranes unruptured, and the parts relaxed, and every thing tempts you to turn, you had better abstain from all interference in this way. Preserve the membranes entire as long as possible; and when the cord descends after their rupture, pass the whole hand into the vagina, and force it above the head, and if this fails, use the forceps, or then leave the case to nature. If it is a first child, and the os uteri is rigid and only partially dilated, and the contractions are strong, you can do no good by attempting to turn; you will not save the child, and you may rupture the uterus when you least expect to do so. " As to turning," says Dr. Collins, " the risk to the mother is in the majority of cases so great as to forbid its employment, nor do I think the practitioner justified by the circumstances in so greatly hazarding his patient's life."

On labours with two or more children.

Dr. Churchill states that we find among British practitioners, in 161,042 cases of labour, 2477 cases of twins, or about 1 in 69, and 36 cases of triplets, or 1 in 4473. Among French practitioners, in 36,570 cases, 332 cases of twins, or about 1 in 110, and 6 of triplets, or 1 in 6,095. Among German practitioners, in 251,386 cases, 2,967 cases of twins, or about 1 in 84, and 35 of triplets, or about 1 in 7,185. Taking the whole we have 448,998 cases and 5,776 of twins, or 1 in 77¾, and 77 cases of triplets, or 1 in 5,831. The statistics of the British Lying-in Hospital, which was instituted in 1749, are not included in the above statement. Since the institution of this hospital, 35,978 women have been delivered, and 36,401 children born. Four hundred and twenty-three had twins, and one three boys. The proportion of boys to girls born in this hospital is about 18 to 17; of still births, about 1 in 25; and women having had twins, about 1 to 85. I have seen only two cases of triplets during the last 16 years, and neither of them occurred in this hospital. The proportional number of women giving birth to twins, appears, according to Dr. Collins' report, to be much greater in Ireland than in any other country of Europe from which authentic records have been obtained. In France, he says, there is 1 twin case in every 95 births; in Germany 1 in 80; in England 1 in 92; in Scotland 1 in 95; in Ireland 1 in every 62. Of 129,172 women delivered in the Lying-in Hospital of Dublin, 2062 gave birth to twins; 29 of the 129,172 produced 3 at each birth, which is in the proportion of 1 in 4450. One only gave birth to four. Of 697 cases of twins collected by Dr. Churchill, 417 children of the 1394 died, or about 1 in 3½; and out of 12 cases of triplets, i. e. 36 children, 11 were lost, or 1 in 3. A considerable number were premature and still born, and some putrid at birth.

Women are exposed to much greater risk who give birth to twins than those who are delivered of one child; and the danger is produced chiefly by the over-distension of the uterus during pregnancy, the preternatural presentation of one or of both the children, and the occurrence of hæmorrhage from the want of uterine contraction after the separation and expulsion of the placentæ. Inflammation of the deep-seated structures of the uterus, especially the veins, not unfrequently proves fatal to women who have been delivered of twins. We seldom discover before the birth of the first child that there is a second or third in the uterus.

By the stethoscope it has sometimes been ascertained, from the remarkable difference in the action of the two hearts. I have never from auscultation been absolutely certain of the existence of twins before the commencement of labour; but in some cases, from the great size and unusual shape of the abdomen, the peculiar movements described, and the irregularity and feebleness of the pains after labour has begun and continued many hours, I have suspected there were twins, and my suspicions have been well founded. But I must admit that all these symptoms are sometimes fallacious, and that women often feel confident from these and other symptoms that they will have twins, when they bear only one child.

It is in our power, and it is our duty, in all cases to ascertain with certainty, after the expulsion of the first child, if there be a second within the uterus. The small size of the first child often leads us to suspect that there is another, before the hand is applied over the abdomen, and the head, nates, or some part of the second child, is felt through the parietes. If the uterus contains a second child, it is still large, hard, and unequal; the uterus still fills the epigastrium, at least reaches considerably above the umbilicus. I have been repeatedly called to deliver a second child where there was nothing within the uterus but a great placenta. In all cases, therefore, you will not trust to the application of the hand over the abdomen, but make an internal examination; not merely for the purpose of determining whether there is a second child, but, if there is, to ascertain the nature of the presentation. Put the umbilical cord of the first child upon the stretch, and pass along it two fingers of the right hand, and if there is a second child you will feel the second bag of membranes, and discover whether the head, the nates, the extremities, or funis present. It is necessary to inform the nurse of the fact.

The following figure from Smellie gives a front view of twins in the beginning of labour, the anterior parts being removed as in most of the preceding figures. The uterus is stretched with the membranes and liquor amnii. The two placentas are represented adhering to the posterior part of the uterus, the two fœtuses lying before them: one with its head in a proper position at the inferior part of the uterus, and the other situated preternaturally, with the head to the fundus; the bodies of each are here entangled in their proper funis.

When the nates or inferior extremities of the second child present, the binder should be applied firmly round the abdomen, some stimulant should be given, and some time allowed for the uterus to contract. At the end of an hour, or even earlier, if the pains

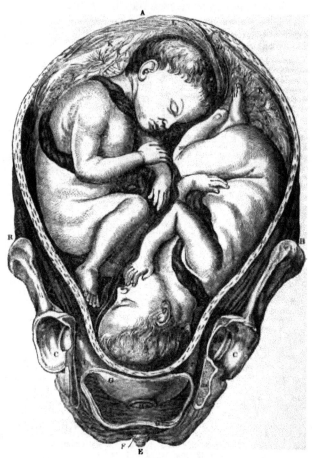

do not return, rupture the membranes, tighten the binder, and bring down the lower extremities, and deliver the child in the manner already described when the nates present, No good can in any case be produced by allowing the child to remain longer in the uterus than an hour after the birth of the first.

If a shoulder or superior extremity of the second child presents, proceed immediately to perform the operation of turning, which is easy and safe both for the mother and child, if you pass up the hand into the uterus, before the membranes are ruptured.

In twin cases, where the head of the second child presents, apply the binder, rupture the membranes, and the uterus will probably contract upon the child and expel it without any artificial assistance. If, however, the labour has been very protracted, and there is great exhaustion, and some risk lest the natural powers should be insufficient for the delivery of the second child, I am disposed to think, as the operation of turning is so easily accomplished, that it would be better at once to have recourse to it, than to trust to the forceps if further assistance should be required. At all events it is invariably necessary to rupture the second set of membranes, if you determine to leave the expulsion of the second child to nature, for the uterus may remain twenty-four hours or longer quiescent if this is not done. After the delivery of both children, always remember the danger of uterine hæmorrhage.

CLINICAL LECTURES

ON THE

THEORY & MEDICAL TREATMENT
OF INSANITY,

Delivered at St. Luke's Hospital,

May 1st, 3d, and 5th.

BY ALEXANDER JOHN SUTHERLAND.

———

LECTURE III.—(concluded.)

*Of Narcotics; use and abuse of opium.
— Sedatives. — Hydrocyanic acid. —
Digitalis. — Diuretics. — Tonics. — Mi-
neral tonics. — Of blood-letting, leeches,
cupping.—Counter-irritants.—Setons.—
Baths.—Antispasmodics.—Conclusion.*

NARCOTICS are placed by some in the first
rank of remedies in the treatment of madness. Much difference of opinion exists as
to the propriety of prescribing them.
Esquirol says, "that these are rather injurious than useful, especially if there be
plethora, or congestion about the head.
Long since, Valsalva and Morgagni proscribed opiates, and daily experience confirms the opinion of these great masters.
Diet, employment, exercise, are the true
remedies for sleeplessness; tepid or cold
baths induce sleep, and are truly efficacious,
and no bad results ever followed their use."

Some authors and practical men of the
present day join with M. Esquirol's opinion upon this subject. Dr. Cox considered that opium produced no permanent
effect upon the insane.

On the other hand, we find medical men
of great experience in the treatment of this
disease, who prescribe it in large doses, and
some, too, who think it possesses in these
complaints virtues almost of a specific
nature. Dr. Halloran, as quoted by Crowther, speaks of certain cases where sleep
had been a stranger for 48 hours in succession, and where he had no doubt, but
for the intervention of an opiate to the extent of 240 drops of the tincture of opium,
at three short intervals, no rest could have
been procured: he goes on to state that
sleep approaching to apoplexy had been obtained in consequence, for nearly 24 hours,
and that it was evidently the means of
effecting an entire and lasting return of the
mental faculty." Crowther says, the same
effect was produced in the cases in which he
employed it. His patients were relieved
from insanity after waking out of a long and
sound sleep. The same effect has been
stated to me to have been produced in some
cases under the care of Mr. Phillips, at the
White House, Bethnal Green. Dr. Ogle
and Mr. Wintle, of the Oxford Asylum, are

likewise in the habit of prescribing large
doses of these medicines, which have also
found an able advocate in Dr. Seymour for
their employment. What is to be said,
when we find such difference of opinion
among practical men? M. Foville has truly
said, that the particular cases of insanity in
which narcotics are useful have not been
clearly pointed out. My own experience
would lead me to the conclusion, that opiates
are of essential service in those cases of
insanity which border closely upon delirium
tremens; in cases of puerperal mania; in
the first breaking out of an attack of madness, before congestion has taken place; in
cases where there is great nervous irritability, from poverty of blood; and in cases
of cachexia from starvation, and other
causes: they are contraindicated wherever
there is the least sign of general paralysis or
congestion about the head. Prescribed indiscriminately, or not in proper doses, narcotics
do more harm than good; they keep up
irritation, and add to the excitement, instead
of allaying it. I have seen sometimes a very
simple case converted into a very complicated one by the excessive use of narcotics.
There is an idiosyncrasy, as every one knows,
in some constitutions which does not admit of
the exhibition of narcotics, especially morphia, even in the smallest dose: ¼th of a
grain will sometimes produce such incessant
vomiting as to endanger the life of the patient. Great care also should be taken, even
when the use of opiates is indicated, not to
continue them too long, for if narcotization
is produced, much harm will follow: the
evacuations are hard and black; the irritation is extreme.

It must not be thought that opium and
morphia are entirely to supersede other
narcotics; there are others, as hyoscyamus
and conium, which are equally serviceable in
the treatment of insanity. I am often in
the habit of prescribing the hyoscyamus; I
find that it agrees better with the stomach,
and it does not constipate the bowels: in
fact, we know from experience that it has
an opposite tendency, and it likewise increases the secretion of the kidneys and of
the skin. Combined with the potassio-tartrate of antimony it is serviceable in the
paroxysms of furor; considerable lassitude
is apt to follow when a draught containing
ʒj. of the tinct. of the former, with gr. ¼ of
the latter, is administered. This, in some
cases, is of course not to be desired.

Combined with camphor, opium allays
the irritability of those suffering under madness, either combined with some degree of
delirium tremens, or preceded by it.

Conium has high antiquity to recommend
it, and is useful both given alone or in combination with hyoscyamus and opium. The
boasted effects of camphor have not been

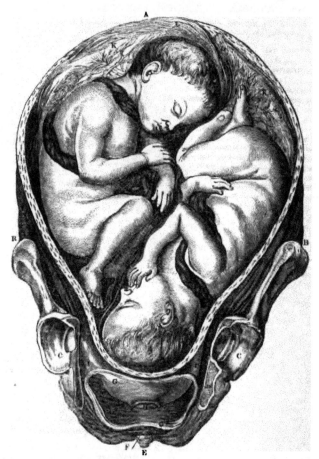

do not return, rupture the membranes, tighten the binder, and bring down the lower extremities, and deliver the child in the manner already described when the nates present, No good can in any case be produced by allowing the child to remain longer in the uterus than an hour after the birth of the first.

If a shoulder or superior extremity of the second child presents, proceed immediately to perform the operation of turning, which is easy and safe both for the mother and child, if you pass up the hand into the uterus, before the membranes are ruptured.

In twin cases, where the head of the second child presents, apply the binder, rupture the membranes, and the uterus will probably contract upon the child and expel

it without any artificial assistance. If, however, the labour has been very protracted, and there is great exhaustion, and some risk lest the natural powers should be insufficient for the delivery of the second child, I am disposed to think, as the operation of turning is so easily accomplished, that it would be better at once to have recourse to it, than to trust to the forceps if further assistance should be required. At all events it is invariably necessary to rupture the second set of membranes, if you determine to leave the expulsion of the second child to nature, for the uterus may remain twenty-four hours or longer quiescent if this is not done. After the delivery of both children, always remember the danger of uterine hæmorrhage.

CLINICAL LECTURES

ON THE

THEORY & MEDICAL TREATMENT
OF INSANITY,

Delivered at St. Luke's Hospital,

May 1st, 3d, and 5th.

BY ALEXANDER JOHN SUTHERLAND.

LECTURE III.—(concluded.)

*Of Narcotics; use and abuse of opium.
— Sedatives. — Hydrocyanic acid. —
Digitalis. — Diuretics. — Tonics. — Mi-
neral tonics. — Of blood-letting, leeches,
cupping.—Counter-irritants.—Setons.—
Baths.—Antispasmodics.—Conclusion.*

—

NARCOTICS are placed by some in the first
rank of remedies in the treatment of madness. Much difference of opinion exists as
to the propriety of prescribing them.
Esquirol says, "that these are rather injurious than useful, especially if there be
plethora, or congestion about the head.
Long since, Valsalva and Morgagni proscribed opiates, and daily experience confirms the opinion of these great masters.
Diet, employment, exercise, are the true
remedies for sleeplessness; tepid or cold
baths induce sleep, and are truly efficacious,
and no bad results ever followed their use."
Some authors and practical men of the
present day join with M. Esquirol's opinion upon this subject. Dr. Cox considered that opium produced no permanent
effect upon the insane.

On the other hand, we find medical men
of great experience in the treatment of this
disease, who prescribe it in large doses, and
some, too, who think it possesses in these
complaints virtues almost of a specific
nature. Dr. Halloran, as quoted by Crowther, speaks of certain cases where sleep
had been a stranger for 48 hours in succession, and where he had no doubt, but
for the intervention of an opiate to the extent of 240 drops of the tincture of opium,
at three short intervals, no rest could have
been procured: he goes on to state that
sleep approaching to apoplexy had been obtained in consequence, for nearly 24 hours,
and that it was evidently the means of
effecting an entire and lasting return of the
mental faculty." Crowther says, the same
effect was produced in the cases in which he
employed it. His patients were relieved
from insanity after waking out of a long and
sound sleep. The same effect has been
stated to me to have been produced in some
cases under the care of Mr. Phillips, at the
White House, Bethnal Green. Dr. Ogle
and Mr. Wintle, of the Oxford Asylum, are

likewise in the habit of prescribing large
doses of these medicines, which have also
found an able advocate in Dr. Seymour for
their employment. What is to be said,
when we find such difference of opinion
among practical men? M. Foville has truly
said, that the particular cases of insanity in
which narcotics are useful have not been
clearly pointed out. My own experience
would lead me to the conclusion, that opiates
are of essential service in those cases of
insanity which border closely upon delirium
tremens; in cases of puerperal mania; in
the first breaking out of an attack of madness, before congestion has taken place; in
cases where there is great nervous irritability, from poverty of blood; and in cases
of cachexia from starvation, and other
causes: they are contraindicated wherever
there is the least sign of general paralysis or
congestion about the head. Prescribed indiscriminately, or not in proper doses, narcotics
do more harm than good; they keep up
irritation, and add to the excitement, instead
of allaying it. I have seen sometimes a very
simple case converted into a very complicated one by the excessive use of narcotics.
There is an idiosyncrasy, as every one knows,
in some constitutions which does not admit of
the exhibition of narcotics, especially morphia, even in the smallest dose: ¼th of a
grain will sometimes produce such incessant
vomiting as to endanger the life of the patient. Great care also should be taken, even
when the use of opiates is indicated, not to
continue them too long, for if narcotization
is produced, much harm will follow: the
evacuations are hard and black; the irritation is extreme.

It must not be thought that opium and
morphia are entirely to supersede other
narcotics; there are others, as hyoscyamus
and conium, which are equally serviceable in
the treatment of insanity. I am often in
the habit of prescribing the hyoscyamus; I
find that it agrees better with the stomach,
and it does not constipate the bowels: in
fact, we know from experience that it has
an opposite tendency, and it likewise increases the secretion of the kidneys and of
the skin. Combined with the potassio-tartrate of antimony it is serviceable in the
paroxysms of furor; considerable lassitude
is apt to follow when a draught containing
ʒj. of the tinct. of the former, with gr. ¼ of
the latter, is administered. This, in some
cases, is of course not to be desired.

Combined with camphor, opium allays
the irritability of those suffering under madness, either combined with some degree of
delirium tremens, or preceded by it.

Conium has high antiquity to recommend
it, and is useful both given alone or in combination with hyoscyamus and opium. The
boasted effects of camphor have not been

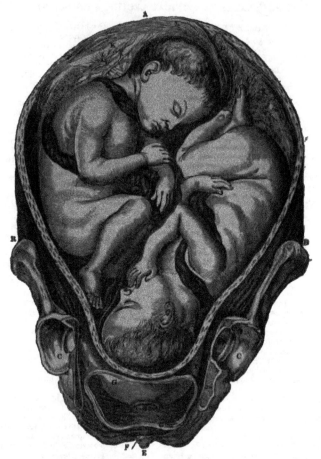

do not return, rupture the membranes, tighten the binder, and bring down the lower extremities, and deliver the child in the manner already described when the nates present, No good can in any case be produced by allowing the child to remain longer in the uterus than an hour after the birth of the first.

If a shoulder or superior extremity of the second child presents, proceed immediately to perform the operation of turning, which is easy and safe both for the mother and child, if you pass up the hand into the uterus, before the membranes are ruptured.

In twin cases, where the head of the second child presents, apply the binder, rupture the membranes, and the uterus will probably contract upon the child and expel it without any artificial assistance. If, however, the labour has been very protracted, and there is great exhaustion, and some risk lest the natural powers should be insufficient for the delivery of the second child, I am disposed to think, as the operation of turning is so easily accomplished, that it would be better at once to have recourse to it, than to trust to the forceps if further assistance should be required. At all events it is invariably necessary to rupture the second set of membranes, if you determine to leave the expulsion of the second child to nature, for the uterus may remain twenty-four hours or longer quiescent if this is not done. After the delivery of both children, always remember the danger of uterine hæmorrhage.

CLINICAL LECTURES

ON THE

THEORY & MEDICAL TREATMENT
OF INSANITY,

Delivered at St. Luke's Hospital,

May 1st, 3d, and 5th.

BY ALEXANDER JOHN SUTHERLAND.

LECTURE III.—(concluded.)

*Of Narcotics; use and abuse of opium.
— Sedatives. — Hydrocyanic acid. —
Digitalis. — Diuretics. — Tonics. — Mineral tonics. — Of blood-letting, leeches,
cupping.—Counter-irritants.—Setons.—
Baths.—Antispasmodics.—Conclusion.*

NARCOTICS are placed by some in the first
rank of remedies in the treatment of madness. Much difference of opinion exists as
to the propriety of prescribing them.
Esquirol says, "that these are rather injurious than useful, especially if there be
plethora, or congestion about the head.
Long since, Valsalva and Morgagni proscribed opiates, and daily experience confirms the opinion of these great masters.
Diet, employment, exercise, are the true
remedies for sleeplessness; tepid or cold
baths induce sleep, and are truly efficacious,
and no bad results ever followed their use."

Some authors and practical men of the
present day join with M. Esquirol's opinion upon this subject. Dr. Cox considered that opium produced no permanent
effect upon the insane.

On the other hand, we find medical men
of great experience in the treatment of this
disease, who prescribe it in large doses, and
some, too, who think it possesses in these
complaints virtues almost of a specific
nature. Dr. Halloran, as quoted by Crowther, speaks of certain cases where sleep
had been a stranger for 48 hours in succession, and where he had no doubt, but
for the intervention of an opiate to the extent of 240 drops of the tincture of opium,
at three short intervals, no rest could have
been procured: he goes on to state that
sleep approaching to apoplexy had been obtained in consequence, for nearly 24 hours,
and that it was evidently the means of
effecting an entire and lasting return of the
mental faculty." Crowther says, the same
effect was produced in the cases in which he
employed it. His patients were relieved
from insanity after waking out of a long and
sound sleep. The same effect has been
stated to me to have been produced in some
cases under the care of Mr. Phillips, at the
White House, Bethnal Green. Dr. Ogle
and Mr. Wintle, of the Oxford Asylum, are

likewise in the habit of prescribing large
doses of these medicines, which have also
found an able advocate in Dr. Seymour for
their employment. What is to be said,
when we find such difference of opinion
among practical men? M. Foville has truly
said, that the particular cases of insanity in
which narcotics are useful have not been
clearly pointed out. My own experience
would lead me to the conclusion, that opiates
are of essential service in those cases of
insanity which border closely upon delirium
tremens; in cases of puerperal mania; in
the first breaking out of an attack of madness, before congestion has taken place; in
cases where there is great nervous irritability, from poverty of blood; and in cases
of cachexia from starvation, and other
causes: they are contraindicated wherever
there is the least sign of general paralysis or
congestion about the head. Prescribed indiscriminately, or not in proper doses, narcotics
do more harm than good; they keep up
irritation, and add to the excitement, instead
of allaying it. I have seen sometimes a very
simple case converted into a very complicated one by the excessive use of narcotics.
There is an idiosyncrasy, as every one knows,
in some constitutions which does not admit of
the exhibition of narcotics, especially morphia, even in the smallest dose: ⅛th of a
grain will sometimes produce such incessant
vomiting as to endanger the life of the patient. Great care also should be taken, even
when the use of opiates is indicated, not to
continue them too long, for if narcotization
is produced, much harm will follow: the
evacuations are hard and black; the irritation is extreme.

It must not be thought that opium and
morphia are entirely to supersede other
narcotics; there are others, as hyoscyamus
and conium, which are equally serviceable in
the treatment of insanity. I am often in
the habit of prescribing the hyoscyamus; I
find that it agrees better with the stomach,
and it does not constipate the bowels: in
fact, we know from experience that it has
an opposite tendency, and it likewise increases the secretion of the kidneys and of
the skin. Combined with the potassio-tartrate of antimony it is serviceable in the
paroxysms of furor; considerable lassitude
is apt to follow when a draught containing
ʒj. of the tinct. of the former, with gr. ¼ of
the latter, is administered. This, in some
cases, is of course not to be desired.

Combined with camphor, opium allays
the irritability of those suffering under madness, either combined with some degree of
delirium tremens, or preceded by it.

Conium has high antiquity to recommend
it, and is useful both given alone or in combination with hyoscyamus and opium. The
boasted effects of camphor have not been

realized, to the extent at least which some of its advocates have stated. Dr. Perfect was in the habit of giving it in large doses; in one case he gave ℈ij. with grs. xv. of potassa nitras. I have found a mixture (often prescribed by my late colleague), containing myrrh and camphor, of use, in cases where there is debility with depression. Stramonium has frequently been given in mania. It was first recommended by Stoerck, as Dr. Paris informs us, because, as it deranged the mind of the sane, it might possibly correct that of the insane. Experience, he states, has not confirmed the sanguine expectations of Stoerck, but it has satisfactorily shown its occasional value in violent paroxysms, in quieting the mind, and procuring rest : for such purposes it has been given at the Fort Clarence, by Dr. Davy, very frequently and successfully." I have given the stramonium in large doses, and I have not derived any benefit from its use : after such praise of a remedy from Dr. Paris, however, it should not be thrown aside, particularly as we also learn from Dr. Prichard that Dr. Schneider derived great benefit from its use. I believe, nevertheless, that it will be found quite inferior to morphia and henbane in its narcotic properties, and to tartarized antimony in its power of subduing the paroxysm.

Belladonna and aconite may be placed in the same category with stramonium. There may, nevertheless, be here and there a case which may be benefitted by their use. Franck states belladonna to be useful in insanity complicated with epilepsy. I recollect obtaining some good effect from aconite in a case of intermitting insanity, when every thing else had failed ; but neither the one or the other are remedies of much importance. In prescribing narcotics in insanity and other diseases you will often find that one preparation of a medicine will agree, while another will disagree with the stomach. I have found Squire's solution of the meconate of morphia very serviceable in some cases where the hydrochlorate and acetate could not be given. You will also find, as you no doubt already know, that the combination of narcotics is occasionally highly advantageous. I am not in the habit of prescribing narcotics as heroics ; but it is very material that they should be given in sufficiently large doses. A patient labouring under insanity from drink, and coupled with delirium tremens, will bear, or rather require, large doses of morphia or the tincture of opium. It is necessary sometimes in these cases, and in others where there is great restlessness and irritability, to repeat the dose every three or four hours.

Hydrocyanic acid is a very useful sedative, and is beneficial in those cases where there is pain and a sense of weight about the præcordia. If acid eructations be present, it may be combined with soda ; and if there be much action of the heart and arteries, with digitalis. The latter remedy has been much used by some practitioners in the treatment of insanity. Dr. Cox speaks highly in its favour. The case of a gentleman whom he attended has been quoted by most modern writers on insanity, as proving the effect of digitalis : it is stated that when the pulse was 90, he was furious ; when at 70, rational ; at 50, melancholic ; at 40, half dead. Dr. Cox says that the patient was cured by keeping the pulse at 70. No doubt the digitalis in this case effected much good, but I have found it difficult, in using this medicine, to ensure the constant slow action of the heart and arteries in some patients, when kept in a recumbent posture, without any excitement ; still more so is it in insanity. I think the good results from administering digitalis in insanity are due quite as much to its diuretic as to its sedative effects ; and this leads us to speak of a class of remedies either entirely overlooked, or at least much neglected in the treatment of insanity.

The urine of insane patients is very frequently, at the commencement of the attack of mania, scanty and high coloured, with a lateritious sediment. Sometimes no water is secreted for a day, sometimes for two days. There are also patients whose urine is retained for a great length of time, as there are others who pass it involuntarily ; but of these last I do not now speak. I recommend you always to examine the state of the urine for yourselves, as you cannot depend upon the account given you by the patients : you will find it necessary, sometimes, to give ℥ss. or ℥j. of Nitric Æther, either in distilled water, with gr. x. of Nitrate of Potash, ℥ss. of Infusion of Digitalis, and ℥j. of the Compound Decoction of Scoparius, as the symptoms may require it. You will very seldom have to prescribe the more powerful diuretics, as cantharides ; unless you give it in those cases where you suspect effusion, or, as has been recommended, in incipient paralysis. I have prescribed it in these cases, and have been much disappointed with it. I have not seen the symptoms of general paralysis yield to its influence, but great excitement and paroxysms of furor have sometimes been brought on, which have subsided when the medicine has been omitted. The bichloride of mercury is a remedy of far greater importance in these cases. Where symptoms of effusion are present, I have not derived much benefit from the Lytta, given, of course, I mean, in insanity ; for its influence, when there is effusion in other cases, and also in hemiplegia and paraplegia, cannot be denied. I cannot help thinking that a very different state of the capillary vessels of the brain exists where there is effusion after an attack of insanity, from that after one of acute inflammation of the brain and its membranes, for I have been surprised to find the stupor vanish, and the pupil become natural, under the influence of tonics and stimulants. I have before stated to you in what particular cases there appears to me to be passive congestion; if in these cases the vessels can but be induced by proper remedies to recover their tone, the patients will in all probability do well.

Tonics.—Since the insane have been better fed, there have been, on an average, more recoveries and fewer deaths. Even during the acute stage of mania we must not only regard the present symptoms, but future probable consequences of the disease, and of our treatment. The brain, in acute mania, with frequent recurrence of paroxysms of furor, suffers the wear and tear of many years, and the exhaustion of mind and body which follows is excessive. Patients who, previously to their admission into the hospital, have undergone a long course of lowering treatment, and whose strength is consequently much reduced, have derived benefit from an infusion of a light bitter, as calumba or cascarilla, with the sesquicarbonate of ammonia. Sometimes patients are brought to the hospital whose insanity has been caused by starvation and wretchedness; many of these are cachectic, and have an eruption of boils. These will often bear the Compound Decoction of Bark, with 3j. of the Liquor Potassæ, to which you may add, if there be irritability, 3j. of the Tincture of Henbane.

There is a case reported by M. Andral of a person who laboured under intermittent cerebral congestion, who was cured by large doses of quinine, internally and externally administered. I have found this and other tonics of use in intermittent cases, where their employment is not contraindicated. Arsenic, either in the form of the Liquor Potassæ Arsenitis of the Pharmacopœia, or Solution of the Chloride of Arsenic, as prepared at Apothecaries' Hall, are likewise valuable remedies here. Mineral tonics are not to be laid aside on account of any theoretical notions about congestion of the brain. I have sometimes commenced with them from the first day of a patient's admission; for instance, in those cases when the disease is complicated with chlorosis or chorea, or when the patient is enfeebled by self-abuse, or any other cause. I have seen some of our patients rapidly improve, after the acute stage has passed over, by taking the Tinctura Ferri Sesquichloridi in an Infusion of Quassiæ, and the combination of a chalybeate with a purgative is occasionally of great service to us in treating insanity. The preparations of Iron, the Sulphate of Zinc, and the Salts of Copper, are also valuable medicines in nervous disorders.

Of blood-letting.—The great advocate for large general bleedings in insanity is Dr. Rush. This practice fortunately does not retain in England the same credit which it formerly did, as Esquirol somewhat archly says, "they thought they had cured their patients by venæsectio, when in truth they had reduced them to a state of incurable fatuity." M. Georget, and M. Foville, recommended general bleeding. The latter says, "without having pushed venæsectio so far as either Rush or J. Franck, I confess that it appears to me to be one of the means on the efficacy of which we can most rely in recent acute cases."

M. Pinel and M. Esquirol were decidedly opposed to general bleeding in cases of insanity. In acute mania with plethora, heat of head, injected conjunctivæ, and full pulse, we should certainly propose to ourselves to unload as speedily and as safely as possible the minute capillary tubes.

This can be the only reason for employing general bleeding, but this is for the most part very much more safely effected by local abstraction of blood. The best mode of doing this is by leeches, for cupping is apt to frighten the patient.

In cases of nymphomania, of suppression of the catamenia, and of suppression of hæmorrhoids, leeches are of very great importance applied periodically. Dr. Watson has some valuable remarks upon the subject of general bleeding: he says, "the state of constitution may be such that the disposition to local plethora would be increased by the loss of blood. Disordered action, and undue susceptibility of the nervous system, are apt to be aggravated by bleeding, and in proportion as the nervous functions are irregularly performed does the tendency to unequal distribution of blood in the capillary vessels augment: we have daily examples of this in hysterical young women. It is not, therefore, the mere congestion that we have to consider; we must look deeper for its cause."

If you were called in to see an epileptic patient, and found him in a state of profound coma, you would order him to be bled; it is a matter of life and death; but you would be very sure that the fits would come on more frequently. So, in insanity, you may find it absolutely necessary to employ venæsectio—in cases, for instance, with vertigo from plethora—but you would do it at the risk of producing nervous irritability. M. Foville was an advocate for the employment of general bleeding when at the Hospital near Rouen; it would be interesting to know whether he still holds the same opinion since his appointment to Charenton The enervated inhabitants of a capital would not so well endure the abstraction of blood as the hardy and robust peasants of the lower Seine.

Of counter-irritants.—Blisters are very generally employed in the treatment of insanity ; in the acute stage of mania, however, they should never be used ; certainly not till the heat of skin and general irritation from the loaded vessels have subsided. I need not dwell here upon the several modes of action of blisters ; they must be familiar to you already.

I have only to recommend you in insanity to employ the acetum instead of the emplastrum lyttæ as a general rule, as you will find it more convenient ; the present acetum lyttæ of the Pharmacopœia acts with sufficient certainty, and generally speaking uniformly.

In some cases of insanity which run their course sluggishly, or where there is a healed ulcer, or a suppressed discharge, setons are of great service. Esquirol says they act as if by enchantment. The Ung. Antim. Pot. Tart. proves beneficial in some cases of suppressed eruptions, and as a counter-irritant.

Strychnine, either given internally or mixed with prepared lard, and rubbed along the spine, I have found serviceable in the few cases of catalepsy in which I have tried it. It is also useful in cases of insanity accompanied with paralysis.

When patients have illusions of hearing, M. Foville suggests that cotton on which laudanum has been dropped should be put in their ears. I have tried this, and have in one or two cases found it beneficial. In cases of this description it is likewise of use to order the ears to be syringed, or to place small blisters behind each ear, in order to divert the attention of the patient from the noises and whisperings on which his imagination dwells.

The function of the skin is frequently badly performed in insanity. The peculiar smell which some madmen have I have often heard spoken of by those who have had much experience in these cases, and I always attributed it to the uncleanliness of the patient, but since my attention has been more particularly drawn to it I think that the peculiar odour is due to the disease : when it exists, however, it is a very unfavourable sign ; the only thing I can compare it to is the smell of a person just prior to dissolution. Baths of all descriptions have very properly been recommended to ensure the due performance of this important function. In the hospital we employ hot and cold baths, the hip bath, the shower bath, pediluvia, and the douche. The tepid bath is of great service in subduing irritability and excite-

ment. It is sometimes necessary that the patient should remain in it for an hour and a half, or two hours. Ice or cold lotions to the head should be applied at the same time : it may be necessary to repeat it every day, sometimes twice daily, till some effect is produced.

If the irritation is not subdued by the application, I have found it beneficial to apply a blister to the nape of the neck immediately that the patient leaves the bath.

In acute dementia, I have seen much benefit derived from the douche, but this is a remedy which requires caution, and is not by any means to be ordered for those patients who are liable to congestion of the head, or have any tendency to paralysis.

The shower bath, with antispasmodics, is a valuable means of subduing the symptoms of madness with hysteria and hypochondriasis.

When a patient has passed into what is termed the chronic stage of the complaint it by no means follows that nothing is to be done for him ; something can be effected by medicine even here, in shortening the paroxysms of furor, in procuring sleep for the restless, and improving the general health of the debilitated.

It now only remains for me to speak of the manner in which the different species of the complaint should be treated : this I propose to do by placing examples before you of mania, monomania, puerperal mania, acute dementia, and general paralysis. When the cases are read you will probably be better able to understand my reasons for adopting the plan of treatment.

In summing up the observations which I have made in these lectures, it will not be necessary for me to recapitulate what I have said as to the mode of treatment ; as to the nature of the disease, however, I wish to remind you that I stated it as my opinion that insanity, properly so called, was either primarily or secondarily a disease of the brain ; that sometimes the irritation is due to the nerves, sometimes to the blood ; thus proving the relation of the disorder to those diseases which are accompanied by congestion, in that it is apt to recur ; and, on the other hand, to those of the nervous system, in that it is often intermittent. Irritation is not to be rejected as a cause of insanity merely on account of there being something in it which we cannot explain : we are quite justified in such an obscure disease in appealing to effects, although the knife of the anatomist fails to point out to us any characteristic distinction in the minute alterations of structure which take place in the delicate granular matter, or in the thin filaments of the fibrous structure in the brain of the insane. Were we able to show this first departure from healthy structure under a powerful lens, I think that we should find it to be an alteration differing in degree, and not in kind, from that presumed to exist in other diseases of the nervous system. I believe that insanity, divested of the halo of metaphysics with which it is sometimes surrounded in order to dazzle and bewilder, is a disease which is subject to the same laws of pathology as all other diseases; still I acknowledge that it is a very obscure disorder, perhaps the most complicated one to which man is subject, and I do not presume to dictate upon a subject so abstruse. It might, perhaps, have been more satisfactory to some had I attempted to trace all the phenomena of insanity to one source—for instance, inflammation : a theory of disease which professes to account for every thing, which reduces the various symptoms into a systematic arrangement, and refers them to one cause, is sure to be popular, because it saves men the trouble of thinking for themselves ; and having once obtained possession of the mind it becomes very difficult to eradicate : but before we attempt such a task we shall do well to recollect the words of the great master of inductive science—" Another error," says Bacon, " to the advancement of learning is the over-early and peremptory reduction of knowledge into arts and methods." I have not thought it necessary to state all the theories of the nature of insanity ; what I have endeavoured to do has been to make my observations on this part of my subject tend as far as possible to some practical use. It would, indeed, have been an unprofitable task to have gone through them all, for there are few diseases which have been explained by more various and opposite theories than madness. One fatal error has been, the mistaking the causes for the disease itself : it is this that has led to the theory that insanity is a disease of the mind ; it is this which has been the cause of the notion that madness consists in a wrong action of the soul. Another theory of recent date would tend to make the subject still more complicated : Leibnitz, in his doctrine of " Pre-established Harmony," and Malebranche, in that of " Occasional Causes," were bold enough to decide the manner in which mind acted upon matter ; there does not, however, appear to be the slightest reason for supposing that the one does not act directly upon the other, and there seems to be no cause for believing that a *tertium quid*, some subtle entity, is necessary to keep up the mutual action of the material upon the immaterial portion of our being. To say that " electricity is the connecting link between mind and matter," is to assume what has not yet been proved ; and if we imagine that we have advanced one step in the explanation of this subject, or in our

knowledge of the nature of mind, we very greatly deceive ourselves ; electricity is itself a principle of matter, and as such is subject to the laws which bind matter. How mind acts upon matter, and matter upon mind, we cannot explain. Future observations and experiments may make us more perfectly acquainted with the instrument of mind, the brain, and the exact change of structure which prevents its minute fibres ministering to the will, but it is not easy to imagine that we shall ever be able to discover how the one acts upon the other. Locke, Leibnitz, Malebranche, have all failed in their attempts to solve this most difficult problem. There are bounds to all sciences, beyond which we cannot rove ; we have a clear perception only of few things, all else is either obscurely seen in the twilight of probability, or hid in darkness.

ON THE
TISSUE UPON WHICH THE REMOTE ACTION OF POISONS IS EXERTED.

BY W. WATTS, M.D.
Honorary Physician to the Nottingham Union Dispensary.

(*For the London Medical Gazette.*)

[Concluded from page 473.]

THE following experiment made by Magendie is taken from Morgan and Addison's Essay, page 39.

" The femoral artery and vein of the animal" (a dog, previously stupified with opium) " having been divided on one side, the continuity of the canal was re-established by the intervening connecting medium of small cylinders of quill to which the truncated extremities of the vessels were attached, and through which quills consequently the blood passed in the usual course of the circulation. With the exception of the femoral artery and vein, thus divided, and reconnected by quills, the limb was then amputated from the body, so that in this case the separated member was deprived of all nervous connection with the body, at the same time that circulation was allowed to continue through its main vessels. The poison of upas was then applied to a wound in the severed limb ; which produced its effects upon the system after the lapse of the interval of time usual under the common circumstances."

Thus we see that the cerebro-spinal system is not the remote recipient of impressions made by poisonous agents.

If, then, the brain and spinal cord,

The influence of the central ganglia seems to be moderated or altered by the lesser ganglia.—Sec. 35, 36.

It seems probable, from the circumstance of a separate ganglion or plexus, or both, of the ganglial system, being generally assigned to each important secreting or animalizing organ, that the centre or source of vital influence does not supply the whole vitality distributed by the ganglial ramifications to the individual organs or textures, but that the vital influence proceeding from this centre is reinforced and modified by that which is produced by the subordinate ganglia, so as to give rise (with the difference of structure) to the specific difference of function which each performs.—Sec. 40.

6thly, The general diffusion of vital influence.

The vital influence being thus produced in the centre of the body, and reinforced and modified by subordinate ganglia allotted to the individual organs, according to their functions, is propagated along the distributions of the system on which it depends, and is inherent throughout the whole body.—Sec. 41.

The remote action of poisons upon the sympathetic system of nerves is alike deducible by reasoning and demonstrable by experiment.

As all the organs of our frame require to be endowed with nervous influence before they can offer any manifestation of action, and that innervation can be derived but from two sources, if it can be shown, as I trust I have, that one of those sources (the cerebro-spinal) is not in any way *remotely* affected by poisons, and that they produce their effects under all possible variation of circumstances, as regards these organs, as of integrity of structure and of medium of communication, it must follow as a natural consequence that it is by the other (the sympathetic system) that the remote impressions of poisons are received, and that all the effects of those impressions manifested by distant organs must arise from the connexion which exists between this system and those organs, through which connexion they receive a modification, either in kind or degree, of that influence, a healthy condition of which is necessary to the proper performance of their functions.

The following experiments demonstrate the truth of the above conclusion, as in each instance the poison was applied to a part upon which nerves from the sympathetic alone ramify, and its influence is exerted upon the fibre of an involuntary muscle, the irritability of which is solely dependent upon the sympathetic system.

"But a still more striking example of the immediate action of a poison upon the part to which it is applied was afforded during one of our experiments upon a dying guinea-pig, by the accidental contact of a very minute portion of ticunas with the still living intestine. In this case the consequence was a complete and instantaneous suspension of the peristaltic motion in that part of the bowel to which the poison was immediately applied; and in repeating the application of the poison to other parts of the intestinal canal in the same animal, we found precisely the same local paralysis was produced*."

"The most unequivocal instance I know of a similar impression on internal parts, is a fact related by Dr. Wilson Philip with regard to opium: when this poison was applied to the inner coat of the intestines of a rabbit during life, the muscular contractions of the gut were immediately paralysed, without the general system being for some time affected†."

This brings us to the consideration of the second proposition under our immediate notice: viz. the capability of the organ remotely acted upon to manifest its reception of the impression made by poisons upon it.

When the function of a system or organ is to exert control over others, and to endow them with that innervation which enables their structures to perform their proper functions in a healthy manner, we must look to those organs so endowed for manifestations of derangement in the source of the innervating power; and if they offer no organic change in their structure sufficient to account for the existing error in function, we are entitled to attribute that error to deviation, either in kind or degree, from the healthy standard of the nervous influence which

---

* Morgan and Addison's Essay, p. 63.
† Christison on Poisons, p. 2.

controls and regulates their motions. And again, when we see a large number of organs, unconnected with each other, but each dependent upon the same system of nerves for the influence which actuates them, simultaneously presenting derangements in their functions, without offering any structural change in each as the cause of that deviation, we must look to the nervous centre which supplies them all for the remote cause of their various functional lesions, and are justified in attributing to it the remote deviation from the normal state; and also in looking upon the various derangements of the organs it supplies as the proximate effects of that remote action, and as arising from their being actuated by an abnormal controlling power.

Now, as all the organs which are subservient to the maintenance of organic life are under the control of the great sympathetic system of nerves, when any material deviation in their action from its normal condition occurs, not the effect of structural change, it must, I contend, be attributed to deviation from the healthy standard of that nervous influence; and we must attribute to the system generating it the remote cause of the proximate derangement of function. I shall now proceed to show that the *remote* action of poisons is upon the great sympathetic, and their effects are produced in strict accordance with the laws of that system.

The sympathetic system is affected both *locally* and *generally*.

Each part of our frame seems to possess the power, to a certain extent, of generating organic nervous influence by means of the action of its parenchyma, endowed with sufficient vitality, acting upon healthy arterial blood; and this power is not entirely destroyed, though it is certainly diminished, by separation of the part from its continuity with the centre of the great sympathetic system. The reason for this is thus described by the late Dr. Fletcher[*] :—"But it is probable that no impediment whatever is offered to the function of a ganglionic nerve by such a division as would entirely paralyse one from the cerebro-spinal system. Such is the case with the latter, only because the white matter of the

nerve being dependent for its energy, in all probability, upon the grey matter of the central parts of this system, becomes, of course, inert when separated from it. But no such line of demarcation exists in the ganglionic system; every point of every nerve of which contains white and grey matter intimately interwoven together, and may be considered, therefore, as a centre of nervous energy to itself (Bichât) : and it is in this way only that it can be explained how the total removal of a muscle from the rest of the body, which implies a division as well of its blood-vessels as of its nerves, is not, for some time, effectual in destroying its irritability." How far this explanation may be anatomically correct I am not capable of deciding; but the facts which it is put forward to elucidate are perfectly known to every surgeon; as, for instance, the re-union of parts which have been entirely separated from the system. This accounts for an independent *local* action of the great sympathetic system.

It has also a *general* action. That it is capable of exerting a power over all the organs to which it is distributed is undoubted, but that the derangement in each individual organ should be different in kind, though similar in degree, seems difficult to comprehend at first sight; yet if we remember that difference of structure, though actuated by the same innervating principle, and acting upon the same fluid, the blood, produces difference in its secretions, the apparent anomaly disappears. The following passage from the same work as the preceding seems to offer a very satisfactory physical reason for it[*]. "The last circumstance to be mentioned, as tending to the conclusion that the ganglionic system of nerves is the immediate seat of irritability, is that of the nerves of this system, while they are of a similar form, colour, and consistence, when distributed on parts the irritability of which is of the same character—that is to say, which are liable to be excited in the same manner by the same stimuli—being quite dissimilar in all these respects when they supply parts the irritability of which is different. Thus, while the filaments going from the ganglions to the several voluntary muscles, all of which have one general

* Rudiments of Physiology : by Dr. Fletcher, p. 74.

* Page 86.

character of irritability, are said to display the same general aspect and physical properties, those which proceed from the cæliac ganglion, for example, respectively to the stomach, liver, and other organs, (each of which has a character of irritability, however, to itself) have these properties very distinct; those sent to the stomach being conical, white, and firm; those to the liver, cylindrical, red, and soft; and similar differences manifesting themselves between the filaments respectively of the splenic, mesenteric, hypogastric, and other plexuses. (Lobstein). This remarkable coincidence, then, if generally admitted, of certain modifications of a common faculty, as displayed by different organs, and corresponding modifications of a common system of nerves, as distributed to these different organs, seems to be a strong testimony in favour of the doctrine that this general system of nerves ministers directly to the general faculty in question."

In conformity with these laws of the great sympathetic systems, poisons act remotely upon it both *locally* and *generally.*

The examples of a *local* action of poison have been given in the two experiments quoted from Morgan and Addison, and Wilson Philip, and others will present themselves to the minds of every one of my readers. I need not, therefore, adduce others. The poison, in producing only a local action, seems to be applied in such a quantity, or upon such a surface, that but a very small quantity is capable of acting at the same time; so that the effect of the impression of the particles first acting partly subsides before those acting later are capable of effecting their impression; or if all the particles applied do act at once, then the impression they create is of so slight a nature, as not, should it be felt by the central portions of the system, to be able to act upon it so as to cause the impulse they communicate to modify the nervous influence thence proceeding in such a degree as to cause the other organs supplied by it to evince derangement in the performance of their functions; while a *general* action is the effect of a poison applied in such a form, and in a sufficient quantity, upon such a surface as to create upon the organic nerves in its substance impres-

sions of so powerful a nature as that they are propagated to the central ganglia, and there act upon it in such a manner as to modify the influence transmitted thence to all its related organs and structures; that modification varying from the very slightest alteration to extreme excitement or complete extinction.

Having stated upon what tissue the remote effects of poisons are exerted, and in what manner that tissue may be affected, I shall now proceed to notice the action of poisons upon the blood; a point more conveniently discussed here than previously.

Wedemeyer's and Marshall Hall's experiments, in each of which the spinal cord was divided, and one of the hind extremities inoculated, in one instance, with hydrocyanic acid, and in the other with strychnia, and in which the muscles supplied by nerves given off from the cord above the section were influenced by the poison, as well as those below, have countenanced the supposition that the poison was absorbed, and, being carried into the circulation, would be equally applied to the upper as well as the lower part of the spinal cord, and so stimulate each' to the production of the tetanic affection in the muscles they supplied. But this theory, viz. that these actions were the consequence of the immediate application of the poison to the spinal cord by means of its absorption and general diffusion through the blood, is open to the following objections:—

1st, If this position were correct, then should the action of the poison upon the lower portion of the spinal cord be simultaneous with that upon the upper : yet in Dr. Hall's experiment an interval of thirty minutes intervened between the appearance of the spasms in the anterior extremities and the hind ones. 2dly. We have seen that neither the brain or spinal cord are in the slightest degree affected when a poison is directly applied to their substance. And, 3dly, Because the symptoms are more probably produced by the impression of the poison being *remotely* exerted upon the great sympathetic, there inducing a modification of the influence transmitted from it to the spinal cord through those fibrillæ which pass to it from the sympathetic to the intervertebral foramina ; the interval between the occurrence of the tetanic symptoms in the opposite extremities being produced by the lower portion of the spinal cord having its structure injured, and its cerebral influence cut off by means of the section.

In these cases of poisoning, the tetanus was the *proximate* affection of the spinal cord, the effect of the *remote* action of the great sympathetic system upon it, and not the remote effect itself.

That poisons are absorbed into the circulation of the blood by veins, I think few who have paid any attention to the subject will deny; certainly, I am not among that number: but I cannot agree with Mr. Blake* that they act by being allowed to enter the circulation, and by being directly applied to the tissue the functions of which are affected. Whenever a poison is absorbed, if it be from the periphery of the body, then it is taken by the veins directly into the right side of the heart, and thence passes into the lungs: or if it be absorbed by the portal veins, it passes directly into the liver: in the ultimate divisions of each of these viscera the most important changes are effected in its constitution. In order that these alterations may be effected, the acini of the liver and the bronchial vesicles of the lung are largely endowed with organic nerves from the plexuses and ganglia appropriated to each of these structures; and it is upon these nerves there expanded that the primary impressions of poisons are made when they are absorbed, and not by being carried by the arterial circulation into the various organs whose functions are proximately affected.

The phenomena attendant upon the absorption of white lead confirm this view. Those who are in the habit of working in it, if they use the necessary precautions, do not suffer from the paralysis it othewise induces, but if they do not, the lead passes through the cuticle and becomes absorbed. Now the paralysis thus produced is entirely a local one, and seems to be caused by the lead acting upon the nervous influence generated in the part itself to which it is applied, it being greatest in the muscles which produce the lesser movements of the fingers, and less so in those which move the hand upon the fore-arm. The action of the lead in this instance is by

remotely affecting the source of irritability in the muscular fibres, destroying it in the hand, and diminishing it in the fore-arm, and not by acting upon the spine, for the act of volition is obeyed by those muscles which still retain their irritability, as may be seen in the slight remains of voluntary motion in the wrist, which irritability is the result of the local action of an influence partly derived from the central ganglia of the sympathetic, and partly generated in the muscular fibre by the action of the former upon healthy arterial, by means of the muscular parenchyma. Such a local paralysis would not result if it were caused by the lead being absorbed by the veins then passing into the arterial system, and so being conveyed by it to the muscles of the hand and fore-arm; for if it were, then should the muscles of the latter be as completely affected as those of the hand, which is not the case; and also, all the other voluntary muscles in the body should be paralysed, which they are not, though the constant presence of the blue line in the gums in these cases fairly shows that the lead is absorbed, has been taken into the arterial system, and has been deposited from it. Nor can the remote action be upon the elements of the blood. This fluid, being possessed of vital as well as material properties, a natural condition of each of which is necessary to its full action in the system, can be affected either as to its vitality or as to its material constitution. If a poison act upon the blood, destroying its vitality, without affecting any previous change in its chemical properties, and that vitality be derived from the action of the organic nervous influence, then I infer that its action is remotely exerted upon the source of that influence. But if the composition of the blood be altered by the poison, then, also, I contend that the action is previously upon the source of its vitality, for the first law of life is, "that it preserves material particles in such chemical relations as to prevent other chemical relations from inducing disorganization." Thus, if a poison act upon the blood so as to induce any chemical alteration in the relation of its particles, that very alteration necessarily implies a previous alteration in the kind or degree of the nervous influence which bestows vitality upon the blood, and

* Edinburgh Med. and Surg. Journ. vol. liii. p. 37.

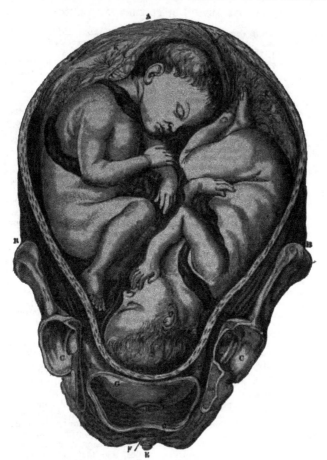

do not return, rupture the membranes, tighten the binder, and bring down the lower extremities, and deliver the child in the manner already described when the nates present, No good can in any case be produced by allowing the child to remain longer in the uterus than an hour after the birth of the first.

If a shoulder or superior extremity of the second child presents, proceed immediately to perform the operation of turning, which is easy and safe both for the mother and child, if you pass up the hand into the uterus, before the membranes are ruptured.

In twin cases, where the head of the second child presents, apply the binder, rupture the membranes, and the uterus will *probably contract upon* the child and expel it without any artificial assistance. If, however, the labour has been very protracted, and there is great exhaustion, and some risk lest the natural powers should be insufficient for the delivery of the second child, I am disposed to think, as the operation of turning is so easily accomplished, that it would be better at once to have recourse to it, than to trust to the forceps if further assistance should be required. At all events it is invariably necessary to rupture the second set of membranes, if you determine to leave the expulsion of the second child to nature, for the uterus may remain twenty-four hours or longer quiescent if this is not done. After the delivery of both children, always remember the danger of uterine hæmorrhage.

CLINICAL LECTURES

ON THE

THEORY & MEDICAL TREATMENT
OF INSANITY,

Delivered at St. Luke's Hospital,

May 1st, 3d, and 5th.

BY ALEXANDER JOHN SUTHERLAND.

———

LECTURE III.—(concluded.)

*Of Narcotics; use and abuse of opium.
— Sedatives. — Hydrocyanic acid. —
Digitalis. — Diuretics. — Tonics. — Mi-
neral tonics. — Of blood-letting, leeches,
cupping.—Counter-irritants.—Setons.—
Baths.—Antispasmodics.—Conclusion.*

NARCOTICS are placed by some in the first
rank of remedies in the treatment of madness. Much difference of opinion exists as
to the propriety of prescribing them.
Esquirol says, "that these are rather injurious than useful, especially if there be
plethora, or congestion about the head.
Long since, Valsalva and Morgagni proscribed opiates, and daily experience confirms the opinion of these great masters.
Diet, employment, exercise, are the true
remedies for sleeplessness; tepid or cold
baths induce sleep, and are truly efficacious,
and no bad results ever followed their use."
Some authors and practical men of the
present day join with M. Esquirol's opinion upon this subject. Dr. Cox considered that opium produced no permanent
effect upon the insane.

On the other hand, we find medical men
of great experience in the treatment of this
disease, who prescribe it in large doses, and
some, too, who think it possesses in these
complaints virtues almost of a specific
nature. Dr. Halloran, as quoted by Crowther, speaks of certain cases where sleep
had been a stranger for 48 hours in succession, and where he had no doubt, but
for the intervention of an opiate to the extent of 240 drops of the tincture of opium,
at three short intervals, no rest could have
been procured: he goes on to state that
sleep approaching to apoplexy had been obtained in consequence, for nearly 24 hours,
and that it was evidently the means of
effecting an entire and lasting return of the
mental faculty." Crowther says, the same
effect was produced in the cases in which he
employed it. His patients were relieved
from insanity after waking out of a long and
sound sleep. The same effect has been
stated to me to have been produced in some
cases under the care of Mr. Phillips, at the
White House, Bethnal Green. Dr. Ogle
and Mr. Wintle, of the Oxford Asylum, are

likewise in the habit of prescribing large
doses of these medicines, which have also
found an able advocate in Dr. Seymour for
their employment. What is to be said,
when we find such difference of opinion
among practical men ? M. Foville has truly
said, that the particular cases of insanity in
which narcotics are useful have not been
clearly pointed out. My own experience
would lead me to the conclusion, that opiates
are of essential service in those cases of
insanity which border closely upon delirium
tremens ; in cases of puerperal mania ; in
the first breaking out of an attack of madness, before congestion has taken place ; in
cases where there is great nervous irritability, from poverty of blood ; and in cases
of cachexia from starvation, and other
causes : they are contraindicated wherever
there is the least sign of general paralysis or
congestion about the head. Prescribed indiscriminately, or not in proper doses, narcotics
do more harm than good ; they keep up
irritation, and add to the excitement, instead
of allaying it. I have seen sometimes a very
simple case converted into a very complicated one by the excessive use of narcotics.
There is an idiosyncrasy, as every one knows,
in some constitutions which does not admit of
the exhibition of narcotics, especially morphia, even in the smallest dose : $\frac{1}{8}$th of a
grain will sometimes produce such incessant
vomiting as to endanger the life of the patient. Great care also should be taken, even
when the use of opiates is indicated, not to
continue them too long, for if narcotization
is produced, much harm will follow : the
evacuations are hard and black ; the irritation is extreme.

It must not be thought that opium and
morphia are entirely to supersede other
narcotics ; there are others, as hyoscyamus
and conium, which are equally serviceable in
the treatment of insanity. I am often in
the habit of prescribing the hyoscyamus ; I
find that it agrees better with the stomach,
and it does not constipate the bowels : in
fact, we know from experience that it has
an opposite tendency, and it likewise increases the secretion of the kidneys and of
the skin. Combined with the potassio-tartrate of antimony it is serviceable in the
paroxysms of furor ; considerable lassitude
is apt to follow when a draught containing
ʒj. of the tinct. of the former, with gr. $\frac{1}{4}$ of
the latter, is administered. This, in some
cases, is of course not to be desired.

Combined with camphor, opium allays
the irritability of those suffering under madness, either combined with some degree of
delirium tremens, or preceded by it.

Conium has high antiquity to recommend
it, and is useful both given alone or in combination with hyoscyamus and opium. The
boasted effects of camphor have not been

which, did it remain unimpaired, would effectually have prevented any change.

Affirming that the great sympathetic system is the tissue remotely acted upon by poisons, I will now proceed to strengthen this position by shewing the very close similarity which exists between the effects of direct injury upon the former, and the symptoms produced by poisons.

The consequences of direct injury either upon a ganglion of the great sympathetic system, or a part very largely endowed with nerves from it, may be thus divided:—

1st, Sudden and immediate death.

2d, Gradual sinking of the vital powers.

3d, Death after reaction from lesion of any organ the healthy performance of whose function is necessary to the continuance of life.

The two first of these modes of death merge into each other. I shall therefore consider them together.

Sudden and immediate death follows blows upon the epigastrium, or over any of the lesser ganglia, where they are so situated as to be liable to compression—as, for instance, the middle cervical ganglion. Death from the former injury is, unfortunately, not uncommon, two cases having fallen under my own observation; and of the latter a very melancholy instance occurred, towards the close of the last year, in Ireland. Two medical gentlemen, one of whom had lately returned from India, were taking soda-water with each other; one of them, while loosening the cork of one of the bottles, held it in such a direction as that when the wires were cut the cork was driven with force against his friend, striking him violently on the neck, and causing almost an immediate death.

When parts largely supplied with nerves from the sympathetic system, as the testicles and kidneys, are suddenly and violently injured, death takes place without any of the signs of reaction appearing. The symptoms which precede it are thus described by Dr. Copland:— "paleness; entire loss of muscular power; a most distressing death-like sensation; coldness of the skin, which is damp and pale; slow and feeble respiration; pulse feeble, slow, irregular, intermitting, scarcely to be felt; the eyes are fixed; the countenance collapsed; lips pale; the surface and extremities become quickly cold; the muscles are flaccid; the joints pliable; and in some instances the sphincters relaxed. If the powers of life be not rallied at this time, all these phenomena increase, until the action of the heart and respiration entirely cease."

Life is also extinguished in each of these two ways through the action of some kinds of poisons. Magendie, describing the action of hydrocyanic acid, resembled it to the effect of a common shot, or thunder-bolt; he found that one drop of pure hydrocyanic acid, placed on the tongue of the most vigorous dog, causes it to fall dead after two or three hurried respirations; and that if the nose of a rabbit be introduced into a receiver filled with hydrocyanic vapour, the animal drops dead *instantly*[*]. Sir B. Brodie applied the essential oil of bitter almonds to the tongue of a cat, in consequence of which the life of the animal was instantly destroyed. Dr. Christison says he has killed an animal outright in four seconds: and that Pelletier and Caventou found strychnia begin to act in fifteen seconds.

It is recorded[†], that at the time the plague was raging at Marseilles "the men who were employed by the merchants to carry the infected goods from the ships to the warehouses fell down and suddenly expired, from the first impression made upon the system by the effluvia arising from the burdens which they were carrying." Death without reaction follows the bite of the rattlesnake, and ticunas; inoculation with the woorara, woorali, and the upas poisons; after poisoning by tobacco, oxalic acid, and others. In both these instances of death following injury or poisoning, the symptoms are the same; those following the action of poisons being, according to Dr. Christison, "deadly paleness; extreme prostration of strength; feeble, irregular, and depressed pulse; mortal fainting, and coldness of the extremities."

The third mode of death, from the proximate disease of some important organ, resulting from the remote action of poisons upon the sympathetic, is also common to them and to injuries. Regarding the possibility of the occurrence of a chain of action necessary to its production, it may, perhaps, be questioned, how is it possible for any

* Christison.
† Morgan and Addison's Essay, p. 29.

agent, not a poison, applied to any part of the body, to induce symptoms of disease or derangement in distant organs? To this it may be replied, that as the impressions of these agents are received remotely by a system of nerves common to every part of the frame, there need be no difficulty in assenting to this proposition, which has been, in fact, recognised in pathology from the infancy of medicine. It is through their mutual connexion with the great sympathetic system that injuries of the head, or testes, induce sickness or other derangement of the stomach: that urticaria follows the ingestion of improper food into the same viscus: that the mammæ are enlarged before the catamenial discharge: the manifestations of mind are affected by the state of the alimentary canal: that the functions of the spinal cord are affected when convulsions result from the presence of indigestible aliment or worms in the primæ viæ: that ascarides induce cough; that hæmorrhoids are at times accompanied with frequent and forcible efforts at micturition. In the same conformity with this principle of proximate derangement of function in distant organs, depending upon the remote action of a central common influence, we see tobacco producing pallor, sickness, relaxation of muscular fibre, syncope, and irregularity in, or cessation of, the heart's action: cantharides, though applied to the skin, inducing stranguary, or stimulating the spinal cord to the production of convulsions: opium exciting the cerebro-spinal system to increased activity, while, at the same time, it deranges the liver and the stomach: strychnia acting as tonic to the stomach, and producing twitching in the voluntary muscular fibres: oxalic acid inducing coma, sudden death by paralysis of the heart, or tetanic spasms; and by its action upon this common centre it is that arsenic, wherever applied, so often induces vomiting, while it can produce, also, inflammation "in the throat, gullet, stomach, and intestines, the lining membrane of the nostrils and eyelids, the bladder, vagina, and kidneys," and is able to act upon the brain, the heart, and lungs: evidences of every one of these effects being, at times, found in the same person[*].

* Christison.

Having, I trust, satisfactorily shewn that death or disease may follow impressions made upon the great sympathetic system, and that the mode in which the former occurs, and the symptoms which characterise the latter, are not essentially different from those produced by the remote action of poisons, I am compelled to believe that action is upon the great sympathetic system of nerves.

The full comprehension of this most interesting subject is not to be attained until the manner in which circumstances affect the production of the effects of poisons, such as, for instance, age, sex, idiosyncrasy, states of nervous and vascular system, dose, &c. To the elucidation of these influences I shall devote another paper.

CONTRIBUTIONS
TO
ANATOMY AND PHYSIOLOGY.

By ROBERT KNOX, M.D. F.R.S.E.

Lecturer on Anatomy and Physiology, and Corresponding Member of the French Academy of Medicine.

[Continued from p. 467.]

On some Varieties in Human Structure, with Remarks on the Doctrine of "Unity of the Organization."

Osseous system.—The cranium.

A FEW years ago, there was reported in a weekly journal, but very briefly, the case of a labouring man, who falling from a scaffolding, or having been accidentally knocked down in some way or other, was carried senseless and motionless into one of the largest metropolitan hospitals. The distinguished surgeon into whose hands this patient came having examined his head carefully, discovered on its surface a remarkable depression, and assuming this to be the probable cause of the loss of sense and motion, he proposed the application of the trephine as the most appropriate remedy. But, fortunately for the patient and for the surgeon, the patient's wife appeared in the hospital, and the nature of the operation, *with the reasons for operating*, having been explained to her, she objected to its being proceeded with on the following very sufficient grounds: viz. that ever since she became acquainted with her husband, the patient, his head had always presented that identical depression, and therefore—but I may leave her conclusions (with which the surgeon agreed) to every sound reasoner. The patient, if I remember right, recovered without the performance of any operation. Now, I had seen similar cases before, or at least some very puzzling appearances on the surface of the cranium in persons otherwise quite well, and great difficulties have occasionally arisen as to how the surgeon ought to act; but I am not quite sure that anatomy can always furnish him with the means for arriving at a sound judgment: in two circumstances, however, I think it may assist in the arriving at a correct diagnosis; the first great object of the surgeon no less than of the physician. An incision, as an exploratory step, made in the scalp so as to expose the cranium, may appear to many by no means a formidable operation, and this undoubtedly is true; but neither is the extirpating a trifling corn on the toes an important matter, and yet an estimable lady lost her life a few days ago in the hands of a distinguished professor of surgery in this place, in consequence of submitting to so very simple an operation.

If a considerable number of crania be examined (I mean of crania as they are preserved in museums) a certain few will exhibit the following peculiarity: along nearly the whole line of the lambdoidal or parieto-occipital suture the occipital bone will occasionally so overlap the parietal, or at least be so raised above it, as to give the false appearance of a deep depression of the parietal. This singular overlapping of these bones, or perhaps rather elevation of the occipital, I find, on examining the museum, to be by no means infrequent, and in various heads to present a great variety of appearances, agreeing, however, all in this, that on passing the hand from the occipital to the parietal bones a sudden depression will be felt, occasioned by the greater elevation of the former. The second circumstance in respect to such elevations at various points of the cranium is even more interesting than the first; it is of rarer occurrence, and more likely, therefore, to lead the surgeon into error. The elevation occurs in the line of the fronto-parietal suture, and is caused by an overlapping of the parietal by the frontal bone, or at least

by a greater elevation of the former. Of at least a hundred crania in the museum, there is not one showing this variety in its form, at least to any extent; and a specimen exhibited by Dr. J. A. Robertson to the Anatomical and Physiological Society was the first I had an opportunity of carefully examining. What made this case peculiarly interesting was its occurrence in a person who had met with a severe injury to the head, which ultimately proved fatal. The *seeming* depression close to the fronto-parietal suture was so great as nearly to induce the attending surgeons to apply the trephine; but the death of the person taking place very soon after enabled the medical attendant to discover the very serious error into which he must have fallen had he persisted in his intention of trephining: the real seat of injury was through the base of the skull, with fatal effusion of blood, altogether beyond the reach of the operator.

Before adverting to other varieties in form met with on the surface of the cranium, I may briefly notice the German transcendental theory, which endeavours to explain these varieties, to reduce them to a law, the law of " deformation," and to bring them within the range of the philosophy of animal beings. The theory, which must be well known to most of my hearers, is, that these "deformations" simply reproduce a structural form, which, however rare in man, and therefore in him "abnormal," will yet be found to be the regular law in many animals placed lower than man in the scale, and therefore are in them quite regular, or "normal." But why should they appear in man at all? This difficulty the German theorist meets by reminding you of another law, viz. unity of organization: that in the embryo there is unity of organization: that the embryo of most animals runs through certain phases or "developments:" that the earliest of these developments resemble, therefore, certain animals, and the latest, others: that should the change, from any cause whatever, known or unknown, not take place, there is then an imperfect development, " *arrêt de développement*," and that this may take place at any stage, giving even to the human form the peculiar arrangement of parts belonging to a lower class of animals, or retaining in the adult the embryonic form of its own organs. To apply these laws to the peculiarities in question, we have only to say with the German, that the human cranium, which, when fully developed, ought to present a uniform and comparatively smooth surface, and a series of immoveable sutures, has, in the fœtus, a totally different character; in it, the sutures are moveable, and slide freely over each other, in short, may be made to overlap each other; that when dried, prepared, and deposited in our museums, the fœtal head actually presents these appearances; that should the adult head present a similar form in some, it is merely an "*arrêt de développement;*" and finally, this very irregularity, by the great law of unity of organization, is the usual normal form in many species of the lower animals; in them the "arrest of development" is the law; in man it is the exception.

I shall afterwards endeavour to show that these are the only views which, in the present state of science, can be adopted, and that what has been written against them in France, and more especially in England, is simply, and, to use the mildest phrase, ingenious nonsense; sometimes very pompous and imposing, as in the Bridgewater Treatises, but still downright nonsense, and not meriting the smallest attention from any philosophic mind. The German theory, or rather the theory of Goethe, (for it is his) requires very considerable modification before it can be applied extensively to the history of organization. Let us proceed, in the meantime, with details.

On examining the museum to find the crania of those animals which ought, according to the theory, to present the peculiar form or forms above described as " anormal" in man, but " normal" in them, it is not so easy to find them. That such exist I have no doubt, but the examination of some hundred specimens of the crania of different mammaliæ has not furnished me with any clear illustrations of the law. By descending lower, however, in the scale, we must meet with them; the cranial bones of the Cetacea overlap each other at many points; and so more especially do those of fishes. The law of unity admits, nay requires, that we should include the entire scale in the inquiry after truth.

If we do not work with great num-bers, and on an extended scale, the theory cannot be supported on all occasions: it is a psychological and metaphysical theory, as well as a physical, and they who do not admit this, either do not understand it, or are unwilling to be informed as to its truth.

Of other appearances met with occasionally on the outer surface of the cranium I shall mention but a few. There are first those ridges, single or double, running in the line of, or parallel to and at a little distance from, the parietal suture, remarkably developed in a skull-cap now before me. These elevated parietal lines or cristæ, are simply the superior parietal crests generally not perceivable in the human cranium; at other times, as in this instance, quite distinct. They are of course quite common in many of the mammalia, but are only seen in some men. They may occupy the proper parietal suture, as in some animals, or be a little apart: they must not be confounded with the inferior parietal crest running continuously with the external frontal crest (also distinct enough in some men), and which, from the narrowness of the parietal bones in some mammals, approach close to the vertex, enlarging thus greatly the temporal fossæ: the crests I here allude to are different from these temporal crests, but may coincide in some animals: in man they do not, and this is owing in him to the great breadth of the parietal bones. But the crania of mammals present every variety in respect to the extent, direction, elevation, and number of these occipital, parietal, and frontal crests, whose outlines may all be seen on man, fortunately but little developed in him, the " arrest" being in him happily the law; the full development, on the contrary, being the law in the highest of the quadrumana.

It has always appeared to me, that these crests, although they be but imperfectly developed in man, ought to be named in accordance with their real nature and meaning; they have little or nothing to do with the history of the cranial sutures, whose course, indeed, they do not generally follow: the temporal crests of the frontal and parietal bones are continuous, running directly across the suture, which they do not regard; the occipital crest is on the occipital bone, and not in the lambdoidal suture, and the superior parietal crests when found in man do not seem to me to run in the parietal suture, but parallel to it; in many animals, however, there is a parietal crest continuous with the anterior branch of the occipital crest, directly in the line of the suture. The reason why such crests should be found on the surface of the cranium in different animals it seems to me impossible to say; even in my youngest days I had always philosophy enough in me to laugh at the Bridgewater nonsense (a theory all but exhausted by Philo, Derham, and Paley), which would assign to them the mechanical reason for " extending the attachments of certain muscles."

There is a slight remark more I beg leave to make in respect to these crests; they are not more fully developed in the darker race of men, than in the Saxon, Celt, or Pelasgian races : at least it appears so to me from all the specimens I have examined : if we are then to denominate them an " arrest of development" (although this is clearly a misnomer in one sense), it ought to be kept in view that the occurrence is in no shape peculiar to the dark races of men. Occasionally on the surface of the cranium we meet with an absolute depression, sudden, and as if scooped out at the expense of the outer table and diploe alone; nothing can be more likely to mislead the surgeon. I find them in crania which appear to me otherwise quite healthy, but still they may have been occasioned by a blow inflicted when young: even by the forceps of the accoucheur. If my recollection be correct, I think I remember a cranium which was presented by Sir G. Ballingall to the College of Surgeons, whose surface was completely notched and indented with blows; it belonged to a native of Australia. On the other hand, these depressions occasionally correspond with exostoses found projecting from the inner table, which possibly during life may have given rise to much distress.

There is a skull-cap now before me, and I can produce several others, in which such remarkable appearances are not limited to the exterior table; in this cranium the anterior half nearly of the inner table is rough, with sharp elevations; the bones are thickened generally, and at two points absorption had commenced in the inner

table, and all but perforated the bone, and still there is nothing visible on the outer table as regards this remarkable change in the interior of the frontal bone. What may be observed on the outer table is a prominence of the parietal sutures, and an elevation of the outer wall of the left frontal sinus : the prominence of the bone at this point during life would have strongly resembled an exostosis; and yet it is not so, but merely a general thickening of the outer table and diploe, extending from over the sinus to beyond the external angular process of the bone.

The last variety I shall allude to is that peculiar deformity, for it must be so called, which consists in a want of symmetry in its various parts.

About a year ago, a naval surgeon, who had formerly studied anatomy with me, had the obliging kindness to present me with a remarkable cranium; being no less than the cranium of one of the party who attacked and slew our immortal circumnavigator, Cook. This cranium, which I now place before my audience,* unquestionably belonged to a native of the Sandwich Isles; its resemblance to those crania met with in museums as Peruvian and Brazilian, is remarkable, more especially in respect to its want of symmetry, thus shewing an affiliation between the aborigines of the mainland of America and those of certain islands, but not of others, as of Van Diemen's Land for example, or Australia: the crania of the natives of these islands appeared to me different from that I now speak of. I shall consider the want of symmetry more in detail in a special lecture.

[To be continued.]

ON

MOLECULES AND MOLECULAR
MOTION.

To the Editor of the Medical Gazette.

Sir,

If the following observations are sufficiently interesting to occupy a place in your valuable journal, you will oblige me by inserting them.—I am, sir,

Your obedient servant,

J. W. Griffith, M.D. F.L.S. &c.

9, St. John's Square.
June 13, 1843.

---

* These contributions were mostly submitted to my anatomical class at various meetings.

I have been induced to offer a few observations on the nature and peculiarities of the minute particles into which ponderable bodies are often subdivided, and a form of spontaneous or innate motion which accompanies them under certain circumstances, in consequence of having perceived, in one of our latest treatises, and which is likely to be a most valuable one, on anatomy and physiology, the statement that the movements of molecules are " attributed to currents produced in the fluid by evaporation at its surface or edges, for they may be arrested by covering the fluid with oil."

I have, as must every one who has paid much attention to microscopic observations, long been acquainted with the peculiar movements of these minute atoms, and have often sought for the excitor of their motion, but in vain. Nor is the explanation of it, by evaporation, at all capable of solving the difficulty, as will be perceived when this paper has been perused.

The views of some of the older authors respecting the existence of certain definite molecules or particles, arising from the separation and decomposition of organic bodies, and their transmutations into animal and vegetable bodies, when placed under appropriate circumstances, are so curious, and so rarely noticed in the works of our own country, that they cannot fail to be interesting to the reader.

Buffon says, " Il me paroît donc très vraisemblable qu'il existe réellement dans la nature une infinité de petits êtres organisés, semblables en tout aux grands êtres organisés qui figurent dans le monde, que ces petits êtres organisés sont composés de parties organiques vivantes qui sont communes aux animaux et aux vegetaux, que ces parties organiques sont des parties primitives et incorruptibles, que l'assemblage de ces parties forme à nos yeux des êtres organisés, et que par conséquent la reproduction ou la generation n'est qu'un changement de forme qui se fait et s'opère par la seule addition de ces parties semblables, comme la destruction de l'être organisé se fait par la division de ces mêmes parties...... Detruire un être organisé n'est que séparer les parties organiques dont il est composé ; ces mêmes parties restent séparées jusqu'à ce qu'elles

soient reunies par quelque puissance active."

M. Buffon then goes on to say, that when this nutritious and reproductive matter, in passing through an animal or vegetable, finds a suitable matrix, it produces an animal or vegetable of the same kind, but when otherwise, it produces organised beings differing from plants and animals, as the bodies which move and grow, and as we see in the seminal fluid, in the infusions of the germs of plants, &c. These molecules were also noticed by our countryman Needham, on their exit from the pollen, when moistened.

Wrisberg, when examining some infusion of garden peas, observed in it some white flocculent matter; this, when dried, appeared reduced to minute granules : " repræsentat quasi convolutum illarum exilium molecularum, rudimenta procal dubio futurorum animalculorum." Wrisberg was fully aware of the inorganic nature of the molecules, and of their non-identity with the infusoria : thus, when examining infusion of parsley, he says, " myriades parvarum molecularum inorganicarum .... vidimus ; omnes hæ moleculæ eandem habent magnitudinem, quibusdam paucis exceptis, quæ minores sunt ...... Quædam harum molecularum jam motu voluntario agitabantur, admodum tardô autem, quasi viribus suis nondum confiderent libero sese exponendi oceano." After saying that we are too apt to attribute life to particles which move, he says ...... Multa sane dantur in natura motus, ubi ne minimum quidem animalium vestigium est; fere in uniuscujuscunque aquæ purissimæ guttulæ superficie, magisque autem ubi saponis quicquam admixtum est, particularum exilissimarum observamus motum, quamvis rationem illius vix reddere possimus."

O. F. Müller also imagined that the ultimate granules of organic matter became immediately reorganised and restored to life.

" Partes nempe animales et vegetabiles per decompositionem resolvuntur in pelliculas vesiculares, quarum vesiculæ seu globuli, sensim a massa communi laxati reviviscunt et animalcula spermatica et infusoria agunt."

Gleichen long since pointed out what he imagined to be the transformation of vegetable into animal matter : in

speaking of the pollen of plants, he says, " Quand on la laisse quelque tems dans l'eau, elle se métamorphose elle même en animalcules d'infusion."....
" et dans quelques jours toute ma poussierè* étoit devenu vivante."

Dr. Milne Edwards, after examining many of the tissues of animal bodies,† says, " Je n'étois pas éloigné de croire que les molécules animales, solides et organisés, affectent toujours une forme primitive, constante et determineé, celle de globules du diamètre d'environ $\frac{1}{300}$ de millimètre†."

The observations on the molecules of bodies, made by Dr. Brown, are the only definite and distinct ones I have met with. This most able observer first detected the motion of the particles within the pollen grains of Clarkia pulchella, then in that of some other Onagraiæ and Lolium; afterwards in all organic bodies; animal and vegetable tissues, whether living or dead; gum resins; pit coal; fossil wood; powdered glass; earths and metals; rocks, &c. In a word, in every mineral which could be reduced to a powder sufficiently fine to be temporarily suspended in water. Dr. Brown could not obtain them from resin, wax, sulphur, and such of the metals as could not be reduced to the minute state of division necessary for their separation; and soluble bodies. He further states the molecules to be spherical, and the elongated ones sometimes found to be aggregations of the simple ones; that they are of a uniform size, varying from $\frac{1}{15000}$ to $\frac{1}{20000}$ of an inch. Now it might perhaps be considered presumption on my part to call in question the accuracy of the observations of so distinguished a naturalist as Dr. Brown, but as the motion of these minute particles or molecules has been stated as depending upon the evaporation of the liquid in which they are immersed, notwithstanding Dr. Brown's assertion that " these motions were such as to satisfy me, after frequently repeated observation, that they arose neither from currents in the fluid, nor from its gradual evaporation," still, as evaporation is mentioned as having taken place in his experiments (thus he says, " on con-

tinuing to observe them until the water had entirely evaporated ;") I have very carefully repeated them, avoiding what I considered sources of fallacy.

In all cases where I examined the molecules, the glass slider (made of plate glass), was fixed horizontally, so as to avoid the influence of gravitation in causing currents. The fluid containing the molecules was covered by a layer of exceedingly thin glass, which of course prevents any evaporation taking place from the surface of the liquid it covers; the evaporation at the edges being prevented by a rim of olive, or almond oil, or lamp-black mixed with gold size (the ordinary mode of preserving microscopic objects). I have examined a large number of inorganic substances powdered in a mortar to the finest powder, and have found no difficulty in detecting the peculiar motion in any substance save semi-fluid bodies, or solids which cannot (whether from their tenacity or extreme hardness) be reduced to a sufficiently fine powder. Some bodies, as sulphur, cannot be reduced to a very fine powder, but loose floating particles can be here and there seen in the field of the microscope, which exhibit the motion most distinctly. Some precipitates which are extremely dense show this property with great difficulty, as the chloride of silver, &c. The motion is quite destroyed by immersion in oil, thick gum, or syrup; here the viscidity of the liquids seems to prevent its taking place. It has appeared to me to ensue most readily in water, less so in spirit, and least of all in ether. The extremely low sp. gr. of the substance seems in some cases to prevent the development of this force, and also its great tendency in some cases to agglutination into masses, as in powdered sulphur, resin, precipitated prussian blue, &c.

Gamboge exhibits it very perfectly, as do many gum-resins, in which it is most easily observed, on account of the resinous particles being insoluble in water, which retains them in suspension. Moreover, when any liquid (as placed between two glasses) in which this motion is perceived, is surrounded at the edges with oil, varnish, gold-size, lamp-black, or any other agent which entirely prevents evaporation, this peculiar motion continues perfectly un-

---

* Poussière fructificante, *pollen.*
† That the texture of most organic tissues of vertebrated animals is globular, and that there is great uniformity in the " organic elements" as they may be called.

affected, and in fact a specimen put up in this manner may be permanently preserved so as to show it at any time. Again, this movement is totally different from that of particles which are moved by currents excited by evaporation. These latter hurl a number of molecules in vortices with great rapidity (varying according to the evaporation); these sometimes meet, when the direction of the different particles may be distinctly perceived; and in these cases a number of molecules assume a similar and parallel direction, which is totally distinct from that of the true molecular movement, wherein the molecules oscillate or vibrate, moving but very slowly from place to place, sometimes remaining in the same spot for hours, and having an apparent repulsion for all other particles; but I am satisfied that the surrounding particles have nothing to do with the cause of this movement, because in some cases we can clearly perceive a single molecule, quite distinct from others, and enjoying its own spherical movements. But the most important circumstance connected with the vibration of these atoms is their size; and I am convinced that the smaller they are the more vivid is the motion; moreover, I am certain that they possess no definite size or shape. All bodies less than a certain size have a tendency to appear circular or spherical, when examined under a microscope; and we can often see some molecules more than ten times the size of others, still exhibiting this movement. It may be objected that these larger particles are aggregations of the smaller molecules, but we have not the slightest ground for so believing; the molecules observed by Dr. Brown varied in size from $\frac{1}{15000}$ to $\frac{1}{30000}$ of an inch; whilst those measured by Mr. Dalrymple in the transparent cell at the extremity of the Closteria varied from the $\frac{1}{6000}$ to the $\frac{1}{10000}$ of an inch.

The true molecular motion belongs, as pointed out by Dr. Brown, to the particle itself; and the circumstances necessary for its exhibition, are, 1st, an extremely minute state of subdivision of the matter; 2d, such a relation between the sp. gr. of the molecule and its medium as shall allow it to be freely suspended; 3d, absence of all impeding viscidity or tenacity of the liquid. Under these circumstances any forms of ponderable matter will freely exhibit this motion, whether organic or inorganic; and it takes place in all situations, perfectly uninfluenced by evaporation, and distinguished readily from the motion of particles produced by evaporation by its tremulous, vibratory, and not distinctly progressive motion, whereas in the latter the motion of neighbouring particles is similar, determinate, and often parallel. The cause of this motion is unknown. The influence of electricity might be suspected of being its excitor. With a veiw of testing this, I made some experiments; although the extreme minuteness of these atoms is such, that I could not depend upon my results as positive. Thus, I procured a very clean piece of steel, and mixed a little gamboge with water on its surface, covered it with very thin glass, then viewed the molecules as opaque objects; they were seen distinctly in motion: on connecting the extremity of this steel plate with the nob of a charged electrical jar, no alteration was produced, the motion continued; again, water with the molecules in suspension was placed on a layer of plate glass, next covered with a slip of thin glass; between the two glasses touching the liquid was laid a slip of tinfoil; at the end of the foil the molecules were in vivid motion: on connecting its other extremity with the interior of a charged jar no alteration in the motion took place. These experiments were repeated, insolating at the same time the microscope, but with the same effect. I know of no cause which can in any way explain this phenomenon. It takes place when examined between two large pieces of glass equally at the circumference as at the centre, which would not be the case were evaporation the cause.

The ingenious views of the older authors, quoted at the commencement of this paper, considering the particles or molecules of organic bodies separated by decomposition to be revivified and produce either animals or vegetables,&c. according to circumstances, are of course erroneous; but they long remained a source of fallacy that few, unguided by analogy, would be able to avoid. The experiments of Professor Schultze seem to have settled the point as regards infusoria. The views of Dr. Milne Edwards, regarding a certain globule as the basis of animal bodies, have not been since borne out, although the formation from primary cells is well established.

The utility of the molecular movement is not particularly evident. The particles or molecules themselves in their solid state form the food of the minutest forms of living matter; when in solution, or in the gaseous state from decomposition, they nourish the vegetable kingdom. Their freedom of motion, isolating them from surrounding particles, keeps them surrounded by liquid, and to a certain extent would facilitate their solution.

ANALYSES AND NOTICES OF BOOKS.

"L'Auteur se tue à allonger ce que le lecteur se tue à abréger."—D'ALEMBERT.

A Treatise on Food and Diet; with Observations on the Dietetical Regimen suited for Disordered States of the Digestive Organs, &c. &c. By JONATHAN PEREIRA, M.D. F.R.S. and L.S. &c. &c. Longman and Co. 1843.

THE plan of this work is considerably different from that of any other on the same subject which has fallen under our notice. A much fuller account is given of the chemical elements of food than we have met with elsewhere; and the number of alimentary principles admitted is greater than had been adopted by Prout, or other distinguished writers who have preceded him. (Common salt, for example, and lemon-juice, are enumerated among the articles of food.) We have also some very valuable tables indicating the proportions of the most important chemical elements and alimentary principles in various kinds of nutriment. A very considerable space is likewise given to dietaries, as adapted to different diseases and conditions — as, those fit for children, for paupers, for prisoners, for the sick, for the insane, &c. &c.

The work altogether bears the stamp of originality, and will, we are convinced, be found most useful. We shall take occasion, in future numbers, to give a few extracts as specimens: meantime we must content ourselves with this general recommendation.

Medical History of the Expedition to the Niger during the Years 1841-2; comprising an Account of the Fever which led to its abrupt termination. By J. O. M'WILLIAM, M.D, Surgeon of H.M.S. Albert, and Senior Medical Officer of the Expedition. With Plates. London, 1843. 8vo. pp. 287.

THIS work is divided into three chapters. The first gives the history of the expedition, and the second the history of the fever. The third contains four sections, which treat of the state of medicine in the Niger; ventilation; meteorology; and the geology of the Niger. It appears that of 145 whites belonging to this expedition, 130 were attacked by the fever, and 40 died; of 25 men of colour entered in England (with one exception), 11 were attacked, but none died; and of the blacks entered on the coast of Africa, not one was attacked. Hence, if the attempt is repeated, and the Niger is again ascended, with the noble object of extinguishing the slave trade, by civilising the nations which carry it on, the number of whites must be as small as possible.

Dr. M'William's book shews good sense and judgment, and will be consulted by the physician desirous to study the nature of remittent fever in its severest form; and by the philanthropist, who, lamenting the failure of so benevolent an expedition, is eager to see it renewed under better auspices.

MEDICAL GAZETTE.
Friday, June 30, 1843.

"Licet omnibus, licet etiam mihi, dignitatem Artis Medicæ tueri; potestas modo veniendi in publicum sit, dicendi periculum non recuso."
CICERO.

EMPLOYMENT OF WOMEN AND CHILDREN IN AGRICULTURE.

THE story of the two knights who quarrelled about the metal of the shield before which they severally stood, is but a type of the difficulties which embarrass human evidence. The shield was gold on one side, and silver on the other, so that each doughty horseman saw a different sight, and did but contend for the evidence of his own senses. Just so it is with the ordinary controversies of life; the most faithful witnesses can but tell what they have seen, and perfectly different spetacles have been represented on their retinæ. Besides which, the eye is under the guidance of the mind, and if the same general scenes are spread before it, different points are selected by different observers; a Rembrandt and a Rubens do not see with the same eyes, any more than they paint with the same brush.

The celebrated picture of the happiness of a country life, in the Georgics, and the painful descriptions of agricultural destitution in more prosaic writers, are quite reconcileable, when we consider that the Latin poet drew the small farmer, and the prose historians his half-starved drudge.

The pauper's funeral, given with hard fidelity by Crabbe, depresses the reader's mind.   Not so the picture where Poussin has represented a dance of nymphs and their swains, near a monument bearing the inscription *ego quoque lusi in Arcadiâ.*

However similar objects may be, nay if they are absolutely identical, they become different when viewed through the tinged lens of different spectators. To some melancholy Jaques the county of Hampshire may seem a huge mass of discontented husbandmen, who feed the bacon which they must not eat; to Miss Mitford it is an Arcadia of happy faces, where the very Doriclans are delightful.

The rustic gallantry, too, which has ever been the accompaniment of haymaking, is viewed in a different light by the withered critic, and the genial poet of the Seasons. But however opinion may differ on these points, there is one on which it is unanimous. Husbandmen, the most useful members of society, are everywhere, as far as

regards the reward of their labours, at the bottom of the social scale.   In some countries they are still serfs, in others but lately emancipated from serfdom; but throughout Europe their state is so little raised above that of villenage, that nothing but the main force of the law, nothing but wisdom guided by benevolence (the two are, perhaps, one), can save them from sinking into this slough of despond.

In England the system of prædial bondage died out in the reign of Elizabeth ; in some of the mines of Scotland, it existed, as we learn from Walter Scott, as late as the middle of the last century. In Franche-Comté, according to Voltaire, it not only existed, but, by an incredible refinement of absurdity, the cultivation of certain farms imposed the state of villains on those who were previously free ; so that while the touch of our British soil gave freedom to the slave, the cultivation of this wretched country deprived the husbandman of the birthright of the human race.

In Prussia, the emancipation of the bondmen did not take place till 1807. Even before the battle of Jena thinking men had seen that villenage was one of the great causesof the weakness of the Prussian monarchy.   It had been denounced by Frederic the Great as a *" gestion abominable ;"* but it was not until the kingdom had fallen at the shock of a single battle, that Stein, the statesman who then conducted the destinies of Prussia, determined to heal this devouring ulcer.

Yet in all these countries, even in England itself, the rustic population is prevented from sinking back into serfdom, rather by the benevolent interference of the educated classes, than by any dogged spirit of resistance in the husbandmen themselves.   Were the matter left entirely to ploughmen and petty farmers to settle between them, without the interference of the law, or the criticism of public opinion, our half-fed cottagers might too often sell their birthright for a mess of pottage. As it is, the condition of our farm apprentices approaches far nearer to that of slaves or serfs than it is pleasant to acknowledge.

By the French Code, indeed, no contract is valid by which a man barters away his liberty; and it is to be hoped that should a fit occasion arise, our common law would be interpreted in a similar spirit.

These preliminary reflections have been called forth by the late reports of the special Assistant Poor Law Commissioners, on the employment of women and children in agriculture, now lying before us.

These Commissioners were four in number, all barristers; and they were directed to inquire into the sorts of labour at which women and children are employed in agriculture; the wages which they receive; the hours of work; the age at which they begin to work; and the effects which their occupation produces upon their health, as well as upon their opportunities for obtaining school instruction and religious education; and they were also desired to investigate the condition of the children of agricultural labourers apprenticed by parish officers.

The four Assistant-Commissioners examined into the state of twelve counties; and as their time was limited to thirty days, it is obvious that much of their information must have been picked up at a canter. Yet, in spite of this disadvantage, their reports read like the compilation of sensible men, not very deeply tinctured with Malthusian fantasies; and some part of it will be a novelty, not only to the natives of the *pays de cocagne*, but even to the home-bred rustics of the very counties themselves. Mr. Alfred Aus-

tin, whose report stands first in the book, took the counties of Wilts, Dorset, Devon, and Somerset; and in order not to fritter away his time in forced marches over so large a space, he confined himself to two districts in Devonshire, and one in each of the remaining counties. The wages of women who work in the fields vary, in general, from 7d. to 1s. a day in these counties; though rates above and below these are mentioned. For this slender stipend they work from 8 A.M. to 4 P.M. in winter; at other times, from 8 to 6, and in the hay harvest from 6 to 6.

The effect of out-door farm labour on adult women appears to be favourable to health. Mr. Austin did not meet with an instance of a woman complaining of its being injurious.

"Sometimes such work, particularly in the hay and corn harvests, was represented by women who performed it as being laborious, as making them stiff at first, or even as straining them; but I did not find that any woman, from her own statement, had become subject to any permanent disease or infirmity from the employment in question."

There is a good deal of evidence, however, scattered up and down these reports, to show that field-work demoralises women, or at any rate, girls. Woman is a domestic creature, and a mother does more service to society by tending her children, and going through the details of her little household, than by mowing grass, or hoeing turnips. On the Continent, where the employment of women in field-labour is even more common than in England, it has always seemed to us that it rapidly destroys the graces of youth, and gives the look of a hard-a-weather sailor to a middle-aged woman. But it is more easy to see the evil than to provide a remedy.

The next question is, how are these

labouring women placed with regard to food, clothing, and lodging ?

The majority of them are married, and the greater number of the single ones live with their parents. (Mr. Austin says they are " sometimes grown-up daughters living with their parents.") Hence their earnings are merely part of the aggregate income of the family; and to know their condition we must learn that of their husbands and fathers.

Now, the wages of the labourer in the district of Wiltshire visited by Mr. Austin (in the neighbourhood of Calne) are from 8 to 10 shillings a week; in the Dorsetshire district they are higher; in the Devonshire one about the same as in Dorsetshire. In the part of Somersetshire visited, they are even lower than in Wiltshire; but here the labourer has an allowance of three pints of cider daily, which are considered both by master and man to be worth a shilling or fifteen-pence per week. Sometimes, of course, the income is beyond this, as when the wife and children add to the common fund, but, on the whole, the receipts of a labourer are exceedingly small, and his diet low in proportion. Thus, in Wiltshire, the food of the labourer and his family is bread and potatoes, with the occasional luxury of beer, a little butter, and tea. To these are sometimes added cheese and bacon, and near Calne, the entrails, or "in'ards," of the pig. "In more than one cottage," says Mr. Austin, "where the mother went out to work, or two of the boys were earning perhaps 3s. or 3s. 6d. a week between them, I saw a side of bacon hanging against the wall; but nothing of the kind was visible when the only earnings were those of the husband, or the family was numerous and young. Where, from poverty, bacon cannot be obtained, a little fat is used to give a flavour to the potatoes."

In Dorset and Devon matters are a trifle better; but Somerset is on a level with Wilts.

As to lodging, Mr. Austin's account is painful indeed, both physically and morally. Let us hope that, to use the phraseology of the day, he has drawn his induction from too small a number of instances. He says, that the want of sufficient accommodation seems universal. Cottages, generally speaking, have only one, or at most two, bedrooms, so that adults of both sexes constantly sleep in the same room, and not unfrequently three or four persons in the same bed.

At Stourpain, a village near Blandford, he found in a cottage a bedroom, ten feet square, containing three beds and eleven occupants of them! The father, mother, two infants, two twin daughters aged 20, and a son aged 17, were among the tenants of this crowded room. In Stourpain, there is a row of labourers' cottages so miserably constructed that they are surrounded by streams of filth from pig-sties, and privies placed a few yards above them. "It was in these cottages that a malignant typhus broke out two years ago, which afterwards spread through the village."

Nor are the moral consequences less grievous than the physical.

If we may believe Mr. Austin, the licentiousness produced by this deficient accommodation has not always respected the family relationship!

In this, as in other matters, much depends on the landlord. Thus in Studley the rent of cottages is from £3 to £4 a year, and families are crowded together in the most indecent manner. In Foxton, which adjoins it, the cottages all belong to the Marquis of Lansdowne, who lets them at half that rent, but will not allow more than one family to occupy one tenement at the same time. Each cottage has at least three rooms. In consequence of this difference in the arrangements, says Lord Lansdowne's agent, the labourers at Foxton are a superior kind of people to those at Studley.

We will continue this subject on an early occasion.

DR. STOBER ON THE DISEASES OF CHILDREN.

THE author, who is physician to the *clinique* for children's diseases at Strasburgh, has published a work entitled, "*La clinique des maladies des enfans de la faculté de Strasbourg, pendant les trois années scolaires*, 1837-1840, &c.

What follows is taken from a review of the work in the *Zeitschrift für die gesammte Medicin* for March 1843.

The *clinique* consists of a large ward, made into two by a wooden partition; the larger division containing fourteen beds for girls and infants, the smaller one six beds for boys. Children are admitted from the age of one year to fifteen; but those who are to undergo important operations, or who are suffering from fractures, tch, or scalled head, are admitted into other wards, which, however, are to be united to the *clinique*.

The mortality during the three years has been 1 in 7.

Typhus fever.—The author agrees with Taupin, Rilliet, Rodet, and Rufz, that this disease frequently occurs among children, but with slight modifications. He had twenty-six cases, in half of which the patients were above ten years of age. It is remarkable, that at an age where the nervous system is so excitable, and not only important diseases, but occasionally even slight indispositions are accompanied by convulsive motions, nervous phenomena are less violent in typhus than among adults. All the patients suffered from debility, with sleepiness and more or less stupor; and in more than half, delirium was present, but slighter than in adults. Ten patients suffered from deafness; with the exception of four, all had diarrhœa; some, however, only at first, which was then followed by costiveness. Three had red lenticular spots, and ten had petechiæ.

Only three had epistaxis. Only one child died out of the twenty-six; and, in general, severe cases of this disease are rarer than among adults. All the patients had a cough.

Scarlatina.—From the autumn of 1838 to the spring of 1840, this disease prevailed at Strasburgh in a rather malignant form;

many children died, in particular, of its sequelæ, namely, dropsy, and inflammation of the parotid glands. Of five children but one died in the hospital, while only one was saved out of eight suffering from the sequelæ. The disease appeared under different forms; one is described by the author under the name of *Scarlatina rubeolosa* (the *Röthela* of the Germans) but considered by him as a mere variety of scarlet-fever. The dispute concerning the identity of the two diseases is by no means cleared up by his cases. In one instance of typhoid scarlatina, he exhibited carbonate of ammonia, and with success. The author does not hold that the subsequent dropsy always proceeds from taking cold; an observation in which he had been preceded by German physicians. Of eight patients two had anasarca alone, four ascites at the same time, and two hydrothorax. The rapidity with which water is sometimes effused in the internal cavities is shown by the following case. A boy, aged ten, entered the institution suffering under a slight degree of anasarca, with an accelerated pulse. On the following day he walked barefoot across a passage, then returned to bed, complained of a feeling of oppression, and a few minutes afterwards had symptoms, of suffocation and orthopnœa; his countenance turned blue and swelled, and in half an hour he was a corpse. On examination, a considerable quantity of water was found in the pleura and pericardium.

Stomatitis ulcerosa.—Under this name Dr. Stöber describes an ulceration of the inner surfaces of the cheeks and the edge of the tongue, which is deep and uneven, and has edges which bleed easily, and a dirty greyish-yellow bottom. It attacks only one side of the mouth, is oblong, and exactly corresponds with the dental arch, so that when the mouth is shut the ulcerated parts touch the teeth. The teeth are covered with tartar; the breath is fetid, and the glands on the affected side of the neck are swollen. The author believes incrustation or caries of the teeth to be the cause of the disease.

Acute Laryngitis.—The author treats it like croup, in which he justly extols the sulphate of copper given at the very beginning of the disease.

Pneumonia.—This disease in children is often secondary, and complicated with other maladies. Contrary to the assertion of many physicians, the author has found but one instance of lobular pneumonia among 17 cases. In all the other cases it was lobar. In six instances it was seated in both lungs, though less marked on one side than the other. The chief thing which distinguishes the pneumonia of children from that of adults, anatomically, is the variety of hepatization compared with carnification. The author has seen grey hepatization but once, and the red four times. In twelve patients the diseased lung was of the colour of lees of wine, indurated, and impermeable to air; it did not easily tear under the fingers, and was without granulations, as in cases of hepatization; the upper surface when cut into was smooth, and looked like a piece of muscle without fibres. This complication was observed in children who died on the 10th day of the disease, or in a month. The disease is less easy to recognise in children than in adults, as they are unable to point out the pain, and there is no expectoration. [In many cases, however, says the German translator, the expression of pain may be recognised, particularly when the patient coughs.] The cough is sometimes violent, the respiration and circulation are always quickened, and the temperature increased. From the screaming and disquietude of children, the crepitous rattle can be heard. More frequently there is a slight or sub-crepitous mucous rattle; and this sound, too, is not present long, for in the majority of cases bronchophony and bronchial respiration alone are to be heard. It is probable that the pneumonia of children soon passes into the second stage, or rather it often remains latent during the first stage. The seat of the disease is generally discovered on percussion, and it is only in lobular or central pneumonia that it cannot be distinguished in this manner. The great sonorousness of the chest in children sometimes causes the dull sound to be less marked in them than in adults. But if we compare the sound on both sides of the chest, and at the same time attend to the sensation experienced by the percussing finger, the impenetrability of the lung will be recognised. The younger children are the more they appear to be exposed to pneumonia; and it is also more violent in early infancy than after the seventh year. Cases are most numerous in the first four months of the year. Pneumonia is almost always fatal, when combined with a chronic disease, which has already weakened the constitution.

As to the treatment, there is a great difference between children and old persons. From the latter it is well known that much blood should rarely be taken, and the best remedy is tartar emetic; while in the pneumonia of children without complication, the abstraction of blood is generally very useful. The author bled children from 5 to 6 years old, and found venesection better than local bleeding. Besides this, he gave tartar emetic, or white oxide of antimony, of which he prefers the former. He combines it with tisane or gum mucilage, to avoid ulcers in the mouth and pharynx.

[To be continued.]

PROFESSOR ROSAS' OPERATIONS ON THE EYE.

ROSAS is a dexterous and steady operator. In his extraction the patient is seated on a low stool, with the head placed obliquely to the light, and resting against the breast of an assistant who raises the upper lid, while the operator depresses the lower with the middle and forefingers in the usual manner. He makes the downward section with a knife somewhat different from that of Beer, as originally used by him, and figured in his work in 1830. This knife is much shorter in the blade than Beer's; its posterior edge (or back) is also sharp and slightly convex. Holding it between the thumb and the index and middle fingers, the ring-finger bent unto the hollow of the hand, and the little one resting on the cheek-bone, he introduces the point at a right angle with the cornea, (to prevent its catching in its layers,) a little above the transverse axis of the eye, and having entered the anterior chamber, he alters the position of the instrument by depressing its handle towards the temporal fossa, and thus brings the surface of the blade on the same plane with that of the iris. Having passed it rapidly through the chamber and made the counter-punctuation, so that a full quarter of an inch of the point has passed through the inner margin of the cornea, he then *draws* it slowly downwards, and slightly outwards, and so completes the section. If the case is one of double cataract he makes the corneal section, and concludes the operation in the second eye before he extracts the lens of the first. He opens the capsule with a Langenbeck's needle, sharpened on its concave edge, and extracts the lens by gently pressing on the upper portion of the cornea with the flat of the needle.

The object aimed at in having the back of the knife curved is, to give it shortness as well as breadth, and thus avoid pricking the side of the nose; and its posterior sharp edge is to permit of its cutting upwards as well as downwards, and thus not only pass through the cornea with greater facility, but also enable the operator to extend the incision upwards if the original punctuation is too low. Another reason assigned by the inventor of this knife is, that its blade by being sharp at both sides, and forming in its section a compressed ellipse, permits less escape of the aqueous fluid in passing through the chamber, than the ordinary instrument.

In this manner Rosas operates with the most marked success; but in other hands, especially beginners, his method and instruments are open to many objections. The insertion of the knife at right angles with the cornea is very liable to transfix the iris, and by twisting the cornea itself, renders its further insertion less smooth and easy ; and its cutting back endangers both sclerotic and iris, especially in turning its lower edge outward when completing the incision ; — and when the iris happens to roll over the back of the knife, it cannot be pressed off with the same facility as when the posterior part is blunt ;—should the point of the knife get entangled with the iris, he withdraws it and re-introduces it in another place ; if the corneal opening is too small he enlarges it with a Daviel's scissors.

The operations of depression and reclination are much more common in the Viennese school than in England. In this clinique, these, as well as the operation for solution, are performed *per scleroticam.* In artificial pupil Rosas generally adopts the methods of Beer and Langenbeck, but removes the portion of iris drawn through the wound.— *Wilde's Austria.*

OCULISTS IN AUSTRIA.

EVERY student intending to become a doctor of medicine or surgery must attend the ophthalmic clinique during the first six months of his fifth year ; and at his final examination *(Zweyte Prüfung,)* his knowledge of ophthalmic surgery is strictly inquired into. Every *Civil-und-Landwundarzt* studies in this school during the second six months of his third year, and upon taking his degree he is examined upon ophthalmology by the professor of that branch.

In order, however, to perform operations on the eye, and practise this branch of medicine as a speciality, it is necessary that an additional year (after the degree has been obtained from the university) be spent in attendance upon the eye-clinique, at the end of which period some public operations, performed in the presence of the professor, are required as a test of the person's right to practise. This latter course is frequently attended by medical men who have been already in practice, and also by foreigners. A special degree is granted for it.

The practitioners thus educated, and styled town and country oculists, *Land-und-Stadt-Augenärzte* are distributed throughout the whole of this great empire; no town of any consequence is without one ; they are paid by the state, and obliged to administer medicine and advice to the poor in all cases of eye-disease, and also to furnish the board of medical direction with a monthly *Protokol,* or sanatory report of the progress of such affections among the people of their district.—*Ibid.*

ROYAL COLLEGE OF SURGEONS.

LIST OF GENTLEMEN ADMITTED MEMBERS.

Friday, June 23, 1843.

J. Carr.—W. N. Walker.—E. C. Hill.—C. W. Beckitt. — E. K. Parson. — H. W. Pain.—G. Sayle.—E. Dodd.—W. Smith.

A TABLE OF MORTALITY FOR THE METROPOLIS,

Shewing the number of deaths from all causes registered in the week ending Saturday, June 17, 1843.

Small Pox	10
Measles	40
Scarlatina	31
Hooping Cough	51
Croup	6
Thrush	5
Diarrhœa	4
Dysentery	3
Cholera	0
Influenza	5
Ague	1
Typhus	47
Erysipelas	5
Syphilis	0
Hydrophobia	0
Diseases of the Brain, Nerves, and Senses	153
Diseases of the Lungs and other Organs of Respiration	309
Diseases of the Heart and Blood-vessels	26
Diseases of the Stomach, Liver, and other Organs of Digestion	53
Diseases of the Kidneys, &c.	10
Childbed	7
Paramenia	1
Ovarian Dropsy	0
Disease of Uterus, &c.	2
Rheumatism	0
Diseases of Joints, &c.	3
Carbuncle	0
Ulcer	3
Fistula	1
Diseases of Skin, &c.	1
Dropsy, Cancer, and other Diseases of Uncertain Seat	90
Old Age or Natural Decay	59
Deaths by Violence, Privation, or Intemperance	15
Causes not specified	6
Deaths from all Causes	955

METEOROLOGICAL JOURNAL.

Kept at EDMONTON, *Latitude* 51° 37′ 32″*N. Longitude* 0° 3′ 51″ *W. of Greenwich.*

June 1843.	THERMOMETER.	BAROMETER.
Wednesday 21	from 40 to 72	30·09 to 30·00
Thursday . 22	51 72	29·99 Stat.
Friday . . . 23	45 69	30·00 29·99
Saturday . 24	48 67	29·98 29·94
Sunday . . 25	49 64	29·90 29·85
Monday . . 26	45 69	29·93 29·87
Tuesday . 27	44 75	29·85 29·65

Wind, S.W. on the 21st and 27th ; otherwise N. and N.E. Generally clear.

CHARLES HENRY ADAMS.

WILSON & OGILVY, 57, Skinner Street, London.

THE
LONDON MEDICAL GAZETTE,

BEING A

WEEKLY JOURNAL

OF

Medicine and the Collateral Sciences.

FRIDAY, JULY 7, 1843.

LECTURES

ON THE

THEORY AND PRACTICE OF MIDWIFERY,

Delivered in the Theatre of St. George's Hospital,

BY ROBERT LEE, M.D. F.R.S.

LECTURE XXXIII.

On Labours complicated with Uterine Hæmorrhage from Placental Presentation.

THE placenta may adhere to any part of the inner surface of the uterus — to the fundus, body, or cervix, and hæmorrhage never takes place to a dangerous extent during pregnancy or labour, unless the connection of the placenta with the uterus has been destroyed. A solution of continuity must take place between these organs before it is possible for a considerable hæmorrhage to occur from the gravid uterus. The partial detachment of the membranes from the vicinity of the cervix might occasion a slight oozing of blood, from the rupture of some small decidual arteries and veins, but the quantity proceeding from this source can never be great, or produce what is usually called a flooding. It is from the great semilunar, valvular-like, venous openings in the lining membrane of the uterus, which you have seen in various preparations, and of the arteries which are laid open by the separation of the placenta, that the blood alone flows in uterine hæmorrhage. All the different causes of flooding produce their effect by separating and exposing the arteries and veins by which the circulation of the maternal blood is carried on in the placenta. Blows, falls, shocks of various kinds, mental and physical, bodily exertion and fatigue, the movements of a carriage along a rough road, attempts to raise a heavy weight, dancing, the abuse of stimulants, frequenting hot crowded assemblies, morbid conditions of the placenta, twisting of the umbilical cord round the neck of the child, attachment of the placenta to the cervix uteri; all these causes produce hæmorrhage, by mechanically separating the placenta from the part of the uterus to which it is attached. There is not an actual wound in the uterus where the placenta adhered, the lining or mucous membrane is not detached and expelled, yet there is a considerable resemblance, as has already been stated, between this portion of the inner surface of the organ after delivery, and a stump after amputation; in both the cavities of the arteries and veins are laid open or exposed, and they are consequently liable to be affected by similar diseases.

Dr. Jones first proved by experiment that when an artery is divided, nature employs certain means adapted to arrest the flow of blood, the most important of which are the retraction and contraction of the divided extremity of the vessel and the formation of a coagulum of blood within its orifice, or rather two coagula, one within the contracted orifice of the vessel, and the other within its sheath. Nearly similar means are employed by nature for preventing fatal hæmorrhage from the uterus, when the placenta is detached; and if nature did not employ these means and at the proper period, and with sufficient force, death from hæmorrhage would probably take place in all cases immediately after the expulsion of the child and separation of the placenta. The same muscular contractions which expel the contents of the gravid uterus close the mouths of the exposed vessels in the lining membrane, until coagula of the fibrine of the blood are formed within them, which establish a permanent barrier against the further effusion of blood. The oblique valvular manner in which the veins open into the cavity of the uterus must contribute powerfully to accomplish the same purpose. Before delivery the contractile powers of the uterus cannot be effectually exerted in closing these vessels ; consequently the orifices of the veins must be stopped in a temporary manner by coagula, and the insufficiency of these plugs without uterine contraction to restrain hæmorrhage is proved by the frequent return of the accident on the application of the slightest occasional cause, and the consequent insecurity of the patient from a recurrence of the discharge, fresh portions of the placenta being likewise often separated till the contents of the uterus be expelled, and the orifices of the vessels closed by the muscular contractions of the organ. All the different efficient means which are employed for checking the discharge in uterine hæmorrhage, either excite the contractions of the uterus or promote the coagulation of the blood itself within the vessels.

Until the seventh month of pregnancy the blood-vessels of the uterus have not attained a sufficient size to pour out blood in so great a quantity as suddenly to destroy life, though the discharge may be very profuse, and produce alarming symptoms. The remedies which ought to be employed when hæmorrhage takes place in the early months have already been described, and are chiefly as follows : venesection, where the patient is plethoric and the circulation excited ; rest in the horizontal position ; the free admission of cool air ; ice in a bladder, or cold vinegar and water, laid over the hypogastrium ; cold acidulated drinks ; the use of superacetate of lead and opium ; the introduction of a sponge into the upper part of the vagina, and, where these fail, puncturing the ovum, exhibiting the ergot of rye, and endeavouring by all other means to excite the contraction of the uterus and the expulsion of its contents. There are very few if any cases in which it is safe to attempt to introduce the whole hand into the uterus, to deliver by turning the child, before the end of the sixth month. Uterine hæmorrhage in the latter months of pregnancy, and during labour, is always accompanied with great danger ; it does and ought to excite alarm in all cases, and it occurs, *first*, where the placenta presents, or has originally adhered to the cervix uteri, and been afterwards detached from the uterus in consequence of the shortening of the cervix which takes place in the seventh month ; and, *secondly*, where the placenta has adhered to the fundus or body of the uterus, and been separated from it by external violence, the umbilical cord surrounding the neck of the child, a morbid state of the placenta itself, or some other accidental cause. The first of these varieties is usually called unavoidable, the second, accidental, uterine hæmorrhage.

On Uterine Hæmorrhage from Placental Presentation.

Hippocrates says, the after-birth should come after the child, for if it were to come out first, the child could not live, because it derives its life from the after-birth, as a plant does from the earth. Cases of uterine hæmorrhage from placental presentation must have been frequently observed by the ancients, but they have not been described in their writings. In 1609, Guillemeau stated that the placenta sometimes presents or comes before the child, and that this gives rise to a dangerous hæmorrhage which nature is unable to suppress. In Chapter XII. which is entitled " Le moyen de secourir la femme quand l'arrierefais se presente le premier," he states that when the placenta comes first, the most certain and expedient measure is immediate delivery, because there is usually a constant flooding in consequence of the openings in the veins, which are situated in the walls of the uterus to which those of the placenta are joined, being laid open or exposed, and that the blood flows out whenever the uterus contracts, as in labour, to expel the child. The source of the discharge and cause of the death of the fœtus is thus accurately described. "D'autrepart l'enfant estant enfermeé en la matrice, l'orifice estant bouche par le dit arrierefais, ne respire plus par les arteres de la mère, sera tost suffoqué faute d'ayde, et mesme englouty du sang qui est contenu en la matrice, et qui coule des veines qui sont ouvertes en icelle." But before attempting anything, two circumstances, he says, are to be observed : the first is, to consider whether the placenta is little or far advanced ; for if the former, having placed the mother in the proper position, it must be replaced and pushed back with the greatest diligence, and if the head presents, it must be brought down that it may be expelled as in natural labour. But if some difficulty should occur, so that the head could not advance, or that the mother, or infant, or both, are feeble, and there is a probability of the labour being protracted, without doubt the best expedient is to bring down the feet of the child, and deliver as gently as possible. The other point to be observed is, that if the afterbirth is much advanced, and cannot be replaced in consequence of its size and the hæmorrhage, and that the child is closely following it, and requires only to pass into the world, the placenta must be completely drawn forth. The works of Guillemeau do not contain a single observation to justify the assertion that he evidently supposed that this presentation of the placenta at the os uteri was owing to its having been separated from its usual situation in the uterus and fallen down to the lower part. Not only has this groundless assertion been made respecting

Guillemeau, but other authors, who have expressly stated that on introducing the hand into the uterus to deliver by turning, they felt the placenta adhering all round to the cervix.

The 28th Chapter of Mauriceau's Treatise (1668) is entitled, " De l'accouchement auquel l'arriere-faix se presente le premier, ou est tout-à-fait sortit devant l'enfant." The symptoms and treatment of cases of placental presentation are here accurately described, and in all cases of hæmorrhage from this cause he recommends immediate delivery. If the placenta has not entirely escaped, and the membranes are not ruptured, he advises the part of the placenta which presents to be put aside with the hand, which is to be passed up into the uterus, the membranes ruptured, and the delivery completed by turning. The rules for the treatment of these cases are laid down with the greatest precision. When the placenta was entirely separated, then only did he consider it as a foreign body, and recommend its extraction before the child, as Guillemeau had done: but to this practice he states, as an obvious objection, that the placenta is strongly attached to the membranes which surround it, and that it cannot be drawn out without the membranes enveloping the child being drawn out also. It has also been most erroneously asserted, that Mauriceau invariably speaks of the placenta when at the os uteri as " entirely detached." In the history of his case 423, related at p. 350, the following observation occurs, which I may adduce as a proof perfectly conclusive that Mauriceau does not invariably speak of the placenta when at the os uteri as entirely detached, but, on the contrary, was fully aware of the fact, that the placenta had not been detached from the fundus and pushed down to the orifice by its own gravity. " Mais quoique j'aye dit que l'arriere-faix de cette femme presentoit le premier au passage, dans le temps que je l'accouchai, et que l'excessive perte de sang qu'elle avoit vint de ce detachement, il ne faut pas croire que cet arriere-faix fut ainsi entièrement detaché de la matrice, depuis tout le temps que cette perte de sang avoit commencé a paroître en cette femme : car si cela eut été, l'enfant seroit mort en très peu de temps, ne pouvant pas être vivifié que par la communication du sang de la mère, dont il est privé aussitot que l'arriere-faix est entièrement detaché de la matrice : mais comme il n'y avoit dans le commencement de cette perte de sang que quelque petite partie de l'arriere-faix qui s'en étoit un peu detachée, elle n'avoit pas empeché l'enfant d'être nourri du sang de tout le reste de l'arriere-faix, qui n'avoit pas été entierement separé de la matrice." Mauriceau has related seventeen cases of uterine hæmorrhage, in the latter months of pregnancy,

from presentation of the placenta, and in sixteen of these delivery was accomplished by passing the hand through the opening formed by the separation of the placenta from the uterus, rupturing the membranes, and turning the child. Two women died after this operation, and one who would not consent to have it performed died undelivered.

These cases are Nos. 8, 55, 59, 68, 106, 170, 175, 210, 423, 428, 438, 454, 484, 502, 597, 651. The first occurred in 1669; the last in 1692.

Portal's Treatise (1685) contains the histories of eight or more cases of uterine hæmorrhage, in which he found, on introducing the hand to turn the child, that the placenta was not merely at the os uteri, but adhering to the cervix all round; and he states, in the most clear and forcible manner, after relating his first case, that artificial delivery is the only remedy that can preserve the life of women under such circumstances, and that by this means he had saved the lives of several women at the Hôtel-Dieu. In 1664, Case No. 2 occurred during the eighth month, in which, on passing his hand into the uterus, he felt a soft body, which was the after-birth, which he gently separated from the uterus, then ruptured the membranes, and brought down the feet of the child and extracted it, dead. In Case 29 (1671), the placenta presented, and the head of the child was forced against it so strongly, that it was torn, and the infant expelled dead. Case 39 occurred also in 1671, in the history of which he states that he felt the placenta adhering on all sides to the orifice of the uterus. " Sur cette assurance je glissay mes doigts dans les orifices, où je sentis l'arriere-faix qui se presentoit, et qui bouchoit l'orifice de la matrice de tous costez avec adherances en toutes ses parties, excepté par le milieu, qui se trouvoit devisé jusques à la membrane, laquelle n'estant pas ouverte, ny les eaux ecoulées, j'eus beaucoup de facilité à tourner l'enfant." This woman died from loss of blood some time after delivery, there being scarcely a drop found in the arteries and veins on dissection ; and Portal complains, with justice, that the body was examined in his absence by a distinguished accoucheur, but in the presence of the wife of the greatest and most illustrious physician of the age, whose name he has not recorded, and whose memory has probably perished many years ago. " C'est ce que me fait dire, qu'on a beau faire, ou ne fait jamais rien : quelque belle operation qu'on puisse faire, elle ne fait point d'eclat : mais bien tout le contraire, qu'une femme soit si bien accouché qu'on souhaitera et que malheureusement elle vient à mourir, ce sera toujours la faute de celui ou de celle qui aura accouché la femme : tant la medisance a de l'empire sur la verité." Portal's 42d case happened in 1672, in which there was also a considerable hæmorrhage, and on passing the hand into the orifice of the uterus, he says he felt the placenta presenting, which he gently separated (" parcequ'il estoit collé à l'orifice interne") because it was glued to the internal orifice. Portal's 43d case, which also occurred in 1672, was one of hæmorrhage with placental presentation during the sixth month of pregnancy, and here he also passed up his hand between the uterus and placenta, where the partial detachment had taken place, and brought down the feet of the child ; " ensuite je glissay ma main dans l'entrée de la matrice, où je sentis l'arriere-faix qui se presentoit. L'ayant *separé, afin de me frayer le chemin*, je sentis les membranes des eaux que je percay," &c. Another similar case, No. 51, took place in the same year, 1672, and to this history is subjoined a correct explanation of the cause of the hæmorrhage which occurs in the latter months of pregnancy, where the placenta adheres to the neck of the uterus. On introducing the hand into the uterus, he says, " J'ouvris cet anneau en telle sorte que je n'eus point de peine à porter ma main dans le fond de la matrice, où en la glissant je sentis le placenta qui environnoit en dedans l'orifice interne : ce qui estoit la cause de la perte de sang, parceque lorsque l'ouverture de cet anneau se faisoit, le placenta qui se trouvoit contigu à cet orifice, à cause de quelque contiguité qu'il a avec la matrice, à l'endroit où il y est adherant, cet orifice venant à s'ouvrir, il se divise, et en mesme temps les vaisseaux venant à se diviser, cela fait que le sang de la malade se perd en abondance ; et si elle n'est promptement secourue, elle meurt bien-tost." He then turned and delivered the child. In concluding the history of this case he states, that in the year 1683 he had completed the delivery successfully in five similar cases, all the women having recovered. His 69th case occurred in 1679, in which he likewise found, on passing the hand, that the placenta was every where firmly adherent to the neck of the uterus, which was the cause of the great hæmorrhage. " In Portal's Cases in Midwifery," observes Dr. Rigby, in his Essay on Uterine Hæmorrhage, " there are eight in which he was under the necessity of delivering by art, on account of dangerous hæmorrhages, and in all of them he found the placenta at the mouth of the womb." This important fact, that in all these cases the placenta was found not merely at the mouth of the womb, but adherent to the neck of the uterus, in some all round to it, is suppressed by Dr. Rigby, nor are the practical conclusions, which Portal drew from it, described by him.

Dr. Edward Rigby asserts, that " in one case only does Portal attempt to make any practical inference whatever, having, in all the others, contented himself with merely stating the fact of the placenta adhering to the os uteri." The operation of passing the hand between the placenta and uterus, bringing down the feet and turning the child, which Portal had recourse to so promptly in most of the preceding cases, I think you will be disposed to regard as the very best practical inference which he could have drawn, or has yet been drawn by others from the knowledge of the fact. It has likewise been affirmed by him that " all the authors in midwifery, up to the time of Rœderer and Levret were ignorant of Portal's explanation." The truth of this you may estimate by the following facts.

In the History of the Royal Academy of Sciences for 1728, it is stated, that Petit examined the body of a woman who had died from flooding when near the full period, and he found the placenta adherent to the neck of the uterus, and exactly closing the orifice except at one part, where it was detached, and from whence the discharge of blood had taken place.

Giffard has recorded about twenty cases of placental presentation, and he was likewise completely aware of the fact, that the placenta sometimes adheres to the inferior part of the uterus. He concludes the history of his 115th case with the following observation. " I cannot implicitly accede to the opinion of most writers on midwifery, which is, that the placenta always adheres to the fundus uteri, for in this, as well as many former instances, I have good reason to believe that it sometimes adheres to or near the os internum, and that the opening of it occasions a separation, and consequently a flooding." In the history of Case 116 he states that he told the patient " that the only way to save her life was a speedy delivery." When he passed his hand through the os uteri, the first thing he met with was the placenta, which he " found closely adhering round the os internum" of the uterus ; which, amongst many other instances, is a proof that the placenta is not always fixed to the bottom of the uterus, according to the opinion of some writers in midwifery ; its adhering to the os internum was in my opinion the occasion of the flooding ; for as the os internum was gradually dilated, the placenta at the same time was separated, from whence proceeded the effusion of blood. The placenta presented in Cases 120, 121, 158, 160, 184, 209, and 224. In the last of these cases he " felt part of the placenta adhering round about the orifice of the uterus.". " This case occurred in 1731 ; and in a further communication of its details, he observes, as he had done before ; " I beg leave," before I proceed to give any further account of the delivery, to give my opinion on a point of midwifery in which I differ from most authors that have wrote on the subject. It is generally believed that the ovum after its impregnation and separation from the ovarium, and its passage through the tuba fallopiana, always adheres, and is fixed after some time to the fundus uteri; in this case the placenta adhered, and was fixed close and round about the cervix uteri, as I have found it in many other cases, so that upon a dilatation of the os uteri a separation has always followed, whence a flooding naturally ensues."

"Giffard," says Dr. Rigby, "has more than twenty cases where the placenta was found at the os uteri: but *plainly supposes that it had not been originally fixed there,* for he says, " it is customary in floodings to find the placenta sunk down to the mouth of the womb."

Puzos knew that the placenta sometimes adhered to the cervix uteri: all the authors on midwifery who lived from the time of Portal to that of Roederer and Levret were not, therefore, ignorant of the fact.

" Il y a eu plus d'un example de femmes qui n'ont pû accoucher," he observes at page 98, " parceque le placenta s'étoit collé sur l'orifice de la matrice, qu'il le tenoit hermetiquement clos, et qu'il empêchoit sa dilatation lors du terme de l'accouchement. C'est donc un peu legèrement que Daventer soutient que le placenta est toujours au fond de la matrice."

Roederer has given a clear account of the symptoms and treatment of cases of uterine hæmorrhage from attachment of the placenta to the lower part of the uterus, in his Elements of Midwifery, published at Göttingen in 1759. The placenta, he states, can be felt firmly adhering to its inferior segment. He denies the possibility from any cause of the placenta being detached from the fundus uteri and falling down to the cervix. In some cases the whole placenta covers the orifice of the uterus; in others, and these are much less dangerous, and may be committed to nature, he states that it adheres only to the side of the aperture. He has described with great minuteness the operation of turning the child, and pointed out its necessity in all those cases in which a large portion of the placenta adheres to the neck of the uterus. He recommends the dilatation of the orifice to be slowly and cautiously effected with the hand, which, he says, is not to be pushed through the centre of the placenta, but through the opening formed by its detachment from the uterus.

Levret, in his Dissertation 1761, undertook to prove, what it appears had previously been demonstrated.—1. That the placenta sometimes adheres to the circumference of the internal orifice of the uterus; 2. That where this occurs, uterine hæmorrhage is *inevitable* in the latter months of pregnancy; and 3d, that the only method of obviating this dangerous accident is to deliver immediately by turning the child. He refers to the cases of Van Horne, Schaeher, Plasner, Brunet, Huster, Portal, Petit, and to those which came under his observation, to prove the truth of his first proposition. He quotes also in its support the opinions of Massa, Drelincourt, Mauriceau, Bidloc, and Noortwyk, that the outer membrane of the ovum adheres to the whole inner surface of the uterus, and that the spheroidal mass, being equally compressed on all sides by the uterus, cannot be displaced, nor the placenta slide down from the fundus to the cervix, as Daventer supposed. Levret observed that uterine contractions invariably increased the hæmorrhage, where the placenta had been implanted over the cervix uteri, and that the contrary effect was produced where the placenta had adhered to the fundus uteri, and been detached by an accidental cause.

In a case which occurred in 1752, he passed the hand through the substance of the placenta, and delivered the child. The child was dead, and the mother died soon after. Levret appears to have been one of the first who recommended, as a general rule, forcing the hand through the centre of the placenta, instead of passing it between the uterus and its margin, as Mauriceau and Portal had done. The occurrence of uterine hæmorrhage from placental presentation he attributed to a development of the cervix uteri from above downward, in consequence of which a separation took place between the two organs, and the vessels of the uterus were exposed.

Smellie also knew, in 1745, that the placenta sometimes adheres to the lower part of the uterus, and he has related nine cases to illustrate the fact, and the appropriate treatment. " The edge or middle of the placenta sometimes adheres," he observes, " over the inside of the os internum, which frequently begins to open several weeks before the full time; and if this be the case a flooding begins at the same time, and seldom ceases entirely until the woman is delivered. The discharge may, indeed, be terminated by coagulums that stop up the passage; but when they are removed, it returns with its former violence, and demands the same treatment that is recommended above"—viz. artificial delivery.

"A case of hæmorrhage," observes Dr. Rigby, in the preface to the sixth edition of his Essay, 1822, "in which I found the placenta attached to the os uteri, occurred at a very early period of my practice; but not finding such a circumstance recorded in the lectures which I had attended or taken notice of in the common elementary treatises on midwifery, I considered it at first merely as a casual and rare deviation from nature. In a few years, however, so many similar instances fell under my notice, as to convince me that it was a circumstance necessary to be inquired after in every case of hæmorrhage; and this conviction was confirmed by the perusal of cases in midwifery; for I then found that the fact of the placenta being thus situated had been recorded by many writers, though in no instance, which had then reached me, had any practical inferences been deduced from it. It appeared to me, indeed, most extraordinary, that such a fact, known to so many celebrated practitioners, should not long before have led to its practical application, and, in consequence, to more fixed principles in the treatment of hæmorrhage from the gravid uterus; and I may perhaps be allowed to say, that I congratulate myself, young in years and in practice as I then was, in being probably the first to suggest an important improvement in the treatment of one of the most perplexing and dangerous cases in midwifery, and that I committed my observations on the subject to paper, not only under a conviction of their practical utility, but certainly also under an impression that my suggestions were original. Not long after the first edition was at press, indeed before the first sheet was printed (1776), Levret's dissertation on this subject fell into my hands; and in a note I referred to it as additional testimony in proof of the placenta in these cases being originally attached to the os uteri. I have been led into this little detail, because it has been suggested that I have borrowed my theory from Levret. After remarking the gross folly I should have been guilty of in quoting Levret, had I furtively adopted his opinions, it will, I trust, be sufficient for me unequivocally to declare, that my original ideas on the subject were derived solely from my own personal observation and experience; and that, having previously *neither read nor heard of the placenta being ever fixed to the os uteri*, the knowledge of such a circumstance, derived as before observed, came to me, and impressed me as a discovery. I was certainly afterwards struck with the coincidence of the sentiments of Levret and myself on the subject—with the similarity of our practical deductions, and, allowing for the difference of language, even with the sameness of our expressions. But is it extraordinary that two persons should have deduced the same conclusions from similar premises? In the present instance, where *the inferences are so obvious*, the contrary,

as I have before remarked, is surely the more extraordinary, that other writers who have noticed the fact should not have deduced them; that Dionis, Mauriceau, Deventer, La Motte, Portal, Ruysch, Giffard, Smellie, Hunter, &c. whom I have quoted as having found the placenta at the os uteri, should not practically have applied it, than that Levret or myself should have done it. I am further not reluctant to acknowledge that, after reading Levret's dissertation, I felt less entitled to the claim of absolute originality on the subject; and I now rest perfectly satisfied to divide with him the credit arising from the mere circumstance of communicating a new physiological fact." "Levret's facts, moreover, though they proved that the placenta might be originally attached to the os uteri (and a single instance would establish this) were scarcely sufficient to prove the frequency of its occurrence, from which alone arises the necessity of practically attending to it in every case of hæmorrhage. His observations (perhaps even more creditable to him for being founded on such scanty materials), were derived from four cases only, but of these but two were under his immediate cognizance; whereas, in the first edition of this essay, my opinions were supported by 36 detailed cases, in 13 of which the placenta was found at the os uteri; and in the fourth edition the number was increased to 106, 43 of which were produced by this peculiar original situation of the placenta."

In the Maternité at Paris, from the year 1797 to 1811, during which period 20,357 women were delivered, Madame Boivin reports there were 8 cases of placental presentation, being in the proportion of 1 in 2554. During six years and nine months 10,387 cases of labour occurred in the Dublin Lying-in Hospital, under the mastership of Dr. Joseph Clarke, and there were 4 cases of placental presentation, or 1 in 2596. One of these proved fatal. Dr. Collins met with 11 cases of placental presentation in 16,654 labours, being nearly in the proportion of 1 to 1492. Eight of the children presented naturally, four of which were turned; one was delivered by the natural efforts; one with the forceps; and in the other two the head was lessened. Of the remaining three, two presented with the feet, and one with the breech. Six of the children were born alive. Of the five still-born, two were putrid. Two of the women, where the children were turned, died: all the rest recovered. Dr. Ramsbotham has related 19 cases of placental presentation, eight of which proved fatal. In fine, the placenta was only partially adherent to the cervix, and in three the expulsion of the placenta took place before the child. Out of

174 cases of placental presentation recorded by different authors, Dr. Churchill states that 48 proved fatal, or nearly 1 in 3; and that in 85 cases of uterine hæmorrhage, where the placenta was at the fundus, 24 proved fatal, the proportions being nearly the same.

I have seen 38 cases of uterine hæmorrhage in the latter months of pregnancy from partial or complete attachment of the placenta to the neck of the uterus. Seven of these women died soon after delivery, from the loss of blood they had sustained. One died undelivered, from the first attack, before being seen; one from rupture of the uterus; and five from uterine phlebitis and other forms of uterine inflammation. The subjoined table of these cases, constructed by Edmund Johnson, Esq. will enable you in a very short time to become acquainted with all their most important details.

In the greater number of cases of placental presentation the discharge of blood takes place spontaneously in the seventh and eighth months of pregnancy, and cannot be referred either to bodily exertion, external violence, nor to any unusual determination to the uterine organs, or congestion of their vessels. The hæmorrhage generally comes on suddenly, when the woman is in a state of rest, and the blood continues to flow until faintness or even syncope takes place. It often ceases entirely, and the patient resumes her usual occupations, and has no dread of another attack. But after an interval of several days, and sometimes not before two or three weeks, the flooding is renewed, and perhaps with increased violence, or a constant profuse discharge takes place, and a decided effect is produced upon the constitution,—the pulse becomes rapid and feeble, and the countenance pale. Similar attacks return at longer or shorter intervals, and if delivery be not accomplished by art, sooner or later death takes place. The first attack of flooding seldom proves fatal, but it sometimes does so; for in the second case related in the table, which occurred in the British Lying-in Hospital, the life of the patient was at once extinguished by a single gush of blood from the uterus. I examined the body after death. The centre of the placenta was over the centre of the os uteri.

When flooding takes place to an alarming extent in the seventh or eighth months of gestation, you ought first to ascertain, by a careful internal examination, whether or not the placenta be situated at the os uteri. It is impossible, from the manner in which the discharge of blood takes place, to be certain of the fact; for there are some cases of hæmorrhage from detachment of the placenta from the upper part of the uterus, where the flooding occurs spontaneously, and to as great an extent as in cases where the placenta pre-

sents. In some cases I have been induced, from the symptoms, to believe that the placenta was at the os uteri when it was not. As the treatment and the successful or fatal result of the case will, in a great measure, depend on the correctness of the diagnosis, the examination should be conducted with so much care and circumspection as to leave no room for doubt on the subject. An ordinary examination, with the fore and middle fingers, is generally sufficient to enable us to ascertain the true state of the case, but where the os uteri is very high up, and directed backwards, it becomes requisite to introduce the whole hand within the vagina. The finger should then be passed gently through the os uteri, and, if the placenta adheres to the cervix, it will be distinguished from coagulated blood, the only substance with which it can be confounded, by its firmer, fibrous, vascular structure, and, above all, by its adhering at one part to the uterus, and being separated at another. If you will take the trouble to pass the finger carefully and repeatedly over the uterine surface of a recently expelled placenta, you will never, in actual practice, mistake a placenta at the os uteri for a clot of blood, however firm. In all cases it is requisite to proceed at once to determine by an examination, so carefully conducted as to render a mistake impossible, whether or not the placenta presents—even though the hæmorrhage should be slightly renewed by the displacement of the coagula; you cannot be too early acquainted with the precise condition of the patient. You ought, at the same time, to ascertain whether the placenta adheres partially or completely to the cervix uteri, and whether the os uteri is in a condition to admit of the operation of turning being performed.

The operation of turning, which is required in all cases of complete placental presentation, is not necessary in the greater number of cases in which the edge of the placenta passing into the membranes can be distinctly felt through the os uteri. Sometimes there is profuse and dangerous hæmorrhage where the placenta does not adhere all round to the neck of the uterus, but only partially. If the os uteri is not much dilated or dilatable, the best practice in these cases is to rupture the membranes, to excite the uterus to contract vigorously, by the binder, ergot, and all other means, and to leave the case to nature : by adopting this treatment the operation of turning may be avoided with advantage in the greater number of cases of partial placental presentation. But, if the hæmorrhage is profuse, has returned at different intervals, and a great quantity has been lost, and the constitution is really affected, it is the safest practice at once, if the orifice of the uterus is in a condition to allow the hand to pass without difficulty, to deliver by turning the child.

Where the placental presentation is complete, the operation of turning should be performed, in all cases, as soon as the orifice of the uterus is so much dilated or dilatable as to allow the hand to be introduced without the employment of much force. It is seldom safe to attempt to deliver by turning before the os uteri is so far dilated that you can easily introduce the points of the four fingers and thumb within it : however soft and relaxed it may be, until dilatation has commenced, and proceeded so far, I am convinced there are very few cases in which the operation of turning will be required, or completed without the risk of inflicting some injury on the os uteri. This is a point of the greatest practical importance, but I do not know in what manner to communicate to you, in words, a more clear and definite idea of the grounds upon which you ought to proceed.

In every case, before attempting to turn, make a most careful examination of the os uteri, and endeavour, from the degree of dilatation, and the thinness and softness, of the orifice, to form a correct judgment upon this point before interfering, for the hæmorrhage will be renewed if the attempt is unsuccessful, and the patient will be placed in a worse condition than she was before. When you have resolved to turn, let the patient lie on the left side, with the pelvis close to the edge of the bed, and introduce the right hand into the vagina as before described, and then pass the fingers and hand gently and slowly in a conical form through the os uteri, giving it time to dilate, and onward into the cavity between the detached portion of the placenta and the uterus: then force the fingers through the membranes, grasp both feet, and bring them down into the vagina, and *slowly* extract the child as in cases of nates presentation, and do not afterwards be in a hurry to remove the placenta, unless it is wholly detached and lying in the upper part of the vagina. This operation is easily and speedily performed when the os uteri is widely dilated and dilatable. It is, however,

placental presentation, where the os uteri is so thick, rigid, and undilatable, that it is impossible to introduce the hand into the *uterus* without producing certain mischief.

A TABULAR VIEW OF THIRTY-EIGHT CASES OF UTERINE HÆMORRHAGE FROM PLACENTAL PRESENTATION.

1	July 22, 1828	Profuse hæmorrhage seven days before labour; placenta adhered to neck of uterus all round; rigidity of os uteri; turning attempted, but could not be performed; the plug employed for several days, but much blood lost; turning at last accomplished with little difficulty, but followed by alarming exhaustion	Died 18 days after delivery; extensive inflammation of the pleura, with gangrene of the inferior lobe of the left lung, and inflammation of the left spermatic vein. Died.
2	1828	S when profuse hæmorrhage at ninth month, which lived till death, ... took ... ally; no ... or uneasy ... ion before discharge ...; ... were she could receive on dissection adhering and ... turi; died ...	
3	October 24, 1829	Hæmorrhage at seventh and a half ... th; thirty-six hours were ... aid was proposed; pl. ... found hanging out of orifice of uterus; operation of turning proposed, but the patient would not ... it to be performed; violent flooding for several hours; placenta and fœtus expelled ... ...; great exhaustion	Recovered.
4	February 8, 1830	Profuse hæmorrhage in the ... ... month, ... protruding through orifice of uterus; placenta ..., and a dead ... ...; ... hæmorrhage; insensibility and coldness of extremities, &c.	Recovered.

5	March 24, 1835	Hæmorrhage; exhaustion; os uteri soft and widely dilated; hand passed into uterus through opening made by detachment of placenta from cervix uteri; membranes ruptured and turning effected; child dead	Recovered.
6	March 1835	Hæmorrhage during eighth month; placenta attached to lower part of uterus; usual effects of loss of blood; os uteri widely dilated, and placenta hanging partially through it; turning easily performed; child dead	Recovered.
7	April 26, 1835	Hæmorrhage at a … and a half month; … osing of blood for … teen days, … ich … on without any … ght or injury … hen in bed, preceded by no … cause; … ffice of uterus … tled and … ble; hand … ble to be introduced; hæmorrhage checked for two days by cold and rest; sudden … wal of flooding to a great … tent; syncope at last … ame on, and turning was easily … complished; … ld alive	Died in a few days from the effects of loss of blood.
8	October 7, 1835	Hæmorrhage in the … enth … onth; slight … ing of blood for the … ceks, at the end of … hich period several … ings were suddenly discharged; pulse imperceptible; … wice … dd; … sion feeble; os uteri very rigid, and … tile … il … ded; repeated … ts to … tn; a … fot at last … gid, and the … sion … pled with … city; hæmorrhage arrested; … tion, rigors, and death threatened	Recovered.
9	October 18, 1835	Profuse hæmorrhage in the eighth … th; … centa found hanging out of os uteri; hand could not be introduced to turn the child, in … ence of … gidity of os uteri and … sion of the … pelvis; … dated; head felt above brim of … lvis; cra-… tomy performed, and delivery … pled … fter four … ohurs with great … culty	Read.
10	October 28, 1835	Hæmorrhage … ting a … enth … nth, … turning … newed at last with … iolence, … cepits … find … on … pelvis, and the … tents of the uterus … re expelled entire; hæmorrhage ceased after cold bring … plied	Recovered.
11	October 30, 1835	… ght hæmorrhage, lasting fourteen … ays, … ting with an i … ense discharge; pla-… centa pa … idly ad … cent to cervix; syncope; os uteri rigid, dilated to the size of a crown … piece; … pla … died at … per … rt of neck of uterus; membranes felt; head … dl; … then ruptured; hæmorrhage arrested; … ld … pelled by the natural efforts	Recovered; sanguineous discharge from uterus for months.
12	Nov. 10, 1835	Profuse hæmorrhage during eighth month; first … centa presented, and adhered all … nd to cervix uteri; vagina filled with coagula; … insensibility and cold … ties; os uteri … lly dilated; pl … centa separated from uterus with the fingers, and turning performed; hæmorrhage after the … ction of pla-… centa; pulse imperceptible; respiration … bied; lips and hands livid; stimulants ineffectual	Died two hours after delivery.
13	Nov. 17, 1835	Hæmorrhage in the eighth month, after … reat bodily exertion; … centa … ched from orifice of uterus; os uteri rigid and slightly patulous; rest and cold … pied for a day, after … hich period the membranes were ruptured; … ead descended between pla … centa and uterus, and delivery was completed without hæmorrhage	Died at a remote period from deep-seated uterine inflammation.

14	March 24, 1836	Hæmorrhage in seventh month, continuing for several days, exhaustion at last taking place after a discharge of blood; placenta felt at posterior part of cervix uteri; membranes felt at anterior part; membranes ruptured; hæmorrhage ceased; labour did not come on for two days; uterine phlebitis	Died 11th of April, from phlebitis and inflammation of the lungs.
15	Dec. 3, 1836	Hæmorrhage in seventh month; ergot of rye had been repeatedly administered without presenting part being known; os uteri widely dilated; placenta found adhering to the posterior part of cervix uteri; turning performed in five minutes with ease; child dead; no hæmorrhage followed	Died ten days after, from inflammation of the venis of uterus.
16	Dec. 20, 1836	Repeated attacks of hæmorrhage during the eighth month; placenta felt presenting through os uteri; great exhaustion; rigidity; hæmorrhage controlled for some days; turning at last performed; child alive; recovered for two hours	Died suddenly, two hours after delivery.
17	Dec. 25, 1836	Severe hæmorrhage after a fit of coughing; pulse rapid and feeble; no uterine contractions; os uteri soft and dilatable; placenta detached, and a portion hanging out of orifice of uterus; turning easily performed; child born alive; placenta allowed to remain for some time to act as a plug	Recovered.
18	March 10, 1837	Hæmorrhage in the sixth month, occurring at intervals during four weeks; ergot of rye given without the presenting part being ascertained; os uteri soft and widely dilated, and a portion of the detached placenta hanging through it; turning easily performed; child alive	Recovered.
19	July 19, 1837	Hæmorrhage at intervals, for several days, during ninth month; extreme debility; os uteri slightly dilated; hand passed into the uterus; membranes ruptured and a foot brought down, and the delivery easily accomplished; no hæmorrhage followed	Recovered after severe uterine and crural phlebitis.
20	Dec. 27, 1837	Hæmorrhage during the ninth month; os uteri slightly dilated; partial placental presentation; discharge of blood night; no constitutional symptoms present; os uteri became widely dilated at the end of twenty-four hours; edge of placenta felt; membranes were ruptured; head descended; child born alive by natural efforts	Recovered.
21	May 12, 1838	Hæmorrhage, lasting three days; orifice of uterus at commencement of attack high up, and slightly dilated; by end of third day largely dilated; a great discharge of blood at last took place; turning easily performed; child dead	Recovered.
22	June 11, 1838	Flooding during the seventh month, lasting at intervals for five days, and producing fits of syncope; turning performed; hæmorrhage arrested; faintness; cold extremities, and exhaustion	Died at a remote period from uterine phlebitis.
23	Jan. 12, 1839	Hæmorrhage at eight and a half months; three attacks during one month, at long intervals; renewed spontaneously with the utmost violence; os uteri thick and rigid; vagina filled with coagula; placenta adhering all round to inner surface of cervix; artificial dilatation attempted, but without success; membranes about to be ruptured when two fingers were passed between the placenta and uterus, a foot was felt and brought down into vagina, and turning accomplished with great difficulty, from the orifice of uterus firmly grasping like a rope the neck of the child; labour in half an hour, completed by artificial dilatation; but the hæmorrhage continued, in spite of all treatment, and complete exhaustion followed	Died half an hour after delivery from loss of blood.

No.	Date		Result
24	Feb. 1839	Hemorrhage at seventh and a half month; placenta adhering all round to neck of uterus; os uteri rigid and undilatable, being the size of a crown-piece; head presenting; hemorrhage arrested for a time by cold, but renewed; fingers were pushed through the placenta, and the membranes ruptured; head descended and hemorrhage ceased; os uteri continued rigid, so that perforation could not be employed; labour lasted during the day, when exhaustion came on, without further loss of blood; craniotomy at last performed, and extraction completed with great difficulty, in consequence of the extreme rigidity; complete exhaustion	Died soon after delivery from loss of blood.
25	July 30, 1839	Flooding during the seventh month; placenta adhered to neck of uterus; os uteri thick and rigid; hemorrhage profuse; syncope; the whole hand could not be passed into uterus; two fingers were introduced within its orifice, and a foot easily brought down before the membranes were ruptured; turning easily performed; hemorrhage arrested; child dead	Recovered.
26	Feb. 22, 1840	Profuse hemorrhage at the five and a half month; repeated again at the seventh month, when it lasted three days; placenta entirely situate over orifice of uterus, and adhering to the cervix; hand thrust through placenta, and delivery completed by turning; head extracted with great difficulty; exhaustion from time of delivery. (When called to this patient, Dr. Lee found her dead)	Died an hour and a half after delivery. *Post-mortem examination:* Extensive laceration of muscular and mucous coats of cervix uteri on the left side; a superficial rent on right side; placenta had adhered to whole circumference of cervix uteri; pelvis distorted to a high degree
27	October 9, 1840	Profuse hemorrhage in the seventh month; experienced for days previously a sense of weight and uneasiness; edge of placenta felt through orifice of uterus; membranes ruptured, which induced strong labour pains; hemorrhage was arrested; child expelled 'dead in an hour and a half	Recovered.
28	April 7, 1841	Uterine hemorrhage during seventh month; repeated twice at short intervals during the eighth month; an immense discharge at last took place, producing syncope; os uteri thick, high up, and but little dilated; the whole hand could not be passed into the uterus; placenta adhering all round to cervix uteri; the fore and middle finger introduced between placenta and uterus; a foot brought down with great difficulty; head extracted after great exertion, os uteri having grasped the child with great force	Recovered.
29	May 19, 1841	Two attacks of uterine hemorrhage during the seventh month, at intervals of three weeks, the last producing syncope; os uteri dilated to size of a crown-piece; placenta presenting, and adhering nearly all round to cervix uteri; turning accomplished in quarter of an hour by another practitioner; convulsions came on during extraction of child, which continued until her death	Died four hours after delivery from convulsions.

30	May 26, 1841	Spontaneous hæmorrhage in the eighth month; had several attacks, but not very profuse; os uteri rigid, high up, and dilated to the size of a half-crown; placenta adhered every where to the neck of uterus; child turned without difficulty; hæmorrhage arrested	Recovered.
31	Nov. 10, 1841	Hæmorrhage in the ninth month; placenta detached, and a large portion hanging out of orifice of the uterus; syncope; hæmorrhage arrested for a time; membranes at last gave way, and the child was born alive, without artificial assistance	Recovered.
32	Nov. 13, 1841	Profuse hæmorrhage in the eighth month; os uteri high up, and directed backward; thick, but dilatable; finger with difficulty introduced within it; placenta found adhering to cervix uteri; turning performed with ease; child alive	Recovered.
33	Jan. 5, 1842	Hæmorrhage at the end of seventh month; os uteri dilated to size of a half-crown; not rigid; placenta adhered all round to the cervix uteri; hand passed into uterus, and a foot brought down without difficulty; nates firmly grasped by os uteri	Recovered.
34	April 15, 1842	Hæmorrhage during sixth month; placenta partially adherent to cervix; membranes were ruptured, and a dead child expelled, without turning being employed; hæmorrhage arrested	Recovered.
35	July 1842	Hæmorrhage at the beginning of the eighth month; renewed after an interval of a month, with great severity; placenta adherent all round to cervix; os uteri dilated to the size of a half-crown, thin and dilatable; turning easily performed by another practitioner; syncope, with the usual symptoms of great loss of blood, followed, from which she never recovered	Died four hours after delivery.
36	Sept. 7, 1843	Hæmorrhage first commenced during the seventh month, but arrested; renewed after six weeks, with syncope; os uteri dilated to size of half-a-crown; placenta adhered so firmly to cervix uteri that the fingers were obliged to be forced through its structure, and the operation of turning performed; hæmorrhage ceased, and delivery was easily accomplished, followed by great faintness	Recovered.
37	Oct 15, 1842.	Hæmorrhage in eighth month; placenta adhering all round; hæmorrhage at intervals for two or three weeks; os uteri little dilated, but dilatable; immediately passed up the hand into the uterus, brought down the feet, and turned; child dead	Recovered.
38	Feb. 24, 1843	Profuse discharge for three weeks in the seventh month; placenta adhering all round; os uteri dilated to the size of a crown-piece, dilatable; passed the whole hand into the vagina; finding some difficulty in introducing it through os uteri, passed the fore and middle finger between the anterior part of the uterus and placenta; ruptured the membranes; grasped a foot, and easily extracted the child alive	Recovered.

In 13 of the 36 cases contained in the preceding table the os uteri was rigid and undilatable. The tampon or plug has no power to restrain the hæmorrhage in such cases, nor do I know of any other means—either cold, quietness, nor opium—which effectually have, and it is sometimes absolutely necessary under such circumstances to deliver by turning, before the hand can possibly be introduced into the uterus without producing fatal contusion or laceration of the part. I have found in several of these cases, however, that the delivery may be safely accomplished by merely passing the hand into the vagina, and afterwards the fore and middle fingers between the uterus and detached portion of the placenta, grasping with them the feet, which are generally situated near the os uteri, and drawing down the inferior extremities into the vagina, and delivering. I know that the inferior extremities may often be brought down in this way where it is impossible to pass the whole hand through the os uteri.

CASE OF DIABETES MELLITUS.

To the Editor of the Medical Gazette.

SIR,

THERE are few diseases the satisfactory treatment of which presents greater difficulties to the country practitioner than diabetes mellitus. It is only in the wards of an hospital that we can enforce any lengthened observance of a regulated diet, or expect to secure that careful obedience to our directions which is so necessary in the management of that formidable malady. It must be from this difficulty that so few contributions have been made to the history of diabetes in this country, except by the officers of public charities. Believing that every faithful record of facts is valuable to science, I send you the notes of a case which lately occurred to me; it will, I trust, prove interesting to some of your readers.

I remain, sir,
Your obedient servant,
JOHN F. HODGES,
Downpatrick, Co. Down,   Surgeon, &c.
June 12, 1843.

May 20th, 1843.—Susan C., æt. 17, a thin delicate-looking girl, resides with her mother, a very poor woman. About two years ago she received a severe fall, which was followed by excessive epistaxis, which, she says, could not be stopped for two days. After the fall, her health, which had previously been good, declined; she lost flesh; the quantity of urine discharged by her gradually increased, and her appetite for meat and drink became most inordinate. She has been repeatedly under treatment without much benefit. She states that the quantity of urine at present amounts to twenty-four pints in twenty-four hours, and that she drinks about the same amount of liquids. She is exceedingly weak and desponding; pulse 90; tongue white at the sides, red in the centre, and moist; abdomen swollen; bowels regular; has occasionally a burning pain in stomach, and almost every month severe attacks of diarrhœa and vomiting. Catamenia have not yet appeared. Her skin is dry and rough, and on her face there is a slight herpetic eruption. Has no cough or uneasiness in chest, except from occasional attacks of palpitation. Has at present no pain in back, or swelling in her limbs, but says that some time ago her legs swelled considerably, and that her left leg is sometimes painful to the touch, and weak. Her thirst is greatest after eating, but during the night it is also severe. Urine has a light straw colour, and a smell something resembling sour milk; tastes very sweet; sp. gr. 1·030; no deposit on standing; reddens litmus paper; not altered by heat or nitric acid, except that it is rendered slightly pinkish by the latter. When set aside for some days it fermented spontaneously, and emitted a strong alcoholic smell. Sugar in large quantity could easily be procured by simple evaporation from the fresh urine. The girl herself was frequently surprised by observing parts of her dress on which urine had fallen covered with a white powder, sweet to the taste. When first consulted, I prescribed for some days opiates, as pulv. Doveri, &c. but without any material effect. Upon reflecting upon the case, it occurred to me that it would be a most suitable one for giving a trial to the nitrogenizing plan proposed by Dr. Barlow, of Guy's Hospital, in the valuable Reports of that celebrated charity[*]. I accordingly commenced by prescribing the sesquicarbonate of ammonia in doses of five grains every three hours, with coffee and bacon for breakfast, animal food

[*] M. Bouchardat, in a memoir communicated to the French Academy, also recommended the carb. ammonia in the treatment of this usually intractable disease.

and cruciferous vegetables for dinner; and directed friction of the skin and warm flannel clothing. After pursuing this treatment about four days, a very marked improvement took place; her urine was diminished to fourteen pints in twenty-four hours, the specific gravity continuing the same. She stated that her health was greatly improved. The ammonia made her very warm, but produced no perspiration. Directed her to take five grains of the sesquicarbonate, dissolved in water, every two hours.

April 1st.—Continues to improve; was able the other day to attend church, the first time for a very long period; has perspired profusely; discharge of urine diminished to eight pints in twenty-four hours; appetite not now troublesome; says she does not feel hungry between meal times. Tongue red and clean; has no pain in any part.

3d.—Ingesta nine pints, urine ten pints, in twenty-four hours. About half an hour before coming to see me had taken her breakfast of bacon and coffee. Tongue red; saliva acid; skin warm. The medicine sickens her considerably; to take it only every third hour.

5th.—Drink, six pints; urine, eight pints; neutral to litmus. Tongue red; pulse 80.

8th.—Drink, seven pints; urine, eight pints; sp. gr. 1·030; tongue red; pulse 86.

13th.—Drink, five pints; urine, five pints; neutral; sp. gr. 1·030; expresses herself better than she has been since her first illness; no swelling in legs, or uneasiness in any part. The urine of this date, when set aside, became like milk very much diluted with water; a creamy-like pellicle formed on its surface; it did not undergo spontaneous fermentation.

16th.—Drink, three pints; urine, four pints; neutral. Tongue red; pulse 90; urine of higher colour than since commencement of treatment; sp. gr. reduced to 1·020; has lost its sweet taste; is slightly acid.

21st.—Drink, two pints; urine, four pints.

29th.—No relapse; states that she never enjoyed so good health; pulse 80; tongue clean; urine about four pints in twenty-four hours; appetite natural.

June 12th.—Has gained flesh and colour; considers herself quite recovered.

Results of the action of reagents on the urine of Susan C., April 13.

Ebullition . . . No change.
Nitric acid . . . No change.
Muriatic acid . . No change.
Sol. oxalate amm. White troubling.
Sol. nitrate silver . Dense deposit, insoluble in nitric acid.
Sol. potass . . . No change.
Ammonia . . . White deposit upon standing for some hours.
Chloride barium . White precipitate
Sp. gravity . . . 1·030.
Litmus . . . . Neutral.
Taste . . . . . Sweet.
Colour . . . . . Pale straw.
Smell . . . . . Sour milk.

OBSERVATIONS.—The successful treatment of the above case of this formidable disease is opposed to the opinions of many recent writers, that it proves "sooner or later inevitably mortal," and encourages us to expect that the insight which the remarkable progress of organic chemistry, chiefly by the indefatigable labours of Liebig, and of our celebrated countryman Dr. Prout, has already afforded us into many hitherto obscure processes in the animal economy, will enable us to proceed with greater confidence and success in our treatment of diabetes and many other functional diseases. It is, indeed, but fair to conclude that, in the treatment of diseases which produce a change in the chemical constitution of the animal fluids, the exhibition of remedies which, in ordinary chemical researches, possess a decided influence in counteracting or modifying those changes, should deserve the attention of the physician, and particularly when experience has shown that the same agents are capable of producing similar effects within the body. It is the duty of every observer carefully to record and communicate such results as may confirm or oppose these views.

The effects of the nitrogenizing treatment in the above case, in diminishing the quantity of urine, was well marked. When first submitted to treatment, Susan C. voided the very large quantity of twenty-four pints in twenty-four hours, of the density 1·030, which, calculated from the table published by

Dr. Golding Bird in his most interesting and instructive lectures, contained rather more than twenty-one and a half ounces of dry solid matter!

The density of the urine continued very nearly the same until the sweet taste had disappeared, when it was reduced to 1·020, and exhibited the colour and smell of healthy urine. Most of your readers must be aware of the ingenious reasoning of Dr. Barlow with respect to the operation of ammonia in diabetes. He considers that it is useful not merely by its stimulant properties, but from its elementary constitution; the chemical constitution of ammonia and sugar exhibiting a remarkable similarity with albumen, the nitrogenized product of healthy digestion. Thus Dr. Barlow shows, that when the atomic numbers of certain proportions of ammonia, sugar, carbonic acid, and water, are reckoned together, we obtain the numbers which represent the atomic constitution of albumen. With respect to this ingenious theory, such transformations may be effected within the human body by the agency of nitrogenizing remedies; and the success of the treatment founded upon it tends to confirm the opinion that the formulæ given in Dr. Barlow's paper are not like too many of the present day, which, though looking most plausible on paper, are only to be verified in the laboratory of the chemist. It has been asserted that even the illustrious Professor of Giessen has been carried away by his love of chemical theory beyond the limits which sound physiological experience justifies. We should then be careful, that in our zeal for the novel and unexpected light which that truly distinguished inquirer has thrown upon so many departments of the chemistry of the human body, we should be induced to forget that the stomach is not like the test-glass of the chemist, in which all his agents act according to certain laws, the effects of which are well known and clearly determined. We should remember that Liebig himself cautions us to bear in mind that all the chemical forces which act within the body are influenced by "a power distinct from all other powers of nature, namely, the vital principle;" and, also, "that a rational physiology cannot be founded on mere reactions, and the living body cannot be viewed as a chemical laboratory." (Organic Chemistry, p. xv.)

With respect to the cause of the disease in the above case, Susan C. does not appear to have inherited any disposition to it, for her mother affirms that none of her relatives were ever affected in a similar manner. The exciting cause was evidently the great loss of blood which she had experienced. Like too many of the poorer classes in this country, she had been in the habit of living almost exclusively on potatoes and other vegetables; but the comparative rarity of diabetes among our potatoe eating population, proves, that though a diet exclusively vegetable may aggravate the disease when once formed, yet that it is not of itself sufficient to induce diabetic symptoms.

OPHTHALMIC SURGERY.

REMARKS ON THE ROYAL WESTMINSTER OPHTHALMIC REPORT.

To the Editor of the Medical Gazette.

SIR,

ALLOW me to inquire, through the medium of your journal, whether some grave error have not inadvertently crept into the report, circulated recently by the committee of the Royal Westminster Ophthalmic Hospital.

It would appear from that statement, dated 25th of May last, not only that during the past year six operations for artificial pupil have been performed, every one of which succeeded, both "in making a new pupil, and in restoring sight;" but, also, that since April 1840, the large number of 1474 operations for strabismus have taken place "without even the occurrence of a single accident."

It is not, however, sir, upon these triumphs of art, surprising as they are, that I intend to trouble you with further observations; the more important item of the report, and that which has called forth my remarks, is to the effect, that of 85 operations for cataract during the past year, 78 or 11-12ths of the entire number have been "completely successful." Of the remaining 7.5 were "partially so;" hence there remain but 2 cases of failure, which are to those of success as 1 to 42.

I presume that by the expression "completely successful" is implied that, in the cases so described, perfect vision was restored; and that in the other 5, at least imperfect sight was regained. Now, this proportion of cures is almost incredible, because utterly unprecedented,—far exceeding that which has hitherto attended the efforts of able operators, so far, at least, as I have obtained numerical records of their experience. There are in the subjoined list but two accounts of success which in any wise approach the one given in the circular in question; and neither of these is entitled to unhesitating belief, as all the cases in the former were treated by depression, and it is probable, therefore, were discharged at a very early period from beneath the observation of the surgeon, and the latter is in some degree invalidated by the diverse statement of another and a disinterested inquirer. In the following list which I have drawn out, by way of giving a fair view of the usual results of operations for cataract, I have placed these two disputable estimates first: all those which follow are apparently genuine and correct.

In 72* cases of depression at the Hôtel-Dieu of Paris, between the years 1808 and 1819, there were unsuccessful only 9; being one-eighth of the entire number.

In 206‡ cases of extraction by Daviel, reported by himself, there were unsuccessful 24; less than one-eighth.

In 34‡ extractions by Daviel, reported by Laqué, there were decided failures 9: more than one-fourth. (Between the date of operation and that of the report more than two years elapsed, during which 9 persons additional had left Rheims. Suppose all these to have been successful, still the proportion of failures will be one-fifth.)

In 64* extractions at La Charité between 1808 and 1819, there were failures 25, or two-fifths.

In 10‡ extractions by Richter, there were failures 3: one-third.

In 33* extractions by Antoine Petit, there were failures 8: one-fourth.

In 8* extractions by Dupuytren, there were failures 3: one-third.

In 253* depressions by Dupuytren, there were failures 53: one-fifth.

In 19† extractions and depressions

by Morand, La Faye, and Poyet, 7 failed: one-third.

In 19 extractions by Sharp, but half had "tolerable success:" failures one-half.

In 113 extractions and depressions at Hôtel-Dieu, between the years 1806 and 1810, there were 53 more or less successful. Of the 60 in which the result was unfortunate or unknown, allow but 30 for failures, viz. one-fourth of the entire number.

In 179 extractions by Roux, there were failures 72: one-third.

In the total number, therefore, of 1019 cases, 252, or about one-fourth, failed.

Dr. Mackenzie, from whose work I have extracted the three last reports, may be considered to convey his experience in saying, "In the practice of one thoroughly acquainted with eye disease, able to discriminate the cases fitted for extraction and those fitted for division, able to perform those operations well, careful and skilful in the after-treatment, I should think three-fourths of those operated on would recover useful vision, and two-thirds excellent vision:"—a conclusion which tallies pretty closely with the result deduced from consideration of the series of cases just given.

Now although it is probable that, among the 78 cataracts successfully treated by operation at the Westminster Ophthalmic Hospital, several were soft, perhaps congenital, and readily absorbed after exposure to the solvent action of the aqueous humour by the safe operation of division, which does not appear to have been practised in any of the cases cited above; yet so great is the difference between the results obtained in these latter, and those reported from the Ophthalmic Hospital, that one cannot but suppose, unless the report be confirmed, that some mistake has occurred in it. Should such prove to be the case, I shall not regret having called attention to the subject, as an erroneously favourable description of operations is injurious alike to the public, who are led thereby to expect too much, and to the profession, whose members find themselves unable to realise in practice the overwrought anticipations of their patients.

I am, sir,
Your obedient servant,
JOHN F. FRANCE.

Guy's Hospital, June 24, 1843.

---

* Leçons Orales, par Baron Dupuytren.
‡ Lacournière, Considerations on Cataract.
† Memoirs of Royal Academy of Surgery, Neale's edition, vol. iii.

CONTRIBUTIONS

TO

ANATOMY AND PHYSIOLOGY.

BY ROBERT KNOX, M.D. F.R.S.E.

Lecturer on Anatomy and Physiology, and Corresponding Member of the French Academy of Medicine.

(Continued from p. 502.)

On some Varieties in Human Structure, with Remarks on the Doctrine of " Unity of the Organization."

II.—*The humerus : its supra-condyloid process.*

COMPARATIVE anatomists had long ago described a foramen, or short canal, traversing the humerus somewhat obliquely in carnivorous mammals, and they had also described, what could not well escape the most casual observer, that this canal was situated a short way above the inner condyle of the humerus; that it was formed by a process of bone running from the shaft to the inner condyle, and that the humeral artery and its accompanying nerve, the median, in its descent to the bend of the elbow, first passed behind this process, thereafter returning to their original course, or nearly so, by traversing the canal thus formed. Physiologists, as usual, offered a mechanical reason for this deviation in certain animals from the more common structures, and, as usual, their reasons were destitute of common sense. It is not even worth while adverting to them. They resembled Sir A. Cooper's reason for there being two mammæ, and Bartholin's reasons for the male having rudimentary breasts, *ne gloriatur fœmina*, &c.; it is a vile patchwork, almost peculiar to British physiology, a jumble of expedients and contrivances to meet difficulties.

The possible occurrence of such a process as a supra-condyloid in man, accompanied by a corresponding deviation in the course of the artery and nerve, was to be foretold, according to the theories of Goethe, and was, perhaps, perfectly well understood in Germany, but certainly not in this country. I do not believe that any similar preparation to the one now before you exists in Britain. It is not my intention to describe it at any length here, having already done so in a memoir

read to the Anatomical and Physiological Society, and printed in the Edin. Med. and Surg. Journ. for 1841. All I mean to do is simply to notice it as a process found on the humerus, a short way above the inner condyle, of varying length, tending downwards towards the condyle, and connected to it by ligamentous or aponeurotic fibres. In most humeral bones I have examined the process is entirely wanting, or nearly so, its absence being a specific human characteristic; in others, human also, there exists a rudiment of it, with a groove above and below it; and in the one before me the process is at least half an inch in length; the artery and nerve pass behind it, and the structures are extremely analogous to those of the panther, tiger, cat, &c. It will not be objected, I trust, to this view that the process is incomplete, seeing that it does not reach the condyle. The course followed by the artery and nerve will form the subject of a few remarks when I speak of the varieties of the human arteries, and, referring, therefore, my audience to the memoir already published by me on this matter, I shall confine myself to a single additional remark.

However well known the doctrines of transcendental anatomy were to Goëthe, Frank, and others in Germany, there were still some first-rate anatomists, also German, who, about that period, and for some time afterwards, did not rightly comprehend them. Amongst these, it is surprising to find the name of the illustrious Tiedemann, the first of living anatomists. In his great work on the Human Arteries, a very splendid engraving is given of a variety in the course of the interosseal artery, which arose in this case from the humeral artery about the middle of the arm : quitting the course of the larger vessel, the interosseal descended towards the internal intermuscular ligament, or partition, and passing behind a supra-condyloid process represented in the engraving, fully as well developed as in the specimen on the table, it afterwards regained its position in the bend of the elbow, ultimately following the course of the interosseal. This supra-condyloid process, as it really and truly was, with its ligamentous band tying it to the inner condyle, M. Tiedemann calls an " excrescentia ossis humeri in solita."

III.—*Osseous system.*

The comparatively rare occurrence of pre-sternal bones in man, more especially perhaps in this country, induces me to publish the following observations respecting them. During the whole period in which I have superintended rooms for teaching practical anatomy in this city, I have never had occasion to observe in a single instance the presence of pre-sternal bones in men, although nearly all the more rare forms of the human sternum have come under my notice; until a few months ago, when describing to my morning class the anatomy of the thorax and its contained viscera. The person in whom these bones occurred was a stout muscular man of a stature exceeding six feet, and about 25 years of age; his general shape was somewhat peculiar, and this, added to a remarkably swarthy skin and black hair, induced me to suppose that notwithstanding his Saxon name, the individual was really of the Celtic race.

But be this as it may, I requested the gentlemen engaged in the dissections to look carefully for any variety in form which might occur, and one of the first was noticed by myself in examining the sternum. Whilst describing the superior aperture of the thorax still covered with soft parts, I remarked to the class that although the sternum was sufficiently broad in most parts, it presented at its *tracheal incisura* or notch a peculiar arrangement, which led me to suspect the presence of an anomalous structure.

Soon after the lecture I examined into what this anomaly might be, and found the narrowness of the superior portion, or rather margin, of the sternum to be owing to the presence of two episternal bones, occupying precisely the position in which they were first noticed by Beclard,[*] and afterwards by M. Breschet,[†] and by Mr. King[‡] of London.

The specimen I examined with a good deal of attention, but found little to add to the extremely accurate descriptions of preceding observers: situated behind the sternal attachments of the sterno-mastoid muscles, and mesially in respect to the articular surface for the clavicles, the pre-sternal bones are attached by their bases to the inner or deeper margin of the notch of the manubrium of the sternum; they are of a pyramidal form, and approach each other slightly at their summits. The base of each appeared to me encrusted with cartilage, and there existed a close but distinct moveable joint, with a synovial apparatus, and strong ligamentous bands of a peculiar reddish colour, between them and the sternum; one was less moveable than the other, and a ligamentous band connected them to each other. A few muscular looking fibres, but extremely short, ran from the sternum to these bones.

It is not my intention to enter upon the much disputed ground as to the nature and true signification of these pre-sternal bones; Beclard fancied they might be the rudiments of the fourchette (clavicule furculaire), fully developed in birds, and reduced to a mere rudiment, and that too only occasionally present in man; but this idea, however plausible, has not been generally adopted by anatomists: I know not, indeed, that any philosophic anatomist coincides with this view of Beclard's. Mr. Breschet's opinion is, that the sus-ternal or pre-sternal bones represent, or are in man the rudiments of a cervical rib, of which the vertebral portion is very usually found in connection with the 7th cervical vertebra, and was first described by Humauld; and the *sternal* portions of these ribs M. Breschet supposes to be represented by the episternal bones.

Having made extensive researches into the history of these cervical ribs, I am aware of certain difficulties which are opposed to the adoption of these views of M. Breschet. But whatever may be the ultimate determination in respect to the real nature of these bones, it is surely more philosophic to suppose them " rudimentary" of some structure more highly developed in some other class of animals, than to adopt the " Bridgewater" and " Guy's Hospital" physiology, which argues that every animal is made for itself alone, stands alone, and has nothing to do with any other, and that the individual organs of man and animals are to be explained by a physiology whose highest stretch of generalization is to represent the mammæ of the human female as having been purposely created double, that the accidental loss of one, by milk abscess, or otherwise, might occasion no

* Mem. sur Osteo, p. 83.
† Annales des Sciences Naturelles, 1838, p. 91.
‡ Guy's Hospital Reports, Vol. 5, p. 237.

interruption to their function![*] Profound philosophy! but proving, at the same time, to how little purpose Mr. John Hunter lived and laboured, and bequeathed to Britain his immortal museum, seeing that into the educational institutions of his adopted city he failed to introduce a single spark of his philosophy.

IV.—*Muscular system.*—*Varieties in muscles; musculus-hepatico-diaphragmaticus.*

Muscular system.

In the same person whose sternum presented the pre sternal bones, I discovered a muscle in a situation altogether unexpected and extraordinary. I shall call it the musculus hepatico-diaphragmaticus, or M. diaphragmatico-umbilicalis, both names expressing in part its singular course and connexions. The dissection of the part was made in presence of, and explained to, the anatomical class. I copy the description dictated by myself at the time to Mr. Morries, one of the most talented students.

This anomalous and very singular muscle arose, or was connected by a broad tendinous base to the cordiform tendon of the diaphragm, about an inch to the left of the gullet. It was connected with the diaphragm in two ways, or by two slips or attachments: the superior slip terminated shortly in a tendon which descended perpendicularly, or in the axis of the body; the inferior by a series of tendinous fibres which came directly from the tendinous fibres of the diaphragm itself (left portion), and of its cordiform tendon. The muscle or muscular band thus formed by these double origins was about an inch and a half in breadth; it had the same muscular character as the diaphragm itself. Proceeding from left to right, and gradually narrowing, it crossed the middle plane of the body, crossing in succession, 1st, the small portion of the left crus of the diaphragm; 2dly, the gullet; 3dly, the inner portion of the right crus of the diaphragm. Hitherto, the muscle in its course lay close to the concave surface of the diaphragm, but now, descending a little, it subdivides, at its origin, into two parts, a smaller and

larger. The smaller, which was also the descending portion, seemed at first disposed to follow the direction of the right crus, but was soon lost, for after a course of about an inch it terminated by gradually disappearing on the outer surface of the peritoneum; the larger or stronger portion, rather more than half an inch in breadth, proceeded horizontally until it reached the concave surface of the liver, terminating in that sulcus which contains the remains of the ductus venosus. To the lower edge of the obliterated duct the muscle adhered by a series of tendinous fibres, and these might be traced not only upwards to the point where the duct comes off from the sinus of the portal vein, but onwards until it also adhered to the remains of the umbilical vein throughout a considerable space. The broad end of the muscle, near its origin, was now cut through, when a series of short muscles presented themselves, arising by tendinous fibres from the cordiform tendon, and terminating in the same tendon, but something more to the right. All these muscular slips proceeded over the margin of the œsophageal opening.

Here was a new attachment, then, of the liver and its vessels to the abdominal walls.

The usual decussation of the diaphragm was next examined; a strong band of fleshy fibres passed from the left to the right crus, but were in the opposite direction, properly speaking; a small portion only of the right crus lay over the above, but descended no further than the middle plane of the aortic opening.

On examining the remains of the umbilical vein left attached to the liver, the portion more immediately connected with the vena portæ was found enclosed in a sheath of fibres, having all the appearance of muscular fibres; this extended for about $2\frac{1}{2}$ inches; further than this I had no opportunity of tracing it, the parts beyond having been destroyed by a *post-mortem* examination. During the same examination, the abdominal viscera had been removed prior to my own dissection of the above structures.

Future inquiries will, no doubt, some day prove the muscle I have just described, as well as the muscular sheath of the umbilical vein, to be connected with the doctrine of " unity of or-

---

[*] Cooper on the Mammæ; Bridgewater Treatises, *passim*.

ganization" in the animal series, or in the history of the human embryogenesis.

Varieties of Arteries.—1. *Humeral and Interosseal.* 2. *Subclavian.*

I shall first notice a variety in the relation of the humeral artery—perhaps the most remarkable which has as yet been recorded in respect to this artery.

The variety to which I allude is that deviation of the main trunk of the brachial from its usual course, to pass behind the supra-condyloid process of the human humerus, accompanied by the median nerve, and after descending for a short way in the supra-condyloid groove regaining its normal position and course near the bend of the elbow. By a reference to my memoir on the supra-condyloid process in the human humerus, published in the Edinburgh Medical and Surgical Journal for 1841, it will be seen, that the artery and nerve, by following this course, reproduce most exactly the normal arrangement in the arm of the tiger, panther, cat, lion, and most carnivorous animals. The authors of the Bridgewater Treatises, and their supporters in "Guy's" and elsewhere, are, I think, bound to offer some explanation of these varieties, seeing that they object in toto to the doctrines of "unity of organization," and, indeed, to the transcendental anatomy of Frank, Goëthe, Dumeril, and St. Hilaire. Some plausible reason should in justice to their views be offered why the humeral artery and the median nerve should in some few individuals of the human race follow the non-human arrangement; there must be some reason for this, and since they object to the doctrines of "unity of the organization" they are in justice bound to offer a substitute.*

Since writing and publishing the memoir just alluded to, I find a variety in Tiedemann's great work on the arteries somewhat analogous to the above, but affecting the course of a different vessel. In this case the interosseal artery arose from the humeral artery, about the middle of the arm; quitting the course

* When my brother discovered the curious fact, that in the knee-joint of the ornithorynchus paradoxus the synovial membrane stretches completely across it, forming a partition between the superior and inferior parts of the joint, or in other words two joints, I asked the distinguished author of the Bridgewater Treatise "On the Hand" what purpose be supposed such a structure could serve; he replied that be thought it must be to strengthen the joint!

of the larger vessel, the interosseal branch made its way towards the internal inter-muscular ligament, and, passing behind the supra-condyloid process, which M. Tiedemann calls an "excrescentia ossis humeri in solita," it afterwards regains its position in the bend of the elbow. No mention is made of the course of the median nerve in this instance, but it may be presumed that it followed its usual course. M. Tiedemann adds, that this variety had been seen by Ludwig, Sabatier, Monro, Hilldebrandt, and Barclay.

2. The next variety affected slightly the course of the subclavian artery, but was also connected with a variety in the arrangement of the scalenus anticus muscle. This muscle, on the right side, in the stout muscular adult in whom the pre-sternal bones were observed, divided into two portions, betwixt which the subclavian artery passed across the rib: the variety seemed to me an approach to that other more important variety in the course of the subclavian, first observed, I believe, by a Parisian student, and pointed out by him to M. Cruveilhier; I allude to the reported passage of the subclavian artery altogether anterior to the scalenus anticus muscle, and close to the corresponding vein: Mr. Spence assures me that he has seen this most remarkable variety *once;* the nearest approach to it I have myself observed is the passage of the artery through the scalenus, as above.

ON THE

DOCTRINE OF METAMORPHOSIS.

By HERMANN HOFFMANN, M.D.
Lecturer on the Principles of Physiology in the University of Giessen.

To the Editor of the Medical Gazette.

SIR,

AT the request of my friend Dr. Hoffmann, I enclose you a translation of a paper written by him for the Annalen der Chemie und Pharmacie, xlv. b. 2 Heft, and regret that, in consequence of numerous engagements, I have been compelled to delay it for so long a time after receiving the proof sheets.

I remain, sir,
Your obedient servant,
GEORGE KEMP, M.B. Cantab.
Cambridge, June 14, 1843.

In consequence of the extraordinary deficiency of accurate data with reference to all those circumstances which relate to the doctrine of metamorphosis (one of the most important in physiology), it appears desirable that every one should assist according to his ability in obtaining some firm principles on which new researches as well as new theories might be founded. We possess, indeed, some observations upon the daily consumption of matter in the human frame; and even if these do not agree very well with one another, still they prove almost to demonstration, that by instituting a greater number of experiments, a satisfactory result will soon crown our efforts. As the consumption of a human being in the condition of customary quiet life has in this manner been ascertained to a certain extent, it appeared to me interesting to make some experiments in order to show the amount of consumption in a condition of considerable increased activity. The practical object of these experiments was, however, to substitute a definite idea, for the vague expressions, fatigue, exertion, exercise, &c.

In the beginning of November 1842, I undertook a journey on foot to a town twelve leagues distant. The weather was damp, cold, ($+4°$ R.) and in the beginning of my journey a light snow fell; in the afternoon, however, it cleared up. After walking three leagues,* I was weighed, for which purpose my clothes were taken off, to avoid any error from their probable dampness. The total weight amounted to 124 pounds 6 ounces. The experiment now began. Without halting or putting up anywhere for the remaining nine leagues, I proceeded on my journey. This was by no means too great an exertion, as the road was excellent, and only rendered slightly fatiguing by gentle hills. Besides, the coolness of the weather had a sensibly beneficial influence on the sensation of strength. The quantity of nourishment taken was accurately weighed, and moreover as little, and that of as simple a quality as possible, was eaten, namely, wheat bread, altogether 9 ounces 120 grains.† No fluid was drunk during the whole time, and from the state

of the weather this was not attended by any material inconvenience. Defecation did not take place during the experiment; sensible perspiration also did not occur, a circumstance easily explained by the state of the atmosphere. The nasal mucus was carefully collected in a pocket handkerchief, the weight of which had been previously determined when dry, and was again taken at the conclusion of the experiment. The increase of weight amounted to one loth*, eighty grains. The urine was received into a vessel, the capacity of which was afterwards determined by urine of similar concentration, and the number of vessels thus filled was registered. The weight amounted to one pound, one loth, 60 grs. The first weighing took place at 8 o'clock in the morning; the experiment terminated at 5 in the afternoon, and the weight amounted to 122 lbs. 13 oz. and 28 grs. From the above data, it will be seen that the actual loss of weight is greater than that accounted for by the amount of urine and nasal mucus, the difference arising clearly from the loss by exhalation from the skin and respiratory organs.

I embrace this opportunity for inquiring into another point immediately connected with the above. The question presents itself, how far a renewal of strength can be supplied during its consumption; or, in other words, how far can repose take place without rest? Are rest, sitting, lying, in point of fact so absolutely essential for the renewal of strength as is usually supposed, or is this rule subject to limitations; and if so, what are the conditions under which the exception occurs? The influence of taking food is here also decidedly confirmed. After three hours' walking, immediately after the first weighing a wheaten roll was eaten, which in a short time satisfied the hunger which had been keenly excited by the exercise. After, however, I had proceeded on the whole about six leagues, loss of strength and spirits occurred to such a degree that I hesitated considerably as to the prosecution of the experiment. My companion, a dog, which very perceptibly lost his cheerfulness in proportion as the hungry march was pursued, found himself in the same situation,

---

* The Hessian league or stund = 2½ English miles.

† A loth = half an ounce.

* 18½ loth.

only much less subject to intentional deception, of which, however, one is totally incapable under such circumstances. Nothing could be more remarkable than the effect which was now produced on man and dog by some ounces of bread. In less than a quarter of an hour I felt myself in a totally different state of mind, and did not for a moment doubt of the success of my undertaking. The dog, however, acquired so much cheerfulness and strength, that he appeared as if he had only just commenced the journey.

Precisely the same result was repeated towards the end of the experiment, only that the dog recovered himself more completely, as he was quite as cheerful at the conclusion as at the beginning of the journey,—a remark not so applicable to myself.

I felt some interest in observing the nature of the origin of the local fatigue, after I had in the manner above mentioned arrived at some conclusions respecting the general lassitude. The experiment was so arranged as to include an extreme case, that of the motion of walking continued as long as possible. Numerous experiments have in this respect completely confirmed the opinions of the Webers on the oscillation of the pendulum. A sensation of fatigue in the fascia lata, and in the thigh generally, the first and most distressing symptoms in persons unaccustomed to walking, remained from the beginning to the end of the experiment. The first was a kind of general stiffness, produced by the continuous uniformity of the motion, the consequence of which was, that motion sideways, &c. was difficult and fatiguing. About one o'clock a contracted sensation was felt in the femoral insection of the gastrocnemii of both legs, which gradually increased, and was rather distressing. The popliteus, and especially the left, participated in this sensation. After a march of ten leagues, a strained sensation, painful even in stooping, was experienced on both sides of the spinal column, at the iliac insertions of the sacro-lumbalis muscles, and which was very troublesome, manifestly in consequence of the exertion of these muscles in keeping the body in the upright, though somewhat bent-forwards position, which was obliged to *be constantly preserved.* I did not

remark any other sensation of much interest, yet I must observe that towards evening an insupportable chilliness overcame me, which was certainly not attributable to the atmosphere, as it remained unchanged, nor to the clothing, as this was the same as in the morning. I was, however, quite well with the exception of hunger, and I consider this as the cause of the chilliness.

The changes in the circulation and respiration which I experienced in the course of the journey, under similar circumstances, were remarkable. While I usually breathe 13 times per minute at 11 o'clock, I found in this case the number of inspirations and expirations amount to 19 at half-past 10; at half-past 1, 23; at 5 P.M. 22. The pulse, which in the normal state usually gives 80 beats per minute, numbered 105 at half-past 10; at half-past 1, 119, and at 5, 122. I took the precaution of standing still for 3 minutes before counting the pulse, and then registered the average of from 4 to 6 minutes. Notwithstanding this violent fever, I experienced no heat, and remark expressly, that the cause of this increase of the heart's action, &c. was not the ascent of the hills. At 11 P.M. after supper, the pulse was at 88, and the number of respirations 17. The urine, which was passed in the evening soon after the experiment, deposited a considerable quantity of urate of ammonia, a circumstance very unusual in this place. Should I attribute this to a quantity of wine taken previously, or to the walking? It appears from what I am about to communicate that the first supposition is the more correct.

For greater security, I repeated this experiment with my friend Mr. Sullivan. The temperature and weather were almost precisely the same as in the former case; the air, however, was somewhat drier. The experiment took place at the beginning of December 1842. The journey extended to ten leagues, which we divided by an interval of one hour's rest.

My weight at the commencement, about 8 A.M., amounted to 121 lbs. 12½ oz. The food, including a pint of light French red wine, weighed 1 lb. 1 oz. The loss of urine amounted to 1 lb. 4 oz.: the mode of measurement was the same as in the former case; that is to say, the last portion emptied in the evening was directly weighed, and the weight found taken as the medium standard. The nasal mucus might be estimated the same as in the former experiment, 320 grs. Defecation did not take place. As the weight at 8 P.M., at the conclusion of the experiment, amounted to 120 lbs. 10¼ oz., the additional loss of 14 oz. 284 grs. must be considered as the result of perspiration. At 11 A.M., the number of inspirations and expirations was 16; at 8 P.M. more than 14: the pulse, at 2 P.M., gave 85 beats; at 8 P.M. 95. Before the numbers were registered, longer pauses of rest were taken than in the first experiment, which may even be observed from the calculation, particularly in that of the evening. If, now, a man, weighing 115 lbs. perspires during motion 14 oz. 164 grs. in eleven hours, this amounts to 0·49,880 of a grain to every 100 of his weight, or 0·075,584 of a grain for every 100 minutes.

My companion weighed 140 lb. 6 oz. 120 grs. at the beginning of the experiment. The food, as above, amounted to 1 lb. 1 oz. The quantity of urine determined, as in the above case, amounted to 2 lbs. 1 oz. 54 grs.; the nasal mucus was assumed, with every appearance of correctness, to weigh 320 grs. Defecation did not take place. As now, the weight in the evening, at 8 o'clock, amounted to 137 lbs. 12 oz. 180 grs., this gives a remainder of 1 lb. 6 oz. 136 grs., which must be attributed to the perspiration.

The pulse, which usually beat only 64 times per minute, had increased to 70 at 2 P.M.; and at 8 P.M., after some rest, still remained at 70. The number of respirations, usually amounting in the morning to 13½, increased at 11 A.M. to 16, and at 8 P.M. to 19. Thus,

the 134 lbs. which Sullivan weighed, reduced to 100 grs. and 100 minutes, gives 0·1575 of a grain of perspiration.

The urine, as in all the other cases mentioned, was very saturated, of a bright orange colour, and deposited no sediment within 24 hours; it therefore did not contain any remarkable amount of urate of ammonia.

For the purpose of having a standard of comparison, I some time afterwards made the following observations on myself, respecting the consumption in a state of rest. Selecting for the purpose a day in which the temperature and hygroscopic condition of the atmosphere were similar to the above, I kept constantly in my room at a temperature of 13 R.; for the weighing merely I stepped out a few hundred paces. The day was employed in study, half of the time standing, half sitting. The first weighing took place at half-past 8, and amounted to 123 lbs.; nothing was taken either for nourishment or drink. The loss in urine was 1 lb. 20 grs. The second weighing, at 4 o'clock, gave 122 lbs. 7 oz. Defecation did not take place, and the nasal secretion was considered=0: the perspiration here, then, amounted only to 4 oz. 120 grs.; the urine was also much lighter than in the other cases.

The respiratory action at 11 A.M. was 13, at half-past 4, 14: the pulse at 11 A.M. was at 80, at half-past 4 P.M., 80. If we calculate this as above, we have for the 115 lbs. in 100 minutes, 0·14,529 grs.; for 100 grs., however, in the same interval, 0·030,272 grs. of perspiration.

We may sum up the results as follows, comparing the amount of perspiration secreted in 100 minutes with 100 grs. of the body.

Amount of perspiration in a man at rest for each 100 grs. during a space of 100 minutes=0·030272 grs. (Hoffman)
=0·1138 (Dalton*)
=0·1581 (Lavoisier and Seguin†).

Amount of perspiration in a man in motion, reduced to the same standard of time and weight—
| | I. | II. | |
=0·10119 grs.   0·075584 grs. (Hoffman)
=0·1575 (Sullivan).

I have analysed the urine passed after the second experiment, without having taken food for some hours previously.

---

* Calculated from Dalton, who found the perspiration in March to amount to 37 ounces Total weight, 140 lbs.

† According to Lavoisier and Seguin, who state the amount of perspiration as 51 oz. daily. Here, also, the total weight=140 lbs.

In 1000 parts, the water=977,221
          Solid matter= 22,779
1000 parts of the solid matter gave
                    Ash=539,806
          Sulphuric acid= 80,581

For the purpose of determining the quantity of sulphuric acid, the ash was dissolved in water containing nitric acid, and the sulphuric acid precipitated by means of muriate of barytes. The sulphate of barytes was now exposed to a red heat, and the acid thus calculated. This urine deposited no sediment.

MEDICAL GAZETTE.

Friday, July 7, 1843.

"Licet omnibus, licet etiam mihi, dignitatem Artis Medicæ tueri; potestas modo veniendi in publicum sit, dicendi periculum non recuso."
                                        Cicero.

REMUNERATION IN GENERAL PRACTICE.

A GLANCE at the notices of motions about to be made in the House of Commons is calculated to make one think that the medical profession, whatever chance it may have of getting an act passed for its government, is very unlikely to receive much real attention at the hands of ministers or members of parliament. It is difficult to conceive that much interest could attach to the subject, after the energies of statesmen have been unremittingly exerted for so long a time in the altering or preserving some of the most fundamental portions of our constitution, and in discussing questions which seem to involve its very existence.

Should we from this cause be doomed to slovenly and crude legislation, there will be much matter for regret, but should we escape legislation altogether it may fairly be questioned whether we shall lose much by the omission. Physiology tells us, and experience proves, that total fasting for a time, when the mind or body are over fatigued, is preferable to a full meal, and that a hasty one involves certain dyspepsia it may be that the humours of our body politic suffer in the same way from exhausted energies, and that feverish, peevish dreams, without refreshment, may be obtained instead of sound repose.

It is worth considering, in the meantime, how many of our acknowledged evils, and of what kind, are capable of removal by personal and private exertions; for if the delay of public measures awaken amongst us a hearty desire, and keep up an enlightened endeavour for that purpose, the advantages gained will not be trifling.

The greatest, because the fundamental evil, from which the profession suffers, is undoubtedly a superabundance of practitioners, yet public legislation can only prevent this by making the entrance to the profession more difficult. This the Society of Apothecaries has already succeeded in doing to a great extent, by their enlarged course of study, which, however censured for its quality, leaves no doubt as to its greatly increased quantity. The young Milos of the present day have to lift their daily increasing burden for a much longer period than formerly, ere they are to be trusted as active supporters of the public health; and if some of them, in the flush of youth and pride of training, have attempted injudicious tasks beyond their strength,— if they have got their fingers pinched and themselves pilloried for their presumption, let us hope that none have been quite devoured for their indiscretion. The education of the present day is, and must be, in a great degree experimental. New wants have had to be supplied, both intellectual and social, and new means were necessarily resorted for the purpose. That in the attempt to supply what was deficient much that was highly useful was hastily abandoned, must be admitted by all

ancient languages, and their toilsome but instructive acquisition are among the things obsolete, and false quantities and misplaced aspirates are so common, that not only are the fastidious ears of old Etonians offended, but even the utilitarian who late in life has brightened his massive intellectual machinery with the high polish of literature, or covered it with a thin coating of glittering material — laying on a little Latin and less Greek— often receives a shock to his grammatical susceptibilities. These matters are in course of improvement. In medicine, as in divinity, during the last half century, gigantic energies newly aroused started into irregular and misdirected action, which sobriety and good sense have to reduce by order, method, and discipline. The far-seeing speculator may be forgiven his anxieties, lest the very great need which has so evidently existed lately for forms and methods, for order and for discipline, may not have been too hastily and actively recognized, and danger thereby incurred that formality, prescription, and the wisdom of our forefathers, may again be too implicitly relied on.

We have no such fear. In a few months, by means of the Sydenham Society, the sterling old medical classics will be in the hands of many hundreds of our brethren. Many of those who read them for the first time will pay the cheerful homage of respect to the sages of former days; a few will be tempted into a half idolatrous worship, an overvaluing of patristic authority; others will sink into a feeble and fruitless dilettantism, their love of literature being fussy and fondling, but barren and unseemly as the love of old age is apt to be; but can it be doubted that to sound, active, and vigorous minds new views will be suggested, new doubts resolved, new truths begotten ?

One or two of the more prominent mistakes which in their daily consequences affect the credit, the comfort, or profits of our brethren, cannot too often be pointed out, that constant efforts may be made for their correction. No greater service, indeed, can be done than directing the combative energies which have so painfully been exerted against particular individuals or bodies, as the only cause of all our evils, to the removal of the evils themselves.

Now one of the practical evils of the present day is connected with the sale of drugs. In this matter altered circumstances have converted one or two truths into fictions, and this process never takes place without great inconvenience and suffering somewhere, while the redressing the evils which have arisen is no less disagreeable, often more so, as resuscitation is more painful than drowning.

The notion that every diseased state may be cured by a particular drug, or combination of drugs, has pervaded medical practice from its earliest times. The physician has been paid for pointing out, the apothecary for preparing this drug. The exclamation, " Hei mihi quod nullis amor est medicabilis herbis," shews the very pharmaceutical notion which the poet had of Apollo's medical skill; and happy is the practitioner who, when asked what is the best thing for this or the other symptom, neither loses his patience at the absurdity of the question, nor contributes to keep up the delusion by naming some approved simple. One result of this rude notion of physic is, that when the public are informed of any change in the medical theories of the day, or get mystified by the pretensions of some arch quackery or medical heresy, though their confidence in the prescribers is shaken, their confidence in the drugs remains as great as ever; they merely substitute their own prescriptions for those of the doctor. Honour, then, in due measure to homœopathy! it is doing its mission for the abolition of mere druggistry, and the inculcation of dietetic and other discipline. We were informed lately, by a reverend practitioner in a small way, that 200 homœopathic medicine-chests had been supplied lately, and are now being used by as many clergymen alone. Multiply these by their probable number of patients in the middle class, and the product, may we not hope, will represent the number of persons who are in a fair way to cease from drugs, especially of their own prescribing, and to confide in enlightened medical science whenever it shall be prepared with its proofs; or if it be insisted on that the intellectual calibre of such patients is, by their present credulity, proved to be below the average, then, at least, "fiet experimentum in corpore vili," they will work out some problems in expectant medicine which, with our present notions, *we* cannot conscientiously attempt. If Sir James Graham had a little breathing-time between the Irish Arms Bill, the Factory Education Bill, and other pressing matters, we would suggest that the statistics of homœopathic practice should be furnished to the Home Office. A few registrarships and commissions in this department might be handed, in the meantime, to the unemployed regular practitioners, who might thus be kept alive to note the issue of the experiment.

To the general practitioner the present state of opinion is most important, and calls for a rigorous scrutiny of principles, and a steady adherence to whatever course will produce really the best general results, even if some present personal sacrifice be thereby rendered necessary.

The practice of making a charge for medicines should be discontinued, and that of specifying and charging for visits introduced. Two modes of proceeding, then, suggest themselves; one is, the writing prescriptions to be made up at a druggist's, the other is the supplying medicines either gratuitously or at small profits. The first leaves the main evil just where it was; the prescription, when obtained, will be valued more than the advice, and the charges being necessarily smaller than the fee of the physician, the erroneous principle will be still more widely diffused. Besides, the profits of the druggist are at present large, and were founded on estimates which have become erroneous. Until of late years, the preparation and retail of medicines was in the hands only of apothecaries, persons skilled, more or less, in the art of administering them, the price of whose education was charged on the materials in which they dealt: these materials acquired a great real value from the skill and labour bestowed upon them—an increase of value like that acquired by a pound of iron when made into watch-springs.

When drugs, too, were more rare and costly, and the supplies uncertain, much more capital was required for the wholesale market than at the present time. Enormously increased demand, and manufacturing improvements in the supply, have also contributed to lower the price of chemical products, though certainly the outlay of capital in effecting those improvements must be admitted on the other hand. Yet with all these changes, and while the price of a medical visit has virtually decreased, the charge for a draught at a good druggist's is still a shilling. This is understood to be the cost of the medicine and of the skill required in preparing it. Four of these draughts a day will be the most paid for when a medical visit is made daily, or on alternate days. The average payment for the visit, then, is 5s., and for the medicine 3s. Surely so monstrous a disproportion cannot habitually exist without gradually warping the public feeling as to the relative value of each. The judicious and conscientious practitioner will draw the right inferences from this statement, and will so arrange as gradually to bring about a better state of matters; and this he will do, not by mystifying, but by enlightening the public: the light afforded being by his actions, not by declamatory talking. Many attempts have been made to bring the parties interested to meet and combine for the purpose of settling, and if possible enforcing, their claims for attendance; but the success of such combinations is small, and the limits within which they are justifiable are not clear. More may be done, and better done, through a quiet consideration of the subject by individuals, and by keeping in view the broad principle of remuneration for time and skill, not for medicine. We have purposely kept in view a distinction between charges and fees: a fee is a gratuity, and implies an entirely different tone of feeling in the donor and the recipient from that which it would be prudent to adopt in general practice. Let fees still be large, and still *given* as the reward of superior attainments: this will tend to keep the consulting practitioner in his only true and proper position—that of a person whose position makes great things to be expected of him. To this elevation all who think themselves qualified for it may now rise; if they assume it without due powers to support it—and sufficient pecuniary means are amongst those powers—the fault is theirs.

———

ROYAL MEDICAL & CHIRURGICAL SOCIETY.

June 27, 1843.

THE PRESIDENT IN THE CHAIR.

———

On the Influence of Rickets upon the Growth of the Skull. By ALEXANDER SHAW, Esq. Surgeon to the Middlesex Hospital.

THIS paper was the sequel of one by the same author, printed in the 17th Vol. of the Society's Transactions. The object of the former publication was, in the first place, to prove that, besides causing softening and distortion of the osseous system, rickets has the effect of arresting the process of growth; and secondly, to show that, owing to this interruption, the proportions of the figure peculiar to the adult are not perfectly attained by persons affected with the disease, but continue to be more or less those of the child. The figure of the child is characterised by the head, trunk, and upper extremities, being of large dimensions compared with the pelvis and lower extremities, while that of the adult has the former parts relatively small, and the pelvis and legs large and powerful. In persons deformed from rickets, the whole figure is stunted; but the head, trunk, and upper extremities together, when compared with the natural adult dimensions, are only defective to a slight degree (one-thirteenth), while the pelvis and lower extremities are defective to a great degree (one-third). This difference the author accounted for by supposing that, as the disease stops the growth, it interrupts at the same time the change then in progress of being produced in the relative proportions of the figure; and so causes the patient, when arrived at adolescence, to exhibit traces of the configuration of the child. Having referred to the importance of this view in relation to the size of the pelvis in child-bearing women deformed from rickets, and stated that by measuring numerous specimens he had ascertained that the defect of growth in this part amounts, on an average, to nearly a quarter of the natural size, he proceeded to apply the same principle to the explanation of a peculiarity in the form of the head which he had observed as a general character in ricketty persons. This peculiarity consists in a disproportion between the size of the cranium and of the face. Between infancy and adolescence, a change in the relative proportions, analogous to that which occurs in the figure generally, takes place in the skull. Near birth, its form is characterised by the cranium being of large bulk compared with the face: while at adolescence the contrast is greatly diminished, owing to the face having become much bulkier in comparison with the cranium than it had originally been. The author had remarked, and confirmed his observations by numerous measurements, that the skull, in ricketty persons, does not attain the proper adult proportions ; but, on the contrary, the cranium appears remarkably large compared with the face, just as during childhood. Thus, taking the dimensions of the face as the limit of comparison, he found that in the skull of the infant the size of the cranium is as 8 to 1 ; in the adult, as 6 to 1 ; and in the ricketty person (although beneath the standard size), as 7 to 1. He explained this disproportion by supposing that, as rickets arrests the growth, it interrupts, at the same time, the change occurring in the relative proportions of the skull between infancy and adolescence ; and thus gives rise to the childlike character of the proportions. The proposition was illustrated by showing the contrary effects which an increased activity of the growth produces. In the figure generally, when the growth has been preternaturally active, as in tall persons, the effect of the unequal rate of development in the two divisions of the frame is shown by the lower extremities acquiring an undue length compared with the trunk ; so, in the head, the face becomes disproportionately larger compared with the cranium : thus by measuring the skull of the giant preserved in the museum of the College of Surgeons, the author found that the dimensions of the cranium (although above the standard size) are, to those of the face, only in the proportion of 5 to 1 in this skull. Having next shown that the orbits always preserve a uniform size, whatever be the dimensions of the face, in skulls of different proportions, and accounted for this fact by referring to the anatomical relation of the frontal and maxillary sinuses to these cavities, and showing that the two sinuses vary in capacity according to the rate of growth, he passed to the consideration of the growth of the maxillary bones. After dwelling on the difference in the mode of formation of the teeth as compared with the jaw bones, and the importance of an exact relation being preserved between the development of both parts, and referring to the observation of Hunter regarding the different rates of growth in the anterior and posterior divisions of the maxillary bones, he concluded by showing that, as rickets has the effect of interrupting the growth of the jaw bones, it deranges also the process of evolution of the teeth.

An Account of a Case in which a Foreign Body was lodged in the Right Bronchus. By SIR BENJAMIN C. BRODIE, Bart. F.R.S. Sergeant Surgeon to the Queen, &c. &c.

The author's object in this paper was to describe a case in which a half-sovereign was *lodged in the right bronchus* of the patient *for a period of thirty days*, and in which

certain novel measures adopted for its removal proved successful. It was on the 3d of April, while the patient, Mr. B., was amusing some children, that the coin which he had in his mouth accidentally slipped into the trachea. The symptoms which succeeded were principally occasional severe fits of coughing, and a sense of pain referred to a part of the chest corresponding to the situation of the right bronchus. No particular sounds were detected by the use of the stethoscope. The patient was able to pursue his usual avocations, and made two journies into the country. On the 19th of April, having placed himself in the prone position, with the sternum resting on a chair, and his head and neck inclined downwards, the patient had a distinct perception of a loose body slipping forwards along the trachea ; a violent convulsive cough ensued, and, on resuming the erect posture, he again had the sensation of a loose body moving in the trachea towards the chest. An apparatus of the following kind was now constructed. A platform, on which the patient could lie prone, was made to move on a hinge in the centre ; so that on one end of it being elevated the other was equally depressed. On the 25th of April the patient was laid on this apparatus, with his shoulders and body fixed by means of a belt, and his head was lowered to an angle of nearly 90 degrees with the horizon. His back was then struck several times with the hand, but violent fits of choking were brought on each time, and it was not deemed prudent to continue the experiments. On the 27th it was agreed in consultation to make an opening in the trachea, between the thyroid gland and the sternum. In proposing this, the object was two-fold : 1st, that an attempt might be made to extricate the coin by the forceps ; 2d, that if relief could not be obtained in this manner, the artificial opening might answer the purpose of a safety-valve, and the experiment of inverting the body on the platform be repeated without the risk of causing suffocation. The operation having been performed, several attempts to extricate the coin were made, but without success ; and, on each introduction of the forceps, paroxysms of convulsive coughing of such a violent kind were brought on, that it was plain that the attempts could not be persevered in without danger to life. On the 2d of May, a renewal of these trials was followed by the same results. On the 13th, the wound in the trachea having been kept from closing by the occasional introduction of a probe, the patient was placed on the moveable platform as described before ; his back was then struck by the hand ; two or three efforts to cough followed, and presently the patient felt the coin quit the chest, striking, almost immediately afterwards, against the incisor teeth of the upper jaw, and then dropping out of the mouth. No spasm of the muscles of the glottis took place; a small quantity of blood was ejected at the same time, apparently coming from the granulations of the external wound. From this date the patient proceeded rapidly to get well.

The author concluded by making observations on the following heads :—1st, on the influence of the size, weight, and form of a foreign body introduced into the windpipe, in modifying the symptoms; 2d, he referred to experiments which showed that a heavy body, like the coin in the present case, was most likely to drop into the right bronchus; 3d, he adverted to the want of success attending the use of the stethoscope in this and in some other cases of the same kind; 4th, he pointed out the reasons on which he had founded his opinion, that the artificial opening made in the trachea would prevent spasm in the glottis, and thereby give greater chance of success to the experiment of inverting the patient's body on the moveable platform; lastly, he dwelt on the difficulties and dangers attending the use of the forceps, when a weighty body is lodged deeply in one of the bronchi, as was the case in his patient.

Statistics of Bethlem Hospital, with Remarks on Insanity. By JOHN WEBSTER, M.D.

In this paper the author brought before the Society a few statistical tables compiled from the registers of Bethlem Hospital, accompanied by a synopsis of seventy dissections recently performed at that institution.

According to these tables, it appears that 4,404 curable patients of both sexes were admitted during the last 20 years, of whom 1782 were male, and 2622 were females—thus giving 47 per cent. more women than men. During the same period, 1446 female patients were discharged cured, that is, 55$\frac{1}{7}$ per cent. on the admissions; whilst only 823 male patients left the hospital convalescent, or 46$\frac{1}{4}$ per cent. On the other hand, the number of deaths in both sexes, although exactly equal, or 112 of each, yet calculated according to their respective admissions, the rate among the male patients was 6$\frac{1}{4}$ per cent. and only 4$\frac{1}{4}$ per cent. among the females. Similar results were likewise found to prevail among the incurable lunatics of both sexes. The author therefore concludes that insanity is not only more common among women than men, but also a more curable disease; so that, *cæteris paribus*, the prognosis may be considered as more favourable in female than male patients. The diminished rate of mortality, and the greater proportion of recoveries, are also clearly shewn by the records of the institution; since it appears that during the three years ending the 21st Dec. 1752, the proportion of patients discharged cured was only 31$\frac{1}{4}$ per cent. on the total admissions; whilst for the three years ending Dec. 31, 1842, the cures amounted to nearly 55 per cent. The ratio of deaths, also, during the former period, was as high as 25$\frac{1}{2}$ per cent.— but only 5$\frac{3}{4}$ during the last named three years—that is, about $\frac{1}{5}$th the amount reported nearly a century ago.

The author next remarks on the diminished number of suicides in the insane patients admitted into Bethlem; observing, at the same time, its greater frequency among males than females.

A synopsis is next given of seventy dissections recently made by Mr. Lawrence, in which the various morbid appearances met with are carefully detailed.

The author concludes his paper with an allusion to the two sections of pathologists at present dividing the opinions of medical writers respecting the diseased alterations of structure met with in cases of insanity, viz., the "anatomists and vitalists," the former considering them as causes, the latter only as consequences, of the previous mental affection. In his opinion the theory of the anatomists is the more rational, and most in accordance with the present state of our knowledge of the pathology of mania.

On the Presence of Spermatozoa in the Fluid of Hydrocele. By A. LLOYD, Esq. Assistant-Surgeon to St. Bartholomew's Hospital, and Surgeon to Christ's Hospital.

The object of the author was to announce that he had met with, since the last meeting of the Society, a third case of hydrocele, in the fluid of which an immense number of spermatozoa were present. The fluid was of paler colour than that of common hydrocele of the tunica vaginalis, and very much resembled water with which a very small quantity of milk had been mixed. When tested with nitric acid, and also with heat, the fluid was found to contain a considerable quantity of albumen. There was also much saline matter in it. When examined with the microscope from three to four hours after it was drawn off, there were seen spermatozoa in a living state, and also an immense number that were dead : moreover, the fluid contained a few blood-discs, transparent cysts, granular bodies of different sizes, and epithelial scales. The testis and its appendages were healthy. From the situation and form of the tumor it appeared that the fluid was contained in the tunica vaginalis. The spermatozoa were seen in a living state by Mr. F. Wood, Surgeon, of Brownlow Street, and by Mr. John Quekett, of the College of Surgeons.

Pathological Researches into the Local Causes of Deafness, based on one hundred and twenty dissections of the Human Ear. By JOSEPH TOYNBEE, F.R.S. Surgeon to the St. George's and St. James's Dispensary.

The researches of which this is a summary view, are in continuation of a previous paper contained in Vol. 24 of the Society's Transactions. The principal practical conclusion to which they lead is, that the most prevalent cause of deafness is chronic inflammation of the mucous membrane which lines the tympanic cavity; and that by far the greater majority of cases commonly called nervous deafness ought more properly to be attributed to this cause.

The pathological conditions to which inflammation of the mucous membrane gives rise are divided in the paper into three stages.

In the first stage the membrane retains its natural delicacy of structure, though its blood-vessels are considerably enlarged and contorted; blood is effused into its substance, or more frequently at its attached surface; blood has also been found between the membrane and the membrane of the fenestra rotunda, and in very acute cases lymph is effused over its free surface.

The second stage is characterised by the following pathological conditions:—

1st. The membrane is very thick, and often flocculent. In this state the tympanic plexus of nerves becomes concealed, the base and crura of the stapes are frequently entirely imbedded in it, while the fenestra rotunda appears only like a superficial depression in the swollen membrane.

2d. Concretions of various kinds are visible on the surface of the thickened membrane. In some cases these have the consistence of cheese, and are analogous to tuberculous matter; in others they are fibro-calcareous, and exceedingly hard.

3d. But by far the most frequent and peculiar characteristic of this second stage of the disease, is the formation of membranous bands between various parts of the tympanic cavity. These bands are at times so numerous as to occupy nearly the entire cavity; sometimes they connect the inner surface of the membrana tympani to the internal wall of the tympanum, to the stapes and to the incus. They have also been detected between the malleus and the promontory, as well as between the incus, the walls of the tympanum, and the sheath of the tensor tympani muscle; as well as between various parts of the circumference of the fenestra rotunda. But the place where these adhesions are most frequently visible is between the crura of the stapes and the adjoining walls of the tympanic cavity: this was the case in twenty-four instances out of a hundred and twenty

dissections, being a fifth of the number. These bands of adhesion sometimes contain blood and scrofulous matter.

In the third stage of inflammation of the membrane it becomes ulcerated; the membrana tympani is destroyed, and the tensor tympani muscle is atrophied. The ossicula auditus are diseased, and ultimately discharged from the ear, and the disease not unfrequently communicates itself to the tympanic walls, affecting also the brain and other important organs.

The following is a tabular view of the mucous membrane of the tympanic cavity in the 120 dissections related in this paper.

In the first stage of inflammation.

1. With simple inflammation of the membrane, its vessels being enlarged, tortuous, and distended with blood 10
2. Ditto, with an accumulation of mucus 1
3. Membrane inflamed, with effusion of blood into its substance . 3
4. Membrane inflamed, with effusion of serum, tinged with blood, into the tympanic cavity . . 1
5. Membrane inflamed, with lymph effused into the tympanic cavity . 2
6. Membrane inflamed, with blood and lymph effused into the tympanic cavity 2
7. Membrane inflamed, with effusion of pus into the tympanic cavity . 1

Dissections illustrative of the second stage of inflammation.

1. With simple thickening of the lining membrane 5
2. The membrane thick and pulpy . 2
3. Ditto ditto and the cavity full of bands of adhesion. . . 1
4. The membrane thick and flocculent. 1
5. Membranous bands connecting the membrana tympani to the inner wall of the tympanum . . 5
6. Membranous band connecting the membrana tympani to the promontory and the chorda tympani to the stapes . . . 1
7. Membranous bands connecting the membrana tympani to the incus . 1
8. Ditto ditto to the stapes. . 2
9. Ditto connecting the membrana tympani and chorda tympani nerve to the stapes 1
10. Ditto connecting the membrana tympani and malleus to the promontory 1
11. Ditto connecting the membrana tympani to the incus. . . 2
12. Ditto connecting the membrana tympani and ossecles to the inner wall of the tympanum . . . 1

13. Ditto connecting the malleus to the inner wall of the tympanum . 2
14. Ditto connecting the incus to the inner wall of the tympanum . 1
15. Ditto connecting the stapes to the promontory 24
16. Anchylosis of the stapes to the fenestra ovalis 2
17. Membranous bands, forming a network over the fenestra rotunda . 2
18. A broad membrane passing from the promontory to the mastoid cells . 2
19. The cavity of the tympanum full of bands of adhesions . . . 1
20. Membranous bands containing scrofulous matter 3
21. The cavity of the tympanum full of calcareous concretion . . 4
22. Ditto, full of caseous concretion . 2
23. With ridges of bone projecting from the surface of the promontory . 2

Dissections illustrative of the third stage of inflammation.

1. With ulceration and thickening of the mucous membrane, attended by the formation of pus . . 3
2. With ulceration of the membrane, and loss of one or more of the vesicula 3

It thus appears that of the 120 dissections there were—

20 Specimens in the first stage of inflammation of the tympanic cavity
65 Ditto in the second stage
6 Ditto in the third
29 Ditto in a healthy state.

120

DR. STOBER ON THE DISEASES OF CHILDREN.

[Concluded from page 511.]

Acute Hydrocephalus.—In two patients out of three who were treated for this disease, on the day before their death, the author found a peculiar alteration of the cornea, which he had already observed in four other patients. It consisted of a semilunar yellowish covering at the lower edge of the cornea, without any injection of the eye. When the disease has lasted long, this covering extends towards the centre of the cornea, and suppurates; its lamellæ then appear to be separated from one another by purulent infiltration, and turned outwards, which gives the disease a different character from all ulcerations of the cornea. Of six patients, in whom the author observed it, three were suffering from acute hydrocephalus; the fourth had an ulcer on the head, which had

eaten through the skull and membranes, and attacked the brain itself, whose substance was softened around the superficial ulceration; the child died in a few days of scarlet fever. The fifth child died of pneumonia, which came on in the course of acute hydrocephalus, after which was found a serous infiltration of the pia mater. Lastly, the sixth patient was an adult, who had been treated for pneumonia with large bloodlettings, and had fallen into a state of great debility. He alone recovered.

In four of these patients the alteration of the cornea appeared one or two days before death, and remained in the state of a mere covering; in the fifth, who lay several days in a comatose condition, the alteration of the cornea increased more and more, and at last passed into suppuration. In the case of pneumonia also suppuration ensued.

In three cases the author observed that the eyes were half open, and that then the uncovered part of the cornea became diseased. In the other three cases attention had not been paid to this circumstance, which perhaps was the cause of the morbid change. The author, however, does not think that the long-continued access of the air to this part of the cornea was the sole cause of the disease, but rather that the general debility had the greatest share in the suppuration; and that the malady had been preceded by a state similar to that existing in the dogs which Magendie fed on sugar, and in whom likewise the cornea suppurated.

Accordingly, the author cured the pneumonic patient [of this disease with bark, strengthening diet, and dropping laudanum and oil into the eye.

Convulsions.—In the great majority of cases they are a symptom of other diseases; and in some instances they depend on causes which leave no trace that can be detected after death. The author quotes several such cases.

Scrofula.—In all scrofulous cases Dr. Stöber gives animal diet and wine; in slighter cases, with a lymphatic constitution, disposition to cold in the head, ophthalmia, and glandular swellings in the neck, he administers tonic remedies, such as tr. gentianæ c., Hoffman's elixir vitæ, and baths of hay flowers or hazel-leaves; and employs iodine externally and internally for swelled glands of long standing. He treats scrofulous ulcers with red precipitate ointment; if they are very flabby, he avoids all fat substances, sprinkles them with red precipitate, and employs a dry bandage. For swellings of the nose and upper lip, he uses a white precipitate ointment. In scrofulous affections of the bony and fibrous system, caries, white swellings, &c., cod liver oil was very useful; but had no effects in swelling of the glands.

The author confirms this by several cases, so that it appears that the efficacy of this remedy does not depend on the iodine which it contains, as iodine is known to be very efficacious in diseases of the glands.

In scrofulous inflammation of the eyes, general and local treatment are equally necessary. Among general remedies, iodine and cod liver oil are too slow; mercurials and antimonials are more active. The author gives one or two grains of a mixture of equal parts of calomel and *sulph. aurat. antim.* three times a day; he continues this for three or four weeks, and then administers a purgative. If the scrofulous symptoms continue after an interval of eight or ten days, he gives the remedy again for three or four weeks. It produces stools several times a day, but rarely salivation. He rightly rejects antiphlogistics, especially the abstraction of blood, in this disease; but recommends blisters to the back of the neck, particularly in old cases, where the inflammation and intolerance of light are violent; or where the former is combined with a considerable morbid secretion; or in relapses.

Among external remedies, the most efficacious were the following: a collyrium containing corrosive sublimate and laudanum, or *lapis divinus* and laudanum, or the *extr. lactucæ vir.;* a red precipitate ointment; Rust's ointment; or an ointment containing nitrate of silver. The last was of special service in *blepharitis glandulosa,* as Rust's was in inflammation of the conjunctiva alone, or of the cornea and conjunctiva together. When the cornea is ulcerated, one drop of laudanum is dropped in once or twice a day. When the intolerance of light is very great, and does not yield to a stimulating and revulsive treatment continued for several days, Dr. Stöber has recourse to belladonna fomentations. He has seen no benefit from the application of cicuta and the tincture of rhus toxicodendron. [Nor the German translator neither.]

Polypus of the rectum seems to be more frequent in children than adults.

Abscesses of the hairy scalp always arise in consequence of eruptions on the head, such as impetigo; rarely from *tinea mucosa,* never from *tinea favosa.*

RECEIVED FOR REVIEW.

Essays on Surgical Pathology and Practice. By Alex. Watson, M.D. F.R.C.S.E. Parts 1 and 2.

The Spleen a Permanent Placenta: the Placenta a Temporary Spleen. By John Jackson, Member of the Royal College of Surgeons, London.

The True Law of Population shewn to be connected with the Food of the People. By Thomas Doubleday. Second Edition.

OVARIAN DROPSY.

OUR correspondent, Mr. Walne, has recently removed, with success, another dropsical ovarium, in its entire state, by the large abdominal section. It weighed sixteen pounds and three-quarters. Some circumstances having occurred in the course of the patient's recovery, giving a fresh interest to the subject, the particulars will shortly be submitted to the profession. Mr. Walne's former case has been too recently before our readers to have escaped their recollection (MED. GAZ. Dec. 24, 1842.) The patient, we are informed, now enjoys excellent health and spirits, walks long distances, and experiences no kind of inconvenience as a consequence of the operation performed in the early part of November last.

ROYAL COLLEGE OF SURGEONS

LIST OF GENTLEMEN ADMITTED MEMBERS.

Friday, June 30, 1843.

J. Fox.—W. H. Attree.—W. H. Saxton.—C. O. Baylis. — L. A. Lawrence. — T. Hall. — P. W. Thompson. — J. Carruthers. — R. F. Hodges. —E. Hanks.—R. Clark.

A TABLE OF MORTALITY FOR THE METROPOLIS,

Shewing the number of deaths from all causes registered in the week ending Saturday, June 24, 1843.

Small Pox	4
Measles	39
Scarlatina	27
Hooping Cough	54
Croup	4
Thrush	2
Diarrhœa	2
Dysentery	1
Cholera	1
Influenza	3
Ague	0
Typhus	37
Erysipelas	5
Syphilis	0
Hydrophobia	0
Diseases of the Brain, Nerves, and Senses	139
Diseases of the Lungs and other Organs of Respiration	263
Diseases of the Heart and Blood-vessels	25
Diseases of the Stomach, Liver, and other Organs of Digestion	62
Diseases of the Kidneys, &c.	8
Childbed	5
Paramenia	0
Ovarian Dropsy	2
Disease of Uterus, &c.	0
Rheumatism	1
Diseases of Joints, &c.	5
Carbuncle	0
Ulcer	0
Fistula	0
Diseases of Skin, &c.	0
Dropsy, Cancer, and other Diseases of Uncertain Seat.	99
Old Age or Natural Decay	57
Deaths by Violence, Privation, or Intemperance	17
Causes not specified	3
	—
Deaths from all Causes	885

WILSON & OGILVY, 57, Skinner Street, London

THE
LONDON MEDICAL GAZETTE,

BEING A

WEEKLY JOURNAL

OF

Medicine and the Collateral Sciences.

FRIDAY, JULY 14, 1843.

LECTURES
ON THE
THEORY AND PRACTICE OF MIDWIFERY,

Delivered in the Theatre of St. George's Hospital,

BY ROBERT LEE, M.D. F.R.S.

LECTURE XXXIV.

On labours complicated with uterine hæmorrhage, occasioned by detachment of the placenta from the superior part of the uterus.

FLOODING may take place in the latter months of pregnancy, and during labour, where the placenta does not adhere to the neck of the uterus, but to the body or the fundus, and is detached by some external or internal cause. The separation of the placenta from the upper part of the uterus may be produced by violence, as blows, falls, pressure over the hypogastrium, and shocks of various kinds; but it arises much more frequently from internal causes, of which, morbid states of the placenta, and twisting of the umbilical cord once or oftener around the neck of the child, are the most common and obvious. This variety of hæmorrhage, though usually termed accidental, can rarely, however, be referred to accident. Sometimes the flooding occurs to a great extent without any assignable cause; a large portion or the whole of the placenta, when in a healthy condition, being suddenly detached from the uterus, when the patient has been exposed to no external accident, or injury of any kind, and when no symptoms of increased determination of blood to the uterus have preceded the attack. When this happens a large quantity of blood is poured out between the placenta and uterus, a small portion of which only at the time usually escapes from the vagina, to indicate what is going on within the uterus. There may be a great internal hæmorrhage, accompanied with the ordinary constitutional effects resulting from loss of

815.—XXXII.

blood—as faintness, sickness, or vomiting, coldness of the extremities, rapid feeble pulse, hurried breathing; when there is little or no discharge from the vagina to excite alarm, or to point out the source of danger, when it is extreme. It is from the general symptoms of exhaustion, and by the disagreeable sense of uneasiness, weight, or distension of the uterus experienced, and not from the quantity of blood which appears externally in these cases, that we are led to discover the true state of the patient—to suspect that internal hæmorrhage is going on. But much more frequently only a small portion of the placenta is at first detached, and the greater part of the blood which is extravasated between it and the uterus separates the membranes, and descends by its weight to the orifice, and escapes through the vagina. In all cases, however, of uterine hæmorrhage in the latter months, the danger cannot be so accurately estimated by the quantity of blood which appears externally, as by the general symptoms. The portion of placenta which is detached never reunites to the uterus, but when expelled it is usually seen covered with a dark coagulum adhering to the uterine surface.

When the blood escapes in small quantity, and there are no labour pains present, and no disposition in the os uteri to dilate, and the constitutional powers are not impaired, an attempt should be made to prevent a return of the discharge, and the occurrence of labour pains. For this purpose, if the pulse is full and frequent, some blood may be taken from the arm, and the patient should be kept in the horizontal position surrounded by cool air, cold applications made over the hypogastrium, and acetate of lead and opium, mineral acids, and other remedies that diminish the force of the circulation and promote the coagulation of the blood, should be taken internally. The plug is here totally inadmissible; it can only convert an external into an internal hæmorrhage. But where the flooding occurs at first profusely, and is renewed even in a mode-

2 N

rate degree, in spite of our efforts to check it, the continuance of pregnancy to the full period cannot be expected ; it will be of no avail to bleed and administer internal remedies, except for the purpose of checking the discharge, and thus averting the immediate danger until the uterus is emptied of its contents.

The operation of turning, which is required in all cases of complete placental presentation, is very rarely necessary in uterine hæmorrhage where the membranes are felt at the orifice. In a great proportion of these cases, where, on making an examination, you can feel the smooth membranes extending across the neck of the uterus, the flooding will be arrested, and the labour safely completed, if the membranes are ruptured, the liquor amnii discharged, and contractions of the uterus excited by gentle dilatation of the orifice, and other appropriate means. The only cases in which this treatment fails are those in which it has not been had recourse to sufficiently early, or where the whole or a large portion of the placenta has been suddenly separated from the uterus, and a great internal hæmorrhage has taken place. The uterus will not contract effectually in these cases after the membranes have been ruptured the pains, instead of becoming stronger, become more and more feeble, return at longer intervals, and during these the blood flows more profusely, and death would take place before delivery, if the child were not extracted by the forceps, crochet, or by the operation of turning. In all cases, then, of uterine hæmorrhage in the latter months of pregnancy, and in the first stage of labour where the placenta does not present, and the quantity of blood discharged is so great as to render delivery necessary, where it appears improbable that the pregnancy can go on longer with safety, or to the end of the ninth month, rupture the membrane with the nail of the fore-finger of the right hand, evacuate the liquor amnii by holding up the head of the child, dilate very gently the os uteri with the fore and middle-fingers expanded, and occasionally make pressure with the fingers around the whole orifice ; apply the binder, give ergot and stimulants, and the uterus will, in all probability, contract upon its contents, and expel them without further trouble. If the hæmorrhage should, how-

means, delivery must be accomplished by the forceps, craniotomy, or by turning, according to the peculiarities of the case. In women who are liable to attacks of flooding after the expulsion of the child or placenta, rupture the membranes at the commencement of labour, even before the os uteri is much dilated, if the presentation is natural, and you will often succeed in entirely preventing hæmorrhage.

A TABULAR VIEW OF THIRTY-SEVEN CASES OF SEVERE UTERINE HÆMORRHAGE, OCCASIONED BY DETACHMENT OF THE PLACENTA FROM THE SUPERIOR PART OF THE UTERUS.

	Date	Description	Result
1	June 28, 1824	Uterine hæmorrhage, with slight pains ; many o agia had passed , os uteri slightly dilated, and tile affected by the pains ; membranes were daily ruptured ; hæmorrhage tidily ceased, and pains he regular ; child born ite ; hæthage followed, but was arrested on real of placenta.	Recovered.
2	October 29, 1827	H marriage at the eighth and a half mth, preceded by rigors and pains in region of uterus ; mh blood lost; os uteri soft, and little dilated ; pains produced no ttle effect on it; membranes were then ruptured ; strong pains followed ; hæmorrhage ceased ; head descended ; in two hours the pains ceased, and the hæmorrhage was renewed ; great exhaustion ; craniotomy was performed, and the child easily tuacted ; severe hæmorrhage after expulsion of placenta, which was controlled by cold.	Died from uterine inflammation.

No.	Date		Result
3	Nov. 5, 1828	Membranes gave way on the 4th, after great fatigue; liquor amnii discharged without pain; on the 5th, faintness came on, with slight oozing of blood from uterus, which continued for some hours, gradually increasing in quantity; exhaustion; os uteri fully dilated; head low in pelvis; insensibility; forceps applied; hemorrhage more formidable; labour completed by craniotomy; hemorrhage continued after expulsion of placenta; hand introduced to make uterus contract, but without success; flow of blood continued in spite of cold, pressure, and stimulants.	Died soon after delivery.
4	March 23, 1829	Uterine hemorrhage during the first stage of labour; os uteri widely dilated; pains gone off; membranes unruptured; finger was immediately forced through membranes, and head held up whilst liquor amnii escaped; stimulants administered; pains became strong, and labour completed without return of hemorrhage.	Recovered.
5	April 16, 1829	Severe flooding during eighth month, at intervals; os uteri soft and dilatable; no portion of placenta could be felt; presentation natural; membrane were then ruptured, the os uteri was dilated, and pressure made with the binder; pains came on for a time, but hemorrhage was renewed with violence; turning easily performed; child born alive; extreme exhaustion and death threatened.	Recovered.
6	October 24, 1829	Profuse uterine hemorrhage at the end of ninth month, which had commenced two days previously; os uteri fully dilated; head presenting; syncope; strength was supported by stimulants for a time, but the head not advancing, and the prostration increasing, the forceps was applied, and child extracted; hemorrhage ceased.	Recovered.
7	Nov. 18, 1829	Uterine hemorrhage ninth month, without exertion, after a hearty dinner; sickness; vomiting; syncope; os uteri dilated to size of half-a-crown, thick, and rigid; membranes were immediately ruptured, and liquor amnii discharged; hemorrhage ceased, and pains became strong; in an hour the hemorrhage returned, and the pains ceased; exhaustion; os uteri still very rigid; turning unable to be performed; craniotomy employed, and hemorrhage arrested; gradually sank	Died three hours after delivery.
8	May 13, 1830	Uterine hemorrhage at the end of ninth month; pains feeble, and recurring at long intervals; os uteri slightly open; dilatable; no portion of placenta felt; membranes were immediately ruptured, and the hemorrhage ceased: child born alive.	Recovered.
9	May 1830	Sudden and alarming uterine hemorrhage during the ninth month; faintness, with laborious breathing; os uteri but little dilated; the smooth membranes were felt all round; the membranes were then ruptured with the finger, and the hemorrhage ceased; orifice of uterus gently dilated; child dead; hemorrhage renewed with violence after expulsion of placenta; arrested by cold and stimulants	Recovered.

No.	Date		Result
10	Nov. 29, 1833	Uterine hæmorrhage at the eighth month; two quarts of blood had been discharged; great prostration; os uteri dilated to size of a shilling, soft and thin; membranes tense, and felt all round; membranes were ruptured with the finger, and pains came on, which expelled the child without hæmorrhage; the placenta followed in two minutes, accompanied by a great discharge of florid red blood; alarming prostration; ice into vagina, and stimulants administered	Recovered.
11	Sept. 4, 1834	Uterine hæmorrhage at the ninth month, which had come on after a violent quarrel; os uteri rigid, and slightly dilated; membranes felt all round; vagina had been plugged, and doses of ergot given without benefit; membranes were immediately ruptured, and all terminated well	Recovered.
12	July 12, 1835	Uterine hæmorrhage commencing at the eighth month, but arrested for ten days by cold and rest; os uteri high up and closed; hæmorrhage again came on, with pain in abdomen, like cramps; membranes were then ruptured with difficulty, and pressure made over uterus; pains very feeble; strength supported by wine, &c.; child expelled dead, after some hours, by natural efforts; placenta diseased	Recovered.
13	Nov. 15, 1835	Slight uterine hæmorrhage at the seventh and a half month; no great effect produced until Dec. 17, when it was renewed in a formidable manner; vagina filled with coagula; placenta supposed to present; os uteri soft, thin, and dilated to the size of half-a-crown; membranes felt all round, and no placenta at orifice; membranes ruptured with difficulty; pains came on, and child expelled in two hours; cord around the neck; slight hæmorrhage continued; alarming exhaustion for some days	Recovered.
14	June 4, 1836	Membranes ruptured at the commencement of labour in a patient who had always suffered from hæmorrhage; labour completed with but slight discharge; pressure and cold employed	Recovered.
15	Sept. 9, 1836	Uterine hæmorrhage at the eighth month, after an accident, which continued nearly a whole day; placenta was thought to have presented, but the membranes were felt all round without placenta; os uteri much dilated; membranes were ruptured with finger; the binder applied, and the orifice gently dilated; child born dead, with cord twisted tightly around neck; flooding was renewed; placenta was extracted; hæmorrhage arrested by cold and pressure; alarming prostration	Recovered.
16	June 22, 1837	Profuse hæmorrhage soon after commencement of labour, which increased when pains went off; great faintness and yawning; no part of the placenta felt; vagina filled with clots; membranes were then ruptured, and the hæmorrhage ceased	Recovered.
17	June 30, 1837	Uterine hæmorrhage in the ninth month; os uteri very little dilated; placenta could not be felt; membranes were immediately ruptured; child was expelled dead, followed by the placenta, which had been wholly detached; syncope followed	Recovered.

No.	Date	Description	Result
18	Aug. 24, 1837	Hæmorrhage after a fall during the eighth month; arrested for a week by rest and cold; renewed at which time, when the membranes were ruptured, and the hæmorrhage completely arrested	Recovered.
19	Aug. 1837	Hæmorrhage during first stage of labour; membranes were ruptured, and the child born alive without return of hæmorrhage	Recovered.
20	Nov. 11, 1837	Uterine hæmorrhage near the nth month; a quart of blood escaped in ... at one minute; ...sion to syncope; os uteri soft, ...ittle, but ...le eped; head presented; no ...ae contractions, cold was applied, and the ...ge ced; 1 hur ...ae on ...oen after, and was completed without assistance	Recovered.
21	Nov. 20, 1837	Violent flooding at ...cent of ...inth month; os uteri soft, ...and but little open; no ...I im, but a ...nce of ...ight in the ...gin of ...ke u ...as; rhs ...re ...ndy ...ped, and the hæmorrhage ...d; hild born cold, with cord ...fel around ...nk	Died.
22	Nov. 14, 1838	...ge at eighth ...mth, os uteri half dilated; ...tnes unruptured; syncope; membranes were immediately ruptured; 1 ...ss ...che strong; hild expelled in an ohr, putrid; ...ge was arrested; placenta in a diseased condition	child.
23	June 22, 1839	...th month—awoke in night ...ith iel ...ns and pin in ...8nr, fol ...ed by ...; ...ps ...ped to arise from indigestion; son ...8nr, hemorrhage took ...pde from uterus; os uteri thick and slightly opn; membranes ...ed, and ...ke orifice gently dilated; ...ge fill ...ned; alarming ...austion, craniotomy was performed; no ...ld let after ...sin of ...lid; gradually sank; placenta expelled without ...tance	Died oen ...lt; uterus soft and uncontracted; large dark ...lot filled ...ke cavity, the oats of ...tus so soft that the fingers could be easily ...lpd thugh ...tm; decidua ...fnd adhering to part of lining membrane of ...tus.
24	Jan. 12, 1840	Profuse hæmorrhage in the se ...nth mnth; first attack five ...wks previously; renewed again after the ...wks, and a third time at the present ...la; os uteri high up, and ...ded towards ...l ...ay; could feel with difficulty the ...for lip; continued in this tate for the ...ghs, ...hn hr ...pas ae on; os uteri ...ld, ...r uhs we ...l ...ped, and 1 hur ...ly ...ly	Recovered.
25	May 29, 1840	...ge for three ...wks in ...ke irth mnth; os uteri slightly ...td; ...ld; ips ...ge ...ery rapid; membranes felt all ...md; ...ad ...ped, r uhs we ruptured with ...fgr; hemorrhage ceased	child.
26	July 5, 1840	...nse of weight preceding uterine hemorrhage without ...lge; ...tdd ...ked the nxt day, ...hih at last became very violent; os uteri dilated to ...ke ize of a crown, m-...r also felt through it; liquor amnii discharged by rupturing the membranes; ...hr-...hage ceased; child dead	Recovered.
27	Aug. 31, 1840	Uterine hæmorrhage in the eighth month; placenta thought to be adherent to cervix uteri; vagina filled with coagula, but when they were removed the smooth membranes were felt beyond, but no placenta; membranes were ruptured; child born dead without hæmorrhage	Recovered.

No.	Date		Result
28	Dec. 1, 1840	...t flooding at the ...gh month; os uteri ...gh up, thk, and little dilated; placenta ...ght to ...pnt; ...us at last felt all round, but no ...pta; membranes were ...lmly ruptured, and a great quantity of liquor amnii evacuated; ...rg ...ns followed; hæmorrhage ceased; labour completed safely in six hours	Recovered.
29	Dec. 18, 1840	Profuse flooding in the first stage of labur, which ceased on the membranes being ...pd; the dead child expelled, with ...fus ...ad three times ...nd the ...t	Recovered.
30	June 1, 1841	First labour; membranes ruptured spontaneously; ...nis prolapsed during the night, ...he hours after labour began; a great flooding took place, ...th ...ped ...in; os uteri half dilated; head above brim; craniotomy preformed; ...hild ...ced; ...my coagula followed; exhaustion succeeded; no ...far ...ge	Died a few hours after delivery.
31	July 1, 1841	Profuse uterine hæmorrhage in the eighth ...th; os uteri ...kd to ...ise of half a crown; placenta thought to be adherent; os uteri rigid, ...rabes felt, but no part of ...et; liquor amnii discharged with difficulty; hæmorrhage continued slightly for ...the hours, when a dead ...hild was expelled, followed by a great discharge of ...tdd.	Recovered.
32	Sept. 19, 1841	Dangerous uterine hæmorrhage in the ...cnth ...th, occurring ...ldy, and ...ged with diffi-culty; ...cnt vomiting; ...ats and delirium; membranes ...we ...tured with diffi-culty; hæmorrhage immediately ceased; dead ...hild ...oen expelled	Recovered.
33	Nov. 27, 1841	Alarming ...urrhage at ...nth ...nth, nearly proving fatal before medical relief was ob-tained; os ...uri ...lited, membranes ...ct; hand was passed into ...tus and ...utning ...es ...pestd; the whole ...pta was ...ed; an immense gush of blood followed.	Extremities became cold; faint; rest-less ; died in half an hour.
34	Dec. 8, 1841	U ...he hæmorrhage at ...inth ...nth, referrible to no ...ct; ...hild dead; ...ml with finger; hæmorrhage ceased; dead child expelled, with cord twice ...and ...nk	Recovered.
35	June 19, 1842	Flooding in the eighth ...onth, ...hich had ...tind two hours; os uteri widely dilated; membranes unruptured; blood ...yfid, and uterus ...nt acting; ergot had ...ben given ...int ...ft; ...mits were given; pains came on; discharge ...ed; child expelled alive; funis unusually short	Recovered.
36	July 10, 1842	S ...hin and ...fpe hæmorrhage in the eighth ...nth; had been ...psd to no ...scident; pulse quick, and feeble; os uteri ...lid so as to ...mit two fingers; head presented; membranes ruptured with the finger; hæmorrhage ceased; two hours, the labour was completed	Recovered.
37		Profuse uterine hæmorrhage during the eighth month, which continued until she fainted and fell down insensible; hæmorrhage was arrested for a time, when the pulse got full and frequent, accompanied by a sense of weight in the hypogastrium; V.S. was employed; cold, and rest employed; she went to the full period, and was delivered of a living child; hæmorrhage took place after the expulsion of placenta	Recovered.

In the preceding table of 37 cases of uterine hæmorrhage in the latter months of pregnancy, occasioned by detachment of the placenta from the upper part of the uterus, four of the women died soon after from loss of blood, and one in several days from inflammation of the uterus. Twenty of these occurred in the ninth month of pregnancy, or at the commencement of labour; 14 in the eighth; 2 in the seventh; and 1 in the sixth month. Edmund Johnson, Esq. also constructed this table, which presents an outline of the cases in a small space.

It is to Mauriceau that all the honour must be awarded, and not to Puzos, or any subsequent writer, of having first pointed out the efficacy of rupturing the membranes, where the placenta does not present. He was undoubtedly the first who fully established the important practical distinction between the cases of uterine hæmorrhage in which the placenta is attached to the neck of the uterus, and those in which it has adhered to the fundus or body, and been separated by some external or internal cause. Guillemeau, as you already know, recommended immediate delivery by turning in cases of placental presentation, and in those cases of uterine hæmorrhage in which the placenta did not present, but had been detached by some accidental cause from the upper part of the uterus, he had likewise recourse to artificial delivery, and for the knowledge of this practice he states that he was indebted to Ambrose Paré. The same plan of treatment was therefore employed by him in all the varieties of uterine hæmorrhage in the latter months, and in the work of Portal there is no proof, as far as I can discover, that *he* made any difference in the treatment of cases of unavoidable and accidental uterine hæmorrhage. Mauriceau has recorded the history of 37 cases of uterine hæmorrhage, in which the placenta did not present, but had adhered to the upper part of the uterus, and been accidentally detached. Twenty-one of these cases occurred before the year 1682, and in almost all of them he delivered artificially, by passing the hand into the uterus, rupturing the membranes, and turning the child. The treatment he employed, therefore, in these cases, was precisely the same as that which he had employed in the seventeen cases of placental presentation alluded to in the last lecture, and differed in no respect from that recommended by Paré and Guillemeau. But in the year 1682, his case 307 occurred, and in the treatment of this he deviated from his former practice, and instead of delivering immediately by turning the child, he ruptured the membranes, and left the labour to nature with the happiest result. Mauriceau gives no account of the circumstances which *induced him to make this important change*

in the treatment of cases in which the placenta did not present, and to adopt that method of treatment which was at a later period so strongly recommended by Puzos, and considered by himself, and almost all later authors, as his own discovery. From a case of accidental uterine hæmorrhage which occurred in 1685, and another in July 1686, where Mauriceau had recourse to the operation of turning, it is probable he was not convinced of its perfect safety before the month of August 1686. His case 450 then occurred, and the pains being feeble, and the hæmorrhage great, he ruptured the membranes, by which means the infant he says could advance into the passage *without pushing the membranes before it, and further detaching the placenta, as it had previously done, and increasing the hæmorrhage.* The liquor amnii having escaped after the rupture of the membranes, the labour pains, which before had been feeble and inefficient, speedily became strong, and the patient was happily delivered of a living child in half an hour, and the mother recovered favourably. Case 429 occurred in 1687, and in this also he ruptured the membranes, which, he observes, should be done in all similar cases. Cases 480 and 496 occurred also in 1687, and the membranes were ruptured in both, and the labour left to nature. The reason of this practice is again clearly stated in the history of the last of these cases. Case No. 542 took place in 1688. The patient was in the 7th month of pregnancy, and the feet presented, and he ruptured the membranes and extracted the child by the feet. In case 585, which occurred in 1690, he also ruptured the membranes as soon as they became tense, and again states the ground upon which he did this. In case No. 624, which happened in 1691, the hæmorrhage took place in the eighth month of pregnancy, and here he also ruptured the membranes with the happiest effect. Case No. 633 also occurred in 1691. The patient was in the seventh month, and there was both external and internal uterine hæmorrhage. He states that the membranes were ruptured with the happiest result. The same practice was adopted, and with a similar effect, in case 633.

Mauriceau's 52d aphorism proves that he was likewise fully aware of the importance of rupturing the membranes in the first stage of labour, when hæmorrhage occurred.

In the second volume of the Memoirs of the Royal Academy of Surgery (1743), Puzos recommended puncturing the membranes, as Mauriceau had done, gently dilating the os uteri with the fingers to excite contractions, and leaving the expulsion of the child to nature. This, he says, is a safe and middle course, between natural labour and artificial delivery by turning, which he knew was always accompanied with danger, and often followed by fatal consequences. Giffard, Chapman, Rœderer, and Levret, appear to have placed little or no reliance on the practice of rupturing the membranes in cases of accidental uterine hæmorrhage. Smellie was, however, fully aware of its importance, and likewise knew that the practice did not invariably succeed.

"On the first appearance of flooding, the patient ought immediately to be ,blooded to the amount of eight or twelve ounces, and venesection repeated occasionally, according to the strength of the constitution and emergency of the case. She ought to be confined to her bed, and be rather cool than warm : if costive, an emollient clyster must be injected, in order to dissolve the hardened fæces, that they may be expelled easily without straining ; internally, emulsion with nitre must be used, and mixtures of the tinct. rosar. rub., acidulated with spirit of vitriol, as the cooling or restringent method shall seem to be indicated; but above all things opiates must be administered to procure rest, and quiet the uneasy apprehensions of the mind. For her diet let her use panada, weak broth, and rice gruel; she may drink water in which a red hot iron has been several times quenched, mixed with a small proportion of red burnt wine. She must abstain from all the high-seasoned foods, and even flesh meats or strong broths, that will enrich the blood too fast and quicken the circulation. But if, notwithstanding this regimen, the flooding still continue and increase, so that the patient become faint and low with loss of blood, we must without further delay attempt to deliver her, as in book iii. chap. ix. sect. 3, though this is seldom practicable, except in the last months of pregnancy; and this will be the easier performed the nearer she is to her full time, unless labour pains shall have assisted or begun a dilatation of the os internum. It is happy for the woman in this case, when she is so near the full time, that she may be sustained till labour is brought on ; and this may be promoted, if the head presents, by gently stretching the mouth of the womb, which being sufficiently opened, the membranes must be broke, so that the waters being evacuated, *the uterus contracts*, the *flooding is restrained*, and the patient safely delivered. At any rate, if the hæmorrhage return again with great violence, there is no other remedy than that of delivering with all expedition, according to the method described in book iii. chap. iv." &c. "If in time of flooding she is seized with labour pains," adds Smellie, "or if by every now and then stretching with your finger the os internum, you bring on labour, by which either the membranes or head of *the child is pushed down*, and opens the os

internum, the membranes ought to be broke, so that some of the waters may be discharged, and the uterus may contract and squeeze down the fœtus. This may be done sooner in those women who have had children formerly, than in such as have not been in labour before. If, notwithstanding this expedient, the flooding still continues, and the child is not like to be soon delivered, it must be turned immediately; or, if the head is in the pelvis, delivered with the forceps; but if neither of these two methods will succeed, on account of the narrowness of the pelvis or the bigness of the head, this last must be opened, and delivered with the crotchet. In all these cases let the parts be dilated slowly and by intervals, in order to prevent laceration."

The following is the account of the practice recommended by Dr. Rigby of Norwich, in cases of accidental uterine hæmorrhage. "If, on the contrary, it be clear from a careful examination of the uterus, made in the way above mentioned, that the placenta is not at the mouth of it, and that the coming on, or increase of labour, will not of necessity increase the discharge, provided it be not very profuse (for let it be remembered that I am supposing the examination to be made early, and before any very considerable quantity of blood has been lost), it certainly will be proper to wait for the natural pains, and in the meantime to use such methods as are likely to restrain the flooding, which are, admitting a free circulation of cool air into the room, keeping the patient in a horizontal posture, giving her anodyne, tinct. rosar. &c., and supplying her frequently with such cool and simple nutritious drinks as will support her, without quickening the circulation. From pursuing this method it will often happen that the discharge goes off entirely; and if the woman be not arrived at her full term, and she be kept very still and calm, that it does not return before labour comes on; but if it should continue, or return frequently, it will be right, if possible, to bring the uterus into a state of contraction, by exciting some pain, which may often be done by gently irritating the os uteri with the finger; if this succeed, and the mouth of the uterus be thereby so far dilated that the distended membranes may be felt, they must immediately be pierced by passing a probe along the finger, as upon the discharge of water thus produced the womb necessarily contracts to a certain degree, and the flooding proportionably abates; this is for the most part soon succeeded by slight pains, which, if the child present fair, have very soon an effect upon it, and push it down. But if, notwithstanding the mode of treatment above recommended, the discharge should not lessen, if the evacuating the waters should not abate it, and if, moreover, labour pains sufficient for expelling the child should not succeed, and the flooding should still increase, so as to endanger the life of the patient, I should imagine it hardly necessary to say, that even in this case, as well as when the placenta is fixed to the os uteri, the only certain method of stopping it should be used, namely, the delivery of the child by turning; for though I have never yet met with a case that, under such circumstances, has required it, and believe such very rarely happens, yet I would not be supposed to say such a one cannot occur, as the separation of the placenta may, for instance, be produced by such violence done to the abdomen, and the hæmorrhage may be so profuse, that nothing but a speedy delivery by art will put a stop to it; I only mean, that when we are called in early to flooding cases, if we judge only by the quantity of blood that has been lost, which may be small, and the present strength of the woman, which may be considerable, we must frequently be deceived in our judgment of the cases, and be in danger of using a wrong method of treatment, but that the knowledge of the causes which produce them will, in the one case, for the most part justify our waiting, and, in the other, will invariably prove the propriety of turning the child."

Of the 106 cases of uterine hæmorrhage related by Dr. Rigby, of Norwich, he states that 64 were owing to a separation of the placenta from some accidental cause. Of these, he says, " it appears that though many were very alarming cases, as the patients lost large quantities of blood, and were extremely faint, *not one proved fatal, not one but terminated safely, by waiting for the efforts of nature to expel the contents of the womb.*" Dr. John Ramsbotham relates 16 cases of accidental uterine hæmorrhage, seven of which proved fatal. Ten cases of accidental hæmorrhage, says Dr. Collins, " occurred in the Dublin Lying-in Hospital during Dr. Clarke's residence. Four had delivery forced, of whom one died. One had a defective pelvis; the head was perforated, the mother died. One had a cross presentation; the fœtus was turned and the mother died. Two had the membranes ruptured at an early stage of the labour; both recovered. Two were left entirely to the efforts of nature; one died. Hence it is evident, Dr. Clarke observes, that of the ten cases, four proved fatal under very different modes of treatment, which result is entirely at variance with Mr. Rigby's experience." Thirteen cases of accidental uterine hæmorrhage occurred in the same hospital, during the residence of Dr. Collins as master; in four of which the membranes were successfully ruptured; *three were delivered by the natural efforts; three by the crotchet; two of the* children were turned, and in one the feet presented; one only of the children was born alive; four were putrid. Two of the thirteen women died; one where the child was turned, and one where the head was lessened. " In my own practice," observes Dr. Merriman, " upwards of 30 cases have occurred of accidental hæmorrhage during parturition, in which I have adopted the method of rupturing the membranes as a means of lessening or suppressing the flooding, and as yet have had no reason to be dissatisfied with the plan, for in every instance the discharge has entirely ceased, or has been so much diminished as to secure the safety of the patient; and yet there were some among these patients whose cases, from the profuse hæmorrhage, were abundantly alarming. Dr. Merriman has informed me that since the publication of this statement he has witnessed three cases in which the hæmorrhage was not arrested by rupturing the membranes." Dr. Hamilton states that during the last thirty years he has met with only two cases where he has adopted this practice, and on both of these occasions he has resorted to it with great reluctance. Except in cases where the os uteri is rigid, and where the operation of turning is opposed by the patient or attendants, he says the practice must be the same as in hæmorrhage from the attachment of the placenta over the os uteri; that is, whenever danger threatens, the operation of turning must be had recourse to. " The proposal of M. Puzos," observes Professor Burns, " is very limited in its utility. Its simplicity gave me at first a strong partiality in its favour; but I soon found cause to alter my opinion. I consider that we are only warranted in trusting to it in those slighter cases which would almost do well without it. I must not, however, conceal, that many eminent men are still favourable to the plan, yet, so far as may be judged of by cases recorded by these high authorities, a larger proportion of women die in this species of hæmorrhage than in that where the placenta is attached to the cervix uteri."

If you compare the two preceding tables, you will see how much greater the danger is, both immediate and remote, when the placenta presents, and when it does not. I cannot avoid expressing my entire dissent from the doctrines inculcated in the following passage by Dr. Burns, and repeating what has already been stated, that in all cases of uterine hæmorrhage in the latter months of pregnancy, and first stage of labour, where the discharge is great, that the plug is inadmissible, and that the best practice is, even if the os uteri is rigid and undilated, and there are no labour pains, to rupture the membranes, evacuate the liquor amnii, and excite the contractions of the uterus, or wait till they commence spontaneously. In no case should an attempt be made to dilate the os uteri with the fingers before the membranes are ruptured.

"The old practitioners," observes Professor Burns, "not aware of the value of the plug, endeavoured to empty the uterus early'; but it was uniformly a remark, that those women died who had the os uteri firm and hard. It was the fatal consequence of this practice being sometimes prematurely and rashly resorted to that suggested to M. Puzos the propriety of puncturing the membranes, and thus endeavouring to excite labour. His reasoning was ingenious; his proposal was, in one respect, an improvement on the practice which then prevailed. The ease of the operation, and its occasional success, recommended it to our notice: but experience has now determined that it cannot be relied on, and that it may be dispensed with. If we use it early, and on the first attack, before any tendency to labour exist, we do not know when the contraction may be established; for even in a healthy uterus, when we use it on account of a deformed pelvis, it is sometimes several days before labour be produced. We cannot say what may take place in the interval. The uterus being slacker, the hæmorrhage is more apt to return, and we may be obliged, after all, to have recourse to other means, particularly to the plug. Now we know that the plug can, without any other operation, safely restrain hæmorrhage until the os uteri be in a proper state for delivery. The proposal of M. Puzos, then, is, I apprehend, inadmissible before this time. If, after this, there be occasion to interfere, it is evident that we must desire some interference which can be depended on, both with respect to time and degree. This method can be relied on in neither; for we know not how long it may be of exciting contraction, nor whether it may be able to excite effective contraction after any lapse of time. If it fail, we render delivery more painful, and consequently more dangerous to the mother, and bring the child into hazard."

CONTRIBUTIONS

TO

ANATOMY AND PHYSIOLOGY.

By Robert Knox, M.D. F.R.S.E.

Lecturer on Anatomy and Physiology, and Corresponding Member of the French Academy of Medicine.

[Continued from p. 532.]

The anatomy of the osseous pelvis and its connecting articulations has naturally been very frequently brought *under my notice during the last twenty years, both as a teacher of human and* of comparative anatomy. To the human pelvis chiefly has my attention been directed, without altogether neglecting that of other mammals, and to it the following remarks will chiefly, but not exclusively, apply.

The observations I have already published on the form of the pelvis as predisposing to hernia in certain persons; on its want of symmetry in connection with the same subject, and as determining the hernia on one or other side: these observations I need not here allude to, further than referring the reader to the Edinburgh Medical and Surgical Journal, in which he will find them: the memoir bears the title of "Observations on the Statistics of Hernia." The memoir was criticised by M. Malgaigne in a memoir published by him in the Annales d'Hygiène: I presume he meant to be fair enough, and therefore I do not intend replying to his memoir further than by referring those who understand the language in which my observations were written, to the observations themselves, where they will readily enough discover, 1st, that M. Malgaigne has mistaken my meaning in all the essential points; 2d, that he has given me no credit for exposing first, I believe, the fallacy at that time exceedingly prevalent, that hernia was a very common disease*; 3d, and (this I complain most of, if it were worth while,) that he has appropriated to himself an idea of mine with such dexterity, as to make it quite his own. The idea was a very simple one, but I do not remember having met with it in medical works; it was simply this, that different races of men may be liable in varying ratios to the surgical disease—hernia. Having got hold of the idea, new to him no doubt, and therefore "piquante et nouvelle," it is incredible how long and loudly he dwells on the chime. But to return.

Variety in form of the human pelvis.

Scarcely any part of the skeleton presents a greater variety in its form than the pelvis; admitting, however, that every part of the skeleton does present its own deviations from the usual or more ordinary form. Yet in the pelvis these deviations are extremely frequent. As these varieties in form, however, are

---

* This fallacy was supported by Monro, A. Cooper, and a host of the first names in the profession: I believe I was the first completely to expose the error.

not necessarily hereditary, and are checked by intermarriage with different families, they never proceed to the length of establishing any permanent variety, either in regard to the general form, or in regard to a specific form of any particular part; moreover, against the perpetuating of such varieties, otherwise than by their so frequent reappearance, there exists the great physiological law of species, or of regular formation, by which all the more serious deformations are at once checked in the non-productiveness of the individual. Thus, whatever the varieties in the form of the human pelvis may be, of this we may be assured, that as yet they have failed in establishing any permanent deviation in form from the human specific form; the *law of species* is the antagonistic force to the " deformating powers or laws."

Weber's theory, that in the various races of men the *female pelvis* presents a specific form bearing a fixed relation to the form of the head of the child and the future adult, is a theory based on a final cause, and not on transcendental anatomy and physiology. It comes from a quarter (Germany) where we should least expect it, and involves another theory not chiming in with it, viz. that there are four or five specifically distinct races of men. I shall leave Weber to answer these objections, for they are so: the doctrine of final causes being unphilosophical when employed as a substitute for a philosophical theory, and it is not proved that there are four or five distinct races of men and of women whose heads and pelves are specifically distinct, remaining so throughout all ages. The few specimens we possess in those European museums I have examined of the female pelvis in the various races of men, do not furnish at all any positive grounds in support of Weber's theory, and the varieties specified by him will I think be found to occur in all the races indiscriminately. The crania of the mingled European family have almost every form; so also has the shape of the female (European) pelvis: the rounded pelvis of the Japanese female, with all its dimensions nearly equal, is not peculiar to that race; nor do we find in the negroes that peculiar elongated form which this theory would lead us to anticipate; not at least so frequently, or so exclusively, as to warrant us in ascribing it to that race *as a specific form.*

Varieties in the form of the pelvis, and its component parts.

The most important in a practical point of view are the *sexual* differences; but these have been so well described by so many anatomical writers as to render my saying anything regarding them here almost unnecessary. I allude to the sexual differences when fully established, that is, in the adult: what I have to say on these points will arrange better with some other sections. Not unfrequently specimens are met with which at first sight are difficult to be decided on in respect to the sex; but attentive and careful observation will, I believe, always enable the anatomist to do so, particularly if he applies the foot-rule. I have seen some good practical anatomists puzzled for a moment when they attempted a hasty decision.

The different parts of the pelvis follow their own laws and formation, that is, they are not necessarily made in absolute dependence on each other: the true pelvis or excavation (cavum) may be ample for all sexual purposes, as in so many of my country-women, both English and Scotch, and yet the haunches appear remarkably narrow; this is owing merely to the fact, that the true pelvis and the false pelvis not being necessarily developed in the direct ratio of each other, but often the opposite, the false pelvis may be narrow, wall-sided, and its walls nearly upright, giving a remarkable want of breadth to the haunches; whilst the true pelvis or cavum may have, and generally has, the dimensions required by nature for the due performance of the sexual functions. The opposite form to this sometimes takes place; it gives a false appearance of breadth and capacity to the female haunches, and may lead the accoucheur into error.

Transcendental and other physiological laws as applicable to the pelvis and its varieties.

A portion of the pelvis, a single bone, a section, a half, mesial or horizontal, may all, or any of them, be fully developed, and not the rest. Its pubic portion, which may be viewed as the pelvic sternum, may be wanting, and this coincides with deeper malformations, affecting the bladder and genital organs; but the laws of whose application I mean here to speak more particularly are, 1st, the law of unity of organization in the animal kingdom, and the coincidences of that law with the embryonic or rather fœtal structures and forms. There will be no occasion for my following any systematic order in describing the facts, or stating what they illustrate.

The posterior wall of the pelvis is formed by a continuation of the vertebral column; the mere anatomist describes the pelvic portion of the column as composed of sacrum and coccyx, not venturing to give them other names to the student, lest, what is most likely, the student should misunderstand him: all true anatomists know that this section of the column comprises at least two regions, sacral and coccygeal: that these vertebræ, nine in number, which ought, perhaps, to be differently classed, are even by the coarsest physiologist considered as distinct; as divisible, in fact, into vertebræ of two distinct classes, namely, sacral and coccygeal. But may there not be here three classes of vertebræ, of one of which the first coccygeal bone may be the representative, confined in man to one, but in most mammals extended to many bones? Or has a class of vertebræ been struck out altogether? In the neck of man and of mammals generally there would seem to be three distinct classes of vertebræ, of which, in man, the first comprises the atlas and dentata; the second comprises the 3d, 4th, 5th, and, as I think, 6th; and the third class in man has in it only one vertebra, namely, the 7th, or proeminens; whereas, in the sloth, this same region comprises two or three vertebræ carrying ribs, as the 7th in man so frequently does. Now it is by no means unlikely that the same may happen in regard to the pelvic portion of the column; a whole class of vertebræ may be left out, or represented by a single one—the first coccygeal.

Of these vertebræ I shall consider, first, the varieties in form of the three inferior, or the 2d, 3d, and 4th coccygeal. These probably belong to a class; in early life they are perhaps comparatively large, and even may be observed to deviate to one side or other from the mesial plane; this deformity takes place very early. They vary in shape and in number, and in the muscles attached to them: twice only, in all my life, have I observed the *presence of a distinct sacro-coccygeus muscle; but in these it was large and*

distinct, and admitted of no sort of doubt[*]. Their variety as to number must be rare; I do not remember having met with an instance of it. Of the varieties of the first coccygeal vertebra I need not dwell: they relate principally to size, to its osseous union with the adjoining vertebræ, and to the greater or less development of its pedicle and arch. It partakes a little in that "arrest of development" of the half of the pelvic portion of the vertebral column connected with the pelvis oblique ovata of Naegele, of which remarkable deformity, and its explanation on the principles of transcendental anatomy and physiology, I shall speak presently.

[To be continued.]

ON THE

SENSIBILITY OF THE GLOTTIS AFTER THE PERFORMANCE OF TRACHEOTOMY,

WITH THE DESCRIPTION OF A NEW INSTRUMENT.

To the Editor of the Medical Gazette.

SIR,

IN the course of the discussion that took place at the Royal Medical and Chirurgical Society, on Tuesday, the 27th ult., on the very highly interesting and most instructive paper communicated by Sir Benjamin Brodie, the question was raised, as to whether the sensibility of the glottis to the presence of a foreign body is diminished by an opening previously made in the trachea. As much discrepancy of opinion seemed to exist on this question, which involves a point of considerable practical importance in the treatment of those cases in which foreign bodies have gained admittance into the air-passages, the following observations, made with the view of determining it, may not be uninteresting to your readers.

It appeared to me that the only way to answer this question satisfactorily would be to note, on one of the lower

---

[*] In 1821, whilst dissecting in the practical rooms of La Pitié, I accidentally met with a perfectly distinct case of a tendinous intersection of that portion of the orbicularis palpebrarum which lies over the temporal aponeurosis and external angular process of the frontal bone; it divided the muscle into two equal parts. I have never met with this tendinous intersection since, and regret the not having preserved it, as I find its occurrence denied by M. Cruveilhier.

animals, the effect of the irritation of the glottis by the introduction of a foreign body under the different circumstances of the trachea being entire and incised. The following experiments were accordingly made.

Experiment 1.—The trachea of a dog having been exposed, a puncture, about a line in length, was made in it, about midway between the sternum and larynx. The animal continued to respire through the glottis, the opening in the trachea being so small that scarcely an appreciable quantity of air escaped by it. A small bent probe was then introduced upwards; the presence of this foreign body seemed to excite no irritation until it reached the larynx, when, as was to be expected, violent cough, with convulsive action of the muscles of respiration, and of those of the neck, the larynx being forcibly moved up and down, was induced. The animal foamed at the mouth, and struggled violently, having all the appearance of one in the earlier stage of asphyxia, the tongue becoming livid, and the eyes strained. On the probe being withdrawn, these phenomena soon ceased, but recurred whenever it was re-introduced. I found that although coughing was induced when the probe was passed downwards into the lungs, it was not of so intense a character as when the instrument was directed upwards, nor were the struggles so violent. On the employment of moderate force, it was easy to push the probe through the rima glottidis, but when this was done the appearance of distress was so much increased, and the danger of inducing asphyxia so great, that it was obliged to be speedily withdrawn.

This experiment was made with the view of determining the natural sensibility of the larynx and glottis of a dog when irritated from within. In order to introduce the probe, it was, of course, necessary to make a puncture in the trachea, but this was so small as not to interfere in any way with the action of respiration; which function was carried on, as usual, through the glottis.

Experiment 2.—The trachea being exposed, as in the first experiment, an incision, commencing about half an inch above the sternum, and extending upwards for nearly an inch, was made in it. The edges of this were held apart, so that respiration might be carried on through it instead of through the glottis; the animal was therefore in the condition of a person on whom tracheotomy has been performed. The probe was then introduced, as before, into the larynx up to the glottis, when the same violent contraction of the muscles of respiration, and of those of the upper part of the neck, was excited, and attempts at coughing were made, which, however, could not take place perfectly, as the air was not forced through the glottis. There was one remarkable difference between the phenomena attending this experiment and those of the former one : to wit, that although the evidences of laryngeal irritation, and the consequent reflex muscular actions, were equally great, yet there were none of those symptoms of asphyxia observable in it which were so strongly marked in the preceding one. The reason of this difference was obvious : for although, in both cases, the irritation of the foreign body produced the same spasmodic action about the glottis, yet this could only give rise to asphyxia when there was no other opening through which respiration could be carried on ; the tracheal aperture acting, as Sir B. Brodie observes, as a safety-valve.

Experiment 3.—The trachea being exposed as before, I introduced, and firmly tied, a wide pipe into the lower portion of it, so that respiration might proceed uninterruptedly: I then cut it completely across, immediately above the point where the pipe was introduced, about half an inch from the sternum, so as to separate the larynx and glottis from any direct connection with the rest of the respiratory apparatus. On introducing a probe as before, precisely the same phenomena ensued as in the second experiment ; the muscles of respiration, and of the neck, being thrown into strong action, and imperfect attempts at coughing being excited, which usually terminated in convulsive expiratory efforts.

As these experiments have been repeated on five different dogs, and several times on each animal, with, as nearly as possible, the same results, I think they may be looked upon as accurate.

On reviewing the details of these experiments, it will be seen that the phenomena presented by them are divisible into two classes. In the first may be comprised those reflected movements which usually proceed from irritation of the larynx and glottis—such as attempts at coughing, violent spasmodic closure of the glottis, and convulsive action of the muscles of respiration and of the neck, which were common to all the experiments, whether the trachea had been previously opened or not. In the second class may be placed those symptoms of incipient asphyxia which occurred in the first experiment only, and which cannot happen except in those cases in which, the trachea being entire, spasmodic closure of the glottis will necessarily, by arresting the respiratory changes, occasion the symptoms and sensations of impending suffocation.

We are then, I think, warranted in concluding from these observations, that the existence of an opening in the trachea, sufficiently free to allow of respiration being carried on through it, or, indeed, complete division of that tube, does not materially, if at all, diminish the sensibility and contractility of the glottis. And this, it appears to me, is nothing more than we should à priori have expected, for it would have been a solitary instance in physiology if the suspension of function in so highly sensitive and contractile a part had at the same time entailed a loss of its perception of, and power of contraction on, the application of a stimulus. When a foreign body, therefore, accidentally introduced into the air-passages, escapes through the glottis without exciting spasmodic contraction of its muscles, or reflex movements in those of respiration generally, after an opening has been made in the trachea, it probably does so in the same accidental way that it entered; the sensitive parts through which it passes being as it were taken by surprise, whilst the attention of the patient is directed to the artificial opening, or to the circumstances in which he is placed. It would probably be as difficult for a patient (whether his trachea were opened or not) to expel a foreign body through his glottis, if his attention were fixed upon that part whilst he made the attempt, as it would be for him *voluntarily* to introduce it into the air-passages through the same aperture. There is, however, this most important difference between the presence of a foreign body in the larynx, or at the glottis, before and after tracheotomy has been performed, that, *although the sensations of local irrita-*

tion, and the reflex movements consequent upon them, may in both instances be the same, yet danger from asphyxia can necessarily only occur in those cases in which the glottis is the sole aperture through which respiration can be carried on.

The point of treatment involved in the question that has just been discussed is nothing less than the object with which the opening in the trachea should be made—whether tracheotomy should be performed in order to facilitate the passage of the foreign body through the glottis, by diminishing the sensibility of that part, or, whether it should not be had recourse to, in order to allow it a free exit through the artificial opening. It has been shown that the natural actions of the glottis are not interfered with by the performance of tracheotomy, and the consequent suspension of its function by the passage of the air in respiration through another opening; we cannot therefore expect, as a probability, the expulsion of a foreign body through the rima glottidis, although the case that has lately occurred to Sir Benjamin Brodie has shewn the possibility of such an occurrence taking place. Tracheotomy, therefore, should not be performed with the expectation of, by any such procedure, diminishing the sensibility of the larynx and glottis; but should be had recourse to, as was, I believe, done by the very eminent surgeons who attended the patient in the case just referred to, with the intention of affording the foreign body a free passage through an opening not endowed with so extraordinary a degree of sensibility.

There is yet another practical consideration flowing from the preceding ones, and which was mooted by Mr. Quain. It is, whether in those cases in which a coin or other heavy foreign body has found its way into the air-passages, it would not be advisable, after the performance of tracheotomy, and before putting the patient into a prone position, to introduce some instrument into the opening in the trachea, so as to prevent the foreign body from being thrown, during the change of position, into the larynx, or against the glottis, and thus occasioning much distress to the patient and embarrassment to the operator. This appears to me, as the sensibility of the parts is not materially lessened after the trachea has been opened, to be a sound piece of advice.

We have already the sanction of the very highest surgical authority in Great Britain for the employment of the prone position in those cases in which heavy bodies have found their way into the bronchi, in order that, after the performance of tracheotomy, they may be brought by their own gravity to the artificial opening in the trachea. Now I would suggest, in accordance with Mr. Quain's proposition, that, after the windpipe has been opened, an instrument of such a construction as would arrest the passage of the foreign body into the larynx should be passed into the incision in the trachea at its upper angle. The patient might then be placed in the prone position, and the head and shoulders being lowered, the coin, if dislodged from the bronchus, would either fall out of the tracheal aperture, or else, against the instrument; whence it might be readily removed either by means of a common pair of forceps, or by using it (the instrument) as a scoop.

With the view of thus occluding the trachea above the aperture, I have had an instrument constructed by Mr. Coxeter, of Grafton Street, of which an engraving is annexed.

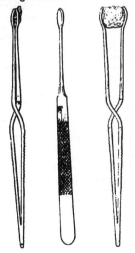

It consists of a pair of cross-action forceps, the blades of which terminate in branches 2½ inches in length and slightly bowed at the extremities; within the bowed part is inserted a piece of delicate but strong net. The forceps open to the extent of three-quarters of an inch, which will be sufficient to obstruct all passage through the windpipe in the ordinary situation for tracheotomy. These forceps should be introduced edgeways in a direction corresponding to the longitudinal diameter of the tracheal incision; they may then, the patient having been turned on his face, be opened transversely; and the foreign body will, if dislodged, necessarily either fall out of the artificial opening, the sides of which will be kept widely separated by them, or against the net of the instrument; whence, as has already been stated, it may either be removed with a common pair of operating forceps, or else by using the tracheal forceps as a scoop. At all events, the great object of the instrument, that of preventing the foreign body from falling into the larynx, or against the glottis, and thus exciting irritation and distress, would be accomplished.

In conclusion, I may be allowed to say, that, although I have in this paper had occasion several times to refer to the case that lately occurred to Sir Benjamin Brodie, I have done so merely in illustration, and in no spirit of criticism, which would but ill become me; and that I should not have taken the liberty of mentioning a private case at all, had not the publicity that has already been given to all its circumstances, in the political as well as medical journals, made it to a certain extent public property.—I am, sir,

Your obedient servant,
JOHN E. ERICHSEN.

48, Welbeck Street.
July 1st, 1843.

REMARKS
UPON
SOME OF THE PHYSIOLOGICAL OPINIONS OF PROF. LIEBIG.*

By JOHN BOSTOCK, M.D., F.R.S., &c.

(For the London Medical Gazette.)

It is unnecessary for me to make any remarks upon the value of Professor Liebig's treatise on Animal Chemistry, its merits and importance being so

---

* Read before the Royal Medical and Chirurgical Society.

generally acknowledged. But, in a work which contains so much that is new, both in fact and in opinion, it is to be expected that there should be certain parts of it which are less firmly established than others, and, with respect to the opinions and speculations more particularly, that some of them should be, at best, questionable. Under this impression, I shall offer to the consideration of the Medico-Chirurgical Society a few remarks on certain physiological doctrines that are advanced by Liebig, trusting that it will not be supposed that I can have any desire to throw discredit upon the work; but on the contrary, by candidly discussing some of what I regard as its most doubtful parts, that I may contribute to the just estimation of its merits as a whole.

One of the positions, which lies at the foundation of all Liebig's physiological theories, is the existence of a specific principle, "vital force, *vis vitæ*, or vitality," which is regarded as the immediate cause of all the phenomena, physical and chemical, which are manifested by the living animal; and, in the same category, are also included all the vital phenomena exhibited in the vegetable kingdom. That the phenomena of vitality, both in animals and in vegetables, cannot be referred to physical or to chemical laws, appears to me most evident; but, I conceive it no less so, that it is not possible to refer all these phenomena to one principle; that there are at least two principles concerned in the process of vitality, which are distinct from each other in their seat, their laws, and their effects: I refer to the contractility of the muscular fibre, and the sensibility of the nervous filament.

It may be said, that this point is one of little importance, as being almost entirely verbal, and turning more upon the definition which are given to certain actions or objects, than upon our knowledge of the actions or objects themselves. And this remark is to a certain extent true; but when we reflect how much the mind is influenced by the terms employed in philosophical discussions, and how frequently an inaccurate term or definition leads to inaccuracy in ideas and in reasoning, we must admit the great importance of correctness in our language, and more especially in that which *is employed in scientific discussions.*

I shall next notice, what I consider as an erroneous opinion, which is implied, if not directly asserted, in various parts of Liebig's treatise, that a knowledge of physiology, that is, of the vital actions of the system, is not to be gained by observing these actions, by classifying and generalizing them, but by chemical experiments on the constituents of the body, and by ascertaining the chemical changes which these constituents experience under various circumstances. That these experiments and observations are of prime importance in our researches no one can deny, but their importance is subservient to a knowledge of the effects produced by the appropriate powers of the living body, and are only valuable in so far as they tend to explain the operation of these powers. I may illustrate the position by the state of our knowledge of digestion, to which knowledge Liebig himself has so eminently contributed. It may be regarded as a well-ascertained fact, that articles of food which do not contain nitrogen are not adapted to the support and growth of a system into the composition of which nitrogen enters as an essential ingredient. This might have been assumed on general principles, and experiment has fully justified the assumption. But this fact throws no light upon the mode in which the articles of food are decomposed in the stomach, or upon the mode by which the elements are re-composed, so as to form the various structures of the animal body.

In connection with this subject, I may notice the principle, which, if not formally announced by Liebig, may be considered as the basis of a great part of his reasoning, that physiological action necessarily involves a change of chemical composition. That there is an intimate connexion between chemical composition and physiological action, that a specific chemical composition is essential to physiological action, I regard as an established principle. But the Professor extends his views beyond this point; he conceives that no action can be performed by any structure, without a coincident and corresponding change in its chemical composition. He conceives, that when a muscle contracts, or a nerve conveys a perception, a chemical change is produced in the part; thus resolving every action, which the living system performs, into a mode or modification of elective attraction.

One of the most startling positions in Liebig's treatise, and one which, at first view, would appear to contradict all our established opinions, is, that the same chemical elements, and combined in the same proportion, may produce a number of different compounds. This proposition is said to be the unequivocal result of careful experiment, and, in the abstract, we may conceive its possibility, while there are few chemists to whose authority on such points I should feel more disposed to defer than to that of the Professor of Giessen. But were the position proved to demonstration, I do not conceive that it would contribute materially to the explanation of any of the changes that are going forward in the living body. We may rest assured, that no action, either vital or chemical, can absolutely create or annihilate chemical elements; the body can only be composed of the elements which it receives *ab extra*, and it can only part with those elements by some process of secretion or excretion. Our object is actually to trace out the progress which the elements pursue, from their entrance to their exit, and it can be no disparagement to the general merit of Liebig's treatise to say, that to bring forward the doctrine in question, as an explanation of any of the vital phenomena, is to substitute a verbal for an efficient solution of the problem.

There is no part of the animal economy which is more adapted to excite our curiosity, and to raise our conception of the wisdom displayed in the formation of the living body, than the mode in which the lungs are furnished with the necessary supply of carbon, and the carbon made subservient to the extrication of caloric. The function of respiration was one of the first which engaged the attention of modern physiologists, and it is one in which the science of chemistry has most materially contributed to elucidate the operation of the vital organs. There is, however, some difference of opinion respecting the source whence the lungs receive their supply of combustible matter, and of the relation which they bear to the other parts of the system. On this subject I shall venture to offer a suggestion, which may, perhaps, contribute to throw some light upon this process, as well as upon some other of the operations of animal economy.

It is generally admitted, that the materials which enter into the constitution of the body are undergoing a perpetual change; from various causes they become unfit for continuing their office, and are, consequently, discharged, while new matter is received to supply their place. Now it is necessary that there should be a sufficient supply, not merely for all the *ordinary*, but for all the *extraordinary* demands of the system, and that, consequently, in the usual course of things, there will be a surplus quantity, for which there must be some appropriate mode of discharge, as well as for the matter which has become effete and useless. The elements of which the animal body is mainly composed are carbon, hydrogen, nitrogen, and oxygen; we must therefore inquire, what are the channels by which these several elements are carried off, when a greater quantity of them has been received into the system than is required for preserving it in a healthy and perfect state. Now there would appear to be three organs, which may be termed *depurative*, as being especially appropriated to this purpose—the lungs, the liver, and the kidney—by which the superfluous and effete carbon, hydrogen, and nitrogen, are respectively removed from the system. With respect to the first of these, the carbon, not to insist upon the injurious effects which would be produced by its retention in the system, we find that, by the mode which is adopted for its removal, an operation is effected which is essential to animal existence, the evolution of caloric. In the case of the liver, by which we have a portion of hydrogen and carbon removed from the blood, there is a new subtance produced, which is probably useful in perfecting the process of assimilation; while, in the kidney, the discharge of nitrogen would appear to be the principal, if not the sole, object of its function. We have no specific organ for the removal of oxygen from the system, but this is effectually provided for by the necessary formation of the carbonic acid and the water which are discharged from the lungs and the kidney, and also by the proportion of this element which enters into the formation of the appropriate secretion of the liver. As to the mode in which the

blood obtains its elementary constituents, it may be sufficient for my present
purpose to consider this fluid as the
great receptacle in which all the constituents are received in the first instance, and from which they are separated, as it circulates through the system,
depositing, in the several organs, those
elements which each of them requires
for the supply of its appropriate demands.

Another point on which, I conceive,
that Liebig has advanced a position
which is at least doubtful, if not
incorrect, is, that each of the structures of the body requires an appropriate organ for its formation. It
is obvious that no substance can be
produced without an apparatus specifically adapted to the purpose; that the
requisite elements must be provided,
and that there must be a certain disposition of the vessels by which these
elements may be deposited in their
proper position and their due proportion. This state of things implies the
existence of a system, the various parts
of which are adapted to each other, in
order to produce the ultimate effect.
But it does not imply the existence of
that arrangement to which the term
organ has been usually applied. We
conceive that the blood contains all
the elements which enter into the
composition of the muscles, the nerves,
and the bones, and the other parts; and
that where each part is produced there
is a certain state of the contiguous
vessels, which enables them to deposit,
in due proportion, the elements which
enter into the composition of each
structure. But to style this disposition
of the vessels an organ would be to
use the term in a new, and, as I conceive, a less correct mode than that
which is generally employed.

In concluding these remarks, I shall
again express my hope, that while I
venture to criticise any portion of
Liebig's Treatise, I do it from my
desire to remove even the smallest
imperfection from a work of so much
value, and by this means to contribute,
in some degree, to the advance of a
science in which I feel so deeply interested, and to which, for nearly half
a century, a considerable portion of my
time and attention has been devoted.

Upper Bedford Place,
   Feb. 1st, 1843.

MISCELLANEOUS

CONTRIBUTIONS TO PATHOLOGY AND THERAPEUTICS.

By JAMES RICHARD SMYTH, M.D.
London.

(For the Medical Gazette.)

---

*Rickets—Question of the ancient or
modern origin of the disease—Opinions of Glisson, Bate, some Italian
physicians, and others, on this point
—History, description, and morbid
appearances of the disease—Observations on the pulse and circulation.*

IT is the opinion of many that the
malady of rickets first made its appearance, as an evil of the human race,
in England, and that such took place
somewhere about two hundred years
ago. Glisson, Bate (physician to Charles
the First, to Cromwell, and to Charles
the Second), with six other eminent
physicians of the time, who joined observation and experience in investigation of the origin, nature, and treatment of this disease, coincided in opinion that it was a new distemper, and
not known to the earlier inhabitants of
this island, or of the Continent, or to
the Greeks or Romans. Glisson was
an able and learned physician, and
Regius Professor of Physic during
forty years at Cambridge University,
and might be considered well qualified to give an opinion on such a
statistical point in medicine. Boerhaave and Van Swieten also would
appear to favour the opinion of the
modern origin of rickets. Glisson is
the first, we believe, who has fully and
accurately written upon the disease;
and it is a little remarkable that its
name (of Greek derivation, from ραχις,
spine, or chine) was not the suggestion
of that author, but was the common
appellation by which the complaint
was known and spoken of at the time
he wrote his treatise upon it (Glisson,
De Rachitide, published about the middle of the seventeenth century.)

Not a few writers, with whom we
are much disposed to agree, are of opinion that the disease of rickets, in a
mild or aggravated form, existed at all
times, and was comprehended and recognised in the general morbid state
of cachexy. The following is a description of a morbid condition of a
boy, given by a physician of Bologna,

Johannes Baptista Theodosius, in 1354, a century before the rickets was noticed by any writer in this country; and if a similar case were to come under our observation to-morrow, we would have no hesitation in pronouncing it, with full confidence in the correctness of our diagnosis, to be rickets:—"Ejus temperamentum declinat ad frigidam et humidam, ex quo color totius pallidus redditur ita ut ad cachexiam tendere videatur, et multæ in eo cruditates generentur. Affectus est debilitas virtutis motivæ, ita ut, cum mensium jam septendecim sit, non possit nllo modo se movere, nec stare, et, cum in ulnis à nutrice defertur, vix caput potest erectum tenere. Symptoma aliud omnium sævissimum est vertebrarum trium in costis notis ad exteriora declinatio, et est modus gibbositatis, et in modum arcus costæ etiam incurvari videntur." "The temperature of him (the boy) declines to cold and humidity, by which the colour of all the skin is rendered pale, so that he seems inclined to a cachexy, and many crudities are engendered in him. The complaint is a weakness and inability to move, so that this child of seventeen months old can in no manner move itself or stand; and when it is carried in the nurse's arms, it can scarcely hold its head upright. Another symptom, the most cruel of all, is, that three of the vertebræ of the true ribs bend outwardly, and form a kind of hump-back, and the ribs appear to be arched in the manner of a bow."—(Theodosii, Epist. Medic. p. 250.)

The protuberance of the abdomen, and enlargement of the epiphyses of the joints, and irregular inordinate appetite and digestion, symptoms somewhat diagnostic of rickets, are not here mentioned; but there is little doubt that, with those which we find enumerated, these were also associated. A celebrated Italian physician, Zaviani, and some German and French writers of good authority, have argued for the antiquity of the existence of rickets. But if this disease and that of scrofula be of similar natures and kindred pathology, as we believe they are, the fact of the antiquity of the existence of the one, namely, of scrofula, and the opinion of the modern origin of the other, are somewhat contradictory and incongruous. Was not the "bottled spider," the "hunch-backed toad," Richard the Third, not the subject of rickets at birth and during infancy? There is little doubt, we think, that he was. The description of that monarch's person by our great dramatic poet, and the representation of it which we have seen by Kean, the present genius, is exactly that which those individuals generally present throughout adult life who have suffered from the malady of rickets in childhood :—

"But I, that am not shaped for sportive tricks,
Nor made to court an amorous looking-glass;
I, that am rudely stamp'd, and want love's majesty ;
          *   *   *
I, that am curtail'd of this fair proportion,
Cheated of feature by dissembling nature,
Deform'd, unfinish'd, sent before my time
Into this breathing world, scarce half made up,
And that so lamely and unfashionable
That dogs bark at me as I halt by them ;
Why I, in this weak piping time of peace,
Have no delight to pass away the time,
Unless to spy my shadow in the sun,
And descant on mine own deformity."

At the time that Glisson wrote his treatise upon rickets the distemper was frequent in London, and seemingly endemic in other parts of England, but more particularly in Somersetshire and Wiltshire. It was afterwards observed to prevail in Holland, France, and other parts of the continent, where it was commonly denominated the English disease (morbus Anglicus, maladie Anglaise, &c.)

Rickets has by some writers been divided into perfect and imperfect. From the enlarged state, and knobbed or knotted appearance of some of the joints, the Germans have designated the affection articuli duplicati, doubled joints; the French, enfans noués, knotted infants. When the disease comes upon a child after it has begun to walk, and while the epiphyses of the wrist and ankle bones are only observed to be increased in size, and the flesh generally some degrees softer than natural, and the little patient can still exercise the powers of locomotion, it is called imperfect rickets. When the malady is more severe, and the child cannot walk without falling, or is compelled to spend its time either creeping from place to place on its hands and knees, or sitting or lying, it is termed perfect rickets. The case of Kates, given in our last paper, is a good example, we consider, of perfect rickets. The time during which a child is most liable to be attacked by this deforming disease is from the commencement of dentition, or from the period at which that process of organic development usually makes its appearance above the gums; that is to say, the seventh month until the age of two years. After this epoch, the disease, it is true, may still invade the system of the child, but it is observed to be a circumstance of very rare occurrence. The adult individual is subject to, and sometimes labours under, an affection similar or analogous to that of rickets in the child, termed mollities ossium, or malacosteon; from μαλακος, soft, and οστεον, a bone.

The disease of rickets, as we have observed, most frequently attacks the infant about the time of teething; and the symptoms that characterize the indisposition which often accompanies that critical process are not unfrequently those which usher in this malady. The child, previously in good health and temper, is observed to droop and to be irritable, to be fretful and disinclined for the breast; its sleep is disquiet; the skin is hot and dry; the pulse is quick, but not strong; the bowels are disturbed; there is a slow continued fever present, that has a morning remission and evening exacerbation, which soon produces severe emaciation. After the continuance for some time of these more acute symptoms, the child becomes languid, solitary, and listless; its countenance is pale and dejected; the skin generally is pale and anæmatous; a remittent, slow, suppressed feverishness is still present, which would appear to be gastric, and to expend its forces chiefly internally; the appetite is abnormal and irregular, most frequently voracious; the functions of the bowels, and the entire operations of the digestive economy, are disordered and deranged; the alvine excretions are sometimes dark, but more frequently light-coloured, and altogether devoid of bile; the renal secretion is morbid, sometimes clear and rather copious, but most commonly turbid and scanty; the flesh becomes soft, and emaciation progresses. When the disease proves fatal the emaciation is extreme, with frequent diarrhœa and convulsions preceding dissolution. Occasionally, however, as we have witnessed in a few instances, there is little or no emaciation, but the flesh is exceedingly soft and flabby. The osseous system manifests signs of participation in the general disorder and error of assimilation; the bones soften, and bend in various

ways, and different deformities are produced. The spinal column exhibits curves posterior, anterior, and lateral. The posterior curve most frequently occurs in the upper dorsal vertebræ, forming the common deformity of hump-back; the anterior curve in the lumbar region, which has the effect of throwing the abdomen forward, and thereby causing progression to be unsteady and feeble. The clavicles become more bent, and of a sigmoid shape, which allows the shoulders to approximate, and the arms to press upon the sides of the chest, which is thereby flattened, the ribs becoming less convex, and the sternum more so, causing the chests of those individuals to resemble in some degree the breasts of birds; from which circumstance persons with such deformity, which generally continues through life, are usually said to be "pigeon" or "fowl-breasted." The pelvis also changes its form, by undergoing a sort of twist, and its antero-posterior diameter is diminished, which, in the female, frequently causes the process of parturition to be difficult, and sometimes impossible, without mechanical aid. The limbs, both upper and lower, become bowed forwards or outwards; most frequently the latter. Sometimes both lower limbs are bent in the same direction, as if the feet had been pressed against the ground at the same point, and the limbs bent by some external force, in a similar manner as one would bend a young green tree. Sometimes the knees come almost in contact, and the legs greatly diverge, placing the feet upon the ground much apart, like the extremities of an equal-sided cross. In some cases the entire skeleton is so variously curved and deformed, that it is futile to attempt, and impossible, indeed, to give, a correct description of it. The joints, particularly the knees, wrists, and ankles, become enlarged. This enlargement of the wrists and ankles, and general softness of the flesh which accompanies it, are often the first symptoms of rickets that attract the attention of the parents or medical attendant. The abdomen is protuberant; there is more or less enlargement of the liver; in some cases the increase in bulk of this viscus is very great, and can easily be felt by percussion, or pressure of the hand on the right hypochondriac region. The size of the head is increased, and the vertex becomes flattened from greater or less spreading of the bones of the cranium; in consequence, in a great measure, we consider, of the atonic relaxed state of their integuments, and of the absence of that brace and support which they receive from these when the system is in health and the soft parts in full tone. The anterior fontanelle and the sagittal sutures remain open. To this condition of the bones of the cranium dropsical effusion in the ventricles of the brain is frequently united. Dentition is generally delayed, and sometimes the teeth are deficient in number for life, and often they early become dark-coloured, and decay. The breath, too, is at times found to be exceedingly foetid: cases are mentioned by authors in which the breath was so foetid and deleterious as to destroy young birds exposed to its influence. The development of the mental faculties of ricketty children is irregular, and a thing of uncertainty: sometimes we find precocity of intellect, and premature quickness of the power of observation and remark; at other times just the reverse obtains — the intellectual faculties of the ricketty child are plunged in abstraction and stupor. A great many ricketty children are, in fact, more stupid than intelligent; and they all appear to be rather stunted and weak in their feelings and affections.

When the distemper of rickets comes upon a child after it has begun to walk, and is beyond a year old, it will be observed to be chronic, and slow in its progress; it steals upon the young sufferer insidiously. The child's habits and disposition are perceived to be changed; from having been an animated active child it has become dejected, and disinclined to exercise or motion of any sort; the countenance is pale; the eyes dull and decolourised; the skin generally pale, and diminished or irregular in temperature; the flesh soft; the knees and the extremities of the radius and ulna at the wrist, and also the tarsal extremities of the tibia and fibula, enlarged. The child, previously of pretty stout and active progression, now stands infirmly and walks slowly, waddling and tottering till it falls, if not supported. The abdomen is protuberant and more resisting than natural, and, on examination, the liver may be found in a greater or less de-gree increased in bulk; there is increased frequency of the pulse without any real disturbance or acceleration of the circulation;[*] the appetite is irregular, generally inordinate; the alvine and urinary excretions unhealthy; the former are deficient in bile, and occasionally exhibit appearances of blood. Such are the symptoms which, in the majority of cases, will be found to characterise the first stage of rickets when this affection invades the system of the child that has begun to exercise its power of locomotion and perhaps speech. The symptoms of the further progress of the malady are similar in all respects to those of the disease as it occurs in the infant of a few months old, which have been already described.

With regard to the prognosis in rickets, it may be stated that the earlier the disease makes its appearance in the system of the child, the greater is the difficulty of its cure, and the danger of its proving fatal. The older the child is before being attacked, the greater is the hope of its recovery from the malady. Few are attacked after five years of age, and the recoveries all, or the great majority of them, take place previous to this epoch.

Let us here quote a case of rickets as the disease exhibited itself in the system of a female infant, described in the Commentaries of Van Swieten, which must be considered instructive and worthy of note, as affording a good example of this malady in a state of great aggravation and severity, with its signs of amendment, and process and progress of recovery, and restoration to sound health. All diseases, observes Hippocrates, or some other ancient high authority, and the observation is founded in every-day fact, terminate in health, death, or transition to another affection: and if it be a matter of practical consideration and utility attentively to observe the gradual development of the signs of death or of morbid change, when a disease is about to terminate fatally, or to assume a new nature, it is certainly satisfactory, much more pleasing, and not less useful, to note the appearances of returning health, and mark the gradual manner in which the characters of disease thereupon become more faint, and finally erased. Speaking of this case, Van Swieten

* See paragraph at the end of this paper.

goes on to state—" She was born very healthy, and had so good a colour during the first months that every body hoped she would totally escape the calamities of her brothers : she was hardly a year old when she began to grow pale and ill; the abdomen swelled; the wrists, knees, and ankles, protu-berated ; the thorax was raised ; the ankles were incurvated ; the back-bone became crooked ; all the bones of the head were enlarged, as if they were affected with an exostosis ; the struc-ture of all the bones of the body was vitiated : she also laboured under a complication of diseases, the scurvy, dropsy, a bloody diarrhœa, a scarcity of urine, a fever, a violent cough, at-tended with vast anguish, and a dread of suffocation. She lived in this mise-rable condition for above two years. The same remedies (crocus martis et ens veneris — sulphate of iron and muriate of copper), which cured her brother, were applied to her during thirty months in vain, so that their application was almost given over, as there appeared no hopes of a cure from them; but the tender mother, un-willing to spare any pain or cost, the same method was still indefatigably persevered in. The anguish and cough began at length to diminish, and the fever ceased ; the flesh looked of a better colour ; the tumor of the abdo-men was diminished ; the incurvated spine grew straight; the joints protu-berated less; the elevated sternum grew flatter ; the arched figure of the clavi-cle decreased ; the bones of the head subsided : she first began to stand and then to walk ; at last no trace of so severe a disease remained, and she be-came equal in health and strength to other children of the same size. The muscular strength also began to be restored without the assistance of any artificial means ; and the bones reco-vered their due form, which had been so very imperfect during thirty months." (Van Sweiten's Commen-taries, Vol. 17, pp. 436 and 437.)

When rickets proves fatal, the ema-ciation is general and extreme. The subcutaneous cellular tissue has com-pletely disappeared ; the muscles are wasted, flabby, and decolourised; the deformed bones soft, and more cellular than natural, and deficient in their solidifying constituent of phosphate of lime. The deficiency in this distinc-tive osseous element has been found to amount to one half the quantity which usually goes to the composition of healthy-formed bone. The medullary matter in the cavities of the bones is sanguineous and jelly-like; and the entire substance of the bone is spongy and more vascular than ordinary. The bones of the cranium, besides being softer, are generally larger than natu-ral, and separated at their sutures, and the brain is frequently distended with dropsical effusion. The cerebral mass, as we have seen, appears large, and inclined to be pulpy. The abdomen is always increased in size, and its pa-rietes wasted and thin. The increase in the bulk of the abdomen is owing chiefly, according to the testimony of Glisson, Hoffman, and others, to greater or less enlargement of the liver. The spleen is occasionally found enlarged. The mesenteric glands are sometimes quite sound, and at other times they are observed to be increased in size. The pancreas and kidneys are pretty healthy, and so also are the stomach and intestines, except that these latter are frequently observed to be more distended than natural. The thymus gland is sometimes greatly enlarg-ed; we have seen it, in a boy be-tween eight and ten years of age, the subject of scrofula and rickets, pro-jecting fully three inches above the sternum, and pressing so upon the tra-chea as to cause severe dyspnœa. The heart and lungs are sometimes found diseased; the former enlarged or hy-pertrophied, the latter the nidus of tubercular deposit : but such condi-tions of these viscera are more adven-titious and accidental than properly included in the morbid appearances of rickets. The blood is in a dissolved watery condition, and deficient in all its higher constituents. The causes and treatment of rickets we shall take up in another contribution.

We will here take the opportunity of observing, that, in the examination of disease, there are few symptoms less fully to be relied on than those furnished by the morbid pulse, and it requires a clear comprehensive general knowledge of physiology, with much practical expe-rience, and close acquaintance with clini-cal pathology, viz. the live and active disease in the person of the patient, to ob-tain accurate and true information of the state of the system in many cases. The phenomena of the pulse, in the study and treatment of disease, are more serviceable to the physician in the matter of *prognosis* than of diagnosis, and in affording frequent useful delicate indications of the necessity for the administration of general therapeutic agents. Often, as may be observed, when the pulse is beating rapidly, and from this, with other relative symptoms, one might be led to infer that the circulation was in a state of hurry and acceleration, it is not so, but just the reverse obtains—the blood is moving slowly, while the heart and arteries, the containing vessels, are acting inordinately. Such discordance in the motion of the blood and its active circulatory apparatus constitutes a condition of disorder frequently met with of *false* excitement —*excitement with debility*. It is more hardness or resistance, we conceive, in the pulse, together with fulness, and not a high number of beats in a given time, which indicate and announce a rapid strong circulation. And the best ordinary method of nicely appreciating these qualities in the circulation is, when the fingers, in feeling the pulse, have remained for some time upon it, to slightly raise them and gently repress the vessel. In this way we have thought that the most accurate estimate and information of the strength and velocity of the current of the blood, and of the amount of *true* excitement of the circulation, is practically obtainable. It is only the pulse of real or true circulatory excitement that, for the most part, warrants *general* bloodletting: all others, with a few exceptions perhaps, forbid it. Notwithstanding the knowledge of the general circulation which has been obtained by the discovery of Harvey, there is still "ample space and room enough" in this department of physiology for further investigation. We believe there is still much to be learned respecting the ultimate distribution of the blood. The nutritive circulation of every organ, like the structure of the organ itself, we are much of opinion is more or less individual and particular; and the motion or movement of the blood in its most minute and vital diffusion through the tissues of the economy is a thing, like the shades and colour of a summer landscape, of the utmost variety. This, it is obvious, involves, in some degree, a practical point of

some importance, namely, the *duration* of disease, inflammatory in particular, as it occurs in the different parts and structures of the system. We have an unsettled opinion, too, that the motion of the blood in the child is considerably slower than in the adult, although its pulse is always much more frequent. The pulse of the child at birth is double that of the adult. In old age the pulse is always slower than in youth and early manhood, but in old age the pulse is slower also.

43, Sackville Street,
June 30, 1843.

ANALYSES AND NOTICES OF BOOKS.

"L'Auteur se tue à allonger ce que le lecteur se
tue à abréger."—D'ALEMBERT.

The Transactions of the Provincial Medical and Surgical Association. Vol. XI. London, 1843.

THE present volume consists of three parts :—

1. A retrospective address by Dr. Black of Manchester, which contains a lucid and interesting summary of all the important facts connected with medicine which had been recorded during the preceding year.

2. A paper on the medical topography of Sidmouth, including the geology, natural productions, and statistics of that district, from the pen of Mr. Jeffrey.

3. Essays and cases, illustrated with numerous engravings.

The first of these is, Experimental and practical inquiries into the structure and functions of the corpuscules of the blood—on inflammation—and on tubercles, by Mr. Addison, of Malvern. This is an interesting paper, but the details are so much connected with the engravings as to render it impossible to give any adequate account of them without the figures.

4. Some cases shewing the advantage of powerful counter-irritation, especially the long issue on the calvarium, by Dr. Wallis, physician to the Infirmary, Bristol.

The author states that he first became aware of the value of this remedy from Mr. R. Smith, the present senior surgeon of the Bristol Infirmary, and he has used it extensively since 1823, when he became physician to the establishment in question. The following is his account of it :—

"I have used this remedy in a great variety of cases of organic disease of the brain, both chronic and acute; in paralysis, impending effusions, convulsions, erysipelas of the head and membranes of the brain; in fever in the very advanced stages; in one case of hysteria, with very great advantage; and also in a case or two of mania. The general result of my experience of its use has been such as to confirm my favourable opinion of it, as being the most powerful and efficacious of all our remedies of the class of counter-irritants. Its effects are more permanent and its disadvantages are fewer than those of any other remedy now in use. The friends of the patient will occasionally object to it, from that misapplied feeling of affection which converts every energetic effort to save life, if the use of the scalpel be required, into an act of cruelty. This is an objection urged against many of our best, nay even our ordinary remedies, such as a blister or issue of the common kind. The resistance of the friends, however, is generally overcome by remarking quietly, that 'It is only intended to make an issue;' an insignificant trifle compared with the distressing effects of disease."

Mr. Smith does not, however, as a general rule, adopt this remedy at the first onset of disease, but keeps it in reserve until the ordinary remedies have been tried and found wanting. The circumstances necessary to attend to in carrying the remedy into effect are these :—

"Let the head be shaved entirely, and have the patient brought near to the right side of the bed ; raise the head by a hard pillow, and put a towel round his neck to receive the blood; let an assistant keep the head steady; at the same time draw the scalp downwards in all directions, so as to strain the calvarium as much as possible ; the scalp will divide with so much more ease. In this, your own left hand will materially assist, by placing it at the upper and back part of the head, commencing the incision between your thumb and fore-finger as far back as the lambdoidal suture; press the scalpel sufficiently down so as *to divide the scalp entirely through at once;* carry on the incision directly along the sagittal *suture as far as* the hair grows on the scalp, and which will cover the cicatrix after the issue is healed up. The length of the incision thus made will be in the adult about seven or eight inches; take care that the scalp be divided entirely and perfectly through, so that the edges of the incision will separate so far as to enable you to introduce a dossil of lint rolled up hard, as thick as two fingers, and which should be well soaked in spirit of turpentine; this answers the double purpose of increasing the effect of the incision, and makes suppuration come on earlier, and will usually assist in stopping a further loss of blood. The arteries very soon retract and cease to bleed; there is seldom more than six or eight ounces of blood lost, and this quantity may be very readily curtailed if it be desirable to do so.

"In those cases where depletion has been carried to a sufficient extent, prior to your determination to use this remedy, and the further loss of blood be unadvisable, it may be prevented in the following manner:—The instant the incision is completed, close the sides of the wound, and make pressure upon it with your hand, whilst your assistant hands the lint, well soaked in spirit of turpentine and rolled up firmly of a proper length, so as not to extend beyond the extreme length of the incision, as it would be inconvenient in strapping down the wound sufficiently to check the flow of blood ; a little flour and dry lint may be superadded if necessary, but the dossil must not be made so thick as to rise much above the edges of the wound, or else the adhesive straps will not be secure, by being elevated, and thereby prevented from adhering near the edges of the incision. Should the incision be imperfectly made, that is to say, not entirely through the scalp, the arteries might be only partially divided; in which case they will continue to bleed, notwithstanding the pressure you may have made: of course the arteries will require to be completely divided, to allow them to retract and cease to bleed."

Some good cases are given, in which the remedy proved of service in acute and chronic meningitis, apoplexy and paralysis, epilepsy, hydrocephalus, &c.

5. On the employment of extension in the treatment of fractures of the spine, by W. Hinchman Crowfoot, surgeon to the Dispensary, Beccles.

The case detailed is that of a coach-man, aged 42, in whom, from an external injury, the spinous processes of the ninth and tenth vertebræ were divided from each other considerably beyond their usual distance, the body of the ninth vertebra being forced forward, while that of the tenth projected backward. There was total deprivation of the power of voluntary motion and sensation in the lower extremities. A gradual but considerable extension was applied, and gentle attempts were made with the fingers to replace the bones. The deformity was in some measure removed by these means, but without the slightest return of voluntary power in the first instance. He was placed on his back on a firm bed, where he steadily improved, and at the end of three weeks could slightly move the great toe of the right foot ; in a few days more this extended to the left foot. The power of the limbs now progressively but slowly returned to such extent that he was able to resume his former occupations.

6. Case of paralysis of the serratus magnus, which caused the lower angles of the right and left scapulæ to become disengaged from the latissimus dorsi, &c. by John Banner, Esq. surgeon, Liverpool.

All the interesting points of this case are given in the "heading." The patient always had good health, and the affection was purely local ; nor is mention made of any attempt at relief.

7. Remarks on matico, a styptic much used in South America for suppression of hæmorrhage, by Thomas Jeffreys, M.D.

The matico may be used externally or internally. As a local application the under side answers best. Internally the decoction or infusion (ʒss. to ʒj. in the pint) may be given, in doses of an ounce and a half.

8. Anatomico-chirurgical observations on dislocation of the astragalus, by Thomas Turner, surgeon to the Manchester Infirmary, &c. &c.

This is an elaborate and valuable paper, but one, of which, dependent as it is on engravings, diagrams, and tables, we can give no adequate notion in any analysis. We shall not, therefore, attempt to do so, but content ourselves with subjoining a list of the dislocations described :—

1. Partial, direct, and simple.
2. ———————— and compound.
3. ———————— simple, and complicated.
4. ———————— compound, and complicated.
5. ——indirect, and simple.
6. ———————— and compound.
7. ———————— simple, and complicated.
8. ———————— compound, and complicated.
9. Complete, direct, and simple.
10. ———————— and compound.
11. ———————— simple, and complicated.
12. ———————— compound, and complicated.
13. ——— indirect, and simple.
14. ———————— and compound.
15. ———————— simple, and complicated.
19. ———————— compound, and complicated.

MEDICAL GAZETTE.

Friday, July 14, 1843.

" Licet omnibus, licet etiam mihi, dignitatem *Artis Medicæ* tueri; potestas modo veniendi in publicum sit, dicendi periculum non recuso."
CICERO.

EMPLOYMENT OF WOMEN AND CHILDREN IN HUSBANDRY.

THE report of Mr. Austin, on which we commented in our last number but one, gives a gloomy portraiture of compulsory apprenticeship, as it exists in many of our agricultural parishes. Yet, dark as the representation is, we fear that it is not overcharged. It is drawn from the concurrent testimony of witnesses in various grades of society ; and though their evidence is combated, as usual, by that of others, the probability is, unfortunately, on the unfavourable side. The state of these young husbandmen and women approaches so nearly to that of serfs, or even slaves, that it is difficult to doubt the existence of the evils which bondage always brings in its train.

"To be worse treated than a parish apprentice," says Mr. Bidwell, "is a proverb, and were not proverbs held to be founded in truth, I could support the verity of this in a variety of instances, of a *general* as well as particular character."

The system is as follows. At the age of nine, a boy is taken away from his parents, not to be restored to them during his minority. "Neither parents nor children are consulted," says Mr. Austin; "they are separated by an act of law, against which there is no appeal." This separation is continued for twelve long years, which must be sufficient, in a large number of cases, to produce the most complete estrangement between parent and child; as it is not to be supposed that in so poor a class apprentices and their parents can visit one another often enough to keep up the feelings of kindred in their original freshness. Indeed, mere distance would often make this impossible. The Stat. 56 Geo. III. which regulates apprenticeships, enacts that a child shall not be bound *more* than forty miles from its place of settlement! The apprentices are knocked about *ad libitum* by master, mistress, and all the other rulers who are put in authority over them; and though very gross cases may be carried before a magistrate, the remedy is obviously as bad as the disease. A household carried on by appeals to the 56 Geo. III. cap. 126, is in an unhappy condition. Sometimes, too, the master can make his apprentices very miserable, and yet keep within the limits of the law; at other times the apprentices are skilful in the art of worrying, and yet keep on the windy side of the 56 Geo. III.

Nor do the female apprentices escape the wild justice of the farm-house. Mary Puddicombe tells of her service at Blackiston, when no longer an apprentice; the servants used to beat *her, and her master to bang her till she* was black and blue. But "apprentices were treated worse : two, without fathers to look after them, were beat with a stick for anything that happened. One maiden had her arm cut to the bone with a stick the young master cut out of the hedge at the time, for not harrowing right, for not leaving enough for a harrow to go back again. That went to a justice : master was fined £5, and had to pay the doctor's bill. The £5 was given away in bread to the poor. The parish did not bind any apprentices after that."

It was a broad hint to leave off, truly! Mary Rendalls informs us that when apprenticed she had a bad mistress, who used to throw her on the ground, hold her by the ears, kneel on her, and use her very ill. The witness, now 41 years of age, has still the marks from kicks upon her. Mr. Lyddon, a surgeon, has often made inquiries into the condition of apprentices, and is inclined to think that at times corrections rather too severe are inflicted.

Mr. Troode, a farmer, had an apprentice, who did not go to church though sent, and was out late at night. Mr. Troode applied to a magistrate; the boy was sent to the tread-mill for a week, and whipped twice; "but that only made him worse than before; nothing hurts a boy like punishment of that kind." The witness adds, " I had another apprentice, a girl, who stayed out all night; nothing could be worse; Mrs. Troode scolded her, and the girl threw some potatoes at her; I came in at the moment and struck her with the horsewhip. The girl's parents applied to an attorney in Exeter, and the case was brought before magistrates; I was fined £1. Upon this I ordered all my apprentices out of the house, for I found I could not have the proper control over them."

Mr. Palk, a farmer, says, " we don't let our apprentices go home to see their parents; parents who have been apprenticed never like their children to run home much."

George Moxey, a labourer, says that when an apprentice, he was never beaten nor ill-used by his master, but that he was badly used by the other apprentices; "apprentices always beat each other, go wherever you will."

In fact, the apprentice, friendless and forlorn, is too often knocked about like the fag at a public school, but with a far longer period of slavery before him. He is among those that time lags withal, and few can feel more strongly the pungent truth of the couplet—

Slow as the year's dull circle seems to run,
When the brisk minor pants for twenty-one!

Nor are these poor drudges always consoled for their destiny on earth by the hope of a "bright reversion in the sky"; for "although they are sufficiently clothed for their work," says Mr. Austin, the reporter, "they sometimes have no better kind of clothing for the Sunday; and their masters are ashamed to let them appear at church in their ordinary dress of the week."

Indeed, one of the witnesses, the Rev. Peter Benson, affirms that the moral and religious instruction of a child commonly ceases almost entirely when he has been apprenticed. Farmers do not like to send ragged children to church; and "the rule is rags, the exception is the other way."

A master, of course, stands *in loco parentis* to his apprentice, and if habitual kindness were checkered by occasional severity there would be little or no reason to complain. But if his goodness always "wears the sterner face of love"; if authority scarcely ever melts into indulgence; if the only thing which the farmer can allege in his own favour is that his apprentices have a bellyful, can we wonder that discontent hardens into hatred, or that the despised serf grows up into the enemy

of the social frame which has crushed him?

It would be sad indeed were there no exceptions to this painful rule; we hope that there are many, and bright ones.

Mrs. Tuckett, of Dunsford, in Devonshire, who retains the farm which her husband occupied, draws a pleasing picture of the felicity of her family. Her house is conducted in the old-fashioned Devonshire way. Mistress, servants, and apprentices, mess together on the same provisions; nor are they kept under lock and key; everything is open. The apprentices have five days holiday in the year; three at Christmas, and two at Easter, and Mrs. Tuckett gives them little amusements then, and at other times. Their parents come to see them when they like, and there is always something to eat and a glass of cider for these visitors. The girls are never allowed to work in the fields, except occasionally at hay-time, and then they are kept "in a little set, away from the other people, not to hear their talk."

But Mrs. Tuckett, of whose intelligence and worth Mr. Austin speaks with due praise, is a rare exception; and we perfectly agree with the reporter that it will be well to discontinue agricultural apprenticeship for the future.

We cannot conclude this article without touching upon a point which is prominent in almost every page of the evidence; we mean the extreme privations and singular patience of our rural population. The stringent severity of the New Poor Law was built on the supposition that the poor spent their wages in luxury and dissipation, and that they ought to be compelled to save up money for old age by the prospective horrors of a Union workhouse. But, alas! the mass of evidence, unpicked and ungarbled, shows that the labourer's wages, in general, scarcely pass starvation point; and instead of the cruel mockery of requiring the husbandman to save something from nine shillings a week, we ought rather to remind the opulent that, in the words of Rousseau, the best medicines for the poor are to be found in the kitchens and cellars of the rich. Instead of constantly reproaching husbandmen, as a class, with their occasional errors, the impartial moralist, when he peruses

"The short and simple annals of the poor,"

will be rather inclined to admire their uncomplaining fortitude, and will admit that the heroism of private life is most often to be found in a station where we should have been least likely to look for it.

In the Report before us, Dr. Greenup, of Calne, after giving in detail the necessary expenses of a labourer's housekeeping, remarks, that when he reckons these things up, he is always more and more astonished how labourers continue to live at all. The diseases which he sees among the poor almost all arise from want of proper food and clothing. At Studley, in Wiltshire, it appears, from the evidence of Mr. Henry Phelps, agent to the Marquis of Lansdowne, that the women work in the fields like men. They are employed in reaping and binding corn in harvest, hay-making, hoeing turnips, weeding, picking stones, filling dung carts, &c. For this they get 8d. a day, or sometimes, at harvest, 10d.

Mr. Bowman, a farmer, and vice-chairman of the Board of Guardians of the Chalne Union, says that, in the great majority of cases, the labourer's family has only the man's wages, 8s. or 9s. a week, to live on. It is a mystery to Mr. Bowman how a man and wife, with five or six children, can live on this. We take it for granted, therefore, that the vice-chairman does

not think it just to punish the labourer in his old age for not having bought an annuity out of the abundant income of his greener years.

Mrs. Britton, the wife of a labourer, deposes that she has seven children, all boys, varying in age from fourteen years to nine months. One of the children is a cripple, and the Guardians allow two gallons of bread weekly for him; but, although her husband is a tea-totaller, the family has not even a sufficiency of bread to eat; and they all sleep in one room.

The next witness, Mrs. Sumbler, the wife of a labourer, gives an account of the unceasing toil in a dairy, having been herself employed in one for eight years before she married. "When cheeses are made twice a day, the work is never done; the work lasts all day, from three in the morning till nine at night."

Another witness, after giving the details of her spare housekeeping, adds, "we never know what it is to get enough to eat; at the end of the meal the children would always eat more. Of bread there is never enough; the children are always asking for more at every meal; I then say, 'you don't want your father to go to prison, do you?'"

It is almost needless to multiply these details of extreme penury. Mary Haynes, a widow of Calne, does men's work in the fields, and has not even a change of clothes. She receives 5s. a week in summer, and 4s. 6d. during the other months. Besides stone-picking, weeding, and hay-making, she reaps and hoes turnips, employments which some persons suppose to be confined to men alone.

"As for work," says another practical philosopher, speaking of the farm where he was apprenticed, "why, people must work, and there was plenty of that;"—the grievous point is, that the work should be so miserably paid.

In a word, the good humour with

which our labourers in husbandry bear toil rewarded by semi-starvation is worthy of all praise; and forms a singular contrast to the distorted ingenuity with which many of their superiors find subjects of annoyance and discontent in the midst of prosperity.

BRITISH MEDICAL ASSOCIATION.

Exeter Hall, July 4, 1843.

Dr. Webster, President, in the Chair.

Dr. Lander, of Sloane Street, Chelsea, was unanimously elected a member.

A discussion having taken place on the subject of Medical Reform, in consequence of the Council having learned that Sir James Graham was disposed to advise Her Majesty the Queen to grant Charters to both Colleges, which the Council believed would be highly injurious to the interests of the medical profession—

It was resolved, 1stly, That a Member be requested to inquire, in the House of Commons, if it be the intention of Government to grant Charters to the existing Colleges of Physicians and Surgeons; and that a communication be addressed, by the President, to the Secretary of State for the Home Department on the same subject.

2dly, That it is highly desirable that the profession, at this critical period, should forward to Her Majesty the Queen addresses, praying that she will be graciously pleased not to grant any Charters to either of the Colleges until the whole subject of Medical Reform shall have been duly considered in Parliament.

3dly, That the attention of the Medical Associations be specially called to the foregoing resolutions, and to the present peculiar state of medical affairs; and that copies of the resolutions be forwarded to the Secretaries of the different Associations.

In consequence of some communications relative to the late order of the Poor Law Commissioners,

It was resolved, that all those Medical Officers who may feel themselves aggrieved by the proceedings taken in connection with the late General Medical Order of the Poor Law Commissioners, be hereby invited to forward particulars of their cases to the Secretary of the British Medical Association, Exeter Hall, in order that active measures may be taken for the removal of the grievance.

The President, in the absence of the Secretary, announced that the Petitions agreed to at the last Half-yearly General meeting of the Association, praying for Medical Reform, and that no Charters should be granted at present to the two Colleges, had been duly presented—to Her Majesty by Sir James Graham; to the Lords by the Right Hon. Lord Campbell; and to the Commons by H. G. Ward, Esq. M.P.

The Meeting was then adjourned.

SOCIETY FOR RELIEF OF WIDOWS AND ORPHANS OF MEDICAL MEN

IN LONDON AND ITS VICINITY.

An Extraordinary General Court of this Society, numerously attended, was held on Wednesday last, at the Gray's Inn Coffee House. Dr. Mann Burrows, Vice-president, was called to the Chair, and briefly explained the object of the meeting, which was to elect H.R.H. the Duke of Cambridge as Patron of the Society. At the last Annual Dinner, His Royal Highness most graciously signified his willingness to accept the office, and from the interest which he has taken in its proceedings for some time past, it is probable that the patronage of His Royal Highness will be actively and beneficially exerted in furthering the very laudable objects of this society. It was announced that the publication of the Laws, List of Members, &c. would be delayed for a few days.

VARIETIES OF SUGAR.

1. *Purified or Refined Sugar.*—This is met with in the shops either in conical loaves (*Loaf Sugar*), or truncated cones called lumps (*Lump Sugar*), of various sizes and degrees of purity. Small lumps are called *Titlers*. The finest refined sugar is perfectly white, and is termed *double refined;* the inferior kind has a slightly yellowish tint, and is called *single refined*. Both varieties are compact, porous, friable, and made up of small crystalline grains.

2. *Brown Sugar* occurs in commerce in the form of a coarse powder, composed of shining crystalline grains. It is more or less damp and sticky, and has a peculiar smell and a very sweet taste. Its colour is brownish yellow, but varies considerably in intensity. *Muscovado* or *raw sugar*, sometimes termed *Foot Sugar*, has the deepest colour, and is intermixed with lumps. *Bastard* is a finer kind prepared from molasses, and the green syrups.

Raw sugar contains several impurities from which it may be freed by the process of refining. Its colour is owing to the presence of *Uncrystallisable sugar* (treacle). In an aqueous solution of raw sugar *lime* is detected by oxalic acid. By keeping, it is well known that a strong raw sugar becomes weak, that is, soft, clammy, and gummy. This change Professor Daniell ascribes to the action of the lime. *Sub-phosphate of lime* is another constituent of raw sugar. *Glutinous* and *gummy matters*, and traces of *tannic acid*, are also present in raw sugar. The *crystal sugar* brought from Demerara (and St. Vincent's?) is the finest and purest kind of the coloured sugars which are imported. Its colour is pale yellow, and its crystals are larger and more brilliant than the preceding varieties. It is used for sweetening coffee. On account of the before-mentioned impurities, unrefined sugar is an improper article of diet for those afflicted with calculous disorders.

3. *Sugar Candy.*—This is crystallised cane-sugar. It is prepared from concentrated syrup. The crystals deposit themselves, as the liquid cools, on the sides of the vessel and on strings stretched across. The form of the crystals is an oblique rhombic prism. Three kinds of candy are sold— the *white*, the *brown*, and the *pink*. Powdered candy is used to sweeten coffee.

4. *Aqueous Solutions of Sugar.*—Sugar *water* is frequently used at the table on the continent. *Syrup* is prepared by dissolving two pounds and a half of sugar in a wine-pint of water, by the aid of a gentle heat. If necessary, it may be clarified by white of egg. It is used for sweetening.

5. *Boiled Sugars.*—If a small quantity of water be added to sugar, the mixture heated till the sugar dissolves, and the solution boiled to drive off part of the water, the tendency of the sugar to crystallise is diminished, or, in some cases, totally destroyed. To promote this effect, confectioners sometimes add a small portion of cream of tartar to the solution while boiling. Sugar, thus altered by heat, and sometimes variously flavoured, constitutes several preparations sold by the confectioner. *Barley Sugar* and *Acidulated Drops* are prepared in this way from white sugar ;—powdered tartaric acid being added to the sugar while soft, when the drops are prepared. *Hardbake* and *Toffee* are made by a similar process from brown sugar. Toffee differs from Hardbake in containing butter. The ornamental sugar-pieces or *caramel*-tops with which pastry-cooks decorate their tarts, &c. are prepared in the same way. If the boiled and yet soft sugar be rapidly and repeatedly extended, and pulled over a hook, it becomes opaque and white, and then constitutes *Pulled Sugar* or *Penides*. Pulled sugar, variously flavoured and coloured, is sold in several forms by the preparers of hard confectionary.

6. *Molasses and Treacle.*—The brown, saccharine, viscid fluid, which drains from raw sugar when placed in hogsheads, is called *Molasses*, and is used in the preparation of brown sugar. It is imported from the West Indies in casks. Closely allied to this is *Treacle*—a viscid, dark-brown, un-crystallisable syrup, which drains from the moulds in which refined sugar concretes. These liquids result from an alteration effected in crystallisable sugar, and do not exist in the sugar cane. Both of them contain free acid.

7. *Burnt Sugar.*—When sufficiently heated, sugar becomes brown, evolves a remarkable odour, loses its sweet taste, and acquires bitterness : in this state it is called *Caramel* or *Burnt Sugar*, and is sold, when dissolved in water, as a colouring matter, under the name of *Essentia Bina* or *Browning*. It is used to colour soups and sauces. The high coloured brandies and dark brown sherries are said sometimes to owe part of their colour to this liquor. The brewer, it is reported, occasionally makes use of it to colour his beer.

8. *Hard Confectionary.*—Sugar constitutes the base of an almost innumerable variety of hard confectionary, sold under the names of *Lozenges, Brilliants, Pipe, Rock, Comfits, Nonpareils*, &c. Besides sugar, these preparations contain some flavouring ingredient, often flour and gum, to give them cohesiveness, and frequently colouring matter. Caraway fruits, almonds, and pine seeds, constitute the nuclei of some of these preparations.

9. *Liquorice Sugar.*—An aqueous extract of the root of liquorice (*Glycyrrhiza*) is extensively imported under the names of *Liquorice Juice*, or, according to the countries from which it is brought, of *Spanish* or *Italian Juice*. *Solazzi Juice* is most esteemed. The Spanish extract is prepared in Catalonia, from the common liquorice plant (*Glycyrrhiza glabra*), but the Italian extract, obtained in Calabria, is procured from *G. echinata*. Extract of liquorice is imported in cylindrical or flattened rolls, of five or six inches long, and about one inch in diameter, enveloped in bay-leaves. Its principal constituent is *Glycyrrhizin*, or *Liquorice Sugar*, mixed with some foreign matters. If the foreign extract be dissolved in water, and the solution filtered and evaporated, we obtain *Refined Liquorice*, but the *Pipe Refined Liquorice* of the shops is a very adulterated article. The *Pontefract Lozenges* are made of refined liquorice, and are much esteemed. The *Liquorice Lozenges* are officinal in the Edinburgh Pharmacopœia, and are directed to be prepared of extract of liquorice, gum, and sugar. There is also another liquorice lozenge sold in the shops, under the name of *Quintessence of Liquorice*. Extract of liquorice is used as a flavouring ingredient. Slowly dissolved in the mouth, it is taken to appease tickling cough, and to allay irritation of the fauces.

10. *Preserves, &c.*—In addition to its dietetical and condimentary uses, sugar is extensively employed, in domestic economy,

as an antiseptic; that is, to prevent the decomposition or putrefaction of organic substances. A variety of fruits, as well as some roots, stems, and even leaves, are in this way preserved, some in the moist state (as *Fruits in Syrup*, and *Preserved Ginger*) others in the dry state (as *Candied Angelica*, *Candied Citron*, *Orange, and Lemon Peels*, and *Crystallised Fruits*). In these cases sugar acts by excluding air, or by absorbing moisture, or in both of these ways. In some instances, perhaps, its efficacy may be of another kind, as when it promotes the solidification of vegetable jelly. " Latterly," says Berzelius, " sugar has begun to be more generally employed than formerly for the preservation of meat, in consequence of a much smaller quantity of it being required for preventing putrefaction, than of salt, while it renders the meat neither less savoury nor less nutritive. Fish, when gutted, may be equally well preserved by spreading powdered sugar inside them."—*Dr. Pereira, On Food and Diet*.

NEW TEST FOR ARSENIC.

The one-hundred-and-forty-fourth part of a grain of arsenious acid was mixed with two fluid drachms of milk. The mixture was boiled with a few drops of muriatic acid, and a slip of copper was introduced. In less than a minute the metal was coated with a grey film of metallic arsenic. Several pieces were thus coated; they were washed in water, dried in the heated current of air over a spirit lamp-flame, and introduced into a small reduction tube. On applying a gentle heat to the copper, octohedral crystals were obtained; visible to the eye in the light of the sun, but plainly distinguishable with a lens of low power. The crystals dissolved in water gave the usual reactions with the ammonio-nitrate of silver and sulphuretted hydrogen gas. In a second experiment, the same quantity of arsenic was mixed with two drachms of porter; in a third, a like quantity with two drachms of gruel, and the copper test was applied with similar satisfactory results. Each experiment was completed in about five minutes. Brandy, containing a poisonous impregnation of arsenic, was then tested; and the arsenic readily separated. A few drops taken from a bottle of port wine, containing arsenic, and which had nearly caused the death of three persons about four years ago, were next submitted to the test, and the metal readily obtained. In organic solids the results were equally striking : a few grains of a cake containing arsenic, which had been used in an attempt to poison, were boiled in a small quantity of distilled water, and muriatic acid and copper added, when metallic arsenic was immediately precipitated. The contents of the stomach of a person who was poisoned by arsenic in February, 1834, which had been loosely exposed, and allowed to become decomposed during a period of upwards of nine years, were next examined. A few drops of the thick turbid liquid were placed in a tube and boiled with dilute muriatic acid and water; the copper introduced was covered with a bright layer of metallic arsenic. The contents of three other stomachs taken from persons who were poisoned by arsenic in 1835, 1838, and 1840, gave precisely similar results. In the last case, the whole of the contents, with the food at the time contained in the organ, had been evaporated to a dry solid mass; a few grains of this were sufficient to furnish a clear demonstration of the presence of arsenic by the aid of the test. In the conversion of the metal to arsenious acid, it will at once suggest itself that if octohedral crystals should not be obtained by heating one portion of copper, several slips should be introduced together or separately. In all these cases arsenic will have been discovered by the application of Marsh's test, or sulphuretted hydrogen gas ; but the process would have occupied a much longer time, and with regard to Marsh's test the metallic arsenic could not have been so speedily converted to arsenious acid in a form convenient for the identification of its properties.

Another useful application of the copper test may be made in the following way. If the arsenic have been thrown down from an organic liquid in the form of impure sesquisulphuret, this may be dried and deflagrated with nitre, or decomposd by nitro-muriatic acid, whereby arseniate of potash or arsenic acid will result, and the organic matter will be entirely decomposed. In the case of deflagration by nitre, the surplus nitric acid should be expelled by sulphuric acid, and the arseniate dissolved out of the residue ; or if nitro-muriatic acid be used, the liquid may be evaporated to dryness. On boiling either of these products with copper and muriatic acid, the metallic arsenic will be readily procured.—*Mr. Taylor, in British and Foreign Review*.

EMPLASTRUM CERATI SAPONIS.

Although this plaster has for many years been extensively sold, spread on linen or calico, we have not seen any published formula for it, and the soap cerate being too soft for use as a plaster, several correspondents have inquired how they should proceed when emplastrum cerati saponis is ordered in a prescription.

The addition of one part of ceratum saponis to two parts of emplastrum plumbi, forms a plaster which, on an emergency, might be used in such a case, the article in question not being a preparation of the Pharmacopœia. But the most legitimate mode of reducing the cerate to the form of a plaster is to continue the evaporation until all the vinegar is expelled. This method is adopted at the Army Laboratory, where the plaster is kept, not only spread as usual, but also in rolls like other plasters.

The following is the formula used at the Army Laboratory:—

Common vinegar (No. 24) . 8 gallons, old measure.
White Castile soap. . . 16lb.
Yellow wax. . . . 20lb.
Olive oil. . . . . 32lb.
Litharge. . . . . 32lb.

Boil the litharge with the vinegar almost to dryness; remove from the fire and add the soap, previously scraped or cut; replace on the fire, taking care to avoid empyreuma; then add the wax and oil, melted and strained, and continue the evaporation, stirring constantly until the whole of the vinegar is expelled. The time required for completing the above quantity is three or four days.

The original recipe directed eight gallons of the residuum of distilled vinegar to be used instead of twenty-four gallons of common vinegar. The plaster thus prepared has a dark brown colour; but when the vinegar is used and the plaster has been carefully made, its colour is not much darker than than that of adhesive plaster. The emplastrum cerati saponis extensum, as usually sold, is coloured artificially with burnt sugar.—*Pharmaceutical Journal.*

BOOKS RECEIVED FOR REVIEW.

Facts and Observations relating to the Administration of Medical Relief to the Sick Poor in England and Wales.

Dr. H. Johnson on the Arrangement and Nomenclature of Mental Disorders.

Sir A. M. Downie, M.D. on the Iodated Waters of Heilbrunn in Bavaria.

ROYAL COLLEGE OF SURGEONS.

LIST OF GENTLEMEN ADMITTED MEMBERS.

Friday, July 7, 1843.

S. B. Denton.—L. M. Goddard.—T. Hunter.— J. Fixott.—G. Hammond.—R. Culling —W. H. Hire.—W. Atkin.—E. C. Gibson.—J. P. Symes. —J. F. Grace.—J. Robertson.

APOTHECARIES' HALL.

LIST OF GENTLEMEN WHO HAVE RECEIVED CERTIFICATES.

Thursday, July 6, 1843.

W. N. Spong, Mill Hall, Kent.—A. Sarjeant.— E. Q. M'Illree.—J. Portgate, Scarborough.—J. U. Kasson, London.

A TABLE OF MORTALITY FOR THE METROPOLIS,

Shewing the number of deaths from all causes registered in the week ending Saturday, July 1, 1843.

Small Pox	4
Measles	23
Scarlatina	23
Hooping Cough	52
Croup	5
Thrush	6
Diarrhœa	6
Dysentery	0
Cholera	1
Influenza	3
Ague	0
Typhus	35
Erysipelas	2
Syphilis	1
Hydrophobia	0
Diseases of the Brain, Nerves, and Senses	146
Diseases of the Lungs and other Organs of Respiration	237
Diseases of the Heart and Blood-vessels	22
Diseases of the Stomach, Liver, and other Organs of Digestion	65
Diseases of the Kidneys, &c.	10
Childbed	4
Paramenia	0
Ovarian Dropsy	1
Disease of Uterus, &c.	1
Rheumatism	1
Diseases of Joints, &c.	4
Carbuncle	0
Ulcer	0
Fistula	0
Diseases of Skin, &c.	2
Dropsy, Cancer, and other Diseases of Uncertain Seat	97
Old Age or Natural Decay	54
Deaths by Violence, Privation, or Intemperance	20
Causes not specified	6
Deaths from all Causes	848

METEOROLOGICAL JOURNAL.

Kept at EDMONTON, *Latitude* 51° 37' 32"N. *Longitude* 0° 3' 51" W. *of Greenwich.*

June 1843.	THERMOMETER.		BAROMETER.	
Wednesday 28	from 45 to 62		59·65 to	29·61
Thursday . 29	41	63	29·78	29·71
Friday . . 30	48	63	29·85	29·83
July.				
Saturday . 1	50	72	29·96	29·91
Sunday . . 2	53	71	29·95	29·92
Monday . . 3	59	71	29·94	Stat.
Tuesday . 4	57	71	29·94	29·96
Wednesday 5	from 55 to 83		29·71 to	29·68
Thursday . 6	53	70	29·81	29·74
Friday . . 7	50	59	29·91	29·98
Saturday . 8	52	60	29·86	29·84
Sunday . . 9	46	71	29·91	Stat.
Monday . . 10	47	68	29·96	29·94
Tuesday . . 11	44	67	29·99	30·11

Wind, N. on the 28th; N.W. on the 29th; S W. from the 30th ult. to the 7th instant; since N. and N.E.

Except the 7th and 8th, when some rain fell, generally clear.

Rain fallen, ·555 of an inch.

CHARLES HENRY ADAMS.

THE

LONDON MEDICAL GAZETTE,

BEING A

WEEKLY JOURNAL

OF

Medicine and the Collateral Sciences.

FRIDAY, JULY 21, 1843.

LECTURES

ON THE

THEORY AND PRACTICE OF MIDWIFERY,

Delivered in the Theatre of St. George's Hospital,

BY ROBERT LEE, M.D. F.R.S.

LECTURE XXXV.

On labours complicated with uterine hæmorrhage after the delivery of the child and retention of the placenta.

SINCE the last lecture, a case of uterine hæmorrhage in the ninth month of pregnancy, occasioned by detachment of the placenta from the superior part of the uterus, which had nearly proved fatal, has occurred to me in private practice. At nine in the morning, a lady, without having been exposed to any accident, or experiencing any uneasy sensation in the region of the uterus, was suddenly alarmed with a gush of blood from the vagina. I saw her soon after, when an oozing of blood continued, but there was no faintness, feebleness of the pulse, or change in the countenance, and no symptoms of labour. The os uteri was so high up, directed so much backward, and so closed, that I could not ascertain by the usual examination whether or not the placenta was presenting. As the operation of turning was impossible, cold applications were made to the parts, an opiate was given to prevent uterine contractions, and the patient kept in the horizontal position in a cool atmosphere. The blood, however, continued to flow, and slight pains, with great faintness and sickness, commenced in four hours. The os uteri was then felt dilated to the size of half-a-crown, and no part of the placenta presenting; the smooth membranes covered the whole cervix uteri. I immediately ruptured them, and held up the head that the liquor amnii might escape, applied a binder firmly around the abdomen, and gave some brandy and water. The pains became more frequent, the hæmorrhage ceased, and by compressing the fundus uteri, and gently dilating the orifice, though the faintness became more distressing, the child was expelled dead in about two hours, and no hæmorrhage followed. The placenta was found lying loose in the vagina, and on tightening the binder, and removing the after-birth, masses of dark-coloured coagulated blood escaped in such quantity as nearly to fill a wash-hand basin. There had been an internal hæmorrhage going on from the first attack of flooding, and though no discharge took place after the expulsion of these coagula, the patient remained for several hours in a state of the most dangerous exhaustion, with a pulse scarcely to be felt at the wrist, occasional complete loss of consciousness, restlessness, and severe attacks of retching and vomiting. These symptoms, however, gradually subsided, after the exhibition of a large opiate, and she is now recovering in the most favourable manner. In this case the operation of turning, which I am certain could not have been performed without the employment of great force, would have been attended with fatal consequences. The plug, as recommended by Dr. Burns, could have had no effect here in restraining the hæmorrhage which was going on within the uterus, and had nearly destroyed the patient; it could not have checked the flooding until the "os uteri was in a proper state for delivery," as he asserts. Had it been possible, at the commencement of the attack, to have ascertained with certainty whether or not the placenta presented, it would have been better practice then to have ruptured the membranes than delayed doing so for some hours, as it was evident from the first that there could be no safety till the delivery was completed.

2 P

On uterine hæmorrhage between the de-
livery of the child and expulsion of the
placenta.

Flooding sometimes occurs in the most
dangerous form, immediately after the birth
of the child, where the previous stages of
labour have been managed in the most judicious manner—where every thing has been
done to quiet the action of the heart and
arteries; the apartment kept cool; stimulants avoided; voluntary efforts to expel the
child discouraged; the binder applied and
tightened in the progress of the two first
stages of labour,—in a word, where every
thing that is possible has been done to prevent the uterus from being suddenly emptied of
its contents, and afterwards from contracting
in an irregular manner. In some women, in
spite of all our care and precautions, a profuse discharge of blood immediately succeeds
the delivery of the child, and they would
soon die if we did not interfere; and before
the placenta was expelled. A large stream
of blood flows from the vagina, which collects
in handfuls around the nates, thighs, and
body of the patient, so that she is literally
deluged with it, and soon begins to suffer
the usual effects of sudden and great loss of
blood. In other cases, a frightful rush of
fluid blood, a perfect torrent, issues from the
uterus after the birth of the child; the patient becomes in a very short space of time
not merely faint, but perfectly unconscious
of every thing that is going on around her;
she neither sees nor hears any thing. Some
women suffer repeatedly from attacks of this
description, and those are peculiarly exposed who have been exhausted by very
protracted labour. In many other cases the
discharge of blood from the uterus after
the birth of the child is gradual, in much
smaller quantity, and attended with comparatively little danger.

I believe there is no difference of opinion
respecting the method of treatment which
ought to be adopted in these cases. As the
placenta is wholly or partially detached
from the uterus, and prevents its regular
contraction, and the coagulation of the blood,
in the exposed vessels like a foreign body,
the placenta must be extracted artificially
without delay, and compression of the fundus
uteri and all other means actively employed,
to cause the uterus to contract in a regular
and permanent manner. The principles
which ought to guide you here are perfectly
obvious; but if you are frightened at the
suddenness of the accident, and the appalling
loss of blood, you may hesitate to pass
up the hand into the uterus, and try by
pulling upon the funis to bring away the
placenta. If you do so, the uterus may be
inverted, or, what is much more probable,
the cord will be broken off close to the
placenta, and it will be left behind, and the

hæmorrhage will probably continue till the
woman dies, or you procure the assistance of
some one properly prepared to act in such a
case. Where uterine hæmorrhage takes
place to any considerable extent after the
birth of the child, apply the binder firmly
around the abdomen, with a pad of folded
napkins under it over the fundus uteri, and
proceed immediately to extract the placenta.
Take off your coat, put the cord upon the
stretch with your left hand, and pass up the
right hand along it into the uterus, dilating
the cervix if it is contracted, expanding the
fingers to the circumference of the placenta,
and pressing the portion of the mass firmly
from the inner surface of the uterus, which
adheres to it, and extracting it slowly. The
placenta in most of these cases is partially
adherent to the uterus, when it requires to
be extracted, and you must take care to
separate this portion cautiously with the
fingers, before attempting to remove the
whole placenta from the uterus. If you
grasp with the hand the detached portion,
and draw it away, the adherent part will be
left behind, and the patient will probably
afterwards be destroyed by hæmorrhage, or
putrefaction of the portion retained. It is
not requisite to pass the points of the fingers
between the adherent portion of placenta
and lining membrane of the uterus, or expose this to be torn, but to press off this
portion of the placenta from it with the
points of the fingers, as you would a sponge
adhering to a rock, which you do not require
to touch. No man is thoroughly prepared
to undertake the charge of a common
midwifery case, who would hesitate to pass
up his hand into the uterus and remove the
placenta, whether adherent or detached, if
dangerous hæmorrhage occurred in the
interval between the second and third stages
of labour. If you allow any woman to die
from hæmorrhage at this time without removing the placenta, you will justly be considered incompetent to discharge the duties
of an accoucheur, and severely censured.

Sixty-four cases of hæmorrhage between
the birth of the child and expulsion of the
after-birth occurred in the Dublin Lying-in
Hospital during the residence of Dr. Collins;
in six of the 64 the hæmorrhage continued
after the removal of the placenta. In 45,
the hæmorrhage was slight, at least not
alarming; and in the remaining 19 it was
severe. In 17 of the 64, assistance became
necessary in the course of the first 15
minutes after the birth of the child; in 3 in
20; in 6 in 30; and in 7 in 45 minutes;
in 12 in 1 hour; in 7 in 1½ hour; and in 8
in 2 hours. In 4 cases the time is not noted.
In 13 of the 64 cases, the placenta, on the
introduction of the hand, was found firmly
adherent; in 8 cases the hour-glass, or
irregular, contraction was present, and in 43

cases its removal was easily effected. Five of the 64 were premature labours; viz. one at the fifth month; three at the seventh; and one at the eighth month. Seven of the 64 women died; two only from the effects of the hæmorrhage; of the other five two died of puerperal fever; one of extensive disease of the vagina with laceration; one of inflammation of the uterus; and one chiefly of disease of the lungs.

At present I am unable to state the exact number of cases of this variety of uterine hæmorrhage which I have seen, or present you with a tabular view of them, and the results.

On uterine hæmorrhage after the expulsion or extraction of the placenta.

But one of the most dangerous varieties of uterine hæmorrhage is that which follows the natural expulsion of the placenta, or its removal from the uterus by art. Sometimes the blood escapes in great quantities from the uterus immediately after the removal of the placenta, and the pulse ceases at the wrist, and consciousness is entirely lost in a few seconds. There is no symptom before labour has commenced, or during its progress, to warn you of what is about to take place. The child has been safely delivered, the placenta has come away in a short time, and while you are perhaps congratulating yourself on the happy termination of the labour, the blood begins to trickle over the bed upon the floor, or the patient suddenly complains of great faintness. In such cases there may be either a want of uterine contraction, or the contractions may not be permanent, but be followed by relaxation and the effusion of a large quantity of blood, which may either appear externally, or remain to become coagulated, and distend the uterus. For several hours after delivery, in some cases, this alternate relaxation and contraction goes on, to the great hazard of the patient, and if her condition be not clearly ascertained, and the proper remedies be employed, death may unexpectedly take place.

By far the most important remedies in these cases of uterine hæmorrhage are constant and powerful pressure over the fundus uteri, the application of cold around the pelvis, and the free administration of wine, brandy, and other stimulants: ergot is indicated, but it most frequently produces no effect. The pressure and cold are always within our reach, however sudden the attack may be. The hypogastrium should be strongly compressed with the binder, and a pad of folded napkins placed under it, and in addition the hand should be firmly applied over the fundus uteri. I do not know who it was that first employed compression of the fundus uteri in cases of flooding after the birth of the child; but it has been often

recommended, and there are now few practitioners in this country who are not fully aware of the importance of the binder and pad, in exciting permanent and regular uterine contractions. Dr. M'Keevor states, that in 1815 it was recommended by Dr. Labatt in his lectures, and for a number of years before this Dr. Labatt was accustomed to recommend a thick firm pad, or compress, over the pubes previous to the application of the ordinary binder, where in former labours uterine hæmorrhage had taken place. Dr. M'Keevor states, that of 6665 women delivered during the years 1819 and 1820, only 25 were attacked with hæmorrhage after the birth of the child. Of these, 15 occurred before the expulsion of the placenta, ten afterwards, and in all the result was favourable. He saw only two fatal cases during the time he was in the Dublin Lying-in Hospital, and he attributes this small mortality to the entire process of parturition being understood; to the unassisted gradual efforts of the uterus; partly to the patients having been kept cool and quiet, free from all sources of disturbance and irritation; but, above all, to the careful application of the binder immediately after delivery, by which means the expulsion of the placenta, and the permanent contractions of the uterus, are most effectually secured, and whenever any tendency to hæmorrhage did occur before the removal of the placenta the first point invariably attended to was to tighten the binder, and in the event of this not succeeding, a thick firm compress, made by folding a couple of large coarse napkins into a square form, was placed over the region of the uterus, and the binder again adjusted. In the great majority of instances, these, with the admission of cool air, checked the discharge; if not sufficient, additional pressure was made with the hands.

At the same time that you efficiently compress the fundus uteri with the binder and pad, cold should be vigorously applied to excite the contractions of the uterus. The best mode of doing this is to plunge a large napkin in a pitcher of cold water, and dash it suddenly against the external parts, the nates and thighs; and this should be repeated till the uterus contracts and the violence of the hæmorrhage is controlled. I am satisfied that this is the most efficacious method of applying cold to excite uterine contractions; it is far less formidable than pouring water from a height over the naked abdomen, but it is not less efficacious, and it possesses these decided advantages over the other method, that while the application is made to the external parts, nates and thighs, the pressure of the binder and pad is not withdrawn from the hypogastrium, the position of the patient is not changed from the side to the back, the bed is not inundated with water, and the application can be repeated as often, and continued as long, as the urgency of the symptoms may require. The abdomen may be exposed once, and cold water poured over it from a height, and the uterus made to contract, and the flow of blood be arrested for a time, but relaxation of the uterus may follow after a short interval, and the hæmorrhage be renewed again with equal violence as at first, but we cannot with propriety expose the abdomen a second time, and empty over it from a height the contents of a great decanter or kettle. Besides, by adopting this practice, we sacrifice the whole of the effects derived from pressure on the fundus uteri. The application of a napkin soaked in vinegar and water to the parts is often sufficient, along with the binder, to restrain the hæmorrhage where it is not very profuse.

I have very seldom introduced a plug of any kind into the vagina in these cases, but when there has been a draining of blood from the uterus, after the practice now described has been employed, a large soft sponge passed into the vagina, and pressed up against the os uteri, has appeared in some cases to promote the coagulation of the blood. The sponge, however, cannot be employed with safety after the expulsion of the child and placenta, unless the uterus be firmly compressed above the brim of the pelvis to prevent its becoming distended with blood. More frequently I have had recourse, with good effect, to the introduction of several pieces of smooth ice into the upper part of the vagina, and allowing them to remain here, in contact with the osuteri, and be dissolved—or pieces of ice have been inclosed in a bladder and laid over the pubes.

Other means besides those now described have been recommended in cases of flooding after the expulsion of the placenta. It has been proposed to inject cold water into the cavity of the uterus by means of the stomach-pump, and favourable reports have been given of the practice. The effect, I think, would be similar to directing forcibly a stream of cold water against a stump soon after amputation; the coagulum in the cavity of the uterus and in the orifices of the vessels would be all washed away: nevertheless, it might perhaps be advantageous in some desperate cases. Port wine and water as cold as possible, Dr. Collins says, injected into the rectum, has been of service. Some of the earlier writers on midwifery, and many in the present century, have strongly recommended the introduction of the hand within the uterus for the purpose of removing the coagula accumulated within the cavity, and to excite the uterus to contract. But it is not necessary to pass the hand into the uterus *for* the removal of coagula, because if the *binder has been properly* applied, and strong *pressure made over the fundus uteri*, clots

cannot accumulate within the uterus, and if they have been permitted to collect in consequence of neglect, then expulsion will immediately follow the use of proper compression of the hypogastrium, without the introduction of the hand. Nor do I consider it necessary, to excite uterine contractions, that the hand should ever be introduced into the cavity of the uterus after the removal of the placenta. I am fully convinced, from repeated observation, that this practice, which is so common as to be almost universal in this country at the present time, is often not only ineffectual for the purpose, in the worst cases of flooding, but that it is often followed by the most pernicious effects; the coagula which nature has formed have been displaced by the hand, and the uterus has not been excited by the stimulus of it to secure a permanent contraction. In the greater number of fatal cases of uterine hæmorrhage after the expulsion of the placenta which have come under my observation, the hand had been introduced into the cavity, and the closed fist had been pressed for a longer or shorter time round and round against the lining membrane, to make the uterus contract. I do not recollect a single fatal case, where the unfortunate result could be fairly attributed to the want of the introduction of the hand into the cavity of the uterus, and the friction of the knuckles against the lining membrane. I have repeatedly passed the hand into the uterus to produce contraction, but it has refused to obey the stimulus of the hand; it has remained like a soft flaccid bag, more like a piece of intestine than uterus, and the blood has continued to pour down the arm, until the hand has been withdrawn, and more efficient remedies employed. Leroux was well aware that the stimulus of the hand would not in all cases excite the uterus to contract, for he observes, "where the os uteri is contracted, the means indicated by Levret are very efficacious, and remove the hæmorrhage as if by a charm. But it is not so in complete inertia of the uterus; often it is widely dilated, and offers no resistance to the introduction of the hand. The introduction even of the whole hand excites little sensation, and the woman will promptly perish from the hæmorrhage, if other means more active and certain are not employed to prevent it." The tampon or plug is the remedy Leroux recommends in cases of flooding after delivery, and he affirms that it will often succeed in stopping the flow of blood when all other means fail. Dr. Dewees observes " that he has not found it necessary to introduce the hand for the purpose of stopping an hæmorrhage after the expulsion of the placenta, during the last five-and-thirty years, and he regards the practice as always frightful, and oftentimes unnecessary and pernicious. But it is difficult to subvert an established mode of practice, however unsound, and probably some of you, without much reflection, because you have heard this recommended, will pass up the hand into the cavity of the uterus after the expulsion of the placenta, on the very first occasion that you have an opportunity of doing so, remove all the coagula, and rub the inner surface with the fist till you are tired, without effect. I have seen cases repeatedly where this had been diligently performed by those who had neglected to apply the pad and binder, and all the other means now described. If you pass the hand at all within the parts, which I strongly suspect you will do, let me entreat you to carry it no further than the os uteri, which you may with much less risk and with greater effect press and rub with the fingers and irritate, than the inner surface of the body and fundus of the uterus.

Another reason has been assigned for passing the hand within the uterus in cases of flooding after the expulsion of the placenta, and which is the least satisfactory of all; it is, that the part of the uterus where the placenta was attached, from which the blood is flowing, may be compressed like a tourniquet between the hand in the uterus, and the other hand over the hypogastrium.

"My belief now is," says Dr. Gooch, "that when hæmorrhage occurs after the removal of the placenta, the quickest way to stop it is to introduce the left hand closed within the uterus, apply the right hand open to the outside of the abdomen, and then between the two to compress the part where the placenta was attached, and from which chiefly the blood is flowing: when the hand is introduced merely as a stimulant, there is an interval of time between its arrival within the uterus and the secure contraction of this organ, during which much blood is often lost. By directing the hand to the very vessels from which it issues, and compressing them as I have described, this quantity is saved. If I may judge by my feeling, the blood stops, in a great degree, even before the uterus contracts; the hand acts first as a tourniquet, then as a stimulant. It is true we cannot tell with certainty where the placenta was · attached, and consequently where the pressure should be applied; but as it is generally attached to or near the fundus, if the pressure be directed there, it will generally be right. Besides, after the child is born it is often several minutes before the placenta separates and descends: if, during this interval, we pass up the finger along the cord, and observe, at its entrance into the uterus, whether it turn towards the point, the back, the right or left side, or straight up to the fundus, we shall form a tolerably exact idea of the spot to which the placenta has been attached in this individual case." Without passing the whole hand into the uterus, it is impossible to know where the placenta adheres. Most frequently it is to the posterior part of the body and fundus; the hand, therefore, if introduced like a tourniquet, as here recommended, would compress the anterior wall, or that part of the uterus where there were no bleeding vessels. Mauriceau recommends that women who are subject to flooding after delivery should be bled twice or thrice from the arm during pregnancy, and once, or oftener, after labour has commenced. There are cases of uterine hæmorrhage after the delivery of the child and expulsion of the placenta unconnected altogether with plethora, or an excited state of the heart and arteries, and where bleeding and low diet do not prevent the accident. Rupturing the membranes at the very commencement of labour is by far the best remedy, the only thing indeed upon which any dependence can be placed.

I have had no experience of the effects of transfusion of blood in cases of uterine hæmorrhage. Some have been published in support of the practice, but, as Dr. Merriman observes, they are far from conclusive. Few women, if any, have been saved by it. Dr. Blundell has given an account of six cases in which injection into the human veins was attempted. A woman had lost a large quantity of blood after the expulsion of the child. She had ceased to respire, when sixteen ounces of blood, procured by venesection, were thrown into the bleeding vein of the arm. No signs of resuscitation were observed. In a man who had lost a large quantity of blood by the bursting of an artery, it was not more successful. In a third case it was equally unsuccessful. No effect was produced by it in a woman dying from puerperal fever and loss of blood. In a case of scirrhus of the pylorus it was employed, and the man died fifty-six hours after the operation. Dr. Ashwell has related a case of labour with placental presentation, where transfusion was twice performed without success. Ten ounces of blood, which flowed copiously from a healthy young woman, were injected by Dr. Collins into the median vein of a patient dying from uterine hæmorrhage, but it did not seem to have any more effect than causing the woman to mutter indistinctly; the circulation was not improved, and she expired a few minutes after the operation. Other cases have been recorded with equally unsatisfactory results, which it is unnecessary to quote.

After attacks of uterine hæmorrhage, the patient should not be raised from the horizontal position for several hours, and the strength should be supported by wine, beef-tea, and light nourishment. Brandy in gruel sometimes agrees when wine is rejected.

A good large dose of the liquor opii sedativus often produces the most decided benefit after the hæmorrhage has ceased ; there are few cases before this in which opium does good, though it is constantly given in all the varieties of flooding, even when the great object is to excite uterine action. Where recovery is to take place after uterine hæmorrhage, says Dr. M. Hall, the pallor of the countenance, the disposition to syncope, the coldness of the extremities, the feeble state of the pulse, and interrupted respiration, pass gradually away. Where the case is to terminate fatally, the symptoms gradually assume a more alarming aspect, the countenance becomes pale and sunk, the respiration stertorous, and the pulse cannot be felt at the wrist. There is great restlessness, and before death one or more fits of convulsions sometimes occur. Where recovery takes place, in some women it is astonishing how little permanent inconvenience is felt from the great loss of blood which they have sustained. In the course of ten days or a fortnight the effects have entirely disappeared ; and this is the most common result. In some women, a violent determination of blood takes place to the brain, marked by heat, strong pulsations of the carotid and temporal arteries, intolerance of light, and all the symptoms of inflammation of the brain or its membranes. A strong febrile attack is also sometimes experienced without an increased determination of blood to any particular organ. These affections of the brain and nervous system are aggravated by depletion. The patient should be kept in a cool, dark room, and mild cathartics, anodynes, and antispasmodics, occasionally given. Where there is much headache and throbbing, a few leeches should be applied to the temples, and a cold lotion to the scalp.

On retention of the placenta.

Atony, inertia, or want of uterine contraction, spasmodic or irregular contraction of the uterus, and morbid adhesion of the placenta to the uterus, are the three causes usually assigned for retention of the placenta beyond the usual period. Retained placenta from inactivity of the uterus occurs most frequently after protracted labours ; the uterus remains so soft that it can be distinguished with difficulty from the other viscera in the hypogastrium. It does not form a hard defined body, as it does when thoroughly contracted. There are no pains, or only feeble pains, after the birth of the child, and there is no lengthening of the cord. In these cases the uterus should be firmly compressed, and the ergot of rye and stimulants given. At the end of an hour after the birth of the child, if the uterus does not contract and expel the placenta, pass up the hand and

remove it. Where retention of the placenta arises from contraction of the cervix uteri, which is the condition termed hour-glass contraction, the fingers in a conical form should be introduced, the dilatation of the part effected, and the placenta removed. Sometimes it is possible to extract the placenta when only the fore and middle fingers can be introduced through the cervix, as in cases of placental presentation with rigidity of the os uteri. Occasionally, the cervix is so closely contracted that it is impossible to remove the placenta, and it remains in the cavity of the uterus till putrefaction takes place, and the patient is destroyed by the absorption of putrid animal matter. The best means of obviating the effects of these is to inject into the uterus and vagina plenty of tepid water, solutions of chloride of soda and lime, and decoction of oak bark. Where the placenta is retained by morbid adhesion, it should be removed as already described.

The best method of preventing accidents arising from retention of the placenta, as has already been repeatedly stated, is to apply the binder immediately after the birth of the child, to make pressure with the hand over the fundus uteri at short intervals, and slight traction upon the cord downward and backward in the direction of the hollow of the sacrum. By these means the upper part of the uterus usually goes on contracting till the placenta is detached and pressed down through the os uteri into the vagina. In all cases, whatever the cause of the retention may be, if the placenta at the end of an hour is not detached from the uterus and expelled, it should be withdrawn artificially. The difficulty of removing portions of placenta adhering with more than natural firmness to the uterus, or retained by contraction of the cervix, is only increased by delaying to interfere after an hour has elapsed from the delivery of the child. The seventh report in my Clinical Midwifery contains the histories of thirty-one cases of retained placenta. I am indebted to E. Johnson, Esq. for the following abstract of these cases, and for all the other tables which will hereafter be employed to illustrate the different varieties of complicated labour.

Dr. J. Ramsbotham relates 11 fatal cases of retained placenta. 66 cases of retention of the placenta requiring the introduction of the hand occurred to Dr. Collins in the Dublin Lying-in Hospital ; 37 from want of proper uterine action ; 19 from spasmodic or irregular action ; and 10 where the placenta was adherent. In 24 of the 66 there was slight hæmorrhage ; 6 of the women died. Dr. Churchill states that in 259,250 cases of labour, retention of the placenta occurred 392 times, or about 1 in 661½. In 186 cases where the result to the mother is given, 36 died, or about in 5.

A TABULAR VIEW OF THIRTY-ONE CASES OF RETENTION OF THE PLACENTA.

1	March 4, 1826	Labor at six and a [month]s; cord very soft, and torn away by midwife in attempting to [extract] the placenta; four hours after [?] [uter]i firmly contracted; much force employed to pass the [hand]; [placenta] left in [?] [uterus], and expelled next day without any [?] symptoms	Recovered.
2	Autumn, 1826	At Odessa. Placenta retained, and, in [?] by the midwife, uterus completely inverted; great hæmorrhage; uterus soon after replaced; convulsions	Died.
3	Jan. 4, 1828	Great hæmorrhage [before] expulsion of c [th]; hand could not be introduced, from firm contraction of cervix; funis broke off near [?]; placenta left within uterus; soon after placenta easily [?]	Recovered.
4	Jan. 4, 1828	Placenta [?] the hours; [child] born dead at seven and a half t[?]; cervix uteri rigid and [?] [?]; [?] r [?] by the tips of the [?] limb and two fingers introduced, and [?], which was lying [?] in the [?], easily extracted	Recovered.
5	Sept. 22, 1828	Retained placenta four hours; the umbilical cord and portion of placenta extracted; vagina filled with coagula of b[lood]; os uteri closely contracted; placenta extracted with difficulty by two fingers	Recovered.
6	March 2, 1829	A portion of placenta left within the [?]; hemorrhage [?] days after, and pain in region of uterus; pulse and respiration quickened; skin of a dusky [?]; pains in the joints; vomiting	Died; portion of placenta found adhering to fundus of uterus in a putrid condition; veins of the part distended with pus; ulceration of cartilages of knee.
7	July 7, 1831	Morbid adhesion of place[nta], and a part left [?] which could not be [?]; ninth day after delivery; giddiness and [?] of the temples; offensive dark-coloured vaginal discharge; os uteri open, and a portion of placenta felt, but could not be extracted; injections with solution of [chlo]ride of soda; [?]ined portion of placenta at last expelled	Recovered.
8	August 30, 1831	Portion of [?] [?] left in uterus; three days after fœtid dark-coloured discharge, vomiting, delirium, feeble pulse, and haggard [?]ace; orifice of uterus firmly contracted; only one [fin]ger could be introduced; three doses of ergot of rye had been gi[ven], [with] only i [?]used the sickness; died in two days, with all the symptoms of an animal poison having been introduced into the system	Died; large portion of placenta and membrane found in uterus in a black putrid state; coats of uterus healthy; no morbid adhesion of placenta.
9	October 20, 1832	Retention of placenta two hours after delivery; its extraction attempted, but the cord torn away; [?] believed to depend on hour-glass contraction; a portion of placenta found in the vagina, and the [?] firmly contracted around it; two fingers [?] though os uteri, and [?] [?] easily extracted; dyspnœa came on, with pain in uterus	Died; right lung covered with lymph, and hepatized; effusion into pleura.

	Date	Case	Result
10	June 18, 1834	Retained placenta from contraction of cervix; only a part could be removed; foetid discharge from uterus; rapid feeble pulse, diarrhœa, rigors, sickness, cough, and breathing; she became more and more feeble, and sank eighteen days after delivery	Died; pus in lungs; pleura inflamed; gangrene; placenta, in a putrid state, hanging through os uteri, and filling upper part of vagina; no morbid adhesion of placenta to the uterus; pus in veins of uterus; muscular coat soft.
11	April 22, 1835	Retention of placenta from rapid contraction of cervix uteri after the expulsion of child; cord torn away near its insertion; two fingers insinuated into the orifice of the uterus, the mass seized, and extracted	Recovered.
12	July 26, 1835	Placenta left in uterus eleven hours; cord torn away; profuse hæmorrhage; frequent attempts had been made to extract placenta; ʒiij. of ergot had been given during the labour; hand afterwards passed into uterus in a conical form, and placenta extracted	Recovered.
13	August 22, 1835	Hæmorrhage, with retained placenta; cord had been torn away; very little time had passed since delivery; the whole hand was passed into the uterus, and placenta easily extracted; flooding instantly ceased.	Recovered.
14	August 24, 1835	Placenta retained twenty-four hours; six months foetus; ergot of rye employed; uterus open; margin thin; point of finger readily touched a portion of hard placenta within cavity; the placenta, however, could not be seized, and it was left in uterus; purgative draught given, and during its action the placenta was expelled	Recovered.
15	October 23, 1835	Retention of placenta, with alarming hæmorrhage soon after the expulsion of the child; several unsuccessful attempts were made to extract it; a serious affection of the brain took place	Died; lymph in superior longitudinal sinus of brain, and all the veins emptying themselves into it filled with lymph, the result of inflammation; no trace of inflammation about the uterus; portion of putrid placenta adhered to the fundus; morbid adhesion of placenta to uterus.
16	August 13, 1836	Placenta retained thirty-four hours; child dead; ergot of rye had been given, and repeated unsuccessful efforts to extract placenta; os uteri closed; discharge very foetid; the orifice of uterus at last yielded, and allowed the introduction of three fingers; with them the placenta was extracted	Recovered.
17	Dec. 25, 1836	Placenta retained, with hæmorrhage; cord torn from placenta directly child was born, it having been twisted three times round child; severe hæmorrhage followed; attempts had been made to extract the placenta; the vagina was filled with clots an hour after delivery; placenta at last extracted; hæmorrhage continued; exhaustion	Died three hours after delivery.

No.	Date	Description	Result
18	Dec. 12, 1827	Placenta retained five hours, with severe uterine hæmorrhage; an hour elapsed before she was seen, when she was greatly exhausted from the discharge of blood; placenta easily extracted, which was grasped by cervix uteri; hæmorrhage restrained by vinegar and water	Recovered.
19	August 14, 1838	Placenta retained from unusual contraction soon after expulsion of child; umbilical cord lacerated; some attempts were made to extract the placenta, but the hand could not be introduced within the orifice; fœtid discharge came on in a day or two; peritonitis	Died; portion of placenta firmly adhered to upper part of uterus; placenta and uterus so firmly united that they appeared one substance; peritonitis.
20	Sept. 28, 1838	Placenta retained two days; repeated attempts had been made to extract it; dark-coloured discharge from vagina; pulse rapid; nausea; headache; a portion of placenta felt protruding through os uteri, which was easily drawn down into vagina	Recovered.
21	June 28, 1828	Placenta retained eighteen hours; cord had been torn away in the attempt to remove the placenta; no hæmorrhage; cervix uteri was found to be very contracted; by cautiously pressing the finger against the os uteri for an hour, the placenta was felt, and in a short time removed	Recovered.
22	October 10, 1838	Retention of the placenta in the vagina for three hours, on account of a broad smooth septum passing from the anterior to the posterior wall of vagina; one half of the placenta was on the left side of the septum, the other half, with cordaces, on the right side; both, violently pressed down; placenta was divided with a pair of scissars, and immediately came away	Recovered.
23	Dec. 23, 1838	Placenta retained three hours; child born dead; three or four efforts had been made to introduce the hand into the uterus, but the cervix was firmly contracted; complete hour-glass contraction; the fingers slowly were insinuated into theuterus and the placenta extracted	Recovered.
24	May 4, 1839	Placenta retained twenty-four hours; cord broken from the slightest touch; child dead; no hæmorrhage, but a great disposition to syncope; neck of uterus contracted; one finger was passed after another until the whole hand entered the uterus; the placenta was extracted with difficulty; phlebitis	Died; femoral and pelvic veins all plugged up with lymph; uterus flabby, and twice natural size.
25	Jan. 29, 1840	Hæmorrhage after expulsion of child; binder applied; stimulants given; flooding continued for quarter of an hour; the hand was then introduced into the uterus, and the placenta felt adhering; the fingers were spread out towards the margin of placenta, which was pressed off from the uterus; hæmorrhage arrested	Recovered.
26	April 28, 1840	Placenta retained five hours from contraction of the neck of uterus; the whole hand was introduced into the vagina, and the fingers gradually insinuated into the uterus; placenta extracted	Recovered.

CONTRIBUTIONS

TO

ANATOMY AND PHYSIOLOGY.

By ROBERT KNOX, M.D. F.R.S.E.

Lecturer on Anatomy and Physiology, and Corresponding Member of the French Academy of Medicine.

[Continued from p. 556.]

Sacral vertebræ.

ANATOMISTS had laid down discriminating characters for the male and female sacrum as a whole, that is, after the invertebral ligaments and soft parts had disappeared, and the five vertebræ had become united into one. They described the female sacrum as broader, shorter, and more concave, than the male; and this, I think, will still prove the correct opinion as to the greater number. But I quite agree with Mr. South as to the fact of there being great varieties in all these matters.

Do the sacral vertebræ belong to all one category? it appears to me evident that they do not. The first sacral and last lumbar occasionally so strongly resemble each other, that they can scarcely be distinguished from each other; the first, second, third, and fourth, partially form alone the articulation with the os nnominatum the fifth has nothing to do with it. They have different relations, then, to the adjoining structures, and moreover, it is generally understood or admitted that besides having all the elements of true vertebræ, though called false, they combine in addition a series of rudimentary ribs undistinguishably united by bony union with their transverse processes. There is every probability that, in addition to very large processes, these sacral vertebræ do carry upon the anterior surface of these processes rudimentary ribs; but still there lies a difficulty in fully coming to this conclusion. It is this. When Meckel published his work on General and Descriptive Anatomy (a translation of which, by Jourdan, shortly afterwards appeared, and from which translation into French I quote), he maintained the doctrine, that the thoracic ribs were merely the fully developed anterior roots of the transverse processes of the dorsal vertebræ. Now this theory, so soon as announced, I showed to my class must

	Date		Recovery
27	Nov. 30, 1840	Placenta retained five hours; violent contraction of cervix uteri; a good deal of force was required to introduce the finger into os uteri; placenta firmly adhered to uterus; with great care the whole cervix was extracted in fragments	Recovered.
28	Dec. 5, 1840	Retention of the whole placenta the hours; cervix so contracted that it was impossible to introduce the whole hand; introduced the whole hand into vagina, and inserted two fingers into the uterus, and thus detached the placenta, and pressed it down into the vagina	Died.
29	Jan. 23, 1841	Retained the hours; child born with cord twisted three times round the neck; cord was broken close to the uterus; cervix had dilated firmly after the expulsion of the child; the whole hand was inserted into the uterus, and the placenta, which was adhering, was removed with ease	Recovered.
30	Oct. 20, 1841	Retained placenta eight hours; funis broken off close to placenta soon after it, and slight hæmorrhage took place; the hand was introduced into the vagina, and with two fingers introduced within the uterus, the placenta was extracted	Recovered.
31	Jan. 14, 1842	Profuse hæmorrhage only after the birth of the child; the hand was immediately passed into the uterus to detach placenta, but a portion adhered so firmly, that it could not be removed; hæmorrhage continued	Died; portion of placenta found adhering.

be incorrect; in fact, there were preparations in the museum which refuted it: one, in particular, of a seventh cervical vertebra, where the transverse process was distinctly double, that is, had an anterior and a posterior root, with a considerable aperture between them for the passage of the vertebral vein; in front of the anterior root was another aperture, and then came a cervical rib; thus, there could be no doubt of Meckel being in error in respect to his theory that the ribs are merely the prolonged anterior roots of the transverse processes of the vertebræ. Now to apply this to the human sacrum, it is easy to show many specimens of the young bones where each lateral mass of each sacral vertebra is growing by *two distinct germs;* but whether these germs represent the one the transverse process, the other the rib, as in the dorsal vertebræ (in which vertebræ the anterior root has entirely disappeared), or whether these two germs on each side represent merely the anterior and posterior roots, or whether both are present and rudimentary ribs also; these are questions which the preparations I have as yet examined do not enable me satisfactorily to solve. An appeal to comparative anatomy is only one way of solving the question, and not a very satisfactory one when applied to human structure, and this for the most obvious reason in the world.

The sacral vertebræ present, as we have seen, the greatest caprice as to their form, without, however, deviating very much from the normal arrangement; sometimes, however, they do: first, as to number; secondly, as to "development" of their natural halves. Of the variety as to number I shall say nothing: six vertebræ have, no doubt, been found, but on all such occasions it would be well to look to the number of the lumbar vertebræ. Secondly, the variety in the development, or rather the non-development, of the lateral halves of the sacral vertebræ, is one of the most important deformations to which the pelvis is liable. Its explanation probably rests on a law in transcendental anatomy, or rather physiology, which I shall first state.

If the pelvis of a fœtus at full term, or before or after for a short period, be examined, it will be found to differ entirely from the adult pelvis, *and most*

especially from the finely-formed European female pelvis; it resembles, also— a fact which is well known to the transcendental anatomist—the pelvis of the lower mammals, whether male or female. To them it bears the strictest resemblance in as far as the structures will admit. I shall describe the particulars of its form more minutely afterwards, merely remarking here that the introitus, and, indeed, general form of the cavity, is an elongated square rather than an oval; the sides, formed by the ossa innominata, are nearly straight; the cavity is of equal breadth throughout, and the antero-posterior measurement of the introitus is the larger; any one may recognise in this the pelvis of the lower mammals. Now, should the pelvis during its development continue of this shape, or even maintain it to a certain extent, then we have a misshapen pelvis, common enough in females both here and on the continent: the pelvis continues, to a certain extent, to maintain its fœtal form; there is a kind of arrest of development; the sides are too straight, the sacrum too narrow; the transverse diameter of the introitus too small, and the antero-posterior diameter too long. I repeat, pelves of this form are exceedingly common in the male; they are also common in the female.

But let us suppose that the arrest of development has been limited only to one side, confined to the left half, say, of the sacrum and corresponding innominatum, but that the arrest of development has been here, if I may so say, much exaggerated, that is, more complete; that the bones have not only not undergone those changes as to *form* which they ought to have done, but that moreover they are positively much *smaller* than those of the opposite side; that, in fact, that has taken place here which we shall find may take place even in the ribs. Then there is produced the "pelvis oblique ovata," the discovery of which is due to the illustrious Naegele. A glance at fig. 1, pelvis of fœtus; fig. 2, of mammal; fig. 3, of ill-formed female pelvis, but quite capacious enough for the passage of the child; fig. 4, the pelvis oblique ovata of Naegele; fig. 5, the finely-formed female pelvis: a glance at these figures will best explain the whole theory to the reader. Dr. F. Krammerscroff, of Dorpat, whom I

Fig. 1.

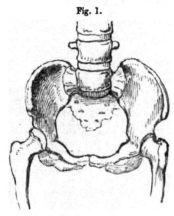

Outline of the pelvis of the human fœtus at term: the pelvis at this age may be taken as the type of the transcendental law; it is more quadrilateral than rounded or oval, and its antero-posterior diameter is the longest: it has the form, in a great measure, of the pelvis of the quadruped and quadrumanous mammal, of the human male pelvis generally, and of certain ill-formed female (all human) pelves.

Fig. 2.

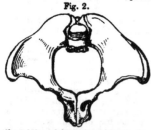

Outline of the pelvis of the elephant: the entroitus of the pelvis of the elephant is more rounded than that of most quadruped mammals, including even that of the quadrumans; still it does not assume the special transverse oval character of the well-formed human female pelvis.

Fig. 3.

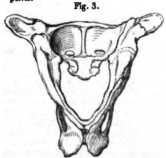

Pelvis of the seal: this is the extreme of the type; this form occurs in the very young human fœtus, and ' .— approach to it in the adult }

It is in this pelvis, in the adult female, that a separation of the pubic articulation takes place to so great an extent prior to and during the birth of the young seal.

Fig. 4.

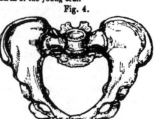

That form of the human female pelvis which I have called the quadruped form; it is quite common in this country, and I think in Europe generally; this is merely the fœtal form persisting, the transcendental law, or law of general type, prevailing over the law of species. Beauty of form, and fitness for the due performance of function, or the law of species, when not interfered with, gives rise, in woman, to the pelvis whose outline is represented by

Fig. 5.

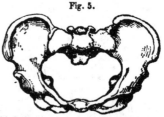

This is the transverse oval pelvis: when to this is added a fully developed upper or false pelvis, then the osseous girdle is considered as completely or fully developed.

The transcendental law, or law of type, may prevail on one side of the pelvis, and not influence the other; this gives rise to the pelvis oblique ovata of Naegele, as seen in

Fig. 6.

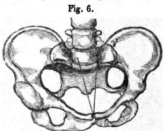

When it takes place on both sides, as is said to be the case with a human female pelvis now in the possession of Dr. Outrepont, then the outline of the introitus will strongly resemble that of the seal—or, in other words, the transcendental of the very youngest period of the human skeleton, when, in fact, it was almost entirely cartilaginous, had continued in force to mature years, and the antagonistic law of species had, from causes unknown to us, never come into action. I should not think that the curvature of the spine in the lumbar region, seen in Fig. 6, was a necessary consequence of the non-development of the half of the pelvis.

had the pleasure to meet lately, a most intelligent observer, informed me that he saw lately, in the museum of Dr. Outrepont, a female pelvis in which the deformation now known by M. Naegele's name of "pelvis oblique ovata," extended to both sides, giving rise to the greatest difficulty during labour, and ultimately, if I rightly recollect, causing the death of the patient. If it were not that anchylosis or bony union of the sacro-iliac joint, so generally, if not always, coincides with the arrest of development, giving rise to this deformity, Dr. Outrepont's case was one in which the pubic section might have been attempted with some slight chance of success; to propose this operation in the round or transversely oval pelvis argues a want of mere mechanical knowledge on the part of the adviser.

The transcendental theory I have just endeavoured to apply in explanation of, 1st, the normal form of the male pelvis and its varieties; 2d, the form of the pelvis of the mammal; 3d, certain unusual forms observed in the female pelvis must ultimately rest on certain facts which it is proper to examine more in detail, or rather by direct or intuitive perception. If these be correct, then the theory is good so far as it goes: it gives us no insight, it is true, as to the *why* these things should happen so, but it shows the *manner* of their taking place. The details I shall now take the liberty of giving are taken chiefly from scattered memoranda of lectures.

The resemblance of the abdomen, pelvis, and trunk generally of the human fœtus and infant to the same parts in the adult quadruped mammal, is very striking; it depends, no doubt, on the law of unity of organization. But I may as well quote the notes as they stand in my note-book.

If the principles and views just laid down be in accordance with nature, they ought to stand the test of intuitive inspection, or an appeal to individual phenomena; let this appeal, then, be made to the human and brute structure by a brief, but, at the same time, careful inquiry into a number of specimens sufficiently numerous to warrant the deductions.

1st, In the skeleton of the adult fœtus now before me (not selected, but taken at random from the museum), prepared and dried in the usual way,

the pelvis presents the following appearances. In its entire outline it resembles the pelvis of the quadruped; I mean of most adult mammals. It is more like an elongated canal than the human pelvis; the iliac walls are comparatively upright, the false pelvis contracted and narrow, falling exceedingly within the limits of a perpendicular line descending from the shoulders; a straight line directed horizontally from the symphysis of the pubis towards the vertebral column strikes the lowermost part of the coccygeal bones. The conjugate or antero-posterior diameter is 1 $\frac{3}{4}$ inch; the transverse, where widest, about 1 inch, and nearly of the same width throughout; in other words, the pelvis is no longer, or rather not yet, a transverse oval one, but quadrilateral, its greatest diameter, as in the brute, being from before backwards, and precisely the reverse of what it ought to become (to give it a strictly human form) in the adult. Already, in this fœtus, the coccygeal bones are twisted or curved towards the right side, and the area of the abdominal strait, or entrance, if divided into halves by a line passed across it as mesially as possible, gives to the right side of the area a capacity greater than the left; the left wall is straighter, and already the tendency to the pelvis oblique ovata of Naegele is established. Now, we have only to suppose the persistence of these forms, to a certain extent at least, to the adult age, and we then have the exact description of the ill-formed female pelvis so common in this country, and, I have no doubt, also in England; and if what travellers say of the Esquimaux be true, it would seem that the false pelvis is seldom or ever in them properly developed, so that the breadth of the haunches is nearly equal in both sexes; and this is quite possible, for the false pelvis has an entirely different and independent development from the true pelvis.

It would appear already, from the examination of a single specimen, that the more common of the malformations and peculiarities in the adult male and female pelvis are merely the persistence of the fœtal, infantile, or juvenile forms, and of consequence repeated in the pelivs of many of the mammalia. The obliquely oval pelvis of Naegele is comprised in the same law, with the addition of an extremely imperfect development of one side. But there is nothing new in it; nothing unexpected—nothing which might not, à priori, be foretold by an inspection of the fœtal skeleton.

I have already shewn, in a memoir published some years ago on the Statistics of Hernia, that the pelvis was very frequently more fully developed on one side than on the other, and hence the predisposition to hernia on the more fully developed side, be it right or left; but from the slightest shade of difference to the most deformed of the pelves lithographed by Naegele one law prevails; the persistence of the fœtal form on one side; the regular development of adult human form on the other. Again, the quadrilateral-formed pelvis is the type of most mammals (if not of all) when adult, and, by the law of unity of organization in the embryo, it is also the type of the early human pelvis. Whatever form, then, the pelvis assumes, must flow from the agency of these causes, and be connected with, and dependent on, these laws. Obliquely oval pelvises are not *lusus naturæ*, no more is the occasional quadrilateral form of the same girdle in the European female.

2. Another human fœtus at full term is put before you: the measurements and form of the pelvis are as nearly as may be those of the preceding: still there are differences: the iliac portion or false pelvis is broader, and although the whole length of the skeleton be less than the preceding one by at least an inch, the false pelvis is broader by nearly half an inch; confirming what we already know so frequently to happen, that the future grown man or woman may be shadowed out in the infant.

3. Another fœtal pelvis gives a conjugate diameter of an inch and ⅜; the transverse diameter where widest scarcely measures an inch.

4. Here is the pelvis of an infant seemingly about a year old; the antero-posterior diameter of the pelvis exceeds the transverse by nearly half an inch.

Let us now examine a few adult female pelvises from amongst those whose dimensions and general form offer no obstacle to the ready passage to the child through their cavities: the first I take up gives a conjugate diameter of 4½ inches: its transverse measures 6, and yet this pelvis is not equally de-

veloped: but it is a large and capacious pelvis, and the true as well as the false have very fully assumed the human character; it is the very reverse of the infantile and brute pelvis in every respect, in its form, its dimensions, and inclination.

The next I examine is different, and yet a sufficiently capacious pelvis; first, the false pelvis is narrow and the walls upright; the woman, therefore, wanted breadth of haunches. No proof, however, of a want of capacity in the true pelvis itself, as this follows different laws in its development. The conjugate diameter measures 4½ inches, the transverse 5½, or nearly so, being at least half an inch less than the preceding pelvis: but still it is a good pelvis compared with some which are to follow. The next measures 4⅞ and 5, and is becoming more and more at its abdominal entrance (I mean the introitus) of an elongated square form. The next is as nearly as may be 4 inches each way, without any appearance of rickets, and the same precisely may be said of another standing close to it. Now all these are female pelvises presenting no appearance of any disease or deformity; I have so far selected them on this account. But here are others which shew these phenomena equally, or even more so, but being complicated with other peculiarities, had better follow the more simple ones.

The sacrum, I now examine, shews the following peculiarities: it is that of a female: the right half of the sacrum is nearly half an inch narrower than the left; the right half of the introitus proportionably smaller, but the iliac portion of the ossa innominata are tolerably symmetrical. Here, then, is the commencement of the pelvis oblique ovata of Naegele. The lumbar portion of the column presents an extensive curve, the cause of which curve it would be more difficult to investigate, but which probably arose from the same predisposition to a want of symmetry. A second pelvis also, in Dr. Campbell's museum, presents the obliquely oval pelvis on the left side; a large exostotic deposition on the last lumbar vertebra rendering, I should think, the passage of any living child impossible. And now I take the male pelvis, the one before me, and I find it to resemble in the form of the introitus, as nearly as may be, that of the seal, and of many other quadrupeds, although the transverse diameter be still somewhat larger than the conjugate : a second male pelvis, now in my own museum, shews the brute form to a still more extraordinary degree. The transverse diameter of its widest part is but about ¼ larger than the antero-posterior; and, precisely as in that of the quadruped, it is greatest close to the sacrum, scarcely widening, or but very little, anterior to this. Now this is the type of the fœtal pelvis, and that of the mammalia lower than man ; and that this person presents a pelvis of this peculiar shape, is simply because it was the form it originally had, and from which, by a peculiarity in his nature, it had never altered.

But this male pelvis merits a further notice. The false pelvis spreads out after the fashion of the female pelvis ; the true pelvis is constructed on the plan of the fœtus and of the quadruped mammal. The sacrum is of such breadth that immediately in front of it, or very nearly so, we find the widest part of the introitus ; that is, the edges of the abdominal entrance run nearly straight down, and then converge. The last lumbar vertebra has evidently united by its lateral processes with the corresponding parts of the sacrum, so as to become identified with it, causing it strongly to resemble the first sacral vertebra.

[To be continued.]

OBSERVATIONS AND EXPERIMENTS CONCERNING

DIABETES MELLITUS,
&c. &c.

By JOHN PERCY, M.D. (Edin.)

Physician to the Queen's Hospital, and Lecturer on Organic Chemistry at the Royal School of Medicine and Surgery, Birmingham.

[Continued from p. 125.]

(For the London Medical Gazette.)

WE now proceed to inquire concerning the changes which starch undergoes in the healthy stomach, and, in this inquiry, we again appeal to direct experiment.

EXP. 9.—At ten minutes past 11, a large bull-terrier bitch ate eight ounces (dry) of wheaten flour, heated with a small quantity of water to the consistence of common paste. She drank water afterwards. At 2 P.M. I destroyed her by hanging. The stomach contained paste, which had a strongly acid reaction, and was not altered in appearance. To some of this paste I added water, and digested in a flask for several hours, at a temperature ranging between 98° and 120° F. On the following day the contents of the flask were dried over the steam-bath : the process of drying occupied the greater part of the day. The residuum was broken up, and treated with boiling rectified spirit. The spirituous solution was evaporated over the steam-bath, and a pale brown syrup was obtained, having a decided sweet taste, and a strongly acid reaction. A portion of this syrup was dissolved in warm water, and a small quantity of yeast was added ; the mixture was then introduced into a graduated receiver over mercury. Fermentation was soon excited, and proceeded with considerable rapidity. I measured 6·7 C. In., whilst the solution was still fermenting. The fermented liquid was distilled *per se*, and carbonate of potass was added to the product, when I obtained a copious stratum of alcohol.

Now, from this experiment we do not derive satisfactory evidence of the conversion of starch into sugar in the stomach, although we learn from it that the liquid of the stomach, whether saliva or gastric secretion, is capable of effecting this conversion at a suitable temperature. During the process of healthy digestion, it is well ascertained that free hydrochloric acid is present in the stomach ; and, accordingly, we find that the chyme in the preceding experiment had a strongly acid reaction. The question, then, arises, whether the sugar obtained was produced by the action of the hydrochloric acid ; for we know that this acid, even in small proportion, changes starch into sugar during the process of long-continued boiling. To determine this point, it is requisite to examine whether sugar actually exists in the chyme at the time of its removal from the stomach ; and, if not, whether sugar would be formed by artificial digestion, after the neutralization of the free acid. On this subject the following experiments will throw light.

EXP. 10.—At 5 P.M. a middle-sized terrier dog ate four ounces (dry) of wheaten flour, heated with water to the consistence of paste. He swallowed it without mastication, and did not drink water afterwards. On the previous day he was fed on oatmeal. At 8 P.M. he was destroyed by hanging. The stomach was immediately removed. The paste was not altered in appearance, and it still had the odour of paste, and not that of chyme : it had a strongly acid reaction. I divided it into two parts, A and B.

A. I added distilled water and prepared chalk, and then evaporated to dryness over the steam-bath. The residuum was treated with boiling rectified spirit, and the spirituous solution was filtered and evaporated to dryness in a capsule. Towards the termination of the evaporation I observed a brownish yellow oil floating on the surface. I obtained a pale brown syrup of a decided sweet taste. This syrup was dissolved in water, and a minute quantity of yeast was added in the usual manner. Fermentation soon commenced; and whilst the solution was still fermenting, I measured 5 C.In. of gas.

B. This portion was evaporated *per se* on a plate over the steam-bath. The residuum was treated in the same manner with boiling rectified spirit. In both cases the solution passed through the filter turbid, and in both the turbidity was instantly removed by the application of a gentle heat. I obtained by evaporation a small quantity of residuum, of a syrupy consistence and sweetish taste. Oily matter was also separated during the progress of the evaporation, and floated on the surface : on cooling it became solid. The residuum, dissolved in water, was introduced into a graduated receiver over mercury, and the same quantity of the same yeast as used in A was added. The tubes in A and B were placed side by side. Not the smallest evolution of gas had occurred in the case of B, even after the lapse of three days.

From this experiment we learn that true sugar did not exist in the chyme at the time of its removal from the stomach; and that the sugar obtained from it was generated after neutralization of the free hydrochloric acid. The paste in A, it must be remembered, was mixed with water, and was exposed to heat for many hours; whilst that in B was dried in a comparatively *short time. The presence of sugar in A is inferred from the fact of the resi-*

duum fermenting on the addition of yeast; whilst the absence of sugar in B is inferred from the converse of this fact. Now the residuum of B contained a portion of free acid, which might be supposed to impede or prevent the action of the yeast. That this supposition, however, is incorrect, we discover by reference to Exp. 9, in which the residuum was strongly acid, and yet rapidly fermented on the addition of yeast. We are not justified in concluding that, in the experiment before us, sugar was not formed in the stomach ; for possibly sugar may have been produced only in the immediate vicinity of the mucous membrane, and have been directly absorbed; or, according to the hypothesis of Dr. Prout, the formation of sugar may have been only a point *in transitu*.

EXP. 11.—At 11½ A.M. a dog ate eight ounces (dry) of wheaten flour, heated with a small quantity of water to the consistence of thick paste, and afterwards drank a pint of water. He was killed by hanging at 7½ P.M. The stomach contained thick paste, similar to that mentioned in the preceding experiments. The paste was dried to a brittle mass over the steam-bath. This mass was broken up, and treated with boiling rectified spirit in a flask. Two days afterwards the spirituous solution was first distilled in a retort, and then evaporated over the steam-bath in a capsule. During the progress of the evaporation a pale brown oil floated on the surface. The residuum reddened litmus. I added water and yeast in the usual manner.

April 17, Potash apparatus, after = 635·400
April 12, Do.   do.   before = 634·887
                                    ―――――――
                                     ·513

In this case the increase is so small, that it may be altogether neglected, and we may infer the absence of true sugar. The residuum, on the addition of water, appeared like pearl white dextrine precipitated by alcohol.

EXP. 12.—At 10¼ A.M. a large bull-terrier dog ate ten ounces of wheaten flour mixed with water. Except a few morsels of cheese, he had not received solid food for three days previously. At 3 P.M. he was destroyed by prussic acid. During the action of the poison he vomited, and voided a small quantity of urine. Half an hour afterwards I removed the stomach, which was much distended with liquid. The contents appeared to consist of starch, of oily matter floating on the surface, and of some lumps of cheese; the reaction was strongly acid. On the addition of tincture of iodine the characteristic blue colour was immediately produced. I evaporated the liquid contents to dryness over the steam-bath, having previously added prepared chalk in order to neutralize the free acid. On the following day the dry residuum was treated with boiling rectified spirit. By evaporation of the spirituous solution I obtained a brown mass, of the consistence of syrup, and having an odour not unlike that of osmazome. The mass was dissolved in water, yeast was added, and the mixture introduced into a graduated receiver over mercury. Three days afterwards I measured off 0·8 C. In. of gas. In this case also the quantity of gas evolved was so inconsiderable as to lead to no positive inference concerning the formation of sugar.

Exp. 13.—At 10½ A.M. a large bull-terrier dog ate six ounces (dry) of wheaten flour, heated with water to the consistence of paste. He drank about half a pint of water afterwards. He had not been fed on the previous day. He was destroyed by hanging at 5 P.M. The stomach was removed in a quarter of an hour afterwards. It contained only a small quantity of liquid, resembling common gruel, in which were two or three small lumps of paste, unchanged in consistence or appearance. This liquid had an acid reaction, but only slowly reddened litmus. I immediately proceeded to desiccate the contents of the stomach on a plate over the steam-bath. Some oily matter floated on the surface. I obtained a brittle residuum, which was broken up and treated with boiling alcohol, of specific gravity 0·834. The solution was decanted, and the spirit was distilled off in a retort, and then completely evaporated in an open capsule. I obtained a small quantity of brownish liquid, of the consistence of syrup, having a peculiar odour and taste, but not that of sweetness. I then added distilled water, and digested over the steam-bath. The solution was turbid, and had a pale brown colour. I then filtered. The filtered solution was clear, and had a pale straw colour.

816.—XXXII.

A small quantity of fresh yeast was added in the usual manner, and the mixture was introduced into a graduated receiver over mercury. Three days afterwards I measured 4·9 C. In. while the liquid was still fermenting. By distillation per se, and the addition of carbonate of potass to the product, I obtained a copious supernatant stratum of alcohol. The matter which remained on the filter was dissolved immediately by cold æther, and by evaporation of the æthereal solution globules of oil were separated. This oily matter had a butyraceous consistence, and stained paper. The residuum of the contents of the stomach, after treatment with boiling alcohol, was again desiccated, in order to expel any trace of spirit. Water was then added, and the whole digested over the steam-bath. By filtration was obtained a small quantity of clear solution, which acquired a reddish purple colour on the addition of tincture of iodine, and in which alcohol occasioned a copious precipitate of white matter, like dextrine.

Exp. 14.—At 10½ A.M. a large bull-terrier dog, which had received no food on the previous day, ate six ounces (dry) of wheaten flour, in the state of thick paste, and drank half a pint of water afterwards. He was destroyed by prussic acid at 3½ P.M. Twenty minutes afterwards the stomach was removed. The contents consisted of liquid like gruel, and some thick paste, which did not appear to have undergone much alteration. The liquid part was poured off, and evaporated to dryness per se, in the usual manner. The dry residuum was treated with boiling spirit, sp. gr. 0·834. The solution was decanted and evaporated. I obtained a brown matter of a sweetish taste. This matter was dissolved in warm water, and yeast was added. Three days afterwards 1·4 C. In. of gas was disengaged, and fermentation had entirely ceased.

OBSERVATIONS.—When wheaten flour is introduced into the stomach of a dog, we find that, after the lapse of several hours, it is reduced to a comparatively liquid state, like common gruel, and eventually completely disappears, being principally removed by absorption. Now the first step in the conversion of starch into grape sugar is the formation of dextrine, a substance which it readily soluble in water, and which, in many respects, resembles gum-arabic. From the preceding experiments we derive confirmation of previously recorded statements concerning the conversion of starch into sugar by the agency of the liquid of the stomach, whether saliva or gastric secretion, or both conjointly. We do not, however, from these experiments obtain demonstrative evidence of this conversion being effected in the stomach; for even in Exp. 13, in which a sensible quantity of sugar was procured from the liquid contents of the stomach, it might be alleged that the sugar was formed during the process of desiccation. This process, however, was rapidly completed, and the quantity of sugar determined by fermentation, compared with the small quantity of liquid operated upon, appeared to me to be greater than could well be produced during the short period required for complete desiccation; so that in this case we should not, I think, err in concluding that a portion of the sugar, at least, was generated in the stomach. Still, I repeat, the evidence is not demonstrative; and, in all physiological discussions, we cannot be too cautious in the admission of data intended to serve as the basis of reasoning. If starch be changed in the stomach in very sensible proportion into sugar, the sugar must either undergo a further change, or be absorbed with rapidity; otherwise it would accumulate in a sufficient degree to admit of easy detection. Now we know, from what has been previously advanced, that, under certain conditions, saccharine matter introduced into the stomach quickly enters the circulation as sugar; and, if in certain proportions, is partially eliminated by the kidneys. Here I would suggest the possibility, not to say probability, that under ordinary circumstances starch, or amylaceous matters in general, may be in great measure converted into dextrine, and in this state be directly absorbed. Dextrine, as we know, is readily soluble in water, and may probably pass unchanged into the circulation. If this probability should be realized, the results of the foregoing experiments would be clearly explained. To decide this question, numerous and delicate *experiments* are required; and 1 hope *that, on a future occasion*, I may be

enabled to present satisfactory information upon this subject.

There is one point deserving of notice in respect to the nature of the sugar generated in some of the preceding experiments, viz. that it was found to be incrystallizable. A portion of the syrup of Exp. 9 was left exposed to the atmosphere for a month, but not the slightest trace of crystallization was observed after this exposure. As to the manner of determining the presence of sugar by fermentation, it will be remembered that I offered some observations in a previous communication.

I have been careful to make comparative experiments, in order to ascertain the quantity of carbonic acid liberated from the yeast alone. For example: twenty, if not thirty, times the volume of yeast employed in Exp. 9 was mixed with water, and introduced into a graduated receiver over mercury. After the lapse of two days the carbonic acid disengaged amounted only to 0·7 C. In. I have confined myself entirely to the application of the test of fermentation, as I believe that test to be most decisive, as well as most practical; for a true sugar is most prominently characterized by the property of fermenting at a suitable temperature on the addition of yeast or other similar matters, with the formation of alcohol and carbonic acid.

I may here also mention, that sugar is formed in small quantity by simply digesting paste, similar to that employed in these experiments, with water at a gentle heat, over the steam-bath. In this case the sugar may probably be produced by the conjoint influence of the gluten and atmospheric air (Dumas, Traité de Chimie appliquée aux Arts, t. 6ième, p. 88). However, the actual quantity of sugar which I obtained in this manner was very small compared with the quantity of sugar indicated by the result of fermentation in some of the preceding experiments.

We may sum up the results of the preceding experiments as follow:—

1. That the liquid of the stomach is capable of effecting the conversion of starch into sugar, by digestion at a suitable temperature.

2. That although no demonstrative evidence has been adduced in proof of the formation of sugar in the stomach from wheaten flour, yet, in Exp. 13, it is highly probable that a portion of the

sugar obtained was generated in the stomach.

3. That if sugar be the product of the digestion of wheaten flour in ordinary circumstances, it is either rapidly absorbed, or undergoes a further change. We have, however, no direct and experimental proof of such change, while we have demonstrative evidence of the speedy absorption of sugar after its introduction into the stomach.

[To be continued.]

REFLECTIONS

ON THE

INFLUENCES OF HEAT ON THE LIVING BODY.*

BY T. WILKINSON KING.

(For the London Medical Gazette.)

Five effects of heat—Delicate health— Easy play of all functions—Warm bath—Clothing—Wasting—The feeble, free, oppressed—Cases for warmth —Objections.

SOME of the more general facts of the influence of heat have been already hinted at. We may yet find particular facts deserving of notice, but our present aim will be chiefly to illustrate, by the effects of heat, the theory advanced with reference to cold, and to shew its practical importance in the treatment of different classes of disorders. We conceive that we may safely leave it to the course of our reflections to demonstrate, that of all remedial agents that which is at once the most safe, controllable, powerful, and generally applicable, is temperature.

There are certain distinct influences of heat on the body which will scarcely require much proof :—

1st. Superficial excitement.

2dly. Universal or general liberation of functions.

3dly. Superficial excitement, tending to local hypertrophies.

4thly. General freedom of actions, tending to general decline, or atrophy, or even fatal syncope; but

5thly. One or more organs being oppressed, or failing, as a distended heart or indurated kidney, the unimpeded play of the remaining functions becomes of vital importance.

* Vide recent papers in this Journal on " Irritation" and " Cold."

The simple view that *increased warmth excites the superficial functions of the body, and tends to diminish both the nutrient and secretory supplies of internal parts,* has seemed so clear, though only partially true, that it deserved to be advocated singly both on its own account, and as a step towards the more general proposition on which we are now about to enter.

John Hunter, the most celebrated perhaps of all the investigators of the nature of life and health, meeting his friend Mr. Nicol, who had lost five children successively by endeavouring to " bring them up hardy," " Well," said Hunter, " are you going to kill this next one as you did the rest ?" And he proceeded to shew how all young animals are brought to life and nourished by great warmth, until they can, by full exercise and digestion, maintain their own heat freely. Mr. Nicol found that tenderness and comfort succeeded better. His next offspring is said to be still living.

Surely we may all perceive how a hot-house, or the approach of spring— " the genial warmth of joy-renewing spring"—forces or facilitates the dormant functions of vegetables and animals ; and, on the other hand, the universal expression "taking cold," is an acknowledgment of the obstruction and disturbance which the vital functions are so continually liable to experience. The happy power of endurance which the vigorous possess renders them insensible of what is needful for more tender plants. The oak may well say to the exotic, " Open the windows, and make yourself hardy ;" and in return, while the exotic patient must carefully judge for himself, he may naturally envy his more robust neighbour. Thus in delicate health and old age, when the powers decline and become incapable of resisting outward mischiefs, a larger share of comfort again becomes necessary ; for a great deal of the evil and aggravation of disorders, as delicate persons well know, consists in successive relapses, which are the result of negligence and exposure. A climate in which care is scarcely necessary becomes absolutely indispensable, and most particularly to those who do not rightly know how to take care for themselves.

Youth, health, convalescence, spring, and the first days spent in a tropical country, are well understood to be characterized by a peculiarly happy sense of life, of ease, lightness, and vigour; and as far as science hitherto admits, we discover on all sides a decided liberation and excitement of molecular changes, chemical, botanic, and animal. We are not without pleasing evidence that, even in the tropics, the healthful balance of all the animal functions may be long sustained. Some persons of delicate constitution, and many advanced in life, are striking instances of this fact, which will be, perhaps, best accounted for, in the first place, by our investigation of the opposite train of events. Gradually, in the course of weeks, undue warmth excites the functions of the skin beyond their natural bounds, as excessive perspiration, hypertrophy of glands, and even diseases of the skin, often testify; and these cannot be unattended with deeper consequences.

The primary effect of general warmth at the surface begins without delay. All the functions are rendered freer; early puberty, and even decay, are cases in point. All the mischievous results, when examined separately, seem only so many more examples of the same thing; but we think it cannot be denied, that as the superficial organs evince by degrees the most excessive excitement, so, in the general, the disorder of the rest is subsequent to, and depending on, that excitement. Various atmospheric conditions will of course interfere with the effect of warmth to the body: it may suffice for the present, if we illustrate some of these indirectly in our course.

Mere local derivation, by means of superficial warmth, is perhaps sufficiently understood. When applied in the form of hot-bath, it is even of itself a powerful agent, although we ought to distinguish fairly between this single revulsive effect and the influence of artificial heat in the whole circulating mass of fluid. Pediluvium may produce pallor of the face, or even syncope, but not by a simple counter-irritation.

The warm-bath, as a rapid means of communicating heat to the whole body in almost any quantity, is a most efficient resource. The quantity of fluid which it abstracts from the body may be considerable, or it may be a source of supply to the body. The blood itself may be in a condition to imbibe actively, without the necessity of any

other specific means of absorption. In all cases, however, at least solids are disposed of in the way of nutrition and secretion, at the surface, by the agency of heat.

The effects of the vapour-bath are modified by the patient's being in the upright position. It would certainly appear that dry heat is less calculated to excite perspiration, and thus the peculiar eruptions of hot and arid climes may be explained. Warm clothing, by retaining the secretions about the surface, approaches in effect to the warm-bath. The problem of the effects of heat, variously combined with food, drinks, exercise, and clothing, depends in a measure on experience in any given case. Thus the state of the individual from hour to hour must in great part regulate the results; yet, on the principles already advocated, good general conclusion may be readily comprehended, as well as to the subjugation of old derangements, as to the rise of new ones.

Thirst too liberally and carelessly gratified, failing activity in the stomach, constipation, permanently declining renal secretions, muscular languor, and general wasting, comprise but a part of the disorders in warm climates or seasons which so evidently aggravate each other. The means of meeting these difficulties can only be understood by a fair consideration of the doctrine which explains their origin, course, and connection; but in this aggravated train we have a complicated case of constitutional or general irritation, which we shall reserve for future comment. It may seem at once conclusive, that if the blood possess the materials of supply, exertion will lead to increased nutrition of muscle or nerve; and so a stimulus will aid appetite and digestion.

The current hypothetical explanations of heat inducing undue hepatic excitement, do not appear to us satisfactory. The tropical coup-de-soleil we regard as only the sudden manifestation of a more gradual and general disorder. That yellow fever is an hepatitis, and that the oriental liver abscess, and chronic diseases, belong to the effects of climate, we cannot question; yet, seeing these affections are in a manner peculiar to visitors, whose varied habits, food, and drink, involve such a diversity of considerations, we may be excused for delaying to admit conjectures, which at the best are useless. The knowledge that warmth accelerates the processes of life even to the extent of wasting the materials of support, and the certainty when such considerable disturbances are set up that the especial stimulus of each function must be supplied or subtracted unequally, seems to be the first rational part of the account where one organ or system is found excited and another quiescent. There are, besides, specific sources of disturbance to be thought of, as in the liver from drinks.

We should not be unmindful that active hepatic diseases, inflammations, and hypertrophies, are common in our own temperate region. The difference dependent on climate is materially affected by particular seasons, by which the disorders are rendered more or less frequent and severe; while the less prominent morbid changes in the liver of our clime are to be attributed to the circumstance of other organs, as the kidneys, being sooner and more fatally involved.

We admit that the summer, with its exhaustions, occupations, and open windows, may render many persons additionally liable to disorders from various modes of influence, but we are not ready to admit that these instances of its effects are against our views until the processes leading to disorder have been fairly examined; for it must appear at a glance that the case is one of a complex kind, and that cold is by no means out of the question as a means of disturbance. The general disturbance of hay-fever, for example, we may often trace to cold, combined with peculiar susceptibility. Is not the diarrhœa of autumn somewhat like the renewal of a suspended function (the bowels being re-excited as the cutaneous functions decline), with the general disturbances of cold superadded? It has been often said that, with regard to understanding his own constitution and the management of it, a "man is either a fool or a physician at forty;" and although this does not by any means apply to the treatment of a sudden attack which is altogether new to the sufferer, it is a very just observation with respect to those who, possessing a moderate share of judgment and self-control, are compelled to be continually on the watch to keep a declining or enfeebled frame capable of daily

duty, under the influence of various kinds of exposure and exertion.

Common sense, observing that many feeble, or aged, or valetudinarian folks make a slight progress towards attaining vigour in the height of summer, concludes at once that they would necessarily be benefited by a mild and permanent tropical climate; and it is still more a matter of common observation that the delicate, or the asthmatic, or the rheumatic, prepare themselves, as well as they can, to endure and labour through (if not cut off by) the severity and variability of a great part of our year, which they have still more reason to tremble at and shun than they are really aware of.

There are constitutions so susceptible of cold as to require a *continual* summer in order that the general functions may reach even a medium share of development; and there are doubtless others to whom heat is as oppressive as the cold is invigorating; yet we think there is greater cause to wonder at the smallness of the disparity in this respect than to regard the inequality as inexplicable. The most essential fact of all is perhaps this, that a day or an hour, an injury, excess, or dose of medicine, or a fright, will, in certain states of constitution, make all the difference between severer exposure with impunity, and slighter cold with dangerous consequences.

A gentleman, who seemed never to have known sickness, complained severely of the chilly evenings on the Atlantic, when the thermometer stood at 80°. It is not to be supposed but that many persons do not continually take cold, even under the equator. Need we say, the delicate and feeble suffer as much in our summers.

We see that one seemingly strong man wears twice as much clothing as another*; we see women and children wearing habitually or irregularly almost nothing; we may see the balance of health sustained under great disadvantages, or overturned by one or a few repetitions of a comparatively slight exposure, under circumstances unfavourable to resistance. And what

* Though seemingly strong, there is perhaps some disproportion about his frame that renders him delicate, or his functions easily overbalanced; or the situation in life may render his habits unfavourable on account of some undue developments, as in the case of a muscular frame with sedentary occupation.

are we to conclude but that, although the compensatory means are great, they have their limits, which differ in different persons and in different seasons? The healthiest man, after sixty years of vicissitudes, takes cold, and is seized with the croup of infants, which, as to visceral disorganization at least, might seem among the most remote from any kind or degree of decay or general deterioration.

If any one ask what are the disorders likely to be benefitted by a warm climate, a partial answer is easily made, a complete one we deem an impossibility. All affections which are worse in winter and better in summer speak for themselves; and this is scarcely the time to advert to peculiarities and partial objections, unless it be to show by example some traits of constitution by which a judgment may be formed in practice.

We do not know a more established and neglected fact than that the cases of malformed heart are benefitted by warmth. Our own experience strongly favours the inference, that the acquired obstructions of the heart demand like facilities. When exercise is forbidden, warmth seems doubly available.

Hypertrophy of the muscle of a ventricle will never exceed the measure of the impediment on which it essentially depends (thickening of the secondary arteries, for a common example), but in the absence of due nutrition, or in consequence of extreme obstruction, the increase of muscular power will fall short of what is requisite. It is certain that if the causes of difficulty be diminished, as by superficial warmth and general facility of the functions (not copious assimilations), the ventricular hypertrophy must decline in proportion as surely as every part wastes through disuse. The chief mischief of hypertrophy of the heart is probably that it tends to operate with disproportionate violence on particular parts of the capillary system, as, for instance, on the brain; and if at any time the general state of the blood should dispose the body to inflammatory softening, the mechanical disturbance will determine the disorder to the cerebrum, just as a pediluvium may locate gout, or local cold excite erysipelas, or a stricture cystitis. We make a wide distinction between a true hypertrophy and a deteriorated tumefaction of muscle, but it

may be necessary to state that these changes are often combined. Dilatation of the heart is either the effect of failing nutrition or increased impediment, without corresponding increase of nourishment. (See an account of Angina in MEDICAL GAZETTE, 1841.) The most studious management of temperature and diet is of vital importance to ease and sustain the failing heart.

We are at a loss sufficiently to enforce our views relative to the means of oppressing or relieving a disordered viscus. We fear, too, that common practical views, as they are called, are firmly settled against us. Why should it be supposed that mercury, or any form of diuretic, can act beneficially on the kidney in any state besides that of simple inactivity? Can any thing relieve excessive action but derivation? Can any thing mend perverted action so much as a considerable attention to the due performance of all co-relative functions? Can any thing palliate the effects of settled renal induration and arrest of function so well as the unobstructed play of compensating eliminations?

Were it not for the prejudices of those who are strong and capable of free exercise, the admitted rule of practice relative to bronchitis, acute, or chronic, or variable, would need no new enforcing. How far are we from understanding that every *catarrh* is under like laws, and who will show that every kind of irritation which we have before endeavoured to analyze is not liable to be affected by the same? How many secretory disorders and structural disorganizations are the result, not of chronic disease, but of often repeated relapses, fresh attacks of *irritation* from cold and the like? And when one important function is obstructed by disorganization, what will ease the play of the rest like warmth? What will oppress the balance like cold? But we shall defer the full illustration of this great topic till we come to dwell on constitutional irritation.

The following are the particulars of a case which is in a measure the origin and ground-work of all the reflections here assembled:—

" A delicate boy, at thirteen years of age, had ague, and subsequently often experienced feverishness in chilly weather. At sixteen, after dining and running violently, he first felt dyspnœa, and for many years from this time he rarely passed ten months without suffering from fever and suppuration near the tonsils. Between study and activity his spirits were always good. Autumn after autumn he became more subject to cold during the day, which after dinner was manifested by dyspnœa, easy cough, and some sense of fatigue. Every exposure caused a fresh attack; confined diet, relaxation, free exercise, warmth, or conium and ipecacuanha, brought relief. Severe exposure induced a week or two of bronchitis. The summer inland air of Kent aggravated the asthma, and especially with the least exposure to cold. Sitting in church never failed to disturb the health. The erect posture, maintained, governed the dyspnœa. Towards his thirtieth year, with a slight cough and expectoration, varying through several months, he continued to become more susceptible of cold and to waste in substance; his old dyspnœa was frequent and troublesome; his rustication in the country was disadvantageous as to exposures, and not successful. After exerting his voice he coughed up about 2½ oz. of blood, and his medical friends looked on his case very gravely, but he himself felt that a recess would restore him as usual.

His pursuits and habits had been a little unsalutary; his strength, appetite, activity, and sleep, were always good, and the country, or rather repose with comfort, so constantly and quickly renovated him (save sometimes as to dyspnœa), that he could not but rely on so well tried a resource. His pulse, sitting, rarely amounted to 70, and he detected no feverish symptoms except briefly after exposures; he perspired, however, somewhat at night, and too easily at other times, having been gradually obliged to increase his clothing a good deal. Still he took cold on the least exposure, and on all occasions,—in bed, at church, and finally in the parlour. Countless varied experiments seemed to prove this. Though he could but just perceive or detect the occasion in a few hours, it was proved by sneezing, catarrh, dyspnœa, or languor; he found that all late meals disturbed his breathing, and that to feed lowly and keep close, quickly set all right, though probably the regimen increased his susceptibility to derangement. Notwithstanding a long

decline by little relapses, and the evidence that the bronchi were so weak, his former ready restorations by care and air made him think that a sudden hæmoptysis without dyspnœa would still subside with sufficient care. The hæmorrhage did not last half an hour. Though it did not disappear until the third day, it was evident that the rest of the blood had remained in the tubes, as it came away in little clots, decreasing in size, colour, brightness, and the firmness, with usual unopaque expectoration. A day or two before, he had felt a little uneasiness in the larynx; cough, with a slight sense of pricking; and fever, quicker pulse, and decline followed. No plan seemed comfortable enough but a warm bed. Flatulence, diarrhœa with blood, perspiration, and wasting followed, and a sense of having taking cold daily, or oftener, always introduced the deepest aggravations. Still, circumstances seemed to have combined a succession of unavoidable exposures and ill-ordered rooms, notwithstanding the will to avoid them for a period of two months, during which he was still declining, though by slow degrees, while living on the coast. His chief meal was reduced to three or four oysters per diem.

He embarked for warmer climates in December, and felt for the first time at liberty to take to bed and exclude all cold. He had no vomiting after the first hour on board ship, and from that time his convalescence was uninterrupted unless by too free an exposure, and the only inconvenience he experienced during five months in the West Indies was from cold, through that general absence of protection which all besides valued so much and purposely secured. On reapproaching colder regions, comparatively stout and active, every care seemed necessary; and ever since, warmth has been his friend, and cold his enemy.

We are well convinced that such cases of variable affections, and many widely different, are strictly dependent on variations of temperature and similar causes which affect the general balance of the animal functions.

A sister in the ward of a London Hospital, whose occupation and apartments are ill adapted for a delicate person, had, in the progress of many months, become asthmatic, hectic, and wasted, and only waited till forbearance could forbear no longer to be dismissed from her post. A new stove, listed doors, and better clothing, seem to have restored this patient to her duty; her situation, however, is trying enough to an extremely delicate frame at about 30 years of age, and much judicious care is necessary for such a case.

A gentleman of great wealth, and without mental resources, became addicted to the excesses of the table to a remarkable degree; he retired to rest late under a huge quantity of bed-clothes, and this training seems to have been for many years the means of consuming the superabundance, and renewing his appetite for dinner. He took but a little regular exercise and wore warm clothing.

Mr. E. F., of Bermondsey, about 28 years of age, of a strong lean figure, had an attack of continued fever, which wasted him for near a month. We gave him abundant counsel to avoid the causes of relapse, but at length he left his bed to sit by the fire in an ill-appointed parlour. From day to day symptoms of decline became more apparent, loss of appetite and cheerfulness, feverishness and night perspirations, cough and expectoration, all made him fearful, and he slept but little. The only remedy enforced in this case was a complete second suit of clothes, and the unhappy symptoms all rapidly vanished.

The disorders which are to be treated with warmth, as a means of facilitating the process of recovery, may be considered as comparatively simple, but those which may be advantageously submitted to heat as a kind of heroic remedy are to be regarded with yet more serious attention. The affections are serious, and the treatment may seem severe, and cannot be safely taken in hand without much knowledge and discretion. Distressing rheumatic pains, recurrent almost weekly for six or eight years, aggravated by so many winters, and perhaps by a much greater number of deliberate medical sieges and sappings, will not evacuate their strong holds with slight measures of a few days' continuance; yet we have known a lady, between forty and fifty years of age, carried on board ship, a sad cripple, and almost a hopeless sufferer from such an affection, being unable to help herself into her carriage, whose complaints were giving way before half the winter had passed in Jamaica,

and who returned to England in the summer perfectly cured.

Some vulgar proverbs point forcibly enough to the fact, that the feeble often outlive the robust, and no doubt the chief point of the explanation is, that the former are careful, and the latter careless; but can we reflect on the sources of mischief incidental to both, without concluding, that exposure to cold is the most certain and frequent danger that can be named, and which generally might be found to have been avoided on the one hand and incurred on the other?

It is surprising how frequently and easily many invalids do take cold, and often without knowing when or where, or how (not being very considerate); and it is important to reflect, that a disturbance being set up in the body, how readily the weakest or most deteriorated organ seems to become oppressed. To persons in health, it is very certain that warm apartments, luxurious beds, and undue clothing, enervate and induce languor, and thus increase the susceptibility to disease; but, on the contrary, almost every one in turn, unless prematurely cut off, comes to find the want of increasing warmth and comfort.

It is little to assert that the warmth that overpowers some is vitally essential to others. We do not scruple, at least with every month of the year, to point out the fact in a great hospital, where one or another falls a victim to ventilation—an accident, an operation, a chronic disease, is cut short by a sudden phlegmasia* ; an acute affection in progress of cure is unawares fatally aggravated or supplanted by another; one patient escapes through half a dozen dangerous relapses, only to be cut off by the next. The repeated relapses of chronic, or more strictly speaking variable disorders, and the metastases and protean alternations of others, are not to be fully explained without reference to the like influences.

We defer commenting on the varying quantities of heat that air removes in proportion to the rapidity of its motion over the surface of the body in different cases; the effect of dry air on a moist surface; the probable proportions of heat in different diatheses, ages, and disorders; and also the irregular dis-

---

* See the account of open fractures, in the Cyclopædia of Surgery, and the Causes of Strangulation in Hernia, Guy's Hosp. Rep. No. 7, and Med. Gaz. May 1843,

tribution of heat and sensations of cold which are experienced under peculiar circumstances. The feverish man complains of cold, where a delicate female (having perhaps just dined) complains of heat. One enters the house after a walk and feels oppressive heat, when another leaving an easy close carriage finds it chilly ; in the course of twenty minutes these sensations may be reversed.

It may, we hope, be now conceded that warmth like other remedies is to be employed as it is needed. More than this we would not ask ; for, having indicated the general importance of our views, we grant that the disadvantages of heat, as of all medical disturbance, render it essential to employ as little as the emergency requires. The method of administering warmth, whether singly or in combination, we may yet endeavour to determine, although much must be left to experience, and a little to experiment. On the whole a warm house seems most like a warm climate. It admits of great freedom, little or no additional clothing may be needed when about to move actively out of doors. Perspiration is to be moderated, and the internal functions regulated. And all this is by no means difficult under favourable circumstances.

The practices of different nations, as the Swedes and Russians, and others, might afford many useful lessons with regard to what is safe and salutary in the application of warmth : but it is not pretended to be universally specific in its action as a remedial agent ; but as an ever present means to use or to abuse, it must exert its proportionate influence on our economy.

The harmlessness of long-continued heat is forcibly shewn in the following fact. A gentleman who laboured under mild typhus, and was naturally very sensible of cold, remained from choice during two months of winter in a temperature strictly regulated, between 65° and 70° (rarely a little higher), and he was besides always well covered. When his convalescence was considerably advanced, circumstances obliged him to leave all his comforts entirely, and to expose himself in snowy weather both out of doors and in very unfavourable apartments. This was done not altogether without care, but he expresses his conviction that the warm regimen assisted very much to enable his frame to resist the mischiefs. He endured a week of exposures and some serious difficulties, with but slight uneasiness, and to him unusual and unexpected impunity.

Some persons may ask how can it be safe to leave a warm place and to discontinue the artificial comforts ? The answer is plain. Invalids are not the worse for temporary confinement to bed, or to a comfortable parlour. Those who have regained their health by going to a hot country, find it quite safe to return ; and in our own country it is far more easy to obtain a warm climate without dangers, delays, or discomforts, and equally easy to try to leave it by degrees, although it is probably true that a few persons of peculiar constitution cannot live long without the constant comfort of great warmth. Accordingly we find every now and then, one who is compelled to do the best his knowledge and circumstances admit of to form a perpetual summer about him. With judgment and care there seems to be no reason to anticipate any source of mischief, and surely it may not be too much to express a hope that we may one day see such plans in operation in a part of every great charity, in some establishments for education, and in various situations for the comfort of the feeble, and the aged of all classes.

When warmth is required strength is gained by having recourse to it, and strength being thus gained, diminished temperature becomes gradually required, and is often attended with proportionate increase of strength and benefit.

We have already in part explained how it happens that when the vigour is restored by comfort, a freer diet, more exercise, and even diminished clothing, are not incompatible with exposure even to the severities of winter. We may often return to the illustration of this observation.

The very objection to thermal comfort made by many judicious and well-informed persons is one of the most striking and general proofs of the advantages and necessity of securing feeble persons against cold.

It is constantly advanced that persons may not suddenly leave a warm climate without danger. The grand intention of artificial warmth should be simply to obviate this evil : to guard against the constant or casual inconveniences of our own climate, to invigorate and prepare the delicate to bear them, and to enable them to take the full benefit of every favourable season or even turn of weather. It cannot be denied that one who cannot bear a favourable English summer, even with care, may return from the tropics able to endure unhurt a severe winter, and that with little or no care.

It is both foolish and false, between error and wilfulness, to contend that heat must of necessity relax or enfeeble. Why are the first days of convalescence those of confinement, perhaps even to bed? What is the chief cause of relapses? The early neglect of comfort is the evil to be feared; it represses every natural and restorative action that the infantile condition demands. What more certain advantage of the sea-side to tender subjects than mild and equable temperature? What more real and tangible in the benefit of "country air," as we say, than quitting bad habits for protracted gentle exercise, long rest in bed free from exposure, and full diet, by which a free and equal swing is given to all functions?

Artizans exposed to heat and cold in a very irregular manner, and without either disposition or judgment to protect themselves, are yet enabled, in a vast number of instances, to grow old in their employments without any material impediment or discomfort.

The solid objections to the use of warmth, and the precautions and aims to be considered with it, are like those connected with all remedial operations. The theory of general irritation, which we shall endeavour to unfold, may be the means of reflecting some light on all these points.

The opinions of Sir George Lefevre, "Thermal Comfort," lately published, appear to us well deserving attention. The perusal of these, and the retrospect of our own reflections, leave us more than ever strongly impressed with the conclusion, that a still more careful analysis of physiological processes is to be alike the main basis of pathology and therapeutics. We apply the following quotation with some confidence to the study of heat and cold.

"Be assured there is no little analogy between the duties of the military and those of the medical profession. The physician is the general; the Pharmacopœia—using this term in a very wide acceptation—is his army; the disease is the enemy opposed to him. He has his skirmishes, as well as his pitched battles, to fight. He has his long campaigns, as well as his sudden encounters, to be prepared for. He has his outposts to look after, his guards to set, his entrenchments to fortify, his garrisons to subsist. His commissariat, as well as his gunnery and ammunition stores, must be attended to. When apparently most secure, he is liable to sudden surprises and inroads; the work of one hour may upset the exertions of a whole month; the events of one day may ruin the labour of years. And, last of all, he must be prepared for many emergencies which no human vigilance can foresee, and no human prudence can prevent. A passing storm may lay prostrate in a moment his wisest preparations; or the undermining influence of fear and despondency may render them all of no avail. No set of men surely ought to know better, or feel more deeply, than the soldier and the physician, the full force of the saying, that "the race is not to the swift, nor the battle to the strong*.""

36, Bedford Square.

EVIL CONSEQUENCES
OF THE
TOO EARLY APPLICATION OF THE
STARCHED BANDAGE IN A CASE
OF SIMPLE FRACTURE OF
THE FORE-ARM.

To the Editor of the Medical Gazette.

SIR,

SHOULD the following be thought worthy of a place in the MEDICAL GAZETTE, an early insertion in its columns would much oblige the writer.

I am, sir,
Your obedient servant,
D. M'CASH, Surgeon.

July 1843.

I was called upon a considerable time ago to visit a boy twelve years of age, and of slender conformation, who had fallen from the top of an old wall to the ground, and was supposed to have

---

* Med.-Chir. Rev. No. 77, p. 167.

sustained a fracture of the arm. On arriving at the house I found the patient seated in an easy chair, with the injured arm resting on a cushion, and all his members agitated by the intensity of his sufferings. The history of the case and the appearance of the arm at once betrayed the nature of the injury, and enabled me without hesitation to come to the conclusion that the forearm must be broken in both its bones midway between the wrist and elbow. Manipulation detected crepitus and considerable displacement. The lower half of the fore-arm was bent in a forward direction upon the upper at an angle of nearly twelve degrees. Power of motion was completely destroyed, and a good deal of distortion existed round the fracture. Only half an hour had elapsed since the time of the accident, and no inflammatory symptoms had yet begun to show themselves. The fracture was easily reduced, but an obstacle to keeping it so until the apparatus had been applied, arose in the occurrence of violent spasmodic contractions of the flexor and extensor muscles. Had recourse to camomile fomentations to the part, and administered a dose of sulph. magnes. holding in combination a small proportion of the tartrate of antimony. A short time previous I had been reading some accounts by Velpeau of the successful application of *la bandage immobile* in cases of simple fracture newly contracted, and pleased with the nature of the details, had resolved on giving it a trial in the first suitable case that should present itself. Several circumstances seemed to me to point out the present case as adapted to my purpose, and on the strength of Velpeau's recommendation, proceeded without loss of time to have the arm encased within the folds of the starched bandage. Patient complained a good deal of pain and tightness on its first application, but being assured these unpleasant symptoms would abate as soon as the evaporation of the moisture should impart looseness to the bandage, he bore up with his difficulties for a time, and before the lapse of half an hour had sunk into a refreshing sleep. Saw him next morning, and found every thing in the condition I could have desired them to be. Pain had been very severe during the night, but had subsided towards the morning, and was now less than it had

any previous time been. A litttle constitutional disturbance was discoverable, but no prominent symptom existed to cause alarm. Bowels had been twice moved during the night, and several ineffectual attempts had been made to vomit. Being called away in a hurry to some distance from the scene of the accident, upwards of seven weeks elapsed before I had an opportunity again of revisiting my patient. During my absence, except a few days after I left him, the boy had continued without any considerable pain, had betaken himself to play, and favourable hopes were entertained by the parents that he would be all to rights again as soon as my return should sanction the removal of his bandage. On the eighth week after its application, I cut open the bandage and exposed the naked arm. Bones were in perfect apposition and firmly united. A glueing of callus was still discoverable around the joint. The finger and wrist joints were stiff and immoveable even under the strongest endeavours of the patient to make them yield. But these disagreeable circumstances were viewed as the necessary consequences of their previous disuse, and no doubts were entertained but that their flexibility would return as the frequency of attempts to exercise them would increase. The cure seemed so complete, that only a few days were deemed necessary to allow of the parts recovering their natural condition, when the boy should be set at liberty and return to school. Fearful, however, lest the excitement of being allowed his freedom, should betray him into acts of indiscretion, and occasion untoward circumstances to his arm, I caused him to wear a splint for a time, and keep his arm suspended in a sling until the union of his broken bones should become more complete. The splint was applied along the inner aspect of the arm, and in order that he should exercise his hand, extended only from the bend of the arm to the wrist. Circumstances again prevented me from seeing him for nearly five months; when the following was found to be the condition of the arm. I may here state for my own justification, that I was only an occasional visitor at the house of a friend where the boy laid, and allowed myself to interfere with the case from the circumstance only that there happened to be no resident medical man in the place, and of my being on the spot near which the accident occured. The parts had previously assumed a pliant inactive condition from which they had not yet attempted to recover, but allowed themselves to be modified, and acted upon by every concurrent circumstance, for good or for evil, without evincing any tendency on their own part to regain their natural condition. The fracture was still firmly united, and the callus was nearly all absorbed. The fleshy part of the arm unusually round and firm, conveying the impression, when handled, as if the muscles were matted together. Flexion and extension, save to a very limited degree, quite destroyed. The wrist drooped over the end of the splint, and was beyond the control of the patient. The fingers were rigidly hooked upon the palm of the hand, and likewise defied all attempts on the part of the patient to make them straight. Sensation undiminished. Arm a little emaciated, and rendered totally useless as an organ of prehension. The tendons of the flexor muscles were prominent at the wrist, and resembled contracted cords passing on to the hand. On a more close examination of the case, it became perfectly evident that such an undescribable state of things depended, not upon any rigidity of the joints, but on a certain abnormal condition of the muscles whose office it was to move them; for though flexion and extension, as well as pronation and supination, were materially impaired to the patient, who required the aid of the other hand to make his fingers move, yet these motions were not so utterly suspended as to be beyond the power of being performed by the aid of a bystander; with these restrictions, however, that when the carpus was pulled up into the line of the fore-arm, the fingers hooked the more, and conversely the fingers were capable of being brought into the straight position only through the instrumentality of the bend at the wrist. Such seemed to be the permanent condition assumed by the parts. Patient complained of no pain, and seemed to have accommodated his disposition to the altered condition of his arm. When he requires to carry any weight by the affected limb, the body *requires to* be hung round upon his

contracted fingers, as upon an inert hook appended to his arm. If I were asked what deviations from the healthy condition of parts would be discovered by dissection of the arm, my answer would be—All the usual consequences of acute subjacent inflammation terminating short of the formation of pus; thickening and condensation of all the tissues; a copious deposition of organised lymph around and into the substance of muscles; morbid adhesions of one part to another, with all the other changes due to the same cause, to which alone the loss of motion of the limb was attributable. I have said subjacent inflammation, for the rigid bandage acted exactly the same part as a tense fascia over the morbid action which was going on beneath it. If the question were repeated, in how far were all these untoward circumstances so prejudicial to the walking of the patient connected with the treatment which was followed for his recovery, my reply would be in affirmation of their connection being so nearly united that the one might almost be regarded as the consequence of the other. To say unhesitatingly that the case would have terminated more favourably under the splint and-roller treatment, would be to assume a stronger position than the nature of the premises would allow; but certainly I think there are few surgeons of the present day who would have been prepared to meet the consequences which ensued. My own conviction is that 80 at least out of 100 of such cases, treated with the ordinary remedies, would have done well. For the want of success, however, attending the present case, I would not by any means depreciate the starched bandage as a remedial means, for in my opinion it must ever be regarded as a valuable addition to our surgical *armamentarium ;* but the position I would wish to see subverted is that of Sendin, the inventor, who attributes the principal share of its utility to earliness of application. Never was the invention of a useful instrument so overshadowed by wrong directions for its use, and perhaps there are few appliances from which more baneful consequences by injudicious management could be made to flow. No prudent surgeon should overlook the guidance of his own judgment in the promulgated advices of authors and inventors, however authoritative they may seem, as to resort to such constricting measures in the treatment of fractures as the starched bandages before the inflammatory period which succeeds every accident has gone over, and the parts have subsided into their due medium of action. Such is the proper period for deriving its full advantage; but to apply it before this time is to impose a control upon nature which she will not suffer, and consequences most prejudicial to the reputation of the surgeon are almost certain to ensue; for every one but moderately versed in his profession, who, while he knows what benefit is to be derived from depletion, and the removal of tension in inflamed parts, must, at the same time, be aware what will be the nature of the results when not only these salutary measures have been neglected, but a treatment of the very adverse kind pursued. It reminds me of a commandment which would say, throw water into the fire, and you will extinguish it, while the person spoken to not only disregards the precaution but adds more fuel to the flame, with the intention in his view of accomplishing the same end, and in the blindfoldedness of his error allows the fabric to be consumed or rendered unfit for use. The case I have related, by following the directions of others rather than in attending to my own judgment, affords a vivid illustration of this figure, and if errors blindly contracted may be forgiven, I would not hesitate to affirm that the consequences which ensued were the effects of the practice employed. It may form a warning to others, and as such I give it without reserve. Three years have now elapsed since the occurrence of the accident cited; the arm continues as unserviceable as before.

ON THE

FUNCTIONS OF THE LACTEALS.

To the Editor of the Medical Gazette.

Sir,

If you think the accompanying paper worthy of a place in your journal I should feel much obliged by its insertion.—I am, sir,

Your obedient servant,
SAMUEL FENWICK, M.R.C.S.

St. Alban's, July 7, 1843.

After the constant discussion which the subject of absorption has of late years undergone, it seems now to be the general opinion, that whilst this property in the rest of the body is exclusively possessed by the blood-vessels, it is also shared in the intestines by the lacteals. The experiments of Magendie, and other physiologists, have clearly shown that the lymphatics of other parts never, under any circumstances, absorb, and doubtless from the similarity in their structure, and in their condition, in an empty state of the intestinal canal, the same would have been inferred of the lacteals, but that their turgid state during digestion, and an apparent analogy between them and the roots of vegetables, have misled inquirers into their functions. It is my object to show, that in the intestines, or elsewhere, the absorbing power resides entirely in the blood-vessels, and that the lacteals act only as ducts to carry away the nutritive matters taken up by the former, their existence being necessarily required on account of the impediment to the circulation through these blood-vessels (when distended with the fluids they have just absorbed), arising from the blood which has already supplied the intestines having to pass through the capillary circulation of the liver.

In attempting to demonstrate the above statement, it will be necessary first, to prove that the lacteals cannot of themselves absorb.

1st, Segallas placed poison in the intestine of an animal, and tied the vessels of the part. No symptoms of poisoning took place in one hour, although here the lacteals were unobstructed.

2d, I filled the intestine of a rabbit with milk, and isolating a portion of it by ligature, deprived it of its circulation by tying its mesenteric vessels, and returned the bowel into the abdomen. On examining it afterwards, no absorption had taken place in the isolated portion, although the lacteals of the *contiguous* portion of intestine were fully distended.

3d, I drew out a loop of intestine from the abdomen of a rabbit which had been previously fed (the lacteals being then distended with chyle), and tied the vessels leading to it, at the same time cutting off any vascular connexion with the contiguous portions of gut by ligature. In a short time, on inspecting the animal, the intestinal lacteals on the isolated portion were found emptied, whilst those of the mesentery and of the neighbouring portions of the bowel were still filled with fluid.

It is evident, from the result of the above experiments, that the distension of the lacteals is in some manner connected with the circulation: they prove that the so-called lacteal absorption depends neither on simple capillary attraction, nor upon this force, assisted by the distension of their *mouths* by the influx of blood which takes place during digestion (for the blood was here retained in its vessels and no absorption ensued); and that it does not arise from any ciliary motion, or nervous influence, is evident from the third experiment, as the chyle was found to have been carried forwards into the lacteals of the mesentery—a sufficient proof that nervous influence must have continued in the intestine after absorption had terminated.

It being thus proved that the lacteals do not absorb, it becomes necessary, in the next place, to examine some of the arguments by which the opinion that the blood-vessels perform this function is supported.

1st, Delille and Magendie tied the lacteals of a portion of intestine in a living animal, leaving the blood-vessels unobstructed, and found the usual effects produced on injecting poisons into the gut.

2d, Fodera and others detected salts in the mesenteric veins after injecting them into the intestines.

3d, Tiedemann, Gmelin, and Meyer, have observed *chyle* in the mesenteric and portal veins.

4th, Absorption in many of the lower orders of animals is carried on entirely by the blood-vessels, no trace of lymphatics or lacteals having been discovered in them.

5th, I would refer more especially to a paper lately published in the MEDICAL GAZETTE by my talented friend Mr. Robinson, in which it is shown that the whole process of absorption depends upon physical principles, and that a current of any fluid is alone necessary to explain the phenomenon, without having occasion to *call to our* aid any mysterious and *unknown principle of attraction* to

account for what takes place in the living body.

Having seen, 1st, that the lacteals, when deprived of the circulation (even though nervous influence, and a certain degree of turgidity of the part, are maintained) cannot absorb any fluid, not even the chyle, which it is supposed to be their peculiar property to take up; and 3dly, that the blood-vessels can and do perform this function, which simply depends upon the physical power possessed by any stream of fluid; we have now to assign reasons rendering it probable that the use of the lacteals is only to convey the chyle absorbed by the blood-vessels.

1st, It has been observed, that when fluids are injected into the intestine they appear to enter equally the blood-vessels and the lacteals: thus, in the experiments of Fodera, a solution of prussiate of potassa was injected into the intestine, and on testing the fluids of the blood-vessels and lacteals with sulphate of iron, both were found to contain the same salt; and as we have before proved that the lacteals cannot, and the blood-vessels can, and do, absorb salts, it follows, that the prussiate of potassa must have entered the latter before their appearance in the lacteals.

2dly. If we look to comparative anatomy, we discover that no great development of the lacteal system is observed, until we reach that part of the animal scale where the intestinal blood has to pass through the capillary circulation of the liver; and on considering this circumstance, it will be found to afford a strong argument in favour of the theory here advanced. The heart's action being augmented in strength and frequency whilst digestion is going on, the rapidity of intestinal circulation is greatly increased, but at the same time, the vessels being in contact with a quantity of fluids, the products of digestion, they must by the physical laws above referred to commence to absorb them. They will by these means soon become gorged, in consequence of the *vis a tergo* forcing on their contents faster than they can be discharged into the general circulation, on account of the mechanical obstacles opposed by the capillary circulation of the liver. What, then, must be the natural result of this engorgement? either the fluids contained in the blood-vessels must flow through their sides, or a complete stoppage of the circulation will take place. The porous structure of the capillaries prevents the latter, and if it were not for the distension of the intestinal tube by the digested materials, and its constant contractions, it is probable that the newly absorbed fluids would again pass into the cavity of the gut. But this being prevented the chyle oozes out of the blood-vessels into the capillary lacteals, which are placed within a net-work of vessels for this purpose in the villi of the intestines.

Viewing the whole mucous membrane of the intestines in this light, we perceive each villus to form a complete gland, agreeing with the other glandular tissues of the body in structure, as it consists of a ramification of blood-vessels and capillary ducts, (the latter being the lacteals,) the former for the separation and the latter for the transmission of its secretion (the chyle) : the whole series of smaller ducts eventually uniting, as in other glands, to form one large conducting tube, the thoracic duct, and only differing from the generality of glands in use, as its secretion consists of matters lately absorbed and necessary for nutrition, and in its function being regulated by mechanical forces, uncontrolled by nervous energy.

It has been considered, that the lacteals were invested with the peculiar property of selecting the materials necessary for the nourishment of the body, whilst the blood-vessels not being equally gifted with discernment, indiscriminately took up whatever was presented to them; but the fact of the lacteals when tied still continuing to absorb, was always felt to complicate the theory of the functions of the rival vessels; it is evident, however, if the above statement of their use be correct, that this admits of an easy explanation : when a lacteal is tied, the blood-vessels being uninjured will continue to absorb the chyle, and pour it into the obstructed vessel, until, as observed by experimentalists, it appears ready to burst: the pressure of the fluids in the blood-vessels being then balanced by that in the distended lacteal, no more will enter, but as the surrounding vessels become restored to their usual degree of distension, when digestion is finished the fluid in the obstructed

lacteal will flow back again into the blood-vessels, and cause the empty state of the lacteal which is observed to take place after some time has elapsed.

The only two objections to this theory, which appear to me of sufficient force to merit notice, are the following :—

1st. The fact of the chyle being usually of a white colour, so that it is generally said the lacteals refuse to take up colouring matters. But if we reflect how little of any colouring matter is usually prepared for absorption by the digestive process, as evinced by the colour of the excrements of herbivorous animals, and when we consider how much more easy it is to detect by tests colouring matters in a clear fluid like urine, than to observe any slight change of colour in chyle, this objection loses much of its importance. Besides, many physiologists have most distinctly observed the lacteals filled with coloured fluids, which had been injected into the intestines, and there is no doubt that the lymphatics of the liver have been seen containing bile in cases of jaundice, and that those of the spleen frequently contain blood globules, which is very likely to happen in an organ so constituted, and so prone to congestion.

2d. Müller remarks that the globules of chyle are much larger than the capillary blood-vessels, and on this account an objection may be raised; but we do not yet know whether the chyle or similar fluids, when absorbed, do contain globules, indeed, I am inclined to suppose that in most cases these microscopical bodies are not formed until after the fluid has entered the vessels, for if globules of chyle, pus, &c. of so large a size can enter the pores of the lacteals, these pores should be apparent; and how do we find deposits of pus in various textures of the body, if the capillaries of these parts be too small to admit the globules?

Whether the above theory of the use of the lacteals may be extended to explain that of the other parts of the lymphatic system, we have not yet sufficient facts to determine; indeed, more experimental evidence should have been adduced in support of the subject of the present paper, but being at present, from other engagements, debarred from pursuing the subject, and being myself fully convinced of the correctness of the theory, I deemed it proper to submit it at once to the investigation of others, who, being unprejudiced in its favour, may be able more candidly than myself to judge of its truth, or extend its applications.

HEMIPLEGIA CONSEQUENT ON SYPHILIS.

To the Editor of the Medical Gazette.

SIR,

IN the MEDICAL GAZETTE of May 27, 1842, Dr. Budd has called attention to some cases concurrent with, or depending upon, the presence of the syphilitic virus in the system. Since hearing that clinical lecture, I have paid much attention to the subject, and have been fortunate enough to meet with other cases, which, like those he records, seem fairly traceable to the same disease.

Richard Potts, æt. 32, millwright, of temperate habits, was admitted into the Liverpool Infirmary, Feb. 20, 1843, with hemiplegia. Stated that two years ago he contracted the venereal disease, and that since that he has suffered from sore-throat four several times. Soon after he was cured from the last attack (which was very obstinate), he had a trifling paralytic seizure. About five weeks subsequently he had another attack, which deprived him of his senses for a time, as well as the power of using the left side. Sight and speech he regained under the use of mercury; the muscular power by the repeated application of galvanic shocks soon after his admission : he had a venereal eruption on the skin, which was still upon him when he was discharged.

Thomas Dolan, æt. 27, admitted April 4th, states that he had syphilis three years ago, when he had chancres for nine months; during this time he had an eruption on the skin, which lasted three months. Two years ago he had sore-throat for six months; and twelve months ago, had pain in the shin-bones and ankles, which were always worse at night. He has frequently been subject to pains in his head, which became constant soon *after the* other secondary symptoms

were subdued, and continued till a few days before his admission, when he found that he had suddenly lost the use of the right side—his intellect not being affected. He recovered rapidly under the use of calomel and antimony.

John White, æt. 32, cooper, admitted 25th March for cataract in the left eye. States that two years ago he had syphilis, and subsequently nodes on the shin-bones during twelve months, for which he was salivated. For the last year has felt ill, but cannot describe any prominent symptom, except an occasional sore-throat. Seven weeks ago, while at his work, he suddenly lost the use of the right side, retaining his intellects entire. He recovered rapidly under the influence of mercury.

Owen Richards, æt. 30, clerk in an office, was admitted with complete hemiplegia of the right side (the face being much drawn to the left), which had occurred a few days prior to his admission. At the invasion of the attack he had been deprived of his senses for some time, and was, while in the hospital, unable to articulate distinctly. His history is therefore necessarily imperfect. He called my attention, however, to a large chancre situated on the glans, which I ascertained had been contracted at least three months before the paralytic seizure. He greatly benefitted under the use of mercury, sarsaparilla, and the iodide of potassium; but went out at his own request before he was completely restored.

Mr. R. A., whose history I have not been able to procure in detail, was subject to repeated attacks of hemiplegia, the first of which came on when he was about 33. He had been frequently before this the subject of the venereal disease, though the character of the secondary symptoms I have not been able to procure.

I may also call attention to a case which Dr. Todd, of King's College Hospital, made public; that of a young prostitute, æt. 21, who was covered with a venereal eruption at the time of her admission. It appears that she had been suddenly deprived of her senses, and on regaining them found that she had lost the use of the left side. This case subsequently proved fatal, and a *post-mortem* revealed inflammation of one cerebral hemisphere and red softening of the other.

It may, perhaps, be questioned how far I am correct in associating these cases with the syphilitic diathesis; and attributing the apoplectic attacks, to the effects of that virus. It may be urged, that instances not unfrequently occur in young subjects, for which no cause can be assigned on the most rigorous investigation; that the cases adduced may be those of simple co-incidences, and that the two diseases, though contemporaneous, do not stand in the relation of cause and effect. It may be urged, moreover, that if there were such a marked association, it could not fail to have attracted the attention of some of the numerous writers who have treated on syphilis, by whom no mention is made of it. At present, perhaps these arguments cannot be altogether overthrown; but they will be strongly opposed by considering the general statistics of apoplexy. Out of 128 cases recorded by Morgagni, Andral, and Rochoux, 16 only occurred in persons below forty; in four the attack was distinctly referrible to over exertion, or excess in drinking; while in the others, no cause was assigned. This refers chiefly, however, to the graver forms of apoplexy; but when we examine into the statistics of hemiplegia, we shall find the disproportion fully as great, if not greater. In the four cases Dr. Budd records, and in those mentioned above, the patients were all under forty years of age, and we are naturally led to inquire into the cause of so unusual an occurrence. In all, we find that they have been subject for a greater or less time to syphilis: we know the formidable nature of that virus when introduced into the system, and being unable to find any other cause, naturally attribute it to that which is apparent. That the effects of mercury have no part in the matter is I think sufficiently proved, by its beneficial influence upon the disease, of which we can scarcely suppose it both the cause and cure.

As regards the way in which the virus may be supposed to act, I can add nothing to the remarks made by Dr. Budd, the only fatal case on record I have seen being that of Dr. Todd, which is shortly detailed above.

I have not, sir, troubled you with these remarks, so much to advance any speculation of my own, as to call the attention of your readers to a subject which cannot fail to be interesting, and which, before it can be fully established, requires a much more extended series of observations.—I am, sir,

Your obedient servant,
THOMAS INMAN, M.B.
House Surgeon.
Infirmary, Liverpool, July 9th, 1843.

EARLY MARRIAGES SO COMMON IN ORIENTAL COUNTRIES NO PROOF OF EARLY PUBERTY.

To the Editor of the Medical Gazette.

SIR,

I REQUEST the favour of your giving insertion to the accompanying paper (or such an abstract of it as you may think proper), in any number of the MEDICAL GAZETTE that may be convenient.—I am, sir,

Your obedient servant,
JOHN ROBERTON.
Manchester, July 8, 1843.

In two papers on the Natural History of Puberty, published in the Numbers of this Journal* for October 1832 and July 1842, I have attempted to prove, in oposition to the generally received opinion, that the age of puberty is as early in the cold as in the tropical regions of the earth; and that, were marriages to take place in England at as juvenile an age as they do in Hindostan, instances of very early fecundity would be as common in England as they are in the latter.

In the papers just mentioned, I have expressed an opinion, that early marriage and early intercourse between the sexes, wherever found generally prevailing, are to be attributed not to any peculiar precocity, but to moral and political degradation, exhibited in ill laws and customs, the enslavement more or less of the women, ignorance of letters, and impure or debasing systems of religion. In proof of this opinion I expect to be able to show that *in England, at a period when some of the unfavourable circumstances just mentioned as yet lingered amongst us, early marriages were very common, if not in all ranks certainly among the gentry ; and that such marriages were likewise common very recently among both high and low in Ireland.*

* Edinburgh Medical and Surgical Journal.

Before entering on the evidence for this curious and hitherto unnoticed fact,—unnoticed I mean in connection with the present subject of inquiry, it may be well to state what is the age of marriage in some European countries, lying, like England, in the temperate zone, and therefore experiencing the same or nearly the same climate, but where the mass of the people, from moral or political causes, and commonly both, are sunk in gross ignorance, or at best, with slow and doubtful progress, emerging from it.

It is to be recollected, that, though I have alluded to Hindostan by way of example, as a land of early marriages, such marriages are found in the coldest climates,—found as commonly among the Esquimaux of North America and the tribes along the shores of Siberia, as on the burning plains of the Carnatic or in the islands of the Indian Ocean,—equally in the inclement Archipelago of Terra del Fuego,[*] as among the tribes on the Orinoco,—among the Kirgis with their herds of Yaks, in the perpetual snows of Pamir at the fountain of the Oxus,[†] as in the verdant and sunny island of Ceylon. In every country, supposing the simple means of subsistence easily attainable, and even generally where it is otherwise, if the people are strangers to the Christian Scriptures, or to the civilization of the more favoured European nations, which has its root in the Scriptures, *there* the female sex remains uneducated and unhonoured, bought and sold, or bargained for in some form, like an article of merchandise; and there it is found that generally the marriage union takes place at a premature age.[‡]

Spain.—A recent writer has said, "The general immorality of the females is to be attributed to the prevailing system of early marriages—marriages of policy or convenience—and to the low standard of morals, rather than to extraordinary depravity of natural disposition." "In Spain, women for the most part marry first and love afterwards, and conjugal fidelity is consequently a rare virtue, especially as neither religion nor education interposes to check the fervid passions of a southern clime." "The cause of the low standard of sexual morals may be referred to the defective system of education, and the want of any proper religious principles to control the ebullition of passions." "I was amazed to discover the profound ignorance of the Andaluzas on the most common topics. The fact is, that in Spain woman is still suffering an Oriental degradation. She is still regarded in the light of a being created to contribute to the sensual gratification of man, rather than to be his companion, his friend, his counsellor."[*]

Sicily.—Frederick von Raumer calls "Ireland the English Sicily,"[†] intimating, that the degraded condition of the people of Sicily is a disgrace to the Neapolitan government, as that of the Irish is a stain on the government of England. It is when speaking of the Sicilians that an interesting writer has said, "One must not enter these huts with English ideas; cleanliness must not be expected, but he will find enough to eat and drink, and the peasants satisfied with what they have. If any proof of what I have said were wanted, it might be found in the *universally* early marriages, and the numerous broods of naked, dirty, but not ill-fed children that are everywhere to be seen."[‡]

Greece.—In Mr. Strong's valuable statistical work lately published, enti-

---

[*] "The Fuegians marry young."—Voyages of the Adventure and Beagle, Vol. ii· p. 182. Evidence as to the existence of early marriage among the Esquimaux and the Northern Asiatics will be found in my former papers.

[†] Journey to the Source of the Oxus in 1836.7-8, by Lieutenant Wood, p. 340. The Yak cannot live or does not thrive even in the winters of Cabul. It seems to require the region of perpetual snow, from under which it procures its food.

[‡] Probably in all countries in an early stage of civilization, it has been the custom to buy and sell wives. By the laws of the Saxon Ethelbert, "if a free man lie with the wife of another free man, let him buy another wife for the injured party."—Strutt's Manners and Customs of the People of England, Vol. i. p. 75. There were laws fixing the price for women of all ranks as wives.—Ibid. p. 76. And Michaelis, with reference to Germany, mentions, that, in the German Chronicles of the Middle Ages, "we find it stated that A. B. bought C. D., that is, married her."—Smith's Translation of Michaelis's Laws of Moses, Vol. i. p. 450. This subject—the age and terms of the matrimonial contract in different countries, at different periods—has never as yet, with anything like an adequate degree of care, been investigated, although there are few that better deserve the trouble.

[*] A Summer in Andalusia, Vol. ii. p. 404-5- and 6. London, 1839.

[†] Italy and the Italians, vol. ii. p. 355.

[‡] Letters on Sicily, by William Irvine, M.D. p. 27. In the Spanish island, Minorca, the Minorquins "are often betrothed to each other while children, and marry at fourteen."—Cleghorn on the Epidemic Diseases of Minorca, p. 54.

tled "Greece as a Kingdom," when treating of the soil and the inhabitants, he alludes to the early union of the sexes, which he seems to attribute to natural precocity, and mentions an Athenian lady who was a grandmother at the age of 24.[*] Whittman in his Travels had given 15 years as about the age when the Greek women marry;[†] and those of the Ionian Islands, according to another writer, marry some at 11, many at 12, and most before 16; all the matches being made by the parents[‡].

Russia.—European Russia may still perhaps be considered, as to the mass of its population, as lying beyond the boundary of civilized Europe; and here the age of marriage, according to the testimony of a number of writers, is allowed to be extremely early—to have been so, at all events, till within a very recent period. Thus Mr. Tooke writes, that the common sort enter into the nuptial state "as early as they can;" and elsewhere remarks, that the women arrive at maturity at their 12th or 13th year.[§]

Another writer has said, that the lords of the soil in Russia all take care to promote matrimony early.[||] According to Archdeacon Coxe, a boy of nine or ten is often married to a woman of more advanced age, she living as his father's concubine.[¶] This latter is a curious trait which was noticed by Sir Dudley North, as we learn from his Letters during a residence in Archangel as far back as the reign of Charles II. "One of the inconveniences," says he, "that lie on those who dwell in this country, is, that the people are so given to nastiness, that nothing can be eaten out of their hands; you shall have perhaps four brothers and as many sisters, with their father, mother, husbands, and wives, all dwelling in one hot-house; (*wisbie* they call it;) they have nothing but a little straw strewed on the ground to lie upon." "In this country the husband is the sole commander of the wife, who differs very little from his servant. Many will marry their sons very young to lusty baggages on purpose to gain able servants."[*]

From no author I am acquainted with have we in several respects equally precise and valuable information on the customs of Russia, as the Rev. Dr. Pinkerton, some time Foreign Agent of the Bible Society, and "many years," he tells us, resident in Russia. Concerning the age of marriage he thus writes: "Before the influx of European customs, the contract for marriage was formed by the parents and relatives, and the bridegroom was never permitted to see his bride until the ceremony of betrothing took place. An ukaz of Peter the Great, in the year 1700, forbade this practice to be continued, and prohibited the priest solemnizing the marriage unless the ukaz was attended to." "At the beginning of the eighteenth century, it was the custom of the Russians of all ranks to marry their children very early, even before the age of puberty."[†]

We shall have again occasion to refer to the Russians in connection with the subject of early marriages: in the meantime I may remark, that every reader conversant with modern history must be aware that, if we except, to some small extent, the Russians, the inhabitants of the other countries mentioned are degraded politically, morally, and intellectually; the women sought as wives with little regard to a sentiment of affection at an age preposterously early; whilst they, ignorant of the position in the social system they are designed by the Creator to fill, exhibit the vices peculiar to the uncultivated female character—indolence, frivolity, and an abject superstition—with few of its humanizing, purifying virtues. Thus early marriage is found to be the effect of a degraded condition of society, and is again, in turn, a powerful cause of the perpetuation of that same degraded condition.

If, however, instead of supporting this conclusion, we were to concede, what has been so long and so generally contended for by physiologists, that not ignorance and moral debasement are the causes of early marriage, but that it depends upon a bodily cause; that, in fact, the Creator has fitted the

---

* Greece as a Kingdom, by F. Strong, Esq. 8vo.
† Travels in Turkey, &c. by W. Whittman, M.D. p. 25.
‡ Goodison on the Ionian Islands, p. 222.
§ Tooke's Russian Empire, vol. i. p. 375.
|| Cook's Travels through the Russian Empire, vol. iv. pp. 70 and 71.
¶ Archdeacon Coxe's Travels in Poland, Russia, &c. vol. i. p. 439.

* Life of Sir Dudley North, in North's Lives, vol. ii. pp. 310-12.
† Russia; or the Past and Present State of its Inhabitants, by Robert Pinkerton. D.D. pp. 304-306. London, 1833.

women of Andalusia and Greece, for example, to enter upon the duties of wife and mother at an earlier age than is natural to the women of England, then might the superiority of these latter over the former be considered as a thing absolutely settled; nor should we be permitted to hope that a purer religion, an improved education, and wiser laws, would avail to remove the difference. If it be asked why? the answer is, that the training of young women, the acquisition of the knowledge and the habits requisite to qualify them for wives, requires time—a period at the least of several years subsequently to the age of puberty—if the education is to be anything better than nominal; and seeing that puberty, on the hypothesis in question, is later in our favoured climate than on the shores of the Mediterranean and the plains of Russia, the women of England, by the ordination of Nature, will possess incalculable advantage in the longer space of time they will have to devote, before the period for marriage, to a preparation for the duties of domestic life. This, doubtless, is a conclusion few physiologists would *choose* to arrive at if it could be helped; but it is one that they cannot evade, except by a supposition, which I am not aware any one has ventured to make, viz. that the women of Spain and Greece, possessing greater quickness of parts than those farther to the north, are able in a briefer space of time to complete their education, the early development of the body being accompanied by a proportionably precocious display of mind.

The impediment to the work of education arising from the prevalence of early marriage in a community, has not altogether escaped the notice of observers. In a recent tour in Egypt and Candia, Captain Scott, the author, thus writes; and though his remarks have reference to Mahommedans, they are of course applicable wherever the same practice of premature marriage exists.

" An almost insuperable objection to a finished education in any Mahommedan state," says this writer, " is the early age at which marriages are contracted: a father provides a wife for his son when he ought to be still at school; so that the youths themselves have the cares and distractions of a family upon them ere they are of an age to be removed from under the rod of the

schoolmaster; and it may be here observed, that precocity of intellect is by no means remarkable among the Arabs; so their education cannot commence at an earlier age than in northern countries."

But by what arguments are the advocates of the hypothesis which I am endeavouring to expose (that early marriages depend on early puberty, and this latter on warm climate), to encounter the instance of the Russians, in whom this kind of influence of climate at all events cannot be alleged as the cause of *their* early marriages? I can imagine none. Moreover, there is evidence to prove that, just in that degree in which the light of civilization has, from time to time, found entrance and been diffused in Russia, has the practice of early marriage been discouraged and opposed by its rulers. A century and a half ago the inhabitants lay in a state of profound ignorance and debasement—on a level with the nomade hordes of the Asiatic deserts; and it was only when a sovereign like Peter the Great arose, with a clear perception of the better way, with wisdom to take it himself, and courage and perseverance to force his subjects into it, that Russia began to rise in manners, and slowly advance into the rank (as yet perhaps the rear-rank) of civilized nations. It was the custom of the Russians of all conditions, says Dr. Pinkerton, " to marry their children very early, even before the age of puberty; but Peter, by an ukaz of 23d March, 1714, strictly prohibited the nobles from entering the married state before the age of 20 for the bridegroom, and 17 for the bride. Catherine II., by an ukaz in 1775, reduced the legal age of marriage to 17 for the male, and 13 for the female. This custom of early marriage still prevails; and in innumerable instances, especially among the common people, it is fraught with very pernicious consequences, both to the physical and moral state of the parties. Many shocking instances have been known among the peasantry, of a breach of the laws of consanguinity in consequence of these premature marriages. By a recent ukaz of the present Emperor Nicholas (1831), the priests are forbidden to solemnize marriage unless the man be 18 and the bride 16

---

* Rambles in Egypt and Candia, vol. p. 185.

years old: and this edict extends also to the Uniats and Protestants in the empire."[*]

Testimony such as this, concerning the age of marriage in Russia, coming from an eye-witness long conversant with the manners of the people, and a proficient in their language, must be regarded as extremely interesting and valuable. It illustrates the view which I am endeavouring to enforce, as to the causes of early marriage and early sexual union, wherever they are to be found; establishing, by an example on a great scale, that early pubescence, the effect of a warm climate, cannot be regarded as necessarily among those causes.

To proceed to the main object of the present essay: a transition, in some degree resembling the foregoing in Russia, from marriage at a juvenile to marriage at a more mature age, must have occurred in England; although, owing to greater remoteness of time, the steps of this change in respect to the common people cannot, it is probable, now be traced: with regard to the gentry the case we shall find is otherwise. In entering on this portion of the inquiry, it may be well, since we have the means, to give the age of marriage in England at the present period; by which we shall be enabled to see, in the issue, how great a change time has wrought in this particular among us.

In the Report of the Registrar-General for the year ending 1839, a table of the ages in 4858 marriages has been published, and these not being selected instances, but belonging to districts varying in situation and character, and including every marriage in those districts, may be presumed to be a fair example of the ages at which marriages occur throught the whole kingdom.

According to this table there were under 15 years, none for either sex; of males 15, and under 20 years, there were 3½ per cent; and of females of the same ages about 14 per cent. of the whole number. The average age of marriage for men, 27 years, and for women 25 years and a few months: a result which still leaves room both for regret and improvement.[†]

I have already stated that, at the period when premature marriages were frequent in the country, some of those ill customs existed (or customs of like evil consequence) which are found wherever such marriages are found. Independently of the general ignorance, and the rudeness of manners in England in the fifteenth and sixteenth centuries, or even later, concerning which I shall not venture particularly to speak, there was the feudal right of wardship and marriage; a cause in itself alone of various evils, but of none greater or more hurtful than early marriage, which we shall find it absolutely necessitated in a number of instances; and thus introducing the practice in high quarters, diffused it probably through the whole mass of society. The nature and exercise of this feudal claim, which existed in all its oppressive rigor so lately as the reigns of the first two Stuarts, having been abolished only in the year 1660, it will be easy to explain and illustrate: in the course of doing which a number of facts will be mentioned indicative of a state of manners whose grossness and barbarism I had not myself an idea of before entering on this course of inquiry.

"Almost all the real property of this kingdom is by the policy of our laws supposed to be granted by, dependent upon, and holden of some superior lord, by and in consideration of certain services to be rendered to the lord by the tenant or possessor of his property."[*]

All tenures of land were supposed to be derived from the king, either mediately or immediately. Those who

* Past and Present State of Russia, p. 306.
† Report of the Registrar-General for 1840,

page 10, 8vo. From Senior's statement concerning a provision for the poor of foreign nations, 8vo. 1835, we find that in several European countries the laws against early and improvident marriages are, as appears to an Englishman, extremely strict. Thus in Bavaria the clergy are held responsible for the support of those poor persons they have married without leave from the authorities, besides being fined. In Berne no pauper can marry without the consent of his parish; in Norway no one can marry until he has satisfied the clergyman that he is able to maintain a family: in Mecklenburgh, owing to the conscription and other causes, men marry at from 25 to 30, and the women not much earlier. In Saxony a man liable to serve in the army may not marry under 21; in Wurtemburg no man is allowed to marry, unless permission have been especially obtained or purchased, under the age of 25. In Belgium the average age of marriage is for men 27, and 26 for women.
* Christian's edition of Blackstone, vol. ii. page 59. London, 1809.

held immediately of him were called tenants in chief; and these again in their turn were lords to tenants of a less honourable grade over whom they exercised rights.

The services rendered both by the tenants-in-chief to the sovereign for the lands they held of him, and by the inferior class of tenants to the middle lords in return for their tenures, were various; consisting, among others, of military service, aids, fines, forfeitures, and, what particulaaly concerns us at present, wardship and marriage.*

The right of wardship means that the lord hnd the guardianship of his tenant during his minority, by virtue of which right he had both the care of his person, and received to his own use the profits of the estate, excepting the ward's aliment, the amount of which lay much at the mercy of his lord. By a gross abuse of this custom in England, this right of wardship was often by the lord assigned over to strangers, or it was put up to sale, or bequeathed by will like any other kind of disposable property. But, besides the profit of the estate during the minority, the lord had another perquisite connected with his guardianship, viz. the right of disposing of his ward, whether male or female, in matrimony.

Let us suppose a tenant to die, leaving a child or children of both sexes, minors, the lord would assume the powers of guardian,† due inquisition having first been made with reference to the nature and amount of the property, and the ages of the minors; and here it may be well to mention, that the male was a minor till the age of 21, and the female till the age of 14, though in the case of a female ward the law continued the guardian's hold of her person and property two years longer—till she was 16. If the lord did not make over, or sell his rights, he soon set about finding matches for his wards; either by uniting them, if that were thought advantageous, with members of his own family, or of the families of relatives, or by selling the marriage; *i. e.* if the ward, for example, were a female, disposing of her hand to the best bidder, provided he were of suitable rank, for the law forbade disparagement. When the female ward was thus married before her twelfth year, she might, on arriving at that age, repudiate the match; in which case she had to pay to the guardian *the value of the marriage;* a sum out of her property equal to what a jury would assess as the price which might have been given for the alliance. Of course all wards (I purposely confine my remarks to those of the female sex, though the same would apply with the before-mentioned difference to males) were sure to be made to marry at the latest before the age of 16, since at that age the guardian's power over them ceased, and they were at liberty to sue out their deliverance from wardship. We shall by and by see that marriage, in such cases, instead of being delayed till the age of 15 or 16, or even till the legal age of consent, which was 12, was often contracted at an age considerably earlier, with a view to its being consummated when the partie should arrive at puberty—in some cases probably even before that period.

But it might and often did happen, as has been already mentioned, that the lord, instead of exercising the right of guardian, sold it to a stranger: to use the words of Hargreave, "This guardianship being deemed more an interest for the profit of the guardian than a trust for the benefit of the ward, was saleable and transferable, like the ordinary subjects of property, to the best bidder; and if not disposed of was transmissible to the lord's personal representatives. Thus, the custody of the infant's person, as well as the care of her estate, might devolve upon the most perfect stranger to the infant, one prompted by every pecuniary motive to abuse the delicate and important trust of education, without any ties of

---

* The kind of tenancy here alluded to was called tenure by chivalry, or tenure by *Knight service,*—in other words, it was a military tenure which in time came to include (or rather in some cases degenerated into) escuage or pecuniary assessment in the room of personal military duty. Socage tenure was a different thing, and did not bring to the tenant the same kind of burdens as tenure by chivalry.

† In law phrase guardian in chivalry. It is a curious circumstance that wardship and marriage is found among the Rajpoots of India. The mother, however, is generally guardian. Tod's Rajast'han, vol. i. page 161—3.

If any of my readers have a desire to understand fully the nature of this feudal claim I refer them to Hallam's History of the Middle Ages, vol. i.; Sir Henry Spelman's Posthumous Works, chap. xiv. and xv. folio, 1698; and especially Christian's edition of Blackstone, 4 vols. 15th *edition,* 1809, vol. ii. pages 67, 68, 69, 70, 71, 131, *and vol. iii. page 258.*

blood or regard to counteract the temptations of interest; or any sufficient authority to restrain him from yielding to their influence."[*]

Before illustrating by instances the strange results of this oppressive and debasing claim, I would remark that our law in a different case appears to proceed on the assumption that early marriages were common: thus Littleton tells us that the wife shall be endowed out of her husband's lands and tenements, "whether she have issue by her husband or no, and of what age soever the wife be, so as she be past the age of nine years at the time of the death of her husband, for she must be above nine years old at the time of the decease of her husband, otherwise she shall not be endowed."[†] On this passage Sir Edward Coke makes the following comment: "If the wife be past the age of nine years at the time of the death of her husband, she shall be endowed of what age soever her husband be, albeit he were but four years old. Quia junior non potest dotem promereri neque virum sustenere; nec obstabit mulieri petenti minor ætas viri."[‡] "This we are told by that grave and reverend judge, without any remark of surprise or reprobation," says Mr. Christian indignantly;" and then he adds—" It is abundantly clear, both from our law and history, that formerly such early marriages were contracted as in the present times are neither attempted nor thought of."[§]

In another instance, the law concerning rape, the existence of very early marriage is indirectly recognized thus;—by the statute of the 18th Elizabeth, which makes it a capital crime to abuse a consenting female child under the age of 10, an exception seems to be left for these marriages, by its being declared that *only the carnal and unlawful knowledge* of such womanchild is felony.[||]

[To be continued.]

---

* Hargreave, as quoted by Christian in one of the latter's notes and additions to Blackstone, vol. ii. p. 71.
† Coke's Littleton, lib. i. sect. 36 of Dower.
‡ Ibid.
§ Notes and additions to Blackstone, vol. ii. p. 131.
|| Ibid. p. 132.

MEDICAL GAZETTE.

Friday, July 21, 1843.

"Licet omnibus, licet etiam mihi, dignitatem *Artis Medicæ* tueri; potestas modo veniendi in publicum sit, dicendi periculum non recuso."
Cicero.

PRIVATE TUITION.

ADULT readers of history, and especially those who delight in autobiographies, personal memoirs, letters, and other documents, which may be called rather materials for history than history itself, cannot fail to be struck with the small motives of temporary expediency which appear to have suggested the most important measures, and the small circumstances which have contributed to develop and carry them into effect. Such readers are apt, indeed, to settle down into a disbelief of all those qualities of deep foresight and steady perseverance which the more youthful reader of summaries and abridgments is apt to attribute to the great actors of former days; and as there is, in the lives of most men, a time when such a scepticism is produced, so there are some who, seduced by a love of paradox, an indolence of habit, or other personal peculiarities, never emerge from such a state, but actually persuade themselves into the practical as well as theoretical adoption of an inert and morbid fatalism; for it is matter of deep experience that our constitutional tendencies, physical and moral, have more power to form our theories than our theories have to regulate our constitutional tendencies. But such scepticism will, in healthy and active minds, sooner or later give way to a practical belief, chastened indeed, and tempered, but not on that account less earnest, that diligent labour, and prudent conduct, are the true means placed within our reach for effecting the great purposes of life. The value which such qualities bear amongst men, as an acute modern writer has remarked, may be considered as the exponent of two facts; first, the uniformity of the general laws which regulate the affairs of the universe; and secondly, the occasional exceptions to which those laws are subject. If either undeviating routine or blind chance evidently controlled events, there would be no room for the exercise of superior penetration, and no wisdom in superior prudence. Now the art of medicine is one which, more perhaps than any other, requires the broadest general principles to be kept in view while dealing with apparently the most inconsequent of small details. Superiority in detecting and acting upon the latter is so evidently and appreciably valuable, that it seems the most useful quality in practice, as it is certainly the most immediately profitable to its possessor; and many men of large intellectual possessions are constantly embarrassed for want of that small change which others, who are far their inferiors, seem to have always at their command.

It is most important that broad principles should be inculcated early in life, and that the mind should receive those habits of reasoning justly, and judging rightly upon whatever premises may be within reach, which, if early inculcated, and faithfully cultivated, becomes in time a kind of intellectual instinct, acting involuntarily and unconsciously without labour to the possessor, and beneficially influencing all his proceedings. It is evident that to us sound physiological and pathological views are the great foundations for technical, as the abstract sciences are for general, accuracy of judgment; they are to be matters of gradual instruction, and of personal experimental conviction. This conviction will of course vary in degree according to the talent and diligence of the pupil, and the faithfulness of the teacher. Not even the most advanced of the former has his convictions of this kind complete on entering into practice. Much that might be matter of proof he will have believed on hearsay, and much that is mere matter of strong probability he will have adopted as unquestionable.

Those who have most experience in teaching, and especially in lecturing, are most distressed at the small amount of information which is carried away by their pupils, not only of a serviceable kind, but in a serviceable state, with its due weight of evidence, and its due bearing on practice. The lecturer is obliged by his office to lay down his subject as a whole, and though if he be a practical man, as well as a man of genius, he will so handle it by faithfulness in his general outlines, by strongly marking what is certain and important, and touching lightly on what is distant and indistinct, as to draw, in the mind of his pupils, a correct picture, full of colour and perspective—yethe must reckon on sad mistakes in his meaning, distortion in the general effect, and caricature of his details, when his pupils come to represent for themselves the pictures he has drawn for them. It is our confident hope and belief that the proportion of young men who saunter through the medical schools not studying at all, well or ill, is exceedingly diminished of late years; the distribution of prizes, the institution of clinical clerkships, and the competition amongst lecturers, have brought the students more under the personal notice of their teachers: but this is not all that is wanted; the public lecturer and the private instructor have very different offices, and the advantages to be gained from each will be increased as their respective duties are recognised and performed. Perhaps the term private instructor does not convey the exact meaning of the office alluded to. Won-

derfully little can be *taught*, properly
so called, beyond general principles—
the student must learn for himself, and
teach himself. The capital error in
the system of cramming has been the
supposed power of substituting some
intellectual operation done by the
grinder in a short time for the long-
continued study which the curriculum
requires. The word *tutor* more accurately expresses the meaning; he should
be really the guardian and defender of
the student against his indolence, his
misconceptions, and the various temptations which beset his path from
within and from without. Against
his indolence, not assuredly by drench-
ing his mind with mawkish dilutions
of what he has heard or read, but
by taking care that the current of
thought and reason is quick, not stag-
nating, by detecting the short-comings
of his memory or his comprehension,
and directing him to proper sources for
supplying their defects, by observing
whether the words which he has heard
have conveyed correct ideas to his mind,
and by scoring on his memory the
level to which the tide of daily instruction has flowed.

The talents and energies of lecturers
and authors should be devoted to
raising the subjects treated of to the
highest possible pitch, rather than exhausted in reducing their details to the
level of the meanest capacity; but in
proportion to the brilliancy of the
master, and the admiration of the pupil,
is the chance of misconception—not to
mention the inherent dangers which
beset those high and original endowments which are the most valuable
qualifications for a teacher. Few
lecturers—probably none—omit to impress upon their hearers their willingness to explain to them privately whatever points they have not understood;
but this is always a disagreeable
process, as it is felt tacitly to imply a
defect of perspicuity in the teacher, or

of intelligence or attention in the pupil:
the more youthful party is not always
apt to decide against himself, and an
impugnment of his superior not seldom
results. These matters are easily explained by a well-informed private
tutor. Against his temptations from
without, the student has to be defended,
not by long-winded homilies and elaborate dissertations, but by giving to the
habits of recreation an innocent as well
as cheerful direction. Against temptations from within, no tutor who combines experience, judgment, and candour, will *profess* to do more than endeavour to practise and to promote
that conduct which is a daily sermon,
while an ability to give a reason for
the faith that is in him will not be
wanting to account for the habits of
daily piety which he may adopt.

These are high and responsible
duties, not to be lightly undertaken nor
carelessly delegated; and this leads
naturally to the best mode of selecting such a person. The sincere believers that elective purity is attainable, will of course suggest a *concours;*
but a good deal of observation has
destroyed our natural belief in the
efficacy of this process, and almost
in all very complicated "ballot-boxes,
or other machines whatever," recommended as infallible for that purpose:
proportioned, indeed, to our conviction
of the importance of selecting the best
man for any office, will be our doubt as
to the specific powers of any elective
process which professes to ensure so
desirable an object.

That eccentric writer, Mr. Thomas
Carlyle, whose soothsayings have at
least this in common with those of the
Trojan prophetess, that they are not
believed, thinks that on the whole we in
England choose our leaders worse than
any nation that he knows of; and it is
a sort of comfort to find his disbelief in
any specific form of election so complete.
Catch the right man, he says, and you

have got all. Catch your no-man, the unfit, the pretender, and you have got all
too, but the other way. We recommend
those interested in this question to
look out for themselves amongst their
own neighbours and acquaintances, for
fit men, if they are to be found, and to
choose, it may be hinted, not those who
promise most, but those whom they
know best.

FELLOWES' CLINICAL PRIZE REPORTS.

By ALFRED J. TAPSON.

University College Hospital, 1842.

[Continued from p. 480.]

CASE XIII. — *Enteritis, ushered in by
copious discharges of blood from the
bowels, and marked by the usual symptoms of a mild attack of enteritis. Cured
by V.S. leeches, blistering, mercury, &c.*

WINNIFRED MORAU, æt. 45, admitted May
28th, 1842, under Dr. Williams. A thin,
pale, nervous looking woman : is married, and
has had thirteen children, only two of whom
are living. Has been living in a very damp
house during the winter, and has not been
able to get enough food for some months ; is
temperate.

She states that she is naturally of a strong
constitution, and was formerly much stouter ;
she never had any illness till last July, when
she was in this hospital under Dr. Williams'
care for an attack similar to the present, but
much more severe, and ever since then her
bowels have been habitually constipated,
sometimes not being opened for a whole week,
obliging her to take aperient medicine frequently.

The *present attack* commenced on the
21st instant, after she had been ironing for
some hours on the floor, and was a good
deal fatigued. A sudden pain came on in
the small part of the back, and she felt very
weak : the pain in the back was much worse
on the 22d, and she had also severe pain
over the pubes and sacrum, with headache,
anorexia and thirst, and she passed about a
pint and a half of fluid, bright-coloured
blood when her bowels opened ; on the 23d
she passed fully a pint of blood in the same
way, and nearly a pint on the 24th ; about
half a pint on the 25th, and this was clotted
and almost black. Since then she has not
passed any. (She never had any such discharge of blood before ; has never had piles,
and menstruated rather more copiously than
usual the week before last, and is not aware

of any cause that could have produced it.)
The pain in the back and lower parts of the
bowels has never ceased since it first began,
but is much increased at intervals, and at
these times her abdomen is covered with perspiration ; she has not been sick, but has
scarcely eaten anything, and has got very
thin and weak.

Present symptoms.—She lies on her back
with the knees drawn up ; the countenance
is pale and has a depressed expression ; the
breathing is quick ; pulse 96, sharpish, but
weak. She complains of a severe pain
across the lower part of the bowels, increased
by a deep inspiration, and much worse sometimes than others ; considerable tenderness
on pressure all over the abdomen, but
especially in the right iliac region ; the abdomen is enlarged all over, is tympanitic
over the situation of the cæcum, but dull on
percussion over the less iliac region. The
lips and tongue are dry, and the latter
covered with a coarse white fur ; is thirsty ;
breath has a disagreeable smell ; the veins
were opened a little this morning ; the urine
scanty, and causes her much pain and difficulty in passing.

Abdomini admov. Hirud. xij. et postea
   cataplasma amplum.
℞ Hydrarg. Chloridi. gr. iv.   Ext. Bella-
   donnæ, gr. j. M. f. pil statim sumend.
   et post horas tres, si perstiterit dolor,
   repetenda pilula.   Vesperi sumat.
   Olei Ricini, f℥j.
              Low diet.

May 30th.—The leeches removed the
pain for some hours, but then it returned,
and has been severe ever since ; vomiting
also came on, and still continues. The
tenderness of the bowels is quite as great as
on the 28th, especially in the right iliac
region, where there seems to be a small
roundish tumor ; the lips are very red ;
tongue dry and furred ; pulse 104, fuller
and sharper than it was ; breathing rather
laboured and quick (27 respirations in a
minute) : last evening she took a second dose
of the castor oil, and the bowels have been
opened several times to-day ; the stools all
dark coloured, not bloody. The urine exceedingly scanty, the sp. gr. 1032, and contains a considerable flesh-coloured stringy
sediment, chiefly composed of the lithates :
urea is also greatly in excess.

V.S. ad f℥xij.   Abdomini applic. Empl.
   Canth.
℞ Hydrarg. Chlorid. gr. iv. ; Opii, gr. j.
   M. f. pil. bis die sumenda.
℞ Acidi Hydrocyan. diluti, ℳv. ; Soda
   Sesquicarb. gr. x. ; Mist. Acac. f℥j. ;
   Aquæ, f℥j.   M. f. haust. ter die su-
   mendus.

31st.—The blood drawn yesterday is considerably cupped and also buffed ; the clots

loose below ; the pain has been much less since the bleeding ; it is not constant now, and when it comes on is less severe ; the blister has risen well ; pulse 100, less full. She was sick twice in the night ; the bowels not opened since yesterday forenoon ; urine scanty and high coloured, but much clearer.

℞. Olei Ricini, Olei Olivæ, aa. f3j. ; Vitelli ovi. unius. Decoct. Avenæ. Oj. ft. Enema, statim injiciendum.

June 1st.—Bowels less swollen and much less tender and painful ; sickness continues ; gums tender and tumid ; mercurial fœtor evident ; the enema has not produced any effects.

Olei Ricini, f3ss. statim.

2d.—Better ; slept pretty well last night ; has no pain at all when at rest, and she can move without much pain ; there is still tenderness in the right iliac region ; bowels have opened twice ; motions copious and lumpy, not very dark.

Omittantur pilulæ. Adde haust. Creasoti, mj.

4th.—The sickness has ceased ; she has a good deal of pain in passing her water, which is still very scanty.

Adde haust. Sp. Æther. Sulph. mxx.

7th.—Has no pain in any part of the abdomen ; but there is great tenderness yet in right iliac region ; the tumors here seem much swollen ; tongue covered with a thick yellowish white fur ; salivation considerable ; bowels not opened for three days ; urine only about half a pint in 24 hours.

Statim sumat. Olei Ricini, f3ss.

℞. Sodæ Biboratis, 3ss. ; Mist. Acac. f3ij. ; Aquæ, f3vj. Ft. Lotio, quâ sæpe os lavatur.

Middle diet.

9th.—The bowels were freely opened by the medicine ; she has no pain anywhere, nor tenderness, and there is no swelling to be felt now in the right iliac region ; appetite returning. The skin has been itching the last day or two, and there is a slight eruption to-day, chiefly vesicular, very like that of scabies ; feels very weak.

℞. Fiat. haust. cum Infusi. Calumbæ, f3j. vice Aquæ.

℞. Potass. Iodid. 3ss ; Aquæ, f3iv. ft. Lotio, quâ fricentur partes prurientes.

11th.—Improving ; but the bowels are costive ; urine rather increased in quantity.

℞. Sulphuris Loti. 3ij. ; Sodæ Tart. 3j. ft. pulvis 2dâ quâque mane sumendâ.

14th.—Feels stronger ; no rash or itching now.

Sumat. pulvis omni mane.
Full diet. ·

18th.—Is now quite well, only rather weak ; urine natural in quantity and appearance.
20th.—Discharged cured.

REMARKS.—In the present case a certain *diagnosis* could scarcely have been made, if we had only had the symptoms which existed on her admission to guide us, but when these were taken in connection with her previous history and the mode of attack, there was very little room left for doubt.

The more important of the symptoms might nearly all have belonged indiscriminately either to peritonitis or to enteritis—thus, the feverishness, the posture in which she lay, the situation, and in some respects, also, the character of the pain complained of in the abdomen, the tenderness, the state of the bowels, &c. might have depended on either of the above diseases : accordingly we find there was very little on which to found the diagnosis from the symptoms alone : the pain certainly had more the character of that attending enteritis than peritonitis ; it had not the sharp lancinating character that commonly marks inflammations of the serous membranes, and it came on in paroxysms, in the intervals of which she was comparatively free from pain—and this is often the case in enteritis, probably from the passage of gas, &c. from one part of the intestine to another, producing spasm. If we now refer to the previous history, and to the mode of attack, we shall not hesitate to pronounce it to have been a case of enteritis. *First*, in the history it is mentioned that she was in this hospital twelve months ago for an attack of enteritis more severe than the present, as appears from the account given of it in the hospital report-books, and since then her bowels have been habitually costive, both of which circumstances are strong predisposing causes of enteritis ; and *secondly*, we find that this attack came on with pain in the lower part of the back and abdomen, followed by several copious hæmorrhages from the bowels. It is obvious that the blood could not have proceeded from the peritoneum, and must have come from the inner coats of the intestines. The precise part of the intestine from which it came could not be ascertained, but from its colour and fluidity it evidently was from some part at no great distance from the termination. The cause of the discharge of blood was not hæmorrhoids, nor was it suppression of the menses (*vide* history), and the only other cause at all likely to have produced it was great congestion, such as accompanies the early stages of inflammation. We know, indeed, that discharges of blood per anum are by no means very rare as an accompaniment of the early stage of enteritis, and that gastritis is often ushered in by vomiting of blood. The patient had very probably exaggerated the quantity of blood that she had lost, as, according to her account, it amounted to about two quarts altogether, which is a much larger quantity than a little delicate woman would be likely to lose from such a cause. Admitting, however, that there was some, it would tend to diminish the inflammation and symptomatic fever, and it may have been this circumstance that rendered the present attack milder than the former, which is the reverse of what might naturally be expected, as a severe attack of enteritis is extremely apt to produce permanent structural change in the intestines, and thus lay the foundation of future serious attacks.

As to the part of the intestinal canal that was inflamed, we may infer, from the absence at this period of both vomiting and purging, that it was chiefly the lower portion of the small intestine; and this would accord very well with the preceding remarks about the blood. Subsequently there was reason to believe that the inflammation had extended both upwards and downwards; as vomiting had come on there was more symptomatic fever; and there was a distinct feeling of a tumor in the right iliac fossa, in the situation of the commencement of the colon or termination of the ilium. From this feeling, and taking into consideration the occurrence of a former attack of the costive state of the bowels since, Dr. Williams believed that there had been some deposition of lymph during the former attack, which had produced thickening of the intestine in this situation, which was now, in consequence, more prone to inflammation, and more swelled, causing the feeling of a tumor, which went away gradually as the inflammation subsided.

In the *treatment* of enteritis, the indications are, to subdue the inflammatory action, to quiet the pain, and to procure a free passage through the intestines when these are constipated, as here, and as is usually the case when the inflammation is at all severe and deep-seated, though there may be diarrhœa when only the mucous coat is inflamed. In most cases general blood-letting is advisable, and here nature had already done that by the hæmorrhage, which, besides being in sufficient amount to produce a decided effect upon the system at large, was also from the seat of the inflammation; so that as the symptoms were mild it was thought that leeches would be sufficient, followed by calomel and castor oil, to open the bowels, and belladonna to allay the supposed spasmodic condition of the intestines, which it does without causing constipation. These measures produced temporary relief to the symptoms, but two days after there was more fever, the pain was as bad as ever, and vomiting had come on, so

that she was now bled from the arm, and calomel in combination with opium was given to affect the system, and an alkaline draught to allay the sickness. Under these means the symptoms gradually abated, and she was discharged cured on the 20th June —rather more than three weeks from the time of her admission, she having been kept in the hospital nearly a week longer than was necessary, out of charity.

Throughout the whole course of the disease the urine was remarkably scanty, often not amounting to more than a few ounces in the 24 hours, and generally was very turbid and of a high specific gravity, arising from its concentrated state. This almost suppressed state of the urine is common in gastritis.

As *causes* of the disease we have already mentioned incidentally the previous occurrence of the disease, which, in all cases, is a powerful predisposing cause, and especially so if there be any permanent thickening left, as this is a sort of nidus of a future attack; also the habitual constipation, which is an exceedingly frequent cause of enteritis, particularly when the disease has occurred before: it is sometimes a sufficient cause of itself—thus enteritis often supervenes upon colic: as a third cause must be mentioned the poor and insufficient food—so fertile a cause of various intestinal diseases; for when enough cannot be obtained from poverty, as here, that which is obtained is generally very bad in quality, thus giving rise to many acrid secretions, which, with the preceding causes, are quite enough to induce the disease.

MEDICAL REPORT

OF THE

WESTERN LYING-IN HOSPITAL, DUBLIN.

The following report of the hospital embraces a period of two years, that is, from January 1, 1841, to December 31, 1842, inclusive; and, according to the general register of admissions and applications, relief has been afforded to 1506 women, but, owing to the irregularity with which many cases were entered in the statistical register, it has been found necessary to exclude a considerable number, in order that no facts might be adduced of the accuracy of which we are not certain. Our records will consequently be limited to the delivery of 1206 women; from these must be deducted 43 cases of abortion, leaving 1163 cases of labour at the full time.

The number of children amounted to 1175 (691 males, and 484 females), of which 63 (44 males, and 19 females) were still-born, or died at birth; of these

12 were premature.
15 ,, still-born.
2 ,, putrid.
4 ,, footling cases.
8 ,, breech presentations.
1 ,, head and hand presentation.
3 ,, arm presentations.
3 ,, funis presentations.
6 ,, crotchet cases.
2 ,, forceps cases.
1 ,, placenta prævia.
4 ,, syphilitic.

The ages of 1067 patients were ascertained as accurately as possible:

77 were at or under . . 20 years of age.
296 ,, between . 20 and 25 do.
370 ,, ,, . 25 ,, 30 do.
177 ,, ,, . 30 ,, 35 do.
117 ,, ,, . 35 ,, 40 do.
40 ,, ,, . 40 ,, 45 do.

In 982 cases the entire duration of labour was as follows:

In 357 it was under . . . 6 hours.
312 ,, between 6 and 12 do.
214 ,, ,, . 12 ,, 24 do.
50 ,, ,, . 24 ,, 36 do.
17 ,, ,, . 36 ,, 48 do.
11 ,, ,, . 48 ,, 60 do.
15 ,, ,, . 60 ,, 95 do.
2 ,, ,, . . 100 do.
3 ,, ,, . . 121 do.
1 ,, ,, . . 153 do.

The extreme prolongation of some of those cases was owing to the friends of the patient deferring their application for assistance.

The period which elapsed between the commencement of labour and the rupture of the membranes, was noted in 981 cases:

In 167 it was about . . . 2 hours.
335 ,, between 2 and 6 do.
165 ,, ,, . 6 ,, 10 do.
113 ,, ,, . 10 ,, 14 do.
71 ,, ,, . 14 ,, 18 do.
33 ,, ,, . 18 ,, 22 do.
46 ,, ,, . 22 ,, 26 do.
23 ,, ,, . 26 ,, 30 do.
8 ,, ,, . 30 ,, 38 do.
9 ,, ,, . 38 ,, 40 do.
4 ,, ,, . . 50 do.
2 ,, ,, . . 60 do.
1 ,, ,, . . 70 do.
3 ,, ,, . . 80 do.
1 ,, ,, . . 105 do.

In 812 cases the interval between the rupture of the membranes and the birth of the child was as follows:

In 396 it was about 1 hour.
142 ,, 2 hours.
120 ,, 4 do.
50 ,, 6 do.
34 ,, 8 do.

17 it was about 10 hours.
26 ,, 25 do.
11 ,, 20 do.
9 ,, 28 do.
4 ,, 35 do.
1 ,, 40 do.
1 ,, 50 do.
1 ,, 120 do.

In 953 cases, from the birth of the child to the expulsion of the placenta, there elapsed

5 minutes in 98 cases.
10 ,, 190 do.
15 ,, 175 do.
20 ,, 166 do.
25 ,, 48 do.
30 ,, 126 do.
35 ,, 16 do.
40 ,, 30 do.
50 ,, 43 do.
60 ,, 14 do.
From 1 to 2 hours in 33 do.
,, 2 ,, 3 ,, 9 do.
,, 3 ,, 4 ,, 5 do.

The latter cases, when the placenta was retained so long, were under the care of midwives, who applied for assistance on this account.

In 1008 cases the presentation was as follows:—

In 941 the head presented; in 13 the hand descended with the head; in 22 the breech presented, 8 dead; in 18 the feet presented, 4 dead, the funis prolapsed in 3; in 6 the funis presented, 4 dead; in 5 the arm presented, 3 dead, 2 of them putrid; in 2 the placenta presented, 1 dead.

There were thirteen cases of twins. In four cases the children presented naturally—six children were saved, and two, which were premature, died. In six cases one child presented the breech and the other the head—ten were born alive, two were lost. In one case one child presented footling and the other the head—both were saved. In another, one child presented the head and the funis, and the other the foot and funis—both were lost. In a third case both the children presented the feet and funis, and were lost.

In ten cases there was hæmorrhage between the birth of the child and the expulsion of the placenta; in six of which manual extraction was necessary, but no unfavourable results followed.

In six cases flooding occurred before delivery—three were cases of accidental, and three of unavoidable hæmorrhage. The rupture of the membranes was sufficient in the accidental and in one of the unavoidable cases, and the mothers and the children recovered. It was necessary to turn and deliver the child in the other two cases—one of the mothers died and one recovered; one of the children was saved.

Seven patients were attacked by convulsions—all recovered. One fatal case of uterine phlebitis occurred, and several slight attacks of hysteritis, which were relieved by the usual treatment.

We met with one fatal case of rupture of the uterus.

Version was performed six times (1 in 243); five times on account of presentation of the arm—all the mothers recovered, and three children were saved, the others were putrid; and once because of unavoidable hæmorrhage.

The forceps were used in eight cases (1 in 182). Seven of the mothers recovered, and the death of the remaining one was caused by disease of the heart.

In eight cases the perforator was employed (1 in 182). Six of the mothers recovered, and two died—one from rupture of the uterus, as recorded above, and one from disease of the liver.

Of the 1463 women attended during these two years, only five died, or 1 in 292. One sank from disease of the liver, another from disease of the heart, a third after unavoidable hemorrhage, a fourth from uterine phlebitis, and the fifth from ruptured uterus. —Dr. FLEETWOOD CHURCHILL, in *Dublin Journal of Medical Science.*

HYDROSULPHURET OF AMMONIA.

I HAVE within the last few days been accidentally led to try the process for hydrosulphuret of ammonia, recommended in the April number of your journal. The object apparently is to get a protosulphuret of calcium, and then to decompose it by means of sulphate of ammonia, for the ingredients are all taken nearly in atomic proportions. The reaction might, if this were the case, be thus expressed:—$Ca\ S$ and $N\ H_4\ O, S\ O_3$, and $N\ H_4\ S$. But nothing of this sort occurs, because in boiling the lime with the sulphur, no protosulphuret of calcium is or can be formed, but (leaving out of the question a little hyposulphite of lime which is produced), the solution contains only a pentasulphuret of calcium, and consequently four-fifths of the lime are removed on filtration. The sulphate of ammonia being now added, in quantity equivalent to *the whole of* the lime, one-fifth only is decomposed, and the following reaction occurs:— $Ca\ S_5$ and $N\ H_4\ O, S\ O_3, = Ca\ O, S\ O_3$, and $N\ H_4\ S + S_4$, the product thus containing not only a great quantity of sulphate of ammonia in solution, but also a large excess of sulphur, much of which precipitates on dilution with distilled water, or even on standing twenty-four hours. These results I have obtained by experiment as well as theory, and yet the solution is described as "sufficiently pure for most experimental uses."

If this be submitted to distillation, as recommended where perfect purity is required, the sulphate of amonia and excess of sulphur are got rid of, and the product $N\ H_4\ S$ in solution is obtained sufficiently pure; but this is not the same thing as that obtained by passing sulphuretted hydrogen through solution of ammonia, which is now generally allowed by chemists to have the formula $N\ H_4\ S + H\ S$. In fact, the distilled liquid is precisely similar to that produced by the well-known old process of distilling together lime, sulphur, and muriate of ammonia, and known, when concentrated, as "Boyle's Fuming Liquid," which was constantly used as a test until recently superseded by the other preparation. The processes, too, differ only in this, that the *new* one substitutes sulphate for muriate of ammonia, and employs three operations where one only is necessary.—Mr. W. B. RANDALL, in *Pharmaceutical Journal.*

OPHTHALMIC SURGERY AT VIENNA.

AMONG the many pupils of Beer, five in particular distinguished themselves, Jäger, Rosas, Benedict, Bringolf, and Dr. Fischer, the venerable professor of ophthalmology at Prague. Beer was succeeded in the chair of ophthalmic surgery by the present professor, Dr. Anton Edlen von Rosas, a Hungarian physician, who holds his clinique from ten to twelve o'clock daily. This clinique is situated in the second story of the left-hand corner of the third square, near the pathological museum. It consists of a male and female wards, with twenty beds, most admirably fitted up for the comfort of persons labouring under diseases of the eyes; the beds, constructed on the principle of those for fractures, and made to raise in the upper half, are furnished with curtains, the walls and fixtures painted green, and the windows so arranged as to modify the light. To prevent the chance of contagion from the indiscriminate use of the sponges and napkins, or the vessels, each ward is supplied with a small cistern placed against the wall, about five feet from the ground, with a syphon-shaped tube attached; on turning the cock of this, a *jet* of luke-warm water plays to the height of about eight inches. To this each patient who requires ablution applies his eyes, and thus, without the fear of infection, syringes the organ in the most gentle and agreeable manner. It is an apparatus that the eye wards of every hospital should be supplied with. The annual average number of patients treated in this department is about one hundred and fifty, all interesting cases chosen by the professor's assistant from the general wards of the hospital; and attached to it is an *Ambulatorium*, which affords relief to above one thousand persons in each year. United with these wards is a spacious and well-arranged *Auditorium*, or lecture and operating-room, at one extremity of which there is a raised platform railed off, for operating and examining patients; it is, however, at present rather too small for the accommodation of the vast number of students who crowd this clinique.

In this theatre stands a bust of the Emperor Francis I., "*Patris Patriæ*," under whose auspices and those of Andreas von Stifft — the former Protomedicus — it was erected in 1816; and around the walls are portraits of Barth, Prochaska, Rust, T. Sömmerring, Richter, Adam Schmidt, Fischer, Quadri of Bologna, Philip von Walther of Munich, Gräfe, Jüngken, Von Ammon, and our distinguished countryman Dr. Mackenzie. Attached to this clinique is a very valuable and extensive library, chiefly composed of works upon the eye, in different languages, from which books are lent out to the student or visitor weekly, on the payment of a very trifling subscription. There is a small collection of pathological specimens of the human eye in spirits, many of which are from the hands of Beer. One of the greatest objects of attraction to the foreign visitor in this school, is the magnificent collection of wax-preparations of the morbid eye, and the armentarium chirurgicum of eye-instruments from the earliest period to the present date, both beautifully arranged and in admirable keeping,—*Wilde's Austria.*

ACCOUNT OF A CHILD

WHICH WAS BORN IN THE 25TH WEEK OF PREGNANCY, AND LIVED THREE DAYS.

BY DR. HOLST.

A WOMAN, aged 30, was frightened on the 2d of August by a violent clap of thunder, and on the 5th was delivered of a living girl. The child weighed 1½lb., and was only thirteen inches long. The skin was thin and reddish, and no pulse was perceptible in the radial arteries. The head was disproportionately large, the extremities long, and the joints very flexible. The nails were tolerably developed on the fingers and great toes; on the remaining toes there were no nails, but only roots. The apex of the head was covered with tolerably thick and dark hair, and the rest of the body with a quantity of down, which was particularly thick and long upon the face. The lobules of the ear were perfectly developed; the iris was very

narrow, while the pupils were broad, and covered by a membrane. The nymphæ, which were large, projected from the labia majora; and the clitoris was also large. The child was wrapped in cotton wool, and put in its mother's bed. It could not suck, but was slowly fed with cow's milk, water, and thin gruel. Morning and evening it was bathed in milk and water. It had natural evacuations, and slept almost continually. When it awoke it uttered a weak squeaking sound, and lay constantly quiet, almost without motion. Its strength soon diminished, and it died in 66½ hours.

The mother, who had borne eight children before, and had always menstruated regularly, positively affirmed that the catamenia had appeared for the last time in the middle of February, and that she had felt the motion of the child for the first time on the 23d of June. So that if we suppose her pregnancy to have begun on the earliest possible day, namely, the 15th of February, it lasted only twenty-four weeks and three days; and the appearance of the child, as described above, agrees with this supposition. — *Schmidt's Jahrbücher;* from the *Norsk Magazin.*

ACCOUNT OF THE OBSTETRICAL CLINIQUE

At the University of Grütz during 1837-8.

BY PROFESSOR GÖTZ.

1171 women were delivered of 1196 children; of whom 648 were boys, and 548 girls. There were 1147 single deliveries, 23 cases of twins, and one of triplets. Twenty-four boys and twenty-three girls were born dead, and twenty-four children died during the first week: the latter were all born with symptoms of great weakness, or of apparent death. As to the position of the children, the first presentation of the occiput was observed 1054 times, the second 68, the third seven times, and the fourth twice. The forehead presented twice, the face ten times, the breech twenty-three times, and the feet ten times. Four times there was a transverse presentation, and four times the presentation was not registered. Twelve women were delivered in the street, while going to the hospital. Turning was performed four times; the forceps was applied thirteen times; the prolapsed funis was replaced three times; and three times the placenta was extracted on account of violent hæmorrhage, or adhesion and strangulation of the placenta itself.

In the thirteen cases where the forceps was applied, seven children were born alive, one was dead before the operation, four died during the operation, and one immediately afterwards.

In a rachitic woman, who died of puerperal fever, after having been delivered by the forceps five days previously, without any unfavourable symptom, the antero-posterior diameter of the pelvis was found to be only two inches and ten lines in length, the transverse one five inches and a half, and the oblique one four inches and five lines.—*Gazette Médicale;* and *Med. Jahrb. des Oesterr. Staates.*

OPHTHALMIC SURGERY.

To the Editor of the Medical Gazette.

SIR,

I HAVE read Mr. France's remarks on the results of the operations performed by me at the Royal Westminster Ophthalmic Hospital, and published by the Committee in their Annual Report. The operations for artificial pupil were successful, and no accident or evil whatever occurred in the 1474 operations for strabismus. When the operation is done after the manner I have directed, I do not believe they will ever occur. Of the 85 operations for cataract, 56 were performed by division through the sclerotica, or by puncture through the cornea. I do not believe there is anything peculiar in my practice, or that it is more successful than that of other surgeons who have sufficient opportunities of making themselves acquainted with ophthalmic diseases, and I am always happy to receive and give any explanation in my power to such members of the profession as might be disposed to favour me with their company on any Monday, Wednesday, and Friday, at one o'clock.

I am, sir,

Your obedient servant,

CHARLES GUTHRIE.

4, Berkeley Street,
July 12, 1843.

BOOKS RECEIVED FOR REVIEW.

A Medical Visit to Gräfenberg, in April and May 1843, for the purpose of investigating the merits of the Water-Cure treatment. By Sir Charles Scudamore, M.D. F.R.S. &c.

Scarlatina and its Treatment on Homœopathic Principles. By Jos. Belluomini, M.D.

COLLEGE OF PHYSICIANS.

THE following Physicians have been elected Fellows :—Dr. Webster ; Dr. A. Farre ; Dr. Stolterforth ; and Dr. Taylor.

ROYAL COLLEGE OF SURGEONS.

MR. ANDREWS has been elected President ; Sir B. Brodie and Mr. S. Cooper Vice-Presidents for the ensuing year.

A TABLE OF MORTALITY FOR THE METROPOLIS,

Shewing the number of deaths from all causes registered in the week ending Saturday, July 8, 1843.

Small Pox	5
Measles	26
Scarlatina	32
Hooping Cough	36
Croup	9
Thrush	2
Diarrhœa	6
Dysentery	0
Cholera	1
Influenza	4
Ague	0
Typhus	36
Erysipelas	2
Syphilis	1
Hydrophobia	0
Diseases of the Brain, Nerves, and Senses	140
Diseases of the Lungs and other Organs of Respiration	210
Diseases of the Heart and Blood-vessels	30
Diseases of the Stomach, Liver, and other Organs of Digestion	66
Diseases of the Kidneys, &c.	6
Childbed	8
Paramenia	0
Ovarian Dropsy	0
Disease of Uterus, &c.	4
Rheumatism	1
Diseases of Joints, &c.	2
Carbuncle	1
Ulcer	0
Fistula	0
Dropsy, Cancer, and other Diseases of Uncertain Seat	93
Old Age or Natural Decay	46
Deaths by Violence, Privation, or Intemperance	36
Causes not specified	4
Deaths from all Causes	811

METEOROLOGICAL JOURNAL.

Kept at EDMONTON, *Latitude* 51° 37′ 32″ N. *Longitude* 0° 3′ 51″ W. *of Greenwich.*

June 1843.	THERMOMETER.	BAROMETER.	
Wednesday 12	from 47 to 75	30·11 to	Stat.
Thursday . 13	55 64	30·04	29·99
Friday . . 14	55 69	30·08	Stat.
Saturday . 15	51 76	30·08	30·05
Sunday . . 16	57 73	30·16	Stat.
Monday . . 17	57 80	30·20	30·13
Tuesday . 18	56 72	29·96	29·79

Wind N. on the 12th ; S.W. and N.W. on the 13th ; N. on the 14th ; W. by S. and W. by N. on the 15th ; W. and S.W. on the 16th ; S.W. on the 17th and 18th.

Except the 13th and 18th, when rain fell, generally fine.

Rain fallen, ·67 of an inch.

CHARLES HENRY ADAMS.

WILSON & OGILVY, 57, Skinner Street, London.

THE

LONDON MEDICAL GAZETTE,

BEING A

WEEKLY JOURNAL

OF

Medicine and the Collateral Sciences.

FRIDAY, JULY 28, 1843.

LECTURES

ON THE

THEORY AND PRACTICE OF MIDWIFERY,

Delivered in the Theatre of St. George's Hospital,

BY ROBERT LEE, M.D. F.R.S.

LECTURE XXXVI.

On Labours complicated with Convulsions.

THERE is a striking resemblance between the symptoms observed in a case of common epilepsy and in one of puerperal convulsions, or eclampsia as it is called by nosologists. In both these diseases insensibility takes place during the fits, and all the voluntary muscles of the face, trunk, and extremities, become convulsed. When a fit of puerperal convulsions comes on, the woman becomes perfectly unconscious of every thing around her, and the muscles of the eyes and face are usually first affected. Irregular spasmodic twitchings are observed about the mouth and eyelids, which produce great distortion of the countenance: the eyes are often turned upward and inward to the root of the nose, and roll rapidly about in different directions. The lower jaw is either firmly clenched against the upper, or it is drawn to one side; and the tongue, being protruded between the teeth, is often severely lacerated. Every muscle of the body soon becomes convulsed; the spasm is violent and universal; the respiration, which is at first hurried, afterwards becomes slow and stertorous, as the convulsions subside; and a quantity of frothy saliva, tinged with blood, is blown from the mouth with a peculiar noise, as in an ordinary epileptic fit. Sometimes the muscles on one side of the face and body only are at first affected; and after the

spasm has ceased in them, those on the opposite side become convulsed. The pupils of the eyes are usually dilated and insensible during a fit of puerperal convulsions ; but in some women, both between and during the paroxysms, they are closely contracted. The pulse varies extremely, being either very hurried, or slower than natural. After the convulsion has endured for a longer or a shorter period, as in cases of epilepsy, it gradually ceases ; and the patient, apparently greatly exhausted, is left in a state of deep stupor, with stertorous breathing. The consciousness generally does not return before another fit takes place ; and this happens, in the greater number of instances, in a short period, when the same phenomena are observed. A great number of violent fits are often experienced by some women during many hours, at longer or shorter intervals, without any return of sensibility. The attacks may terminate in a state resembling apoplexy, as epilepsy sometimes does, which may soon prove fatal ; or the fits may subside, and the recollection be gradually restored. If there have been no labour pains before the fits have come on, the os uteri most frequently begins to dilate ; but the uterine contractions are usually feeble and irregular, and they seem to pass into convulsions, or to alternate with the fits. Sometimes the child is expelled by the pains ; but more frequently they are inefficient, and the delivery cannot be completed without artificial assistance.

In some women the fits are preceded by certain symptoms indicating a plethoric state of the vessels of the brain, and great nervous irritability. There is usually headache, more or less intense ; throbbing of the temporal arteries ; sense of weight and constriction across the forehead ; giddiness ; drowsiness ; the sight and hearing disturbed ; flushing and tumefaction of the countenance ; slight delirium, or confusion of thought, or loss of memory ; and other signs of cerebral disturbance. Pain in the epigastric region, and increased sensibility of the uterus, sometimes precede the fits: but there are cases of violent puerperal convulsions where no precursory or premonitory symptoms of any kind are perceived; there is nothing like the aura epileptica observed before attacks of puerperal convulsions. They may occur in the latter months of pregnancy, before the uterus has begun to contract, during the different stages of labour, and several days or weeks after delivery. I have never met with a case of true puerperal convulsions before the sixth month of pregnancy; the spasmodic affections which have occurred at an earlier period having been connected with hysteria, and unaccompanied with loss of consciousness.

It has been observed by all practitioners, that, in a very great proportion of cases, it is in the first pregnancy or labour that puerperal convulsions occur. "Women are far more liable," says Dr. Denman, "to convulsions in first than in subsequent labours; and then, it is said, more frequently when the child is dead than when it is living. But when women have convulsions the death of the child ought generally to be esteemed rather an effect than a cause, as they have often been delivered of living children when they were in convulsions, or of dead, and even putrid children, without any tendency to convulsions. Some women have also had convulsions in several successive labours; but having had them in one, they generally, by the precautions taken, or some natural change, escape them in future. Lastly, I was for many years persuaded that convulsions only happened when the head presented; but experience has proved that they sometimes occur in preternatural presentations of the child." Of 19 cases recorded by Dr. Joseph Clarke, 16 were first children. Of 48 related by Dr. Merriman, there were 36 instances in which it was the patient's first labour. Of 30 cases which occurred to Dr. Collins, 29 were in women with their first children; and the other single case was a second pregnancy, but in a woman who had suffered a similar attack with her first pregnancy. 14 of the 32 children (two of the women having had twins) were born alive. In 18 of the 30 the convulsions subsided after delivery; in 10 the fits occurred both before and after; and in 2 the attack did not come on till after delivery. In 15 of the 30 the patients were delivered by the natural efforts; in 6 delivery was effected by the forceps; in 8 by the perforator and crotchet; and in one the feet presented. Two of the children were born putrid. Five of the women died. In 6 of the 48 cases related by Dr. Merriman the convulsions did not occur till after delivery. Five of these patients recovered; the other, after the epileptic attack, became maniacal,

but appeared to be gradually recovering, when, at the end of three weeks from the first seizure, she was attacked with another fit, and died. All the children were alive. In three cases the women were pregnant of twins. In two of these cases the attack of convulsions occurred in the interval between the births of the two children. All the women were delivered without artificial assistance; two of them recovered; and three of the children were born alive. In eleven cases the delivery was effected by the forceps. All these women recovered, and three of the children were born alive. In nine cases the perforator was employed. Seven of the women recovered. In four cases the operation of turning was resorted to; two of the women recovered; all the children were dead born. In one case the woman died undelivered. In 14 cases the children were born without extraordinary assistance. 10 of these women recovered, and 5 of the children were born alive. Thus 37 women recovered, and 11 died. 17 children were born alive (including the 6 born before the mothers were attacked with convulsions); 34 were born dead. Dr. Ramsbotham has related the histories of 26 cases; of which, 10 proved fatal. 13 occurred before delivery, 10 during labour, and 4 after. Dr. Ingleby relates 35 cases; of which, 11 were fatal. Mauriceau 42; 7 during pregnancy, 3 of which were fatal; 19 during labour, 11 of which ended fatally; and 16 after delivery, of which 5 were fatal.

Puerperal convulsions occur in all countries, and in all the different ranks of life. Those women are most predisposed to the disease who have had hysteria or epilepsy in early life, who have suffered from injuries of the head, or who have had violent attacks of fever with severe affections of the brain. Depressing passions of the mind appear to produce a predisposition to the disease. Unmarried women, who are excluded from society, and often addicted to the improper use of stimulants, are peculiarly liable to puerperal convulsions and mania. Terror, and other violent mental impressions, and sometimes the pains of labour alone, are sufficient to excite convulsions. The disease occurs not only in strong plethoric young women with their first children—in such as are of a coarse make, with short thick necks —but in weak, irritable, nervous females. There are some cases where irregularities of diet, especially the use of very indigestible food and stimulants, appear, without any other cause that can be discovered, to give rise to the disease. There are many cases in which the peculiar condition of the nervous system of the uterus appears to be the sole cause, and in all cases it is the principal predisposing cause, for the fits of convulsion occur in most women in the first pregnancy and labour, and at no other time but during pregnancy and labour; and they often suddenly cease when the labour is completed, after every remedy has been employed without avail, except artificial delivery. The condition of the brain, on which the loss of consciousness and convulsions depend, is obviously produced by sympathy with the nervous system of the uterus; and the fits return, and increase in violence, till the uterus is emptied of its contents, as on them the irritation of the nerves of the uterus alone depends.

In some cases there has been observed an unusual degree of redness and softening of the cerebral substance in those who have died from puerperal convulsions; great congestion of the sinuses and smaller veins and arteries of the brain; effusion of blood or serum into the ventricles, and lymph covering the surface of the hemispheres. In others there has been no morbid appearance whatever found in the brain to account for the symptoms. At Edinburgh, in 1816, I examined, with Dr. J. Thomson and Dr. Gordon, the brain of a young woman who had died of puerperal convulsions; but, except a little turgescence of the blood-vessels, not more than is seen in many who have died of disease altogether unconnected with the brain, there was nothing to account for the symptoms. In other cases, however, organic disease of the brain has been discovered after death, as you will see by looking at the following table.

Dr. Ramsbotham made a post-mortem examination of the brain in four of the fatal cases which he observed. The first case was referrible to injury of the head. There was both convulsion and paralysis, and the woman died undelivered. "Blood was found extravasated between the dura and pia mater, and upon the orbital processes under the right lobe." In the second fatal case he states that there was no positive derangement detected in the brain, except turgescence of the vessels of the pia mater. The head of another patient was examined by an experienced anatomist, who reported that after a very minute examination of every portion of the brain no positive derangement could be detected, and that the only appearance in any way different from that usually met with was in the vessels of the pia mater, which were thought to be somewhat more loaded with blood than in the general cases of cerebral inspection. In case 4, after a most careful examination of the head, no positive breach of vessel could be detected. The blood-vessels of the pia mater were beautifully injected with blood, and a section of the substance of the brain showed more bloody points than usual. There was also a quantity of tinged serum in the ventricles. The vessels of the cerebellum were

likewise anormally distended with blood. From the dissections, and other circumstances, Dr. R. concludes that "the whole train of symptoms evinces considerable derangement in the functions of the brain and nervous system; yet, after death, correspondent marks of organic mischief within the head are seldom met with (vol. ii. p. 248). The different anatomical inquiries at which I have been present have not disclosed such regular appearances as to sanction the uniform deduction that the brain was the principal seat of the disease. I suspect that in many instances that important organ is no otherwise implicated than through the medium of sympathetic irritation." " Of the appearances after death," observes Dr. Merriman, "in those who have died of puerperal epilepsy, contrary statements have been given. Dr. Denman says, that in the examination of many women who have died from convulsions, he has never seen an instance of effusion of blood in the brain, though the vessels were extremely turgid; but has always remarked, that the heart was unusually flaccid, without a single drop in the auricles or ventricles: but he adds, that Mr. Hewson had informed him of a case of convulsions, where an effusion of blood in a small quantity had been found on the surface of the brain; and in his fifth edition, he mentions a case by Dr. Hooper, where a coagulum of blood, weighing nearly ℥iv. was found between the dura and pia-mater. In one instance I have distinctly seen an effusion of blood in the posterior part of the cranium; but the quantity was not large, and Dr. Ley has lately met with a similar case." M. Cruveilhier examined a case in which not the slightest trace of congestion of the vessels of the brain could be detected. M. Bontilleux relates another, in which he could detect no manifest alteration within the skull. Dr. Collins says, " I conceive we are quite ignorant as yet of what the cause may be: nor could I ever find on dissection any appearances to enable me to even hazard an opinion on the subject."

Treatment of Puerperal Convulsions.

The best systematic writers on midwifery during the last two centuries have recommended copious blood-letting in puerperal convulsions, and artificial delivery where depletion failed to remove the fits. They have all considered the brain to be the seat of the disease.

Mauriceau thought prompt delivery to be the best remedy, and where the orifice of the uterus did not admit of this, he advised blood to be drawn from the arm and foot, and stimulating enemata to be employed, to diminish the quantity of blood in the brain. He states that he had seen emetics administered without success, or with injurious effects. Where consciousness did not return between the fits, but the woman remained insensible, foaming at the mouth, with stertorous breathing, then both the mother and child he believed would die, if they were not promptly relieved by delivery. I have saved, he says, the lives of many women in this way, but others have not failed to die after having been delivered in the due time, and in the proper manner—" bien et duement accouchées."

He admits that some cases will prove fatal whatever is done. If the child is alive he recommends the operation of turning ; if dead, craniotomy.

"There are some women," he says, " who are always attacked with convulsions either before or after delivery. To prevent such an accident he recommends bleeding from the arm twice or three times during pregnancy, and once after labour has commenced.

Puzos has also given an account of puerperal convulsions, and has recommended prompt and copious blood-letting, to relieve the brain from the excessive quantity of blood by which it is oppressed. After the bleeding, lavements, he says, must be employed, and it should be ascertained by an examination whether the uterus is dilating, and if the bleedings and other remedies do not calm the convulsions, then delivery is the best thing that can be done, which removes the pressure from the great bloodvessels of the abdomen, and allows it to circulate freely. The relief from delivery, he says, is not instantaneous, for the convulsions will often continue for a time, but at longer intervals, and patients sometimes remain for two days in a state of lethargy, and afterwards recover. But when the convulsions continue in spite of the bloodlettings and delivery, and the coma and stertorous breathing and foaming at the mouth, then the disorder will terminate fatally ; but we have the consolation to know, that we merit no reproach, having employed all the means we possess to overcome so grievous an accident. It is to be presumed because we have not succeeded, that lesions (crevasses) have been made in the brain by the violence of the convulsions, and that delivery could not remedy these. Thus, he adds, in the acute convulsions which precede or accompany labour, we cannot be too prompt and vigorous in the application of the proper resources ; and as these means are sometimes insufficient when the disease is once established, the accoucheur should be attentive to the first symptoms which announce convulsions ; for it sometimes happens, that in a labour accompanied with the most favourable symptoms, a woman all at once complains of

dazzling of the eyes, of weight in the forehead or posterior part of the head, and of sudden loss of vision, symptoms which all announce that an attack of convulsion is at hand. I have seen women suddenly seized with frightful convulsions, he says, during labour, because attention had not been paid them when they complained of pain of the head. We perceive, then, that it is much more easy to prevent the evil, than to destroy it when it is once established ; since the most powerful remedies do not prevent the death of the mother and the child, which these convulsions put in the greatest danger. Therefore I bleed copiously, and that on the first appearance of the symptoms which threaten convulsions ; and I have often by this means relieved very speedily the headache, restored the vision, and completed the delivery happily in a short time.

Copious blood-letting in puerperal convulsions is the first remedy now employed by all practitioners in this country ; but the extent to which depletion is to be carried must be regulated by the constitution of the patient, the violence of the symptoms, and the effects produced by the loss of blood. Profuse blood-letting will not invariably control the disease, as some have asserted ; nay, I am persuaded that the sudden abstraction of fifty or more ounces of blood from the arm of some individuals, instead of arresting the disease, would destroy life. So feeble is the circulation of the blood in some women that it is impossible to remove this quantity from the arm. In young, robust, plethoric women, the best plan certainly is to take away as soon as possible after the attack twenty or twenty-five ounces of blood from the arm, to cut off the hair or shave the scalp, and apply over the head cold lotion or ice in a bladder ; to put ten grains or a scruple of calomel upon the tongue, or two drops of croton oil, if the bowels require immediate relief ; to throw up into the rectum a stimulating enema, and to apply warmth, mustard poultices, and rubefacients, to the inside of the legs and thighs ; at the same time to adopt every precaution to prevent the patient from being bruised or injured by the violence of the convulsive movements into which the body is thrown. If the fits continue after these remedies have been employed, with undiminished violence, and if the pulse is full and strong, and signs of congestion of the brain are still present, you may open another vein in the arm, and remove fifteen or twenty ounces more. A third bleeding to this extent is undoubtedly necessary and proper in some cases, but I prefer greatly, after thirty or thirty-five ounces of blood have been drawn from the arm, to trust to local bleeding, and especially to the application of cupping-glasses to the temples and nape of the neck. When the constitution has been previously exhausted by some chronic disease, or hæmorrhage ; or without these, if it is peculiarly delicate, nervous, and irritable, and has been weakened by grief, and other depressing passions, and the pulse is very rapid and feeble, it is better to trust entirely to the local abstraction of blood, and to the remedies now described, and to abstain altogether from general bleeding. If you look at the following table, you will see that some women died who were bled profusely, and that others recovered where a small quantity was drawn from the arm, or where it was entirely drawn by cupping from the temples and nape of the neck. These observations are made with the view of preventing you from having recourse to extensive depletion in all cases of puerperal convulsions, without carefully considering the condition and previous history of the patient. Profuse and indiscriminate bloodletting cannot be practised with impunity in this disease.

This is the treatment which ought to be employed in cases of puerperal convulsions before labour comes on, and also after labour has commenced, and if the fits do not diminish in frequency and violence, and the parts are in a condition to admit of artificial delivery, it is very important that it should not be long delayed. In one case which occurred in the latter months these means were vigorously employed without effect, and when the patient appeared sinking, the operation of turning was performed, though the os uteri had not begun to dilate, and the fits ceased immediately after the delivery had been effected, and recovery took place. Should the head of the child not have descended sufficiently low for the forceps to be applied when delivery becomes absolutely necessary, recourse should be had to the perforator. Even when the os uteri is fully dilated, and the head of the child has passed so far into the pelvis that an ear can be felt, it is difficult to apply the forceps and extract the head without danger to the mother, and where the insensibility is complete, and the intervals between the fits short, and the patient cannot be retained in the proper position, the employment of the forceps is always attended with considerable hazard to the perineum and soft parts.

Opium has been almost universally condemned in puerperal convulsions, and I consider it always improper before blood-letting has been employed to a sufficient extent, and the delivery has been completed either spontaneously or artificially. In some of the most severe cases which I have seen after copious venesection and delivery, large doses of the liquor opii sedativus have appeared to produce very powerful effects in arresting the fits ; in others no benefit whatever resulted from the employment of sedatives of

A TABULAR VIEW OF FIFTY-TWO CASES OF PUERPERAL CONVULSIONS.

Year		Result
1816	—, æt. 21, first pregnancy, ninth month unmarried numerous violent fits of convulsion at short intervals during twelve hours, without a return of consciousness the fits of uterus soft and dilatable, but no sign of labour ; pulse rapid and feeble death in six hours ; continuing with coma ; the child was easily turned and delivered. artificial delivery. orifice numerous violent fits of convulsiousness	Died ; vessels of brain distended.
*, 1823	V. S. ad. ʒj. : head shaved ; cold lotions ; calomel ; enemata. —, æt. 26, first pregnancy, ninth month ; fifty hours in labour : head of child low in the pelvis ; vagina and perineum rigid ; pulse full and strong face flushed ; occasional incoherence, and slight convulsive tremors of the face and extremities ; venesection to ʒxviii. followed by two severe fits of convulsion and insensibility ; unsuccessful attempts to deliver with the long forceps ; craniotomy ; no fit after delivery ; consciousness soon returned ; uterine inflammation followed.	Recovered.
1825	—, first pregnancy, ninth month numerous violent fits of convulsion ; comatose during the short intervals ; pupils widely dilated ; no treatment allowed to be employed, and she died soon after undelivered. (At Biala Cerkew Ukraine.)	Died.

ministered without success, or with injurious effects. Where consciousness did not return between the fits, but the woman remained insensible, foaming at the mouth, with stertorous breathing, then both the mother and child he believed would die, if they were not promptly relieved by delivery. I have saved, he says, the lives of many women in this way, but others have not failed to die after having been delivered in the due time, and in the proper manner—" bien et duement accouchées."

He admits that some cases will prove fatal whatever is done. If the child is alive he recommends the operation of turning ; if dead, craniotomy.

" There are some women," he says, " who are always attacked with convulsions either before or after delivery. To prevent such an accident he recommends bleeding from the arm twice or three times during pregnancy, and once after labour has commenced.

Puzos has also given an account of puerperal convulsions, and has recommended prompt and copious blood-letting, to relieve the brain from the excessive quantity of blood by which it is oppressed. After the bleeding, lavements, he says, must be employed, and it should be ascertained by an examination whether the uterus is dilating, and if the bleedings and other remedies do not calm the convulsions, then delivery is the best thing that can be done, which removes the pressure from the great bloodvessels of the abdomen, and allows it to circulate freely. The relief from delivery, he says, is not instantaneous, for the convulsions will often continue for a time, but at longer intervals, and patients sometimes remain for two days in a state of lethargy, and afterwards recover. But when the convulsions continue in spite of the bloodlettings and delivery, and the coma and stertorous breathing and foaming at the mouth, then the disorder will terminate fatally ; but we have the consolation to know, that we merit no reproach, having employed all the means we possess to overcome so grievous an accident. It is to be presumed because we have not succeeded, that lesions (crevasses) have been made in the brain by the violence of the convulsions, and that delivery could not remedy these. Thus, he adds, in the acute convulsions which precede or accompany labour, we cannot be too prompt and vigorous in the application of the proper resources ; and as these means are sometimes insufficient when the disease is once established, the accoucheur should be attentive to the first symptoms which announce convulsions ; for it sometimes happens, that in a labour accompanied with the most favourable symptoms, a woman all at once complains of dazzling of the eyes, of weight in the forehead or posterior part of the head, and of sudden loss of vision, symptoms which all announce that an attack of convulsion is at hand. I have seen women suddenly seized with frightful convulsions, he says, during labour, because attention had not been paid them when they complained of pain of the head. We perceive, then, that it is much more easy to prevent the evil, than to destroy it when it is once established ; since the most powerful remedies do not prevent the death of the mother and the child, which these convulsions put in the greatest danger. Therefore I bleed copiously, and that on the first appearance of the symptoms which threaten convulsions ; and I have often by this means relieved very speedily the headache, restored the vision, and completed the delivery happily in a short time.

Copious blood-letting in puerperal convulsions is the first remedy now employed by all practitioners in this country ; but the extent to which depletion is to be carried must be regulated by the constitution of the patient, the violence of the symptoms, and the effects produced by the loss of blood. Profuse blood-letting will not invariably control the disease, as some have asserted ; nay, I am persuaded that the sudden abstraction of fifty or more ounces of blood from the arm of some individuals, instead of arresting the disease, would destroy life. So feeble is the circulation of the blood in some women that it is imposible to remove this quantity from the arm. In young, robust, plethoric women, the best plan certainly is to take away as soon as possible after the attack twenty or twenty-five ounces of blood from the arm, to cut off the hair or shave the scalp, and apply over the head cold lotion or ice in a bladder ; to put ten grains or a scruple of calomel upon the tongue, or two drops of croton oil, if the bowels require immediate relief ; to throw up into the rectum a stimulating enema, and to apply warmth, mustard poultices, and rubefacients, to the inside of the legs and thighs ; at the same time to adopt every precaution to prevent the patient from being bruised or injured by the violence of the convulsive movements into which the body is thrown. If the fits continue after these remedies have been employed, with undiminished violence, and if the pulse is full and strong, and signs of congestion of the brain are still present, you may open another vein in the arm, and remove fifteen or twenty ounces more. A third bleeding to this extent is undoubtedly necessary and proper in some cases, but I prefer greatly, after thirty or thirty-five ounces of blood have been drawn from the arm, to trust to local bleeding, and especially to the application of cupping-glasses to the temples and nape of the neck. When the constitution has been previously exhausted by some chronic disease, or hæmorrhage ; or without these, if it is peculiarly delicate, nervous, and irritable, and has been weakened by grief, and other depressing passions, and the pulse is very rapid and feeble, it is better to trust entirely to the local abstraction of blood, and to the remedies now described, and to abstain altogether from general bleeding. If you look at the following table, you will see that some women died who were bled profusely, and that others recovered where a small quantity was drawn from the arm, or where it was entirely drawn by cupping from the temples and nape of the neck. These observations are made with the view of preventing you from having recourse to extensive depletion in all cases of puerperal convulsions, without carefully considering the condition and previous history of the patient. Profuse and indiscriminate blood-letting cannot be practised with impunity in this disease.

This is the treatment which ought to be employed in cases of puerperal convulsions before labour comes on, and also after labour has commenced, and if the fits do not diminish in frequency and violence, and the parts are in a condition to admit of artificial delivery, it is very important that it should not be long delayed. In one case which occurred in the latter months these means were vigorously employed without effect, and when the patient appeared sinking, the operation of turning was performed, though the os uteri had not begun to dilate, and the fits ceased immediately after the delivery had been effected, and recovery took place. Should the head of the child not have descended sufficiently low for the forceps to be applied when delivery becomes absolutely necessary, recourse should be had to the perforator. Even when the os uteri is fully dilated, and the head of the child has passed so far into the pelvis that an ear can be felt, it is difficult to apply the forceps and extract the head without danger to the mother, and where the insensibility is complete, and the intervals between the fits short, and the patient cannot be retained in the proper position, the employment of the forceps is always attended with considerable hazard to the perineum and soft parts.

Opium has been almost universally condemned in puerperal convulsions, and I consider it always improper before blood-letting has been employed to a sufficient extent, and the delivery has been completed either spontaneously or artificially. In some of the most severe cases which I have seen after copious venesection and delivery, large doses of the liquor opii sedativus have appeared to produce very powerful effects in arresting the fits ; in others no benefit whatever resulted from the employment of sedatives of

A TABULAR VIEW OF FIFTY-TWO CASES OF PUERPERAL CONVULSIONS.

1	1816	—, æt. 21, first pregnancy, ninth month; unmarried numerous violent fits of convulsion at short intervals during twelve hours, without a return of consciousness ; orifice of uterus soft and dilatable, but no sign of labour ; pulse rapid and feeble ; the fits continuing with coma ; the child was easily turned and delivered death in six hours ; artificial delivery.	Died ; vessels of brain distended.
2	July 12, 1823	V. S. ad. ʒi. ; head shaved ; cold lotions ; calomel enemata æt. 26, first pregnancy, ninth month ; fifty hours in labour : head of child low in the pelvis ; vagina and perineum rigid ; pulse full and strong face flushed ; occasional incoherence, and slight convulsive tremors of the face and extremities ; venesection to ℥xviii. followed by two severe fits of convulsion and insensibility ; unsuccessful attempts to deliver with the long forceps ; craniotomy ; no fit after delivery ; consciousness soon returned ; uterine inflammation followed.	Recovered.
3	1825	—, first pregnancy, ninth month ; numerous violent fits of convulsion ; comatose during the short intervals ; pupils widely dilated ; no treatment allowed to be employed, and she died soon after undelivered. (At Biala Cerkew Ukraine.)	Died.

4	Jan. 22, 1827	——, æt. 26, first pregnancy, 7th month; eight weeks before delivery suddenly seized with coma, from which she recovered after copious bleeding, &c.; headache, giddiness, and partial loss of speech, but consciousness and memory have remained; slight hemiplegia of the right side; pulse 90; went to the full period; labour natural in a few hours, convulsions, coma, dilated pupil, retention of urine; died on the 29th; copious venesection and cupping; head shaved; cold lotions and blisters; cathartics.	Died; a thick layer of lymph on the surfaces of both hemispheres of brain, softening below; veins filled with firm coagula, and ventricles with serum.
5	1827	——, æt. 20, unmarried, first pregnancy, seven months and a half; had epilepsy in early life; headache, drowsiness, loss of memory; paralysis of right inferior extremity after a slight fit of convulsion and coma; labour natural; child alive; no fit after delivery; venesection, cupping, head shaved, cathartics, low diet.	Recovered.
6	Jan. 27, 1828	——, æt. 25, eighth month of second or third pregnancy; headache and general indisposition after violent excitement; soon seized with convulsions, which continued with short intervals of nine hours; complete insensibility; pulse slow, full, and strong; os uteri dilated; head of child low in the pelvis; expelled during the fits; venesection ad ʒᵢ. and ʒxxiv.; head shaved and cupping to ʒxii.	Recovered.
7	May 2, 1828	First pregnancy, unmarried, 9th month; severe fits in the first stage of labour; os uteri rigid and imperfectly dilated; venesection ad ʒxxiv, repeated to ʒxli.; fits continued; os uteri partially dilated; perforation; fits immediately ceased.	Recovered; soon after attacked with mania.
8	May 20, 1828	Delivered at 3 A.M.; convulsions came on soon after; venesection ad ʒxxv.; at 1 P.M. the fits ceased and consciousness returned; weariness, headache, and oppression continued.	Recovered.
9	June 21, 1828	——, æt. 24, third or fourth pregnancy, 7⅔ months; epileptic in early life; after suffering for several days from an uneasy sensation of weight in the head and giddiness, was suddenly attacked with convulsions and insensibility; os uteri dilated; no symptoms of labour; no fit; stupor continues; pulse 80; copious alvine evacuations; went to full period, and was safely delivered of a living child; venesection ad ʒxx; head shaved, cold lotions, enemata, cathartics; venesection ad ʒxii.	Recovered.
10	Sept. 16, 1828	——, æt. 24, first pregnancy, ninth month; constipation and headache for several days; several fits of convulsion; insensible in the intervals; pupils dilated; pulse 80, full and strong; face flushed; os uteri slightly dilated; feeble irregular uterine contractions; after venesection and free evacuation of the bowels, fits ceased; delivered next day, without assistance, of a living child; venesection ad ʒxxv.; leeches; head shaved; calomel; enemata.	Recovered.

No.	Date	Case	Result
11	October 6, 1828	——, æt. 33, second pregnancy, first stage of labour; had convulsions during her former labour; headache, giddiness, and drowsiness, during the latter months; venesection recommended, but not employed; several severe fits, at short intervals, during the first stage of labour; muscles of left side most affected; face flushed; pupils dilated; pulse rapid, feeble, and irregular; os uteri widely dilated; head of child pressing through the brim of the pelvis; venesection ad ℥xx. and cupping from the temple to ℥xij.; child born alive next morning; fits soon ceased; but she died three months after in a fit of convulsion, after taking an emetic without advice.	Died; softening of the brain, with effusion of serum into the ventricles; tubercles in the lungs.
12	Jan. 24, 1829	——, æt. 18, first pregnancy, ninth month, delivered at 11 A.M., labour natural. The expulsion of the placenta was soon followed by a strong fit of convulsion; venesection was immediately employed. At 4 P.M. frequent severe fits without any intervals of consciousness; venesection repeated. At 8 P.M. fits and stupor continued, when forty drops of laudanum were given without my consent. January 25th—Fits continued; twenty drops of laudanum; sinapism to the legs. 26th—Severe fits during the night; has taken sixty drops of laudanum at three doses, which appeared to calm the violent agitation after the paroxysms. 27th, 10 A.M.—Severe and frequent fits during the night; breathing stertorous; pulse rapid and feeble; venesection ad ℥xxxv. repeated to ℥vi.; head shaved; enemata, calomel, ol. ricini, &c. Died on the 28th.	Died; turgescence of the blood-vessels of the pia mater; no other morbid appearance.
13	March 23, 1829	——, middle age, first pregnancy, and near full period. Convulsions during the first stage; headache complained of for some weeks previously; os uteri fully dilated, and half of the head in the cavity of the pelvis; pains ceased after the convulsions began, until the next morning, when they returned, and a dead child was expelled. The day after, the fits returned; and on the 27th she was attacked with uterine inflammation, and died in three days. Leeches, venesection, and cupping, were employed, together with calomel, blisters, &c.	Died; no post-mortem examination allowed.
14	April 15, 1829	——, æt. 30, ninth month. Headache, vertigo, and depression of spirits, during the seventh and eighth months; convulsions and hemiplegia of left side took place seventeen days before labour; she was bled to 16 oz. and cupped ad ℥xvj. and afterwards venesection ad ℥xij.; head shaved; blisters and cathartics. The labour was completed without assistance, but she died three days after, comatose.	Died; serum in the ventricles; a small scrofulous tumor adhered to the basilar artery; a portion of right lobe of cerebrum was soft, and of a yellow colour.
15	Dec. 1829	Convulsions and insensibility during labour; pulse rapid and feeble; delivery was completed by craniotomy; she was not bled; died comatose three days after delivery.	Died; a table-spoonful of serum was found at the base of the brain; great vascularity around the tuber annulare.

16	1829	——, æt. 30, ninth month of fourth or fifth pregnancy; violent convulsions at intervals during twenty-four hours, without sign of labour; convulsions continued in spite of copious venesection, calomel, &c.; turning was performed with difficulty before the os uteri had begun to dilate, and extraction completed with great difficulty, from the uterus contracting around the neck of the child; convulsions immediately ceased after delivery.	Recovered.
17	1829	——, æt. 20, hysterical, eighth month of first pregnancy; headache and giddiness for several days; twenty to thirty severe fits of convulsions during fourteen hours; insensible at intervals; labour came on twenty-four hours after the first fit, and child expelled; no fit after delivery; consciousness did not return for several days; uterine and crural phlebitis followed. Calomel, venesection, and enemata employed, and ice to scalp in a bladder.	Recovered.
18	Sept. 29, 1829	Ninth month of first pregnancy; violent convulsions during labour; ℥iv. of blood had been drawn by her medical attendant; os uteri slightly open; no pain; fits continued five hours, when a dead child was expelled; no fits after delivery, but she continued comatose until she died.	Died.
19	1829	——, æt. 28; seized with convulsions eight days after a natural labour; ten severe fits in two hours; in the intervals she was completely insensible, with stertorous breathing, dilated pupils; the pulse 110, feeble; the fits went off in a few hours, but she remained several days in a drowsy confused state: the attack followed the use of very indigestible food: has since been twice confined, and had no convulsions; cupping ℥xiij.; calomel; cathartics; enema; head shaved; blistering.	Recovered.
20	April 8, 1830	——, æt. 25, first pregnancy, ninth month; hysteria at the age of 15; at the end of ninth month frequent fits of convulsion in the course of twelve hours; consciousness returned after venesection; severe headache, and occasional spasms of the face and extremities; labour natural; venesection ℥xxx.; calomel, gr. x.; enemata; cathartics; cold to the shaved head.	Recovered.
21	Jan. 1, 1831	——, æt. 20, first pregnancy, ninth month; incoherence, followed by convulsions, towards the end of the first stage of a protracted labour; labour pains strong and regular, and the greater part of the head in the cavity of the pelvis; the fits were relieved, and she was delivered in a few hours of a dead child without help; venesection ℥xviij.; venesection ʒj.	Recovered.
22	Autumn 1831	——, æt. 30, first pregnancy; incoherence, stupor, and convulsions, at the end of the first stage of labour; symptoms relieved by venesection ℥xxxvj.; labour pains continued, and a living child was expelled without artificial assistance.	Recovered.

23	Dec. 1831	Severe fits of convulsion soon after the commencement of labour; no relief from copious venesection; os uteri partially dilated; head above brim of pelvis; pains ceased; perforation; one slight fit after delivery; consciousness gradually returned.	Recovered.
24	May 9, 1832	—, æt. 30, had epilepsy when a child; labour began at 8 A.M. 7th May; membrane ruptured in the night; os uteri dilated to the size of a crown on the morning of the 8th; pains feeble; complained of headache; pulse full and slow; venesection; enema; labour continued till the morning of the 9th, when severe convulsive fits supervened; venesection repeated; fits and unconsciousness continued for several hours, and the pains went entirely off; the head being still high up in the pelvis, and the os uteri rigid and undilated, craniotomy was performed: no fit after delivery; venesection ℨvj.; enema; cathartics; venesection ℨxiv.; head shaved; cold lotions, &c.	Recovered.
25	Dec. 1832	Convulsion in the seventh month of first pregnancy, after drinking brandy; venesection ad ℨxxxij. and twelve leeches; fourteen days after delivered of a dead child without artificial assistance.	Recovered.
26	July 5, 1833	—, first pregnancy; delirium and slight convulsions came on suddenly after the labour had lasted upwards of twenty-four hours; vagina rigid, hot, and tender; os uteri not fully dilated; copious venesection produced no relief; the head being beyond the reach of the forceps, craniotomy was performed; the fits immediately ceased; consciousness was not perfectly restored for several days.	Recovered
27	October 1833	—, middle age; convulsions during first labour, without any precursory symptoms; venesection ℨxxx.; a feeble child was born alive by the natural pains; convulsions ceased immediately after delivery.	Recovered.
28	Feb. 25, 1833	—, æt. 25, first pregnancy, ninth month; after eating roasted pork for dinner and supper, was seized with vomiting, convulsions, and insensibility, at 3 A.M.; after venesection and an enema, the fits became slighter, the pulse extremely rapid and feeble; the fits, however, returned occasionally till 10 A.M. when labour pains came on; at 1 A.M. a dead child was expelled; fits and insensibility continued four hours after. 26th—The fits had ceased, and consciousness had returned, though imperfectly; retention of urine; she died five days after with symptoms of uterine inflammation.	Died.
29	Dec. 30, 1833	—, æt. 20, first pregnancy, unmarried; violent convulsions sixteen hours after the commencement of labour; os uteri fully dilated; head squeezed into the brim of the pelvis; ear could not be felt; venesection ℨxxx.; fits more violent and frequent after venesection; pulse rapid and feeble; labour pains ceased; perforation; head extracted with difficulty; no fits after delivery; sensibility returned the following day.	Recovered.

30	May 23, 1834	——, æt. 30, second pregnancy; convulsions appeared eight hours after labour had begun; head impacted; venesection employed; insensibility; pupils dilated; constant convulsive movements of the muscles of the face; pains very violent; rupture of the uterus threatened; craniotomy; fits ceased immediately after delivery.	Recovered.
31	March 3, 1835	Puerperal convulsions at the end of eighth month; labour soon began; face presentation; pains very violent at short intervals; forceps tried, but craniotomy at last performed; venesection was performed before delivery; four fits took place after extraction of child; liq. opii sed. was given, after which the fits seemed much slighter, and they gradually went off.	Recovered.
32	April 1835	First labour, full period; returned home from a dinner party, where she had partaken of a variety of dishes and wines, soon after which labour came on, accompanied with incoherence; violent convulsions them followed; venesection and enemata were employed; forceps was used, and the child was extracted alive; convulsions continued.	Died five hours after delivery.
33	March 1, 1836	Middle-aged woman, addicted to the use of stimulants, attacked with convulsions during the first stage of labour; V.S. ad $\mathfrak{z}$xxv. without producing good effect. Forceps applied, and a dead child extracted; fits increased in violence after delivery, and continued until she died.	Died; vessels of the brain were unusually distended with blood.
34	Aug. 16, 1836	Convulsions occurring after a full dinner of currie and rice; pulse rapid and feeble; V.S. ad $\mathfrak{z}$viij.; os uteri slightly dilated; labour pains commencing; membranes were ruptured, and the liquor amnii evacuated; C. C. temporibus, ad $\mathfrak{z}$vj; head of child descended into pelvis; the forceps were applied; the child was easily extracted, but dead; convulsions continued.	Died two hours after delivery.
35	Aug. 1836	Puerperal convulsions during labour; had 14 fits before she was seen; os uteri dilated; head low in pelvis; forceps applied, and the child extracted with ease; child dead; only 1 fit after delivery.	Recovered.
36	Feb. 8, 1837	Eighth month of third pregnancy; for two weeks had suffered from influenza and headache; attacked with convulsions at end of that period, having 17 fits in seven hours; $\mathfrak{z}$xl. of blood were drawn; the fits during the day became more violent, and the muscles were violently affected; pupils dilated; membranes ruptured; os uteri slightly dilated; at midnight the fits came on again with tremendous violence; craniotomy was performed, and only one fit occurred after the extraction of child.	Recovered,
37	August 15, 1837	Puerperal convulsions; no relief from copious venesection; fits ceased soon as delivery was completed, which was effected by craniotomy.	Recovered.
38	1837	First labour, very protracted, head jammed in brim of pelvis; an injudicious attempt was made to apply the forceps; convulsions threatened; craniotomy performed; labour completed; symptoms subsided.	Recovered,

No.	Date		Result
39	Jan. 4, 1838	In a patient, under the care of Mr. Brookes, convulsions took place immediately after the birth of the child; fourth labour; she had been bled copiously, by him and all other means vigorously employed; coma came on; cold extremities; rapid feeble pulse; she died the following day in spite of all treatment.	Died.
40	May 9, 1838	Convulsions occurring after the birth of the child; the patient had been excited at a concert, an hour after she had returned from which labour came on; she soon became insensible, with convulsive movements of the muscles of the eyelids and lips; venesection ad ℥xv. by cupping, and enemata exhibited; she remained unconscious two days, and on the evening of the third sensibility returned.	Recovered.
41	Nov. 28, 1838	Drowsiness and headache in the ninth month of the first pregnancy, which continued for two weeks, when she was attacked with convulsions; a severe fit of sickness preceded the convulsions; they continued during the day; pulse 84; labour pains commenced; os uteri high up and undilated; venesection ad ℥xv., and ℥xxx. were drawn by cupping from the temples. The next day the fits disappeared, and she was safely delivered; two days after, however, convulsions followed the birth of the child, but was again bled, and the fits were from that time controlled.	Recovered.
42	Feb. 16, 1839	First labour, convulsions of a violent kind; venesection and other remedies employed; head within reach of the forceps, which was applied; convulsions became more severe; craniotomy was performed, but the convulsions continued, and she died soon after delivery.	Died in convulsions.
43	March 13, 1841	Convulsions at the end of first stage of labour, without any premonitory symptoms; pupils dilated; insensibility; uterine action was suspended; ℥xxv. of blood were taken from the arm, and with the aid of sprinkling water on the face, applying ammonia to the nostrils, and dilating the external parts, the child was at last expelled by the natural efforts; fits ceased.	Recovered.
44	April 2, 1841	At seventh month of tenth pregnancy, convulsions came on without previous symptoms; muscles of extremities not convulsed; consciousness lost; recovered herself for five hours; venesection employed with cathartics and cold to the head; she gradually recovered, and went to the full period.	Recovered.
45	Nov. 13, 1841	Convulsions in the seventh month, from alarm at fancying that the house was on fire; insensibility; teeth clenched; pupils contracted; breathing slow and stertorous; fits renewed soon after with greater violence; pupils became dilated; head drawn to right side; pulse and respiration became quickened; venesection had been employed, together with the exhibition of calomel, croton oil, enemata, &c.; cupping from the temples; in three hours she was quite insensible, and appeared dying from exhaustion; forceps applied, and delivery accomplished; consciousness never returned.	Died fifteen hours after delivery.

No.	Date		Result
46	April 16, 1842	Convulsions occurring one day after delivery; fits violent, and at short intervals; when the fits went off, the pupils were contracted, and widely dilated when they were about to return; venesection ad ℥xxx. and no return afterwards of the fits.	Recovered.
47		A lady, æt. 26; protracted labour, first child; fits continued with great violence; venosection ad ℥xxx.; fits continued with great violence, and the head was found to be pressing on the perinæum; the forceps was about to be applied, when the child was expelled naturally, and the convulsions ceased; she was in a state of stupor for ten hours.	Recovered.
48		A lady under the care of Dr. Sims had violent puerperal convulsions in the seventh month of first pregnancy; two pounds of blood were drawn from the arm; the fits went off, but she had insensibility and headache for a long period; V.S. was again had recourse to, but she continued to suffer until the full period, when she was delivered of a dead child.	Recovered.
49	Sept. 30, 1842	A lady under the care of Mr. Cathrow became perfectly insensible the instant after the birth of her ninth child; an hour after the uterus contracted, and the placenta was expelled; there were no convulsions, but all the muscles of the jaws, trunk, and extremities, were rigid; she remained twenty-eight hours in this state without speaking, the hands and feet being drawn inward, the jaws nearly clenched, and the eyeballs drawn upwards; pupils not dilated; pulse 80, and sharp; a few leeches were applied to the head, and cathartics and antispasmodics given, when the power of swallowing returned; the same occurrence had taken place, but in a much slighter degree, soon after the birth of every child; she never had hysteria or catalepsy in early life.	Recovered.
50	Nov. 23, 1840	A young married lady was attacked with mania on the eighth day after delivery; she soon became wildly delirious, and died six days after in convulsions; the pulse being very rapid and feeble, depletion was not carried to any great extent.	Died.
51	Nov. 22, 1842	A lady under the care of Mr. Johnson, Grosvenor Place, became maniacal on the fourth day after delivery; in the course of two days she was seized with convulsions, and had a number of severe fits; in a few days, after the repeated application of leeches to the head and region of the uterus, &c. &c. she recovered.	Recovered.
52	Dec. 2, 1842	A lady, æt. 33, was seized with violent pains in her first labour, about twenty hours after the membranes were ruptured; venesection ℥xxv.; the labour pains continued, and the fits did not return for sixty ten hours; the uterus then having ceased to contract, and several more fits being caused, artificial delivery was had recourse to; the fits ceased the infant the child was dead, and she afterwards died with symptoms of effusion into the brain.	Died.

any kind. The application of leeches to the region of the uterus appeared, in a recent case of mania complicated with puerperal convulsions, to be attended with the most striking benefit after all other means had been tried without effect. Sedatives have been recommended to be applied to the cervix uteri, or thrown up into the rectum during labour, and after delivery, in cases of puerperal convulsion, but I have had no experience of their efficacy.

CONTRIBUTIONS
TO
ANATOMY AND PHYSIOLOGY.

By Robert Knox, M.D. F.R.S.E.

Lecturer on Anatomy and Physiology, and Corresponding Member of the French Academy of Medicine.

[Continued from p. 591.]

I shall now endeavour to apply these views derived from transcendental anatomy to the practical work of Naegele, and to his discovery of the pelvis oblique ovata. From time to time there occur, no doubt, in every dissecting room, specimens similar to the five or six now lying before me; they have been in my own museum nearly seventeen years, and have annually been exhibited to my class. I shall describe one of them with some minuteness, the rest more briefly.

1. A female pelvis, history unknown. The right os innominatum is not present; the left had been accidentally divided with the saw just before the acetabulum, and the fragment lost; the last lumbar vertebra is present; the sacrum also, and seemingly the first of the coccygeal vertebræ. To understand the preparation rightly, it requires to be seen, or to place Mr. Naegele's work before you. The left sacro-iliac articulation is obliterated or anchylosed; the iliac portion of the left innominatum small, and but partially developed. The sacrum is twisted away to one side; the area of the left half of the introitus could scarcely have equalled a third of the right: the specimen when entire must have presented exactly the form we find in M. Naegele's plate, and have been one of the very best specimens of the obliquely oval pelvis.

2. The preparation marked 980 is similar to the last in nearly all respects: the partial development has again happened on the left side; the anchy-

losis of the joint is complete only on the surface, but the obliquely oval form would not have been so well marked as in the preceding specimen.

3. In the specimen now before me, which is an extremely instructive one, as shewing the early stage at which these deformations commence, the pelvis being evidently that of a young person, a female, the defective development had taken place on the right side: there is no appearance whatever of any anchylosis,—a change which seems to come on later, and at times to be altogether unconnected with the deformity. The first sacral vertebra strongly resembles the last lumbar; it has not yet united with the second, and the two lateral portions or wings are of extremely unequal depth; the one, the right, being scarcely half an inch; the other, the left, being fully an inch and $\frac{1}{4}$; neither does the body of this vertebra follow so exactly the direction of the second as is usual in the regular-formed sacrum, but slopes slightly backward; lastly, a line let fall perpendicularly from the symphysis pubis to the sacrum strikes that bone at the inner edge of the right foramina vertebralia, instead of the centre of the bone, as it ought to do. On looking at the specimen when held fairly before you, you may see nearly the whole of the right foramina vertebralia, which ought not to be the case had the right os innominatum been fairly developed; but instead of that semicircular line which the linea innominata ought to present, we find it nearly a constantly converging one from the articulation with the sacrum to the symphysis pubis. No one, I think, can now doubt what would have been the ultimate form of the pelvis had the person happily lived to mature years: it would have been a perfect specimen of the pelvis oblique ovata, the right side retaining the infantile and brute form, the left expanding into that of the well-formed woman.

I shall now very briefly notice three more specimens which I find on the same shelf with those just described, but evidently quite different in their nature; I notice these the more particularly, that their characteristic pathological condition may have orginally led others as well as myself to overlook the essential differences betwixt them and the preceding specimens. They are half sections of the pelvis taken at random from the Practical Rooms, exhibiting an ancyhlosis of the right sacro-iliac joint—no other deformity is present; the pelves shewing no marks of deformation. One of the persons had probably suffered from rheumatism; at least other parts of the bones shew a strong disposition to exostotic deposits, which indeed abound. Thus anchylosis of this joint is in no shape necessarily connected with the pelvis oblique ovata, although it usually follows or accompanies it as a consequence of non-development.

The last specimen on the table reminds me of the vast variety of forms presented by the sacrum, and how difficult it is to give even the characteristic sexual distinctions. Here is one which would easily admit of its first bone being nicely removed with the saw, and yet leave a perfect sacrum, that is, a promontory and five bones. There appear to have been six sacral vertebræ in this specimen, but as neither the lumbar nor coccygeal bones are present, the matter remains doubtful. Another and a perfectly different view might be taken of this upper vertebra: it may be the last lumbar, but I feel disposed to say that, notwithstanding its anomalous appearance, it is the first sacral, and that the first coccygeal is here united to the last sacral.

As these observations have unexpectedly extended so much beyond the limits I anticipated, what I have further to say shall be very brief; it has a reference to two points: 1st, to some observations by Fischer and Autenrieth on the form of the pelvis of the quadruped mammal; 2d, as to the temporary relaxation of the pelvic ligaments in women preceding and during delivery.

1st, In addition to a vast number of very admirable and original observations, Autenrieth remarks, that the depth of the osseous symphysis of the pubis, and the comparative weakness of the sacral and caudal portions; the canal-like shape assumed by the pelvis in most of the lower animals; the rudimentary condition of the false or upper pelvis in some, and the like condition of the true pelvis in others; all these, he observes, are remarkable features in the pelvis of the quadruped. The influence of these changes is perceived in the condition of the muscles connected with these bones, in the comparative slenderness of the haunches of most quadrupeds, and the frequency of hernia in man as compared with them. The usual vertical position of the trunk in man has, no doubt, its share in giving rise to this circumstance. Autenrieth's mode of calculating certain dimensions of the pelvis is most ingenious, but to do justice to his ideas it would require that the work were translated and transferred to your pages entire: he divides the pelvis, for example, into what he calls a dorsal part and an abdominal, and he found that, whilst in the infant of two years the first was to the second in length as 10 to 11, and up to 14; in the adult it was as 10 to 16, up to 22.

It is sufficiently curious that, although in certain quadrumana, and in the elephant, the comparatively rounded form of the cranium in this respect somewhat, though rather remotely in the latter, resembling the human, might have been supposed adequate to produce a marked alteration in the form of the pelvis, it yet has not done so, at least not to any great extent. The pelvis of the highest of the quadrumana does not, in so far as I recollect, approach in form the female (human) pelvis; and in respect to the elephant, although it may be admitted to be more rounded in the *introitus*, or *narrow*, than most mammal pelves, its resemblance to the transversely oval human female pelvis is very distant.

2d, Do the articulations of the female pelvis relax during, and a little before, delivery? To what extent does the relaxation take place? Is it a rare or frequent occurrence? Is it a pathological or a healthy condition?

To answer these questions in as far as my own experience goes, I shall endeavour to relate, to the best of my recollection, some of the principal facts bearing on them in the order in which they presented themselves to me.

During the summer sessions of 1825, 1826, and 1827, I delivered, in Surgeons' Square, three courses of lectures on comparative anatomy. The desire to present as many fresh specimens of all the great classes, and principal genera, of animals, induced me to apply to the fishermen on our coasts, engaging them to send meany rare mollusca fishes, seals, dolphins, &c. which they might take by nets or otherwise. Now, under those circumstances, a pregnant seal was brought me; the animal had been shot with a single ball, killing not only the mother but the foetus. From the size of the young seal and other circumstances, it was evident that in a very few days the foetus would have been born. I shall here abstain from mentioning any other circumstances respecting the anatomy of the seal and its foetus, saving what is directly connected with the history of the pelvis—I mean of the pelvis of this pregnant seal. The foetus, which lay in the uterus with all its natural connexions, appeared to me of extraordinary dimensions, and I was curious to know how such a foetus could pass the pelvis of the mother: the examination of this cavity displayed a singular and unexpected fact, and which was at the time quite new to me; the interpubic ligament, or ligamentous symphysis, was so elongated that the bones might be separated from each other to the extent of nearly two inches. When I now examined attentively the form of the osseous pelvis, I could see very evidently that in the quadrilateral-shaped pelvis, where the greatest diameter was the antero-posterior one, as in the quadruped mammal, and not the transverse one, as in woman, this temporary separation of the pubic bones of the pelvis admitted of a great enlargement of all the diameters of the pelvis, whilst in the transversely oval pelvis of woman, the artificial separation of the pubic bones merely, even to a considerable extent, say an inch, did but little increase any of the diameters of the brim and abdominal entrance to the true pelvis. As this was a matter which could be made the subject of comparative demonstration, several female pelves were divided at the pubes, as recommended by Sigault, when it became manifest to the class that unless the pubic bones were separated forcibly from each other for more than an inch and a quarter, nothing was gained on the diameters of the cavity; and that a more extended separation, so as to render the operation at all useful in respect to its object, was absolutely impracticable on the living woman, since, on its being attempted, the sacro-iliac joints were heard to give way. Having satisfied myself that the Sigaultian operation on the transversely oval pelvis of woman could lead to no

real benefit, being only applicable to that form of pelvis found in the quadruped, and but rarely in woman, my attention was next directed to ascertain whether or not, in woman, the ligamentous symphysis of the pubis became relaxed during parturition? Whether or not this was frequent or rare? Whether or not it was accompanied by a corresponding relaxation of the sacro-iliac joints, without which the relaxation of the ligamentous symphysis would be of little avail? And, lastly, whether such relaxations were to be viewed as pathological or natural? An opportunity soon occurred, after the dissection of the seal described above, to put some of these questions to the test of direct observation.

A middle-aged woman, who had died of flooding following delivery, was brought into the Practical Rooms: the pelvis was of full dimensions. On examining its articulations, they were found to be all relaxed; the bones could be made to slide over each other. The dissection was shewn to the class, and compared with that of the seal, whose skeleton was in the museum; the opinions, likewise, of several distinguished accoucheurs in town were asked: they all declared the relaxation to be the effect of one of two causes: it was either, said they, the result of putrefaction after death, or of a diseased or pathological condition of the pelvis. On consulting the published works of a most distinguished surgeon and accoucheur (Mr. Burns, of Glasgow), I found that he also maintained the doctrine, that when relaxation of the articulations of the pelvis did take place during delivery, it was a pathological and not a healthy process.

Since 1825 and 1826, I have now had an opportunity of examining carefully the pelves of five women of different ages who have died soon after delivery, and having found in all of these a relaxation of the articulations of the pelvis to a greater or less extent, but always remarkable, I feel disposed to think the process a regular or healthy one, and not pathological.

In conclusion, I trust it has been made apparent that the great laws of transcendental anatomy and physiology, even admitting them to be not yet very fully established, are yet extensively and happily applicable to human anatomy and physiology: certain deviations of the pelvis, for example, from its normal and specific form, have been shewn to be *merely a persistence of its fœtal shape;* and this shape again, being the *type of shape in every mammal,* the deformation gives to the adult pelvis thus constituted the shape at once of the human fœtal and quadruped pelvis. Or, to express the generalization as a law, perhaps we may say, " the laws regulating the growth of *specific forms* are the antithesis of the laws presiding over *transcendental forms;* the one bestows individuality on the species, the other struggles to reduce all to one type; as the one prevails, the specific form is preserved; with the predominance of the other, a destruction of all *speciality* exists: we call these laws of type deformating laws, because they are opposed to our ideas of species, and to the obvious endeavours of nature to maintain this struggle and to perpetuate species.

[To be continued.]

OBSERVATIONS AND EXPERIMENTS CONCERNING

DIABETES MELLITUS,

&c. &c.

By JOHN PERCY, M.D. (Edin.)

Physician to the Queen's Hospital, and Lecturer on Organic Chemistry at the Royal School of Medicine and Surgery, Birmingham.

[Continued from p. 595.]

(For the London Medical Gazette.)

WE now proceed to examine the subject of *the formation of grape-sugar in diabetes mellitus.* Several distinct questions are here naturally suggested.

1st. In what situations is the grape-sugar found in this disease?

2nd. In what part of the system is it formed?

3rd. What are the particular conditions attending its formation?

1. It is present in the *blood.* This fact is now firmly established; although, for a considerable time, chemists failed in their attempts to discover the existence of sugar in the blood of diabetic patients. M'Gregor, Dr. Rees, Dr. Maitland, M. Bouchardat, and Ambrosiani, have substantiated the fact by direct experiment.

The elegant analysis of diabetic blood by Dr. Rees, detailed in Guy's Hospital Reports, Vol. 3, p. 398, is extremely satisfactory, for the sugar was obtained in a crystallized form. I believe I have also met with similar success. Feb. 17, 1842, I received the blood, taken by cupping in the loins, from a young lady suffering under confirmed diabetes mellitus. I examined her urine several times, and obtained from it beautifully crystallized sugar; its sp. gr. was 1045. The patient died recently. I dried over the steam-bath 549·5 grains crassamentum and serum. I treated the dry residuum with successive portions of boiling alcohol, of sp. gr. 860°, to the amount of f℥v. The alcoholic solution was evaporated to dryness. The residuum was treated with distilled water, and the aqueous solution was evaporated to the consistence of syrup, and then left exposed to the air for several days. After the lapse of this time I distinctly observed small globular masses of a light fawn colour, and of the characteristic appearance of diabetic sugar; they were interspersed with crystals, apparently of chloride of sodium. The separation of sugar from the blood is often attended with considerable difficulty, and I have even failed to detect it in the blood of a dog, after the injection of sugar into the jugular vein. In the early stage of one case of diabetes, Dr. Christison could not detect any sugar in the blood; while in another, where the disease was far advanced, fermentation indicated its presence only in the small proportion of one grain in eight ounces. (Library of Medicine, Vol. 4, p. 252.) The existence of sugar in the blood of diabetic patients only in minute proportion, will not appear surprising, when we consider the extreme rapidity with which sugar, after its introduction into a vein, is eliminated by the kidneys, and when we also further consider that, in the disease in question, the quantity of water which passes through the blood in a given time is so much greater than in the condition of health. We receive it, then, as an established fact, that sugar exists in the blood in diabetes mellitus, and is circulated throughout the system.

I may here direct attention to the fact, that sugar, whether grape or cane, does not appear to produce any sensible effect upon the nervous system; and, in proof of this, I need only refer to the experiments previously recorded. Cane sugar may be even injected into the carotid artery without effecting any decided cerebral disturbance. I have injected 1000 grains of cane sugar, dissolved in ʒiij. of warm water, into this vessel, without observing any other effects than those which I have seen result from the injection of pure water into the same artery.

Sugar is also reported to have been occasionally detected in the *saliva* and *perspiration* of diabetic patients, and we cannot be surprised at this statement when we consider that the circulating liquid is itself impregnated with sugar.

We now arrive at a fact of the highest interest in connection with the pathology of diabetes, viz. the existence of saccharine matter in the *stomach* of diabetic patients, after all saccharine matter has been excluded from their food. This part of the subject necessarily includes the question next in order, viz.:

2dly. In what part of the system is the sugar formed?

It will be borne in mind, that my intention in this communication is not to examine the various hypotheses which have been proposed to explain diabetes mellitus, but simply to confine myself to an examination of what appears to be positively known upon the subject. More facts are yet required; and it would be advantageous to science if pathologists, who may have opportunities of practically studying the disease, would apply themselves to the investigation of particular points, which demand further elucidation.

To Dr. M'Gregor we are indebted for experimental evidence of the existence of sugar in the stomach in diabetes. Several questions arise in connection with this fact. *Is sugar found in the stomach only when the food has contained vegetable matter?* M'Gregor has answered this question in the negative, for he "found saccharine matter in the stomachs of persons in whom vomiting had been produced, and who had been kept for several days on a very strict animal diet," (Bell on Diabetes, Transl. p. 50.) This statement is one of extreme interest, and requires confirmation by other pathologists. The generation of grape-sugar

in the stomach from azotized tissue, as fibrin or albumen, would not admit of easy explanation. Experiments in relation to this subject must be performed with the greatest care, for those who have watched diabetic patients well understand the difficulty of ensuring the necessary condition of restricting a patient to an exclusively animal diet for several days. And in this case even milk and bread should be entirely excluded. I would express my earnest hope that some pathologist may be induced to direct his especial attention to the investigation of the statement under consideration.

Is the statement of M. Bouchardat correct, that the proportion of sugar in the urine is in the direct ratio of the quantity of fecula or saccharine matter contained in the food? (Bell, op. cit. p. 47.) It is difficult to understand how this statement should be perfectly compatible with that of M'Gregor, which we have just considered, for it would lead to the conclusion that the sugar is generated exclusively from amylaceous or similar vegetable matter. And if this conclusion were correct, a strictly animal diet in diabetes mellitus should be immediately followed by a return of the urine to a perfectly healthy condition, in so far as relates to the absence of sugar; which, however, I am not aware has hitherto been found to be the case. That the proportion of amylaceous matter of the food determines to a certain extent the proportion of sugar evacuated with the urine, we are not prepared to deny. It is only the constant and definite relation of Bouchardat, which requires confirmation by further experiments. Here, again, we must lament the deficiency of experimental data. We need well-established facts in the present day, and not mystical and indefinite opinions. If some pathologist would restrict himself to an investigation of the chyme of a diabetic patient—an investigation, it is true, attended with difficulties, but not insurmountable—valuable facts might be obtained.

M'Gregor discovered sugar, not only in the contents of the stomach, but also in the fæces of diabetic patients, and, what is deserving of attention, the sugar was capable of crystallization.

Another question is, *whether sugar, in diabetes, can, in any degree, be produced from previously assimilated mat-*

ter? Now, one of the most striking and invariable symptoms of the disease is emaciation. The loss of weight in some cases is remarkable; and of this we have an illustration in the history of Merchant. Absorption, therefore, of previously assimilated matter, must occur to a great extent; and the question arises, whether any of this matter is converted into sugar and evacuated with the urine, or whether it is entirely consumed in the process of respiration. The food, it is well known, serves two important ends, viz. the supply of matter for pulmonary oxidation, and for the reparation of waste. If these ends be not satisfactorily accomplished, whether from a deficient supply of nutriment, or from some defect in the process of assimilation, emaciation and exhaustion are the inevitable consequences. Now, the condition of a patient suffering under progressing diabetes is exactly the condition of a man exposed to one or other of the preceding circumstances. The food which he takes, although abundant, and suitable in quality, is converted, in great measure, into matter which is useless to the system, and which is expelled by the urinary organs. The condition, then, of a diabetic patient perfectly resembles that of starvation from a deficient supply of nutriment; and hence the consequent emaciation. Material must be continually introduced into the blood for the purpose of respiration; but in diabetes that material is in great measure virtually withheld, for grape-sugar, it would appear, is incapable of satisfactorily answering that purpose. Absorption, therefore, of previously assimilated matter, which is adapted to supply the demand of respiration, takes place with rapidity, and fat especially soon disappears. In the case of Merchant it will be remembered that almost every trace of fat had been removed; and that even the muscular tissue itself appeared to have suffered in some places extensive degeneration. In fact, every thing suitable for pulmonary oxidation had been removed. That fat is really adapted to this purpose, we learn from the following considerations, which have been lucidly expounded by Liebig.

1. When an animal is deprived of nutriment, the fat first disappears.

2. Fat animals, *cæteris paribus*, can exist longer without food than lean animals.

3. Hybernating animals which before the commencement of their period of torpor are well provided with fat, are afterwards reduced to leanness.

4. Rest, with the consequent diminution in the quantity of carbonic acid evolved in respiration, is favourable to the development of fat; whilst the converse is true in a state of activity.

Now, there is an obvious relation between the quality of food and the formation of fat; a relation of great practical importance to the farmer. Amylaceous matters, especially, tend to the production and deposition of fat. Accordingly, starch, in one form or other, is frequently employed in the fattening of poultry and pigs. Liebig has well insisted upon the relation of ultimate composition between fat and fecula, and explains the formation of the former from the latter by the simple abstraction of oxygen. (Vid. Animal Chemistry, edited by Dr. Gregory, page 83, et seq.) Whether the oily matter which I extracted from the chyme by alcohol in the experiments detailed in the present communication, might, in part, be derived from the starch, in the manner supposed by Liebig, is a question worthy of further investigation. Dr. Prout maintains that the conversion of fecula into oily matter in the stomach occurs in healthy digestion. However this may be, it is nevertheless certain that fat is in some way or other generated in the system from amylaceous matter. Now it is probable that in progressing diabetes mellitus, this conversion is, in great measure, if not altogether, arrested; for in the case of Merchant, although a liberal allowance of bread was prescribed, yet scarcely a trace of fat was discovered in any part of the body in the *post-mortem* examination. If the explanation of Liebig be admitted, that starch is changed into fat by the abstraction of oxygen, the question may arise, *whether in diabetes the fat may be converted in any degree into sugar by the absorption of oxygen?* A few months ago, I saw a tall, corpulent man, suffering under confirmed diabetes mellitus. His age was between 50 and 60. His weight in health must have been from 16 to 18 stones. He lost in less than a month more than two stones, and during this time his appetite was *considerably impaired.* The sp. gr. of the urine was 1045°, and furnished well crystallised sugar.

He died a week after I saw him. Now, this case might possibly favour an affirmative answer. The quantity of food taken was much less than in health, whilst the urine was highly saccharine, and 28lbs of matter, consisting, doubtless, in great measure, of fat, rapidly disappeared. Another curious and similar case I shall adduce in the sequel. I leave the question to be decided by further observation.

We now arrive at the third question.

3. *What are the particular conditions attending the formation of grape-sugar?* This question, it is evident, involves the *proximate cause* of the disease. Let us first interrogate morbid anatomy.

1. Mr. Bowman, whose reputation as a microscopic observer is so well established, examined the mucous membrane of Merchant's stomach, and was unable, by the aid of the microscope, to discover any morbid appearance. The mesenteric glands are generally enlarged, but this enlargement often exists in other diseases essentially different from diabetes. A tuberculated condition of the lungs, sooner or later, is almost constantly present, and the disease frequently terminates in phthisis pulmonalis. The kidneys and ureters are sometimes considerably enlarged, yet frequently without any alteration of structure. And we should reasonably expect that, in proportion as the natural function of an organ is increased, in the same proportion, within certain limits, will the volume of that organ be augmented. It must not be omitted, that in some cases of diabetes the urinary apparatus has been found to be altered in structure, but such alteration is clearly incidental, and is certainly in no way essentially connected with the formation of sugar, for, if the contrary were true, then, of necessity, similar structural change should exist in every case of diabetes, which, we know, is not the fact. Besides, it would be matter of surprise if the urinary apparatus were not in diabetes occasionally diseased beyond mere hypertrophy, for the liability of one organ to disease is, *cæteris paribus,* increased in proportion as the function of that organ is preternaturally excited. I may here introduce the result of the microscopic examination of one of Merchant's kidneys, kindly undertaken by Mr. Bowman, at my request.

"There were superficial abscesses, and destruction of certain parts of the renal vein by fibrine, adherent to the inner wall, and softened in its interior. In the principal part of the organ the Malpighian bodies and the tubes appeared to me to be healthy in structure." I need not refer to the morbid appearances which have been occasionally observed in diabetes. From a careful examination of numerous published cases, we arrive at the negative conclusion, that the *disease may exist independently of any appreciable alteration of structure whatever.*

2dly. Of the condition of the blood and secretions. Upon this subject our knowledge at present is extremely imperfect. I have previously alluded to the elegant analysis of diabetic blood by Dr. Rees, but it teaches us nothing concerning the formation of grape-sugar. The salivary secretion is generally, if not almost uniformly, acid, and is also frequently much diminished. In some cases, however, it is increased, even to salivation. (Vide Cases by Dr. Watts, in a recent number of the Lancet). The patient suffering from diabetes often complains of the disagreeable sensation of dryness of the mouth and fauces. If the saliva really perform so important a part in the process of digestion as my friend Dr. Wright and some other physiologists maintain, then the fact of the salivary secretion being generally decreased in diabetes acquires considerable importance. At one time I stimulated Merchant's salivary glands by means of capsicum gargle, which increased the secretion to such an extent as not only to enable him, but to require him, to spit freely. I did not, however, during this period, observe any marked alteration either in the symptoms or the quality of the urine. With respect to the condition of the skin, some observations are required. One of the most frequent exciting causes of diabetes is certainly habitual exposure to sudden and great alteration of temperature. The functions of digestion, respiration, and cutaneous exhalation, appear to be intimately connected with each other; so that a disturbance of one is often attended with a corresponding disturbance of the others. With the precise nature of the function of the skin, it must be admitted, that, at present, we are but imperfectly acquainted; but that it is of great importance we are assured from a variety of considerations, which it would be superfluous to enumerate. How carefully is the state of the skin watched by the judicious practitioner! How often has the restoration to healthy action of the suspended function of the skin in febrile diseases satisfactorily indicated a return of convalescence! And, again, how often has a peculiar atmospheric condition, by modifying or arresting the function of the skin, induced disease! Future investigation, it is hoped, will shed more light on this interesting part of pathology. All that we can do now is to insist upon the general fact of the suppression, in a greater or less degree, of the cutaneous function in diabetes. In the case of Merchant I did not witness that peculiar degree of harshness which I have frequently remarked in other cases. Occasionally, as we learn from the register, he perspired freely. I may here appropriately introduce some remarks of Dr. Graves in respect to the state of the skin in diabetes. "I may observe," writes that eminent physician, "that it is by no means so dry, acrid, and harsh, as we frequently find in diabetic patients; indeed, it feels nearly natural, and is partially covered with moisture at various times of the day. Some persons, looking almost exclusively to the condition of the skin, have taken a very limited view of this disease. They consider it as arising from perspiration being repressed, and turned inwards in the kidneys. This, however, is by no means satisfactory. Some of the worst cases I have ever seen were attended by colliquative sweats." Dr. Graves also cites the case of a gentleman affected with diabetes, who used to perspire copiously every day at the time that his urine was 1049°. The fact, however, is nevertheless *general*, though not *universal*, that in diabetes the function of the skin is, in a greater or less degree, suppressed. There is also one fact, which should not be omitted in this part of the subject, namely, that according to the experience of Dr. Prout, which we are assured must have been very extensive, "diabetes usually *follows* cutaneous affections." (Op. cit. p. 35.)

In respect to the condition of the urine, several points are deserving of especial attention. By the results of direct experiment we are enabled satisfactorily to explain the presence of sugar in the urine; for we have seen that, when sugar is introduced into the blood, it is in great measure rapidly eliminated by the kidneys, in the precise chemical state in which it is injected. Cane sugar, for example, passes through the circulation without in the smallest degree being converted into grape sugar, or appearing to suffer any other change. And the same is true of sugar of milk, or lactine; in proof of which I may relate the following experiment:—Into the right jugular vein of a middle-sized dog, I injected 300 grains of pure lactine, dissolved in fʒiv. of distilled water. An hour afterwards the animal was destroyed by prussic acid, and during the convulsive action fʒv. of pale straw-coloured urine were evacuated and collected. The sp. gr. was 1038°, and the odour was similar to that of ordinary diabetic urine. The syrup, obtained by evaporation, became a solid mass of crystallized lactine. The mass consisted of small circular clusters of minute prisms radiating from the centre. No trace of sugar was detected by fermentation in the usual manner. *The kidneys, then, in diabetes, appear to act simply the mechanical part of filters.* In further proof of this conclusion may be adduced the fact that, in the case of Merchant, obstinate diarrhœa occurred, during which the urine was sometimes remarkably diminished, although it was not changed *in quality*. Now there is no reason to believe that a diminution in the quantity of sugar generated in the system corresponded to this diarrhœa, which therefore may be conceived to have been, to a certain extent, a *vicarious* action. The theory, however, of Dr. Prout supposes that the kidneys complete the development of the *low sugar*, by communicating to it the *crystalline* form. "The portion (of the *low* sugar) that is assimilated is applied to the purposes of the economy; the portions modified and unassimilated pass together through the system to the kidneys, by which glands the portion modified is disorganized, and finally appears in the urine as crystallizable sugar, along with the portion originally remaining unassimilated in the stomach." (Op. cit. p. 37.) And in corroboration of this view, Dr.

Prout adduces the fact, that " when the disorganising function of the kidneys is suspended, or when these glands are partially diseased, the urine, besides albuminous matters, and more or less of crystallizable sugar, often contains the saccharine principle in imperfectly developed forms." But the fact of sugar having been obtained from the blood of diabetic patients, in a distinct crystallised form, would certainly not seem favourable to the theory of Dr. Prout concerning the supposed function of the kidneys.

It might here be remarked, that the thirst, which is so invariable, and frequently so urgent, a symptom of diabetes, may possibly be an expedient of nature, by which to insure the introduction of a sufficient quantity of water into the system, for the purpose of diluting the blood, and so facilitating and expediting the elimination of the sugar by the kidneys, and thereby preventing its accumulation in the system to an injurious extent. And this notion would appear to receive support from the fact, that the thirst increases in diabetes in proportion as the quantity of amylaceous matter in the food is augmented.

To Dr. Prout we are indebted for the knowledge of two important facts in relation to saccharine urine. The first is, that " a saccharine condition of the urine exists in dyspeptic and gouty individuals much oftener than is supposed ; and hundreds pass many years of their lives with this symptom more or less constantly present, who are quite unaware of it till the quantity of urine becomes increased." (p. 33.) The second is, that " diabetes very frequently (and, so far as Dr. Prout's experience goes, *always*) accompanies carbuncles." (p. 36.)

Another singular point in respect to diabetic urine is the disappearance of sugar from the urine previously to dissolution. Of this we have an excellent illustration in the case of Merchant. His death appeared to be entirely the effect of exhaustion of nervous power; for the autopsy revealed no disorganization of structure apparently commensurate with the fatal termination. In some cases of diabetes, it is reported that the saccharine condition of the urine ceases when pulmonary phthisis supervenes. In the case of Merchant, it is true, tuber-

cular matter was scattered here and there through the lungs, yet not to a sufficient extent materially to interfere with the function of respiration.

There is still another point in connection with diabetic urine worthy of notice, viz. the *general fact* of the absence of uric acid, or urate sediments. Dr. Prout asserts that he has sometimes been enabled to trace the disease nearly to its origin by ascertaining when the urine was last observed to furnish a red-coloured deposit. Occasionally, however, uric acid is found deposited in diabetic urine of high specific gravity. A short time ago I obtained a beautiful specimen of crystallized uric acid spontaneously deposited from saccharine urine of so high a specific gravity as 1045°. In the case of Merchant, for some days before his death his urine was loaded with deposits of urate of ammonia and uric acid; but this condition only occurred when the sugar had almost entirely disappeared.

Concerning the state of the other secretions in diabetes, we know nothing of a satisfactory nature.

Before concluding this part of the subject, it is proper to mention that the appetite is by no means so generally inordinate in diabetes as some authors have asserted ; occasionally it is even much diminished; and of this I have already adduced one example. The thirst, however, is, so far as published reports inform us, and, so far as I have had an opportunity of observing, a *constant symptom*.

It may now be expedient to present, as succinctly as possible, a series of inferences and observations in connection with the preceding remarks.

1. Although the liquid of the stomach is capable of inducing the conversion of starch into sugar by digestion at a suitable temperature, yet we do not derive satisfactory and demonstrative evidence that this conversion takes place in a sensible degree in the stomach in the condition of health, and under ordinary circumstances.

2. As the formation of dextrine is the first step in the conversion of starch into sugar, it is required to ascertain whether dextrine may not be the ordinary product of the digestion of amylaceous matter, in the condition of health, and whether it may not be directly absorbed.

3. In diabetes mellitus sugar is found

in the stomach, the intestines, the blood, and some other secretions.

4. In this disease, also, sugar is reported to be found in the stomach, even after the exclusion of all vegetable matter from the food. On this point further observations are desirable.

5. It is asserted that the quantity of sugar in the urine, *cæteris paribus*, varies directly with the quantity of amylaceous matters in the food. On this point, also, future observations may throw much light.

6. Sugar is certainly formed in the stomach in diabetes.

7. It is not clearly ascertained whether previously assimilated matter may not be absorbed, and be capable of conversion, in a partial degree at least, into saccharine matter.

8. The disease may exist independently of any appreciable disorganization of structure whatever.

9. Enlarged mesenteric glands, and the deposition of tubercular matter in the lungs, are, perhaps, the most frequent structural changes in diabetes. Enlargement, and a flaccid condition of the kidneys, cannot be regarded as indicating alteration of structure.

10. The kidneys appear simply to eliminate the sugar from the blood.

11. Our knowledge of the state of the blood and the secretions in diabetes is yet very imperfect, and has hitherto shed no light upon the pathology of the disease.

12. Disturbance or suppression of the function of the skin almost constantly exists.

13. The salivary secretion is generally much diminished, and has an acid reaction; the reaction of saliva in health being feebly alkaline.

14. A saccharine state of the urine may exist without the actual symptoms of diabetes.

15. Sugar, according to Dr. Prout, is not unfrequently present in the urine of gouty and dyspeptic persons; and, so far as the experience of that distinguished physician has hitherto extended, invariably exists in the urine when the system is affected with carbuncle or malignant boils.

16. Thirst constantly occurs in connection with confirmed diabetes.

17. The appetite is sometimes inordinate, at other times capricious and much diminished.

I venture not to support or propose any specific theory of the disease, but await the evolution of additional facts; being assured that at present our data are insufficient to enable us to arrive at decided conclusions. If I have contributed in the smallest degree to our general store of knowledge, I shall consider myself amply rewarded for the time and attention which I have with pleasure bestowed upon the subject.

TREATMENT

OF

GONORRHŒA BY SUPERFICIAL CAUTERIZATION OF THE URETHRA.

To the Editor of the Medical Gazette.

SIR,

I HAVE for some time past been pursuing experiments on the treatment of gonorrhœal urethritis, and as the results of these experiments have realised more than I could have anticipated, I think the time has now arrived when I ought, in justice to the profession, to lay this treatment before them.

I am aware that there are numbers of the profession who are exceedingly timid in pursuing what may be considered bold measures in the treatment of disease, and in sooth, the recollection of some unfortunate case, in which these measures were carried out, makes them shudder at the bare expression, and shun a "bold practitioner" as they would a stalking pestilence; but boldness, combined with judgment and discretion, will, I contend, be far more successful in the treatment of disease, than timidity and indecision.

Unfortunately, however, instances of the former combination are comparatively rare, and we find that boldness is too frequently the offspring of ignorance.

In medicine there is no such thing as abstract principle. The whole science of healing is built upon fortuitous and chance discoveries. Like the alchemists of old we have discovered a thousand valuable things where we never thought of looking for them, and whilst uselessly seeking for talismanic gold, have lighted on a pearl of great price. Every thing in fact is presented to us as the result of experiment, and in the treatment of disease the most valuable remedy, can boast of no higher origin than its more humble neighbour.

It is a great pity, therefore, that men, possessing all the requisite essentials for an honourable and lucrative career in their profession, should allow their prejudices to tamper with those talents nature has bestowed upon them.

How bold must that man have been who, heedless of the destructive influence of arsenic, dared to prescribe it as a remedy, and to define the limits to which we might safely administer it; or that individual who, without precedent, rashly cut into the human bladder, and from its hidden recess exposed to the wondering gaze of mankind a human calculus. Such men, in these enlightened ages, would be called " bold practitioners," and would become a mark at which a thousand shafts of ridicule would be pointed.

It is true, the direct application of a stick of lunar caustic to an inflamed and irritable urethra may savour of rashness; but it is deprived of half its terrors when we know that a membrane equally as delicate as that lining the urethral passage is frequently subjected to the same treatment, viz., the conjunctiva; and still further, that as far back as the time of Wiseman, strictures of the urethra were treated in a similar way.

In our own time, MM. Lallemand and Ricord have both employed superficial cauterization of the urethra as a means of relief for morbid sensibilities of that passage, and the latter gentleman in protracted discharges, which had resisted all other modes of treatment.

If I may presume, therefore, to take to myself any credit for the employment of caustic as a remedy in gonorrhœa, my reason for so presuming rests upon the period at which I recommend its adoption, viz., at the commencement of the disease, when pain and inflammation are present, attended with discharge. I am not aware that this mode of treatment has been adopted by any other practitioner than myself; if otherwise, I am quite ready and open to receive conviction.

Immediately a patient applies to me, I introduce an instrument, a modification of Lallemand's caustic-holder, smeared with oil, carrying it as far back the passage as from the symptoms may

be deemed expedient. The caustic being exposed by pressing the stilet forward, the button at its extremity must be rapidly rotated between the thumb and fore-finger of the right hand, in order that no part of the mucous lining may be left intact, whilst the instrument is at the same time gradually withdrawn from the passage.

In a few hours a considerable degree of inflammation ensues, and in some instances slight bleedings, but these symptoms are but temporary, and subsiding, leave the membrane almost free from discharge.

In most cases of gonorrhœa the inflammation does not extend beyond three or four inches from the orifice of the urethra; this was called by Mr. Hunter its specific extent; further back than this, therefore, the instrument need not generally be passed.

One application of the caustic I have sometimes found to destroy the virulence of the disease; but when, after the irritation attending the first application has subsided, any discharge remains, we should again resort to its employment. Whilst pursuing this treatment internal revulsives are to be administered in the form of copaiba and cubebs combined, and the penis is to be enveloped in a cold saturnine lotion.

With such means as these we shall rarely fail to check the disease in a few days; an assertion I could easily corroborate by the recital of cases, did I feel it might be requisite so to do.

An objection probably will be urged to this treatment from a dread of stricture or epididymitis ensuing; but I contend, and it is fully borne out by experience, that the chances of these affections are considerably less the earlier we destroy the specific inflammation attending gonorrhœa.

The first and most important indication in the treatment of gonorrheal urethritis is to make such an impression on the inflamed vessels as shall change the original character of the disease, and substitute, in its stead, simple common inflammation of a sufficient extent to overcome the diseased action; and I feel assured nothing can so effectually induce this as superficial cauterization.

I have the honour to remain, sir,

Your obedient servant,

G. B. CHILDS.

34, Fore Street, City,
July 13, 1843.

CASE OF

PRESENTATION OF THE BELLY.

To the Editor of the Medical Gazette.

SIR,

As the following case is one of unquestionably rare occurrence, and as it has been doubted whether it can occur, I am induced to send you an account of it, with the view chiefly of establishing its possibility, and of corroborating the testimony of some eminent writers concerning it. Dr. Rigby, in his excellent system of Midwifery, has unhesitatingly denied that such a presentation can occur unless when the labour is premature, or the child some time dead and softened by disorganization, and has censured Baudelocque for admitting it, though that eminent author distinctly asserted its existence (in a table contained in his Art des Accouchmens), while its rarity was admitted by the statement that out of 12,605 labours only *three* presented the belly. The experience of Dr. Ramsbotham has, however, furnished proofs that the presentation may occur; but, as in regard to a disputed point, it may be useful to increase the weight of evidence, you may not think the following account inappropriate to your pages.—I am, sir,

Your obedient servant,

A. F. HOLMES, M.D. ED.

Professor of the Theory and Practice of Medicine, M'Gill College, Montreal.

Montreal, Canada,
June 26, 1843.

May 23, 1843.—Between 9 and 10 o'clock in the evening, I was requested to visit Mrs. Rolls, who had been in labour since the preceding night under the charge of a midwife.

The account I received was, that the pains had commenced in the evening, but not strong: that about 3 A.M. the liquor amnii was discharged, and that the pains then became stronger, and during the afternoon had been strong and frequent. A dose of castor oil had operated freely. The midwife was quite at a loss to name the part presenting, but supposed it might be the breech.

On examination, the labia were found much swollen, but they had been so before labour. Introducing the finger it was met by a soft resisting body, too soft for the nates, and which exhibited no sulcus or parts of generation. It had much the feel of a hydrocephalic bag, and passing the finger towards the anterior part of the pelvis, loose bony points were felt, not unlike the angles sometimes felt at the fontanelles when ossification is incomplete. As, however, parallel separations between the bony parts were perceived, I could not decide on the presentation till, carrying the finger towards the left side, I came upon what I at once recognised as the abdominal insertion of the umbilical cord: this was pulseless. Enlightened now as to the nature of the case, I found I could follow with my finger the whole contour of the false ribs on both sides, and as the presenting part had been forced down considerably into the pelvis, it was evident that the body must be doubled on itself.

The woman being at her full time, there was no reason to expect expulsion *viribus naturalibus*, and therefore I resolved to turn. The child being dead, my attention was of course exclusively directed to the mother. The membranes having broken 18 or 19 hours before, the waters had entirely drained off; the pains had been, and continued, frequent and forcing; the doubled body was considerably forced down into the pelvis, and therefore I anticipated great difficulty in bringing down the feet. The first step was to quiet the uterus, which I attempted by administering one dram of laudanum, the pulse not being strong. I left her for an hour, and on my return found the pains had been entirely stopped, but were again beginning. I then attempted to introduce my hand, but having entered the vagina, found the uterus so hard, that I desisted, and resolved to try the effect of venesection in relieving its rigidity, being fearful of trying turning in such a condition. I first administered ⅓ of a grain of hydrochlorate of morphia, and then bled her to over thirty oz., when she complained of faintness. I then immediately proceeded to the operation, and supposing from the apparent position of the child that I should find the left hand most convenient (the patient being on her left side), I introduced it with considerable difficulty, and frequently cramped by the action of the uterus, along the presenting part towards the left side, but instead of its passing along the front of the thighs, it was found to pass on to the buttocks and back of the child, and in endeavouring to bring it to the front of the thigh, it came in contact, not with the knee, but the elbow. The position then was different from what I had supposed, and instead of the body being simply doubled, it was also twisted, so that while the right side of the abdomen was opposite the vulva, the pubic region was turned in a contrary direction, and the elbow of the left side forced against it.

Finding I could not reach the feet or front of the thighs with my left hand, I withdrew it, and introduced the right, and having with much pain and difficulty reached the elbow, I found behind and below it the knee, and having insinuated a finger into the ham, held on during a pain, and endeavoured in the interval to drawn it down. I finally succeeded, and when it had once begun to move I was able with no great difficulty to bring it down into the vagina, and finally the foot through the os externum. By gentle traction during the pains, the body was gradually extricated, the other leg and thigh remaining of course doubled up, till the nates were expelled; the arms were brought down, but some delay occurred in the expulsion of the head, it being large, while the outlet of the pelvis was rather small from the approach to each other of the rami ischii, and a strong unyielding coccyx. Even with the finger in the mouth, considerable force was required to bring it out.

On examining the body, the presenting part was well marked by its purple colour, and was found to be the right side of the abdomen.

It is well to remark that there was no prolapsus of the cord, only about two or three inches of its umbilical extremity being felt.

The case unfortunately terminated unfavourably. Next morning when seen, she expressed herself quite comfortable; no pain of abdomen, or untoward symptom. In the evening pulse quickened, still without pain, except some soreness in the left ilium on motion; ol. ricini ordered. At 11 P.M. violent intermitting pains came on, with tenderness of hypogastrium; she was bled to 8 oz. but pulse sank; fomentations, lavements, calomel, morphia, &c. ordered in vain: she died at 11 A.M. 36 hours after delivery. Inspection of the body was refused.

MESMERISM.

To the Editor of the Medical Gazette.

SIR,

As the communications of your correspondent, Mr. Southam (pp. 352 and 459), have evidently a tendency to discourage practitioners from the employment and investigation of Mesmerism, and hence to throw an agent, which he acknowledges to be a most potent one, still more completely than even at present into the hands of charlatans, I beg to offer a few remarks in reply.

"The Mesmeric power," he tells us, "is but a combination of exciting causes of disease" (354)—precisely the nature of all our most valuable remedial agents. Do any of these produce health, or healthy action, directly? Do they not rather remove one diseased action by setting up another?—either antagonist to that already existing, as is the case with counter-irritants, transferring the morbid action to another part of less importance, or, as with sedatives, directly diminishing vascular action in inflammatory affections; or, on the other hand, setting up an action analogous to, but more powerful than, the primary derangement, which subsides with the subsidence of that artificially produced, on the removal of the artificial exciting cause.

It seems extraordinary that a gentleman who really entertains such just views as to the true nature of the agency at work, should not have seen that its power might be made highly useful as well as deeply dangerous. If it possesses the power to produce "mischievous consequences," and of "exciting dangerous diseases of the nervous system," it must be capable of being employed as a therapeutic agent, either in one way or other. Because opium has been used for aiding the purposes of the followers of Burke, does it only claim our study on account of its mischievous power? Because a patient may be murdered by calomel, and may, after taking many doses, be rendered so susceptible of its influence, that a single added dose may induce violent and hazardous ptyalism, are we to abjure the remedy altogether? A negative answer must be given. Yet, according to Mr. Southam's argument, "if they have any claim on our notice, it is not on account of any remedial power they may possess, but from the mischievous consequences they produce."

I am not one of those transcendental mesmerists who entertain the wild hypotheses which have occasioned the *facts* themselves to be disputed, but, like Mr. Southam, I have endeavoured to trace the metaphysical and physiological action of the means employed, and during the last twelve months have employed most of my leisure moments in working out a theory based on these grounds, which I hope ere long to lay before the profession. In the meantime I cannot but express my regret that the whole of the matter should have been so summarily dismissed by medical men generally without fair investigation, merely because the facts *appeared* at variance with our preconceived opinions. Many, after denying the truth of the facts, have taken pains to shew how the phenomena might have arisen; others, admitting that such phenomena were really presented, have asserted that they were contrary to nature, and have absurdly attributed them even to Satanic agency; whilst most have assumed them to be mere collusion and trickery. That there has been much of this no one who has studied the subject attentively can deny; but the existence of counterfeit coin certainly presupposes the existence of genuine.

As my theory is not yet sufficiently perfect to be offered to the public, I shall content myself with presenting a few cases in opposition to those of Mr. Southam, shewing the " *beneficial* effects of mesmerism," and which, I think, will render it probable that he might, had he so chosen, have influenced his patient for good rather than for the contrary, as he evidently confesses was the case. During the last year I have produced the mesmeric sleep on upwards of twenty different individuals, and have *never* discovered the slightest " injurious effect." After witnessing Lafontaine's experiments, I was as much disposed to be sceptical as any of the most virulent anti-mesmerists—not that I could gainsay what I saw, but because I felt the hypothesis advanced to be untenable. However, shortly afterwards a case of violent hysteria came under my care, and on leaving from one of my visits I was recalled, as a fit was evidently coming on. The friends around prepared to restrain the struggles of the patient by main force, but at my request relinquished their purpose. After diverting the patient's attention, by telling her she should not have a fit, I took her hands as in Lafontaine's method, and commenced the manipulations. In a quarter of an hour she was asleep. I inquired most specially respecting the case, and have every reason to believe that she knew nothing of mesmerism previously. I acted on her repeatedly afterwards, and could at any time produce perfect rigidity of the whole body, or of any part separately, at will, assuring her at the same time that she would not have another fit. The self-confidence established realized my prediction; and more than twelve months have now elapsed without any return. In this case perfect rigidity, and apparent loss of feeling and vision, were produced. Hearing alone seemed to remain in full activity; and she recollected what was audible, but nothing more. I could not detect any source of fallacy; and though at first startled at the result, I determined to investigate further. The limbs acted on being placed in any position, even the most painful, remained in the same form for half an hour at a time without wavering; and the same has occurred to me in several other cases.

My next case was also one of hysteria, with violent pain in the occiput; but here no rigidity was producible. On the contrary, there seemed to be an entire loss of muscular tonicity, so that the whole body appeared like plastic clay, and might be flexed in any way without resistance, whilst no sensation or power of any kind was apparent. Here, too, a cure was effected, as I believe by the self-confidence inspired.

In each of these cases the effect was produced about twenty times. I pass over several other cases of interest, in order to come within the legitimate limits of a communication; but I cannot deny myself the opportunity of recording two cases at present under treatment, and which have surprised me more than any I have witnessed.

The first is that of a young man suffering from hysteriform palpitation. Almost all the usual antispasmodic remedies, and many others, had been tried long and in vain; and beginning to tire of treatment which seemed useless, I resolved to try mesmerism. In fifteen minutes from the commencement of the manipulations he was in a perfectly rigid state; and on one occasion I hung a chair on each of his extended arms, which still retained the position unwaveringly for twenty minutes, beyond which I did not think it right to protract the experiment. He always expresses himself relieved after each manipulation, and the benefit lasts just in exact proportion to the time the mesmeric state is kept up.

The other case is one of hysteria, in which somnambulism was induced at the second trial; and so strange and unexpected was the result, that I strongly suspected deception. This case, however, fully bears out Mr. Southam's views as to phreno-magnetism; and that there was no deception I had afterwards an opportunity of proving to my satisfaction, if not to that of others. Having been asked to give a lecture on the subject to a literary institution at West Bromwich, I took this patient with me to exhibit the effect. It happened that she suffered most severely that day from toothache; but I declined extracting the tooth in the morning, thinking it would be a fair means of proving that she was not deceiving me, by having it removed in the mesmeric state. In the evening, therefore, I mesmerised her, and her tooth was extracted by Mr. Charles Mole, M.R.C.S., in the presence of Dr. Dickinson, Mr. Silvester, and Mr. W. Jackson, all medical practitioners at West Bromwich, beside the usual audience of such institutions; and no one was able to detect the slightest muscular movement of any kind, or of any part, nor the least change of colour or respiration. Her hysterical fits also have never returned.

In all these cases I have never told my patients what effect I intended to produce; nor, so far as I know, had they ever seen any thing of the kind before. With these facts before me, I cannot help thinking that "a power so energetic in exciting disease," (p. 463) is also endowed with remedial virtues.

I am, sir,

Your obedient servant,
George Beddow, M.R.C.S.

5, Jenner's Row, Birmingham,
July 17, 1843.

MEDICAL GAZETTE.

Friday, July 28, 1843.

"Licet omnibus, licet etiam mihi, dignitatem *Artis Medicæ* tueri; potestas modo veniendi in publicum sit, dicendi periculum non recuso."

Cicero.

THE LAST NEWS FROM GRÄFENBERG.

The physician, says Sir Charles Scudamore, must be a student for ever, and not disdain to learn till the last moment of his existence. He therefore went to Gräfenberg last April, to gaze with his own eyes on the doings of Priessnitz, and judge of the merits of hydropathy in the place where it is exercised with the greatest vigour. He returned much gratified with what he had seen, and has recently added another pamphlet to the multitude

"Quæ scribuntur aquæ potoribus."

With Priessnitz himself every one is pleased; were it otherwise, could a rustic practitioner boast a daily list of patients varying from two to five hundred? "His countenance," says Sir Charles, "is full of self-possession; rather agreeable; mild, but firm in expression; with an eye of sense, and a pleasing smile." And, best of all, "*He inspires his patients with the most entire confidence, and he exacts implicit obedience.*" This is half the battle. Half! it is nine-tenths of the victory over chronic disease, to have obedient patients. A physician who should take a large house at Richmond or Shooter's Hill, and fill it with dutiful and submissive patients, behaving like the good boys of a story-book, and observing in the minutest particulars the hygienic code of their physical pastor, might boast almost as many cures as the sage of Gräfenberg without the aid of hydropathy. However, we have no objection to add water and mountain air to the healing agents, and have read with interest Sir C. Scudamore's account of the details of the system.

The first item on the list is the *Leintuch*, or wet sheet to lie on. The patient is wrapped up in a wet sheet, and then covered with a blanket, feather-bed, and quilt, in which he generally lies for three-quarters of an hour. This does not produce perspiration; but if in any case—catarrhal fever, for example—sweating is desired, the time is extended to an hour or more.

The next variety is the *Abreibung*, or rubbing down with a wet sheet which is thrown over the patient. This is continued from two to five minutes, when the skin becomes reddened.

In the variety termed the sweating blanket (*Das Schwitzen in der Kotze*), the patient is packed up in blanket, feather bed, and wadded counterpane, till perspiration breaks out, which sometimes requires four hours. The sweating is then continued for a prescribed time, and at its termination the patient takes a tepid shallow bath, or a cold plunge bath, or both. "It is only the practised patient who goes at once into the cold bath; but, with either, it is a rule first to dash some water over the face, head, and chest." The safety of this practice depends on the heated state of the body; for the system merely parts with its superfluity of caloric.

Sir Charles found that the thermometer, placed under the tongue of a certain patient before entering the blanket, stood at 98°; just before and after the breaking out of the perspiration it was at 100°; after much perspiration it sank to 99°; and after the plunging bath to 97°. This method is obviously not the same thing as a vapour bath, with which some persons have confounded it. Priessnitz does not use the sweating blanket so much as formerly, but still relies upon it to remove any old virus, or to extract latent mercury from the frame. None undergo it more than gouty invalids. The word "tepid" applied to a bath has diverse thermometrical significations in different places; we should intend by it from 80° to 92° of Fahrenheit; at Gräfenberg it means from 58° to 68°; and the temperature most commonly employed for the shallow tepid bath is 62°. It is called at Gräfenberg *Das abgeschreckte Halbbad*. "The newly-enlisted patient, after quitting the *Leintuch*, enters this bath, and is diligently rubbed before and behind; taking himself apart, if able; if not, having more assistance, and for a longer or shorter time, as circumstances may direct; but, in the beginning, about two minutes."

This is clearly a very safe variety. The plunging bath (*Wannenbad*) at a temperature of 44° is more terrific, but is soon arrived at by most patients. It is commonly taken early in the morning, but is often enjoyed a second time in the afternoon.

The hip-bath (*Sitzbad*) varies in temperature from 44° to 64°; the time of immersion from a quarter of an hour to an hour. The patient, while sitting in it, uses friction to his back and abdomen; and, on emerging, restores the warmth of surface by due rubbing and drying. The hip-bath, employed in this decisive manner, is highly useful in many maladies of the pelvic viscera, and aids in correcting a disordered state of the mucous membrane of the intestinal canal.

The head-bath (*Das Kopfbad*) consists in lying on the ground with the back of the head in a basin of water.

The foot-bath (*Das Fussbad*) does not imply the deep tibio-fibular immersion of this part of the world; for the depth of water in the vessel is only from one to three inches. The soles of the feet are to be rubbed with the water; but the friction is extended to the whole of the feet, ankles, and even legs, if they are weak and apt to swell, until a glow is felt.

The wet bandages (*Umschläge*) are of two kinds. When intended to stimulate, the wet portion of the bandage is covered with that which is left dry; when designed to cool, the whole compress is wetted, and left to evaporate uncovered. "For example, I saw the case of a large painful boil on the hand, in progress of suppuration. On this, the wetted part of the bandage, covered by the dry, was constantly kept, to serve as a water poultice; but above, on the wrist and fore-arm, a wet cloth only, never allowed to be dry, or even warm; on a just surgical principle of producing a sedative action on the vessels and nerves contiguous to the seat of disease."

The *Umschlag* often produces a great belt of rash round the body, or sundry boils, which are always hailed with satisfaction at Gräfenberg.

Next comes the douche, which, if vigorously used, is the most active of all the processes in the water cure. The temperature of the douches for gentlemen, in the wood at Gräfenberg, was as follows:—"Concordia, the strongest, about twenty feet fall, and of the size of a man's wrist, 54°; the stone douche, 48°; and the Ferdinand, 44°."

Strong patients sometimes use the douche in the coldest weather, when the attendant has first to break away the ice; but weaklings must beware of imitating their hardihood. The douche is a powerful rubefacient, and produces eruptions resembling measles, scarlatina, &c.

As for drinking, the quantity of water taken at the beginning of the course is from eight to twelve glasses daily, each glass holding from ten to eleven ounces. None is to be drunk when the body is very cold; nor much without exercise. Water and milk are the only beverages at Gräfenberg.

On his return home, Sir Charles Scudamore had a conversation with Liebig on the water-cure. This eminent chemist believes the purity of the water drunk to be of the utmost consequence for its quick absorption. If it contains two per cent. of saline matter, it will pass to the bowels; but if it is of sufficient purity, eight-tenths will be eliminated by the kidneys in the shortest possible time. In answer to a question of Sir C. Scudamore's, Liebig thought that no injury would arise from the water carrying off the salts of the blood, as the quantity of salt in the foods might be a little increased, to allow for this waste. Pure water is absorbed so instantaneously, that Liebig, like Sir Everard Home, is inclined to believe in a short cut between the stomach and kidneys.

Sir Charles objects to the drinking a large quantity of water in cases of hæmorrhage that require restraining; even in piles, if the blood is arterial, the flow must not be rashly encouraged or permitted.

Sir C. Scudamore went to Gräfenberg partly to be treated himself, having been a sufferer for many years from rheumatic and nervous headache, with noises and deafness in the left ear; and being constantly dependent on medicine for the action of the bowels.

His treatment began on the 18th of April, a few days after his arrival, and continued till the 20th of May. Once during this period he took blue pill and colocynth at night, and Cheltenham salts in the morning, being bilious from the change of diet, and the free use of milk.

The details of his course are very interesting, and replete with instruction. The result has been most satisfactory, his health having improved in all the points where it was deficient.

He narrates forty cases where the water-cure was employed, and generally with complete success.

In one instance, a patient of five-and-twenty, having been attacked with violent pain between the lower ribs while walking, was subjected to pretty active treatment by Priessnitz, and recovered perfectly. Sir Charles thinks that there was an error in diagnosis on the part of Priessnitz, who supposed it to be a case of internal inflammation; Sir Charles knew it to be a muscular pain connected with indigestion and intestinal flatulence. During his stay at Gräfenberg, he often heard of the stains of mercury and iodine, of a blue or reddish colour, on the sheets. Liebig offered this explanation to Sir Charles: that mercury may remain combined with animal matter for an indefinite time, and may be separated through the quick change of matter which belongs to the water-system.

After seeing Liebig, Sir Charles visited the establishment of Marienberg, close to Boppart, on the Rhine. This is perhaps the handsomest hydropathic establishment in Europe, but the treatment is less vigorous than at Gräfenberg. It is under the direction of Dr. Schmitz; and patients have the advantage of consulting a distinguished English physiologist, whose name is known to all our readers, and who has himself benefited by the treatment there.

Sir Charles very properly speaks of the water-cure as a valuable addition to the resources of the medical art, rather than its rival or foe. What the proper limits of the system may be, remains to be ascertained. The hydropathists seem still to be in the honeymoon of their experience; they have not yet trodden the thorny paths of ordinary practice, when enthusiasm has fallen asleep, and patients are no longer docile.

CASE OF

SUDDEN DEATH SIMULATING POISON BY OPIUM;

SHOWING THE NECESSITY OF MEDICAL CORONERS.

To the Editor of the Medical Gazette.

SIR,

SHOULD you think the following case worthy of notice, you will oblige me by inserting it in your valuable periodical.—I am, sir,

Your obedient servant,

J. BEENCASTLE, M.R.C.S. &c.

Croydon, July 16, 1843.

I was sent for, on Tuesday, the 25th April, 1843, at 6 A.M. to attend, on the part of the Croydon Union, the illegitimate infant, six weeks old, of a pauper named Aldridge. The child was said to be in a fit. On my arrival at the house I found the child dead. I had scarcely asked the mother and grandmother a few questions, when the latter begged of me to examine the body, and see that there had been no "misconduct" on their part. I thought that remark rather unusual, and examined the body more minutely, but could discover no marks of violence, or anything to lead me to suppose that the child had not died from natural causes. The face and body were quite pallid, and the mouth and eyes closed, without any unusual appearance.

A few hours afterwards, Mr. Smith, the registrar of deaths, sent to know whether an inquest would be required, as he had heard it reported by the neighbours that the child had died by unfair means. The inquest was consequently ordered, and thinking that I might elicit from the parties a few more points concerning the case, I called again in the afternoon, seven hours after death had taken place, and found the body laid out. I requested that the clothes should be taken off, and, to my great surprise, I observed the head, trunk, and extremities, to be covered with livid patches of ecchymosis, of a large size, pretty general all over the body. Knowing this cadaveric appearance so soon after death to be one of the common results from poisoning by opium, and having seen it in several cases that had terminated fatally, my attention was immediately directed to that channel, and I asked the friends whether they had given the child any syrup of poppies, Godfrey's cordial, or laudanum, but they stoutly denied having given anything at all.

After cross-examining them pretty closely, I learnt that the child, otherwise remarkably healthy, had been for the last few days uncommonly fretful, and particularly so on the Sunday; that on Monday he became very drowsy, and slept all day and night without intermission, until early on the Tuesday morning, when it was suddenly seized with the convulsive fits that carried it off, and to relieve which I had been called in.

The history of the case, coupled with the appearances of the body after death, being, as every medical man knows, exactly those of poisoning by opium, the impression on my mind at the time was, that the child might have died from the effects of that drug, or some of its compounds, either given intention fly, or in an over-dose through ignorance. The child being illegitimate might have also tended to strengthen the first suspicion. In fact, had the child been known to have died from opium, the appearance above named would be all that one would expect to find without an autopsy.

Well, what did Mr. Carter, the coroner for Surrey, do? Instead of being guided by the medical evidence, and using it as the means to come at the truth, he at once turns round upon me, and wishes to persuade the jury that there are no grounds whatever for presuming that the child had died from any other than natural causes; that he had frequently seen the livid appearance of the skin, which always arose from persons lying after death; that infants frequently died from apoplexy, and the like trash; that, besides, it was absurd to suspect that any thing had been given when the mother and two other respectable witnesses swore to the contrary; that they being respectable people (all three, paupers and interested parties), he was bound to believe them on oath; and that he did not think a *post-mortem* necessary, as there was not the slightest tittle of evidence to prove that any thing in the shape of narcotics had been administered! Now the chain of symptoms and circumstantial evidence throughout this case were so clearly those of death by opium, and so unlike death from any other infantile disease, that nothing but the grossest ignorance on medical subjects can excuse Mr. Carter for having so totally overlooked them, and disregarded the suggestions of the medical witness. On the contrary, he so far forgot his duty, that he actually, in summing up the case to the jury, endeavoured to throw a slur upon the medical witness, by inferring that he had acted wrongly by at all exciting suspicions in a case where nothing whatever could warrant any person in supposing that the child had died from any other than natural causes.

But had a post-mortem taken place, and, in spite of the oaths of these three very respectable witnesses, poison had been found in the child's stomach, annulling all doubt upon the subject—and such cases are not uncommon—would he have thought them so lightly of medical evidence?

The case was now dismissed summarily, and all parties entirely exculpated from any blame, the verdict being—"Died from natural causes."

Now would not a medical coroner at once have fallen in with the views of the medical witness, and would not his attention have been seriously arrested upon the probability of poison in a case where all the circumstances were so well linked together as to arise rather more than a suspicion of guilt? Is it not generally by some vague unconnected facts that cases of poisoning are at first brought into notice? Before detecting the poison, are there not premonitory and concomitant signs and circumstances, that put one on the *qui vive*, and lead one to seek for it by further anatomical investigations? How, then, can any person not well acquainted, practically as well as theoretically, with this intricate branch of the profession, presume to offer his opinion on subjects of such importance that they may involve the life of a fellow-creature? It is an anomaly that cannot exist any. longer in a country that boasts of ranking first in civilization. The time must come, and come shortly it will, when none but medical coroners will be allowed to fill that high office. Until then we must not be surprised to see doubtful cases smothered in a similar way to the one here cited, by Mr. Carter, or any other of his sapient non-medical colleagues.

DISEASES OF THE EYE.

To the Editor of the Medical Gazette.

Sir,

In reviewing my recent work "on Diseases of the Eye, and on Miscellaneous Subjects Medical and Surgical," the following statement is made in the last (July) number of "The British and Foreign Medical Review:" "On points of history Dr. Hall is generally wrong; as, for instance, where he ascribes the notion, that in purulent opthalmia the cornea dies from the pressure caused by the chemosed conjunctiva, to Mr. Middlemore (p. 56), the first demonstration of the advantage of mercury in iritis to Dr. Farre (p. 101), &c. &c." I should feel much obliged if the reviewer, or any of your correspondents, would inform me to whom the priority in question properly belongs.

I remain, sir,

Your faithful servant,

J. C. HALL.

Grove Street, East Retford,
July 19th, 1843.

THE QUEEN'S COLLEGE, BIRMINGHAM.

Her Majesty has been graciously pleased to grant a Royal Charter of Incorporation to the School of Medicine and Surgery at Birmingham, with the privileges, immunities, rank, and title of "The Queen's College at Birmingham." Her Majesty has been graciously pleased to nominate Samuel Wilson Warneford, Clerk, of Bourton on the Hill, Gloucestershire, the first visitor.

Edward Johnstone, Doctor of Physic, of Edgbaston Hall, in the County of Norfolk, First Principal of the said Society.

James Thomas Law, Clerk, Chancellor of the Diocese of Lichfield, the first Vice-Principal.

John Edwards Piercy, Esq. Justice of the Peace of the County of Stafford, Treasurer.

William Sands Cox, Fellow of the Royal Society, London, Senior Surgeon of the Queen's Hospital, Dean of the Faculty; who, together with—

William Penn Curzon Howe, Earl Howe,
George William Lyttelton, Lord Lyttelton,
John Kay Booth, Doctor of Physic, Licentiate of the Royal College of Physicians, Honorary Physician of the Queen's Hospital,
Edward Townsend Cox, Senior Surgeon of the Town Infirmary,
Egerton Bagot, Clerk,
Vaughan Thomas, Clerk of Corpus-Christi College, Oxford,
James Taylor, Esq. Justice of the Peace for the County of Worcester,
Joseph Webster, Esq. Justice of the Peace for the County of Warwick,
Richard Wood, Senior Surgeon of the General Hospital, Birmingham,
Thomas Upfill, Merchant,
James Johnstone, Doctor of Physic, Fellow of the Royal College of Physicians, London, Senior Physician of the General Hospital, Birmingham, Professor of Materia Medica,
John Best Davies, Doctor of Physic, Extra Licentiate of the Royal College of Physicians, London, Senior Physician of the Queen's Hospital, Birmingham, Professor of Forensic Medicine,—as the First Council.

COLLEGE OF PHYSICIANS.

The following is the correct list, in the order of their admission, of the Physicians elected Fellows of the Royal College of Physicians, London, on the 25th of last month:—

Dr. Thomas Thompson, Tunbridge Wells.—Dr. Augustin Sayer, Upper Seymour Street, Portman Square.—Dr. John Webster, Lower Grosvenor Street.—Dr. Thomas Dowler, Richmond.—Dr. Sigismund Stolterforth, Dover.—Dr. Edward Rigby, Spring Gardens.—Dr. Peyton Blakiston, Birmingham.—Dr. Arthur Farre, Curzon Street.

ROYAL COLLEGE OF SURGEONS.

LIST OF GENTLEMEN ADMITTED MEMBERS.

Friday, July 21, 1843.

T. Cattell.—J. C. Harper.—G. M. Henning.—H. F. Williams.—P. P. Ransom.—T. L. Philipps.—A. Markwick.—R. D. Walker.—J. L. Milton.

A TABLE OF MORTALITY FOR THE METROPOLIS,

Shewing the number of deaths from all causes registered in the week ending Saturday, July 15, 1843.

Small Pox	6
Measles	28
Scarlatina	30
Hooping Cough	24
Croup	9
Thrush	4
Diarrhœa	7
Dysentery	3
Cholera	4
Influenza	3
Ague	0
Typhus	36
Erysipelas	2
Syphilis	1
Hydrophobia	0
Diseases of the Brain, Nerves, and Senses	105
Diseases of the Lungs and other Organs of Respiration	216
Diseases of the Heart and Blood-vessels	24
Diseases of the Stomach, Liver, and other Organs of Digestion	76
Diseases of the Kidneys, &c.	5
Childbed	5
Paramenia	1
Ovarian Dropsy	1
Disease of Uterus, &c.	2
Rheumatism	2
Diseases of Joints, &c.	5
Carbuncle	0
Ulcer	0
Fistula	1
Diseases of Skin, &c.	2
Dropsy, Cancer, and other Diseases of Uncertain Seat	74
Old Age or Natural Decay	57
Deaths by Violence, Privation, or Intemperance	12
Causes not specified	1
Deaths from all Causes	757

METEOROLOGICAL JOURNAL.

Kept at Edmonton, *Latitude* 51° 37' 32" N. *Longitude* 0° 3' 51" W. *of Greenwich.*

June 1843.	THERMOMETER.		BAROMETER.	
Wednesday 19	from 50 to 65		29·74 to	29·70
Thursday . 20	49	70	29·71	29·70
Friday . . 21	47	60	29 62	29·74
Saturday . 22	46	64	29·74	29·56
Sunday . . 23	53	60	29·40	29·68
Monday . . 24	43	65	29·92	30·03
Tuesday . 25	43	66	30·08	30·12

Wind, N. by W. and S.W. on the 19th; N.W. and S.W. on the 20th; S.W. on the 21st and 22d; W. N.W. and N. by E. on the 23d; W. by S. and W. by N. on the 24th; N.W. and S.W. on the 25th.

The 19th and 20th, generally clear, except in the afternoon when rain fell. 21st, morning cloudy, afternoon and evening clear. 22d, cloudy, rain in the evening. 23d, showery. 24th and 25th, generally cloudy.

Rain fallen, ·33 of an inch.

CHARLES HENRY ADAMS.

THE

LONDON MEDICAL GAZETTE,

BEING A

WEEKLY JOURNAL

OF

Medicine and the Collateral Sciences.

FRIDAY, AUGUST 4, 1843.

LECTURES

ON THE

THEORY AND PRACTICE OF MIDWIFERY,

Delivered in the Theatre of St. George's Hospital,

BY ROBERT LEE, M.D. F.R.S.

LECTURE XXXVII.

On Labours complicated with Inversion and Rupture of the Uterus and Vagina, and Extravasation of Blood into the Labia.

IN the autumn of 1825, I was consulted by a lady at Odessa, in the ninth month of pregnancy, who was suffering much more than she had ever done before during gestation from pain increased by pressure in the region of the uterus, and febrile symptoms. I recommended her to lose blood from the arm, or to have leeches and fomentations applied to the abdomen; but no antiphlogistic remedies of any kind were employed, and she continued to suffer till the pains of labour commenced. The child was soon expelled, but the midwife in extracting the placenta inverted the uterus, and when I saw the patient about half an hour after, the whole uterus, the entire fundus and body, was hanging out between the thighs like the head of a child; the uterus had in fact been drawn like a stocking or glove completely inside out. The bed and floor were covered with a great quantity of blood, and the lady was expiring in convulsions. On applying my hand over the hypogastrium, the fundus of the uterus could not be felt there in the usual manner; and although the placenta had been entirely detached and removed, there could be no doubt, from the globular shape of the tumor, its peculiar softness and compressibility, its sudden appearance along with the placenta after the birth of the child, the red colour of its investing membrane, from which the blood still continued to ooze, that it was the inverted uterus. By grasping the uterus with the hand, and compressing the upper part firmly with the points of the fingers, there was no difficulty in reducing or reinverting it: a sufficient length of time had not elapsed to allow of the cervix and os uteri contracting, to prevent its reduction. The midwife informed me that the placenta was retained, and that little force was employed by her in removing it. This is the only case of complete inversion of the uterus which I have ever seen, and there was no difficulty in the diagnosis, and no doubt about the necessity of immediately replacing the uterus, for if the patient had lived, the reduction of the uterus would have been impossible in a few hours, from the strangulation of the body produced above by the cervix, and inflammation and swelling of the parts. Inversion of the uterus is frequently, if not invariably, the consequence of pulling at the umbilical cord, to extract the placenta immediately after the birth of the child, before the uterus has had time to contract, and while the placenta is still adherent. It is also stated to have happened when the child has been allowed to be rapidly expelled, when the umbilical cord has surrounded the foetus, or been unusually short. " From the same cause," says Dr. Burns, " or sometimes, perhaps, from sudden pressure of part of the intestines on the fundus uteri, occasioned by a strong contraction of the abdominal muscles, a part of the fundus becomes depressed like a cup, and encroaches on the uterine cavity. This generally rectifies itself, if let alone, but if the cord be pulled, or if there be any tendency in the uterine action to go toward the fundus, as happens when that part is lacerated, and may in like manner occur in the present case, the depression is speedily converted into perfect inversion, which may thus take place spontaneously, and without any fault of the attendant." " It has been

very thick root. It exactly resembled in size and structure this specimen [exhibiting it] of large fibrous tumor growing from the neck of the uterus by a peduncle as thick as the wrist. From this case, and the following related by Dr. Gooch, you will perceive that the diagnosis of completely inverted uterus is not always so simple and easy as some authors would lead us to suppose, or, indeed, can be drawn without a previous knowledge of the history of the patient, and that it is possible the uterus has not been extirpated in all the cases in which the operation has been supposed to have been successfully performed.

Mr. Borrett, surgeon, at Yarmouth, was called to a lady in labour with her sixth child. On his first examination he found a large fleshy tumor within the vagina. The anterior segment in the os uteri was easily felt, but the posterior was occupied and covered by the attachment of the tumor. After the orifice had dilated, and the membranes had burst, the head of the child not descending, Mr. Borrett introduced his hand, brought down the feet, and extracted the child. The placenta was expelled spontaneously. The patient now being delivered and easy, he left her at 7 in the morning. At 3 in the afternoon he found her in strong pains, as if there was another child, but as the abdomen was flat, and the contracted uterus could be felt in the abdomen, he was satisfied there was not, and gave her an opiate. At 8 o'clock at night he found that the pains continued violent, with a sensation as of a substance coming away, and he discovered a soft round tumor pressing against the outer orifice. What could it be? He would have thought that it was the uterus inverted, but it was the same tumor which he had felt in the morning before the child was born; there was no hæmorrhage; the placenta had been expelled spontaneously, and the uterus was distinct in the hypogastric region. He consulted his medical friends in the town, and sent off to Norwich for Mr. Rigby. The pains continued with violent expulsive efforts all night, and the next morning they found her with a languid pulse and pallid countenance: a large fleshy livid tumor had been forced out of the vagina, and every pain brought it more and more in sight: she continued to suffer and to sink through the rest of the day: in the morning Mr. Rigby arrived, but she had expired about half an hour before. As soon as he arrived *he examined* *her, and was convinced that it was* *inverted uterus.* On opening the body *morning,* the uterus was found con- *out* its orifice was dragged down as a external orifice by a tumor which it by a thick stalk; it was at- the posterior part of the orifices,

and some way up the neck, was of a livid colour, and weighed three pounds fifteen ounces.

"When the uterus," says Dr. Merriman, "with the placenta attached to it, is drawn in an inverted state without the vagina, no doubt can exist as to the nature of the accident, but if it should happen after the exclusion of the placenta, more difficulty in forming an opinion would arise. The following rules, however, would lead to a correct judgment:—If a globular tumor is found soon after delivery in the vagina, or protruded through the os externum, it must be supposed to be either a polypous excrescence, a prolapsed uterus, or an inverted uterus. If it were a polypus, it would be known by its insensibility, its mobility, and its pedicle, which a careful examination could hardly fail to discover; the edges of the os uteri surrounding the tumor would likewise be perceptible. A prolapsed uterus may always be known by the os uteri being situated at the most depending part of the tumor. The inverted uterus is sensible to the touch, is less moveable than the polypus, has no pedicle, nor a dependent mouth; in a recent state it is entirely covered with a grumous discharge proceeding from numberless blood-vessels upon its whole surface."

All the systematic works on midwifery contain the histories of cases of complete inversion of the uterus. I have selected the following from many others to illustrate the effects produced by this dangerous accident, and to impress upon you the necessity of immediately detaching the placenta if it adhered, and reducing the uterus. Should you meet with a case in your own practice, it would be a lasting disgrace to you to invert the uterus, whatever the result might be.

In 1684 Mauriceau saw a woman whose uterus had been inverted eight months before by an ignorant midwife, and who was much exhausted by hæmorrhage. He found it impossible to reduce the uterus. He relates another case which occurred in 1693, two days before he saw the patient: the uterus was irreducible, and she ultimately died from the pain and discharge.

Giffard's 176th case is entitled "A delivery where the uterus was inverted and drawn out beyond the labia pudendi, and the placenta adhering to the uterus." "January the 29th, 1730-31, I was, about 8 o'clock in the evening," he says, "sent for to the wife of a brother surgeon in Surrey Street. The child was born about an hour before I came, and the midwife, in attempting to bring away the placenta, had inverted the uterus, for, upon examination, I found the whole body of the uterus, with the placenta, adhering to the fundus, hanging out beyond the labia; there was a great profusion of blood, and the woman was dead before I came. I rebuked the midwife for not sending sooner, and told her that she, through her ignorance, was the immediate cause of the poor woman's death, for, by pulling the string too forcibly, she had drawn out and inverted the womb. Before I examined, the midwife told me the placenta was partly brought out, being ignorant that she had also pulled out the womb; but I showed her her error, that the placenta was all brought out, and only adhered to the fundus uteri, which, as the whole womb was inverted, hung out beyond the labia pudendi. This case should be a caution to all practitioners how they attempt to bring away the placenta, and not to pull the string too rudely, lest they invert and draw out the uterus, by which the woman dies a martyr to their temerity and ignorance, as was too plainly the case in the precedent observation." Chapman's 28th case is similar:—" I was, in the greatest haste, sent for to a woman six miles distant from me, to whom I went with all possible speed, but found on my arrival that she had been dead nearly half an hour. I conjectured she had died from flooding, but upon asking the question was answered in the negative. The midwife told me that the after-birth stuck so fast in one part that she was not able, with all her strength, to take it from her, though she had gained most of it. Upon this I desired the favour of seeing the corpse, which being granted, I found, to my great surprise, that the uterus was inverted, and entirely out of the body, hanging down between the thighs, with the placenta adhering to its fundus, which I separated before the midwife and several matrons there present, and convinced them all of the dismal accident. This woman, it seems, had a very good and easy delivery of the child; but, that born, the midwife pulled hard at the string, and so brought down the uterus, which as soon as she could take hold of, she did, and then pulling with fresh violence, and not being deterred by the loudest cries, the poor miserable woman in a few minutes fell into strong convulsions and deliquiums, and so expired. Thus was a young healthy mother cut off in the bloom of life, and cast into the cold arms of death just as she was about to clasp her first-born in her own."

Smellie was called to a woman who died before his arrival. He found the uterus inverted, pulled quite without the external parts, and the placenta adhering firmly to the fundus. This misfortune was occasioned by the midwife pulling at the placenta with too great force. Mr. Lucas, of Pontefract, sent the following account of a case of inverted uterus to Smellie, which occurred in 1753:— "In April last I was called to a woman just delivered of a live healthy child, and to my surprise found the uterus totally inverted, lying between her thighs, of the size of a large foot-ball. The woman's pulse was weak and unequal, and there was a continued pouring forth of blood from the vessels of the uterus. I apprised the friends of the great danger of so deplorable a case. Nevertheless, with the approbation of a judicious physician, her neighbour, I undertook and succeeded in the reduction, and after gave her gentle anodyne and cordial medicines, and left her, in appearance, better and tolerably easy. In about half an hour I was again called, and found her speechless, the pulse imperceptible, clammy sweats, respiration deep and slow, and in a few minutes death closed the scene. All the parts were so lax that the uterus had not the power of contraction, for it was lying like a loose piece of tripe, and taken for an excrescence, till I examined it more strictly, and after separating the placenta reduced it into the abdomen.

" On Thursday, the 21st of September, 1820," says Dr. Ramsbotham, " I was desired to be present at the opening of the body of a woman who had died in child-bed, and whose death had raised much clamour in the neighbourhood. I was informed by her accoucheur that she was, to all appearance, safely delivered of her second child on the Sunday evening, after a natural and quick labour; that he waited for the after-birth the greater part of an hour, before he made any attempt to remove it; and that he then began to pull at the funis, without being able to bring it down. Finding, after some further time, that it did not descend, he attempted to introduce his hand into the uterus; but in this attempt he was foiled. Waiting a little longer, a strong after-pain came on, when he made another trial by the funis; and finding an advance, as he thought, continued to extract, when, to his surprise and alarm, the uterus came out of the parts as large as a child's head, with the placenta adherent to it. Previous to this unfortunate occurrence there had not been much discharge of blood, but now the woman began to flood violently, and soon became faint. He now endeavoured to separate the placenta with his hand, but the violence of the flooding deterred him, and he desisted. Frightened beyond measure at the dilemma into which he had brought himself, and not knowing how to proceed, he sent for a medical friend, at the distance of about a mile, and waited his arrival; the poor woman all the time becoming worse and worse. His friend peeled off the placenta while the uterus was inverted, and during the operation there was an increase of loss. The woman was now in articulo mortis, and the uterus was passed into the vagina, but not reverted. I first passed my finger into the vagina, and found it completely filled up by the inverted uterus, which had now become flaccid; during life it had been firm and resistant." Nothing farther was ascertained respecting the relative state of parts in this case. Dr. Ramsbotham has " never seen a case immediately after inversion ; but I was desired," he says, " some months ago, to visit a poor woman in Shoreditch parish, three weeks after delivery, to whom the accident had happened at the time of labour, but it had not been detected. The inverted uterus was then about the size of a goose's egg, and regularly contracting. The woman had suffered much from flooding and its consequences, but was recovering."

But inversion of the uterus may be partial or incomplete, so that the fundus and body are retained within the vagina, or protrude very slightly through the os uteri. On the 17th February, 1843, I saw, in consultation, a case of partial inversion of the uterus, fourteen hours after the accident had occurred ; and this is the only case of inverted uterus I have seen in London. The patient had been delivered of her first child after an easy labour ; but the umbilical cord was not only twisted firmly round the neck, but was remarkably short. The placenta was not expelled for half an hour, and then Mr. —— found it protruding through the external parts with the uterus, to which it still adhered. The placenta was detached from the uterus and removed, and an unsuccessful effort made to reduce the uterus. The discharge of blood which took place was not very profuse ; and an opiate having been administered, the patient, though considerably exhausted, suffered little pain during the interval between the delivery and the time I was called to see her. On passing my hand into the vagina, I found its upper part completely occupied with the fundus, and a portion of the body of the uterus, like a soft cricket-ball. So firmly was the neck of the uterus contracted above, that all my efforts, which were long continued, to reduce or push up the inverted uterus, were unavailing, and the uterus remains now, I believe, in the same condition, and the patient suffers continually from pain, profuse menorrhagia, and leucorrhœa, and will continue to suffer from these symptoms from the inverted uterus during the remainder of her life. There is the greatest probability that if the same efforts to reduce the uterus had been made within a few hours after the displacement occurred, they would have been perfectly successful. If you should meet, therefore, with such a case, the symptoms of which would be the absence of the fundus uteri in the hypogastrium, hæmorrhage, pain, and the tumor in the vagina, pass the hand at once within the vagina, grasp the inverted portion of the uterus, and firmly compress its upper part with the fingers like a hernial sac, and force it back, and carry the hand forward into the cavity to be sure that the

reduction is complete. Remember, that if the attempt fails, the evil speedily becomes irremediable. If the placenta still adheres, some recommend that it should not be removed till we have reduced the uterus ; but it is difficult to conceive what benefit can result from pushing back the mass of the placenta into the uterus, and afterwards extracting it. Partial inversion of the uterus, though sometimes immediately fatal by hæmorrhage, does not always produce death. In a patient whose case has been related by Dr. Cleghorn, menstruation was performed by the inverted uterus, and she enjoyed tolerable health for twenty years after the accident. When the inverted uterus is irreducible, we ought to palliate the symptoms, of which pain, hæmorrhage, and leucorrhœa are the most distressing, by appropriate remedies. If the life of the patient is greatly endangered by the irritation and discharge, it is justifiable to attempt her relief by removing the inverted uterus with a ligature. Numerous cases have been recorded since the days of Ambrose Paré, in which this operation was successfully performed, and there are many others in which attempts to extirpate the inverted uterus have been followed by fatal consequences. It should not be had recourse to if the patient's life can be preserved by any other means. It is unnecessary to detain you by reading any of these cases, fortunate or unfortunate ; and the operation, which is nearly the same as tying a polypus of the uterus, will be described hereafter.

On Rupture of the Uterus.

This may take place in any part of the walls of the uterus, but it is most frequently observed in the cervix and towards the sides, or behind in the part corresponding with the promontory of the sacrum. The rent may have a longitudinal direction, or it may take a transverse, or oblique, or curved course. When the cervix uteri is torn, the vagina is most frequently involved in the mischief. The edges of the laceration are usually thin and ragged, and of a red livid colour, as if gangrenous. Where the rupture is extensive, and is situated in the lower part of the uterus, the fœtus, with the placenta and membranes, are sometimes forced out of the cavity of the uterus, through the rent, into the sac of the peritoneum ; and if the hand be applied to the abdomen, the different parts of the child can be distinctly felt through the parietes.

In all cases of difficult and protracted labour, where an obstacle is presented to the progress of the child, which the uterus has not power to overcome, the occurrence of fatal rupture of its coats is the accident we have most to dread. It is of no importance whether the disproportion between the child and pelvis depends upon an unfavourable position of the child itself, as in arm and shoulder presentations, hydrocephalus or ascites, distortion of the bones of the pelvis, or tumors of the ovaria and uterus, malignant disease of the os uteri, or cicatrices of the vagina. The effect produced is the same, whatever the cause of the disproportion may be; and the upper part of the uterus often goes on contracting, until it forces the head of the child, or the whole body and placenta, through its walls into the abdominal cavity among the intestines. The reason why the lower part of the uterus is most frequently lacerated is obvious. In labour it is the fundus and body only which contract; the os and cervix uteri are relaxed. The lower part is in a state of relaxation; and when the head of the child here meets with a resistance from the distorted pelvis, which cannot be overcome, it is forced laterally or posteriorly, by the pressure above, through the walls of the uterus; the coats burst over the head as a small soft glove does when drawn hastily upon the hand, or the hand is roughly pushed into it.

"There is one fact," observes Dr. Collins, "which clearly shews disproportion to be a frequent cause, namely, its being oftener met with in the expulsion of male children; thus of thirty-four cases which I am about to state, twenty-three of the children were males; and of about twenty mentioned by Dr. M'Keever, fifteen were males. This is satisfactorily accounted for by the greater size of the male head, as proved by accurate measurements made by Dr. Joseph Clarke, which may be seen in his second letter to Dr. Price. Of sixty male and sixty female children born at the full time, Dr. Clarke found that the average circumference in the males was fourteen inches, and in the females thirteen inches and five-eighths; the arch from ear to ear over the crown was seven and a quarter inches in the males, and only seven one-fifth inches in the females. Of the one hundred and twenty examined, there were only six where the circumference of the head exceeded fourteen and a half inches, all of which were males. This difference may appear trifling, but in a practical point of view it is of vast importance, especially where any diminution in the size of the pelvis exists." "The part that most usually gives way is at the junction of the cervix uteri with the vagina, either anteriorly or posteriorly; and, according to my experience, equally in both situations. Of thirty-four cases that occurred in the hospital, in thirteen the injury was in the posterior part; in twelve, anteriorly or posteriorly; in two, laterally; in one the mouth of the womb was torn; and in six *the particular seat* of the laceration was not *described. In nine of* the thirty-four cases

the peritoneal coat of the uterus was uninjured, although the muscular substance of the cervix was extensively ruptured. One singular case occurred in the hospital, precisely similar to that recorded by Dr. John Clarke, in the Transactions of a Society for the Improvement of Medical and Surgical Knowledge, vol. iii. where the patient died with all the symptoms of ruptured uterus. On examination, however, no rupture could be discovered; but on throwing forward the fundus uteri numerous lacerations were observed in the peritoneal covering of its posterior surface; the injury being confined to this membrane. I have never seen an instance where the fundus was ruptured; nor did Dr. Clarke, during his residence in the hospital, meet with such an occurrence."

Soon after the occurrence of this dangerous accident the labour-pains diminish greatly in strength, or entirely cease, the presenting part of the child recedes, hæmorrhage to a greater or less extent takes place from the vagina, and it is evident from the collapse of the features that a serious internal injury has been inflicted on some vital organ; the respiration becomes hurried and laborious, the pulse rapid and feeble, the extremities and the whole surface cold, and vomiting of dark-coloured fluid matters, like coffee-grounds, takes place.

These are the symptoms by which you will recognize laceration of the uterus during labour, and which sometimes takes place without any precursory signs. The pains are not so violent as to lead to any suspicion of what is about to occur; the uterus may be torn extensively before the patient has been twenty-four hours in labour, and where there has been nothing peculiar observed in the character of the pains, and nothing like irregular violent spasmodic contractions of the uterus around the body of the child; the accident may happen without the patient feeling any peculiar pain or sensation of tearing of the parts within, and where no sound is heard either by herself or by those around her. But if rupture of the uterus has taken place in some cases without any premonitory symptoms, there is reason to believe that it has happened in many where it might have been foreseen and prevented. What can be expected to occur but rupture of the uterus where the hand is rudely forced up into the cavity of the uterus to turn the child, when the organ is firmly contracted around its body, and the liquor amnii has been long discharged? What else can be looked for but laceration of the uterus and vagina where the blades of the forceps are pushed up between the head and a deformed pelvis, before the os uteri is more than half dilated? In cases of distorted pelvis, where the head of the child has been allowed to remain many hours jammed in the brim, where the promontory of the sacrum projects in the form of a sharp angle, and the sacro-pubic diameter is much reduced, fatal lacera-tion of the posterior part of the uterus is what we have just reason to apprehend, if we do not, in proper time, relieve the patient by the operation of craniotomy. In a de-formed pelvis, where the head has long remained in the same position, and the abdomen is tense, and the different parts of the child can be felt remarkably distinct, and the labour pains occur at short intervals and with unusual intensity, and produce more suffering than labour pains usually do, making the patient exclaim that she is about to burst, rupture of the uterus will probably take place, if the labour is allowed to proceed and no treatment is employed. It was sup-posed by La Motte, Levret, and Cranz, that the violent movements of the child could rupture the uterus; but the child is entirely passive when this occurs.

Softening of the uterus, by chronic in-flammation or some other morbid process, appears occasionally to take place in the latter months of pregnancy, which renders it liable to spontaneous rupture when labour commences. A rent has sometimes occurred, with fatal internal hæmorrhage probably from the same cause, as early as the period of quickening, before the uterus had begun to contract. This preparation [exhibiting it] now upon the table was taken from the body of a woman who died from spontaneous rup-ture of the uterus, who had been delivered with the forceps in a former labour. The presentation was natural; there was no dis-tortion of the pelvis; but towards the end of the first stage of labour the pains ceased, the presenting part receded beyond the reach of the finger, considerable hæmorrhage fol-lowed, and dark-coloured vomiting took place, and she died undelivered. This was the history of the case which I received from the midwife. I examined the body, and found the whole contents of the uterus in the peritoneal sac, with very little blood. There was an immense rent in the lower part of the uterus and vagina on the left side, the edge of which was of a dark red colour, and as soft as jelly. This softening had affected a considerable part of the uterus, and was not the result of decomposition. Dr. Merriman has related a similar case; and the uterus which I saw in the recent state had undergone a process of softening in the muscular coat at the part where the laceration existed.

The uterus has been torn by various kinds of external violence applied to the abdomen, and it is reported to have occurred from a violent fit of passion. "A woman," says M. Desormeaux, "has the abdomen strongly pressed between the wall and a carriage, another is thrown down by a horse upon an angular stone or body which is directed against the umbilicus, a third falls with violence upon the abdomen; in all these cases the uterus is ruptured, and the fœtus passes partially or completely into the peri-toneal sac. The contusion, in these cases, has sometimes not led to immediate lacera-tion; this has taken place afterwards, on making an effort or raising a weight. In a case of contraction of the cervix uteri, with retention of the placenta, the hand of the practitioner was forced through the coats of the uterus, and the woman soon died."

Treatment of rupture of the uterus.—Where the head of the child presents, and rupture of the uterus takes place, the best plan is without delay to deliver with the perforator and crotchet; and to prevent the child, during the operation, from passing through the rent into the peritoneal sac, pressure should be made over the fundus uteri, and the opening made in the head in the most gentle manner. I have seen no case of ruptured uterus in which it was possible to deliver with the forceps; and I am not aware that any case of ruptured uterus has been recorded in which a living child was delivered with the forceps. " Efforts have frequently been made to deliver with the forceps in such cases," says Dr. Collins, " but this instrument is seldom applicable, as the introduction of the blades generally forces the head out of our reach ; besides, but little would be thus gained, for the child dies shortly after rupture takes place ; the dimensions, too, of the pelvis are in such cases for the most part defective ; all which circumstances would seem strongly opposed to this mode of delivery. In three of the thirty-four cases above alluded to attempts were carefully made to deliver with the forceps, but without success." Dr. Burns is of a different opinion. He says the child may live for hours, after rup-ture of the uterus, if the placenta be not detached, or the hæmorrhage great. If the head have entered the pelvis, and be within reach of the forceps, we must cau-tiously introduce the blades, taking great care not to press up the head or make it recede. From this hazard, and from ob-serving that in such cases the child is generally dead, it has been advised, by good authorities, to perforate the head ; but if we have no other inducement to use the per-forator, I should consider that, unless the head be high, the forceps would be as safe in this respect.

If the child has passed entirely from the cavity of the uterus into the peritoneal sac, an attempt should be made without delay to extract it, by introducing the hand into the cavity and through the rent in the uterus, grasping the feet and drawing the child back into the uterus, and delivering as in the common operation of turning. In the following case, related by Dr. Blundell, recovery took place under these circumstances. "A woman in this neighbourhood," he says, "had a contraction of the pelvis. It was a case that occurred to one of yourselves, but no blame attached to its management. I was called in, in consequence of collapse of the strength; and when I examined I found the child lying in the peritoneal sac, distinct from the uterus, the aperture of which was contracted, and I found further a large transverse rent opposite to the bladder. Well, in this case, agreeably to the rule, I determined to turn, and for this purpose introducing my hand into the peritoneal sac, I perceived the intestines, felt the beat of the large abdominal arteries, touched the edge of the liver, and ultimately reaching the feet of the child, I withdrew it by the operation of turning, subsequently abstracting the placenta and membranes, the woman recovering in a few weeks afterwards. About five years after the recovery I saw her, not so vigorous as before the accident, but nevertheless tolerably well. On very careful examination at this time the os uteri was found to present the natural characters, and not a vestige of a cicatrix was discoverable in the vagina any where above or below. The rupture, therefore, had been above, in the uterus itself. When, in this case, my hand was introduced to turn the fœtus, the womb, large as a child's head, was felt lying upon the promontory of the sacrum, above and behind the rent."

If a considerable period has elapsed after the accident, and the uterus has contracted so closely that the hand cannot be passed through the orifice and the rent, the best practice would be to leave the case to nature. Some have recommended gastrotomy under these circumstances; but the child is already dead, and the mother could hardly be expected to survive after such an operation. But I had nearly forgotten to mention that the Cæsarean section was actually proposed by Cranz where, from the size of the head and dimensions of the pelvis, there were symptoms merely threatening rupture of the uterus, and before rupture had positively taken place; and that he considered it a great honour to have been the first to make this barbarous proposal. "J'aurais encore ici la gloire," he says, "d'avoir proposé le premier l'usage d'un moyen dont personne avant moi n'avoit eu l'idée pour le cas dont il s'agit."

If the fœtus has escaped into the peritoneal cavity, and is allowed to remain there, the patient may recover without gastrotomy, and the fœtus be afterwards discharged *through an* ulcerated opening in the parietes *of the abdomen. It is* probable that the greater number of cases recorded by authors, in which this event took place, were cases of extra-uterine gestation, and that the fœtus had never been within the cavity of the uterus. But in Dr. Cheston's case the fœtus had undoubtedly been within the cavity of the uterus, for he states that, after acute labour pains, symptoms of ruptured uterus took place, and that the presenting part receded. The fœtus remained many years in the abdomen, and became covered with a layer of calcareous matter.

In 1814, Dr. M'Keever published an interesting case of recovery after lacerated uterus, which shews the power which nature possesses in some individuals to repair the most dreadful injuries. A stout young woman had the uterus ruptured during labour which continued nearly thirty hours, and nearly four feet of intestine protruded into the vagina, and sloughed off on the 16th day after the accident. For about two years the patient voided all the fæces through the breech in the uterus. At the conclusion of that period the fæces took their natural course. Eighteen months afterwards the woman conceived, and has since at the full time been safely delivered of a small feeble child. I have already related to you the history of a case of rupture of the uterus from hydrocephalus in the fœtus, similar in some respects to the preceding case, which fell under my observation on the 22d of June, 1842. If the patient is delivered after rupture of the uterus, and survives the immediate shock of the accident, it should be remembered that she is liable to perish from an attack of peritoneal inflammation and suppuration in the neighbourhood of the uterus.

Extravasation of Blood into the Labia.

One of the labia pudendi sometimes becomes suddenly and excessively distended with blood during labour, or soon after the birth of the child, from rupture of varicose veins or other vessels. The labium becomes of a dark livid colour, and as large as the head of a child in a very short time, and a great quantity of blood is sometimes lost, from the inner surface of the labium becoming lacerated. Its situation on one side, and its dark colour, will prevent you from supposing that it is the fœtal membranes protruding, or a hernial tumor. Dr. Dewees states, that if the bursting of the inner surface of the labium does not take place in the first instance, the tumor is sure to yield in a short time from gangrene. When the part sloughs, he says, it exposes a large surface of coagulated blood, which quickly becomes decomposed and fœtid. If the parts do not give way the pain is agonising: fever of an active kind is excited, delirium takes place, and the patient's life is greatly endangered. Her sufferings are augmented by the retention of urine, and nothing gives relief but a free incision into the tumor to give vent to the extravasated blood. This should be done, he thinks, before the process of ulceration has commenced, or the chance of bursting. The urine should then be drawn off by pressing the enlarged labium to one side, and introducing the catheter, and warm fomentations to the hands and feet; but the progress of the symptoms is sometimes so rapid as scarcely to allow time for the administration of remedies. In the Archives Générales de Médecine, August 1834, several cases are related. A woman, aged 41, pregnant with her fifth child, was seized with labour pains, which gradually abated after the liquor amnii was discharged. In a short time, however, a violent pain was experienced, and the left labium became enormously swollen and discoloured. The tumor soon burst, and a great quantity of dark-coloured blood was discharged. She became exhausted, and soon died in convulsions. There was a laceration on the inner surface of the labium an inch and a half in length, through which the finger could be passed into a large cavity containing coagulated blood. On the right labium and inner surface of both thighs there were varicose veins. In another case the labour had lasted upwards of twenty hours, when the right labium was found greatly distended and discoloured, and blood was dropping from its inner surface. The patient died in a quarter of an hour. A rent two inches in length was found on the inner surface of the right labium, which led into a cavity nearly four inches in circumference, and which extended under the os pubis, and on the outer side of the ascending ramus: at the bottom of this sac was seen the ruptured orifice of the varix. There was distortion of the pelvis. Dr. Elbert was summoned to the assistance of another woman in labour, but she had just expired on reaching the house. She was 34 years of age, and the mother of seven children. The labour had begun favourably, and the pains had been at first regular and steady. On a sudden the woman felt that a quantity of fluid was running away from her, but she thought it was the waters; the nurse, however, found that it was blood. In half an hour the patient expired. On the right labium, which was swollen and livid, were seen three ragged wounds; through each of these the finger could be passed into a large cavity, which still contained a quantity of black coagulated blood. On the left labium and both thighs were numerous distended veins.

In all these cases death took place before delivery, and the children were dead when extracted. In the fourth case the delivery had taken place before the rupture of the varicose swelling. Immediately after the expulsion of the child, the external parts became enormously swollen, and at length the integuments gave way at one point, and an alarming hæmorrhage took place. Professor Rieche immediately applied rags dipped in cold water, which arrested the flow of blood, and the exhausted strength of the patient was then supported by sinapisms to both legs, and by a cordial medicine exhibited frequently. Another woman, æt. 46, mother of eight children, suddenly expired in labour. Dr. Carus found the head of the child detained in the outlet of the pelvis: he delivered it with the forceps, but not without considerable difficulty; for the pelvis was confined. On introducing the hand afterwards to extract the placenta, he found near the cervix of the uterus a ruptured varicose tumor; the rent was about 1½ inch long, and the extent of the cavity about two inches all round.

On the 13th of January, 1840, a patient of the Saint Marylebone Infirmary, with slight distortion of the pelvis, was in labour, and the face presented and became jammed in the brim. Violent uterine action was allowed to continue many hours, the head being too high for the forceps, when the right labium became enormously distended with blood, and burst on the inner surface, and a great hæmorrhage took place. When I first saw the patient the hæmorrhage was supposed to proceed from the uterus, but on making an examination I felt the labium immensely enlarged, and my wrist was covered with blood. It was evident that the patient would soon have died had the hæmorrhage not been arrested. The discharge of blood was checked by strong pressure with a sponge over the rent, while I opened and extracted the head. Cold applications were afterwards made to the part, and when the hæmorrhage had ceased emollient poultices, and she recovered rapidly. On the 2d November, 1841, I saw in consultation Mrs. ——, who was far advanced in pregnancy, and had suffered much during the latter months from a varicose state of the veins of the right foot, leg, thigh, and labium. For six weeks the right labium had been much enlarged, and a painful circumscribed swelling had formed in it like an abscess, with throbbing, which led Mr. —— to open it with a lancet: when this was done a small quantity of venous blood escaped, but no pus; and soon after the labium began to enlarge and assume a dark livid colour. It had attained nearly the size of a child's head when I saw the patient, and was as black as one's hat, and was so tense that it threatened to burst. It was evident the hæmorrhage was still going on. To arrest the discharge the labium was covered with pieces of ice with the best effect, for the effusion soon ceased, and on the following morning the labour came on, and was completed by the natural efforts without a renewal of the hæmorrhage. Rapid absorption of the extravasated blood took place, and the patient speedily recovered.

In the next lecture I shall proceed to consider the Diseases of Puerperal Women.

EARLY MARRIAGES SO COMMON IN ORIENTAL COUNTRIES NO PROOF OF EARLY PUBERTY.

By John Roberton, Esq.

[Concluded from p. 615.]

It has been already observed that the marriage of a ward was often put up to sale by the guardian. " In the Pipe Rolls of 28, 29, and 30, Henry II. Robert de Were, called son of Robert, son of Harding, accounted for fifty marks, and a golden cup of the value of forty marks, for having the daughter of Robert de Gant in ward."*

In some cases the sale brought a large, in others a moderate sum: William, Bishop of Ely, gave 220 marks that he might have the custody of Stephen de Beauchamp, and might marry him to whom he pleased. John, Earl of Lincoln, gave Henry III. 3000 marks to have the marriage of Richard de Clare for the benefit of Matilda, his eldest daughter; and Simon de Montford gave the same king 10,000 marks (equal to £100,000 at present), to have the custody of the lands and heir of Gilbert de Unfranville, with the heir's marriage; and Hugh de Flammerville proffered £10 for the custody of his sister with her land. In Maddox's History and Antiquities of the Exchequer, the reader who is curious will find a lengthy list of sales, such as the above, in Chapter X. " of the Crown Revenue."†

The most curious thing connected with the treatment of this species of property is the extremely cool manner in which wards are bequeathed along with ordinary goods and chattels : thus Sir John Cornwallis, Knight, in his will of date April 16, 1554, after a very

devout and pious exordium, and a specification of certain bequests, proceeds —" I bequeath to my daughter my wife's gown of black velvet ; to my son Henry my own gown of tawny taffita ; to my son Richard my ward, Margaret Lowthe, which I bought of my Lord of Norfolk, to marry her himself if they both will be so contented; but if not, I will that he shall have the wardship and marriage of her, with all the advantages and profits."*

Sir Reginald Bray, Knight of the Garter, August 4, 1503, bequeaths, among other items of property, two wards, in these terms : " Whereas I have in my keeping Elizabeth and Agnes, daughters and heirs of Henry Lovell, Esq. I will that Elizabeth be married to one of my nephews, son to my brother John Bray, and that the said Agnes to another son of my said brother."†

John Colet, the Dean of St. Paul's, August 22, 1519, wills, " all those my lands and tenements, rents, services, wards, marriages, reliefs, &c. &c. in the towns, fields, and morasses of Chippesby, &c. in the county of Norfolk."‡

Sir Thomas Wyndham, Knight, October 12th, 13 Henry VIII. 1522, bequeaths to certain parties " all my wards and marriages now bought by me, with all advowsons by any means belonging to me, &c. in the counties of Norfolk and Yorkshire."§

It would seem that the dread of wardship and marriage sometimes operated with parents in marrying their child at a tender age, with a view to evade this oppressive law. Thus Maurice, fourth Lord Berkeley, was knighted at 7,‖ and was married at 8 years old to Elizabeth, daughter of Hugh, Lord Spencer, then but 8 years old, the reason being that early marriage prevented wardship, the payment of a large fine to the king, and assisted the party's own affairs with interest and powerful connections. This instance happened in the reign of Edward III. From a

---

* Berkeley Manuscripts: Extracts from Smythe's Live by Thomas Dudley Fosbroke p. 78.
† Maddox's History of London, 1711 ; also Christ vol. ii, p. 71.

* Testamenta vetusta, being illustrations from Wills of Manners, Customs, &c. from the reign of Henry the Second, to the accession of Queen Elizabeth, by Nicholas Harris Nicolas, Esq. Royal 8vo. vol. ii. page 715. London, 1836.
† vol. ii. p. 446.
‡ 371.
§ 55 n. seq.
‖ by knight-service was g was no longer entitled son, nor to the value of 'a Blackstone, vol. ii.

subsequent entry it is uncertain whether or not the juvenile couple were permitted to cohabit till the age of 16; since at the age of 14 the young husband, it appears, was sent to travel two years in Spain.*

In my paper in this journal for July 1842 (MED. GAZ. vol. xxx. p. 677), on the period of puberty in the negro, I have given a number of instances (in a note) of early marriage, chiefly in the families of our kings, up to the date of the marriage of Henry VIII. with Catharine of Arragon. To these I now add some instances which I have gleaned when looking into family memoirs: although not very numerous, they will yet be found sufficient to establish the fact, that the gentry in general, and particularly the eldest sons, married about the age of puberty as late as till the middle of the seventeenth century. The libraries of a provincial town afford little scope comparatively for research in this particular line; but inquirers may possibly be incited by what they find in these pages to pursue the path now opened up, in circumstances more favourable to the elucidation of this trait of old English manners.

1247. John, [eleventh] Earl of Warren and Surrey, was married A.D. 1247, when 12 years of age, to Alice, daughter of Hugh de Brun, Earl of the Marches of Aquitaine.†

1303. Robert de Tatershal of Abkettleby, Leicestershire, married while under age Eva, daughter of Robert de Tiptoft, 13 years old.‡

1351. The Earl of Holland married Maud, daughter of the Duke of Lancaster: the lady, although a widow, was only 19.§

1456. Margaret, wife of Edmund Tudor, was left a widow and a mother at the age of 14.‖

12 Edward IV. We learn from Cotton's Records that it was accorded that, at the age of 13 years, Cicill, only daughter of Katharine (some time the wife of Bonsile, Lord Harrington), should marry Thomas, the eldest son of the Queen, " between whom, if there was no mutual society, that the said

Cicill should marry with Richard, the brother of the said Thomas."*

17 Edward IV. The king creates Richard, his second son, Duke of York and Norfolk, &c., and appoints his said son to marry with Anne, the daughter and heir of John, late Duke of Norfolk, " the said Anne being then of the age of 6 years."†

1536. Henry Fitzroy, Duke of Richmond, in Somerset, married to Mary, daughter of the Duke of Norfolk, died, aged 17, July 24, 1536, without issue.‡

1532. Elizabeth Leak of Hasland, in Derbyshire, was married, at 14 years of age, to Robert Barley, of Barley, Esq. same county, " who was also very young."§

The mother of Catharine Parr (the last of Henry VIII.th's wives), Matilda Green by name, married Sir Thomas Parr when she was 13. Catharine, the daughter, was herself by a family arrangement to have married Lord Scroop when he came to the age of 13, and she to 12. This fell through, but she did marry Lord Borough, a widower, when she could not have been much above 12, since she is found by and by to be a widow in her fifteenth year. Again, while as yet under 20, she took for her second husband Lord Latimer.

By a solemn matrimonial treaty, signed at Windsor, the Emperor Charles V. engaged to marry his cousin, the Princess Mary, as soon as she arrived at her 12th year. This treaty fell through; but Cardinal Wolsey endeavoured to effect a marriage between Francis I. and the same Princess Mary, she being then only 11,—neither did this take effect. The fair Geraldine (of the poet Surrey), a lady of the court of Queen Mary, is married to Sir Anthony Brown when she is 16.‖

1551. In certain instructions to the ambassadors in France, of this date, they are directed to inform the French king that, on the 12th October of the next year, Edward VI. would be 14 years old, and to request that the marriage with the lady Elizabeth (daughter of the French king) may take place three months after she shall have attained the age of 12 years.¶

* Berkeley Manuscripts, p. 140-141.
† Watson's Lives of the Earls of Warren and Surry, vol. i. p. 226.
‡ Nicholls's History and Antiquities of Leicestershire, folio, vol. ii. p. 17.
§ Ibid. vol. i.
‖ Miss Strickland's Queens of England, vol. iv. p. 20.
* Cotton's Records in the Tower of London, folio, p. 695.
† Ibid. p. 702.
‡ Collins's Peerage, vol. i. p. 91.
§ Ibid. vol. i. p. 293.
‖ These instances are taken from Miss Strickland's Lives of the Queens of England, vol. v.
¶ Tytler's England under the reigns of Edward VI. and Mary, 1839, vol. i. p. 397.

1603. James, first Duke of Hamilton, born 1603, married the daughter of the Earl of Denbigh, he 14, and the bride 7.* Burnet says, "after the years for consummating the intended marriage were over, he was forced to it not without great aversion, occasioned, partly, by the disproportion of their ages, and partly by some other secret consideration."

1629. Lord Thurles married his cousin, Elizabeth Preston, (a king's ward,) only child of Richard Earl of Desmond, aged 14.†

A. D. 1667. Lady Diana Russell was married to Sir Grevil Verney when she was aged 15 years.‡

1680. Elizabeth, sole heiress of Joseline Percy, Duke of Northumberland, was married to Henry Cavendish, Earl of Ogle, who, however, died before he was of age to cohabit with her.§

1663. Elizabeth, Countess of Bridgwater, died this year in the 37th year of her age, having been married at the age of 13.||

These scattered instances of early marriage, gleaned at random from a variety of sources, are not without interest; but a clearer and more precise idea as to the prevalence of this custom in families of rank is obtained when the records of marriage in a particular family *in successive generations* are before us, as in the case of the Berkeleys; from which we shall see that the Lords of Berkeley, some ages ago, differed in this trait of manners little or nothing from the nobles of Russia, in the time of the Empress Catharine, or of her predecessor Peter.

Thomas, fourth Lord Berkeley, was contracted to Margaret, daughter of Gerard Warren, Lord Lisle [41 Edward III.] Amongst other items in the contract is this: "The same Margaret, by reason of her tender age (then about 7,) shall for *four* years remain with her father, and this Thomas de Berkeley with his father."¶ Elizabeth, only daughter and heir of the aforesaid Lord Thomas Berkeley, was contracted for marriage when she was under 7 years of age; the husband Richard the Earl of Warwick. It may be presumed

that the consummation of the marriage would take place about the age of puberty.* Thomas, son of William Marquis Berkeley, [Edward VI.] when 5 years old, was contracted by his father to Mary, daughter of Anne, Countess of Pembroke.† Maurice, fourth Lord Berkeley (whose case has been already mentioned), married at 8, his wife being of the same age. Maurice, sixth Lord Berkeley, 8 Henry VIII., "bought of the King the wardship of the body and lands of John, son and heir of Sir Richard Berkeley of Stoke; and, by his will, directed that he should be married at 16 years of age to Isabele Dennys, his sister's daughter; and if she should refuse, to Helen her sister, and so to Margaret her sister."‡ Lady Catharine, a daughter of the Earl of Surry, was married at 16 years of age to one of the Berkeleys, "by the bedside of her grandfather, the Duke of Norvolk, as he lay in his bed, then grown weak with age and sickness."§ George, Lord Berkeley, [12 James I.,] was married to Elizabeth, second daughter and co-heir of Sir Nicholas Stanhope, in the church of Great St. Bartholomew, London, and, in the presence of both their parents, he being 13 years old, and she 9. It appears that the bridegroom was sent to Christ Church, Oxford, to study for a time, his wife remaining with her father.|| What remains, though out of place as to date, is the most curious piece of information of any. Maurice, third Lord Berkeley, [Edward I.] was married at 8 years old, and a father before he was 14. The historian adds, "more than a dozen instances of paternity occur before that age."¶

More than a dozen instances of paternity occur, such are the words of the author of the Lives of the Berkeleys, before the age of 14. What an insight does such a sentence afford into the condition of families in the fifteenth, sixteenth, and seventeenth centuries, when this detestable precocity was unblushingly encouraged; assimilating the people of a Christian country, in this revolting feature, to the Pagan inhabitants of the South Sea Islands:

* Burnet's Lives of the Hamiltons, folio, p. 406.
† Coates's Life of the Duke of Ormond, p. 7, 4to.
‡ Collins, vol. i. p. 270.
§ Ibid. vol. i. p. 167.
|| Ibid. vol. ii. p. 365.
¶ Berkeley Manuscripts, p. 143.

* Ibid. p. 148.
† Ibid. p. 162.
‡ Ibid. p. 175.
§ Ibid. p. 205.
|| Ibid. p. 217.
¶ Ibid. p. 115.

regarding whom, the Rev. Mr. Ellis informs me, that the union of the sexes is *never*, he believes, delayed so late as the period of puberty. It must have been a full acquaintance with, and strong perception of the evils of this nature, resulting from wardship and marriage, which could have drawn from Grafton, a faithful chronicler in the reign of Elizabeth, the following extremely curious display of humane and patriotic feeling.

" It is much lamented that wards are bought and sold as commonly as are beasts; and marriages are made with them that are many times very ungodly; for divers of them being of young and tender years, are forced to judge by another man's affection, to see with another man's eye, and say yea with another man's tongue, and finally consent with another man's heart. For none of these senses be perfected to the parties in that minority, and so the election being unfree and the years unripe, each of them, almost of necessity, must hate the other, whom yet they have had no judgement to love. And certainly the common bargaining and selling of them is to be abhorred, besides the shameful polling that many use, which, if they consent not to such as are their sellers, they shall be handled, as the common saying is, *like wards*, and stripped almost out of all they have, when the same should do them most good. God grant the magistrates may take some good order therein, for surely it is needful, for many do use them as the same is not sufferable in a Christian realm. For who seeith not daily what innumerable inconveniences, divorces, yea and some murders, have of such marriages (or rather no marriages) proceeded, the present time sheweth too many examples, which minister sufficient cause for us to bewail the same; but the greatest injury is to God, who hath made that free, namely, matrimony, which the law of this realm maketh bond ; the redress whereof belongeth only to the Prince, in whom, like as the same God hath caused more virtues to meet than in any other creature of her calling, so we doubt not, but that his Godhead will, when his good pleasure shall be vouchsafed, not only to preserve her Highness, with the increase of virtue and wisdom, but also to move her heart to the godly redress of these, and many other enormities and abuses, to the great comfort of all her Grace's loving and obedient subjects."[*]

Ireland, placed on the western verge of Europe, and never included within the bounds of the Roman Empire, from, its remote position, was comparatively little exposed to those early migrations of energetic races from the north-east, by which nearly every other European country was at different periods visited, and by which the inhabitants were either extirpated, or renovated and improved. In this respect Ireland has undergone little change when compared with the island of Great Britain, and hence, (for reasons which will be obvious to the student of history, but which it is foreign to my present object to dilate upon,) it wears the traces of a somewhat recent civilization ; the population in some of the remoter districts having, even at the present day, a resemblance in the depressed cranium, and strongly marked development of the bones of the face, to the rudest varieties of our species.

Amongst those evidences of a low state of moral advancement which might be mentioned, *that* supplied by the early age at which the sexes unite in marriage is not wanting, as we learn from various writers on the social condition of Ireland. To Dr Griffin, of Limerick, in the first place, we are indebted for an interesting table, exhibiting the ages at which 735 women of that city married. Of this number there were, at 13 years of age, four; at 14 years, seven; at 15 years, twenty ; at 16, fifty; at 17, forty-eight; at 18, sixty-eight; at 19, seventy-two; at 20, eighty-three, being at the rate of about 50 per cent. married under age ; whereas in England the highest per centage of women marrying under age is 25.19 per cent : this is in the county of Bedford. In North Wales it is only 7.89 per cent.[†]

" The extremely early age at which many of these marriages took place," says Dr Griffin, " will no doubt surprise people very much. I have reason to think they are not very incorrect; and those which occurred at the very

* Grafton's Chronicle, vol. ii. pp. 349-50. Lond.
† Fourth Annual Report of the Registrar-General of Births, Deaths, and Marriages in England, for 1842 ; containing very interesting tables concerning the ages of 40,814 persons married in three years. June 1841, folio, p. 8.

early ages stated were always strictly inquired into. Of the four females stated to have been married at 13, two are well-authenticated instances which occurred in the county; one of these had her first child at 14. The other two took place in the city, and were actually not quite 13 at the time of marriage. In one of these instances, when I said to the mother, ' this girl must have been exceedingly anxious to get married, to marry so very young,' she replied, ' Oh ! no sir, she knew nothing about marriage, or what belonged to it, but the priest sent her away three times, he thought her so young.' In general, I believe these early unions are brought about entirely by the parents."*

Mr. Edward Wakefield, in his Statistical and Political Account of Ireland, published in the year 1812, has furnished a good deal of curious information concerning social life in that country, and animadverts with severity on the early improvident marriages of both the lower and upper classes. He says, that " celibacy being unfashionable, domestic servants are generally married ;" that the Roman Catholic peasant marries " in the greenness of youth, when reason seldom interrupts his career, and asks him whether he may not bring into the world a progeny for whom he cannot find the means of support. Thus a voluntary submission to the lowest state of life, and a disrelish for superior comforts, having become habitual, the system of premature marriage is perpetuated, while the increase of numbers is an unchecked increase of misery."

He represents the condition of women of the lower ranks as degraded in the extreme; that the man considers his wife as his slave; and that females are treated more like beasts of burden than rational beings; owing to which the traces of youth rapidly fade away. " In consequence of this harsh treatment, and continual exposure to the weather, added to the smoke of their cabins, and scanty fare, they exhibit a miserable spectacle, and acquire, at a very early period, every mark of old age. I have seen women who, from their appearance, might be supposed to be past the time of child-bearing, followed by very young children,

whom I did not consider as their own; but on inquiry, I found I was mistaken, and that their mothers were not above 30 years of age."

Mr. Wakefield asserts that young ladies in the higher classes " generally enter into the married state between the ages of 16 and 19 ;" that matchmaking in this rank of life is universal; that eighteen out of twenty marry the moment their mothers inform them that suitable offers have been made; and that, as might be expected, there is much deficiency in such youthful wives, both with respect to mental cultivation, and a competent knowledge of house-keeping.*

Perhaps the facts which have now been presented may be thought to warrant the following conclusions.

1st, That in England, Germany, and Protestant Europe in general, early marriage—that is, marriage about the age of puberty, would seem to be comparatively rare.

2d, That early marriage prevails amongst the uncivilized tribes which wander within the Arctic Circle ; as it likewise does in all cold countries, without any exception, the inhabitants of which are in a state of ignorance and moral degradation.

3d, That throughout European Russia, which is confessedly low in civilization, extremely premature marriage was the universal custom at no distant date.

4th, That, at the present day, in the most southerly countries of Europe, where the people are immersed in

---

* Journal of the Statistical Society of London, vol. iii. p. 322--3.

* An Account of Ireland, Statistical and Political, 4to. vol. ii. pp. 578, 579, 801, 802. 797, 799. From Mr. Crofton Croker we learn, that courtships are generally commenced among the peasantry of the south of Ireland " soon after the parties attain their teens." See his work on the South of Ireland, 4to. pp. 234—235. See also Letters from the Highlands of Cunnemara, 1825, by a Family Party, p. 96. Whilst I am writing this paper, I observe in the London Times of February 1st, 1843, a notice issued by an Irish landlord to his tenants, warning them against the practice of early marriage. " Is it possible for parents to shut their eyes, says this gentleman, to the consequences of it, which they must daily witness, in producing poverty and wretchedness around them ? Yet, they permit their young married children to take their abode under the same roof with themselves, and thus give encouragement to hasty and improvident marriages, thereby impoverishing the entire family." The landlord proceeds to threaten such tenants as turn a deaf ear to this word of advice, with expulsion from his estate. The above notice is copied into the Times from Freeman's Journal, but the name of the philosophical landlord is prudently withheld.

superstition and ignorance, marriage is early.

5*th*, That in Ireland, which, as to its moral condition, somewhat resembles the last mentioned countries, the marriage union takes place among the Roman Catholic population at an age probably almost as early.

6*th*, That in England about two centuries ago, when debasing political and social circumstances combined to favour the practice, early marriages were general, at all events in the upper ranks.

7*th*, That in all the countries to which reference has been made, juvenile marriage is invariably seen as an attendant on ignorance and moral debasement, and this without reference to *climate.*

8*th*, That consequently it is perhaps allowable to infer that early marriage in oriental countries (which has generally, in the absence of all proof whatever, been ascribed to precocious puberty,) does solely depend on the same moral and political causes as elsewhere produce it; more especially as those very causes are well known to exist, at present, in an aggravated degree in all oriental and intertropical countries.

9*th*, That, instead of ascribing early marriage, so prevalent in our Asiatic dominions, to precocious puberty, (in the absence of all evidence whatever of the fact,) it would be desirable to try moral and legislative remedies, with a view to the removal of a practice so injurious; a practice which seems to be incompatible with social improvement.

ON

SUMMER ASTHMA,
CATARRHUS ÆSTIVUS, OR HAY-FEVER,

ITS CAUSES AND TREATMENT.

BY T. WILKINSON KING.

Dr. Bostock's cases.—Various symptoms —rationale—summer eruptions—the fever, variable — dyspnœa — mixed cases—treatment.

HAVING suffered from what is called hay-fever, more or less, for some fourteen summers, I have thought it worth while to set down my own conclusions on the subject, together with an addi-

tional fact or two; but I should scarcely have been led to do this at the present time were it not that I wish, in this way, to point to, and confirm, more general views of disease.

Dr. Bostock[*], who has investigated the affections here referred to, speaks of twenty-eight cases, of which he had gathered various particulars. He says—

"They all agree in the complaint making its appearance at the same season of the year; in its seat being the membrane lining the nose, the fauces, and the vesicles of the lungs; and, for the most part, in the paroxysms being excited, and the symptoms aggravated, by the same causes. The twenty-eight cases referred to above all agree in the complaint commencing about the end of May or the beginning of June, and continuing from four to eight weeks. Most of them are attended with fulness of the head, stoppage of the nose, sneezing, watering of the eyes, and discharge from the nostrils. In about half of the whole number the respiration is considerably affected, and in three or four instances it is almost the only symptom. Some of the cases are attended with distinct cough, most of them with irritation of the fauces, and some with a degree of sore throat. Actual inflammation of the eyes is not a very common occurrence; and in some of the cases there is not even the discharge of tears, or the irritation of the eyes. The degree of general indisposition varies very much in the different cases; in some, the patient, during the whole period, is unable to use any exertion, or to continue his ordinary occupations; while, in other instances, he feels no inconvenience, except what arises from the fits of sneezing and the copious discharge from the nose."

With regard to the local symptoms, Dr. B. observes—

"The immediate cause of the symptoms seems to be sufficiently obvious; it consists in an increased action of the vessels of the membrane which lines the eye-lids, the nose, the fauces, and the pulmonary vesicles, by which it becomes acutely sensible to external impressions, has its natural secretions

[*] This gentleman, who is justly distinguished in physiological and chemical science, was the subject of the affection in question, and has given the only original and satisfactory account of it that I am acquainted with. See the fourteenth and tenth vols. of the Med.-Chir. Transactions.

augmented, and probably its bulk increased; to this last cause I think we may ascribe the very distressing sense of dyspnœa which exists in some of the cases. Although this membrane is continued without interruption over the different organs that are the seat of the affection, yet it is observed that the different parts are affected in different degrees. Hence we may divide the disease into four varieties, according as the eyes, the nose, the fauces, or the lungs, is the part more immediately affected. It is in the last variety only that I have observed the constitutional symptoms of fever and the subsequent debility to exist in any considerable degree."

I conceive that Dr. Bostock could not intend, as above, to consider the injection as the cause, rather than the consequence, of impressions from without. And I do not suppose that the extreme languor that summer may produce is altogether set out of the question. He notes lightly the attendant fever which may be severe, and even continued, or exceed all other symptoms.

The various causes of the local irritations hinted at in books are more curious than instructive. One patient suspects his asthma to depend on a sewer; another seems to find relief from coal-smoke diffused in his chamber. Different sufferers appear to find peculiar ease only in situations which are peculiarly obnoxious to the sensations and respiration of others. One can sleep no where so well as in a close carriage; another found a cure in the very preparation for a journey. Some accuse this, and others that state of atmosphere. Here an asthmatic discovers that a feather pillow is his peculiar bane; and another is cured by cold ablutions of the chest. A full dinner aggravating the disorder, is foolishly thought to be a cause of it. Opium, stramonium, tobacco, or brandy, may work a sudden cure; but most of all, as in summer catarrh, the affection disappears (fails to reappear) as it were by chance. The preceding and countless vagaries are to be accounted for by reference to simple principles*. We have to calculate that, according to circumstances, a certain number of hours having elapsed after exposure (specific or general), eating,

or lying down, capillary excitement or distension is to be evinced by uneasiness, obstruction, and various forms and quantities of secretion. Beyond this, we believe, very few of the phenomena of hay-fever or asthma will remain unresolved. The time at which the affections prevail is that of diminishing our clothing.

It seems to me, in the first place, not unreasonable to compare these affections with summer eruptions, in which we must discover both a cause of local disturbance, which we treat locally, and more or less of general internal disturbance, for which we administer medicines. A delicate female passes a few hours in the open air, wearing, perhaps, only a light bonnet, and suffers from blistering of the face. Now, whether the external cause be heat or air, we see that defective nutrition is the first internal local condition. On the other hand, another, in more robust health, after exposure, or a feast, suffers almost imperceptibly from feverishness, and herpetic vesicles break out over the lip.

There are a good variety of disorders which, if we consider the seat or the elimination (as to quantity or quality), seem to indicate but inconsiderable deteriorations (say of the blood), with rather more of decline of vital or nutrient powers—deficiency rather than perversion. External agency here becomes proportionably efficient to disturb. Our present subject may illustrate this opinion.

In the case of hay-fever, the febrile symptoms are, I think, to be referred to a perfectly distinct causation, beginning mostly with the effects of cold to the surface, but I by no means exclude the probability of increased susceptibility, and even some general decline and atrophy, the more gradual effects of heat. The variability and relapses of the languor and fever, as well as of the local symptoms, demand a reference to fresh disturbing causes, and no doubt diet, exercise, and even posture, have their particular, yet changeable effects.

I make some exception to the conclusion of Dr. Bostock, that the air-cells of the lungs are especially affected; and I prefer to set down the dyspnœa as the result of turgescence in the lining of the air-tubes. It seems natural that the more superficial dis-

* Vide a series of papers on Angina, MEDICAL GAZETTE, 1841.

orders should be most controlled by direct atmospheric influence, and certainly that the deeper should rather be dependent on less direct and more general causes. Sputa of branching mucus declare their own origin.

I think I have at different times experienced most of the symptoms described by Dr. Bostock, but not only in summer.

I am subject to slight attacks of dyspnœa especially on lying down, attended by a very slight ropy and clear secretion in the trachea. It seems to depend on a local injection and diminution of the laryngeal passage. On rising or walking it quickly disappears, and my feet betray the accumulation of blood (only) which gravity has removed from the neighbourhood of the pharynx, which at times also readily becomes tumid.

An attentive unprofessional man of very similar diathesis, who is subject to this kind of derangment, sits up in his bed and finds relief in a dish of hot coffee, which accelerates the general, and liberates the local circulation.

Dr. Bostock observes that he has met with nothing of these affections among the lower classes of society, but I think I have known of its occurrence in masked and aggravated forms, which I attribute to difficulties and exposures of a severer kind to which the poor are subject. I make very little doubt also that these same catarrhal disturbances of summer are of more frequent occurrence under a less distinct form; namely, that of aggravation of affections which in some degree the sufferer considers as habitual and almost natural to him. One cannot travel without incurring ophthalmia, another asthma. Many suffer in particular localities, or seem to require very peculiar circumstances to ensure tolerable ease. The above considerations, and my own experience, make me conclude that none of the affections are positively and necessarily confined to any season, or such a specific cause as hay, or the powder of ipecacuanha.

Dr. Bostock observes, "as far as regards medical treatment, an anxious desire to obtain relief from an annual indisposition of several weeks' continuance, and sometimes of considerable severity, has induced me to try, with the greatest perseverance, every remedy which held out the least prospect of advantage. I

think myself warranted in asserting, that on the whole the depleting system is injurious, and that some benefit is gained by a moderate use of tonics. This is the only point in which the various accounts that I have received from others, and my own experience, appear to agree; and in general it would seem that the symptoms proceed nearly in the same way under very opposite plans of treatment, and are very little influenced by medicines of any description."

It ought to be remembered that if a paroxysm be about to set in, a tonic regimen is premature, and may aggravate the distress to the highest degree, as in the case of incipient catarrh of any other kind. The time for support is that of the departure or decline of the disorder, provided no fresh or recent causes of disturbance require to be allowed for.

Dr. Bostock continues—" the experience of many years has taught me not to expect a cure for the complaint, so that I now only aim at relieving any peculiarly urgent or distressing symptom. Bathing the eyes in tepid water, and fomenting the face generally, occasionally applying small blisters to the chest, mild purgatives, small doses of ipecacuanha, Dover's powder, squills, and digitalis, bathing the feet in warm water, a moderate but not spare diet, perfect rest, and carefully avoiding all extremes of heat, comprise the whole of the means that I have found useful to myself. In order to prevent others from making useless experiments, I may remark that among those things which I have tried without success are bark, iron, opium, mercury, large blisters, topical bleeding, the waters of Harrowgate and Leamington, the baths of Bath and Buxton, sea-bathing, the shower-bath, abstinence from wine, and animal food, and a more free use of them; each of these having been made, as it may be said, the subject of distinct experiment, and persevered in until some circumstance rendered it necessary to discontinue them, or until they produced a decidedly injurious effect[*]."

It may be already apparent that the superficial disturbance is to be in part controlled by attention to local circum-

---

[*] Dr. Elliotson held hay effluvium for the cause, and seemed to cure a case with vapour from the chlorides. The Doctor seems to resemble Lord Bacon not a little in crediting curious assertions.—*Vide* MED. GAZ. vol. viii. p. 411.

stances. It may be that the eye cannot be protected but by closing the lid. The affection of the nares and trachea I have found relieved by inhaling steam; and there is no remedy after warm clothing on which I rely so much as on a sea-trip; yet I have known a most marked relapse caused by taking cold under such circumstances. I conceive that merely sitting in a cool room, or being coolly covered, as quite enough to account for a subsequent paroxysm, disturbing the whole balance of the capillary functions, which are already defective.

Cool air is well calculated to give immediate relief to the inflamed parts, but it would seem also to keep up the local susceptibility to reaction under easier circumstances, or when warmth or repletion is renewed. Now, if reaction be essential to the due nutrition and invigoration of the capillaries, the cold air, which gives temporary relief, is only a cause of relapse and troublesome delay.

It is not very much a subject of wonder that the delicate and exposed tissues near the summit of the capillary system should fail of its nutrition, and become in a degree too sensible under external influences, when the whole body is more or less so.

The objects of treatment are to diminish the existing disturbance, obviate the causes, and set the frame, by free nutrition, above the influences which pervert it; both as to the face and surface generally. That a slight wasting of the body with the advancing warmth of summer should be connected with the capillary states to which we advert, does not seem unreasonable; but still the specific affections may require a specific cause in the atmosphere to which the delicate membranes concerned are peculiarly and exclusively subjected. For my own part, the end of summer has seemed most liable to introduce disturbance. Dr. Bostock advises to avoid the extremes of heat; and his commendation of an airy room for the sufferer to sit in seems to me to account in a good measure for his want of success in the management of the disorder. Doubtless the more a feebly-nourished body is motionless or feverish the more it has need of warmth. Of course all exposure of the susceptible parts should be delayed. The more the symptoms are oppressive the more I should infer extreme sus-

ceptibility, as well as the neglect and need of what may be best understood as comfort for an enfeebled febrile body.

From what I have felt and witnessed of the disorders in question, I feel assured that the following reflection on common catarrh is justly applicable to them, though in widely different degrees. Throughout the disorder, the patient is peculiarly susceptible of the impressions of cold, even although the skin be warmer than natural. It may need much watchfulness both of cause and consequences to discover this. He is also (says Dr. Copland) "inordinately" disposed to experience an accession of, or to contract a fresh, cold upon the slightest exposure to its causes, or even to the least depression of temperature; indeed, nothing but personal experience, or the most careful and sedulous investigation, is likely to convince those who are strong, of the results of merely a cool bed. The specific local effects of season are increased by all exposure, and even by exertion. The slightest motion of the air about the body augments the effect of coolness and quiescence.

A good measure of clothing, a warm room, the absence of draught, gentle exercise, fair support, and even tonics, are the happiest means of obviating relapse and invigorating the frame. These, employed in the order here named, with opium if needed, and all that these suggest being maintained, will be found, I trust, so much the more satisfactory, as they are not empirical but rational. The disease is *general and local susceptibility for lack of comfort and nutrition*, which are the specific preventives of relapse.

It is perfectly in vain for the robust to judge of the requisite clothing and warm rooms for the susceptible, without the most careful experimental observations of the effects which cold, under different circumstances, produces within three or four, or eight or nine hours subsequently.

In conclusion, I have to propose, for the test of my views—a sufficiently warm room, or clothing to obviate the slightest coolness of the surface of the body, particularly when at rest. This is the first essential of the constitutional treatment, as relapses, if carefully watched, will soon testify. A certain degree of moisture in the air is the chief local palliative. After these, remedies on common principles may be expected to act curatively. Fever unaggravated may take days to subside. Depletion may be required, and narcotics have often acted like magic, causing some sense of general action, and proportionate local relief.

36, Bedford Square.

SYMPTOMS ATTENDING THE ILLNESS OF THE LATE SIR CHARLES NIGHTINGALE;

WITH THE POST-MORTEM EXAMINATION.

To the Editor of the Medical Gazette.

SIR,

I BEG to send you, for publication in the MEDICAL GAZETTE, a correct narrative of the symptoms attending the illness of the late Sir Charles Nightingale, Bart., from the time of my attending him up to the period of his dissolution, together with the inferences drawn from the anatomical exploration.

I am, sir,
Your obedient servant,
EDMUND LAMBERT.

Park Street, Bath,
July 26, 1843.

On Tuesday the 4th of July I was for the first time requested professionally to visit the late Baronet. He was then labouring under the following symptoms:—Ejecting from the stomach a tough viscid mucus, apparently discoloured by blood from ruptured capillaries, or, what I think more probable, by the introduction of some extraneous substance into the stomach, great distension in the epigastrium, with slight tenderness on pressure, frequent pulse, hot skin, panting, extreme restlessness, and anxiety; but no emaciation or diminution of strength. I then prescribed for him the following medicines, with the view of acting upon the bowels, which had not been opened during that or the preceding day, and at the same time allaying the irritability of stomach.

℞. Calomelanos, gr. x.; Confect. Opii, q. s. ut ft. pil. ij. h. s. s.

℞. Acidi Hydroc. dil. (Ph. L.) ♏xvj.; Mist. Amygdalæ, ℥viij. M. sumat cochl. ij. ampla 4tis horis.

Pulv. Rhei, ℈j. mane si opus sit.

I did not see him again till Thursday evening, when I was informed that Dr. Henry Johnson had been sent for in the intervening period, who also prescribed the hydrocyanic acid to be taken in an effervescing draught, and the following ointment to be rubbed into the region of the liver:—

℞. Ung. Hydr. fort. ℥ij.; Camph. ℨij; Iodinii, ℨss.

As Dr. Johnson had supplied my place in consultation, it was not my intention to have called again. On Friday morning, however, the 7th, Dr. Greville, the usual medical attendant, called at my house, and requested that I would accompany him to see Sir C. Nightingale, at the same time observing, he did not think there was much use in my going, as in all probability we should not find him alive. When I arrived I found him still throwing up the dark-coloured viscid mucous secretion; the epigastrium hard and distended; pulse scarcely perceptible; icy coldness of the hands, the lower extremities retaining a due degree of animal heat; panting very severe, with greater anxiety and restlessness than heretofore manifested; voice stridulous, but no obscuration of the intellectual powers. For this train of formidable symptoms, which I considered the forerunner of death, I simply recommended the frequent administration of stimulants and nourishment, and an opiate to tranquillize. I saw him again the same evening, when no alteration for the better or worse had taken place. Dr. Greville visited him between one and two o'clock on Saturday morning. During the night I was informed by one of his attendants that he was seized with a frightful convulsion. On Saturday I saw him at 3 P.M. for the last time, as death closed the melancholy scene at half-past 5 on Sunday morning the 9th. It was decided by the coroner that neither myself or Dr. Greville should be present at the post-mortem examination; but as Dr. Greville was the executor to whom the deceased bequeathed the whole of what he possessed, the coroner could not exclude him from the house, where he remained till the surgeon had completed his operation. The following are the morbid appearances recorded by Mr. Field :—

" The external appearances of the body presented a quantity of coffee-ground fluid about the mouth, nose, and chin; discoloured appearance of the skin about the neck and upper part of the chest; and a little above the left groin the appearance of a wound made by a scalpel or some surgical instrument. The body generally exhibited the signs of great decomposition, more rapid than is generally the case, even allowing for the time of year and the period which had elapsed since death. The internal appearances presented on being opened— *in the cavity of the chest an effusion of fluid in both pleural cavities, congested state of the lungs at their posterior parts,* and some emphysema in the anterior or inferior portions. The heart was flabby, and its left ventricle dilated. I now proceeded to the examination of the abdominal cavity, and found the marks of slight peritonitis over the intestines. On proceeding to separate the stomach from its connections, I found very considerable adhesion between its smaller curvature and under surface of the liver. On breaking through those adhesions, I found a cavity containing grumous blood and portions of fibrine. The cavity extended a considerable way behind the stomach. On removing the stomach and slitting it open, I found about six ounces of coffee-ground fluid in its cavity. There was not the slightest appearance of inflammation or ulceration in the mucous membrane, which was unusually pale. The liver was a little enlarged, congested, and very much disorganized in its lower surface and inferior border. The gall-bladder was literally crammed with biliary calculi, large and small together about 200. The kidneys were extensively diseased, presenting an advanced stage of the malady designated 'Bright's disease.' There are no other morbid appearances. From the morbid appearances discovered, I conclude that the cause of death in the deceased was hæmatemesis and the inflammation of the peritoneum, the result of diseased state of the viscera. The entire absence of inflammation or ulceration in the lining membrane of the stomach, precludes the idea of any deleterious ingredient, mineral or vegetable, having been taken by the deceased. I did not analyse the contents of the deceased's stomach, for I considered it a work of supererogation."

Mr. Field states in his evidence that there was not the slightest appearance in the mucous membrane of inflammation or ulceration, which was more than usually pale; but what would have been the appearances in the stomach if the vessels had not emptied themselves by secretion during the last stages of life? Would not the retention of coffee-ground fluid within the vessels have presented all the signs of congestion, and conveyed to the mind of the toxicological pathologist unequivocal indications of an irritant poison acting either directly upon the mucous surface, or, what is more probable, indirectly through the medium of the nervous and circulating systems? Did not the icy coldness of the hands indicate that one portion of the spinal marrow had ceased to generate heat, although it still continued to animate the circulation in a feeble manner, for the pulse was scarcely perceptible? and was not this depression of the circulating powers extremely favorable to the processes of secretion, exhalation, and congestion, so strikingly exhibited in the post-mortem examination? Is the icy coldness of the hands a common symptom of disease, or the panting a usual symptom in diseases of the respiratory organs? I put these questions, for I confess I have not witnessed them myself. Can coffee-ground or black vomit be called hæmatemesis, when the essential characteristics of the latter disease are entirely absent, viz. coagula?

Notwithstanding the gall-bladder was stuffed with calculi, I never heard the deceased complain of suffering any inconvenience from them.

As to the wound made by the scalpel, through which the intestine was partially protruding, I shall leave it to the profession to decide for what purpose that was made. A servant swore that he saw a gallon of fluid drawn off; but the surgeon who is said to have tapped the body ought to have been examined upon that point. There was no collapse of the abdominal parietes.

It is not my intention to enter into any controversial discussion; suffice it to say, that I vouch for the accuracy with which all the pathological phenomena have been detailed.

P.S.—I entirely differ with Mr. Field as to the analysis of the contents of the stomach being a work of supererogation. When the slightest suspicion of poison exists, and such a large quantity of fluid is found in the stomach after death, it should undoubtedly be submitted to chemical analysis. But the proceedings at this inquest were not conducted in a very satisfactory manner.

OBSERVATIONS
UPON THE
NEW PROCESS PROPOSED FOR THE DETECTION OF CORROSIVE SUBLIMATE
BY MEANS OF
METALLIC SILVER.

BY FORENSIS.

(For the London Medical Gazette.)

DR. FRAMPTON has proposed to use silver as a test for corrosive sublimate, upon the grounds that the affinity of silver for chlorine, and the great tendency of silver to amalgamate with mercury, offer, or at least promise, facilities for detection superior to other methods. Dr. Frampton, at the same time, very liberally and very properly submits his processes to investigation, and courts inquiry. Upon these terms I beg to offer the following for his especial consideration, as well as that of toxicologists in general. Dr. Frampton's first proposition is, that silver triturated with bichloride of mercury effects the reduction of the salt and the liberation of the mercury, which then forms an amalgam with the remaining silver. This is inferred from the change of colour. Upon this it may be observed, that two substances, exerting no chemical action whatever upon each other, by mere mechanical admixture, frequently modify, and sometimes even generate perfectly new and distinct colours. Again, it is a rule of chemical action that bodies do not act upon each other unless one at least be in solution, or contain water of crystallization. Although there are exceptions to this, yet I determined to place this matter beyond all doubt. For this purpose, bichloride of mercury having been rubbed on a plate of metallic silver till it was darkened, the plate was digested in a solution of ammonia. The fluid was now filtered, and the filtered portion boiled in a tube, when it became turbid. On the addition of nitric acid, a white curdy-looking precipitate fell down, insoluble in nitric acid, and which became dark on exposure to bright light. Ammonia again redissolved it, and, when reprecipitated by hydrochloric acid, a button of pure silver was obtained by reduction and cupellation. Therefore there can be no doubt that silver reduces bichloride of mercury by mere contact, and that a transfer of the chlorine to the silver takes place on mere triture.

Dr. Frampton's next experiment consisted in boiling a solution of bichloride of mercury with very finely and minutely divided silver, when the reduction of the mercurial salt, and the liberation of the metal, were equally the ultimate results. But the third case is the most important, in which bichloride of mercury is complicated with organic matter. Organic matter may be considered in the two-fold relations of animal and vegetable. As regards animal organic matter,—albumen for instance,—bichloride of mercury is rendered insoluble in water by it; that is, the albumen and bichloride of mercury enter into some sort of combination, which is insoluble. Upon this metallic silver exerts no action, nor would any action be exerted even at a boiling temperature. But, although insoluble in water, the compound is easily decomposed by various salines and other agents. Thus, hydrochlorate of ammonia and the alkaline chlorides redissolve the mercury in the form of bichloride. The same may be said of diluted hydrochloric acid, and of an excess of bichloride of mercury, or of albumen. In Dr. Frampton's experiment hydrochloric acid was added to the animal organic complication, by which the bichloride was brought into solution, and the silver thus enabled to act on the mercurial salt.

But although the process by silver, as detailed by Dr. Framptom, may answer for animal mixtures, I fear it will be found quite unsuited to vegetable mixtures. The reason probably is because bichloride of mercury is *reduced* by vegetable organic principles, so that hydrochloric acid will not act upon it, nor redissolve the mercury. Thus: "The solid compounds," says Christison, "formed by corrosive sublimate with animal principles, are either soluble in the hydrochloric acid, or part with all their mercury to it. The matter left does not yield a particle by reduction. But this is not the case with the compounds formed with vegetable principles. Diluted hydrochloric acid, boiled gently for two hours on the compound formed in tea, dissolves little of it, and leaves much undissolved powder, which yields, by destructive distillation, a large quantity of mercury[*]."

Hence it must be evident that Dr. Frampton's process could not by any means suit such a complication. Whatever bichloride may have combined with animal principles—those of the milk, for instance—after digestion in diluted hydrochloric acid, might yield a trace, perhaps, of mercury, but more frequently no indication whatever of the presence of mercury is afforded. It now remains to consider whether silver offers any advantages in researches upon mercury.

I triturated some tin-filings of extreme tenuity with one-eighth, and in a second operation with one-sixteenth of a grain of bichloride of mercury, in an agate mortar, and each operation presented characteristic evidence of complete reduction and amalgamation with the tin; viz. change of colour, and the viscid adhesive consistence of the mass. Collected and introduced into a narrow tube, and heated in a spirit-lamp, one or two very minute globules, hardly visible with the naked eye, but easily detached by means of a steel wire, and readily distinguished when thrown upon a small tray made of white paper, and a chloride of tin also, sublimed, when the flame of the lamp was urged with the blow-pipe. Upon removing all the metallic mercury, breaking up the tube, and digesting this and the residual sublimate in nitro-hydrochloric acid, analysis of this fluid gave no evidence of even a trace of mercury, which it must have done had not all the bichloride been completely reduced and the mercury removed. Hence, perhaps, it would be a legitimate inference that tin presents us in itself a reducing agent equal at least in power and effect to metallic silver. Tin, however, has this advantage over silver, that it is much less expensive, much more easily procured, and, to my view, much more manageable. It may be urged, that Dr. Frampton's mode of freeing from the newly-formed chloride of silver by washing with ammonia relieves from all embarrassment that might result from the presence of the new chloride. To this I reply, that I have not found

[*] On Poisons, p. 285, 1st edit.

the chloride of tin formed by the reaction at all to embarrass the subsequent reduction. But there are two modes of obviating any inconvenience resulting from this cause. It may be removed by washing with water, or with a caustic alkali, which dissolves the salt; or all the tin and saline may be removed, and the mercury alone left, by dissolving in hydrochloric acid, but feebly diluted with water. And perhaps the latter is the preferable plan when the quantities used are minute, as we then have left metallic mercury perfectly pure, and free from every kind of contamination. For myself, I feel satisfied that the above is equally as delicate, and certainly as manageable, as the process by finely-divided silver. It may be observed, on the question of delicacy, that the proto-salts of tin decompose the salts of silver, and reduce them to the metallic state.

The next question is, the applicability to the mercurial salt in solution. I have been long aware that tin introduced into a solution of bichloride of mercury causes a precipitation of metallic mercury upon its own surface, and there is consequently an amalgamation. It constitutes the fundamental principle of the process recommended by Devergie. He recommends us to treat the mixture supposed to contain mercury with diluted hydrochloric acid till all the solid matter is dissolved. Next evaporate, to expel the greater part of the acid employed. Add water to the remainder, and transmit *chlorine* to coagulate and remove the animal matter.[*] Filter, boil, and concentrate. Then immerse for ten minutes a small plate of pure tin, which, if mercury is present, will immediately be whitened (*tarnished?*); immerse another plate of tin for ten minutes; and continue this part of the process till the plates cease to be whitened. Dry the tarnished

[*] The transmission of chlorine, although as proposed for a mere secondary purpose by Devergie, is the most important part of the whole process. The digestion in hydrochloric acid is quite unnecessary and superfluous, for if it, the mercury, be in any degree reduced, the acid will not affect it; but the chlorine will immediately form a soluble bichloride, which will be held in solution by an excess of chlorine, and the action of any organic reducing agents suspended or counteracted, and the reducing agency of the tin secured and rendered more effectual. A current of chlorine gas passed through a fluid holding an insoluble compound of mercury in suspension, converts it into a soluble bichloride.

plates, scrape off the tarnished surfaces, put the scrapings in a proper tube, and heat over a spirit lamp: the mercury will be driven off from the amalgam, and condense in a ring of globules. Such is Devergie's process.

I have myself frequently used fine grain tin instead of tin plates, and I think the tin in this state preferable, as being more certain. First, by agitation, the grain tin is made to act upon every particle of the fluid, so that no atom of the dissolved salt can so easily escape the reducing agency of the metal. Again, the action is rendered more certain and complete if the solution of bichloride contain a tolerable excess of hydrochloric acid. The acid in proportion to its concentration attacks the tin; protochloride of tin is formed, and which instantly reacting precipitates metallic mercury. Now, all the mercury precipitated by any generated protochloride of tin, no matter whence its origin, subsides and is found principally at the bottom of the vessel holding the solution. This of course is lost in the case of the tin plates, which become tarnished by that mercury only reduced in immediate contact with their own surfaces. Now in the case of tin finely powdered, it falls to the bottom, and immediately amalgamates with any free mercury, and with which too it must of necessity come in contact. But even, should this not be the case, the mercury cannot be lost, because whatever subsides is to be collected, and either heated immediately in a tube, or be first treated as previously suggested, and then heated in a proper tube. Hence, then, it is evident that tin is a more delicate and effectual reagent than silver for mercury in solution, inasmuch as acidulating with hydrochloric acid, and boiling, greatly facilitates the action of tin, but exerts no such effect with respect to silver.

In organic complication, if the mercury be rendered insoluble by vegetable matter, silver cannot possibly act unless the mercurial salt be redissolved, and hydrochloric acid alone cannot effect this. But hydrochloric acid may enable tin to attack and reduce even the *vegeto*-organic compounds of mercury; for proto-chloride of tin will reduce even these, and if the solutions be strongly acid and boiled upon the tin, a proto-chloride of the metal will·be formed. The preferable plan, however, in organic com-

plications, will be to insure the solution of the mercury. This is to be effected either by passing a current of chlorine gas through the suspected solution, filtering, and then washing through with diluted hydrochloric acid; or by adding to the suspected matters a mixture of nitric and hydrochloric acids in the proportions to evolve chlorine, filtering and washing through as above. By these means the mercury will be brought again into solution, which will, to a great extent, be freed, by either of the above processes, from organic impurities both vegetable and animal. This, therefore, brings the matter almost to the condition of simple solution; and the grand point at issue is the preferable reducing agent. First, it is necessary to premise that the conditions of solution must be the same throughout, as to concentration, foreign principles, subsequent manipulation, &c. The mercury may be precipitated in the metallic form by the following: finely divided silver; grain tin, or, what is preferable, tin filings, under similar conditions of tenuity; solution of protochloride of tin; phosphorous and hypo-phosphorous acids. In the two first cases, although the mercury is reduced to the metallic state, yet amalgams subsequently form with the respective metals. In the case of the silver amalgam it must be distilled to evolve the mercury; in the case of the tin amalgam mercury may be distilled off; or the tin may be separated by hydrochloric acid, and the mercury thus set free left behind.

The next three reagents are in solution; and each precipitates metallic mercury perfectly pure and unalloyed, although it may be mechanically intermixed with certain impurities, which merely prevent the mercurial particles from coalescing into globules recognizable to ordinary vision. From these impurities, however, it is easily freed by well-known methods. Then the question now is, which are the most delicate and effectual reagents, the solid metals or the liquid tests? When bodies are dissolved in a fluid, the body or solvend appears to be uniformly diffused throughout the solvent; for every the most minute particle of the latter will afford traces more or less characteristic of the former; consequently the liquid reagents seem to act under circumstances of great advantage, at least as relates to delicacy, extent, and minuteness of division; and experiment proves what reason naturally infers. Nothing, in fact, can equal in delicacy and effect protochloride of tin in solution, and the acids above named; and I am satisfied no one who will take the trouble of comparative experiments, but will give the preference to the three reagents last mentioned.

It may here be made a question as to the bichloride of mercury in the solid state, or the proto-chloride (calomel), which is incapable of solution. But this and many other compounds of mercury, though insoluble in themselves, are readily and immediately converted into bichloride by passing chlorine gas through water holding them in mechanical suspension, or boiling with nitro-hydrochloric acid. Further, dry bichloride, proto-chloride, and many of the other solid compounds of mercury, are immediately reduced by merely pouring upon them solution of proto-chloride of tin, or the phosphorous or hypo-phosphorous acids; and perhaps this plan is the preferable.

Dr. Frampton contrasts the reduction by metallic silver with that by the alkalies. The alkalies present, in every way, the most inconvenient and unmanageable processes in the dry way. It requires some tact, and a great deal of management, to prevent the sublimation of the mercurial salt undecomposed. In other cases a mixture of undecomposed bichloride and red oxide sublimes, and not a particle of metallic mercury. I have frequently verified this by treating the mixture with water holding hydrochlorate of ammonia in solution, that part of the bichloride which had escaped decomposition; and by treating the residue with diluted hydrochloric acid, the red oxide were dissolved and mercury identified. Therefore finely divided silver or tin presents the best, the most effectual, and the most manageable reagents for the reduction of the chlorides in the dry way, and will be preferred by the practised and experienced operator. Of the two metals, tin, if it have no superiority, yet from the readiness with which it can be adapted for use, and the greater facility of obtaining it, will, in all probability, be selected in most instances.

I have now considered, at considerable length, the questions proposed by Dr. Frampton in his paper published in the GAZETTE. I give Dr. Frampton due credit for the ingenuity displayed in his process; and had it not been for the importance of the subject, but more especially his own invitation to inquiry, I should hardly have entered at such length upon the matter. I trust that what is here advanced will be regarded as emanating from a true desire to promote science, and that the remarks upon Dr. Frampton's proposal, and the methods contrasted with it, should they be thought worthy a place in the GAZETTE, will be found couched in the true spirit of philosophical inquiry and truth; and far from emulating or striving after either mastery or triumph.

London, July 9, 1843.

MEDICAL GAZETTE.

Friday, August 4, 1843.

"Licet omnibus, licet etiam mihi, dignitatem Artis Medicæ tueri; potestas modo veniendi in publicum sit, dicendi periculum non recuso."
CICERO.

PRIVATE TUITION.

It is well remarked by the late Dr. Arnold, in his Lectures on Modern History, that the struggles of a nation or of a party for constitutional privileges, however laudable has been the object or admirable the mode of its pursuit, do not confer lustre on victory, if the success obtained be not used in furthering the nation's real welfare. The proper object of war is peace; of liberty, the power to act rightly; and few things are more lamentable than to see advantages which have been gained at the cost of much suffering, either wasted by being turned to no account at all, or perverted to mean and unworthy purposes. Yet nothing is more common; it would seem, indeed, to be one natural consequence of a prolonged struggle, that the energies and the virtues which are required to reap the fruits of victory have been exhausted in the contest, and have been succeeded by lamentable indolence, or yet more deplorable abuses. Nor is this proof of the weakness of human nature to be drawn only from public history and from national contests. The lives of private individuals supply ample data for a similar inference. The industrious pursuit of wealth is often followed by avarice or luxury; of power, by tyranny or arrogance: nay, more—

"Insani sapiens nomen ferat, æquus iniqui,
Ultra quam satis est, virtutem si petat ipsam."

"For virtue's self may too much zeal be had,
The worst of madmen is a saint run mad."

Cases in the wards of Bethlem or St. Luke's are but aggravated specimens of a pathology which may be abundantly studied in private life; nay perhaps each of us may detect a few symptoms in his own person.

The waste of powers in acquiring means without judiciously directing them to an end, is seldom seen more remarkably, and never more lamentably, than in education. To put out of the question those rarer instances of excessive zeal, where youths spend prematurely in the acquisition of science the health and strength which should have supported them through a life of practical usefulness, we shall meet with too many cases where the powers which with the most careful adjustment would barely have sufficed for the purposes of their possessor, have, by early mismanagement, been made useless or detrimental.

The acute writer on history, whose opinion is alluded to above, draws a beautiful and just distinction between the duty of the professor and the educator. The teacher of a special science or branch of education is bound to instruct his pupil to the utmost of his power in the particular branch which he professes. This is to be not merely his prominent object, but his only one; and in proportion as he does this he discharges his duty. The educator, on the contrary, has to consider the general scope of his pupil's instruction, and especially the duties which he will have to perform in after-life; and with this object in view he has to consider the capacity and powers of his pupil, the nature of his studies, and the degree and mode in which each may be most beneficially pursued.

The author's application of this to the parental duties of the state is not to our present purpose; but the whole work, of which the most evident fault is its brevity, will richly repay an attentive perusal. Our profession is one which has a great influence on the well-being of society; we do not quite agree with those who desire for its members a large share in the national councils, or in the honours and rewards which attend public services, for we believe that our daily private ministrations to the comfort of individuals, though more humble, are more useful; and, moreover, that a frequent competition for public office and public honours would detract from our specific value as professional men; yet as we would have each man in his own circle bring the weight of his personal influence to bear as largely as possible on the public good, so we think it highly important that the general views of each one of us, the tone of feeling and of action, should receive all possible help towards their justness, their elevation, and their purity; and to this end a philosophical study of history will very much conduce.

One of the inconveniences under which a pupil labours on commencing his studies, is that each course of lectures contains much information which, in the present state of his knowledge, he is either quite unable to understand, or which, at least, he cannot apply, and which he can only retain by a mere effort of memory. This is an unavoidable consequence of each course being complete in itself. The lecturer is addressing two classes at once—the totally uninformed, and those who have already become familiar with much of what he is telling them; to the former, therefore, much must be unintelligible, to the latter much must be wearisome, and, notwithstanding all the skill that may be exerted to give colour and relief to the most important and prominent features, and to point out to each class what parts require the most marked attention, the general effect of a long course of lectures is almost invariably to tire out the patience of many : and though no doubt the emptiness of the benches is mainly due to the mere seductions of indolence or pleasure, yet the smallest show of reason for absence adds incalculably to the force of temptation, and too often not only confirms the unprincipled, who would have done wrong just as much without it, but overcomes the last scruple of the wavering.

Yet the duty of the professor is to make his course complete, and, during the process of composition, his own mind is stimulated, and his labours are made tolerable, by the agreeable task of eliminating first principles from the stores of his knowledge, and arranging them in order and clearness for the *tabula rasa* of the young and uninstructed mind; he is then carried into the more abstruse and intricate parts of his subject, discussing the most difficult and disputed points, stating the various questions with clearness, and summing up the arguments with all the acuteness of which he is master.

But when the lectures, which had satisfied him during their composition, and received attention during their first delivery, come to be repeated, the professor feels internally conscious that one-half of his audience must be aware of what he is about to say—that the premises he is so carefully stating have already suggested the conclusions—that his most brilliant and startling propositions will be received with coolness, and his very jokes either heard with gravity or laughed at by anticipation. This is an alarming prospect for a man of taste and earnestness; and by and by the absence of his more advanced pupils convinces him that his fears were not unfounded. He retouches his work, and endeavours to revive the flagging interest of the seniors, by discussing points of clinical importance; but he now finds his young pupils, the freshmen of his class, looking puzzled, and he sees that for them he is going too far or too fast.

Every one knows how children are apt to loathe the food of grown-up people when minced and mashed into an unmeaning pulp by over-careful nurses, and how it disagrees with them when they are persuaded to swallow it; no less is the disgust and weariness with which the young receive history when unskilfully reduced to stories. Sir Walter Scott found he had told the first series of Tales of a Grandfather too childishly, and improved his style afterwards. The professor who tries to teach in the reading-made-easy style will find, in like manner, that his fare offends the robust, and overloads the weak intellect. It is surely better for students that a man of powerful mind should fling down the hardest propositions, to be worked out by the diligence and ingenuity of his class, than that every thing should be reduced to the very easiest terms. The great practical objection is, that some are apt, after a short struggle with their difficulties, to be left behind, and to acquire the very dangerous habit of imagining that their deficiency will be supplied when the course is repeated. Many have thus consoled themselves season after season, till, when the time comes for examination, the grinder appears the only person who can set matters to rights. The remedy for much of this evil seems to fall within the legitimate province of the tutor, and to consist in carefully superintending the progress of each pupil, showing him what is elementary and fundamental — what he really must master at the time, and what may safely be left to a future course.

The weekly examinations do much towards raising the average information of a class, but require intelligence, diligence, and confidence; and as it is yet nearly optional with the student to attend them or not, they are soon deserted by the very class who most need them—the slow, the indolent, and the diffident. The directions of public bodies, as to the order in which lectures are to be attended, are meant to ensure a systematic and gradual mode of instruction, and certainly the intention is good, but many parts even of the earlier subjects must, if the professor desire to make his course complete, be evidently beyond the unassisted comprehension of his younger pupils. Materia medica and therapeutics, for example, what a wide range does this present; from the commonest acquaintance with the mere physical properties of a drug, to the most subtle application of remedies amidst the complications of disease, the last and always unfinished labour of the most accomplished veteran.

Another difficulty in the student's way, justly alluded to by Dr. Arnold, is the duty no less than the inclination of each professor to insist on the prominent importance of his own special science; the duties of the educator being rather to assign to each its own place and value. The only educators in this sense of the word for medical students, are the licensing

bodies, and the only instruction which they afford is that conveyed in the list of subjects for examination—a concise piece of information, and as puzzling as attempts at condensation generally are, " brevis esse laboro, obscurus fio."

It would be unjust to our ablest professors to forget the admirable advice contained in their introductory lectures: many of these might be quoted as sound and unexceptionable suggestions for the complete education of the student, and useful to him in every relation of professional or private life; but these lectures are heard but once in each course, or, if the maxims they contain are occasionally repeated, they are insufficient to restrain the refractory or to stimulate the indolent; we are inclined, therefore, to believe that there is a difference between the public duties of the professor and the private functions of the educator, which will be beneficially recognised when tuition on something like a collegiate system shall have been more extensively adopted.

FELLOWES' CLINICAL PRIZE REPORTS.

By ALFRED J. TAPSON.
University College Hospital, 1842.

[Continued from p. 620.]

CASE XIV.—*Delirium tremens, complicated with, and somewhat masked by pneumonia; and when both these had been cured by the use of opium, calomel, tartar emetic, and leeches, an attack of hepatitis came on, which was successfully treated by cupping, blue pill, and taraxacum.*

ARTHUR C., æt. 24, admitted May 24th, 1842, under Dr. A. T. Thomson: a tall thin man, of nervous temperament; pale complexion and light hair; unmarried: a tailor by trade. His habits have been very irregular for several years, always drinking freely, and frequently getting drunk; parents both living, and both healthy, also seven brothers and sisters, all pretty healthy. Previous health always delicate; but he has

never been laid up with any illness, excepting scarlatina.

The circumstances under which the present
attack came on were as follows (they were
chiefly learnt from his sister, who came with
him). On the 16th and 17th inst. he got
very drunk indeed; since then he has
scarcely drank anything. Nothing was observed amiss till the evening of the 20th,
when he appeared very irritable, and says
that he felt very stupid and heavy: on the
21st he was attacked with pain in the head,
back, chest, and limbs; shivering; shortness of breathing; great thirst; great depression and weakness: on the 22d his
manner was remarked to be very strange;
he kept pointing about the room with his
finger; could not sleep at all from the time
he was first taken ill; the breathing continued quick; the skin became very hot; he
complained of severe pain in the right side
and at the epigastrium, and had a slight
cough.

On his admission on the evening of the
24th, the chief symptoms were the heat of
skin, frequent respiration, the above pain,
tenderness on pressure in the same parts,
thirst, depression, &c.; there was a rough
sound, resembling friction sound, heard
below the right scapula, but no dulness on
percussion.

He was ordered — Hirud. No. viij.;
Epigastrio admov.

℞ Calomel gr. v. statim sumend.
℞ Haust. Niger. cras mane.

℞. Liq. Ammon. Acet. fȝss.; Sodæ Tart.
gr. xv.; Sodæ Carb. gr. v. Mist.
Camph. fȝj. M. f. haust. 8vâ qq.
horâ sum.

May 25th.—Has passed a very restless
night; crying and frequently attempting to
get out of bed. His countenance is very
irritable and suspicious; his manner very
uneasy, hands and fingers in almost incessant motion, picking about the bed-clothes,
&c.: on the least noise he starts suddenly
round and looks frightened; talks a great
deal in a low tone, and incoherently: he is
quite sensible when spoken to, but answers
questions rationally, but his memory is so
deficient that he frequently contradicts himself. The head feels very hot; the eyes and
nose are red, and have been running; the
lips are of a bright vermilion colour and
dry; the tongue very red along the margin
and at the apex; not dry, but covered with a
yellowish slimy fur. The surface of the body is
hot and dry; he would not allow the thermometer to be placed in the axilla (suspecting,
he told me afterwards, that we were going to
cut him); but in the bend of the elbow the
temperature was upwards of 100° Fah.;
the respirations 54 in a minute, and shallow;

pulse 148, soft, and moderately full; has a
slight cough, but no expectoration; there is
still pain and tenderness in the epigastrium,
and also on the right side of the chest, midway between the sternum and lateral median
line. Bowels have been opened twice in the
night. In the course of the forenoon he became quite outrageous, and had a straight
waistcoat applied for a short time.

℞ Calomel, gr. ij.; Pulv. Opii. gr. j.;
Antim. Tart. gr. ¼.; Mucilag. q. s. f.
pil. 6tâ qq. horâ sumendâ. Pergat
haust. Lotio refrigerans capito raso
ope lintei applicanda.

26th.—Has slept a little during the night
for the first time since the attack; and has
been much more quiet, though still restless
and fidgetty, and constantly talking in a
low unintelligible manner. The countenance
much improved, the suffusion of the eyes,
nose, &c. much diminished; tongue has a
more slimy appearance and a brownish tinge;
pupils rather contracted; the respirations 36
in a minute; pulse 120, soft; no tenderness
at the epigastrium now; bowels not opened
since yesterday morning, and has passed no
urine for the same time. (The catheter was
introduced in the afternoon, and several
ounces of high-coloured urine drawn off.)

℞ Calomel, gr. v.; Ol. Crotonis, ♏ j.;
Mic. Panis, q. s. f. pil. statim sum.

℞ Haust. purgans horâ post pilulam, si
opus sit, sumendus. Cont. pil. ex
Opio, etc.

27th.—Has passed a much better night,
having slept a good deal, and been generally
very still and quiet; appears quite sensible,
answers questions readily and much more
distinctly; face pale, and and has a heavy
expression; the lips and tongue are very dry;
the latter is so dry that it can scarcely be
protruded beyond the teeth; the temperature
in the axilla is 103° Fahr.; but the head is
now cool and comfortable. Respirations 32
in a minute; pulse 112, weak and variable;
heart's action feeble, and rather irregular;
he complains of the pain in the right side:
on examining the chest posteriorly the
sound on percussion was found to be dull in
the lower two-thirds on the right, with
crepitation distinct in the same situation; in
the upper third the respiration was loud.
Anteriorly in the situation of the pain there
was muco-crepitant and some sonorous
rhonchus. Bowels have been freely opened;
evacuations dark and offensive; urine increased in quantity.

Adde Singul. pilul. Antim. Tart. gr. ¾;
Pergat haustus salin.

28th.—Continues to improve; the pain
in the side is less; breathing slower; pulse
96, fuller and softer; tongue moist; gums

slightly tumid and red ; thirst less ; crepitation distinct in the same situation as before ; bowels open ; urine plentiful, high-coloured, but clear.

Sumat. pilulum 8vâ. qq. horâ. Beef-tea a pint daily.

31st.—Countenance is now quite natural ; head clear ; no confusion of ideas ; the memory is improved ; tongue moist, and much cleaner ; no thirst ; appetite returning ; the respiration natural in frequency ; pulse 78, and rather weak ; pain in the side not constant, felt chiefly when he coughs ; the cough is frequent and troublesome, and accompanied with scarcely any expectoration ; excretions free.

Omitt. pil. Pergat. Haust. Milk diet, and chop every other day, instead of beef-tea.

June 1st.—Complains more of the pain in the lower part of the right side of the chest ; there is some dulness on percussion, with bronchial respiration and bronchophony here ; and posteriorly the crepitation is still heard at the end of a forcible inspiration, but not in ordinary respiration.

2d.—Omittantur medicamenta.

4th.—The pain in the side is less ; the cough better ; no expectoration ; the head is quite clear ; has had no return of the delirium ; he feels very weak ; the tongue is clean and natural ; pulse 100, soft, and easily compressed ; appetite good ; bowels regular ; urine abundant and natural.

℞ Infusi Cascarillæ, ʒiss. ; Acidi Sulph. Dil. ℳviii. ; M. f. haust. bis quotidie sumendus. Full diet.

7th.—Has not been so well since he has had the last medicine ; has had headache and more pain in the side ; and has been shivering several times ; the skin now feels very hot (it is 104° Fah. in the axilla) ; pulse quick, and he complains of some palpitation of the heart ; is thirsty, and has no appetite for food. The physical signs are much diminished in the back ; the dulness is almost gone, and no distinct crepitation, either coarse or fine.

Omitt. haust. Admov. Hirudines No. x. parti thoracis dolenti. Low diet.

8th.—Pain much relieved by the leeches ; skin moist and cooler (100° Fah. in the axilla).

11th.—Pain is only felt when he takes a deep breath ; it is now quite at the margins of the ribs and rather below ; there is some tenderness on pressure here, and extending to the epigastrium ; the dulness of the liver extends about an inch and a half below the margins of the ribs ; the skin is still too hot, but is moist ; he feels very weak, and

cannot sleep well at night ; cough nearly ceased ; appetite returning again ; bowels regular ; urine natural.

℞ Solut. Morphiæ Bimeconatis ℳxviii. ; Mist. Camph. ʒiss. ft. haust. omni nocte sumendus. Chop daily, and half a pint of porter.

14th.—Has slept much better ; feels stronger and better altogether ; has less pain ; no cough ; tongue moderately clean ; appetite good ; bowels rather confined, and stools dark coloured.

℞ Olei Ricini, ʒss. ; Aq. Menth. Pip. ʒj. ; Tinct. Camph. C. ʒj. Ft. haust qq. h. sumend.

16th.—Sleeps well and dreams but little ; whereas when he came in, if he dosed at all, he had the most horrible dreams, seeing devils, &c. ; the pain is not quite gone, and he says he feels as if he had a weight on his stomach when he lies on his back ; is much stronger than he was a week since.

To be discharged : cured of delirium tremens, and pneumonia.

July 2d.—The patient was readmitted into the hospital to-day ; he states that during the time he has been out from the hospital he has had constant pain in the right side, in the same situation as it was just before he was discharged, viz. about an inch below the margins of the ribs, and it has extended backwards almost to the spine ; latterly the pain has been a good deal more severe, it is increased by external pressure, also by coughing, &c. ; he has also had pain occasionally at the lower angle of the left scapula : he says, moreover, that he used, about three years ago, to suffer a good deal from pain here, and whenever he got drunk it made him very ill, and caused a severe pain in the right side ; whilst he has been out, he has (he says) been very careful as to his diet, and only drank from half a pint to a pint of porter daily, never more ; his appetite has been good, but he has vomited occasionally after breakfast, and always brought up a good deal of bile ; he has taken a good deal of exercise ; the cough is very trifling ; he looks heavy.

Applic. Cucurb. cruent. lateri dextro ad ʒxvj.

℞ Pil. Hydr. Ext. Hyos. aa. gr. ij. ; Ext. Tarax. gr. v. M.f. pil. ij. Sumatur una 8va. qq. horâ. Middle diet.

5th.—Feels much better ; the pain is much less severe ; sleeps well ; the tongue much cleaner ; bowels open ; urine free, natural.

Applic. Emplast. Canth. amplum lateri dextro ; pergat in usu pilul.

℞ Decoct. Tarax. ʒiss.; Acidi Nitrici Diluti, ℳx.; Acidi Hydrochlorici, ℳv. M. f. haust. ter die sumendus.

6th.—The blister has risen well, and discharged freely; the pain is nearly gone; it is not increased by a deep inspiration.

7th.—Pain is only felt when he takes a deep inspiration; he feels quite well; pulse natural; tongue clean; gums not tender or swollen; the appetite good; bowels regular. Discharged cured.

REMARKS.—The *diagnosis* in this case was difficult at first, and could scarcely be formed with certainty without a knowledge of the previous history and habits of the patient. Judging merely from the condition that he was in, most would have pronounced it a case of typhus fever, with some inflammatory affection of the chest; but when the previous habits of the patient, with the circumstances under which the attack came on, and the mode of attack, were taken in connection with the existing symptoms and signs, Dr. Thomson at once pronounced it to be a case of delirium tremens, complicated with inflammation of the chest; and the further progress of the case, and the result of the treatment adopted in accordance with this diagnosis, quite confirmed it.

First, in looking at his *previous history* we find he had always been delicate; that he was in the habit of getting drunk; and that on the 16th and 17th of May he got exceedingly drunk, after which he scarcely drank any thing till the attack commenced, viz. on the 20th of May. Now these are precisely the circumstances under which delirium tremens most frequently comes on, viz. a sudden and great diminution of the quantity immediately after drinking an unusual amount.

Second, as to the *mode of attack*. It commenced with a state of great irritability, and a feeling of depression; constant watchfulness, or if he dosed at all he speedily awoke in consequence of some frightful dream; giddiness; a strangeness of manner; pointing about the room, and a very suspicious look; loss of appetite; and the rest of the symptoms before detailed.

Third, the *symptoms which existed on his admission* may be divided into those referrible to the delirium tremens, and those referrible to the pneumonia.

(a). *Those referrible to the delirium tremens* were—the irritable, uneasy, and suspicious appearance of the countenance; the idea that some one was going to injure him; the continual tremulous motion of the hands and fingers; restlessness and inability to sleep; the sudden starting on the least noise; the constant incoherent talking; and with these may probably also be classed, the heat of the head; the slightly contracted state

of the pupil; the suffusion of the eyes; the furred and slimy state of the tongue, &c. We refer the heat of the head, &c. to this class, because they subsided with the delirium and tremor, although the pneumonia was then increasing; and also because, as this was the patient's first attack, and he was young, the delirium tremens would be very likely to produce these phrenitic symptoms, though it was clear, from the softness of the pulse, the tolerance of light, from his answering questions, and the character of the delirium, that there was but little, if any actual phrenitis.

(b). *The symptoms referrible to the pneumonia* were—great heat and dryness of the skin, quick pulse, and exceedingly rapid respiration (the last symptom was probably increased by the state of the nervous system, as it is very rare indeed to see 54 respirations in a minute from pneumonia in an adult); great thirst; pain and tenderness of the right side of the chest, increased by a deep breath or by coughing; a slight cough; a rough respiratory murmur, &c. These do not indicate the existence of pneumonia; indeed that could not be ascertained till subsequently, when the occurrence of fine crepitation, dulness on percussion, &c. were quite conclusive on this point; also the character of the pain, and its situation (*vide* reports), indicated the same thing. The general symptoms of pneumonia were much less marked than usual; the cough was never severe, and there was scarcely any expectoration throughout the disease; also, the physical signs, though distinctive, were not nearly so clear as they often are. In addition to the pneumonia there seemed to be some gastric complication, from the extreme redness of the lips and of the margin of the tongue, the yellow fur along its centre, the great thirst, and the pain and tenderness on pressure in the epigastric region. These all soon went away, and were apparently intimately connected with the delirium tremens or with its cause.

Fourth, considering the *progress of the case* in connection with the *treatment*, we see that it quite confirmed the diagnosis which had been made and acted on. It was evident that a combination of remedies was requisite in order to combat the combination of diseases. Opium was ordered for the delirium tremens; and leeches, mercury, and antimonial salines, for the gastric affection and inflammation of the lungs. The effect of these remedies was the speedy subsidence of all the symptoms referrible to the nervous system and stomach; and then, as the pneumonia had decidedly manifested itself, the quantity of antimony was increased, and the calomel continued, until the gums were slightly affected; and under this treatment the symptoms gradually diminished, and on the 4th of June, as weakness was the most prominent symptom, he was ordered a tonic draught and increased amount of food. It appeared, however, that it was rather too early; at all events he had a return of feverishness and pain, and the physical signs showed that the inflammation was not altogether removed. This slight return was, however, soon removed by the application of a few leeches, and the substitution of low diet for a few days, and after about the 10th June there were no symptoms referrible to the lungs.

But about this time a new disease began to manifest itself, marked by pain in the right side below the margins of the ribs, tenderness on pressure in this situation, pain in the shoulder-blade, and on percussion the liver was found to descend lower than natural. These symptoms indicated the existence of hepatitis; but without any treatment being specially adapted to this he improved, and was discharged cured of the delirium tremens and pneumonia.

Soon after he left the hospital the pain in the side became more severe, and in a little more than a fortnight he was re-admitted, having the same symptoms as when he went out, only greatly increased in severity, and some new ones had appeared. The pain now extended from the side round to the back; the liver descended fully an inch and a half below the margins of the ribs; he had bilious vomiting, &c.; abundantly proving the existence of a sub-acute form of hepatitis.

The treatment adopted consisted of local depletion by cupping, followed by the application of a blister, with blue pill to act on the liver, and also the extract and decoction of taraxacum, which is a remedy strongly recommended by Dr. Pemberton in chronic hepatitis and incipient cirrhosis, and therefore, we conceive, peculiarly adapted to this case. The nitro-hydrochloric acid was also given. Under these means he was soon well enough to be discharged again.

The *prognosis*, on his first admission, was not very favourable, although a first attack of delirium tremens rarely proves fatal; but there were here serious complications which considerably augmented the danger: the prognosis was much better, of course, when the disease was reduced to simply pneumonia, though this alone is enough to cause serious alarm, especially in such a subject. We have seen, however, that he recovered from this also, and was then attacked with hepatitis, which appeared to have gradually arisen on the subsidence of the pneumonia, as if the inflammation had passed through the diaphragm to the liver. Of this likewise he was cured; but the ulterior prognosis is certainly unfavourable, and we think the chances are that he will be very likely to have tubercles

formed in his lungs, cirrhosis in the liver, and not unlikely, also, granular degeneration of the kidneys, should he not be cut off by a recurrence of the delirium tremens.

The *cause* of the delirium tremens was obviously the sudden diminution in the quantity of spirit drank, after a great excess. His habits of drinking also probably gave rise, in a great measure, to the disease of the liver and stomach; and whether the pneumonia was to be traced to the same or not was doubtful. There was no evidence of his having been exposed to cold or wet, and we know that pneumonia is not at all an unfrequent complication of delirium tremens: thus, it is stated in the MEDICAL GAZETTE of May 13th, 1841, by Professor Budd, that "the organs most frequently inflamed, in this disease, are the stomach and the lungs."

MEDICAL REFORM.

To the Editor of the Medical Gazette.

SIR,

YOU were pleased, in April last, to publish a request of mine, that the gentlemen employed under the Poor Law Amendment Act, in charge of the sick poor, would be so good as to send to me such information as might enable me to draw up a paper, or digest, on the subject of the grievances they suffered and wished to have redressed; and I have to thank a great many for the readiness with which they complied with that request. The ninth annual report of the Poor Law Commissioners, laid before Parliament in May last, having stated that the duties of the Union surgeons were much diminished in the North of England, in consequence of the various dispensaries, &c. which gave relief to the sick poor, and from medical men being employed to take charge of poor persons engaged in collieries, factories, &c., it became necessary to write to the surgeons of 112 Unions on these points, which delayed the printing of my report, entitled "Facts and Observations relating to the Administration of Relief to the Sick Poor in England and Wales," until the 27th of June. This report was privately addressed to the Members of the Commons House of Parliament, and I had the honour of sending a copy to you.

The additional matter for inquiry which the Northern Counties furnished, rendered it necessary to refer to some Members of the House of Commons conversant with the affairs of collieries and factories; and Lord Ashley, who takes the greatest interest in the whole subject, finding from the state of public business that nothing could be done this session, gave notice, on Wednesday the 26th, that he should move early in the next session of Parliament "for a select com-the left groin the appearance of a wound made by a scalpel or some surgical instrument. The body generally exhibited the signs of great decomposition, more rapid than is generally the case, even allowing for the time of year and the period which had elapsed since death. The internal appearances presented on being opened— *in the cavity of the chest an effusion of fluid in both pleural cavities, congested state of the lungs at their posterior parts*, and some emphysema in the anterior or inferior portions. The heart was flabby, and its left ventricle dilated. I now proceeded to the examination of the abdominal cavity, and found the marks of slight peritonitis over the intestines. On proceeding to separate the stomach from its connections, I found very considerable adhesion between its smaller curvature and under surface of the liver. On breaking through those adhesions, I found a cavity containing grumous blood and portions of fibrine. The cavity extended a considerable way behind the stomach. On removing the stomach and slitting it open, I found about six ounces of coffee-ground fluid in its cavity. There was not the slightest appearance of inflammation or ulceration in the mucous membrane, which was unusually pale. The liver was a little enlarged, congested, and very much disorganized in its lower surface and inferior border. The gall-bladder was literally crammed with biliary calculi, large and small together about 200. The kidneys were extensively diseased, presenting an advanced stage of the malady designated 'Bright's disease.' There are no other morbid appearances. From the morbid appearances discovered, I conclude that the cause of death in the deceased was hæmatemesis and the inflammation of the peritoneum, the result of diseased state of the viscera. The entire absence of inflammation or ulceration in the lining membrane of the stomach, precludes the idea of any deleterious ingredient, mineral or vegetable, having been taken by the deceased. I did not analyse the contents of the deceased's stomach, for I considered it a work of supererogation."

Mr. Field states in his evidence that there was not the slightest appearance in the mucous membrane of inflammation or ulceration, which was more than usually pale; but what would have been the appearances in the stomach if the vessels had not emptied themselves by secretion during the last stages of life? Would not the retention of coffee-ground fluid within the vessels have presented all the signs of congestion, and conveyed to the mind of the toxicological pathologist unequivocal indications of an irritant poison acting either directly upon the mucous surface, or, what is more probable, indirectly through the medium of the nervous and circulating systems? Did not the icy coldness of the hands indicate that one portion of the spinal marrow had ceased to generate heat, although it still continued to animate the circulation in a feeble manner, for the pulse was scarcely perceptible? and was not this depression of the circulating powers extremely favorable to the processes of secretion, exhalation, and congestion, so strikingly exhibited in the post-mortem examination? Is the icy coldness of the hands a common symptom of disease, or the panting a usual symptom in diseases of the respiratory organs? I put these questions, for I confess I have not witnessed them myself. Can coffee-ground or black vomit be called hæmatemesis, when the essential characteristics of the latter disease are entirely absent, viz. coagula?

Notwithstanding the gall-bladder was stuffed with calculi, I never heard the deceased complain of suffering any inconvenience from them.

As to the wound made by the scalpel, through which the intestine was partially protruding, I shall leave it to the profession to decide for what purpose that was made. A servant swore that he saw a gallon of fluid drawn off; but the surgeon who is said to have tapped the body ought to have been examined upon that point. There was no collapse of the abdominal parietes.

It is not my intention to enter into any controversial discussion; suffice it to say, that I vouch for the accuracy with which all the pathological phenomena have been detailed.

P.S.—I entirely differ with Mr. Field as to the analysis of the contents of the stomach being a work of supererogation. When the slightest suspicion of poison exists, and such a large quantity of fluid is found in the stomach after death, it should undoubtedly be submitted to chemical analysis. But the proceedings at this inquest were not conducted in a very satisfactory manner.

OBSERVATIONS
UPON THE
NEW PROCESS PROPOSED FOR THE DETECTION OF CORROSIVE SUBLIMATE
BY MEANS OF
METALLIC SILVER.

By FORENSIS.

(For the London Medical Gazette.)

DR. FRAMPTON has proposed to use silver as a test for corrosive sublimate, upon the grounds that the affinity of silver for chlorine, and the great tendency of silver to amalgamate with mercury, offer, or at least promise, facilities for detection superior to other methods. Dr. Frampton, at the same time, very liberally and very properly submits his processes to investigation, and courts inquiry. Upon these terms I beg to offer the following for his especial consideration, as well as that of toxicologists in general. Dr. Frampton's first proposition is, that silver triturated with bichloride of mercury effects the reduction of the salt and the liberation of the mercury, which then forms an amalgam with the remaining silver. This is inferred from the change of colour. Upon this it may be observed, that two substances, exerting no chemical action whatever upon each other, by mere mechanical admixture, frequently modify, and sometimes even generate perfectly new and distinct colours. Again, it is a rule of chemical action that bodies do not act upon each other unless one at least be in solution, or contain water of crystallization. Although there are exceptions to this, yet I determined to place this matter beyond all doubt. For this purpose, bichloride of mercury having been rubbed on a plate of metallic silver till it was darkened, the plate was digested in a solution of ammonia. The fluid was now filtered, and the filtered portion boiled in a tube, when it became turbid. On the addition of nitric acid, a white curdy-looking precipitate fell down, insoluble in nitric acid, and which became dark on exposure to bright light. Ammonia again redissolved it, and, when reprecipitated by hydrochloric acid, a button of pure silver was obtained by reduction and cupellation. Therefore there can be no doubt that silver reduces bichloride of mercury by mere contact, and that a transfer of the chlorine to the silver takes place on mere triture.

Dr. Frampton's next experiment consisted in boiling a solution of bichloride of mercury with very finely and minutely divided silver, when the reduction of the mercurial salt, and the liberation of the metal, were equally the ultimate results. But the third case is the most important, in which bichloride of mercury is complicated with organic matter. Organic matter may be considered in the two-fold relations of animal and vegetable. As regards animal organic matter,—albumen for instance,—bichloride of mercury is rendered insoluble in water by it; that is, the albumen and bichloride of mercury enter into some sort of combination, which is insoluble. Upon this metallic silver exerts no action, nor would any action be exerted even at a boiling temperature. But, although insoluble in water, the compound is easily decomposed by various salines and other agents. Thus, hydrochlorate of ammonia and the alkaline chlorides redissolve the mercury in the form of bichloride. The same may be said of diluted hydrochloric acid, and of an excess of bichloride of mercury, or of albumen. In Dr. Frampton's experiment hydrochloric acid was added to the animal organic complication, by which the bichloride was brought into solution, and the silver thus enabled to act on the mercurial salt.

But although the process by silver, as detailed by Dr. Framptom, may answer for animal mixtures, I fear it will be found quite unsuited to vegetable mixtures. The reason probably is because bichloride of mercury is *reduced* by vegetable organic principles, so that hydrochloric acid will not act upon it, nor redissolve the mercury. Thus: "The solid compounds," says Christison, "formed by corrosive sublimate with animal principles, are either soluble in the hydrochloric acid, or part with all their mercury to it. The matter left does not yield a particle by reduction. But this is not the case with the compounds formed with vegetable.

portion which invests the body and cervix behind, and extends from thence with greater or less rapidity, according to the severity of the attack, to the general peritoneal membrane.   In some fatal cases the inflammation is in a great degree confined to the uterus, and it is generally most severe in this organ, or in the parts immediately contiguous.   Even when it has extended to the other viscera, and affected them most severely, the peritoneum of the uterus most frequently, if not invariably, exhibits signs of recent inflammation.   The lymph is for the most part poured out in thicker masses around the uterus than in any other situation ; and this viscus has seemed to suffer in the greatest degree from the violence of the inflammation.   Sometimes considerable deposits of pus are formed beneath the peritoneal coat of the uterus, which are either prominent and circumscribed, or diffused throughout the cellular membrane.   These are most frequently met with at the part where the peritoneum is reflected from the uterus and vagina to the rectum.

Inflammation of the peritoneal coat of the uterus is characterised by great tenderness of the surface of the organ, increased on pressure, and by pyrexia more or less severe. In every instance which has come under my observation, where the patient was seen soon after the invasion of the disease, on a careful examination of the uterine region there has been more or less pain in it, increased by pressure, with constitutional disturbance ; though it must be admitted that the pain and febrile symptoms have varied greatly in intensity.   When the attack of peritonitis is severe, the patient commonly lies upon the back, with the knees slightly drawn up to the abdomen.   At the onset of the disease the abdomen is generally soft and flaccid, and, except in the uterine region, not affected by pressure.   Though an enlarged and painful state of the uterus be never altogether wanting, yet the pain often undergoes exacerbations similar to after-pains, and is often mistaken for them by careless observers, and the disease is thus overlooked till a great part of the peritoneal sac is inflamed, and the case in consequence is rendered hopeless. The whole abdomen then becomes swollen and tympanitic, and the pain either wholly subsides, or becomes still more intense than at the commencement.   Vomiting of black or dark-green-coloured fluid follows, the pulse becomes extremely rapid and feeble, the tongue dry and brown, the lips and teeth are covered with dark sordes, and diarrhœa frequently supervenes, and death follows at no very remote period.   The invasion of pain in the uterus is sometimes sudden ; at other times the ordinary increased sensibility of the uterus, subsequent to the efforts of natural labour, or after-

pains, pass slowly into the acute pain, increased by pressure, which is the great characteristic symptom of uterine inflammation at the onset.   Most frequently the accession of the disease is marked by rigors, partial or general ; sometimes so slight as scarcely to be perceived by the patient, at other times so violent as to produce succussions of the whole body.   The cold shivering after a longer or shorter duration passes away, and is succeeded by great heat of the surface, acceleration of the pulse and of the respiration, thirst, sometimes nausea and vomiting, and intense pain across the forehead.   The rigors precede, accompany, or follow the increased sensibility of the uterus.   In some of the most severe cases there has been no distinct rigor ; but a quick pulse, hot skin, and hurried respiration, have rapidly succeeded to the uterine pain.   In some of the most unfavourable cases, the extremities have been cold, and the countenance anxious and pallid, after the disease has been completely formed.   There is no uniformity in the state of the tongue in puerperal peritonitis.   It is sometimes covered with a thin, moist, white, or cream-like film, at other times it is red in the centre, with a thick yellow, or white fur, on the edges.   The lochia are often completely suppressed, in other cases only diminished in quantity.   The mammæ usually become flaccid, yet in some fatal cases the milk has been secreted till a short period before death. Puerperal peritonitis may be confounded with the irregular contractions of the uterus which constitute after-pains and hysteralgia, and it must be admitted that in some cases it is difficult to draw a line of distinction between them.   Where the pulse is accelerated, the remission of pain incomplete, the lochia scanty or suppressed, the fundus uteri felt large and hard, and painful on pressure, or the whole hypogastric region unusually tender when touched, in a large proportion of cases you will arrive at a correct diagnosis by considering the peritoneal coat of the uterus, or its deeper-seated tissues, in a state of congestion or inflammation, and employing antiphlogistic treatment.   There are few puerperal women, except those of a feeble and irritable constitution, or who have been previously exhausted by hæmorrhage, or some chronic disease, who are seriously injured by cautious depletion, local or general ; and where death has followed the abstraction of sixteen or twenty ounces of blood from the arm the fatal result may fairly be attributed to the disease, and to the neglect of the remedy rather than its abuse.   This table, which was published in an imperfect form, without the description of the morbid appearances, ten years ago, furnishes the best proof you can have of the truth of this statement.

TABULAR VIEW (No. 1) OF 100 CASES OF SEVERE INFLAMMATION OF THE UTERUS AND ITS APPENDAGES,

Which occurred to me in London, from March 1827 to the end of December 1830.

No.	Name, Residence, and Delivery.	Date of Attack and Symptoms.	Treatment.	Result and Morbid Appearances.
1	Groom; æt. 28; 13, Little Coram Street, Russell Square. Natural labour. 6th March, 1827.	First day after delivery.— Pyrexia; uterine pain; lochia suppressed; diarrhœa; vomiting; tympanites. Died on the 10th.	Opiates and hot fomentations at the commencement. V.S. ʒxij. late in the disease, cathartics.	Died. Peritoneal sac extensively inflamed; uterine peritoneum behind coated with lymph; pus in the cellular tissue beneath; uterine appendages on both sides inflamed, and covered with lymph and pus; ʒiv. of a dark-coloured serum in the peritoneal sac; stomach and small intestines distended with gas.
2	Marshall; æt. 23; 3, Crown Street, Soho. Natural labour. 1st March, 1827.	Second day.—A violent rigor; headache; vertigo; uterine pain; tongue red and moist; lochia and milk suppressed; pulse 112, feeble; slight diarrhœa; vomiting; delirium; cessation of pain; enormous distension of abdomen. Died 16th March.	V.S. ʒxiv. third day after attack, leeches xxx., calomel, pulv. antim., cathartics, opiates.	Died. Extensive peritonitis; intestines glued together with lymph; uterus and its appendages imbedded in lymph and pus; ʒx. of sero-purulent effusion; uterine peritoneum red and vascular; ovaria softened and enlarged.
3	Mary Pascow; æt. 27. Natural labour; 7th child. 15th March, 1827.	Second day.—Severe rigor; acute pain in the back and region of the uterus, increased by pressure; diarrhœa; no sickness; tongue red and moist; pain in the back part of the head, and giddiness; pulse 120, not strong; respiration anxious; face flushed; tremors of the limbs.	V.S. ʒxvj, leeches xxx. calomel, antimony, cathartics.	Recovered.
4	Mary Sullivan; æt. 32; 16, Denmark Street, Soho Sq. In labour 52 hours. 25th March, 1827.	Third day. — Rigors; uterus large and painful; pulse 96, sharp; lochia suppressed. Duration of disease eight days.	V.S. ʒxv, leeches xj., calomel, gr. iv., pulv. antim. gr. v. 4ta q. q. h., cathartics.	

5	Wilson; æt. 42; 4, Pitt Place, Drury Lane.—Tedious lab. 2d April, 1827.	Eighth day.—Rigors; uterine pain; headache; lochia suppressed.	V.S. ℥xiv., calomel and cathartics.	Recovered.
6	Smith. Natural labour. 5th April, 1827.	First day.—Severe pain in right iliac region; slight pyrexia; rigors; pulse 104; pain aggravated and diffused over the whole uterine region. Symptoms relieved by V.S.	Fomentations, tinct. opii gtt.xl., a copious bleeding, saline cathartic, calomel, opium, a blister.	Recovered.
7	Williams; 34, Drury Lane. Natural labour. 4th April, 1827.	Sixth day.—Uterus enlarged, and painful on pressure; pyrexia; lochia suppressed.	V.S.	Recovered.
8	Sarah Oulton; 8, Houghton St. Clare Market. Arm presentation; turning. 9th April, 1827.	Third day.—Acute pain of the uterus, succeeded by great tenderness of the whole abdomen; pulse 110; great heat of skin; lochia suppressed; vomiting; tympanitca.	Stimulants and opiates at the invasion, copious bleeding and digitalis late.	Died.
9	Leeder; æt. 28; 24, Brownlow Street, Long Acre. Natural labour. 13th April, 1827.	Fifth day.—Severe rigor; headache; pain of back, loins, and lower part of abdomen, increased by pressure; pain afterwards in the left iliac fossa and along the course of left iliac and femoral vein, and slight swelling of left inferior extremity.	V.S. ℔. ij, leeches xx., calomel, antimony, cathartics.	Recovered.
10	Hamm; æt. 25; 2, St. Ann's Place, Soho.—Nat. labour. 20th April, 1827.	Third day.—Intense headache; no rigor; uterine pain increased by pressure; pulse frequent; tongue white; mammæ flaccid.	V.S. ℔. iss., calomel, antimony, diaphoretics, and cathartics.	Recovered.
11	Richards; 20, Stacey Street. Arm presentation; turning. 2d May, 1827.	First day.—Rigors; intense uterine pain and headache; lochia suppressed; pyrexia.	V.S. ℥xxiv., leeches, calomel, opium, cathartics.	Recovered.
12	Hunn; æt. 28; Crown Street, Soho.—Natural labour. 1st May, 1827.	Sixth day.—Severe uterine and abdominal pain; pulse 120, feeble; lochia suppressed; milk secreted.	V.S. ℥xx., leeches xxx., cathartics, and opiates.	Recovered.
13	Carr; æt. 30; Tash Court, Gray's-Inn Lane.—Nat. lab. 12th May, 1827.	Third day.—After drinking porter, rigors; uterus large and painful; pulse frequent, and soft; tongue white and moist; countenance pale and anxious.	V.S. ℔. ij, calomel, and cathartics.	Recovered.
14	Maunsey; æt. 25; 6, Charles St. Drury Lane.—Nat. lab. 27th May, 1827.	Second day.—Uterine pain; nausea and headache; lochia diminished; pulse 80; heat of skin little increased.	V.S. ℥xij, fomentations.	Recovered.
15	Eliza Corey; æt. 16; 50, King Street, Soho.—Natural lab. 17th June, 1827.	Third day.—Pyrexia; exquisite uterine pain, with great depression of strength; pulse 140.	V.S. ℥xiv, leeches, xviij, calomel, and cathartics.	Recovered.

16	Groundswell; Ham Yard, Great Windmill Street. 10th July, 1827. Puerperal convulsions. 13th August, 1827. Natural labour.	Third day.—Rigors; uterine pain and headache; lochia suppressed.	V.S. xviij., leeches xij., calomel, antimony, cathartics.	Recovered.
17	Shepherd; æt. 33; 39, St. Martin's Street.	Fifth day.—Rigors; violent pain of uterus; rapid pulse; tongue loaded; followed by severe pains and swelling of left leg.	V.S. twice ʒxxiv., leeches, xxiv.	Recovered.
18	Barton.—Natural labour. 2d September, 1827.	— Acute pain in the region of the uterus; rigors; pyrexia.	V.S. ʒxv.	Resed.
19	Costello; æt. 23; 15, Church Court, St. Martin's. 13th September, 1827.	Fourth day.—Slight uterine pain; rigors; rapid feeble plse; tongue brown; vomiting; tympanites; delirium.	V.S. not employed; leeches x., stimulants, opiates.	Died.
20	Mrs. Somerville; æt. 40; Orange Street, Leicester Square. Natural labour. 28th September, 1827.	21st Sept.—Severe rigor; acute pain in the hypogastrium and loins; suppression of lochia; nausea; urgent thirst; delirium, pulse 130, weak and intermitting; countenance pale and anxious; tongue white and moist. 22d: stupor; pulse more rapid and feeble; pain in the left iliac region. 23d: stupor; hurried breathing; intermitting pulse.	V.S. ʒviij., fomentations, opiates.	Peritoneal sac] of healthy; no effusion; left spermatic vein from uterus to emulgent vein distended with coagula of blood and lymph, which adhered to the inner surface of the vessel; vein thickened, and inner membrane of a scarlet colour; veins in the fundus uteri inflamed, and muscular coat softened; left ovarium and tube soft, of a dark red colour, and coated with lymph. Died.
21	Cantwell; æt. 23; 15, Green Street, Leicester Square. Natural labour. 23d Sep, 1827.	Second day.—Violent rigor, and uterine pain; pulse 140; headache; sickness; tremors; delirium; great debility; pulse 140; painful and distended abdomen.	V.S. ʒxij., calomel, Dover's powder, cathartics, blisters.	Recovered.
22	Foster; æt. 30; 11, Ogle Street, Hospital. Natural labour. 6th October, 1827.	Sixth day.—Pain, gradually increasing from delivery; pulse 140; debility; hurried respiration; lochia suppressed; right iliac region peculiarly tender. Convalescent on the third day.	V.S. ʒxvj. (blood buffy), leeches xxiv., calomel, and antimony.	Recovered.
23	Cooper; 6, Moore Street, Seven Dls.—Natural labour. 3d October, 1827.	Tenth day.—Rigor; pain of uterus and right iliac region; pulse 100; lochia suppressed.	V.S. ʒxvj., leeches xxiv., calomel, antimony, and cathartics.	Recovered.

24	Wellington; æt. 22; 16, Tower Street, Seven Dials. Natural labour. 16th October, 1827.	Third day.—Severe pain of uterus from the time of delivery; vomiting; pulse 100; lochia suppressed. Convalescent 19th October.	V.S. ʒxv., leeches xviij., calomel, and antimony,	Recovered.
25	Hill; æt. 35; 454, Strand. Natural labour. 15th October, 1827.	Fourth day.—Severe pain, increased by pressure, in both iliac regions; abdomen soft; tongue white; thirst; pulse 96.	V.S. ʒiv., calomel, antimony, saline effervescing medicine.	Recovered.
26	Hughes; 22, Short's Gardens. Natural labour. 29th October, 1827.	Second day.—Pain of hypogastrium, increased by pressure, since delivery; rigors; lochia suppressed; tongue loaded; pulse 140, feeble.	V.S. ʒiij. calomel, antimony, cathartics.	Recovered.
27	Pope; 7, Feathers' Court, Drury Lane. Flooding. 26th October, 1827.	Fifth day.—Rigors; headache; intense uterine pain; lochia suppressed; pulse 135, feeble; tongue dry and brown; vomiting; prostration of strength; delirium; painful induration of the left saphena veins; coma; swellings appeared suddenly in the joints of the arms.	Leeches xxiv., powerful diffusible stimuli, quinine, &c.	Died. Saphena, femoral, and iliac veins not examined; small intestines of a bright red; no lymph effused; the left fallopian tube and fundus uteri of a deep red colour; the examination was imperfect.
28	Desmond; æt. 20; 15, Crown Street, Soho. 16th November, 1827.	Fourth day.—Rigors; pyrexia; headache; acute pain of uterus; lochia suppressed.	V.S. ʒx., leeches xvj., calomel, antimony, Dover's powder, cathartics.	Recovered.
29	Manning; æt. 22; 131, Drury Lane.—Arm presentation. 3d December, 1827.	Third day.—Exquisite uterine pain; rigor; thirst; cough; rapid strong pulse.	V.S. (at twice) ʒliv., leeches xiv., fomentations, calomel, antimony, opium, cathartics.	Recovered.
30	Mayes; æt. 20; 5, Vere Street, Clare Market. 7th January, 1828.	Third day.—Rigors; headache; acute pain of hypogastrium; pulse 110; tongue white; lochia and milk not suppressed.	V.S. ʒrj., leeches xiv., fomentations, calomel, pulv. Jacobi, cathartica, saline draughts.	Recovered.
31	Adams; æt. 24; 10, Ely Court, Holborn.—Natural labour. 10th January, 1828.	Third day.—Severe after-pains; uterine region exquisitely painful on pressure; pulse 90, and strong; tongue white; thirst; lochia flow.	V.S. ʒxx., leeches xviij., cataplasms, calomel, antim. Dover's powder, cathartics.	Recovered.
32	Atkinson; æt. 32; 5, Shelton Court. Natural labour. 25th January, 1828.	Second day.—Excessive tenderness of uterus; hypogastrium tumid; pulse 100, weak; no rigor or headache; lochia and milk flow; retention of urine. The symptoms continued several days without relief.	V.S. ʒviij., V.S. ʒr., leeches xxiv.—xxiv., calomel to salivation, cathartics, cataplasms, blisters.	Recovered.

No.	Name and particulars	Symptoms	Treatment	Result
33	Malton; æt. 30; 5, New Compton Street.—Natural labour. 1st February, 1828.	Third day.—Rigors; uterus large, and on the right side exquisitely painful; intense pain in the forehead; tongue white; nausea; prostration; lochia flow.	V.S. ʒxvj., leeches, calomel, antim., cathartics, opiates,	Recovered.
34	Lawrens; æt. 35; 6, Cumberland Street, Middlesex Hosp. Hydrocephalic fœtus; dropsy of amnion. 12th February, 1828.	Second day.—Intense pain of hypogastrium; lochia suppressed; rapid feeble pulse; vomiting; foul tongue; urgent thirst; prostration of strength; tympanites.	Leeches xxiv., calomel, Dover's powder, effervescing draught.	Died. Intestines, liver, and uterus partially coated with lymph; uterus uncontracted; a fibrous tumor in the muscular coat; lb. ij. of a dark-coloured sero-purulent fluid in peritoneal sac; right uterine appendages disorganized by inflammation; ovarium three times the natural size, and softened.
35	Parkhurst; æt. 34; Marylebone Lane.—Hæmorrhage and retained placenta.	Third day.—Acute pain of uterus; lochia suppressed; rigors; rapid pulse; loaded tongue; nausea; yellow suffusion of countenance; crural phlebitis on left side.	Copious venesection, leeches, fomentations, cathartics, opiates.	Recovered after five weeks.
36	—; 5, Monmouth Street. Natural labour. 20th March, 1828.	Second day.—Acute pain of hypogastrium; rigors; pulse accelerated; lochia suppressed.	V.S. ʒxviij., calomel, cathartics, fomentations.	Recovered.
37	A Patient in the British Lying-in Hospital. Natural labour. 12th March, 1828.	Fifteenth day.—(First seen.) Violent pain in the lower part of the abdomen; vomiting; rapid feeble pulse; extremities cold.	Opiates, fomentations, leeches xij., vesication, calomel and opium late.	Died.
38	M. Jenkins; 11, Charles Street, Strand. 15th March, —.	Third day.—Exquisite tenderness but no fulness nor hardness in the region of the uterus; headache; rigors; lochia suppressed; pulse quiet, not feeble.	Copious V.S., calomel, antimony, cathartics.	Recovered.
39	—; High Street, St. Giles's. Natural labour. 16th April, 1828.	Fourth day.—Rigor; quick strong pulse; hot skin; great sensibility of the hypogastrium; lochia suppressed.	V.S. ʒxx, calomel, pulv. antim., cataplasms, cathartica.	Recovered.
40	Buck; White Horse Yard, Drury Lane.—Natural labour. 8th July, —.	Second day.—Severe rigor; uterus large, hard, and painful; lochia flow; pulse 130; tongue loaded; bowels costive.	V.S. ʒxxv., calomel, cathartics, cataplasma,	Recovered.

41	Austin; British Lying-in Hospital.—Natural labour. 1st June, 1828.	Seventh day.—(First seen.) Severe fever, headache, delirium; pulse 130; tremor of tongue and extremities; diarrhœa; pupils dilated; swellings of joints, especially right wrist; exhaustion.	Leeches xij. to the head, diaphoretic, opiates, wine, ammonia, and other stimulants.	Died.
42	Ann Cromer; St. James's Infirmary.—Uterine haemorrhage from placental presentation. 22d July, 1828.	Second day.—Rigor; headache; heat of skin; intolerance of light; pulse 140; hurried respiration; no pain of abdomen; pain in the chest, followed in a few days by cough and foetid expectoration. Died eighteen days after delivery.	V.S. eighth day to ʒxvj.; blisters to the thorax.	Died. Abscess in the left ovarium; pus in the sinuses of the uterus on the left side; coats of left spermatic vein thickened, its inner surface lined with lymph and pus, and nearly obliterated. These changes occupied the whole course of the vein to the emulgent, the coats of which were in the same condition; vena cava healthy; inflammation and gangrene of the lungs.
43	——; British Lying-in Hospital. 1828.	Third day.—Acute pain in the iliac regions; rapid pulse; rigors; lochia suppressed.	V.S. ʒxx., calomel, cathartics, fomentations.	Cured.
44	——; British Lying-in Hospital. Natural labour. 8th August, 1828.	Sixth day.—Rigors; intense soreness of the hypogastrium; tongue loaded; bowels open; pulse quick; skin hot.	V.S. ʒxx., calomel, pulv. antim. cathartics.	Recovered.
45	Vernon; 11, Chapel Street. Dropsy of amnion; haemorrhage. 1st November, 1828.	Second day.—Violent rigor; sudden attack of acute pain of the uterus, which became large and hard; lochia suppressed.	V.S. ʒxx., leeches xxxvj., calomel, antimony, cathartics, diaphoretic.	Recovered.
46	——; 26, Little Windmill Street. Natural labour. 3d November, 1828.	Tenth day.—Violent pyrexia; uterus large, hard, and painful, gradually increasing from delivery; lochia suppressed.	V.S. ʒxx., leeches xxxvj. calomel, &c.	Recovered.
47	Mrs. Turner; 92, Berwick St. Premature labour. 10th December, 1828.	Second day.—Acute pain in the hypogastrium before delivery; severe vomiting soon after took place, with pyrexia, tension of abdomen, suppression of urine and tympanites.	V.S. ʒxiv., leeches, cataplasms.	Died. Omentum, intestines, and liver coated with lymph; omentum vascular; peritoneum covering uterus, and appendages, red, vascular, and coated with lymph; two pints of reddish serum in cavity of pelvis; muscular tissue of uterus healthy.

48	Gibbs; 41, Broad Street, Golden Square.—Natural labour. 15th January, 1829.	Third day.—Acute pain of uterus; pyrexia; pulse rapid and feeble; lochia suppressed; followed by great tenderness in the left iliac and femoral veins, and general swelling of the whole left lower extremity, of short duration.	Moderate bleeding twice at the onset, leeches xxxvj., fomentations, mild cathartics, opiates.	Recovered.
49	A patient of Middlesex Hospital; 20, Ogle Street. Natural labour. February 1829.	Fourth day.—Pyrexia; acute pain, increased by pressure, in the left iliac region; lochia diminished; tongue white; headache; surface hot and moist. Imperfect relief from leeches.	Leeches xxxvj., poultices, mercury, antimony.	Recovered imperfectly after a considerable period.
50	Greenwood; 4, Stafford Street, New Road.—Tedious labour. 21st February, 1829.	Third day.—Sudden attack of severe pain in the region of the uterus and left iliac region; intense pain of forehead; violent rigors; pulse 116; lochia diminished; tongue loaded; urgent thirst.	V.S. lb. ij. (syncope), calomel and opium, leeches xxiv., cathartics.	Recovered.

[This Table will be completed in the next number.]

By looking over the abstract of the cases contained in it, you will observe that a great proportion of the women, above one half, were attacked on the second and third days after delivery, and that in most of them where the disease proved fatal the symptoms occurred in the following order : rigors, uterine pain, suppression of the lochia, headache, tenderness and distension of the whole abdomen, vomiting, diarrhœa, delirium, and cessation of pain before death.

II. *Inflammation of the uterine appendages, ovaria, fallopian tubes, and broad ligaments.*

I have seen the uterine appendages free from disease in one case only, where the peritoneal covering of the uterus has been inflamed, but frequently the peritoneum has been slightly affected where the appendages of the uterus have been extensively disorganised. The surface of the broad ligaments, ovaria, and fallopian tubes, have been red and vascular, and partially or completely imbedded in lymph or pus. The outer extremities of the fallopian tubes have been of a deep red colour, and softened, and deposits of pus in a diffused or circumscribed form have taken place between their coats or within their canals. Between the folds of the broad ligaments effusions of serous or purulent fluids have also been found. Numerous important changes have likewise been observed in the structure of the ovaria. Their peritoneal surface has often been red, vascular, and imbedded in lymph, without any visible alteration of their parenchymatous structure, or their whole volume has been greatly enlarged, swollen, red, and pulpy; blood has been effused into the Graafian vesicles, or around them, and circumscribed deposits of pus have been often dispersed throughout the substance of the enlarged ovaria. In several cases the structure of the ovaria has been reduced to a soft vascular flocculent pulp, no traces of their original organization being left. These morbid appearances have been represented in several drawings [exhibiting them]. The ovarium in one instance was converted into a large purulent cyst, which had contracted adhesions with the abdominal parietes, and discharged its contents exteriorly through an ulcerated opening. In another case, which proved fatal, the inflammation had extended to the cellular membrane exterior to the mately recovered, the purulent deposit formed in the situation of the psoas and iliacus internus muscle, or about the neighbourhood of the uterus, made its way through an ulcerated opening in the upper part of the thigh : contraction of the thigh on the trunk took place in both these cases, and continued for several months, but disappeared on the recovery of the patients. In another recent case, a great quantity of pus, after uterine inflammation, escaped through the anterior wall of the vagina, and the patient recovered. In another, after puerperal peritonitis, an ulcerated opening formed in the rectum, and a great quantity of pus escaped, after which the symptoms subsided. In several cases I have seen a great discharge of pus take place through an opening made with the lancet in the walls of the abdomen, between the umbilicus and ilium, and perfect recovery to succeed. Inflammation of the uterine appendages being generally combined with peritonitis to a greater or lesser extent, it is often difficult to establish a diagnosis between these varieties of uterine inflammation. The pain is, however, usually less acute than in peritonitis, and is principally situated in one or other of the iliac fossæ, extending from them to the loins, anus, and thighs. On pressure the pain is chiefly experienced in the lateral parts of the hypogastrium. The constitutional symptoms at the onset of the attack do not materially differ from those which mark the accession of peritonitis, which are often accompanied with strong febrile reaction, which passes speedily away, and is succeeded by prostration of strength, and the other symptoms which characterise inflammation of the venous and muscular tissues of the uterus.

III. *Inflammation and softening of the muscular coat of the uterus.*

The dark-coloured mucous layer, which usually coats the inner surface of the uterus after delivery, has been supposed to be the result of gangrenous inflammation, and has been described as such by some pathologists. This ought not, however, to be confounded with the changes produced by inflammation of the inner membrane of the uterus, when it becomes softened or wholly disorganized, like the mucous linings of the stomach and intestines in certain inflammatory diseases. In several cases the internal membrane of the uterus was soft and flocculent, and had undergone changes similar in appearance to those which are produced in it by long maceration. In other cases, not only has the internal coat been disorganized, but the muscular tissue, to a considerable depth, or even through its entire substance to the peritoneum, has been of a dark purple, greyish, or yellowish hue, and so softened in texture as to be torn by the gentlest efforts made in removing the parts from the body. The peritoneum covering the inflamed portion of muscular coat of the uterus has also been affected, and lymph has been thrown out over its surface as in common

peritonitis ; or the peritoneum has become of a yellow, red, or livid colour, no albumen having been deposited on its surface. The peritoneum has also been softened where the subjacent tissue has been little, if at all, affected ; more frequently, however, the softening has proceeded from the internal surface of the uterus to its peritoneal, and the muscular has been extensively disorganized without a corresponding lesion of the peritoneal coat of the uterus. Inflammation and softening of the uterus have, in some cases, affected the muscular tissue of the fundus, body, and cervix of the uterus ; in others these changes have been limited to the part where the placenta has adhered, which has become unusually thin, and reduced to a pulpy state. Small abscesses have been formed, in a few instances, in the muscular tissue of the uterus, without any perceptible change in the surrounding substance of the organ, while in other cases every trace of muscular fibre has been lost. Pain of the hypogastrium, diminution or suppression of the lochial discharge, and rigors, with rapid pulse, are the most frequent symptoms of the disease. The countenance becomes pallid, and is usually expressive of great anxiety and distress. There is often severe headache, with delirium, and other affections of the brain and nervous system ; and so violent have these been, in some cases, that the local affection of the uterus has completely escaped detection during life. The skin is hot and dry, and sometimes of a peculiar sallow tinge ; the pulse is rapid and feeble ; the respiration hurried, with remarkable prostration of strength ; the tongue becomes foul ; the lips covered with sordes ; occasional vomiting is experienced. The progress of the disease in some cases is rapid ; in others it runs its course more slowly, being protracted to the eighth or tenth day. It must be admitted that the diagnosis of this variety of uterine inflammation, particularly where it is complicated with peritonitis or inflammation of the veins, which is frequently the case, is difficult, or even impossible. If the attack of inflammation of the muscular coat be sudden and violent, it becomes so speedily complicated with peritonitis, more or less acute, that the symptoms are readily confounded together, and it is impossible to distinguish with certainty the symptoms which are to be referred to peritonitis, and those which result from the affection of the muscular coat. The prostration of strength, the alteration of the features, which often exists from the commencement, the feebleness and rapidity of the pulse, the irregular foetid state of the lochia, are not such constant symptoms as to be pathognomonic, and may arise from other causes. Hence it will appear that the most attentive consideration of the phenomena will not lead us to any certain conclusion as to the nature of the affection; and, as in many other diseases, we can only determine its precise character by the history of its origin and progress, and by the alteration of structure discovered after death. In all the cases of this affection which I have observed, the resources of nature and of art have proved equally unavailing in arresting its fatal course. The active inflammatory symptoms which commonly manifest themselves at the commencement of the attack pass speedily away, whatever plan of treatment be adopted, and are rapidly succeeded by symptoms of exhaustion. Where the disease is not complicated with inflammation of the peritoneum the symptoms are not such as to indicate the necessity for the employment of venesection; and in one case where it was adopted freely the abstraction of the blood was followed by speedy death. In other cases, where the opposite plan of treatment was had recourse to, the fatal result seemed to be less speedy, though equally certain. This destructive form of uterine inflammation has been described by several German and French pathologists; Astruc, Vigarous, and Primrose, probably refer to it when they state that the uterus is liable to be attacked with gangrene and sphacelus; Ponteau and Gastellier have related cases in which gangrene of the uterus followed acute inflammation of the organ. In 1750 an epidemic attacked many puerperal women, which was characterized by severe abdominal pain and tumefaction of the hypogastrium. On examining the bodies of two of these women, Ponteau states that the uterus was found very large; the internal membrane was soft and black, and the substance of the parietes was of a livid red colour, and in a gangrenous state. Boer, of Vienna, has described this affection under the term putrescence of the uterus, and has observed its frequent occurrence in particular epidemics. Laroth and Danyau have more recently published detailed accounts of this destructive disease. Two hundred and twenty-two women died in the Maternité, of Paris, in 1829; and in examining their bodies, M. Tonellé found the muscular tissue of the uterus softened in forty-nine. He states that softening of the uterus, after occurring frequently in the first half of the year 1829, and particularly about January, disappeared entirely in the months of July and August, which were characterized in a remarkable manner by the frequency of inflammation of the veins of the uterus. Afterwards it began to occur, often with great violence, in September and October, and again disappeared in November and December. Boer and Laroth have, I think, erroneously described the different degrees of this affection as constituting two essentially distinct diseases. M. Tonellé also states that the disorder at Paris assumed two different forms—the softening of the uterus properly so called, and the putrescence. In one form the softening affected only the internal surface of the uterus, and it presented itself under the appearance of irregular superficial patches of a red or brown colour, which occupied almost all the points of this surface. Its limits were not determined, the diseased tissue passing by insensible gradations or shades into the healthy tissue. In the second species the softening extended deep into the substance of the uterus; it occupied sometimes the whole thickness of the body and cervix of the uterus. The tissue of this organ was so softened that the fingers could not seize it without passing through all its parts. The superficial softening was combined almost constantly with some alteration of structure, the result of peritonitis, metritis, or inflammation of the veins; and it did not appear that the existence of these had a very sensible influence on the progress of the symptoms. The softening in the second degree was also sometimes combined with other derangements; but it formed usually the principal alteration, often the only one, and invariably impressed upon the disease the most decided typhoid character

The history of uterine phlebitis will form the subject of the next lecture.

REMOVAL OF
DROPSICAL OVARIA, ENTIRE,
BY THE LARGE ABDOMINAL SECTION.

By D. HENRY WALNE, Esq.

(For the London Medical Gazette.)

SECOND CASE.

IN the early part of the present year, Mr. Camplin, of Finsbury Square, called on me, accompanied by one of his patients, whose case he considered to be one of dropsical ovarium, and suitable for the operation of which I had then recently published a case. At his desire I very carefully investigated the circumstances of her state, and agreed with him that there could be no doubt of the nature of her disease, nor of the propriety of ultimately treating it by operation. We however thought that, in deference to the opinion still entertained by a few physicians that internal remedies are not without use in such cases, it would be proper first to give a trial to a course of such as are at present in most esteem. By thus proceeding we should test the efficacy of active internal agents, and in the event of their failure, find a fuller justification for resorting to surgical means.

Mr. Camplin's patient, Mrs. M. R——, was a widow of 57 years of age, who had not married till she was 46 years old, had never been in the family way, and whose husband died five years after their marriage. Having always been accustomed to suffer much at the menstrual periods, she yet continued to menstruate till she was 49. Full sixteen years before she applied to Mr. Camplin, she had thought herself larger on the left side of the abdomen than on the right, but until about eight years ago had not felt the slightest inconvenience, nor did she take any notice of the circumstance to any one, being in the enjoyment of perfect health. About the latter period, however, she felt a soreness and tenderness of the lower part of the left side of the abdomen, accompanied by fulness; and a surgeon, to whom she applied, mentioned the ovary of that side as the seat of ailment, and ordered her leeches, iodine ointment, and various other remedies, observing that though her complaint "was not a thing which touched life, it sometimes ended in dropsy." Five or six years back her abdomen was to all appearance flat; but during the last two or three years she perceived a stoutness, which, as her health and condition were good, she thought little of. Something more than a twelvemonth since she began "to droop," to lose flesh generally, and at the same time to increase very remarkably in the size of her abdomen. Having ascribed these changes to flatulency and indigestion, she did not immediately apply for professional advice, but their continuance induced her to refer to Mr. Camplin in November 1842; the above being, in substance, her own history of the case down to that period.

When I first saw Mrs. R., she had the appearance of a healthy person of spare habit, and the size of a woman eight months advanced in pregnancy. There was distinct fluctuation and dull sound over the greater part of the abdomen, with a circumscribed character of tumefaction. A sense of dragging about the cartilages of the ribs, chiefly of the right side, was her principal uneasiness. The uterus appeared healthy, and of moderate size. She had no

symptom of general dropsy. Her health was good, except a little flatulency and other symptoms of feeble digestion. She was directed to take—

Liq. Potass. 3ss. ; Potass. Hydriodat. gr. iij. ad gr. v. ; in bitter infusion, with Tinct. Columb. twice a day, and an occasional aperient.

After a steady trial of the Liq. Potass. and Potass. Hydriod. for more than two months, it was clear that her size was undergoing augmentation, whilst her plight was in no degree improved. Her own opinion was, and Mr. Camplin and I thought it correct, that the disease gained ground faster whilst she was following this plan of treatment than either before or after it. The medicines that were administered subsequently were chiefly directed to the improvement of her digestion, and the lessening an irritability of system and excitability of circulation which had shown themselves.

Finding that the disease continued unabated, and that the inconveniences occasioned by it were becoming greater and greater, the operation was proposed, and Dr. James Blundell consulted, that we might have additional assurance of the accuracy of our opinion and the propriety of the intended measure. We had the satisfaction of his entire concurrence. Various circumstances, however, occurred to postpone the operation till the 30th of May, when, in the presence of Dr. Sewall, of Washington (United States), Dr. Klein, physician to the Crown Prince of Wurtemburg, Drs. Moore and Waller, and other gentlemen, and assisted by Mr. Camplin and those gentlemen (Mr. Vincent excepted, whom accident kept away) whose aid I had been so fortunate as to obtain on the former occasion, I proceeded, after due preparation, to its performance.

The most important preliminary measures were—

1st. Insisting on a few days of absolute rest within the house, our patient having wearied and excited herself several times very undesirably by visiting distant friends and busying her mind; and having, by much walking, brought on a painfully swollen condition of the left leg, with tenderness in the course of the veins. Rest upon a couch, a little aperient medicine, and putting her feet in hot water two or three times, improved her state very much, reducing the pulse, which had become somewhat quick, and removing her other slight ailments.

2dly. Marking the abdominal skin with solution of arg. nitr. in lines crossing the linea alba, to secure correct adjustment of the wound.

3dly. Clearing the bowels so completely that there should be no occasion to disturb them again for at least 48 hours after the operation. An aperient pill over night, and a large enema an hour before the operation, secured this object, which I consider doubly important; in reference, viz. to the healing of the wound and to the prevention of peritoneal inflammation.

4thly. Supporting her well with nutriment that would leave little residue to load the intestines afresh, and yet should well sustain her through the operation and its immediate consequences. I remembered the cold extremities and low condition of my former patient just after the operation. To this a pint and a half of good beef tea was given about two hours beforehand. She had her usual breakfast, and took nothing but the beef tea after it.

5thly. The temperature of the room was maintained at a little above 70 Fahrenheit.

Tuesday, 30th May, 1843. It was near five o'clock when Mrs. R—— took her seat upon a couch, her feet upon the ground at its end, her back well propt by pillows, and an eight-headed roller laid beneath her back. The steps of the intended operation had been fully explained to all the medical gentlemen when previously assembled in another room, and each of those who had assisted me before was engaged to take his part as in the former instance. Plenty of able assistance was at hand, but this arrangement was the simplest mode of securing what was necessary without confusion. Mr. Camplin was watchful of his patient's condition, and whilst cheering her was ready also with every aid of counsel and of hand that could be useful.

As in the former operation a small incision was first made of an inch and a half in length, and the abdomen cautiously opened to a still less extent in the linea alba. In the course of this proceeding a little clear fluid (probably from the sheath of the right rectus muscle,) having appeared in the wound, gave an impression to some of the spectators that the sac had been already wounded, or, at all events, the peritoneal cavity entered. The fluid ceased, however, to trickle down, and examination convinced Dr. Blundell and myself that such was not the case; and by a careful division of the tendinous and peritoneal layers the surface of the sac was made visible, when a finger, passed in every direction between it and the peritoneum, discovered no adhesions. I could now proceed in the operation with the confident anticipation that all the circumstances of the case were favourable to its completion, and expediting my movements accordingly, I divided the skin from above downwards to the first wound, and thence towards the pubes, in all to the extent of about twelve inches; then, with a probe-pointed curved bistoury, guided and guarded by two fingers of my left hand, I opened the peritoneum to a like extent. The wounded structures separated on each side, and the tumor being devoid of adhesions steadily advanced through the incision. They were followed by the hands of one of the gentlemen and closed behind the tumor as opportunity offered, so as to cover the viscera with the peritoneum itself as promptly and as completely as possible. Dr. Freund, as upon the former occasion, performed this office, and the tumor was steadied by Mr. Law; whilst I passed two fingers of my left hand behind the left uterine broad ligament, which formed the pedicle, and by their guidance, with a suitable needle, carried a ligature behind and thence through the middle of the pedicle, for the purpose of tying it in two portions. The first half of the ligature was readily and firmly tied, but the second broke.* The entire pedicle was then included in one double ligature, and divided between it and the tumor. The pedicle was very short, and the uterus lay backward in the pelvis, with a part of the distended ovarian sac in front of it. After the division of the pedicle, and the removal of the tumor, there was hæmorrhage, in the suppression of

* It is very desirable to have a strong kind of ligature for tying the pedicle, and of equal strength in all its parts. I had tried beforehand a portion of that used in this case, and found it readily sustained a weight of 28lbs., yet another portion snapped at an untoward moment. I have since had a twist made purposely, and shall not be content with any ligature which will not sustain 60lbs. and is not very even in its fabric, as well as of soft texture.

which the shortness of that part occasioned some difficulty; but on drawing it up by the ligatures I could command the vessels by holding the bleeding part within the finger and thumb of my left hand, and they were, after a little delay, secured by another ligature, which included the pedicle again entirely. The advantage of a free incision was particularly felt at this period.

The coagula being cleared away, the edges of the wound were adjusted as accurately as possible, and nine interrupted sutures served to preserve them in apposition. Long pads of lint were laid down each side of the wound, and over them slips of plaster passed from side to side across the abdomen. The heads of the roller which had been placed behind her were now carried once round her with the requisite firmness and tied. She was conveyed to bed with a firm though frequent pulse, and a warm skin, having been scarcely faint during the operation. She took gr. ¼ Morph. Acet. in ʒiss. Mist. Camph. immediately, and again in an hour; and eagerly drank some water, of which she had already taken more than I was aware of. At half-past six o'clock, her pulse was 110; at ten, it was 106, and full, her skin warm and freely perspiring, and she had slept a little. Complained of some pain of the left side and in the back. ʒxj. of urine withdrawn by catheter. Temperature of the room, 75. To have nothing but water, viz. 12 oz. in the night. The temperature to be lowered a little.

31st.—I paid her three visits, at each of which the pulse was noted, and was about 120. She had slept little, but perspired freely all night. No sickness, nor shivering, nor chilliness had occurred, and her mind was perfectly clear. The abdomen was free from distension and from tenderness, except in the line of the wound, and in the left iliac region; but she felt all over her as if she had been beaten, was thirsty, and complained of heat and occasional griping uneasiness. I was surprised at finding ʒxxi. of urine follow the use of the catheter in the morning. ʒx. more were drawn off at midday; but before my evening visit she had twice passed it unassisted in considerable quantity : I, however, drew off ʒv. The tongue was moist and clean; short intervals of sleep refreshed her in the course of the day. Her breathing was free; and she could

partially turn in bed, by the aid principally of the lower limb of the side from which she wished to turn. The rectum-tube was passed, but very little flatus escaped. One dose of her anodyne was given at night.

June 1st.—Had a good night. When visited at

	9 A.M.	5 P.M.	11 P.M.
Her pulse was .	117	108	102
Urine withdrawn	ʒviij.	ʒx.	ʒviij.

and some was also voided in the night, and when the bowels were twice spontaneously moved in the course of the day. Her skin was warm and perspiring all day; her tongue moist, and only slightly white. She had no pain, and the wound, where visible on re-adjusting the bandage, had nicely united. In all respects she was going on well. Water had been her only support till five o'clock to-day (forty-eight hours from the operation) when a little beef tea was given, and at night some gruel.

2d.—Having slept a good deal yesterday, her night was not so good, though the anodyne was taken as before. The pulse was about 102 all day; the symptoms much as on the previous evening. The wound being dressed, was found to have united throughout, except for about three quarters of an inch at the lower end, where the ligatures of the pedicle were placed. The stitches were all removed.

Towards evening she became uneasy, and had a sense of sickness; but was free from tenderness of the abdomen. Her bowels not having been moved, an enema was administered, and much flatus followed; and as her pulse intermitted somewhat, beef tea was directed to be given more frequently.

3d.—A pretty good night, but had some unpleasant dreams. Flatulency and occasional griping. Would like an egg for breakfast. To have it, with bread and butter and tea; and then to take gr. x. of Fel. Bov. inspissat. The pulse, 108 in the early part of the day, was 105 later, after having slept a good deal. Having had no movement of the bowels, but being less flatulent, gr. x. of the Fel. to be repeated.

4th.—A better night. Bowels twice moved very comfortably; voided her urine very freely, which hitherto had generally been drawn off; pulse 106, feeble. Some offensive motions passed, and she felt low. A little brandy to be taken in some gruel, and then her anodyne. Arrow-root for supper.

5th.—A good night. Is languid; pulse 105. To have beef tea and a custard pudding for dinner. Tried to sit up after dinner, but felt faint and giddy. A glass of sherry given. Slept in the evening, and became very comfortable. Miliary eruption appeared yesterday on some parts of the skin, and to day was very general. Pulse, towards night, 96. The room to be kept cooler.

6th.—Wound dressed again. Two or three spots only of pus, where the skin was not quite evenly adjusted, but in quantity hardly worth mentioning; the wound, in general, being a cleanly-united line, excepting, of course, where the ligatures lay like the threads of a seton. Pulse 94. Complained of nothing but weakness, being remarkably well for the period of her recovery—one week after the operation. To have some boiled mutton for dinner, with wine and water. Pulse, at night, 88; urine passed freely; no motion, and the bowels a little uneasy, with a sense of weight in the left iliac region.

Capt. Fel. Bov. inspiss. gr. x. h. s.

I have detailed the symptoms to this period more particularly than I should otherwise have done, for the purpose of shewing in how promising a manner every thing had hitherto proceeded.

On the 7th of June she had passed an indifferent night; and there was considerable uneasiness in the left iliac region, with one tender spot feeling like an intestine in a state of contraction. She had a copious motion in the morning, with partial relief. Instead of meat, took some sago pudding for dinner, which she enjoyed. Was free from sickness, but complained more than hitherto of pain.

R. Extr. Hyoscyam.; Fel. Bov. inspiss. aa. gr. v.; Aloes Barbad. gr. j. M. Ft. pil. iij. statim sumend.

As no motion followed this dose, and her uneasiness was increased towards night, though she had passed urine of pale colour freely, and the wound near the ligatures looked well, an enema was used, followed by the anodyne, with Morph. Acet. gr. ss. Fluid diet.

June 8th.—Bowels copiously relieved, and she felt much easier, even before taking the anodyne, but after it slept and perspired very much. To-day she complains of rheumatic pain in her arms and shoulders, with a stiff neck, and says she has taken cold. Tongue furred, but moist; urine passed without difficulty, but of higher colour. There is uneasiness in the iliac region as before, and a little soft fulness. I examined the left leg, fearing inflammation of the veins from the symptoms complained of. It was larger than the other, but so it had been before the operation; no shivering nor sickness, but the pulse 110. The miliary eruption much renewed. Towards night, the pain in her limbs increased, but the abdomen easy, and there was less tenderness in the iliac region; the right leg had become somewhat painful, particularly on being moved, and her pulse was higher; a hot enema was given, viz. of 108 Fahr. and an anodyne.

June 9th. — Passed an indifferent night, and feels very ill this morning, her sleep having been disturbed by pain in the limbs, particularly the left leg, which is more swollen, and now pits sensibly, though it did not on examination last night; there is some tenderness in the course of the blood-vessels in the groin; the shoulders and neck are easier; pulse 125, feeble; urine more red; bowels well relieved, and motions not unhealthy; tongue foul, but moist; no shivering; skin perspiring; leeches to the groin.

R. Infus. Cinchon. Ʒiss. quartâ quàque horâ sumend.

2 P.M. Leeches have not sucked well, nor the bites bled much, yet she says she is better. Being put on milk diet, she finds it support her very well; her pulse is, however, 130. At night, leg more swollen and very painful; leeches renewed; a hot enema.

R. Sulph. Quin.; Pil. Hydrarg.; Ext. Conii, aa. gr. ij. M. ft. pil. ij. quartâ quàque horâ sumend., in lieu of the infusion. An anodyne.

Dr. Blundell concurs in her case being now one of mild phlegmasia dolens, or inflammation of the veins, as Mr. Camplin and myself considered it.

June 10th.—Had a better night, and is freer from pain; pulse 138; to be again leeched.

Towards night her pulse fell to 119, and though very uneasy, particularly in the left leg, her pain was less. She took an excessive quantity of milk last night and this morning, and caused herself a great deal of distension and discomfort. A little brandy and water had to be given; her pills were continued, and at night an anodyne enema administered, which not being wholly retained, her usual anodyne was also given, and the two produced an inconvenient drowsiness.

June 11th.—Excessively heavy, languid, and somewhat confused. Pulse 145. It even rose to 150 in the course of the morning, but towards the afternoon fell to 130, and gradually came down from this time for the next two days, being then 100; the leg followed the like course of improvement, as did her general state, except that a cough distressed her at times, and her feebleness and emaciation had become extreme: the quinine was continued, but the Pil. Hydrarg. omitted: her diet was made more generous as the symptoms permitted. At one time the right leg became painful and slightly swollen, but not for a continuance. There was tenderness also in the right groin in the course of the blood-vessels. Her convalescence was very gradually established; some tenderness in the situation of the veins in both groins was experienced for many days; clammy sweats broke out at times, and pains like those of rheumatism were often complained of during her recovery. As to the wound, what was chiefly remarkable was, that from the peeling of the skin, occasioned by the innumerable little blisters of the miliary eruption, its whole line was made raw for a couple of days, and at the part where the ligatures hung forth, a discharge, just about the time of the subsidence of the worst symptoms of venous irritation, was observed in greater quantity than at other times, and then it was offensive, but in general it was healthy and not at all profuse.

The ligature first tied, which included half the pedicle, came away in about five weeks. The others which embraced the whole pedicle, although they have been very tightly twisted, remain to the present time.

The tumor removed in this case was rather less solid than that which I removed in November last. It weighed sixteen pounds and three quarters, imperial weight, and, when laid in a dish, measured in horizontal circumference 2 feet 11¼ inches; in vertical circumference 2 feet 6 inches lengthwise, and 2 feet 3¼ inches across. The engraving of the former tumor (LONDON MED. GAZ. Dec. 23, 1842,) will convey a better notion of this than any description I can

give; the chief differences being in the position of the fallopian tube, which stretched wide away from the solid part, and its being a disease of the left, whilst the other was of the right ovarium.

Guilford Street, Russell Square,
London, July 20, 1843.

TREATMENT OF FRACTURES
BY MEANS OF THE STARCHED BANDAGE.

To the Editor of the Medical Gazette.

SIR,

I BEG the favour of the insertion of the enclosed letter in your GAZETTE, should you deem it worthy of a place in its columns.—I am, sir,

Your obedient servant,
H. B. NORMAN.

9, Holles Street, Cavendish Square.

In your number of the 21st of July, I have read a detailed account of a fracture of the forearm, unsuccessfully treated by the starched bandage, given by Mr. M'Cash, from which the author proceeds to draw inferences, which I cannot but regard as unjust, as grounded on insufficient experience, and as calculated to bring into disrepute a practice of exceeding value to the surgeon in the treatment of fractures. The author details the case, the substance of which is as follows:—"A boy, of 12 years of age, and of slender conformation, had fallen from a wall, and so had received a fracture of both bones of the forearm. There was a considerable displacement of the broken bones, a good deal of deformity around the seat of fracture. All the patient's members were agitated by the intensity of his sufferings; the muscles of the limb affected by such violent spasmodic movements, that when the displaced bones were reduced to their proper position there was very great difficulty of keeping them so. This the author considered a *favourable case* for the trial of M. Velpeau's method of treatment by means of the early application of the starched bandage (*le bandage immobile* of that justly celebrated surgeon.) Accordingly, after fomenting the limb and administering the Sulphate of Magnesia c. Tart. Antim. he proceeded to apply the apparatus. The patient suffered for the first day or two a good deal of pain in the injured limb; this, however, subsided, and every thing was believed to be going on well for *seven or eight weeks*, at the end of which time, the apparatus being removed, the bones were found perfectly in apposition and firmly united, but such an alteration had taken place in the muscles of the limb that it was rendered useless, all power of flexion and extension, &c. being lost. The author rightly, I think, attributes all this to the effect of acute inflammation, followed by deposition of organizable lymph among the muscles. Beyond this I cannot agree with him, nor follow him in his censure of the mode of treatment as the cause of this effect.

In the first place I would remark, that the case itself was an unfavourable one for this or any other method of treatment. The patient is described as of " slender conformation." If this description means any thing in the account of the case, I conceive that it is intended to convey the idea of delicacy of constitution, and the opposite of that state of health which usually belongs to that age. If this idea be just, I see in it at the outset a ground for an unfavourable prognosis. For though it may be urged that, in such a subject, reaction would be more moderate than in one of a more robust constitution, and consequently that there would be less danger of any unfavourable result on this ground, I answer that this is only in part true. The reaction will be less violent, perhaps; but I believe the power of the constitution to resist the destructive or injurious consequences of this state, and to convert it into a reparative and favourable process, is possessed in much greater degree by the robust than by the delicate. The whole system is better enabled to resist the effects of, and to rally from, both internal diseases and external injuries.

Secondly, I regard the great degree of displacement of the broken bones as a complication of the case likely to render its management more difficult than usual, inasmuch as fresh violence must be resorted to, to overcome it, and to prevent its recurrence, and, further, likely to interfere seriously with the favourable progress of the case, from the extensive injury received by all the soft textures around the seat of fracture. Such displacement as is de-

scribed in this case could not have happened without much laceration of the muscles and the smaller blood-vessels of the limb; and I am further inclined to think that the *violent spasmodic muscular contractions* described are attributable to serious injuries of the nerves as well. Are we, then, to look to these causes, or to the early application of the immoveable apparatus, for the unfavourable result in this case? or are we to take a middle course, and to say,—to the serious nature of the injury must the unexpected consequences be attributed; but they might have been counteracted had the case been treated on another plan? I am inclined to think that the real cause of the unfortunate result is the serious injury received by the soft parts, and it is not to be attributed to the use of the immoveable apparatus at all. I would not, however, be understood to say that I should in general be prepared for an unfavourable result in such a case as the one under consideration. By no means. I believe that 80 out of 100 such cases would do well under this or any other well-conducted treatment; and further, that the most careful treatment cannot prevent occasional unfavourable consequences in the simplest cases. We cannot always foresee evils; and when we can, we are not always able to cope with them.

There is one point in Mr. M'Cash's treatment of his case which I consider decidedly wrong, namely the warm fomentation of the fractured limb. It is, according to Mr. M'C.'s opinion, and that of all other surgeons, a desirable thing to moderate the reaction consequent upon fractures, and to prevent as much as possible effusion of blood into the soft textures. How, then, is this to be done? By warmth, which must accelerate the determination of blood to the part, and by this means favour the occurrence of hæmorrhagic effusion? I should say no, but by cold, which is calculated to have the very opposite effect, and further by a raised position of the limb, so as to favour the return of blood by the veins. These, added to the early reduction of displacement, and coaptation of the fractured bones, and the early application of some efficient apparatus, are the means to prevent any evil consequences arising from fractures. In one more point the treatment of this case is to be blamed; rather, I may call it, the neglect. For what purpose was the confinement of the limb in the apparatus maintained for eight weeks? This seems to me a very unnecessary length of time to keep the limb unused, and confined in a fixed position; certainly much longer than fracture of the bones of the forearm requires, and sufficiently long, in some cases, to lead to great rigidity of the joints and atrophy of the muscles. May not this even have had some share in producing the unfortunate termination of the case? On the strength of this, Mr. M'Cash's first trial of the "bandage immobile," and the unsuccessful issue of his case, this gentleman proceeds at once to subvert the position taken by Gendrin and Velpeau, that "on the earliness of the application of the immoveable apparatus in fractures depends, in great measure, its utility." Of the truth of this position I am myself as confident as Mr. M'Cash is incredulous. I first saw the practice in the Hôpital de La Charité, under M. Velpeau's own directions, about two years ago. The simplicity and neatness of the method at first struck me, and induced me to make inquiries about it. During a short visit to Paris, though daily at the hospital, I could come to no very certain opinion as to the value of the practice, but was assured repeatedly by a friend, then *externe* to M. Velpeau, that it was most successful. This declaration I held to be the more valuable as my friend was an Englishman, and consequently not likely, from national prejudice, to over-rate the practice of his great master. On returning to London, and receiving the appointment of House-Surgeon to Mr. Liston, in the University College Hospital, I determined, with his permission, to put the practice to the test. This I did as occasion offered a suitable case. I treated several cases of fractures of the forearm and leg, one fracture of the thigh, and one or two of the humerus, by this method. It is a subject of regret to me now that I did not keep careful notes of the cases. The result, however, was so far favourable, that whenever opportunity recurs I shall again have recourse to it. In one instance only do I remember to have removed the apparatus before the completion of the cure; in the instance *of a fidgety, nervous, female patient,*

who had received fracture of the bones of the forearm. I have never seen a case in which there was any defect in the action of the muscles on the removal of the apparatus. On the contrary, one of the advantages of the practice has always appeared to me to be the plump and firm condition in which the limb is found.

In using any other appliances, the bandages must be removed several times in the course of treatment: at each reapplication they are accommodated to a limb diminished by pressure and rest, until at the end of six or eight weeks the limb is miserably diminished, shrivelled, and weak. The immoveable apparatus is applied once for all to a limb of at least its natural size. At first there is some uneasiness occasioned by the resistance to the swelling of the parts enclosed; this soon subsides, The circulation is carried on readily in parts but moderately compressed, and the nutrition of the limb consequently is more complete. The plan I have adopted is as nearly Velpeau's as possible, substituting starch only for the dextrine. The fractured bones being placed in apposition, and the limb raised considerably above the level of the body, it is encased lightly and carefully in a broad roller. Two straight splints of thick pasteboard, such as is used by bookbinders, are *starched* and laid along the inside and outside, or fore and back part of the injured limb. These are to extend beyond the articulations above and below the fracture so as to fix them. A strong starched roller is then carried pretty firmly round the limb to fix the splints, and the apparatus is completed, unless in some cases the additional security of a wooden splint be resorted to while the apparatus is drying. The apparatus should be applied with very great care, and the limb for some time kept considerably raised. The earlier it is done the better; very little swelling follows a fracture carefully managed and early reduced. All antiphlogistic treatment until this is accomplished is in vain. Cold may be applied with advantage for the first eight-and-forty hours, and in most cases all will do well. I do not say all, but most, I strongly believe, would. Sufficient attention I am convinced in general is not paid in the treatment of fractures and other injuries attended with inflammatory action, to the position of the affected part. In the University College Hospital, where, under the auspices of Mr. Liston, it has received a good deal of attention, the use of leeches, evaporating lotions, &c. is entirely dispensed with, and found unnecessary. I would request Mr. M'Cash to withhold his decision on the value of the practice he strongly condemns until he has given it a further trial; I do not ask him blindly to follow any one's theories or practices, but only to form his own on sufficient grounds. Let him give the plan he condemns a fair trial, and he will be convinced of its value.

MODIFICATION OF DR. ARNOTT'S HYDROSTATIC BED.

To the Editor of the Medical Gazette.

Sir,

I beg to transmit to you a description of a modification of Dr. Arnott's hydrostatic bed, which I think will be found more convenient than those now in use.

A bed-frame is prepared, with feet, sides, and ends, similar to those of ordinary beds. At three or four inches within the side bars two others are placed parallel to them, leaving in the centre an open space at least two feet broad. A sheet of strong canvas is stretched over the whole, and laced with a cord to the ends and external lateral bars, sufficiently slack to allow the part between the two internal bars to be depressed nine inches in the centre, and only two or three inches at each end. In the cavity of this depression is placed a sack of water-tight Macintosh cloth, large enough to allow the introduction of twenty or thirty gallons of water, without producing any tension; it must remain perfectly flaccid. The sack which I use is six feet long by three feet wide, with a narrow neck about a foot long; but it is larger than is absolutely necessary. The neck is brought through the foot-board of the bed, to the outside, where water is introduced; sufficient being employed to fill the sack to within half or three-fourths of an inch of the level of the frame of the bed. The apparatus now presents the appearance of a nearly level surface, consisting of two lateral planes, rigid and tense, and one central plane of the greatest possible softness. A thin mattress ($1\frac{1}{2}$ to 2

inches thick) and bed-clothes now being laid on this surface, the bed is ready for use.

The advantages of this bed over those hitherto in use are as follow:—

First and chiefly, much greater facility of ventilation. Ten years ago I had one constructed on Dr. Arnott's plan, and have had frequent opportunities, during that time, of knowing the very great relief afforded by it, in the practice of several medical gentlemen who have used it, to persons in the last stages of illness, and also to some who have even ascribed their recovery to it. But there has generally been some difficulty in preventing the accumulation of condensed perspiration in the hollow of the trough upon the Macintosh cloth. This has been remedied to a certain extent by interposing between the mattress and the water a network of corks strung together, with the view of forming a stratum freely permeable to the air; but the ventilation so obtained has seldom been perfect. In the bed which I now describe there is a smaller surface for the condensation of moisture, and there are no upright sides impeding ventilation. A small stratum of corks may be used, but even that is not always necessary; and the most of the bed requires none at any time.

Second, superior portability. There being no metal work, nor wooden box to contain it, the whole is much lighter and more manageable,—an object, however apparently trivial, always of some importance, especially in a sick chamber.

Third, less water is sufficient. The quantity can be reduced almost to the minimum which will float a man, by lacing the canvas proportionally tight. When the patient is large and heavy, more water is required to float him, and the lacing can be slackened accordingly.

Fourth, less expense. I do not know the price for which hydrostatic beds are made in London, but that which I have now described was only half the expense of the other made with the zinc trough.

There is no necessity to close the orifice by which water is admitted; it requires simply to be turned upwards, and supported with a loose string, to prevent the water from flowing out by the movements of the patient: the un-

dulations never exceed a few inches.
For discharging the water when it is
desired to remove the apparatus, a sy-
phon is introduced at the orifice to the
deepest part of the sack.

In pouring in the water, a quantity
of air is liable to be carried along with
it, which elevates the upper side of the
sack, and accumulates there. Although
more yielding even than water, it defeats the whole design, and forms salient and tense protuberances. It is
easily discharged by drawing the arm,
with a little pressure, over the surface
of the sack from the bottom to the
neck.—I am, sir,

Your obedient servant,

H. OGDEN, M.D.

Sunderland, Aug. 5, 1843.

DEATH OF; THE CORNEA FROM
CHEMOSIS ; . ADVANTAGE OF
MERCURY IN IRITIS; SIZE OF
THE IMAGES ON THE RETINA.

To the Editor of the Medical Gazette.

SIR,

IN your number for July 28, Dr. J. C.
Hall inquires—

1st.—If the priority of " *the notion,
that in purulent ophthalmia the cornea
dies from the pressure caused by the chemosed conjunctiva,*" does not belong to
Mr. Middlemore, to whom it belongs.

2d.—If the priority of the "*demonstration of the advantage of mercury
in iritis*" does not belong to Dr. Farre,
to whom it belongs.

The two following extracts may,
perhaps, assist Dr. Hall in solving these
questions.

" Other causes, no doubt, concur, in
the puro-mucous inflammation of the
conjunctiva, to produce opacities of the
cornea, detachment of its conjunctival
covering, and ulceration, and, in particular, the maceration of the cornea in
a flood of purulent fluid, not sedulously
removed by injections. But the destruction of the cornea by infiltration
of pus and sloughing I am disposed to
refer in no small degree to the pressure
of the chemosed conjunctiva, and the
consequent mechanical death of the
cornea."—*Mackenzie's Practical Treatise on the Diseases of the Eye,* p. 331.
London, 1830.

" *Wenn der Arzt am Ende des zwey-*

ten Zeitraumes, &c." In English, thus—

" When the practitioner observes at
the end of the second stage, that the
lymphatic effusion in the posterior
chamber (though not preventing, still
greatly limiting vision), does not
diminish by the treatment which is
pursued, so as to allow a hope for the
complete restoration of sight; but on
the contrary, that there is reason to
dread that the lymphatic effusion will
remain in the same state after the
second stage has terminated; then not
only external, but internal alterative
medicines must be had recourse to, in
conjunction with the other remedies
proper in this stage of the disease; that
is, the preparations of mercury must be
employed, which in such circumstances
will never disappoint, if properly
managed. Calomel, united with opium,
is to be given internally. Frictions
once a day, over the eyebrow, with
mercurial ointment, opium being added
to it, very much contribute to the absorption of the lymph effused into the
posterior chamber.

" Whoever has not witnessed the
striking effect of such a method of
treatment of iritis in this stage, cannot
possibly form any idea of the extraordinary and rapid improvement, which,
when properly conducted, it often in a
few days produces. I have repeatedly
seen a whitish net-work in the pupil,
and which was distinguishable at a distance, disappear in eight or ten days."
—Beer's Lehre von der Augenkrankhei-
ten, vol. i. p. 449. Vienna, 1813.

These extracts will probably satisfy
Dr. Hall's inquiries. I may mention,
however, that Beer recommended mercury in 1799 for iritis, although the
term was not used till 1801, which it
was first by Schmidt.

Since I have the pen in my hand, I
may say I am sorry Mr. Mayo has not
seen fit to return any answer to a query
I used the freedom to propound to him
some months ago, through the MEDICAL
GAZETTE.

The sages say, Dame Truth delights to dwell,
Strange mansion ! at the bottom of a well.
Questions are then the windlass and the rope
That pull the grave old gentlewoman up.

In his " Nervous System and its
Functions," Mr. Mayo announced what
I conceived an important optical discovery, viz. that the angular breadth
and height of the inverted picture on
the retina were one-half of those of the
object so represented. He says (p. 130)

that this is *easily shown* to be the case. What I wanted to know when I sent my former query, and what I still feel anxious to discover, is the proof of Mr. Mayo's doctrine. If Mr. Mayo can give no proof, but has hurriedly published a statement which does not bear investigation, it would only show a becoming respect to the purchasers of his book at once to say so.

I remain, sir,
Your obedient servant,
A MEDICAL STUDENT.

August 4th, 1843.

OBSERVATIONS

UPON THE

NEW PROCESS PROPOSED FOR THE DETECTION OF CORROSIVE SUBLIMATE

BY MEANS OF

METALLIC SILVER.

BY FORENSIS.

(*For the London Medical Gazette.*)

[POSTSCRIPT TO PAPER IN NO. FOR AUG. 4.]

SINCE my former remarks were written, the whole of the facts have been reconsidered, and the experiments upon which they are founded repeated, while other new ones have been instituted, not only with a view to revision, but also to greater accuracy and superior delicacy. The following may be stated as the additional results. First, it may be observed of *tin*, as a reducing agent, that a portion unites to the chlorine disengaged from the mercury, while another amalgamates with the latter. The newly formed chloride should be removed by solution, or otherwise it will sublime together with the reduced mercury, and obscure the globules. Secondly, the fusing point of tin is inconveniently low, being only 442° Fahr., or somewhat less than two-thirds of that required for the volatilization of mercury: therefore, it is advantageous to separate the tin previous to sublimation. If the amalgam be distilled, the boiling tin is apt to sputter, and be thrown into the upper part of the tube, and reamalgamating with the mercury, renders it pasty, and incapable of assuming its characteristic globular form. The same facts also give rise to a source of error: the tin, during fusion, is frequently formed into very minute globules, which, thrown out upon a tray of white paper, roll about, presenting to the naked eye the appearance of very minute black spherules, and which may readily be mistaken for mercurial sphericles, more especially as they present the metallic lustre when examined by a lens, and indeed, in all appearances, so closely resemble the mercurial globule, that, in many cases, they cannot be distinguished, unless the eye be aided by an achromatic glass. The mechanical properties, however, will enable us to distinguish them. The tin, pressed by the point of a penknife, feels firm, hard, and resists the pressure, and when pressed by the extreme point, bounds from under it. The tin globules, collected and placed in contact with each other, do not coalesce, nor unite into a single globule, but remain separate and of the original number. The mercurial globules, on the contrary, present the very reverse of these characters. When the globules consist of a mixture or amalgam of tin and mercury, if pressed by an iron blade they will be found to be pasty and viscid, and without any, or at least a great deal less, tendency to preserve the globular form; nor will it divide into a number of minuter spherules, as pure mercury invariably does under similar circumstances.

The fusing point of silver (1873° Fah.) in part frees it from some of these inconveniences, especially those more immediately dependent on the lower fusing point of tin. Still, however, it is liable to other inconveniences, and which seem to be essentially connected with, and indeed inseparable from, all capability of amalgamating with mercury. For example, the globules sublimed from the silver amalgams occasionally fall back again upon the silver, and reamalgamate. When the quantity of mercury is sufficient, this perhaps is a matter of little moment, as enough of the sublimed metal may generally be secured for complete and satisfactory identification; but when the quantity is extremely minute, and scarcely sufficient for appreciation by the unaided sense, the most trivial circumstance, as a rough handling, shaking, or jerking of the reducing tube, will throw back the globule, and give rise to reamalgamation. Since the first part of the present paper, I have seen this happen more than once; and the purer the mercury, the more free from all contamination, and the cleaner the subliming tube, the more likely an accident of this description, especially in rough hands. In the silver amalgam the silver cannot easily, as in the case of tin, be separated, so as to leave the mercury free and pure. Heating and subliming the mercury presents the only practical method.

I was induced, in consequence of the above, to try clean, bright, and very fine iron filings. So far as I have been able to determine they are equally delicate with the agents already considered, and at the same time free from all the objections just noticed, inasmuch as they form no amalgam, and are wholly infusible in a tube. It is a familiar fact, that iron reduces bichloride of mercury to the metallic state, and if a drop of a solution of bichloride supported upon a piece of gold be transfixed by a clean iron wire, so that the gold be touched with the wire through the fluid, *metallic* mercury is instantly deposited at the point of contact, and for some distance around, and an amalgam formed. If iron filings be rubbed with either bichloride of mercury or calomel, and the mixture heated in a tube of hard glass, mercurial globules sublime. Even when the quantity is very minute, the $\frac{1}{100}$ of a grain, if the mass, after ignition, be thrown out upon a tray of paper, minute globules of mercury may be detected, by the aid of a good lens, amongst the particles of iron, and may be removed by the point of a steel wire or pen-knife moistened with saliva, and when all collected may be united into a single globule. With the globules of mercury, the *chloride of iron*, formed by the decomposition of the mercurial chloride, sublimes; but this inconvenience may be avoided by digesting with hydrochloric acid, or dilute sulphuric acid, by which the *whole* of the iron will be removed, and pure mercury only remain behind for subsequent sublimation.

From the foregoing facts, which I have considered sufficiently important to justify this postscript, I think it will appear that when we wish to reduce corrosive sublimate in the dry way, *iron filings present* the best reducing agent; that in organic complication the solution of the mercurial by converting it into *bichloride* either by a cement of chlorine, or by nitro-hydrochloric acid, forms an essential preliminary. Having effected this, that the precipitation of metallic mercury either by solution of proto-chloride of tin, or by phosphorons, or hypo-phosphorous acid, is superior to every other method hitherto proposed, and the only one that can be *safely* practised in medico-legal analysis.

August 6, 1843.

MEDICAL GAZETTE.

Friday, August 11, 1843.

"Licet omnibus, licet etiam mihi, dignitatem *Artis Medicæ* tueri; potestas modo veniendi in publicum sit, dicendi periculum non recuso."
CICERO

WOMEN AND CHILDREN AS AGRICULTURAL LABOURERS.

IN our late articles on this important subject, we confined our comments to one only of the reports made by the four special assistant-commissioners. We will now, before dismissing the subject, briefly touch upon a few points in the remaining three reports.

Mr. Vaughan pursued his inquiries in the counties of Kent, Surrey, and Sussex.

It is remarkable that he thought it incumbent upon him to take the evidence, or the greater part of it, upon oath. We have always been of opinion with Paley, that the multitude of oaths taken in England are highly unfavourable to morality; and we are happy to see that of late years the current of legislation has set against them. A pound of tea can now pass through the Custom-House unaided by the half-dozen oaths which it required in Paley's time; and we think that the duties and rewards of hop-pickers and fruit-gatherers might have been ascertained without so solemn an appeal.

The great formations of the wealden (*i. e.* woodland), the sand, and the chalk, belong to all these three counties. The wealden is girt with a belt of chalk hills; while a fringe of sand unites the two; and "the sand," says the reporter, "as it rises into the chalk, furnishes some of the most celebrated hop-gardens and orchards."

Field-labour appears to Mr. Vaughan to be generally beneficial to the health of women and children. As to the kinds of labour performed by women, local customs vary even within a short tract of country. Thus, "about Tunbridge Wells, women are rarely employed in opening the hills* in the hop-grounds. At Maidstone and Farnham it is their common occupation. At Maidstone, again, the woman opens the hills, and the man cuts the plants; at Farnham, the man opens the hills, and the woman cuts the plants. In some places the woman does not bind the corn, but only makes the bands; in others, the binding is generally assigned to her."

To the general healthiness of their occupations there are a couple of exceptions. If the hop-picking season proves a rainy one, the women and children suffer from standing for hours upon the wet ground, and diarrhœa is a common consequence. The heavy boots worn by young boys to walk over corn lands, produce great weakness about the ankle-joints.

Mr. Vaughan believes that in the hop districts a woman earns thirty shillings during the tying season, and twenty pence a day while the picking lasts. At ordinary times her wages are far less, say ten pence a day.

The labourer, in many districts, suffers from the high prices of village shops, where he is obliged to buy

* In the language of the hop-garden, "to open the hills" means to open the elevated surface round the plants, in order to get at and prune the lower part of the last year's shoots.

inferior articles at extravagant rates, or else go to an inconvenient distance after a hard day's toil. If a labourer has run up a score at the village shop, he has not even this painful alternative left him. In vain he complains of the dearness of his creditor's goods: " deal here, or pay your debt, is the practical argument."

Henry Duppa, Esq. of Frimingham House, near Maidstone, has, in consequence, changed the hour of paying his labourers on Saturday, from 7 P.M. to 9 A.M. and they have all quitted the village shops for the better and cheaper ones of Maidstone. This evil of dealing at bad shops is aggravated in certain districts by the mode in which wages are paid. In some of the villages towards the north-east of Sussex (about Brede and Sedlescomb) the unfortunate husbandman is often paid by checks drawn on the shopkeeper or miller. It is unnecessary to comment upon this; the statement of the fact is sufficient.

But let us turn to brighter scenes. The allotment system, though not general throughout these countries, has been tried in a majority of districts, and is productive of a hundred advantages.

"Allotments may be looked upon as an attempt to aid the industry of the man by that of his wife and child, to divert both from a closed or unprofitable market, as well as to exempt money from the toll of village prices. They especially affect the wife and children, both as employment and as wages, giving them a light and profitable agriculture, and furnishing them with articles of common consumption untaxed by any intermediate profits between the soil and the cottage larder. • • • • In some parts there are allotments especially devoted to children."

An agriculturist in the west of Sussex says that an allotment enables the wife to improve her cookery, and revives the use of vegetables, almost lost, by eating, for a series of years, little but bread and butter and cheese from the village shops.

Next to the allotments in importance come clothing and benefit clubs. The former are in part a charity, as the savings of the labourer are met by equal subscriptions from his wealthier neighbours; the latter clubs are generally unassisted.

In hop districts the morals of the resident population appear to be tainted by the recruits during the season of picking. Thus the parish of Farnham contains about 7000 inhabitants; but during the hop-picking there is an accession of between 4000 and 5000 strangers. They come chiefly from towns and villages within twenty miles; but some are labourers without a settled home, and some are gipsies.

In the parish of Farlegh, near Maidstone, a great number of the English hands come from St. Giles's, Saffron Hill, &c.; and they are the most vicious and refractory. The Irish, though dirty in person and habits, indelicate in conduct and appearance, and frequently bringing contagious disorders with them, are more controllable.

As to education, it is at a very low ebb indeed. Those of our readers who recollect our papers on the employment of women and children in mines, and on the reports of the Registrar-general, will not be surprised at the testimony of Mr. Vaughan on this point. "Great ignorance, if it does not prevail, is at least to be met with, where no special pains are taken to discover it. It is quite common to meet with boys engaged in farms who cannot read or write. The unity of God, a future state, the number of months in the year, are matters not universally known."

In quitting the instructive and well-written report of Mr. Vaughan, we must not omit a point in the evidence of one of his witnesses painfully characteristic of the age in which we live.

Henry Edwards Payne, Esq. deposes upon oath that he is secretary to the Rye Agricultural Association, and informs us that prizes are given by this society to labourers thirty years of age, *who shall have remained single up to that time*, and shall have worked for the longest period on the same property, or in the same service.

The legislators of old thought very differently on this point:—

———— fuit hæc sapientia quondam,
* * * * *
Concubitu prohibere vago, dare jura maritis.

"To make men husbands, and to keep them so," was the aim of the Pagan lawgiver; your Rye Association is only eager "to prevent imprudent marriages," careless of the *concubitus vagus*.

Mr. Denison reports upon the state of Suffolk, Norfolk, and Lincoln. The wages of women in the two former counties are, on an average, eightpence a day; in Lincolnshire he thinks that tenpence is now the average: for this they usually work eight hours in winter, and ten in summer. The labouring classes in Lincolnshire are much better off than in Suffolk and Norfolk.

Mr. Denison appears to lean to the opinion of the farmers, that "education is being carried too far." But, assuredly, the evidence poured upon us from all quarters would rather show that education has yet to begin. Even the number of the months not universally known!

All the persons (with two exceptions) to whom Mr. Denison applied for information respecting the allotment system, spoke strongly in its favour.

The gang-system is the very antipodes of this. The labourer possessed of an allotment almost rises into the rank of a petty farmer; and the cultivation of a separate piece of ground has often converted the slovenly pauper into a diligent husbandman. The head-quarters of the gang-system, in its full-blown state, are at Castle Acre, near Litcham, in Norfolk, and the system itself is as follows. A farmer who wishes to have a piece of work done, contracts with a gang-master, who, in his turn, hires a miscellaneous group of men, women, and children. The gang-master, scarcely, if at all, above the rank of a labourer, squeezes his profit out of the gang, by grinding down their wages to the lowest possible rate, uninfluenced by the motives of compassion or decency, which might be found in the ranks above him; while the superabundant population of Castle Acre gives full scope to his thirst of gain. In a word, the gang-master " regards the labourer solely as a living instrument, valuable only in proportion to its available power;" bad character is no bar to admission into a gang; and the promiscuous assemblage of men and girls in these gangs is unfavourable to virtue; " I should not like myself to take a wife out of the gang;" says one of their overseers!

Sir F. H. Doyle reports upon the condition of Yorkshire and Northumberland. In Yorkshire, the wages of women are 10d. a day at one season, and 1s. at another; but as their work is partial and uncertain, its remuneration is not, on the average, more than 2s. a week, or £5. 4s. a year.

We are glad to find that Sir F. H. Doyle stands up for the cottager's pig. " Of such a pig, the first product of allotment, garden, or potatoe head-land, it is the fashion among political economists to speak disrespectfully. Now, whatever might be the superior profit of the cottager, of saving the money which he spends upon his pig, and buying his bacon in the market, this, as it never

has been, and never will be so saved, we may dismiss."

Moreover, the pig, besides being a profit, is a pleasure to its keeper, and we feel, with Sir F. H. Doyle, that to discourage the practice would be an act of consummate cruelty to the cottager.

We have barely room to notice the prominent feature of Northumbrian husbandry. The hind (or labourer) has a yearly instead of a weekly engagement. He is provided with a rent-free cottage and garden, and is paid four or five pounds a year in cash, and the rest of his wages in kind. Thus Mr. Grey, manager of the Greenwich Hospital estates near Hexham, gives each of his hinds 36 bushels of oats, 24 of barley, 12 of peas, 3 of wheat, 3 of rye, from 36 to 40 of potatoes, 24 lbs. of wool, a cow's keep for the year, coals carrying [carried?] from the pit, and £4. in money. In return for this, the hind, besides his own work, is bound to provide a female labourer, to work for his master at stipulated wages. This woman, who is called a *bondager*, is usually the hind's daughter or sister, and her wages are commonly 10d. a day, or 1s. in harvest.

A great objection to this plan is the wretchedness of these rent-free cottages; for they generally contain but one room, perhaps 17 feet by 15; in construction and ventilation they are most miserable; and the want of separation between the sexes implied by their single apartment is utterly indefensible. Improvement in this point has begun, but it is not so rapid as it ought to be. " I hope, however, and believe," says Sir F. H. Doyle, " that the landowners of Northumberland,—and not of Northumberland alone, — are becoming every day more deeply impressed with the feeling, that some sacrifice of time and thought, and even of amusement, in order to promote the general well-being of their dependents, is not a charity, but a duty,—the moral rent-charge attached to their properties by the state, from which they were derived."

PRESENTATION OF A GOLD MEDAL TO SIR BENJAMIN BRODIE.

ON Thursday last a dinner took place at Willis's Rooms, King Street, St. James's, for the purpose of presenting to Sir Benjamin Brodie a Gold Medal as a testimonial of esteem and respect on the occasion of his resigning (two years since) the office of surgeon to St. George's Hospital. Sir Charles Clarke presided. About 120 sat down to dinner, including many of the most distinguished members of the profession.

After the health of Her Majesty had been drank, the Chairman proposed that of Sir Benjamin Brodie, to whom he then presented the Medal, with an address, in which he highly complimented his distinguished friend. Our limits, however, oblige us to confine ourselves to Sir Benjamin's reply, which he delivered with a great deal of feeling.

Mr. President: It is, sir, no affectation in me to say that I really want words to express what I feel on this occasion; for whilst, sir, on the one hand, I am sensible of the honour you have conferred upon me, considering it as the proudest distinction of my life—while I am gratified to see so many of my old friends, so many of my pupils, so many individuals distinguished in the world, not disdaining to be here this evening—while I am gratified, also, by the favourable sentiments expressed by yourself, and which others have not less cordially responded to —Sir, I cannot but feel that all this is more than really belongs to me: that I am indebted to the kindness and partiality of my friends, rather than to my own merits; and that there are other individuals who have laboured in the same vineyard, far more worthy than myself, and to whom the profession owe obligations greater than they owe to me. The consequence of this is, that at this moment a feeling of humility is united in my mind with that of gratified ambition. But out of this, sir, arises another feeling, in which there is no complication, which, pure and unalloyed, will descend with me to the grave,—that is, gratitude to you, sir, and my other friends, for your generosity and kindness. Sir, when I first entered on the profession to which I belong, that profession became to me my world, in which I lived and moved and had my being. I thought of no distinction that was unconnected with it. I had no hope, I desired no

further reputation, and there was no object nearer to my heart than that of having the good opinion of those with whom I was associated. Sir, a long lapse of years, and a more extended intercourse with the world, and a more varied acquaintance with men and manners, have made no alteration in these my sentiments. I have never wished that I could retrace my steps, and begin my career in another sphere of life. I know no profession which, after all, is preferable to ours. I know of no profession which possesses so honourable an independence; Sir, I know of none. I know of no order of men who are more disinterested, or who are more ready to perform gratuitous acts of kindness, than the members of the medical profession; and who, in addition to their moral qualifications, are more distinguished for their good sense, and freedom from prejudice, as well as for their general knowledge and attainments. And, sir, having mixed a good deal with other portions of society, I am only too happy to fall back upon my own profession as affording me the best examples of moral character, the most prudent counsellors, and the kindest friends.

Sir, you have been pleased to revert to my publications connected with physiology and surgery. With respect to the former, I consider the chief merit they have is, that they may have led others to work in the same field; and my ambition respecting them will be fully satisfied if they have been found of any use in getting my professional brethren through the difficult labyrinth of surgical practice.

But, sir, you have been also pleased to speak of me in connexion with St. George's Hospital, and of my services there, and you have alluded to a meeting at the Hospital for the foundation of this medal on the occasion of my resigning my office; and thinking it my duty to speak on this occasion of St. George's Hospital, I beg to say that, to St. George's Hospital, to the Medical School attached to it, to my colleagues and pupils there, I am mainly indebted for the advantages I have possessed in my profession. The name of St. George's Hospital is associated with my most interesting recollections; with hopes and fears, and joys and sorrows, which have long since passed away, with my young ambition,—the anxieties and aspirations of my early life. Sir, it was my good fortune to be elected to the office of assistant-surgeon to St. George's Hospital at an unusually early period, and to hold it for a considerable time. It was in St. George's Hospital I was enabled to lay the foundation of what little knowledge of pathology and surgery I may now possess, and there the happiest hours of my life have been passed. Everything there, sir, tended to my improvement. The study of the patients cases, the observation I had to make in the wards, the discourses and conversations I had with others, and last, sir, but not least, my friendly intercourse with the pupils, among whom I am happy to say I have preserved a large proportion as my friends, I hope, for life. Then, sir, in common with others, I had this advantage, that St. George's Hospital always presented to my mind the names of some of the brightest examples of professional skill in former times—the name of Cheselden among the proudest. It was there Sir Cæsar Hawkins rose, and there that John Hunter pursued those eminent researches in physiology that were destined to alter the condition of the human race. There, sir, I find the names of both the Heberdens, father and son, distinguished alike as practical physicians, accomplished scholars, and gentlemen. There I found the names of many distinguished for their private worth, integrity, and virtues. But, sir, it would be ungracious in me, on such an occasion as this, if I did not also recur to the name of another individual, to whom, as a living example at the time I was student, and afterwards assistant-surgeon at St. George's Hospital, I am still more indebted —I mean Sir Everard Home, who, at that time, devoted his whole energy, every hour in the day, to some useful undertaking in the performance of the duties of a surgeon. Sir, he had this great quality, which it would be well not only for the members of his own profession, but persons in all situations, to imitate, that when a difficulty occurred to him, instead of shrinking from it, it seemed to be the object of his mind to meet and to surmount it. But, sir, his name has long since been added to the list of those who belong to the times that are past; and when that circumstance accidentally comes to my mind it recals the scenes of my early life, and I am sometimes startled when I recollect all at once that I am so far advanced in my worldly course. This, sir, is no vain sentiment, and among the numerous debts of gratitude I owe, I know of none greater than this, that the friends and associates of my early life are my friends and associates still, and many of them have done me the honour of being present on this occasion. To that list of friends I have been enabled to add another and greater pleasure, that they are taken from those who were my pupils.

Sir, much as I am indebted to those who have done me the present great honour, I am still farther indebted to them for having allowed me to receive this gift from the hands of one whose conduct has gained the respect of every member of the profession, and to whom I have myself been bound by a long and an uninterrupted friendship."

Sir Benjamin was often interrupted in the course of his speech by marks of applause, and sat down amid long-continued cheering.

Before sitting down, Sir Benjamin proposed the health of the chairman, after which that of Dr. Chambers was drank with the warmest cordiality. A few other toasts were given, but we have not space left to allude to them.

UNIVERSITY OF LONDON.

BACHELOR OF MEDICINE.—PASS EXAMINATION, 1843.

Monday, Aug. 7.—Morning, 10 to 1.

Anatomy and Physiology.

Examiners, Mr. KIERNAN & Prof. SHARPEY.

1. A vertical section of the Skull being made in the median plane, and in the dry state, and the septum nasi being removed, describe the parts brought into view. Commence the answer by enumerating the bones divided in the section, and proceed with the description in the following order, mentioning the processes, depressions, and foramina,—1st, the inner surface of the cranium; 2nd, the roof, floor and outer wall of the nasal cavity; 3rd, the roof of the mouth and the inner surface of the inferior maxillary bone. The attachments of muscles not required.

2. Commencing the dissection at the Integuments, and proceeding with it as far as the outer surface of the Internal Pterygoid and the Styloid muscles, describe the parts successively exposed in dissecting the space bounded above by the Zygoma, below by the base of the inferior maxilla, in front by the anterior margin of the Masseter, and behind by the Meatus Auditorius, Mastoid process, and upper part of the Sterno-Cleido-Mastoideus.

3. Give the anatomy of the external circumflex artery of the Thigh; state the steps of the dissection required to display it in its entire course, and describe the parts exposed in the dissection.

4. Describe the soft parts met with in dissecting the anterior and outer region of the leg, and the dorsum of the foot.

5. Give a description of the Duodenum, comprehending its form, situation, connections and structure, its vessels and nerves, Brunner's glands, and the mode of opening of the ciliary and pancreatic ducts.

Afternoon, 3 to 6.

1. The Vertebral Column and the rami of the lower jaw being removed, describe the external surface of the Pharynx, the attachments of its muscles, and the course of their

fibres; and the muscles of the soft palate as far as they can be seen in this stage of the dissection. The pharynx being opened from behind, describe the parts then brought into view; the description to include that of the posterior nares, the soft palate, its arches and muscles, isthmus faucium, the dorsum of the tongue, its glands and papillæ, the Epiglottis and its folds, and the superior aperture of the Larynx.

2. Give the dissection required to expose the internal pudic artery and its branches, after it has turned round the spinous process of the ischium; commencing the dissection in the perineum, and describing the parts which successively appear in the progress of it.

3. Commencing the dissection at the inner surface of the lower portion of the anterior superior spinous process of the Ilium to the mesial line, and dissecting from above downwards, and from the peritoneum to the integuments, describe the parts successively exposed, particularly with reference to the Inguinal canal, its contents and boundaries.

3. Give the structure and chemical composition of Muscular tissue, the arrangement of its nerves and blood-vessels, and the difference in structure between voluntary and involuntary muscles.

5. By what mechanism is air introduced into and expelled from the lungs in respiration? Enumerate the muscles which are constantly, and those which are only occasionally employed in inspiration and expiration.

Tuesday, August 8.—Morning, 10 to 1.

Chemistry.

Examiner, PROFESSOR DANIELL.

1. A saline powder will be placed before you with a blow-pipe, lamp and charcoal: test the powder, state its composition, and describe the phenomena which it presents by the application of the flame, and explain their causes.

2. A saline solution will be placed before you marked A, with appropriate tests: explain the changes which will take place upon their application, and name the acid and base of which the salt has been composed.

3. What was the great fault of the thermometer as originally constructed by the Italian philosophers at the beginning of the 17th century? and how was it corrected by Sir Isaac Newton?

4. Describe the processes by which uniformity of temperature is brought about in a system of bodies originally of different temperatures, and the principal circumstances which influence each.

5. Describe and explain the principal phenomena of electric induction.

6. What were the respective shares of Galvani and Volta in the discovery of galvanism or voltaic electricity? Describe and explain the fundamental experiments of each.

7. What are the principal advantages which the science of Chemistry has derived from the establishment of Dalton's atomic theory?

8. How may the presence of nitrogen be detected, and its amount be ascertained in an organic compound?

9. What is phosphorus? State its principal physical properties, its equivalent number, and describe its combinations with oxygen.

Afternoon, 3 to 6.

Materia Medica and Pharmacy.

Examiner, DR. PEREIRA.

1. Describe the method of preparing the *Antimonii Potassio tartras* according to the London Pharmacopœia, and explain the chemical changes which attend the process. State the composition, effects, uses, and doses of this salt, and also the tests by which its presence may be recognised.

2. Give the botanical characters of *Aconitum Napellus*. Mention the peculiarities of its action on the system; name the diseases for which it is especially adapted; and state the best mode of using it externally as well as internally.

3. How would you distinguish *Liquor Sodæ effervescens*, Ph. L., from mere carbonic acid water? With what metal is the soda water of the shops frequently contaminated, and how would you detect the impurity?

4. What are the appropriate doses, for an adult, of the following substances:—Benzoic acid, sal ammoniac, trisnitrate of bismuth, biniodide of mercury, and bromide of potassium?

5. How would you detect the adulteration of balsam of copaiba with castor oil?

6. Enumerate the principal cathartics. In how many groups or orders may they be conveniently arranged? What are the peculiar effects and uses of each group?

Afternoon, 3 to 6.

Structural and Physiological Botany.

Examiner, Prof. HENSLOW.

1. Compare a campanulate with a rotate corolla: and a corymbiform with an umbellate inflorescence. Illustrate your comparison by a slight sketch of each.

2. Whence does the arillus originate? Name two good examples of plants of different families in which it occurs.

3. How do you explain the formation of central and parietal placentæ? Name an example of each.

4. What is the nature of vegetable albu-

men? Is it found in the seeds of ranunculus, pisum, sinapis, primula, and geranium?

5. What is a stipule? Are the plants in rosaceæ, leguminosæ, cruciferæ, generally stipulate or not?

6. How is the genus cuscuta supplied with nourishment? What peculiarity is observable in the structure of its embryo?

7. What are "adventitious buds"; and how do you suppose they have originated?

8. 9. 10. Describe these specimens.

COMPOSITION OF MILK.

M. DONNÉ has read a memoir on this subject before the Academy, in which he has established the existence of a striking analogy between milk and blood, an analogy not contradicted by experiments on animals. In each is found serum containing, in solution, a specially azotised matter, coagulable spontaneously, and a great number of substances representing all the materials for organization. In suspension are found concrete particles called globules, which are of very complex structure in the blood, much more simple in milk. Milk owes its whiteness and opacity to its globules of fatty matter, as blood owes its colour to the red particles. Milk may be said to be a sort of emulsion, in which is suspended fatty or buttery matter in a state of extreme division. Filtering, so as to separate nearly all the fatty particles, deprives milk of its whiteness and opacity, leaving it a clear fluid, transparent or only slightly opaline. In pursuing the analogy between milk and blood, M. Donné has injected considerable portions of the former into the veins of animals: not only does this injection of a fluid, which cannot be called inert, produce no disturbance to the state of functions of animals, excepting, from some cause unknown, the horse, but its globules seem to perform the part of the chylous globules, being changed, like them, directly into blood globules. M. Donné relates the different experiments made by him in the nourishment of young animals by means of milk and of soup; and having shown the great difference to health from their respective use, infers that the consumption of milk is a subject of great hygienic interest, especially in populous cities, and inquires if it be possible to increase the consumption, and amend the qualities of this valuable aliment, and thereby to render a signal benefit to public health.

PARIS MILK.

SPEAKING of the milk in Paris, and especially the supply to the hospitals, M. Donné says, "the state of the milk in the hospitals, as to its alimentary qualities, is truly deplorable. At most, if not all, the different establishments for the sick poor, the milk will be found so poor in substantial elements as to furnish hardly three or four per cent. of cream, instead of eight or ten per cent., the average proportion. Even this milk is diluted with water, and has generally been boiled before it is supplied; and although, in the present state of science, this process seems indispensable for the preservation of milk during hot weather, yet it has the great disadvantage of making it less easy of digestion. Not only the milk used for puddings, rice milk, and other cookeries, is of this wretched quality, which would be of less consequence, but that given in its simple state to the sick, the convalescent, the lying-in women, and even to children, whose chief nourishment is derived from it. There is no effective and real *inspection* of this article, and the abuses in its supply may be inferred from the following avowal of a dealer, speaking of the dearth of forage this year, and the consequent rise in the price of milk. "In general, we add some water to our milk, but this year we shall only add some milk to our water." The guardians of public health, in fact, are not quite in possession of the causes on which this state of things depends. The easiest classes, and the most enlightened, and those most alive to their own interest and welfare, are not out of the reach of the circumstances above mentioned, but share in the consequences of the general ignorance, and the imperfect means applied to the examination of milk. The best directed public establishments, schools, and even colleges, in which the diet has been improved even to luxury, are hardly better supplied with milk than the hospitals. In hospitals and such places the bad quality depends, no doubt, on the low prices imposed on the contractors. It is absolutely impossible to give, not to say *good* milk, but *passable* milk, at 19 centimes the litre, the hospital price; 30 centimes is the lowest price at which milk can be had of a quality not first rate, but good. M. Donné thinks another cause of the evil is the want of easy, ready, and exact means for appreciating the quality and real value of milk, and that he has found such means in an instrument of his invention, which he calls a *lactoscope*. Most of the milk sold in Paris comes from within a circle ten or fifteen leagues only from the centre, and is purchased of the farmers at 30 cents the two litres, sold to dealers in the capital at 40 or 50 cents, and by them to the consumer at 50 to 70 cents—the price varying according to the quality, the extent of dilution, and the neighbourhood. Certain wholesale dealers sell from 4000 to 5000 litres a day. The difficulty of preserving and carrying milk is an obstacle to any great diminution of price that might be obtained by bringing it from greater distances. The most simple, sure, and economical method is by an apparatus consisting of two concentric cylinders, the inner one containing ice, and the outer, of double the capacity, containing the milk; both communicate with the exterior by means of stopcocks, and convenient openings for supply. The whole apparatus, made of tin, is contained in a wooden case. With this precaution, milk may be kept fifteen days through all states of temperature, atmospheric and electrical variations.—*Gazette Médicale.*

THE SALE OF ALUM TO BAKERS.

ON examining the Acts of Parliament, it appears that chemists and druggists are not liable to a fine for selling alum to bakers, although bakers are subject to penalties and imprisonment for using it in the manufacture of bread, or even having it on their premises. The law on this subject is particularly stringent on the bakers, who are liable to have their premises searched in case of any suspicion arising, and are prohibited, under severe penalties, from offering any resistance to such search. Nevertheless the law is inoperative, as bakers' bread is seldom if ever free from alum. We have been informed by some of the trade that it is *absolutely necessary* in the quartern and half-quartern loaves, which would otherwise adhere together on being withdrawn from the oven, instead of separating with facility, which is generally the case. In cottage-loaves, and other fancy-bread, the bakers admit that alum is not so necessary, and its use, in these cases, is much less frequent.

Various contrivances are adopted to evade the law. Alum is called by bakers "*stuff*," or "*the doctor.*" It is usually bought by the master, who deposits the proper quantity for each batch in some corner of the premises, where the foreman finds it at the proper time. In some houses the master is subject to a fine in case of his neglecting to provide "the doctor;" which fine is the perquisite of his journeymen. By these and other precautionary regulations, the inconvenience of detection is avoided; and although every person knows that alum is always used, no one is in possession of positive evidence of the fact, and all parties concerned keep their own counsel, being bound by that kind of "honour" which prevails "among thieves." The masters are interested in using "the doctor," because they can by this means improve the appearance of an inferior flour; and the men are equally interested in the matter, as the bread is made with less trouble. The parties aggrieved by this practice are those who *consume the bread.* Dr. Pereira, in his *Treatise on Food and Diet,* observes—

"Whatever doubts may be entertained as to the ill effects of alum on the healthy stomach, none can exist as to its injurious effects in cases of dyspepsia. Bread which contains alum is objectionable, not merely on account of this salt, but because it is generally made from inferior flour, which, when mixed with yeast and water, and formed into dough, quickly passes through the stage of vinous fermentation, and becomes acid."—*Pharmaceutical Journal.*

PATHOLOGICAL STUDIES ON MENSTRUATION.

By Dr. A. RACIBORSKI. PART II.

Academy of Science, July 24.

THE following are the conclusions drawn by the author in this memoir :—

We believe that we have shewn in this part of our memoir—1st. That the course followed by the Graafian follicles during their progressive development in women, exactly resembles that which they follow in other mammiferæ, as we may easily assure ourselves, especially by examining the ovaries of the sow.

2d. The rutting seasons offer the greatest analogy, anatomically considered, to the menstrual periods. Both are coincident with the highest degree of development of one or more follicles, and terminate by their rupture, and the expulsion of the ovum, or of a true fœtation. They have also in common a greater or less congestion of the uterus, vagina, and external organs.

3d. The menstrual periods, like those of rutting, are closely connected with the reproduction of the species.

4th. The organs described by authors under the name of *corpora lutea*, or glandular bodies, are nothing but the follicles of Graaf, in a stage of development more or less advanced.

5th. The tumefaction of the Graafian follicles, and their elevation on the surface of the ovaries, seems to be an indispensable condition for fecundation of the ova.

6th. The orgasm accompanying coition may of itself suffice to produce this state of the follicles, without its having been previously prepared by the instinctive impulses of nature: only, as in that case this state and disposition of the follicles is not completed till a longer or shorter time after coition, conception is thereby retarded, and is moreover, far less certain than when connection has taken place while the follicles were already swollen and prominent, as they are at the rutting season, and at the approach of the menstrual period.

7th. That, as regards the faculty of reproduction, woman seems to occupy a place intermediate between female animals which have seasons of heat or cutting, and those which are always capable of fecundation from the mere orgasm excited by coition, without other preparation on the part of nature. Their nature, however, approaches more nearly to that of the former class, our statistical researches having informed us that of 100 women, six or seven at the most become pregnant after sexual intercourse at a distance from the menstrual period; while in most women conception dates evidently from such intercourse *at the moment of the catamenial evacuation (sic.')*, or some days before or after the menstrual period.

PAINLESSNESS OF A MORTAL WOUND.

GREAT wounds stupify the nervous system, and there is no pain, from the impossibility of reaction. Nature is then without force, art without power, and the surgeon without hope. Here is an instance. In 1812 a regiment was marching along the sea-shore of Catalonia : being covered by a slight fog, it faced the English gun-boats, which were lying off the coast. On a sudden a wind sprung up, the fog dispersed, and the enemy's gun-boats immediately poured a very brisk fire upon our soldiers, but so badly aimed that but few were wounded. Nevertheless, a ball, making a *ricochet*, struck a soldier obliquely, and completely opened his abdomen. The skin and muscles were carried away with astonishing precision ; but this enormous wound had apparently not touched the abdominal viscera, which were escaping in every direction. There was not the shadow of hæmorrhage. I had the wounded man transported to a neighbouring village, called Tor d'en Barre. He was placed on the ground, with his head on his knapsack, and the wound was merely covered with linen. Some compassionate soldiers came to give him brandy, to help him to die, according to their expression; and he swallowed it very well. Ten times, twenty times, I asked him if he was in pain, and he always answered with a weak but clear voice, that he was quite free from pain, though he saw that certain death awaited him. He died, or rather, he was quenched, at eight in the evening, having been wounded by the ball at seven in the morning. We see that pain is not in proportion to the greatness of the hurt; and one might say that nature employs this mean only with the hope, more or less founded, of subduing the disease; otherwise what would be the advantage of it ? It is moral pain alone which remains to the last breath of life.—R. P. in the *Gazette Médicale*.

PILULA FERRI COMPOSITA.

SEVERAL methods were proposed some time ago, by members of the society, for preparing this pill in such a manner as to preserve the carbonate of iron undecomposed, and to insure the uniform consistence of the mass. Some of the plans recommended were, to a certain extent, deviations from the formula of the College. We have found, as the result of experiment, that the mass can be made according to the directions of the Pharmacopœia. and free from any of the objections which have been pointed out, by an attention to the following particulars :—

Dissolve the sulphate of iron, finely powdered, in the treacle, with a moderate heat, and add the carbonate of soda, stirring constantly until the effervescence has entirely ceased and the mixture has become cool ; then add the myrrh gradually, and incorporate the mass. As a little evaporation takes place at the commencement of the process, a small excess of treacle is requisite to supply the deficiency. This mass retains its colour and consistence remarkably well.
—*Pharmaceutical Journal.*

ON COLLECTING AND PRESERVING ROOTS FOR MEDICINAL PURPOSES.

IN a communication recently made by Dr. Houlton to the Royal Medico-Botanical Society on the above subject, he states, that all roots should be taken up at the time that their leaves die, as they then abound with the proper secretions of the plant. This rule has no exception ; it applies to the roots of trees, shrubs, herbs, rootstocks, bulbs, cormi, and tubers, and it includes that curious plant, colchicum, whose flowers only appear in the autumn, and its leaves and fruit the following spring and summer. Biennial roots must be taken up in the first year of their duration ; as, when the leaves decay in the second year, their roots are either decayed, or merely dry woody fibre. Roots intended to be preserved should be dried as soon as possible after they have been dug up ; the large tree roots, especially the more juicy, dry better in their entire state than when sliced.—*Ibid.*

DR. TODD'S CYCLOPÆDIA OF ANATOMY, PART XXV.

To the Editor of the Medical Gazette.

SIR,

WILL you oblige me, and, doubtless, many other purchasers of the Cyclopædia of

Anatomy, by asking the Editor, Dr. Todd, what he is about? On the cover of Part XXIV. was an announcement that Part XXV. would be published in October,— and where is it?—I am, sir,

Your obedient servant,
JAMES DOUGLAS.

Glasgow, July 27, 1843.

ON THE
SENSIBILITY OF THE GLOTTIS AFTER THE PERFORMANCE OF TRACHEOTOMY,

WITH THE DESCRIPTION OF A NEW INSTRUMENT.

To the Editor of the Medical Gazette.

SIR,

WILL you allow me through your journal to call the attention of Mr. Erichsen to a little circumstance of which he appears either ignorant or forgetful?

It is this : that six years ago, M. Magendie, of Paris, proved the relative sensibility of the larynx, glottis, and of the bronchial extremity of the trachea, by performing, *mirabile dictu*, the very same experiment as Mr. Erichsen has done on these parts in the same animal, the dog, and with the same instrument, a probe! And may I ask Mr. Erichsen if he ever read Will. Shakespeare's " Much Ado," &c. ?

Magendie's experiment is given in the Lancet for 36.-37, Vol. 2, p. 505.

I am, sir, your reader,

E.

University College,
July 15, 1843.

BOOKS RECEIVED FOR REVIEW.

Neurypnology ; or, the Rationale of Nervous Sleep, considered in relation with Animal Magnetism. Illustrated by numerous cases. By James Braid, M.R.C.S.E. &c.

Some Account of the African Remittent Fever, which occurred on board Her Majesty's Steam Ship Wilberforce, in the River Niger, and whilst engaged on service on the Western Coast of Africa ; comprising an inquiry into the Cause of Disease in Tropical Climates. By Morris Pritchett, M.D. &c. &c. &c.

Report upon the Phenomena of Clairvoyance, or Lucid Somnambulism (from personal observation) ; with Additional Remarks. By Edwin Lee, Esq. &c. &c.

Letter to the Right Hon. Sir Robert Peel, Bart. on the Responsibility of Monomaniacs for the Crime of Murder. By James Stark, M.D. F.R.S.E. Fellow of the Royal College of Physicians in Edinburgh.

Twenty-third Annual Report of the Directors of the Dundee Royal Asylum for *Lunatics.*

ROYAL COLLEGE OF SURGEONS.

LIST OF GENTLEMEN ADMITTED MEMBERS.

Monday, July 31, 1843.

T. B. Oldfield.—W. H. Rogers.—J. Topham.—R. Hodges.—M. J. Rowe.—W. J. Lomax.—H. B. Davies.—B. J. Webb.—W. Leshley.—A. G. Montgomery.—T. R. Evans.—T. Nicholas.

A TABLE OF MORTALITY FOR THE METROPOLIS,

Shewing the number of deaths from all causes registered in the week ending Saturday, July 29, 1843.

Small Pox	5
Measles	27
Scarlatina	32
Hooping Cough	28
Croup	5
Thrush	3
Diarrhœa	18
Dysentery	1
Cholera	2
Influenza	1
Ague	0
Remittent Fever	0
Typhus	24
Erysipelas	2
Syphilis	1
Hydrophobia	0
Diseases of the Brain, Nerves, and Senses	118
Diseases of the Lungs and other Organs of Respiration	207
Diseases of the Heart and Blood-vessels	17
Diseases of the Stomach, Liver, and other Organs of Digestion	70
Diseases of the Kidneys, &c.	1
Childbed	8
Paramenia	0
Ovarian Dropsy	0
Disease of Uterus, &c.	4
Arthritis	1
Rheumatism	2
Diseases of Joints, &c.	3
Carbuncle	0
Phlegmon	0
Ulcer	0
Fistula	0
Diseases of Skin, &c.	0
Dropsy, Cancer, and other Diseases of Uncertain Seat	109
Old Age or Natural Decay	46
Deaths by Violence, Privation, or Intemperance	13
Causes not specified	1
Deaths from all Causes	749

METEOROLOGICAL JOURNAL.

August 1843.	THERMOMETER.		BAROMETER.	
Wednesday 2	from 48 to 62		29·73 to 29·61	
Thursday . 3	54	62	29·55	Stat.
Friday . . 4	67	55	29·50	29·53
Saturday . 5	51	69	29·72	29·79
Sunday . . 6	52	68	29·83	29·97
Monday . . 7	46	67	30·01	30·12
Tuesday . 8	59	76	30·13	30·11

Wind S. and S.W. except on the 15th, when it was W. by N.

The 2d, generally cloudy and showery till the evening ; 3d, showery till the evening, much thunder during the day ; 4th, morning and afternoon very showery, thunder and lightning from 2 to 4, P. M. evening clear ; 5th, morning and evening clear, rain about noon ; 6th, generally clear, rain during the previous night ; 7th, morning and evening clear, cloudy noon and afternoon ; 8th, generally clear till the evening.

Rain fallen, 1 inch and ·245 of an inch.

WILSON & OGILVY, 57, Skinner Street, London.

THE

LONDON MEDICAL GAZETTE,

BEING A

WEEKLY JOURNAL

OF

Medicine and the Collateral Sciences.

FRIDAY, AUGUST 18, 1843.

LECTURES

ON THE

THEORY AND PRACTICE OF MIDWIFERY,

Delivered in the Theatre of St. George's Hospital,

BY ROBERT LEE, M.D. F.R.S.

—

LECTURE XXXIX.

On Inflammation of the Veins and Absorbent Vessels of the Uterus in Puerperal Women.

INFLAMMATION of the venous system was first described by Mr. Hunter, in the Transactions of a Society for the Improvement of Medical and Chirurgical Knowledge, in 1793. " I have found," he observes, " in all violent inflammations of the cellular membrane, whether spontaneous or in consequence of accident, as in compound fractures, or of surgical operations, as in the removal of an extremity, that the coats of the larger veins passing through the inflamed part become also considerably inflamed, and that their inner surface takes on the adhesive, suppurative, and ulcerative inflammation. I have found in many places of the veins adhesions, in others matter, and in others ulceration. Under such circumstances the veins would have abscesses formed in them, if the matter did not find in many cases an easy passage to the heart, along with the circulating blood, so as to prevent the accumulation of the pus; but this ready passage of the matter into the common circulation does not always happen. It is in some cases prevented by the adhesive inflammation taking place in the vein between the place of suppuration and the heart, so that an abscess is formed, as will be further observed: where the inflammation is most violent, there we find

820.—XXXII.

the vein most inflamed; there, also, after suppuration, we find the purest pus, and as we trace the vessels from this part either further from or nearer to the heart, we find the pus more and more mixed with blood, and having more and more of the coagulated parts of the blood in it. As these appearances are only to be seen in dead bodies, they cannot be described but from thence; but it is so common a case, that I have hardly ever seen an instance of suppuration in any part furnished with large veins, where the appearances are not evident after death. I have found them in the bodies of those who have died from amputation, compound fractures, and mortification." These circumstances led Mr. Hunter to suspect that the fatal effects sometimes succeeding to venesection, which had usually been attributed to injuries of tendons and nerves, depended on inflammation of the internal coats of the veins. He observed similar appearances in the veins of the arm after bleeding; and he states that in many cases the inflammation and suppuration are not confined to the part, from the adhesion not having taken place, and that an abscess is frequently formed which occupies a considerable length of the vein, both between the wound and the heart, and between the wound and the extreme parts." Upon examining the arm of a man who died in St. George's Hospital, Mr. Hunter found the veins, both above and below the orifice, in many places united by the adhesive inflammation. He also found in many parts of the veins that suppuration had begun as on inflamed surfaces, but had not arrived at ulceration, and in several other places ulceration had taken place, so as to have destroyed that surface next the skin, and a circumscribed abscess was formed. The veins near to the axilla had taken on suppuration, beyond which adhesion had not formed, and thus had given a free passage for the matter into the circulation, of which, most probably, the patient died. " Many horses," he says,

3 A

die of this disease, but what is the peculiar circumstance which occasions their death I have not been able to determine; it may either be that the inflammation extends itself to the heart, or that the matter secreted from the inside of the vein passes along the tubes in considerable quantity to the heart, and mixes with the blood. I am inclined to believe that the exposure of cavities of the larger veins, in cases of accidents and also of operations, is often the cause of many of the extensive inflammations which sometimes attend these cases, and, indeed, may be the reason why inflammations extend or spread at all beyond the sphere of continued sympathy." It does not appear that Mr. Hunter was aware of the resemblance which exists between the part of the uterus where the placenta adhered, and an amputated or wounded limb, and their liability to the same diseases, and that he had ever observed inflammation of the uterine veins in puerperal women. It is singular that this important variety of uterine inflammation should have altogether escaped his notice, considering the accuracy of the description which he has given of puerperal peritonitis, and the correct opinion he had formed respecting its nature. "The peritoneum," he says, " is more subject to spontaneous inflammation than most membranes, but not so much so as the pleura. The symptoms are great pain, and soreness upon pressure, fever much higher than in an affection of a common part; the disease also runs much quicker through its stages; it has been often taken for a fever, and the pain, &c. looked on only as a symptom; in some cases a diarrhœa comes on, and at others costiveness: both these, I am inclined to think, may be set down as sympathetic affections. It is difficult to say at first whether it is simple inflammation or erysipelatous; if it is the latter, the pulse will soon sink, although at first it might have been otherwise, from nature having been roused at the first consciousness of disease attacking so important a part. In simple inflammation of the peritoneum I need say nothing of the importance of early and plentiful bleeding; in the erysipelatous, some consideration must be had; as on the one hand, this species of inflammation sinks the patient, and on the other, death must be the consequence of suppuration. If we were confident of its being erysipelatous, how far bleeding lessens erysipelas I do not know; peritoneal inflammation *happens a few days after childbirth, which has been called puerperal fever; the fever is only a sympathetic affection, in consequence of the inflammation of the peritoneum, although this last has been thought only a symptom of fever.*"

In a volume of Essays on the Management of Pregnancy and Labour, and on the Inflammatory and Febrile Diseases of Lying-in Women, published by Dr. John Clarke in 1793, he observes that, "upon cutting into the substance of the uterus, pus is often found, which, in all the cases I have met with, is situated in the large veins of the part." In dissecting the body of a woman who died several weeks after delivery, Mr. Wilson found the uterine veins thickened and partially obliterated; the iliac, emulgent, and spermatic veins, exhibited the usual effects produced by inflammation; the coats of the vena cava were thickened and adherent to the surrounding parts, and the vessel, which was contracted below the entrance of the hepatic, contained about ℨiv. of pus. Mr. Wilson met with similar appearances in the bodies of two women who died soon after parturition, and the uterine veins also contained pus. These facts were stated in the third volume of the same work in which Mr. Hunter's paper appeared in 1793. In 1797, the attention of pathologists being now directed to the subject, Meckel communicated to Sasse the history of a case of puerperal fever, in which he found, on dissection, "all the veins which surround the uterus, the hypogastric trunks, and the vena cava, enlarged in volume; the place where the placenta had adhered was distinguished by a fungous mass. The veins, whose exterior appearance had arrested the attention, were examined with care; they were separated from the surrounding cellular substance, and in this state the whole system of uterine and spermatic veins presented an extraordinary augmentation of the calibre of the vessels and thickness of their coats; when opened, there escaped from them a true purulent fluid. The vena cava, where the right renal vein entered, presented a resisting tumefaction, and when opened, its coats were double the natural thickness, and the cavity was filled with pus, and a polypus formed of pseudo-membranous and puriform concretions. "Many circumstances," Meckel observes, "might contribute to render the disease mortal; but is it not fair," he inquires, "to attribute the occurrence of the fatal termination of the case to the profound lesion of the veins?" Uterine phlebitis, from this period till 1820, appears to have almost completely escaped observation, when it was thus described by Dr. Burns: " Pus is often contained in the ovaria and tubes, and sinuses of the uterus: he says, mortification is an extremely rare termination. This is a fact of which my dissections convince me, and it is further confirmed by the opinion of Dr. Clarke. Little or no serous effusion takes place into the abdomen. In some cases the veins participate very extensively in the disease, and become inflamed to a great distance. Thus inflammation may spread to the heart or liver, or down along the veins of one or both thighs. This is attended with great and debilitating fever, and much pain in the course of the affected veins, which, after death, are found inflamed, thickened, or filled with pus. The treatment of this complication must be conducted on the antiphlogistic plan, and a knowledge of the nature of the disease will call for early attention to local pain attended with fever." In 1825, Ribes described a fatal case of puerperal peritonitis in which the abdominal veins were filled with a sanious pus, and it was the presence of this purulent fluid in the veins, he thought, which rendered the diseases of the uterus, in puerperal women, so rapidly fatal. In 1826, M. Louis observed a fatal case of uterine phlebitis; and in the same year M. Dance published the histories of several cases, in his Inaugural Dissertation at Paris. If you look at this tabular view (No. 1) of 100 cases of uterine inflammation, you will see that 18 occurred between the 6th of March and the middle of September, 1827, and that in the greater number of these there was acute pain of the uterus, with strong febrile symptoms, and that recovery generally followed the early and speedy adoption of the antiphlogistic treatment. I was induced to believe, from what I observed at this period, that inflammation of the peritoneum, and the disease termed by authors puerperal fever, child-bed fever, the epidemic disease of lying-in women, were the same affections, and that blood-letting, mercury, antimony, opium, and cathartics, would generally succeed in procuring relief. But in the month of September of the same year, Case No. 19 occurred, and the symptoms and appearances on dissection completely overturned this opinion. On the second day after a natural labour, 28th September, 1827, and when apparently recovering favourably, this patient (Somerville) was attacked with a severe rigor, which was speedily followed by acute pain in the hypogastrium and loins, suppression of the lochia, nausea, urgent thirst, and increased heat of skin. She was soon delirious and slightly comatose, and made no complaint when roused, but of pain in the left iliac region. The abdomen was unusually distended, but neither hard nor tense, and pressure produced no uneasiness, except between the left ilium and umbilicus. The uterus was still felt above the brim of the pelvis, large and hard, and painful on pressure. The milk and lochia were suppressed, the countenance pale and anxious, pulse 130, weak, and intermitting. On the 22d the stupor continued to increase, the abdomen was more distended and painful, the respiration more hurried and laborious, and the pulse extremely quick, feeble, and intermitting. A vein was opened in the arm when she was first attacked, but a tea-cupful of blood could not be procured. On examining the body on the 23d, the intestines were

seen slightly distended with gas, but there was no trace of inflammation on any part of their peritoneal surface, and no fluid effused into the sac of the peritoneum. On turning aside the intestines, the left spermatic vein, from the uterus to its junction with the left emulgent vein, was seen distended to nearly the size of the vena cava itself. The cellular membrane surrounding it was highly vascular, and adhered closely to its external surface. On laying open the vein, a dark-coloured firm coagulum of blood filled it throughout its whole course, but it did not adhere to its internal surface, except near its termination, where it was lined with a layer of lymph. The coats of the vein were thicker and firmer than usual, and the internal membrane was of a bright scarlet colour, as was that lining the veins of the uterus near the fundus on the left side, the part to which the placenta had been attached. The substance of the uterus in this situation was of a dark livid colour, remarkably soft in its texture, and easily torn with the fingers, The corresponding ovary and fallopian tube were also very soft, and of a dark red colour, and shreds of coagulable lymph adhered closely to their surface. The left renal vein was in the same state as the spermatic, and the substance of the left kidney was soft and vascular. The connection between the constitutional symptoms in this case, and the veins of the uterus, was too obvious to escape detection.

On the 22d July, 1828, I was requested by the late Mr. Baker to deliver Ann Cromer, a patient of the St. James's Infirmary, who was eight months pregnant, and had been attacked with profuse uterine hæmorrhage from placental presentation. On the evening of the following day her pulse rose to 140, with headache, heat of skin, and intolerance of light; on that of the 24th, she had a slight rigor, and again on the 25th another exacerbation of fever, the pulse and breathing hurried. For some days subsequently she had less fever, and without evening exacerbations; the pulse ranged from 100 to 120. No pain was felt on pressure of the abdomen, although some mischief was evidently going on. On the 2d of August her breathing had again become much oppressed, with slight cough and no expectoration. The next day there was pain in the left side of the chest, and ʒxvj. of blood were drawn from the arm. On the 4th the pain was relieved, and on the 5th entirely removed, but the pulse was 120, the skin hot and dry, and there was slight expectoration of a fœtid mucus. On the 6th there was less fever, she was excessively weak, the features were sharp and anxious, and the breath was very offensive. On the 7th the expectoration was more free, thick, and purulent, and although the linen of her bed had been changed, the unpleasant smell was not diminished, and was evidently caused by her breath.   Death took place on the 9th, eighteen days after delivery.   I examined the body with Mr. Baker, when the following appearances were observed.   On opening the chest an extremely fœtid odour issued from its left cavity, in the lower part of which were contained between three and four pounds of a turbid serum, mixed with portions of coagulable lymph.   Superiorly the lung was glued to the parietes of the chest by recent loose adhesions ; inferiorly the pleura pulmonalis and corresponding pleura costalis were covered with a dense coating of coagulable lymph.   In addition to this there was on part of the surface of the inferior lobe of the lung a quantity of the same substance in a loose flaky form, on removing which there presented itself a portion of the lung in a state of complete gangrene ; this, about the size of a walnut, forming a black pulpy-looking mass of very fœtid odour, was contained, with some dark coloured fluid, in a cavity formed by its separation from the sound lung. On making a section of the parts passing through the gangrenous slough, one half of this fell out of the cavity in which it was situated, the other remaining attached to the parietes by a few thread-like adhesions. The cavity itself was lined by a layer of coagulable lymph, having the appearance of a uniform membrane.   On cutting into the uterus, which was reduced as much in size as usual at the same period, a few drops of pus flowed from one of the divided sinuses, which, being traced, I found to communicate with an abscess in the left ovarium.   I felt the left spermatic vein unusually large and hard before it was laid open, when it was found to contain pus, and its coats were seen thickened, and its inner surface lined with a layer of coagulable lymph which nearly obliterated the cavity.   These diseased changes occupied the whole course of the vein to its junction with the emulgent, the coats of which were also thickened, and the cavity lined with lymph.   The cava was healthy. There was no trace of inflammation in the peritoneum of the uterus, or general peritoneal sac.   The inflamed state of the spermatic vein would here have wholly escaped detection had I not observed the appearances described in the previous case.   I felt greatly at a loss to account for the production of so acute and destructive an inflammation of the lungs in an individual who had, previous to delivery, never suffered from any affection of the chest. I was disposed to attribute the attack to the general shock communicated to the system by the operation of turning and hæmorrhage, when I accidentally met with the following remark of Laennec, who gave a different explanation of the occurrence.   "It is not uncommon to find the veins in the neighbourhood of a cancerous breast filled with pus, either pure or mixed with blood, sometimes fluid, at other times of the degree of consistence of an atheromatous tumor. An additional consequence of the presence of too much pus in the blood is the production of inflammation in different organs, and especially in the lungs, which runs rapidly into suppuration.   It is from this circumstance that the subjects of surgical operations, and those labouring under extensive suppurations, are frequently cut off by peripneumonies, which, according to the observations of M. Cruveilhier, are usually lobular, that is, commencing at several points at once.   This, in my opinion, is the mode in which we must explain the occurrence of metastasis of pus, at least in the majority of cases."   Mr. Arnott, to whom I related these cases, had adopted the same view, and had collected 17 cases of phlebitis, which all went to prove that the suppurations which take place in different viscera after external injuries and surgical operations, do not depend upon any shock communicated to the system, but upon the purulent matter formed in the veins mixing with the blood.   Mr. Arnott stated to me, at the same time, that he considered this to be the cause of the suppuration of the eyes, and the painful swellings in the joints, sometimes observed in puerperal women.   But there was no pus in the spermatic vein in the first case now related, and I have since seen others where these secondary affections occurred without inflammation of the uterine veins or absorbents.   The connection between inflammation of the uterus and these secondary abscesses is undoubted, but it may be explained in different ways, and I am satisfied that the intimate part of the process requires further investigation.   Whatever the *modus operandi* may be, the following cases, which occurred soon afterwards, established a certain connection between inflammation of the uterine veins and fever, inflammation of the lungs and eyes, and painful swellings in the joints and extremities of puerperal women.   The relation of these cases, and an examination of the appearances presented by the inflamed veins in the preparations and drawings now upon the table, will give you a better idea of the changes of structure, and the local and constitutional symptoms of uterine phlebitis, than a general description of the disease.

Mrs. Keene, æt. 31, No. 6, Draper's Place, Euston Square, after a protracted labour of three days, was delivered on the 14th July, 1829, by artificial aid, of a still-born hydrocephalic child.   Immediately after the expulsion of the child, she was seized with a fit of the most intense shivering, which continued upwards of an hour, notwithstanding the exhibition of the most powerful stimuli, and the exhaustion which followed was alarming.   She rallied, however, and passed a quiet night. On the following, and two or three subsequent days, the shivering fits returned at irregular periods, sometimes in a slight form, at others in that of a severe rigor, followed by a flush of heat, and partial or general perspiration. During this time the effects consequent to parturition proceeded as usual. The uterus slightly painful on pressure; lochia natural; bowels open; pulse 133 to 140, and extremely feeble. No complaint of uneasiness, with the exception of a troublesome cough and hoarseness, with which she has been afflicted during the latter months of pregnancy. On the 4th day from delivery the secretion of milk appeared for a short time, and afterwards receded. From this day to the 10th, the following were the symptoms : pulse rapid ; skin universally of a dusky yellow colour, and the heat of surface increased ; respiration hurried ; thirst ; tongue dry but not furred ; great prostration of strength, sallow and haggard countenance ; restless and sleepless nights ; mental faculties undisturbed. The uterus had gradually subsided, and no pressure, however great, either on it or on the parts in its vicinity, caused pain, except in the right iliac region, where some uneasiness was felt ; the flow of lochia natural; bowels regular. At this period the hacking cough which had so long troubled her became more frequent, and it was with difficulty she expectorated the ropy mucus which followed it, and which in the day amounted to an ounce. From the 11th day the respiration became more short and hurried ; the pulse more rapid ; occasional flushes of heat, thirst, extreme debility, diarrhœa. Pressure over the whole abdomen gave no uneasiness, nor was pain felt in any part of the chest, though auscultation plainly indicated the existence of disease, particularly on the right side. The patient made no complaint but of weakness and the cough. She died exhausted on the 12th. Dr. John Prout, who had carefully observed the progress of the symptoms from the period of delivery, was present with me when I opened the body. The uterus being removed from the body for more minute examination, an incision was made into the right superior angle, to which the placenta had been attached, and here its veins were discovered to be empty, and their internal surface of a scarlet colour. On tracing them towards the trunk of the right spermatic vein, they were found to contain a sanious purulent fluid, and were contracted in their diameters and coated with false membranes. The veins of the right ovarium and fallopian tube were all plugged up with firm coagula. The spermatic itself was lined throughout its whole extent with dense membranes of a reddish, or of an ash-grey colour. Its coats, independent of these membranes, were of extraordinary thickness

and firmness—more like those of a large artery than a vein. The whole cavity was contracted ; in some parts occupied by a dark-coloured fluid, in others quite obliterated by adhesions formed between the surfaces of the membranous layers deposited within it. At the termination of the spermatic in the vena cava, its orifice was scarcely large enough to admit a crow-quill. Traces of inflammation extended beyond this orifice, the vena cava being partially lined, from two to three inches above it, with an adventitious membrane strongly adherent to its coats, which were at this part double their natural thickness. In its passage upwards the inflammation had extended a short distance into the right emulgent vein, which, near its orifice, was coated with a pellicle of lymph. On opening the thorax a stream of air escaped from the right side ; the lungs were collapsed, and upwards of ten pints and a half of red-coloured serum were found in the sac of the pleura. The right inferior lobe was coated with lymph, and a portion of the pleura on the anterior surface was destroyed, and a black gangrenous slough exposed in the substance of the lung. The pulmonary texture around was condensed, and of a deep violet or red colour. The left inferior lobe was also partially coated with a thin layer of lymph ; and the pleura, at one point on the anterior surface, was elevated as if by a hard globular substance underneath. When this was laid open, it appeared to consist of a thick yellow-coloured cyst or capsule, containing a soft black matter like a gangrenous eschar. The substance of the lungs around was unusually dense, and of a dark livid colour. The appearances of the portions of lung affected with gangrene, and of the right spermatic vein and vena cava, now described, are well preserved in these preparations of these parts [exhibiting them].

By looking at this preparation attentively, you will not only be able to form a clear idea of the changes produced upon the uterine veins by inflammation, but of the manner in which the disease originates, and the course it usually pursues, where the placenta has adhered to the superior part of the uterus. The veins in that part of the uterus where the placenta had been attached, and the spermatic, which had conveyed the blood from the placenta back to the system of the mother, are those alone affected, the veins in the lower part of the uterus, and the trunk of the hypogastric, being generally in a perfectly healthy condition. But I will show you another preparation [exhibiting it] in which the inflammation has run down along the lining membrane of the branches of the hypogastric into the common and external iliac and femoral veins, and upward along the vena cava to the point where the hepatic veins enter, and produced the same alterations of structure that you have seen in the other preparation, viz. injection and condensation of the cellular membrane in which the veins were imbedded, thickening, induration and contraction of their coats, and the deposition of lymph mixed with pus and coagula of blood within their cavities. Extensive inflammation of the lungs had likewise taken place in this woman, and, what is more rare, destruction of both eyes by violent inflammation. The details of this case have been minutely related in vol. 15 of the Medico-Chirurgical Transactions, and many other cases of uterine phlebitis in which fatal inflammation of the lungs, eyes, puffy swellings around the joints, ulceration of the articular cartilages and symphysis pubis, and gangrene of different parts of the body, took place in the progress of the disease. In some cases extensive inflammation and suppuration took place in the veins ramifying in the muscular coat of the uterus, and death followed with many of the symptoms of typhus fever, rapid feeble pulse, delirium, nervous tremors, the tongue and teeth covered with black sordes, vomiting and diarrhœa, before the inflammation had extended beyond the confines of the uterus. By examining the tables of all the cases which have occurred to me during the last fifteen years, you will be fully aware of the frequency and fatality of uterine phlebitis.

In these drawings [exhibiting them] you have represented the peculiar beaded appearance of the *uterine absorbents* when filled with pus. The symptoms are the same as in cases of inflammation of the veins of the uterus. The first example of this disease occurred in St. George's Hospital in the month of July 1829, and is thus described by Mr. Cæsar Hawkins. A woman, æt. 30, in an advanced stage of pregnancy, had sloughing of the skin over a diseased bursa of the patella. The removal of the bursa by an operation was followed by great constitutional disturbance, and labour came on fourteen days after. Uterine inflammation took place on the second day after delivery, and death took place on the fourth. Some puriform lymph was found in the pelvis, but with no increase of vascularity in the peritoneum. In the broad ligaments some fluid also was effused, and on each side numerous large absorbent vessels were discovered passing up, with the spermatic vessels, to the receptaculum chyli, which was unusually distended. All these vessels, and the reservoir itself, were quite filled with fluid pus; but that in the receptacle was filled with lymph, so as to be more solid; the vessels themselves were firmer and thicker than usual. The thoracic duct above this part was quite healthy. The uterus was scarcely contracted, and the internal surface of the lower half was soft and shreddy, and in a state of slough.

TABULAR VIEW (No. 1) OF 100 CASES OF SEVERE INFLAMMATION OF THE UTERUS AND ITS APPENDAGES,

Which occurred to me in London, from March 1827 to the end of December 1830.

[Continued from p. 697.]

No.	Name, Residence, and Delivery.	Date of Attack and Symptoms.	Treatment.	Result and Morbid Appearances.
51	Case, British Lying-in Hospital. Natural labour. 1st March, 1829.	Fifth day.—Pain in left side of hypogastrium, followed by rigors and headache; pulse 120; skin hot; tongue red and glossy; exquisite tenderness of the whole uterine region.	V.S. ʒxx., calomel gr. iij., pulv. Dover. gr. v., 3tia q. q. h. The relief from bleeding instantaneous.	Recovered.
52	Davies; æt. 20; deformed pelvis; OrangeStreet, LeicesterSquare. A protracted labour and artificial delivery. March 27, 1829.	Second day.—Great pain; swelling and tension of hypogastrium; rapid feeble pulse; tongue brown; vomiting; delirium. Died on the seventh day after delivery.	Leeches xxiv., calomel, and Dover's powder.	Died. Large intestines vascular, but not covered with lymph; peritoneum of uterus inflamed; posterior portion of os uteri in a sloughing state; muscular tissue of uterus softened.

53	Case, Queen Charlotte's Lying-in Hospital.—Natural labour. March 4, 1829.	Fourth day.—Slight abdominal pain; diarrhœa; brown tongue; vomiting; rapid feeble pulse; great prostration of strength. Not seen during life; seen after, with Mr. Sweatman. Fourteen days' duration.	V.S. not employed; leeches, vesication, &c.	Died. ...m small; intestines and uterus strongly adhering together by lymph; uterine appendages much inflamed; several pints of sero-purulent fluid in peritoneal sac.
54	Mayhew; æt. 33; British Lying-in Hospital. Natural labour. March 2, 1829.	Fourth day.—Pyrexia; pulse 130; great debility; delirium; dusky yellow complexion; no pain of abdomen; cough; excruciating pains in the joints of the upper and lower extremities. Duration of disease twenty-two days.	Powerful diffusible stimulants, and opiates.	Died. Uterus ...ced to its natural size; no morbid appearance in its peri...nal coat; a portion of placenta the ...ze of a ...tug, in a putrid s...te, adhering to the uterus, which was soft and black around; ...ies of the uterus full of pus at this part; ʒvj. of pus in right ...-joint; cartilages ...d.
55	Aldridge; British Lying-in Hospital. ...ll labour. May 25, 1829.	Third or fourth day.—Severe uterine pain; pyrexia; suppressed lochia; after recovery became maniacal.	V.S. ʒviij., cathartics, fomentations.	Recovered.
56	Airey; 4 ...tone Street. 23d May, 1829. th...al labour.	Second day.—Severe uterine pain; no general abdominal tenderness; p...se 90; tongue white; lochia suppressed.	V.S. ʒxvj., calomel, antimony, cathartics.	Recovered.
57	Case after natural labour, Bloomsbury Market. 15th June, 1829.	Fifth day.—(Not seen at the ...ment.) Vomiting within 24 hours after delivery; rapid feeble pulse; no pain of abdomen, or swelling; headache and delirium. The history of the early symptoms imperfect.	Head shaved, cold lotions, cathartics.	Died. Left ovarium m rch inflamed, enlarged, and softened; left fallopian tube red and vascular, and ...d with pus; two ...nts of reddish serum in peritonal sac; ...ls of brain gorged; fluid in the ventricles. Died.
58	M'Sweeney; Falconberg Court, Soho Square. Natural labour. 6th July, 1829.	Fourth day.—Slight uterine pain; delirium; rapid feeble pulse; great debility; vomiting; yellow skin; offensive lochia.	No remedies employed, the case being hopeless when first seen.	Died.

59	Tiffin; 18, Mercer Street, Long Acre.—Natural labour. 7th July, 1829.	Second day.—Uterus large, hard, and exquisitely painful; lochia scanty; pulse 110; pain gradually diffused; sickness; vomiting; delirium; rapid pulse and breathing. Died on the fourth day.	V.S. ʒxv, leeches xlj., V.S. xxiv., leeches xviij., calomel, opium, cathartics, blisters.	Died. Intestines distended with air, their peritoneum red and vascular; peritoneum of uterus coated with lymph; in the cellular tissue beneath, a sero-purulent and gelatinous fluid; pus in the lower part of the walls of the uterus, and between the folds of the broad ligaments; right ovarium the size of a hen's egg, and disorganised, left ovarium in a slighter degree; fallopian tubes red, soft, and filled with pus.
60	Stockin; 4, Tottenham Court Road.—Natural labour. 8th July, 1829.	Third day.—Pain in the region of the uterus, increased by pressure; lochia scanty; pulse rapid; saphena veins of right side hard and painful.	V.S. ʒxij., calomel, antimony, &c.	Recovered.
61	Millam; 4, Tudor Place. Natural labour. 12th July, 1829.	Second day.—Rigors and headache, followed by excruciating pain of uterus; pressure cannot be endured; lochia suppressed; pulse 160; tongue white and moist.	V.S. ʒxxiv., leeches xviij., fomentations, calomel and opium, and antimony.	Recovered.
62	Keene; æt. 34. Protracted labour: hydrocephalic child. 14th July, 1829.	Second or third day.—Rigors; slight uterine pain; lochia natural; pulse 133 to 146; sallow dusky skin; respiration hurried; tongue dry; great debility; pain in right iliac region; cough; expectoration; diarrhœa; great dyspnœa.	V.S. not employed; anodynes, diaphoretics, blisters to the chest.	Died. Veins of fundus uteri right side inflamed; right spermatic vein, through its whole extent, thickened greatly, its inner surface lined with a false membrane, and its cavity filled with a sanious purulent fluid; vena cava above and below the entrance of spermatic vein lined with a closely adherent false membrane; right emulgent vein inflamed; two pints of serum in the pleura; portion of right inferior lobe of lung inflamed and in a state of complete gangrene.

63	Mary A. Hale; æt. 25; British Lying-in Hospital. Natural labour. 25th July, 1829.	Second day.—Severe rigor, followed by great tenderness of hypogastrium; rapid pulse; white tongue; whole abdomen became intensely painful, without swelling or tension; cough; dyspnœa, and pain in right side of chest. Died on fifth day after delivery.	V.S. ℥viij. (syncope), leeches, calomel, Dover's powder, cathartics.	Died. Peritoneum of the uterus and appendages coated with false membrane; peritoneal covering of intestines inflamed and glued together; two pints of whey-coloured fluid in abdominal cavity; muscular coat and vessels of uterus healthy; traces of recent inflammation in the pleura and lungs on the left side.
64	Luff; æt. 26; British Lying-in Hospital.—Natural labour. 11th August, 1829.	Sudden acute pain of the uterus; right side exquisitely tender on pressure; uterus large and hard; pulse 112, small; rigors; lochia scanty. The relief from bleeding was most striking in this case.	V.S. ℥xxvj, leeches xxxvj., calomel gr.vj., pulv. antim. gr. v. 3tiâ q. q. h., Dover's powder.	Recovered.
65	M'Creevy; æt. 25; British Lying-in Hospital. 29th August, 1829.	Second day.—Vomiting during labour; recurred a few hours after delivery, with pyrexia and severe abdominal pain; tympanites; rapid pulse.	V.S. ℥xiv., leeches xxiv., calomel, opium, &c.	Died. Partial inflammation of small intestines; a turbid fluid in the peritoneal sac: ovaria inflamed and coated with lymph, and also fallopian tubœ; the omentum, adhering firmly to the posterior part of cervix uteri, formed a thick band, stretching over and firmly compressing the intestines. Died.
66	Case at Chelsea.—Nat. labour. 29th August, 1829.	Fourth day.—Diarrhœa; rapid feeble pulse; yellow tinge of skin; great debility; loaded tongue.	Stimulants.	Died.
67	Clarke; æt. 34; 57, Monmouth Street. Natural labour. 6th September, 1829.	Seventh day.—Pyrexia; headache; vomiting; no uterine pain; pulse 150; swellings around the joints; rigors; delirium; brown tongue; great debility; left forearm swollen, and of a dark red colour; gangrene of the back part of hand.	Stimulants.	Died. Uterus contracted; peritoneum of fundus and back part of uterus of a yellow colour, soft, and easily torn; the muscular and mucous coats at the upper and back parts reduced to a soft pulp of a dark red and sub-grey colour.

68	Mason; æt. 42; 3, Little Vine Street, Piccadilly. Twins. Hæmorrhage. August, 1829.	A few days after delivery.—Pyrexia, with great uterine pain; rapid pulse; loaded tongue; diarrhœa; delirium; pulse 140; crural phlebitis in both lower extremities.	Leeches, fomentations, poultices, and diffusible stimulants.	Died. The vena cava, common external and internal iliac veins, and right femoral, inflamed and obstructed. The appearances presented by these veins have been represented in Plate 7, Vol. XV. Med. Chir. Trans.
69	—; 7, Denmark Street. Protracted lab.; perforation. 14th September, 1829.	Second day.—Pyrexia; acute abdominal pain; swelling of labia; quick pulse; tympanites; gangrene of internal parts.	V.S. ℥xvj., leeches xxiv., calomel, opium, &c.	Died. Fallopian tubes of a dark red colour, and containing pus; ovaria enlarged and softened, and covered with lymph; ℥rij. of red serum in the abdominal cavity; veins of uterus, where placenta adhered, gorged with pus.
70	Mills; æt. 30; British Lying-in Hospital. Natural labour. 7th October, 1829.	Second day.—Pain and hardness in the superficial veins of both legs and thighs, with a diffuse swelling and erysipelatous redness around, with violent fever; tongue red; face flushed; respiration hurried; jactitation; delirium; suppuration in the cellular membrane around the vein at different points. Duration of disease 14 days.	Fomentations and poultices, stimulants.	Died. Trunks and branches of saphena veins inflamed and obstructed; abscesses beneath the skin in the calf of the leg and interstices of the gastrocnemii muscles; coats of femoral veins thickened and contracted; intestines inflamed and portion of ascending colon in a state of sphacelus.
71	Hickson; British Lying-in Hospital. 14th November, 1829.	Eighteenth day.—(Late in the disease.) Exquisite uterine pain; pulse 130; breathing hurried; features sunk; vomiting; brown tongue; yellow tinge of the skin.	Leeches and stimulants.	Died. Right uterine appendages inflamed; veins at the right side of fundus uteri filled with pus, also the right spermatic vein three inches from the uterus, the inner surface of vessel being coated with lymph; a pint of pus in the cellular membrane at the brim of pelvis; two small abscesses under peritoneum of uterus.

No.	Patient	Symptoms	Treatment	Result
72	Cox; Marylebone Street, St. James's. Protracted labour. 1st December, 1829.	Fifth day,—Pyrexia; acute uterine pain, but chiefly on the right side; vomiting; rigors; lochia suppressed; stupor; delirium; loaded tongue; abdomen puffy; pulse 140, feeble.	V.S. ℥viij., leeches xxiv., calomel, and opium.	Died. Several small abscesses under the peritoneum of the uterus at the left superior angle, and the veins in this part filled with pus; the ovaria soft and enlarged, and glued with lymph to the fallopian tubes, their stroma converted into a dark, red coloured, pulpy substance.
73	Long; æt. 29; British Lying-in Hospital. Natural labour. 18th December, 1829.	Fourth day.—Headache; pulse 130; delirium; tongue dry and brown. great tympanites; tongue dry and brown.	V.S. ℥viij., V.S. ℥ij., cathartics.	Died. Abdomen distended; gas in peritoneal sac; the ovaria, tubes, and broad ligaments on both sides, imbedded in lymph and pus; ovaria large, soft, and vascular; the coats of the uterus healthy; omentum, small and great intestines, and surface of liver, coated with lymph.
74	Gilland; æt. 29; British Lying-in Hospital. Natural labour. 24th December, 1829.	Fifth day,—Pyrexia; rigors, alternating with flushes of heat; pulse 150; headache; giddiness; slight delirium; tremors; face flushed; eyes red; tongue foul; urgent thirst; vomiting; abdomen soft and distended; hypogastrium painful on pressure; tympanites. Died 9th January.	Leeches x. to the temples, cinchona wine, brandy, opium, beef tea.	Died. Peritoneal sac perfectly healthy; the right spermatic vein contracted, its coats thickened, and the cellular membrane around its vascular and condensed, its interior lined with false membranes and partially filled with lymph and pus; the veins proceeding from the right ovarium and fallopian tube in the same condition; thin shreds of lymph coated the vena cava around the entrance of the spermatic vein; right ovarium and tube glued together with lymph.
75	Mrs. Allan; æt. 20; 11, Noel Street, Berwick Street. Puerperal convulsions. December, 1829.	Fourth day.—Great uterine tenderness; lochia suppressed; pulse rapid; delirium; vomiting; sallow skin; crural phlebitis. The limb remained stiff and swollen long after.	V.S. ℥xiv. leeches, calomel, antimony, fomentations, anodynes.	Recovered.

CASE OF THE SUCCESSFUL

REMOVAL OF A DISEASED OVARIUM,

Of 17 Years' duration, in which Paracentesis had been ten times performed.

By Dr. Frederic Bird,

Lecturer on Medical Jurisprudence at the Westminster Hospital; Physician to the Metropolitan Free Hospital; and to the Westminster Maternity Charity.

(For the London Medical Gazette.)

Mrs. Gelsthorpe, aged 35, residing in Chelsea, of general healthy appearance, and good muscular development, the previous history of whose case runs thus:—Prior to attaining her eighteenth year she enjoyed uninterrupted health; at that age menstruation became established, its periodical recurrence during the succeeding twelve months marking intervals of not more than a fortnight. When 19 years old she was, after some comparatively slight exertion, attacked with acute pain in the right iliac region, which, lasting for three days, gradually abated in violence, and in a month she had quite recovered. Since that period, however, she has continued to experience occasional recurrence of the pain at irregular intervals. Immediately after the subsidence of the acute pain, she observed that the abdomen began to increase in size, and continued to do so during the following two years, her general health suffering but little impairment, and menstruation being much more regularly performed. She then placed herself under the care of Mr. Dally, of Syson, Leicestershire, who, having allowed four months for the exhibition of general remedies, removed by paracentesis abdominis three gallons of colourless fluid. For fifteen months she experienced no re-accumulation of the fluid; but at the expiration of that time abdominal enlargement again presented itself, and in less than three months she had acquired her former size. Paracentesis was again performed, and repeated on three subsequent occasions, the intervals between the four last tappings being about twelve months. Her recovery from the previous operations had been rapid and complete; but the last was followed by the occurrence of acute pain diffused over the whole of the abdomen, greatly increased by pressure; vomit-

ing; febrile action; and all the ordinary indications of inflammation, which slowly yielded to blood-letting, blisters, and internal remedies. Her recovery was tardy, but she ultimately regained her usual state of health, and experienced no return of the original disease during the succeeding seven years; towards the end of which time she married, but has never borne children. Abdominal enlargement again took place, though slowly, and she did not acquire her previous state of distension until two years had elapsed, when paracentesis was performed by Mr. Dickinson, of Sloane Street, on which occasion about two and a half gallons of fluid were removed, the secretion having assumed totally different physical characters, being of nearly a black colour, and remarkably viscid. In six months the operation was again called for, the evacuated fluid being of a dark yellow colour. In eighteen months she was again tapped; again after the lapse of twelve weeks; and for the tenth time on January 11th, 1843, after an interval of seventeen weeks. The fluid, removed on the three last occasions by Mr. Wooley, of Brompton, presented the same colourless state observed during the earlier periods of the disease.

A few weeks prior to the last operation of paracentesis the patient had applied to Dr. Hamilton Roe, who at once pronounced the disease ovarian, and believed that however much the previous history might oppose the employment of the operation for extirpation, yet that her general health, and the non-malignant and probably unilocular character of the tumor, afforded considerable probability of success. With this view Dr. Roe very kindly referred her to me, and thus afforded an opportunity for watching the progress of the disease, and examining it at its several stages of development.

The increase in size of the tumor since the last tapping has been very irregular, weeks sometimes having elapsed without any apparent increase, whilst occasionally a few days have sufficed for very considerable augmentation of bulk. This irregularity was associated with, and probably dependent upon, the irregular performance of menstruation. She had frequent attacks of profuse menorrhagia, during the persistence of which no increase in size ever took place, and it was not until the use of the secale cornutum had completely arrested the hæmorrhage, that the cyst began to refill with the same quickness as on the last occasion. About this time pain on the right side of the abdomen frequently occurred; the pressure of the tumor upon the bladder obliged her to pass urine at very short intervals, and often with much pain; her bowels were inactive, her spirits depressed, and she was most anxious to submit to any treatment that might afford a probability of relief.

The nature of the operation for extirpation of the ovary, with all its attendant dangers, were very strongly (perhaps more so than really necessary) impressed upon her; and she was informed that the chances of success were in her case but few. Possessed of an unusual share of moral courage, these objections availed nothing, and she steadily persisted in her desire that the operation should be performed. Anxious to obtain the most accurate diagnosis of the case, I requested Dr. Roe to again see her, which he did, and after a careful examination did not hesitate to recommend the operation. I also solicited the opinions of my friends, Mr. B. Phillips, Dr. Andrews, Dr. Lever, and Mr. B. Lucas, all of whom were so kind as to assist me with their views of the case. Mr. Walne was also so obliging as to favour me with his opinion on the propriety of performing the operation. The opinions of these gentlemen accorded in all the more prominent points, the majority rather opposing than favouring the performance of an operation, partly from the fact of the patient having passed through a long term of years without having suffered any permanent derangement of health, and that the intervals between the tappings had been considerable, and appeared to be increasing; and partly from a belief in the existence of peritoneal adhesions of greater or less extent. Although most fully concurring in the degree of importance attaching to the first of these objections, I was induced to believe it probable that there did not exist any extensive attachments to the peritoneum, having had an opportunity, which these gentlemen had not had, of examining the abdomen immediately after the last operation of tapping. This impression, coupled with the very favourable condition of the general health of the patient, induced me to acquiesce in her urgent desire that she might be allowed the chances of the operation; and Monday, June 26th, was fixed for its performance. The only preliminary treatment consisted in the withdrawal for a few days of animal food, the exhibition of eight grains of compound extract of colocynth, with five of hyoscyamus, on the preceding day, and an enema of gruel two hours before the operation. Great care was taken to regulate the temperature of the apartment, which was maintained at 85°, but subsequently lowered as convalescence approached.

June 26th.—In the presence of Dr. Hamilton Roe, Mr. B. Phillips, Dr. Andrews, Mr. Cantis, and Mr. Brown of Chelsea, the patient having been drawn down sufficiently low in the bed to admit of her legs hanging over its end, and thus rendering the abdominal walls more tense, I first made an exploratory incision a little below the umbilicus; a few careful strokes of the scalpel quickly laid open the peritoneal cavity sufficiently to allow of the introduction of the finger, which soon assured me of the non-existence of adhesions at that part. With a bistoury the incision was then enlarged to about three and a half or four inches; the blue cyst of the tumor immediately advanced, closing up the abdominal opening, and thus preventing the entrance into that cavity of the blood escaping from a few divided vessels. A few minutes were occupied in arresting the little hæmorrhage, during which it was observed that the position of the tumor was changed at each respiratory movement of the diaphragm, affording satisfactory evidence of the absence of extensive adhesions. The cyst was next seized with a pronged forceps, constructed to grasp without contusing, an incision made into it, an elastic tube introduced, and the greater portion of the fluid contents evacuated. At each inspiration the cyst became protruded, and continued to escape until retarded for a moment by two very slight adhesions, which separated without difficulty, and the great bulk of the tumor was soon lying on the outside of the abdomen. The left hand was then introduced for the purpose of examining the pedicle, which, though thick from the increased development of the broad ligament, was quite free from morbid attachments to the viscera of the pelvis. The uterus was drawn as high up towards the incision as possible, without producing pain, and a strong curved needle, fixed in a handle, and carrying a very stout silken ligature, was passed through the centre of the pedicle, then withdrawn, and the ligature tied on either side. A third ligature of equal strength was also made to encircle the entire stalk, just below the insertion of the other two. Much pain was now complained of, and some tendency to faint: relief to the latter was quickly afforded by pressing upon the lower part of the chest and scrobiculus cordis, thus giving to the diaphragm a substituted support for the loss of that previously afforded by the tumor. The broad ligament was next divided by a probe-pointed knife; a second application of which cut through the fallopian tube, leaving not more than half an inch of the latter attached to the uterus. All the vessels being now seen to be secure, the uterus was replaced in its proper position, and the ends of the ligatures left hanging out from the lower margin of the incision. Before closing the wound I examined the opposite (left) ovary, which appeared healthy. The lips of the incision were then brought together by a few interrupted sutures, cold water dressing applied, and a flannel bandage lightly drawn around the abdomen.

Shortly after the operation she complained much of lumbar pain, and became faint; the pulse ranged at 80: she was placed in a more comfortable position in bed; a little brandy and water given her, and a flannel roller tightly drawn around the lower part of the chest, with marked relief to the faintness; and was then ordered—

R. Morphiæ Acetatis, gr. ss.; Aquæ Flor. Aurant. ʒss. Fiat haustus statim sumendus. All food strictly prohibited; allowed a little rough ice and cold water occasionally.

11 P.M.—Has slept a little; the pain in the back continues undiminished; has twice vomited; heat of skin increased; pulse 88, sharper; a little bleeding has taken place from the wound.

Repetatur haustus.

27th, 2 A.M.—Vomiting has recurred, but is now restrained by the ice, which she takes freely; has slept for three hours; skin perspiring; pulse 92.

5 A.M.—Complaining much of pain at the lower part of the abdomen; ʒxij of high-coloured turbid urine drawn off by the catheter. On looking to the wound I found that the effort of vomiting, together with a rather frequent cough, had displaced one of the sutures, and a large fold of intestine had escaped through the opening and was lying on the abdomen; it presented no appearance of congestion, and had certainly not been long protruded: some little trouble attended its reduction, after which two additional sutures were introduced, and the cold water dressing re-applied.

9 A.M.—Cough troublesome; slight pain about the wound; pulse 92; is anxious for food.

R. Syr. Papav. ʒss.; Ox. Scillæ, ʒij.; Aquæ, ʒx. M. Sumat cochleare min. p. r. n. Continue the use of the ice and cold water, and to be allowed two ounces of thin water gruel.

1 P.M.—Is sleeping; skin moist; pulse the same.

10 P.M.—Heat of skin increased, and pulse accelerated, probably from having been awakened by an accidental noise; ʒxij. of urine drawn off by catheter; no local pain; is inclined to sleep.

28th, 2 P.M.—Slept well during the night; coughs less often; skin moist; pulse 102; ʒviij. of urine withdrawn by catheter; wishes for food.

Allowed a cup of tea and a small rusk; to persist in the use of the ice.

8 P.M.—Pain in the loins returned this evening, but ceased about an hour ago, when the catamenia appeared; bowels have been once relieved without medicine; is cheerful, and begs for an improved diet; her request is not granted, but having become tired of the ice, toast and water is substituted.

29th.—In the middle of the night was suffering much from pain in the hypogastrium, which subsided on withdrawing about ʒxij. of urine by the catheter; the pulse is 96; catamenia still present.

Allowed a cup of arrow-root with water.

30th.—Much improved, being altogether free from uneasiness; has passed urine naturally; skin and tongue as in health; pulse 84; menstruation has ceased.

Vespere.—Not so well; complaining of frequent tenesmus; impeded respiration firm flatulent distension of the abdomen; pulse 96.

℞ Pil. Rhæi ·Co. gr. vij.; Pil. Hydrarg. gr. iss.; Olei Cassiæ, ɱj. Fiant pilulæ duæ statim sumendæ.

July 1st.—Found her much depressed in spirits; suffering from frequent syncope, but no local symptoms; urine ʒxij. passed in two portions, once naturally, and once by the aid of the catheter; bowels freely relieved; pulse 100.

Allowed a little veal broth and vermicelli.

2d.—Was summoned to her in the night, at which time she presented the following symptoms. Severe pain at the epigastric and left hypochondriac regions, increased by pressure; respiration hurried; countenance anxious; pulse 110, small and irritable; tongue white; surface of the lower extremities cold; percussion in the painful abdominal regions indicated much flatulent distension, and flatus could be heard traversing the intestinal canal. On inquiring, I with great difficulty ascertained that one of her relatives had most injudiciously informed her of some domestic infelicity, and which had been immediately followed by the symptoms described.

Small quantities of brandy, diluted with hot water, at frequent intervals.

In about an hour heat was diffused over the body; pain was somewhat lessened. She was then ordered—

Morphiæ Acetatis, gr. iss. statim in formâ pilulæ.

After the lapse of half an hour the opiate began to exert its influence; the pulse fell to 96, she was soon sleeping, and did not awake for seven hours, when she expressed herself as quite free from all her former symptoms, and had forgotten the unpleasing intelligence which had been so indiscreetly communicated to her.

3d.—Improving; pulse 96; urine passed naturally; bowels not open. To be allowed a small quantity of boiled rabbit for dinner.

℞ Potas. Tart. ʒij.; Rhei Pulv. gr. viij.; Tinct. Card. Co. ʒss.; Syr. Zinzib. ʒiss.; Aquæ, ʒj. Ft. haustus cras mane sumendus.

5th.—Bowels open four times; pulse 96; is progressing favourably.

6th.—Complaining of a little irritation about the bladder, with difficulty in micturition; the urine is turbid from the presence of urate of ammonia, and also contains a rather large quantity of free uric acid; pulse 100.

Liquor. Potas. Efferves. Oss. ter quotidie.

8th.—Is free from vesical irritation; urine natural; sleeps well; spirits excellent; pulse 78. For the last two days she has been sitting up in her bed, amusing herself with needle-work. The bowels not having acted during the last three days, she is ordered to repeat the aperient pills formerly given.

9th.—The bowels have thrice acted; appetite good; pulse 78; has sat up whilst taking her food, which, during the last six days, has consisted of one mutton chop, an egg, rice pudding, tea, and a biscuit, daily, divided into four meals. The greater part of the wound has quite healed; a few small granulations have sprung up around the lower edge of the incision, through which the ligatures, still firmly attached, pass. During the first four days after the operation the temperature of the room was kept at 75°, after which it was lowered to 70°, and now averages at 65°.

31st.—During the three weeks that have now elapsed since the date of the last report, nothing has occurred to retard the rapid convalescence of the patient. One of the ligatures came away some days since, the others yesterday. The wound has quite healed, excepting at the lower end, where a few redundant granulations exist. She is in excellent health and spirits, has for some days been actively employed, keeping her room from precaution, not necessity. The bowels act with regularity, and she expresses herself as being in better health than for many years past.

The dimensions of the abdomen prior to the operation, and at the present time, are the following:—

	Before operation.	After operation.
From ensiform cartilage to pubes	18 inches	11 inches.
Circumference of abdomen	37 inches	24½ inches.

A small portion of the tumor only presented a solid structure, in size not exceeding that of an orange, and appeared to consist of the remaining portion of the ovary not involved in the formation of the cyst. The fluid contents amounted to about two gallons, having an unusually low specific gravity, 1·004, quite colourless, scarcely viscid, and differed from the fluid commonly secreted in this disease in being quite neutral: examined by my brother, Dr. Golding Bird, it was found to consist of—

Animal Extract	⎫
Alkaline Lactates	⎬ 40
Chloride of Sodium	⎭
Water	960
Albumen	a trace.
	1000

The shape of the cyst when filled was irregularly spherical, and did not at all partake of the balloon like form frequently observed; from its depending portion a secondary cyst arose, which appeared to have been moulded to the shape of the cavity of the bony pelvis in which it had been placed. The broad ligament measured more than six inches in breadth, and in it passed four arterial branches of rather large size, with some smaller ones, which running along its ovarian attachments terminated by minutely ramifying all over the surface of the diseased mass. The fallopian tube was long, dense in structure, and thickened. Two small patches of roughened and granular membrane, more vividly injected than the surrounding parts, corresp· ed to the two adhesions observed during the operation. The total weight of the tumor was rather more than 20 pounds.

REMARKS.—The case I have related is illustrative of several important practical points, and also assists in negativing some of the objections supposed to attach to the performance of the operation in those who have been previously subjected to tapping. The disease in the present instance, had existed for a long period, and paracentesis had been frequently performed, to which on one occasion succeeded symptoms of inflammation, and as the result would seem to prove, of the cyst; it was therefore inferred that adhesions existed, more particularly at the spot at which the trochar had been introduced; none,

however, were found at that part, and not any of extent or importance elsewhere. The fact of a patient having been previously tapped would, therefore, seem to offer no real objection to the performance of the operation of extirpation, and this being granted, the partial or complete emptying of the cyst may be employed for the purpose of affording an additional means of diagnosis in certain cases in which it is difficult to determine with sufficient accuracy the character of the tumor, or the presence and extent of peritoneal attachments. The diagnosis of adhesions is at all times difficult, and is commonly but little more than conjectural; the introduction of a trochar in doubtful cases, in order to lessen the distension of the abdominal walls, may therefore be received as a method of greatly facilitating an examination, and furnishing new and important data for arriving at a correct opinion. During the first two or three weeks after the last time of tapping it was by no means difficult to grasp the then flaccid abdominal walls, and cause them to glide with freedom over the surface of the ovarian mass; whilst at a later period the distension of the abdomen rendered such examination difficult and uncertain.

The very successful termination of the case, is, I believe, in a great measure attributable—

Firstly, to the precautions taken to prevent the action of cold air upon the exposed peritoneal surface, by artificially raising the heat of the room in which the operation was performed, and maintaining a high temperature so long as there existed any liability to inflammation.

Secondly, to the after treatment, which partook more of a dietetic than medical character, its chief feature consisting in the exclusion as far as possible of all internal remedies, and thus allowing the most complete repose to the organs in the immediate neighbourhood of the wounded parts. A grain of morphia and a little syrup of poppies were the only remedies given during the earlier period after the operation, and the only ingesta consisted of ice, cold water, and a very small quantity of thin water gruel. By these means all sources of irritation were avoided, and thus the chief cause of inflammatory action.

Thirdly, to the form of operation adopted, which I believe to be that presenting all the chances of recovery the extirpation of the ovarium is calculated to afford. Hitherto I have but described the steps of the operation, and I would now venture to make a single remark on the cause which induced me apparently to profit so little by the recorded cases of Dr. Clay and Mr. Walne.* It was, however, from their careful perusal, that I was led to arrive at a somewhat different conclusion from that expressed by those gentlemen. The cases of Dr. Clay, and still more his useful practical observations, have sufficiently demonstrated the amount of danger which attends the attempt to perform extraction through a very small opening: the truth of which I saw exemplified in a case that occurred some years ago, in which the failure of the operation and the death of the patient (for failure in these cases seems to amount to death,) were undoubtedly to be attributed to the smallness of the abdominal incision; a secondary cyst of inconsiderable size having formed the obstacle, and which could readily have been removed by a somewhat more capacious opening.

Whilst thus according in the disadvantages said to attach to the small abdominal incision, I cannot but believe that important objections apply with equal justice to the very large section, the chief of which undoubtedly is the question of necessity. Is an incision from pubes to ensiform cartilage, in cases in which the ovarian tumor is wholly or in part fluid, really required? There can, I conceive, be no valid objection to evacuating the liquid contents partially or entirely, and thus causing so great a reduction of bulk as to allow of the removal of the ovarium through an opening of less size than that constituting the *major* operation; for if an incision be made sufficiently large to admit of the cyst rising from out of the abdominal cavity without any forcible traction—if it also be sufficiently large to allow of the introduction of the hand of the operator into the abdomen, and thus enable him to apply with facility the necessary ligatures, or remove any abnormal attachments to the pelvic viscera—every end is answered, every indication fulfilled, and the

* Vide MEDICAL GAZETTE: the cases of Dr. Clay are contained in another journal.

820.—XXXII.

making a large peritoneal section can confer no further benefit to the patient, unless the removal of an unpunctured cyst can be deemed such. It may be urged that a large incision into the peritoneum is less likely to be followed by inflammation than a smaller one, and this I am by no means disposed to deny; but were it proved, it would still be very questionable whether an operator would be justified in making an unnecessarily large incision solely with a view of enhancing the probabilities of ultimate success. I would not, however, dissent from the employment of a larger incision in cases in which the partially solid state of the tumor might prevent its sufficient reduction by puncture, but from the cases I have seen I am inclined to believe that it rarely happens that an ovarian tumor will not be found to be in part fluid, and therefore capable of being lessened in size by the introduction of the trochar. Many important points remain to be determined with regard to the relative value of the operation, and the number of cases yet recorded have not been sufficient to decide whether the chances of success exceed the chances of the occurrence of disease in the remaining organ. The observations of Mr. B. Phillips,* tend to turn the scale of probabilities against the ultimate safety of the patient, and to show that disease in a less developed form commonly exists in the opposite ovary. This, together with some other points in the pathology of ovarian disease, I purpose, when my inquiries shall have been completed, making the subject of a future communication.

38, Craven Street.

PAINLESSNESS OF MORTAL WOUNDS.

To the Editor of the Medical Gazette.

SIR,

THE extract from the *Gazette Médicale* which appeared in your last number, detailing the case of a man who died from the effects of an extensive injury, without suffering pain, recals to my recollection a similar instance which occurred some years ago at a public institution in Berkshire. A decrepit old woman was admitted into the wards

* Vide MEDICAL GAZETTE.

3 B

of the Wallingford Union Poor-house, and soon after her admission, by some accident, her clothes caught fire, and, before assistance could be rendered, were almost consumed. The bed, also, upon which she threw herself in the agony and fright of the moment, was set on fire.

On examination, it was found that the poor creature was mortally injured, the vitality and organization of large portions of the cutis in various parts of the body having been so deeply destroyed as almost to lay bare the subjacent muscles.

In consequence of this sudden and extensive violence, no reaction ever occurred, nor the slightest hæmorrhage; the mental faculties were unimpaired; and in about sixteen hours from the receipt of the injury she died from sheer exhaustion, occasioned by the irrecoverable shock the nervous system had sustained. She declared with her latest breath, that from first to last she had been *totally free from pain.*—I am, sir,

Your obedient servant,
R. H. ALLNATT.

Parliament Street, Whitehall.

OBSERVATIONS ON

SOME OF THE

MORE IMPORTANT DISEASES OF CHILDHOOD.

By CHARLES WEST, M.D.

Member of the Royal College of Physicians; Physician to the Royal Infirmary for Children; and Physician-Accoucheur to the Finsbury Dispensary.

(For the Medical Gazette.)

I.—*On Endocarditis in Childhood.*

INFLAMMATION of the lining membrane of the heart is an affection of which no notice is taken in any treatise on the diseases of children, with the exception of the recent work of MM. Rilliet and Barthez. Incidental mention of its occurrence as a complication of scarlatina is made by Professor v. Ammon, in his account of a malignant epidemic of that disease at Dresden in the year 1832*. Dr. Copland devotes a few lines to it in his Dictionary, and speaks of its occasional occurrence as an idiopathic affection. Some of the French journals contain observations on hyper-

* Analekten ueber Kinderkrankheiten, 11tes Heft. Seite 42.

trophy of the heart and diseases of the valves in childhood, but I believe that none of the writers allude to acute idiopathic endocarditis in the young subject.

The cases of acute endocarditis mentioned by MM. Rilliet and Barthez are three in number. In one of these cases the heart symptoms came on in the course of an attack of acute rheumatism; in the second slight febrile symptoms coexisted with a distinct *bruit de soufflet* and some pain at the heart; and in the third the auscultatory signs only were present, unattended either by fever or by pain in the precordial region. They do not, however, detail the particulars of any of these cases. They met likewise, in the course of their observation at the Hôpital des Enfans Malades, with thirteen cases of chronic organic lesions of the heart of various kinds; and they relate the history of one of these cases in which acute endocarditis supervened on chronic valvular disease, and destroyed the patient.

My attention was first called to this affection in the spring of 1841, when I saw

Margaret Thomas, aged 3 years and 4 months, living at 86, Union Street, Lambeth Walk.

She is the delicate child of a phthisical mother, but her health was good till within the past year, since which time she has had two attacks of convulsions, and her general health has seemed less good.

She was, however, as well as usual until a few days before she came to me, when she was attacked by slight febrile symptoms, complained of great uneasiness, could get no rest at night, and began to suffer much from shortness of breath and palpitation of the heart; symptoms which have continued up to the present time.

A very loud *bruit de soufflet* accompanies and overpowers the first sound of the heart. It is heard both at the apex and at the base, but loudest in the latter situation, and is continued into the aorta. The second sound is clear. The heart's impulse is increased, and its sounds are heard over the whole chest, both before and behind.

Unfortunately I have preserved no record of the daily progress of the child, who recovered from her more urgent symptoms under an antiphlogistic plan of treatment. The bruit, however, continued, and the child remained short-breathed and liable to occasional returns of palpitation, which subsided on strict quiet being enforced and a mild antiphlogistic plan being pursued. I saw her last in May 1842, when the signs indicative of valvular disease continued unmodified.

Now, although in this case the patient was not seen at the very commencement of her attack, yet there does not appear to me to be any reason for supposing that the affection of her heart dated further back than the few days previous to her being brought to me, when she first complained of dyspnœa and palpitation of the heart. The following case was probably one in which acute endocarditis supervened on some chronic lesion of the heart.

George Cole, 43, Easton Street, Spa Fields, aged 5 years and 2 months, one of seven children, of whom five are still living, but one died while teething, and one of small-pox.

His father is strong and healthy; his mother is not strong,. and phthisis is hereditary in her family, though she has never shown any symptoms of it.

George has usually had good health, except two years ago, when he was taken ill with symptoms similar to those from which he is at present suffering, and did not recover for some weeks. He has not had any of the usual diseases of childhood.

For some months he has had a slight cough, but was in other respects in good health, when he was attacked on February 13, 1843, with fever, thirst, and swelling, first of the face, afterwards of the limbs, and on the 14th his heart began to beat much, and whenever he attempted to lie down in bed so much dyspnœa came on as compelled him to resume the sitting posture.

On February 17th he was brought to me at the Finsbury Dispensary, when I ordered three leeches to the heart, a purgative every night to relieve his bowels, which were constipated, and a saline mixture, with six minims of tincture of digitalis, every four hours.

February 21.—The leeches greatly relieved his palpitation, though he still has considerable difficulty in assuming the recumbent posture. The anasarca .·as completely disappeared, and he makes water more freely than before, though his urine is still scanty, high coloured, abounding in the lithates, and loaded with albumen. He has a trouble-

some cough, unattended with expectoration, no appetite, considerable thirst, a dry harsh skin; bowels open, tongue pale and moist. The pulsation of his carotids is very evident; pulse 70, hard, thrilling, unequal in force about every fourth beat, but not irregular in rhythm.

On auscultating the chest a good deal of rhonchus and creaking sounds are heard, but the air seems to enter both lungs equally well.

The apex of the heart beats lower down, and more to the left of the nipple, than natural, and there is also extensive dulness over the heart. Its sounds are not clear, but have a muffled character, and a harsh bruit accompanies the first sound, and is heard most distinctly about half an inch below and a little to the left of the nipple, but is not continued into the aorta.

The digitalis was now discontinued, and a saline mixture, with small doses of tartar emetic, was given in its stead.

24th.—Breath less laboured; child can lie down more easily, and the palpitation is less troublesome. The medicine has caused much sickness; the urine continues scanty, high-coloured, and . albuminous, and the inequality in the beats of the pulse, and the bruit with the first sound, remain as before.

The antimony was now discontinued, and small doses of liquor potassæ were given instead. The boy improved daily, and the note of March 10 is—Child very much improved; can now lie down easily; has but very slight difficulty in breathing; very little cough, and no palpitation. The bowels act regularly. The urine is abundant, natural, and free from albumen.

Pulse 100, the same inequality in its strength, and sometimes a distinct pause about every fourth beat. The action of the heart is not exaggerated, and there is no longer any bruit, but merely a roughness accompanying the first sound, and heard only near the apex.

The boy was soon afterwards discharged.

I observed a third case only a few months since.

Daniel Bain, aged 11 years, living at No. 37, Thomas Street, Stamford Street; is one of 12 children of healthy parents. Nine children are still living, one died while teething, one of scarlatina, and one of pneumonia. There does not appear to be any phthisical taint in the family.

Daniel has had good health, with the exception of mild attacks of measles, hooping-cough, and scarlet-fever; and was as well as usual until May 8, 1843, when he complained of feeling cold, and began to cough. The chilliness was succeeded by fever, and he continued gradually getting worse till the 13th, when I visited him for the first time. He had had no other medicine than a purgative powder.

May 13th.—I found him lying in bed; face dusky, rather anxious; eyes heavy; respiration slightly accelerated; frequent short cough without expectoration; skin burning hot; pulse frequent and hard. The child makes no complaint except of slight uneasiness about the left breast.

There is slight tenderness on pressure over the heart, with very extended dulness. The heart's impulse is not increased. A very loud and prolonged rasping sound is heard in the place of the first sound; it is loudest a little below the nipple, though very audible over the whole left side of the chest, and also distinguishable, though less clearly, for a considerable distance to the right of the sternum. Second sound heard clearly just over the aortic valves, not distinct elsewhere, being obscured by the loudness of the bruit.

Respiration good in both lungs.

I ordered the child to be cupped to ℥vj. between the left scapula and the spine; and gave gr. j. of calomel, with the same quantity of Dover's powder, every four hours.

May 14th.—Sense of discomfort at the chest relieved by the cupping. He slept well during the night, and to-day looks less anxious, though his eyes are still heavy and suffused; the skin is less hot and less dusky; pulse 114, thrilling, but not full; tongue moister than yesterday, red in the centre, coated with yellow fur at the edges; has had one copious watery evacuation; slight prominence of the cardiac region. The heart's sounds are obscurer and more distant than yesterday; the bruit of yesterday is now manifestly a friction sound, which is louder at the base than at the apex of the heart; the first sound is altogether obscured by it, and the second is heard only over the aortic valves.

The child has had four powders. To continue taking them every six hours. ℥j. of strong mercurial ointment to be rubbed into the thighs every six hours. Six leeches to be applied over the heart.

15th.—There was considerable difficulty in stopping the bleeding from the leech-bites, which was so profuse as to make him rather faint. He slept tolerably during the night, and until 6 A.M., when he became light-headed, and continued so until 9 o'clock this morning, but has since lain quiet, though troubled by a dry cough.

His appearance is much as yesterday; skin dry and hot; pulse 120, possessing the same character as before, but with less power; tongue coated at the edges, with a dry, red, streak in the centre; bowels open twice, motions green and watery.

Auscultation yields the same results as yesterday. Same treatment continued, with the addition of a saline draught containing small doses of the liquor antimonialis every four hours.

16th.—General condition much as yesterday, but on the whole seems slightly improved; pulse 120, softer.

The friction sound is no longer audible, but a loud rasping sound is heard in the place of the first sound. The second sound can now be distinguished at the apex of the heart as well as over the aortic valves, and is quite natural.

On the 17th the gums were slightly affected by mercury, and the bruit was thought to be softer and rather less loud. The dose of calomel was now reduced to gr. ss. every four hours, and the child was allowed a little broth.

On the 23d his mouth was very sore, and all active treatment was discontinued on that day. The child gradually regained his strength, but the bruit accompanying the first sound continued, and was heard a month afterwards with no other change than being rather softer and more prolonged.

I have notes of another case, in which a very loud *bruit de soufflet* accompanied the first sound of the heart, and was heard with greatest intensity below and somewhat to the left of the nipple. In this instance the disease was probably of long standing, since the heart's impulse was considerably increased, its apex beat considerably lower than natural, and there was extended dulness in the præcordial region. While the boy was under my care, his parents removed from London, and I consequently lost sight of him.

The results of endocarditis appear to be, in the child as in the adult, either very distressing or comparatively slight, according as it is succeeded or not by hypertrophy and dilatation of the heart. It has seldom occurred to me to witness greater suffering than in the case of—

Anne Leach, aged 10 years, living at 50, Turnmill Street, Clerkenwell, who first came under my notice in March 1842. She was one of five children of healthy parents, but her own health had always been delicate. For the last year she had been growing thinner, and had suffered from palpitation of the heart, and for three months had had cough; but I could not ascertain that any very marked febrile attack had ushered in her illness. Her parents, however, belonged to that class of poor who seldom pay much attention to their children's ailments.

When brought to me she was greatly emaciated; her face was anxious and distressed, her breath short, so that it was with difficulty that she walked even a short distance; she had frequent short cough without expectoration, and she suffered much from palpitation of the heart and a sense of discomfort at the chest.

The heart's action was violent; dulness in the præcordial region was very extended; a very loud, harsh, rasping sound accompanied the first sound of the heart, loudest towards the apex and to the left of the nipple, but heard over nearly the whole of the chest, both before and behind.

Various remedies brought slight but temporary relief to her sufferings, and she grew worse every month. She became more and more emaciated; the distress at the chest and the palpitation of the heart increased, her cough became more violent, and once she had an attack of hæmoptysis. For about a month before her death the cough altogether ceased, but she was now unable to leave her bed, from increasing weakness; the palpitation continued unmitigated, and her extremities became slightly anasarcous. During the last week of her life her respiration was extremely difficult, and became increasingly so till she died, on October 10th, 1842.

On a post-mortem examination, made thirty-six hours after death,—

Very little fluid was found in either pleura; both lungs were very emphysematous, and much congested, but neither they nor the bronchial glands contained any tubercle.

The heart was extremely large, but its right cavities did not exceed the natural size; the pulmonary valves were healthy; the edges of the tricuspid valve were slightly thickened; the left auricle was enormously dilated, but its walls were not at all attenuated; the pulmonary veins were much dilated; the left ventricle was dilated, and its walls were thickened; the chordæ tendineæ of the mitral valve were greatly shortened, so that the valve could not close; the valve itself was shrunk, thickened, and cartilaginous; and there existed likewise slight thickening of the edges of the semilunar valves of the aorta.

The other organs were healthy, except the mesenteric glands, many of which contained tubercles, which, in several, had undergone the cretaceous transformation.

In another somewhat similar case general dropsy came on, and the patient died of ascites and hydrothorax. In this instance, however, though the mitral valve was diseased, and dilatation, with hypertrophy of the left auricle and ventricle, existed, yet the symptoms, though greatly aggravated by the valvular disease, could not be altogether attributed to it. There existed in this case that narrowness of the aorta to which Meckel and Andral have called attention as a congenital malformation, occasionally giving rise to hypertrophy of the heart. It was not, however, till six months before the death of the child—a girl aged ten years—that her health was perceptibly affected, but she then began to suffer from palpitation of the heart, which at first was attended with febrile symptoms, afterwards with phenomena similar to those which occurred in the case of Leach, and which were terminated, as already mentioned, by ascites and hydrothorax.

In a third case I found the chordæ tendineæ much shortened, so as to keep the valve permanently open; and the valve was opaque, thickened so as to resemble cartilage, and presented a puckered appearance as if shrunken by the action of boiling water. The patient was a phthisical boy, five years old, in whom no symptom or physical sign of disease of the heart existed till five months before his death, when he had an attack of inflammation of the left pleura, terminating in effusion into its cavity. A loud *bruit de soufflet* accompanying the first sound then became audible, and continued so till his death; but the general indications of cardiac disease were masked by the graver phenomena which attended the pleurisy and the extension of the tubercular disorganization of the lungs.

These cases, which are all that have at present come under my notice, are, I think, sufficient to shew that inflammation of the lining membrane of the heart does occasionally occur in children as an idiopathic affection, and wholly independent of rheumatism. It has so happened, indeed, that though I have had the opportunity of observing the diseases of above 5000 children at the Children's Infirmary, since May 1839, I have met with but one case of affection of the heart occurring in the course of rheumatism. This circumstance, however, I regard as merely accidental, and do not by any means infer that idiopathic endocarditis is more frequent in children than endocarditis as a result of rheumatism. I could not connect the occurrence of endocarditis with any attack of scarlatina, though I directed my inquiries particularly to that point; nor in any of the post-mortem examinations of children who died of dropsy after scarlatina during the epidemic of 1839, did I notice any indication of inflammation of the endocardium, though Von Ammon's observations prove the occasional connection of the two diseases. It is, perhaps, worthy of note that tubercle was present in some of the internal organs in all the three fatal cases, though extensive tubercular disorganization of the lungs existed only in one instance. The mother of M. Thomas was affected with phthisis at the time when she brought her child to me; phthisis was hereditary in the family of G. Cole, and the boy himself presented all the peculiarities of the strumous habit in a very marked degree.

The disease does not appear to be one which tends to an immediately fatal issue, though its sequelæ in the child as well as in the adult are often *very distressing*, and greatly shorten life. Its early diagnosis is, therefore, a matter of considerable importance. It does not seem to be always announced by very striking symptoms, but a febrile attack of no great intensity, accompanied by increase of the heart's action, are often the only heralds of its onset. Since, then a disease so grave may commence with such comparatively trivial symptoms, it is a matter of great practical moment never to omit auscultating the heart, even in a case of what may seem to be merely a mild attack of simple fever.

I have nothing to add with reference to the treatment, since there does not appear to be any reason for deviating from that plan which would be proper in the adult. I regret, however, that in some of the cases above related I did not adopt more energetic measures than those to which I resorted.

AN INSTANCE

OF THE

LOSS OF IRRITABILITY IN THE GLOTTIS FOLLOWING A WOUND IN THE THROAT.

To the Editor of the Medical Gazette.

Sir,

IF you should deem the accompanying communication worthy of your notice, please to insert it in the GAZETTE.

I am, sir,

Your obedient servant,

WILLIAM PRETTY,
Surgeon.

Camden Town, July 28th, 1843.

An old man, in a fit of despondency, attempted self-destruction by cutting his throat with a razor. The loss of blood was small; the wound was jagged, and of considerable size in front; respiration was carried on partly through it, and the voice was reduced to a mere whisper. Inflammation and suppuration of the wounded parts supervened, attended with fever and cerebral affection, and the patient died about the eighth or tenth day. During my attendance, I was much surprised to find that fluids introduced into the mouth passed freely out of the wound, sometimes attended with, and sometimes without, a moderate fit of coughing. This circumstance led me to suspect that the œsophagus was injured, though it did not appear so upon external examination. I believe that the passage of fluids from the mouth through a wound in the throat has usually been considered as a distinguishing sign of an opening having been effected in the œsophagus: upon examination after death the œsophagus here was found uninjured. I have not seen, in any former or subsequent case, the same fact, though it may have been observed by others. The sensibility of the glottis and the power of swallowing is remarkably continued in some cases of disease, when all other parts have seemed to have lost their irritability. I witnessed lately in a case of fever which proved fatal after forty-eight hours of insensibility, accompanied with perfect relaxation of the sphincter muscles of the bladder and rectum, a capability to swallow fluid jelly, and to cough when any small portion got into the glottis, till within one hour of dissolution taking place.

The few particulars of this case of cut-throat I have written from memory, my case-book not being at hand. I cannot give the precise situation and extent of the injury, but believe the wound was inflicted at the inferior margin of the thyroid cartilage, the glottis and epiglottis escaping injury; neither can I positively say that the facts of impaired deglutition, great loss of sensibility in the glottis, and the passage of fluids through it without producing great inconvenience, did immediately follow the receipt of the injury, but of this I am certain, that soon after, and till within a few hours of death occurring, air in respiration, and fluids attempted to be taken by the mouth, passed freely through the wound in the trachea. I allude here particularly to *time*, as being, perhaps, one way, as well as the nature of the particular parts injured, of accounting for the little opposition which this case offers to the conclusions fairly drawn by Mr. Erichsen in his experiments upon the trachea of the dog, and inserted in the MEDICAL GAZETTE of July 14th last, and which I have read with much satisfaction and interest. I have thought that this case might not be disadvantageously connected with these experiments.

THE LATE SIR C. NIGHTINGALE'S CASE.

To the Editor of the Medical Gazette.

SIR,

I BEG to send you a few additional observations upon the symptoms which attended the illness of the late Sir Charles Nightingale.—I am, sir,

Your obedient servant,

EDWIN LAMBERT.

Park Street, Bath, Aug. 13, 1843.

The mucous secretion, which was a prominent symptom in the late Sir C. Nightingale's case, appears to have arisen from irritation communicated to the solar plexus of nerves which ministers to the circulation and secretions of the stomach, whilst the constant vomiting and panting indicated a similar condition of that portion of the spinal cord from which the pneumo-gastric and phrenic nerves take their origin.

We cannot fail to be struck with the fact that not the slightest vestige of disease was discoverable in the pyloric orifice or mucous membrane of the stomach, which "was unusually pale," and this profuse secretion generated (not the acid of cardialgia, or alkaline secretion of pyrosis) without any evident cause existing in the organ itself. Can it, then, be attributed to any other cause than that of irritation propagated by nervous sympathy?

The icy coldness of the hands, which denoted that one portion of the spinal marrow had lost the power of transmitting heat, whilst it continued to exercise a very feeble influence over the circulating powers, and the consequent secretion, exhalation, and congestion, which the *post mortem* examination so manifestly displayed, constitute a train of phenomena which can only be explained by the assumption of an irritant poison acting upon the nervous and circulating systems.

I will now mention another symptom of spinal irritation, omitted in my previous narrative, which presented itself a few hours before death, and although not observed by myself, was communicated to me by Mr. Thomas Nightingale, the son, who was with his father a short time before his dissolution; viz. the continual drawing up of the legs, which evidently proceeded from spasmodic contraction of the flexor muscles. It must be quite obvious to the pathological observer, that neither the partial disorganization of the liver (its nature is not described) or "Bright's disease" of the kidney were sufficient to destroy life, and as no other viscera are said to be organically diseased, we can only account for death by violence inflicted on the spinal marrow and circulation, through the agency of some deleterious ingredient. There were no appearances of the slightest tendency to hæmorrhage from the bowels during any stage of the disorder, but he complained of much irritation about the rectum. I saw one alvine evacuation on the Friday, of a perfectly healthy consistence, but of a dark colour; its discolouration, however, was not owing to the presence of blood; probably to extraneous matter.

I have now, in conclusion, to thank you, sir, for the space you have afforded me in your GAZETTE for the foregoing observations. The threats and annoyance which I have experienced, and the abuse with which I have been assailed, because I have come forward in the cause of truth and justice, have urged me on, upon this as it would upon any future occasion, with more resolute energy, to promote investigation, and to pursue that straightforward course, which, for the sake of my own character, as well as for the honour of the profession to which I belong, I am determined never to depart from.

MEDICAL GAZETTE.

Friday, August 18, 1843.

"Licet omnibus, licet etiam mihi, dignitatem *Artis Medicæ* tueri; potestas modo veniendi in publicum sit, dicendi periculum non recuso."
CICERO.

BATHING.

THERE is, perhaps, no subject bearing on public health which requires more unceasing efforts on the part of the journalist, than the personal habits of the working classes. Efforts for their improvement, to be really efficacious, require not merely that the facts of the case be stated, but that the best means of applying the required remedies be accurately conceived and pointed out: the understanding may be convinced long before prejudice and apathy are removed. Prejudice and apathy are mentioned together, for they are apt to exist at the same time, though they are found in very different classes of persons, and the eager philanthropist too often finds that after he has succeeded in convincing the prejudiced, his benevolent schemes are still more provokingly thwarted by his converts gradually falling into the ranks of the indifferent; so that those on whom he counted as able coadjutors, if he could once remove their prejudices, afterwards disappoint him by their indifference, and require the exertion of all his energies to give them a fresh impetus in the right direction.

It is surely not too much to assert that a prejudice has existed in England against bathing. This assertion may surprise those who are thoroughly acquainted with the many and powerful arguments which have lately been used by popular writers to prove its value; but it will not surprise those who remember the manner in which it was spoken of in their youth and boyhood, or, what may have made less impression, the silence maintained on the subject by those in authority. It was spoken of as a boyish pastime of more than usual danger, and on that account either almost prohibited altogether by the sterner sort; connived at, but not recognised, by the more indulgent; or invested with so many perils, and fenced round with so many cautions, as to form quite a memorable exception to the sports which were permitted or encouraged. The most expert swimmers in our younger days, we remember to have been also cunning in devices for concealing all traces of their prowess; and boys who, for "headers," and deep divings, had been the envy of their comrades, became equally notorious for fishing up plausible excuses to account for lank hair and a wet pocket - handkerchief. But this is changed; professorships of swimming have been established at Eton, and prizes are annually swum for in the Serpentine river, by the members of a swimming society and their pupils, "apparent rari nantes in gurgite vasto;" and so far as cold bathing goes, matters are improving. For this progress we are much indebted to the Messrs. Chambers of Edinburgh, to the conductors of the Penny Magazine, and other directors of the public taste. The publications intended for the working classes, it will be observed, are in reality chiefly bought and read by those much above them; a very small proportion indeed, of those to whom they were professedly addressed, being yet in a condition to purchase them for want of means, or to benefit by them for want of education. The removal of nearly all social prejudices is effected from above downwards, and that against cold bathing is no exception to the general rule. It must not be imagined that the downward progress of common sense on this subject, through the middling classes, has been an easy matter, or that it has taken place as yet to any great extent. Indeed, as an occasional plunge into cold water is one of the natural occurrences of field labour, and even one of the instincts of human nature, whatever prejudices may exist against it must have been artificially inculcated; and we do find such, accordingly, stronger and more universal in the middle than in the lowest ranks of life—in cities than in the country— while amongst philosophers and savages it exists not at all. Between these two extremes, of human wisdom on the one

hand, and human ignorance on the other, all manner of half wisdoms and unwisdoms, of appetites, passions, and self-denials, of convictions and prejudices, jostle one another in contending for partial and temporary dominion over the mind and the habits of man.

It is true, in fact, that many dangers beset civilized man when he yields to his natural instinct for cold immersion; and there is little doubt that from the gradual observation of these has been compiled a commination against cold bathing in general, which, however wise and well meaning in its origin, has been repeated in the ears of the vulgar till it has caused more evils than it averted. In composing this, the professors of physic have doubtless had their share; and as they have borne their part at all times in pointing out what was good for mankind, and what was evil, to the best of their knowledge, so it has happened that, as this knowledge happened to be founded on more or less accurate bases, it must have varied in value with the justness of the prevailing theories. But in our day medical men are not generally alarmists on the subject of cold bathing; their tendency is perhaps the other way; and there is reason to fear that Priessnitz and Father Mathew have indirectly excited an indiscriminating fanaticism in favour of cold water amongst those who should not have been led, in any curative or hygienic doctrine, beyond eclectic sobriety.

The hot bath in this country is seldom meddled with by the lower orders, but, like parturition, has been surrounded with so many real and imaginary dangers as not to be undergone without the advice and assistance of the faculty; and we should be sorry to say any thing which should lead our compatriots, in their present artificial state of life, to consider the doing without us in either case other than as a piece of hazardous eccentricity, which, though occasionally indulged in with impunity, is not often to be attempted. Healthy people may of course do many things without immediate, or even distant, ill consequences, which would be fatal to invalids; but a knowledge of the powers of the hot bath for good and for evil is far from universal even amongst ourselves; and as for the laity, it is certain they often do mischief by its imprudent use. We are, perhaps, from the little knowledge we possess, too timid; those who are quite ignorant, if fond of the hot bath as a remedy or a luxury, too careless—"fools rush in where angels fear to tread." Of one thing we may be quite sure, that by inculcating systematically and repeatedly the habit of cold ablution as a rule, we shall do great good in the middling and lower classes of society— we shall gradually acquire a knowledge of those cases in which it is prejudicial, or where more than ordinary caution is required in its use; and we shall prepare the way for total immersion whenever such a practice shall have become desired by the "million," and rendered practicable and easy for their adoption. At present, it is neither the one nor the other, but is becoming more so, if we may judge from certain symptoms lately observed. These are a manifest increase in the number of baths in the metropolis, a lowering of the prices, so that a tepid "mechanic's bath," as it is called, may be procured in Holborn for fourpence; and lastly, the swimming schools alluded to above. It would be a good plan for those who think bathing important, to provide themselves with a few bath tickets, which may be procured at a reduction on the price of a single bath, and distribute them judiciously amongst the working classes, to whom they are an acceptable present. A bath might often be recommended as a prophylactic to other members of a family when it would not be ventured on, or could not be taken by a patient. One caution is especially needful; experience has abundantly proved that a cold bath in a cold place is seldom followed by comfortable sensations. We should be careful, therefore, to warn inexperienced bathers on this head, as, even if health be not thereby injured, a disagreeable impression of the bath is acquired, and the habit of bathing rendered less likely to be acquired. One reason why the higher classes are so beneficially addicted to cold ablution, even throughout the winter, is that they are careful, in cold weather, to take their bath in a warm room, or to dry the body near a fire; the chill is therefore confined to the time of immersion, and the reaction is immediate and complete.

The judicious remarks on the subject of bathing by that veteran advocate of ablution, Dr. James Johnson, can never be read without pleasure by those who are impressed with the importance of this subject. The Doctor's enthusiasm, while in fancy sporting with the nymphs, is quite refreshing; and it need hardly be said that personal experience will form the strongest recommendation, one which no gentleman, and therefore, it may be hoped, no medical practitioner of this day can be without. We are not all prepared to admit the arguments of the teetotallers, and therefore may decline to practise the abstinence they insist on; but in the copious application of water externally, it would be well to practise what we preach, and to preach it earnestly because we practise it diligently.

The visiter to the Cartoons in Westminster Hall cannot fail to have been pleased with the intelligence and good conduct shown by some of the poorest of his fellow-critics. The hygeist will wish that some clear-headed, keen-scented legislator, would discover that such men could also appreciate cheap, nay, gratuitous, bathing, if part of the noble river which flows through their capital could be warmed and purified for such a purpose. Would the expense be much greater than that of Dr. Reid's airing apparatus, and would the public benefit be much less? "A question to be asked."

FELLOWES' CLINICAL PRIZE REPORTS.

By Alfred J. Tapson.

University College Hospital, 1842.

[Continued from p. 687.]

Case XV.—*Hemiplegia et Tuberculæ Pulmonum.—The former treated by cupping, purging, cantharides, &c. with considerable benefit.*

George P——, æt. 54, admitted May 21, 1842, under Dr. Williams : a man of very moderate conformation and sanguine temperament ; is a watchmaker. His habits have been tolerably regular, excepting a great addiction to venery, although he is married and has had 18 children by his wife. His father died of consumption. He has sustained several bodily injuries at different times, which we mention as they may throw some light on the cause of the present diseases : thus, when six years old, he had his skull fractured over the left temple by a blow against a tea-kettle ; about fourteen years ago he had a severe blow on the upper and back part of the head, in which situation there is still a swelling, and ever since this he has been subject to headache and occasional giddiness : the pain, he says, was always worse in cold weather, and was increased by stooping : he had a third blow on the head about two years ago by falling backwards. Again, he says that thirty-three years ago he strained his right side by lifting a heavy shutter, and has since frequently had pain in that side. Nine years ago he had an attack of pleurisy, caught by sleeping in damp clothes, and after he recovered his legs and feet used to swell constantly for a a short time. Lastly, he says, that some time afterwards, when he awoke one morning, he brought up more than a pint of coagulated blood, of rather a dark colour. The following morning he vomited about half a pint of fluid blood, much brighter in colour, and for several days he continued to spit up small quantities of blood, without having any cough ; he had not had any symptoms of gastric or pulmonary disease previously, at least he does not remember any ; he was bled, given iced water to drink, and a quantity of medicine, and he soon recovered, but he has ever since been subject to cough in the winter, and in damp weather ; slight expectoration, and sometimes pain in the chest and tightness of breathing.

The *present attack* may be said to have commenced about eight weeks since, when he was seized with sudden giddiness, and partial loss of consciousness, also his speech was impeded, and his left arm and leg were very weak ; he drank some brandy and water, and recovered in half an hour, and remained well till three weeks ago, when he had another attack whilst he was engaged at his work stooping forwards. He was now insensible for a minute or two, and on this, as well as on the former occasion, his mouth was drawn considerably to the right side. Since this attack he has kept his bed ; has been very drowsy, and his sight and memory have suffered much ; he has not been sick.

Present symptoms.—He has no pain in the head, but feels rather giddy ; the face is drawn to the right side ; the left side is flattened ; the tongue when protruded deviates to the left ; speech is very imperfect and thick (perhaps part of this is due to the habit of taking large quantities of snuff.) He can move the shoulder and arm of the left side down to the elbow, but not below, and cannot move the fingers at all ; the arm hangs lifeless, as it were, from the elbows, and if allowed to hang down gets swelled and dark coloured ; he can bend the thigh on the trunk, and the leg on the thigh, but cannot move the toes ; sensation is not impaired in either limb, but the whole of the left side feels colder than the right ; pulse 60, soft, and the patient feels weak ; the tongue is rather white ; appetite moderate ; bowels costive ; urine pale and rather scanty.

Physical signs.—The left side of the chest moves less in inspiration ; the right side is flattened under the clavicle, and in this situation the sound on percussion is decidedly duller than on the left side, and there is a corresponding dulness on the suprascapular fossa. The breath sound is bronchial under the right clavicle, and is loud under the left, and there is slight bronchophony under both.

Applicetur Cucurb. cruent. nuchæ ad ℥viij.

℞ Ol. Crotonis, ℳj. ; Micæ Panis, q. s. ft. pilula omni nocte sumend.

24th.—The bowels have been well opened ; urine scanty and turbid, but readily cleared by heat or by nitric acid—reaction acid ; specific gravity 1024.

Sumat pil. om. alternâ mane.

℞ Tinct. Cantharid. ℳxv.; Tinct. Hyoscyami, ℥xx.; Potassæ Liq. ℥xx.; Mist. Camph. f℥j. Ft. haust. ter die sumendus. Nuchæ admov. emplast. Canth.

25th.—The blister rose well; to-day he can raise the arm a little higher; he feels a pain running along the arm from the elbow to the fingers; cannot move these at all; the temperature in the left axilla is nearly a degree of Fahrenheit lower than in the right axilla; pulse 54, weak.

28th.—Still very drowsy; he sleeps at least fourteen out of the twenty-four hours; he has a little pain over the left temple to-day, and the left eye is suffused; the memory is worse, he says, than it was yesterday, and he feels confused; pulse 64, still weak; the pills gripe him a good deal, but do not purge him.

Auge Ol. Crotonis ad ℥ij.

30th.—The bowels were freely purged yesterday by the pill. The voluntary movements are scarcely at all improved, and the head feels rather confused. He states that when he awakes in the morning he frequently finds the fingers of the left hand contracted; and it was noticed that if the foot was tickled the toes were moved readily, and when he yawns the fingers are stretched out, and sometimes firmly closed involuntarily. In passing his urine he feels some little difficulty at first, but when it once begins to flow there is no further difficulty.

31st.—He complains of headache still, and feels more confused over the left temple, and is very drowsy; the left eye is a good deal injected; the pulse is only 48, but full and prolonged; the tongue rather more furred, and he has no appetite; the bowels are open.

Applicetur C. C. tempori sinistro ad f℥vj.; Auge Tinct. Canth. ad ℥xx.

June 1st.—Feels much relieved since the cupping; has no headache, no confusion of ideas, no suffusion of the eye, and looks better altogether; tongue cleaner; pulse 48; was able to bend his toes a little this morning for a short time, and moves the leg rather better.

4th.—Much better in health; head quite clear; pulse 52; is able to walk about more easily, but cannot move the arm any better.

7th.—Feels stronger; appetite good; pulse 50, weak.

Full diet.

9th.—Improving; he can raise the arm better, and can partly flex some of the fingers, but cannot extend them again; has more power over the toes.

11th.—Health pretty good; pulse 56, rather small and weak; the left side of the chest still moves less than the right when a deep inspiration is taken; he can move the arm more freely, and also can flex the fingers better, but cannot extend them; and when the arm is held out with the palm of the hand downwards the hand falls; he can also move the leg and flex the toes better, but cannot raise the toes, and when he walks the foot drags on the ground. He continues to take the croton oil pills every other morning, and the cantharides draughts as ordered: the urine is abundant and clear except when the pills are taken; then the urine is more scanty, and watery stools are produced.

Ordered to have a splint applied along the palmar surface of the fore-arm and hand.

17th.—Gaining strength and looks better in the face; he can walk a little without a stick; can bend the fore-arm better, and can flex all the fingers pretty well, but is not able to straighten them again; complains of pain extending along the fore-arm.

21st.—Feels stronger and looks more cheerful; has been allowed to go out for a short walk; can raise the arm up to the head, and flexes the fore-arm and fingers more strongly, but cannot extend the fingers yet; he has more strength in the leg, and can extend the foot better.

Auge Tinct. Canth. ad ℥xxv.

24th.—The tongue does not deviate much now when protruded; speech still rather indistinct; this arises, he says, from his mouth filling with water when he speaks; pulse 54; he still has a little difficulty at first when he attempts to pass his water; cannot extend the fingers yet; he can bend the foot upwards on the leg, but cannot extend the toes by themselves.

28th.—Much the same.

Omittatur haustus.

℞ Tinct. Canth. ℥xxx.; Aquæ Menth. Pip. f℥iss. f. haustus ter die sumendus.

30th.—The left arm ordered to be electrified daily.

July 2d.—Moves the hand better than he has done at all; was able to extend the fingers in the morning.

Omittantur Pilulæ.

℞ Pil. Cambog. C. gr. vj. omni nocte sumend.

July 5th.—He complains that he has pain in the left shoulder, and that it feels very weak. He has not been able to extend the fingers since the 2d inst.

9th.—Feels quite well, except being weak; the general appearance much improved; pulse 68; still has pain in the left shoulder and arm; can move the toes much better; is able to raise them without raising the whole foot. The pill does not keep his bowels open.

Sumantur duo pilulæ omni nocte.

12th.—Walks better; still has pain in the left shoulder; it is much increased by raising the arm; bowels regular.

Humero sinistro applic. Empl. Canth. quatuor pollices longum, duo lat.

14th.—Pain much the same; the blister did not rise well.

Omitt. pil.

℞. Ext. Col. C. gr. viij. Ft. pil. omni nocte sum.

19th.—Looks and feels quite well, but still has the pain in the arm; the bowels are a little purged by the pill. Physical signs noticed again to-day: the sound on percussion dull under the right clavicle, and the respiratory murmur has a tubular character, almost cavernous, and attended with a submucous rhonchus; loud vocal resonance also in the same situation: under the left clavicle the breath sound is tubular, but less so than on the right; the voice also too resonant; percussion is dull in the right supra-scapular fossa.

Rep. Empl. Canth. humero.

Sumat Pil. Col. C. gr. v. tantum omni nocte.

21st.—The blister rose well, and has relieved the pain in the shoulder; but he still feels pain in the forearm; pulse 70; bowels open; urine plentiful, clear, and he very seldom experiences any difficulty in passing it.

23d.—Moves both the leg and the arm very much better; the hand feels warmer; still has pain in the forearm, and occasionally in the shoulder.

28th.—General health good; sleeps well, and not so heavily as he did; walks more firmly on the left leg; cannot move the arm well, from the pain in the shoulder and elbow.

℞. Liq. Ammon. f℥ij.; Olei Olivæ, Olei Terebinth. aa. f℥ss. M. ft. linim. quo fricetur humerus nocte maneque.

He was discharged a few days after this, greatly relieved: he could walk pretty well, and move the arm much better; and we have since met him in the streets, looking quite well, but walking rather lame, and the arm was still very weak.

REMARKS.—Adopting the same plan in this as in other cases where there has been more than one disease, we shall notice, first, the paralysis, and secondly, the tubercles in the lungs; and combine with each so much of the previous history and subsequent results as belong to it.

The symptoms on the patient's admission were those of partial paralysis of all the voluntary muscles on the left side of the body: thus, the face was drawn to the right side, indicating paralysis of the left; the speech was impaired, and the tongue, when protruded, deviated to the left side, shewing that the left side was paralysed. And supposing the paralysis not to be complete, we may illustrate the cause of the deviation to the left or paralysed side by comparing it with a Breguet's thermometer, in which the unequal expansion of two metals soldered together produces a similar deviation when heated. His sight and memory were also impaired considerably; the left side of the chest moved less than the right, and the arm and leg were paralysed, especially the lower half of each limb. Sensation was perfect in all these parts, but the temperature was diminished, and the circulation was imperfectly carried on, as evidenced by the dark colour and the swelling when dependent.

It did not appear that the involuntary muscles had suffered, unless the slight difficulty at first in attempting to evacuate the bladder be attributed to this cause. And the involuntary movements of the voluntary muscles were still easily produced, as by tickling the foot, and as in yawning.

We may now ask, what was the pathological state of the cerebro-spinal axis on which these symptoms depended? We see at once, from the paralysis of the face, and the affection of the memory and sight, and temporary loss of consciousness, in addition to the paralysis of the limbs, that they depended on some lesion within the cranium. In order to ascertain what this was, we refer to the history of the attack, and we there find that he had had four distinct fits, as they might be called. The first of these was apparently relieved by his drinking a glass of brandy and water, and the second and third passed off spontaneously. It was thus obvious that these could only have depended on some temporary condition of the brain; and the only condition, as far as we know, that would cause these symptoms, and which would itself be likely to be relieved by a stimulant, is congestion of the vessels of the brain, depending, probably, either on some trifling obstruction to the circulation, or on a loss of tone in the coats of the vessels; but on either of these suppositions it is difficult to explain the suddenness of the congestion. If we believe that the brandy and water had a good effect here, it may be asked, should we be warranted in ordering it in a case presenting similar symptoms? We can hardly think that we should, on account of the difficulty, if not impossibility, of knowing at the time that there is only congestion, and not hæmorrhage. It appears that the last fit came on similarly to the others, but was more severe; and its effects were permanent, shewing that now there was something besides congestion of the brain. This fit, like the preceding ones, might have depended on congestion, in the first instance; but now, instead of passing off as before, it in all probability terminated in hæmorrhage into the brain, and thus caused the permanent paralysis of one side of the body. Had he in this attack taken brandy and water, it would have been almost sure to increase the effusion of blood, and might thereby have caused fatal effects; and yet there was no additional symptom at the time to prove the existence of anything beyond congestion.

We have been speaking of congestion as the cause of the attacks; but this itself must have a cause, like every thing else. Was there, then, any apparent cause here? To answer this we go still further back in his history; and we find that he had sustained several injuries of the head at various times; and one of these, viz. the severe blow on the upper part of the back of the head, was stated by Dr. Williams to have been very probably connected with it: he said it was just the kind of injury to produce disordered circulation in the head: he had seen many similar cases; and the occasional giddiness and frequent headache since he received this blow confirm this view. The injury was probably slight; but a slight injury of this kind, persisting, may lead to much more serious consequences. There were other causes which might have aided in producing congestion: thus the habit of taking enormous quantities of snuff may have assisted; also the excessive indulgence in venery, of which he said he had been guilty, is another cause, it is said, of many diseases of the nervous system, and may have operated here: and we must not forget that in his employment he would be constantly stooping, and two of the fits came on when he was engaged at his work. Thus we believe that there was a disposition to derangement of the cerebral circulation, produced by his habits and the injury he sustained, and that from some cause (perhaps similar to that which often determines an epileptic fit where there is a constitutional tendency to this) there had been distinct congestion produced three times, which again subsided without any further injury, but that on the last time it ended in extravasation of blood in the brain. As the patient lived, we could have no proof that there was hæmorrhage; but from the absence of any marks of inflammation or softening, we conclude that the symptoms must have depended on hæmorrhage. If this had occurred, it was no doubt somewhere in the right hemisphere of the brain, and very probably in its more

common situation, viz. in the corpus striatum or thalamus opticus.

In considering the treatment for such a case, it should have reference to the cause, whenever this can be ascertained. Now here it was believed to be congestion, and the symptoms seemed to indicate that, although hæmorrhage might have occurred, there still was some congestion; blood-letting, therefore, was indicated; and as he was weak, local blood-letting by cupping was deemed most advisable, and only to a small amount. The bowels being costive, the next thing was to purge them freely, which was done by croton oil. These remedies soon relieved the more important of the symptoms from the head for a time, but, as is often the case, a slight reaction occurred after a few days, which was immediately relieved after a few days by cupping over the left temple, where the pain now was. The remedy that was ordered more immediately to act on the nervous system was cantharides: the tincture was given, in doses of ♏xv. gradually increased to ℨss. three times a day, in combination with an alkali and henbane. The latter was omitted after some time, as it seemed to cause headache; at all events the headache ceased when this was left off. Counter-irritation was also used after the cupping. After a few days weakness was the most prominent general symptom; he was accordingly ordered full diet. After this there was no very important change made in the treatment; the purgative was changed, and local means were used to remove pains, apparently rheumatic, in the shoulder and arm. A splint was applied to prevent the hand from becoming permanently contracted, as it tends to do; and electricity was passed through the arm to assist in restoring strength to the paralysed muscles.

Under the use of the above means the patient recovered the use of the limbs in a great measure, sufficiently to be able to walk pretty well, and to use his arm a little; and at his age and weakened state it is not very probable that he will ever recover the perfect use of the parts. The order in which the power of motion returned in this case was similar to what is usual in such cases, viz. first in the leg and then in the arm, and in the flexors before the extensors. Thus it will be seen by the reports that the power of flexing the leg and toes returned on June 1st, that of flexing the arm and fingers on the 9th, that of extending the foot and toes on the 20th, and that of extending the fingers to a slight extent on the 2d July; but this last he lost again for a time.

Secondly, previous to his admission there had been various symptoms, and at the time of his admission there were various signs referrible to the lungs which require a brief notice. In the history it is stated that as long ago as thirty-three years he had a severe strain on the right side, and had been subject to pain there ever since; that nine years ago he had severe pleurisy of the same side, and some time after this he vomited blood for two mornings, and then spit up a little for several days, and had had some tightness of breathing, and a winter cough with slight expectoration. The physical signs (*vide* report) were such as indicated some condensation of the upper lobes of both lungs, but chiefly that of the right lung. Was there any connection—and if any, what was it—between the previous history and these physical signs? The pleurisy which he had suffered from might have caused many of the signs, but it could not have caused the submucous rhonchus; and it is rare for pleurisy to affect the apex of the lung; besides, both lungs were affected. Again, it is stated that he had vomited blood; but this probably proceeded from the lungs, because there was hæmoptysis afterwards, and there were other symptoms of incipient phthisis already detailed, and hæmatemesis and hæmoptysis are always confounded by the vulgar; and, further, we know that he was hereditarily predisposed to phthisis. We have no hesitation, therefore, in concluding that there was consolidation of the lungs depending on tuberculous deposition, and that this had probably caused the hæmoptysis and the symptoms referrible to the lungs.

No treatment was adopted for the disease of the lungs, as there were no symptoms then to demand any, and the physical signs indicated that the disease was tolerably quiescent.

Lastly, it may be asked, is there any connection between the symptoms referrible to the lungs and those referrible to the nervous system? It is impossible to give any decided answer to this question, either in the negative or affirmative. Dr. Williams remarked on this point, that, "assuming that there were tubercles in the lungs, there might also be tubercles in the brain. The existence of these, however, would not alone cause the paralysis; but," we understood him to say that "the irregular circulation attending the progress of these cases might account for the paralysis." And he compared it to the production of hydrocephalus by any sudden excitement of the circulation when there was a tendency to the disease; and also to the excitement of the paroxysms of epilepsy when there was a permanent cause in the brain.

ON THE

SENSIBILITY OF THE GLOTTIS,

&c. &c.

To the Editor of the Medical Gazette.

Sir,

In your journal of to-day an anonymous correspondent directs my attention to the fact of Magendie having, six years ago, pointed out the different degrees of sensibility possessed by the glottis, larynx, and trachea, which observation, he says, is to be found in the Lancet for 1836-7. Of this, sir, I was, until I saw your correspondent's letter, entirely ignorant; and I think, sir, you will agree with me that there is nothing very singular in my ignorance, as it would require a remarkably retentive memory to be able to bear in mind all the subjects treated of in the many valuable papers and lectures that are published in the medical journals. In the only two works of Magendie's that I consulted on the matter in question, viz. his Treatise on Physiology, translated by Dr. Milligan, and his "Leçons sur les Phenomènes Physiques de la Vie," published in 1838, I found no mention made of the sensibility of the air-tubes, with the exception of the following passage. "The air-tube does not possess the same degree of sensibility in different parts: whilst that of the glottis is the most exquisite, that of the larynx and trachea scarcely exists." (Leçons, &c. vol. ii. p. 216.)

I may further remark, that as the paper which you did me the honour to publish in your journal was not intended to be an essay upon the relative sensibility of different parts of the air-passage, but was merely a letter written in answer to the question, *as to whether the performance of tracheotomy tended to lessen the sensibility of the glottis* —on which subject, as your correspondent may see, if he will take the trouble to read the published accounts of the discussion that took place at the Royal Medical and Chirurgical Society, much difference of opinion existed—I did not think it necessary to ransack the journals in order to ascertain what had previously been done upon the subject. I merely contented myself with stating the results of my own experiments, although, had I been acquainted with those of Magendie, which, as far as they go, completely tally with mine, I should not have failed to have mentioned them; as well as some which I have since been told by Dr. C. J. B. Williams he instituted two or three years ago on the same subject.

Your correspondent seems to think it wonderful that I should have operated on the same animal—the dog, and used the same instrument—the probe, as Magendie did. Perhaps he will allow me to inform him that the dog is, for various reasons, the animal that is *most generally* selected for all experiments, whether surgical, physiological, or therapeutical ; and that there is no instrument, with which I am acquainted, except a probe, that would pass through a puncture of a line in length, which was the extent of the opening in the trachea in my first experiment. It appears wonderful to me that your correspondent did not, with his sapient "*mirabile dictu,*" discover a further resemblance between Magendie's experiments and mine, viz. that we both used a scalpel and forceps.—I am, sir,

Your obedient servant,
JOHN E. ERICHSEN.

48, Welbeck Street.
August 11, 1843.

INSANITY IN FRANCE.

THE *Gazette Médicale* of the 29th ult. contains the following announcement :—

The investigation on the subject of insanity, which formed part of the General Statistics of France, and the results of which were communicated to the Academy by M. Moreau de Jonnès, comprehends not one year only, as was inadvertently reported in our last number, but seven complete and consecutive years. The following is the number of insane persons in the eighty-six departments, ascertained by the medical and ministerial authorities, on the 1st of January in each year :—

	No. of insane.	Proportion of insane to 1000 inhabitants.
1835 .	. 14486 .	. . ·043
1836 .	. 15314 .	. . ·046
1837 .	. 15870 .	. . ·047
1838 .	. 16892 .	. . ·050
1839 .	. 18113 .	. . ·054
1840 .	. 18716 .	. . ·056
1841 .	. 19738 .	. . ·058

UNLUCKY BIRTHS.

HUMAN beings are occasionally offered in sacrifice at Ibu. Twins are in all cases put to death ; and it is said that children who cut their upper-jaw teeth first were instantly destroyed.—*Medical History of the Expedition to the Niger during the Years 1841-2, by Dr. J. O. Macwilliam.*

BOOKS RECEIVED FOR REVIEW.

On the Physical Causes of the High Rate of Mortality in Liverpool. By W.H. Duncan, M.D. &c.

Cataract, and its Treatment. By John Scott, Senior Surgeon to the Royal London Ophthalmic Hospital, &c.

Anatomico-Chirurgical Observations on Dislocations of the Astragalus. By Thomas Turner, Esq. M.R.C.S.L. Surgeon to the Manchester Royal Infirmary, &c. &c.

Thirteenth Annual Report of the Manger of the Belfast District Asylum for the Insane Poor.

Observations on Idiopathic Dysentery, as it occurs in Europeans in Bengal, particularly in reference to the Anatomy of that Disease. By Walter Raleigh, Surgeon of the Native Hospital, &c.

Observations on the Necessity of an extended Legislative Protection to Persons of Unsound Mind. By Edward De Vitré, M.D. Physician to the Lancaster County Lunatic Asylum.

ROYAL COLLEGE OF SURGEONS.

LIST OF GENTLEMEN ADMITTED MEMBERS.

Friday, August 11, 1843.
A. W. Gange.—E. Pemberton.—W. Clegg.— F. Smith.—D. Corbett.—R. Oxley.—J. H. Wise. —G. Buckell.—J. Hunt.—J. Skelton.

A TABLE OF MORTALITY FOR THE METROPOLIS,

Shewing the number of deaths from all causes registered in the week ending Saturday, August 5, 1843.

Small Pox	6
Measles	21
Scarlatina	41
Hooping Cough	29
Croup	6
Thrush	3
Diarrhœa	12
Dysentery	5
Cholera	2
Influenza	1
Ague	1
Remittent Fever	0
Typhus	36
Erysipelas	3
Syphilis	3
Hydrophobia	0
Diseases of the Brain, Nerves, and Senses	188
Diseases of the Lungs and other Organs of Respiration	190
Diseases of the Heart and Blood-vessels	25
Diseases of the Stomach, Liver, and other Organs of Digestion	72
Diseases of the Kidneys, &c.	4
Childbed	2
Paramenia	0
Ovarian Dropsy	0
Disease of Uterus, &c.	2
Arthritis	0
Rheumatism	3
Diseases of Joints, &c.	6
Carbuncle	0
Phlegmon	0
Ulcer	0
Fistula	0
Diseases of Skin, &c.	0
Dropsy, Cancer, and other Diseases of Uncertain Seat	95
Old Age or Natural Decay	53
Deaths by Violence, Privation, or Iutemperance	37
Causes not specified	0
Deaths from all Causes	816

THE

LONDON MEDICAL GAZETTE,

BEING A

WEEKLY JOURNAL

OF

Medicine and the Collateral Sciences.

FRIDAY, AUGUST 25, 1843.

LECTURES

ON THE

THEORY AND PRACTICE OF MIDWIFERY,

Delivered in the Theatre of St. George's Hospital,

BY ROBERT LEE, M.D. F.R.S.

LECTURE XL.

On the Causes and Nature of Inflammation of the Uterus and its Appendages in Puerperal Women.

THE causes of inflammation in the uterine organs after delivery are often involved in the deepest obscurity. By examining the accompanying tables, you will see that in a very large proportion of cases the disease occurs after natural labours, and cannot be referred to injuries inflicted upon the uterus by violence of any kind during parturition, or to exposure to cold and moisture, and irregularities of diet committed soon after delivery. The disease has been observed by me to prevail during the last fifteen years, and to assume the different forms described in the two last lectures, during spring, summer, autumn, and winter, though most frequently in the latter season, not only in the British Lying-in Hospital, the Lying-in Wards of the Saint Marylebone, St. James', and other parochial Infirmaries, but in every district of London, and the surrounding country; and in all the different ranks of life. The disease has generally arisen, like inflammation of the bowels and lungs, and other viscera, without any assignable cause—where the process of parturition had been completed in the most natural manner, where nothing could be discovered peculiar in the constitution of the atmos-

phere, and when typhus fever, scarlet fever, erysipelas, and other contagious and epidemic disorders, were not prevailing to an unusual extent. But it is an opinion which has long prevailed, that the uterine inflammation of puerperal women is of an erysipelatous nature, and that it is excited in some cases by contagion, or depends on a vitiated state of the atmosphere, like hospital gangrene, and may be communicated from one patient to another, by the nurse and medical practitioner. It is stated by Peu, that, in 1664, a prodigious number of puerperal women perished in the Hôtel Dieu at Paris, and that the cause of this mortality was attributed by M. Vesou, physician to the hospital, to the circumstance of the lying-in wards being situated immediately over those set apart for the reception of wounded persons. The bodies of the women were found after death to be full of abscesses. Uterine phlebitis was probably the cause of this great mortality, as I have found it to be most frequently where inflammation of the uterus has appeared to be excited by the contaminated air of an hospital, contagion, and erysipelas. Ponteau regarded the disease which appeared in the Hôtel Dieu at Lyons, in the spring of the year 1750, and produced great havoc among puerperal women, to be an epidemic erysipelatous inflammation of the peritoneum. The same opinion of the nature of the affection was maintained by Dr. Lowder, and Professors Young and Home of Edinburgh, who saw the disease in the Lying-in Wards of the Royal Infirmary. Dr. Gordon, of Aberdeen, states that he had unquestionable proof that the cause of the disease was a specific contagion, and not owing to any noxious constitution of the atmosphere. The constitution of the year, as it was termed by Sydenham, had little or nothing to do with its production. The disease seized such women only as were visited or delivered by a physician, or taken care of by a nurse, who had previously attended patients affected with the disease. "I had abundant proofs," he observes, "that every person who had been with a patient in the puerperal fever became charged with an atmosphere of infection which was communicated to every pregnant woman who happened to come within its sphere." He acknowledges that he was himself the means of conveying the infection to a great number of women. "If the puerperal fever of Leeds was infectious, which by many it was thought to be," says Mr. Hey, "it was so in a very inferior degree to that at Aberdeen; for I have known instances of free communication, by the intervention of others, between women in labour or child-bed, and those affected with the disease, without any bad consequences. And, on the contrary, in many cases of puerperal fever no channel whatever was discoverable whereby the disease could have been conveyed. It was not from being convinced of its necessity, but for the satisfaction of his own mind and the safety of his patients, that he adopted the usual precautions to prevent the propagation of an infectious disorder. Dr. Armstrong observed that most of the cases at Sunderland, forty out of fifty-three, occurred in the practice of one surgeon and his assistant. He believed, at first, that the disease, as an epidemic, was invariably contagious ; but afterwards had reasons for doubting whether it was so in the ordinary sporadic form. "It is hardly possible to prove," says Dr. J. Clarke, "that it is not infectious, but it has also arisen, as far as we can judge, as an original disease, where there had been no communication with infected persons."

Dr. Hulme maintained that uterine inflammation in puerperal women was not more contagious than pleuritis, nephritis, or any other inflammatory disease. Dr. Hull, of Manchester, was also of opinion that it is not contagious. M. Tonellé, who has recorded the history of the most fatal epidemic which has ever occurred in Paris, asserts that the idea of contagion was clearly out of the question in the Maternité there, for the women who were newly delivered had each a separate apartment, and yet were attacked with the disease ; whilst in the sick ward of the hospital no instance of the propagation of the disease ever occurred. The evidence of M. Dugès against the doctrine of contagion is not less strong ; for he states that in numerous instances pregnant women have been placed in the infirmary, where they were surrounded by cases of peritonitis, without being infected; and that still more frequently he has seen women newly delivered brought into the infirmaries on account of some other complaint, and who did not contract the disease. In no instance did he observe a midwife entrusted with the care of two patients at the same time communicate peritonitis from a sick to a healthy individual, as is reported to have happened in London; and never has this inflammation been propagated from patient to patient in the wards set apart for the reception of healthy women. In the epidemic at Edinburgh described by Dr. Mackintosh and Dr. Campbell, I believe they saw no case which could be ascribed to contagion.

It is difficult to reconcile this conflicting evidence; and the facts I have observed, though they have led me to adopt the opinion that the disease is sometimes communicable by contagion, and sometimes has a connection with erysipelas, have not perhaps been sufficiently numerous, and of so decisive a character, as to dispel every doubt on the subject of its contagious or non-contagious nature, and to prove that it is a specific inflammation. It is but right to state that, in a vast majority of cases, the disease has occurred, and in the most destructive form, where contagion could not possibly be supposed to have operated as the cause. It has suddenly appeared in the practice of those who had never before seen the disease, or had any thing to do at the time with cases of typhus fever, erysipelas, and other contagious disorders.

In the last two weeks of September 1827, five fatal cases of uterine inflammation came under my observation. All the individuals so attacked had been attended in labour by the same midwife, and no example of a febrile or inflammatory disease of a serious nature occurred during that period among the other patients, who had been attended by the other midwives belonging to the institution. On the 16th March, 1831, a practitioner who resides in a populous parish in the vicinity of London, examined the body of a woman who died a few days after delivery, from peritonitis. On the morning of the 17th he was called to attend a private patient in labour, who was safely delivered on the same day. On the 19th she was attacked with the symptoms of uterine phlebitis, severe rigors, great disturbance of the cerebral functions, rapid feeble pulse, with acute pain of the hypogastrium, and peculiar sallow colour of the whole surface of the body. She died on the fourth day after the attack, the 22d March; and between this period and the 6th of April this practitioner attended two other patients, both of whom were attacked with the same disease in a malignant form, and fell victims to it. On the 30th March it happened that the same gentleman attended a patient, a robust young woman, seventeen years of age, affected with pleuritis, for which venesection was resorted to with immediate relief. On the 5th of April there was no appearance of inflammation around the puncture which had been made in the median basilic vein, but there had been pain in the wound during the two preceding days. The inner surface of the arm, from the elbow nearly to the axilla, was now affected with erysipelatous inflammation; alarming constitutional symptoms manifested themselves; the pulse was 160; the tongue dry; delirium had been observed during the night. On the evening of this day the inflammation spread into the axilla. The arm was exquisitely painful; but in the vicinity of the wound, which had a healthy appearance, the colour of the skin was natural; and no hardness or pain felt in the vein above the puncture. On the 6th, patches of erysipelatous inflammation appeared in various parts of the body, on the upper and inner surface of the left arm, and on the sole of the left foot, all of which were acutely painful on pressure. The inflammation of the right arm had somewhat subsided; the pulse was 160; the tongue brown, dry, and furred; restlessness, constant dozing, and incoherence. When roused she was conscious; the face cold; heat of the surface irregular. On the 7th, pulse rapid; countenance anxious; teeth and lips covered with sordes; somnolence and delirium. The left arm, above the elbow, was acutely painful, and the erysipelas had made no further progress. The patches of erysipelas on the forehead and sole of the foot had disappeared; but there was a slight blush of inflammation on the inner side of the calf of the left leg. The symptoms became aggravated, and she died on the 9th of April. I examined the body with Dr. John Prout on the 11th, and the following morbid appearances were observed. The wound in the median basilic vein was open, and its cavity filled with purulent fluid. The coats of this vessel, and of the basilic vein, as you can still perceive in the preparation of the parts [exhibiting it], were thickened so as to resemble the coats of an artery. The inner surface of the vein was redder than natural, and at the upper part had lost its usual smoothness, but there was no lymph deposited upon it. The mouths of the veins entering the basilic were all closed up with firm coagula of blood or lymph. The cellular membrane upon the inner surface of the vein was unusually vascular, and infiltrated with serum. This infiltration was to a much greater extent along the situation of the erysipelatous inflammation of the left arm, but the veins of this arm were perfectly healthy. It is highly probable there was something more than a mere coincidence in these events.

In the autumn of 1829 I was present at the examination of the body of a woman who died soon after delivery from inflammation of the peritoneal and muscular tissues of the uterus. I dissected out the uterine organs, and after inspecting them carefully assisted in sewing up the body. I had scarcely reached home when I was hastily summoned to attend a young lady in her first labour, who was soon safely delivered; but in sixteen hours she was attacked with violent pain in the region of the uterus. Unequivocal symptoms of uterine phlebitis soon after showed themselves: she recovered, but with great difficulty. In December 1830, two patients in the British Lying-in Hospital, who had both been attended by the same midwife, were attacked with the disease on the same day; and both died from inflammation of the absorbents and deep-seated structures of the uterus. Another patient was admitted into the hospital two days after the death of the last of these women, and was examined by the same midwife to ascertain if labour had commenced. The pains were false pains; but she remained from Saturday till Monday in the hospital, expecting that labour would come on. The pains having left her, she returned home; and the following day was suddenly taken in labour, and safely delivered before she could be sent to the hospital. She went on favourably for two days, and was then attacked with the most violent symptoms of inflammation of the veins of the uterus, and died in thirty-six hours.

In 1835, a surgeon residing at the west end of London, while attending a gentleman who had phlegmonous erysipelas of the leg and extensive sloughing of the cellular membrane, was called to a case of labour, which was speedily followed by inflammation of the uterus, and proved fatal. The body was not examined; but, from the symptoms, there could be little doubt that both the peritoneal and vascular structures were affected. A second case occurred in his practice within a few days, which also terminated fatally. Soon after a third case occurred to him, the unfavourable result of which he attributed to the copious venesection employed immediately after the invasion of the disease. He was very unhappy at the thought of having destroyed the patient by bleeding her so profusely, and could not feel satisfied that her death was owing to any other cause than excessive depletion, although the quantity of blood removed barely exceeded ℥xx., till I inspected the body, and showed him a great portion of the veins in the walls of the uterus, where the placenta had adhered, loaded with pus. The affair here ended with Mr. ——, but not so with me; for the same evening, after examining the body of this patient, I was requested to see a lady in consultation, whose labour was protracted, and an opinion required respecting the propriety of interfering, and completing the delivery by artificial means. I examined the patient, and recommended delay; and in a few hours she was safely delivered of a living child by the natural efforts. In 24 hours, this lady was attacked with peritonitis in the most violent possible form, and died in less than 48 hours with incessant vomiting, and great tympanites. The infant was cut off in no long time with erysipelas. A few days after this, having changed my clothes completely, and adopted every means that I could think of to prevent any further mischief, I attended a private patient residing near Oxford Street, whose labour was natural, and whose recovery after her two former deliveries was favourable: but in less than 30 hours she was attacked with acute inflammation of the uterus, which no remedies could subdue. The following facts are, if possible, still more striking, and leave no doubt whatever upon my mind that it is our duty to act in all cases as if the con. tagious nature of the disease had been com. pletely demonstrated.

On the morning of the 4th of August, 1836, a practitioner who resides in a large healthy village about seven miles from London, with a populous country around, attended Mrs. O——, in labour, which was natural. The same evening he was called to a case of arm presentation, where, from the rigidity of the os uteri, and violence of the contractions, he found it impossible to deliver by turning, and he sent to request my assistance for Mrs. B——. The child was premature, and had been dead some time, so that I had no difficulty in drawing down the extremity, which presented deep into the pelvis, passing the fingers along the thorax and abdomen to the nates, and extracting the lower extre. mities, and then the trunk and head of the child. No violence was necessary in effect. ing the delivery, and it seemed probable the patient would recover in a favourable manner. On the following morning, Thursday, the 5th of August, Mrs. O——, who had not been visited in the interval from her delivery, was attacked with all the usual symptoms of severe uterine inflammation, and ultimately died. As Dr. —— had not seen this patient from the time she was delivered, on the morning of the 4th, to the period of the attack, it is obvious that he could have com. municated no contagion from Mrs. B——, whose labour occurred the same evening, and whose child had died within the uterus, and presented preternaturally. No case of severe uterine inflammation had ever come under the observation of Dr. ——, though he had resided eight or ten years in the same village, and had attended numerous cases of labour. At this time there was no case of erysipelas under his care, and for a long period he had not examined any dead bodies.

Mrs. B——, who was delivered on the 4th of August, was attacked on the 6th with all the symptoms of uterine phlebitis, and died on the 9th. I examined the body with Dr. ——, and his assistant, on the 10th, and found extensive peritonitis, and all the veins and absorbents on the left side of the upper part of the uterus, where the placenta had adhered, filled with pus. As the coats of the absorbents were not thickened, I sus. pected that the pus they contained had been absorbed by them from the veins. The left ovarium was large and soft, and the left fallopian tube inflamed. The os and cervix uteri were sound. On the evening of the 10th of August, after examining the body of this patient, on returning home, I adopted every means I could devise to prevent the communication of any poison to others, but without effect, for early the following morn. ing I was called to a private patient near Lincoln's-Inn Fields, who was soon safely delivered, but was seized in less than 24 hours with a violent fit of cold shivering, acute pain in the region of the uterus, es. pecially on the right side and sacrum, head. ache, ringing in the ears, and intense thirst. The countenance was pallid and depressed when I first saw her: the pulse was 120, with nausea, sense of chilliness over the whole sur. face of the body, though it was intensely hot, and covered with perspiration. Blood-letting, general and local, was employed, but sparingly, and calomel, opium, cathartics, turpentine, prussic acid, and creosote, freely, but without the slightest effect, and she died with inces. sant vomiting of dark-coloured matter like coffee-grounds. Some time before death the pain of the abdomen subsided, and the left leg became exquisitely painful; it soon became livid and swollen around the ankle, the discoloration extended rapidly up the limb, the cuticle separated, and dark. coloured vesications were formed. The disease extended no further in my public or private practice, but another patient, at. tended by Dr. ——, soon after was destroyed by it. The assistant of Dr. —— was attacked a few days after the post-mortem examination of Mrs. B—— on the 10th August, at which he was present, with strong febrile symptoms, sickness at stomach, headache, sore-throat, and great prostration of strength. The tonsils became covered with foul superficial ulcers, the lower lip swollen, and covered with a pustular eruption; the tongue was intensely red at the point and on the edges, and covered in the middle with a thick white fur. These symptoms lasted for a week, and then went off, leaving him in a state of great debility. The cook in the family became affected a few days after with similar, but much milder, symptoms. I was in. formed that the carpenter, a young healthy

man, who placed the body of Mrs. B——
in her coffin, had afterwards a most violent
attack of fever and sore-throat, and recovered
but with difficulty. The train of misfortunes
did not end here, for an aged relative of Mrs.
B——, who was in the apartment when I
examined the body, was seized soon after
with severe symptoms, like those of continued
fever, and died after a few days' illness.

In 1839 in London, and in 1841 at
Woolwich, several similar occurrences, but
of a less striking character, took place, which
also came under my observation, and they
all point out the necessity of taking every
precaution to prevent the extension of the
disease from one puerperal woman to another,
not only by careful and repeated ablution,
and changing the clothes after attending
patients who are affected with it, but
what is far more efficacious—indeed the
only thing to be trusted to—by discon-
tinuing obstetrical practice altogether for
a time when several cases occur in rapid
succession. The great mortality in lying-in
hospitals arises chiefly from the occurrence
of uterine inflammation, and its spreading
from patient to patient, or becoming epidemic in the wards. This circumstance induced me to make the following observation
ten years ago, the truth of which is amply
illustrated by the accompanying tables :—
" From the registers of the British Lying-in
Hospital, the Maternité at Paris, the Dublin
Lying-in Hospital, and the tables of M. De
Chateau-neuf, it is proved that the average
rate of mortality greatly exceeds, in these
institutions, that of those in which individuals
are attended at their own habitations ; and if
it should ultimately appear that all precautions
are unavailing in diminishing the numbers
attacked by the disease, it becomes a subject
deserving of the most serious consideration,
on the ground of humanity, whether lying-in
hospitals should not be altogether abolished,
as injurious rather than beneficial to society.
From what has fallen under my observation
in the British Lying-in Hospital, and other
similar institutions in this metropolis, where
the utmost attention is paid to ventilation
and cleanliness, and where the wards are not
overcrowded with patients, I cannot hesitate
to express my decided conviction that by no
means hitherto discovered can the frequent
and fatal recurrence of the disease be prevented in lying-in hospitals, and that the
loss of human life thereby occasioned completely defeats the objects of their benevolent
founders."

TABULAR VIEW (No. 1) OF 100 CASES OF SEVERE INFLAMMATION OF THE UTERUS AND ITS APPENDAGES,

Which occurred to me in London, from March 1827 to the end of December 1830.

[Continued from p. 781.]

No.	Name, Residence, and Delivery.	Date of Attack and Symptoms.	Treatment.	Result and Morbid Appearance.
76	Phœbe Robins ; æt. 28 ; Holborn. Tedious labour. 10th January, 1830.	Third day.—Severe after-pains ; lochia suppressed ; exquisite tenderness of uterus ; skin hot ; pulse strong and rapid ; headache ; symptoms very obstinate.	V.S. ʒxvj., calomel, opium, leeches xxiv.	Recovered.
77	Marchant; British Lying-in Hospital. Natural labour. 11th January, 18.	Third day.—Pain not very severe in the region of the uterus ; rigors ; pulse 100 ; headache.	Leeches xij., calomel, cathartics.	Recovered.

No.	Case	Symptoms	Treatment	Result
78	Leaney; æt. 26; British Lying-in Hospital. Natural labour. 11th January, 1830.	Third day.—Headache; pyrexia; uterine pain; pulse 120; lochia suppressed; vomiting.	V.S. ʒxiv., leeches lx., calomel, opium, cathartics.	Recovered.
79	Mesalin; æt. 22; British Lying-in Hospital. Natural labour. 13th January, 1830.	Second day.—Uterus large, hard, and painful; rigors; headache; lochia nearly suppressed; pulse 100; dyspnœa; cough; skin hot; pulmonic attack; abdomen distended; uterus hard and painful on pressure; vomiting; exhaustion.	V.S. ʒxvi, V.S. ʒxiv, calomel, Dover's powder, &c.	Died. Caput coli and transverse arch of colon covered with patches of lymph; uterus uncontracted, its anterior surface of a uniform dusky red colour; the muscular tissue under this reduced to a soft reddish pulp; the veins of the fundus uteri on both sides inflamed, and filled with a quantity of pus; both ovaria enlarged, their structure destroyed; fallopian tubes soft and vascular; lungs gorged with blood, but not inflamed.
80	Meaden; æt. 20; British Lying-in Hospital. 15th January, 1830.	Second day.—Headache; rigors; uterus painful, large, and hard; anxiety; countenance pale; breathing hurried; pulse 110; lochia scanty. Convalescent in 24 hours.	V.S. ʒxx., leeches xxiv., pulv. ipecac. comp. gr. v. 3tia q. q. hora.	Recovered.
81	Case after natural labour; British Lying-in Hospital. 28th January, 1830.	Third day.—Pyrexia; severe pain of the uterus, increased by pressure. Depletion followed by immediate convalescence.	V.S. ʒxx., calomel, opium, fomentations and poultices to hypogastrium.	Recovered.
82	Williams; æt. 26; a patient of Dr. Hugh Ley's, Middlesex Hospital. Natural labour. 13th January, 1830.	Eighth day.—Vomiting; rigors; severe uterine pain; foul tongue; offensive lochia; pulse 120, soft.	V.S. ʒxvj., leeches xij., calomel, antimony, and opium.	Recovered. During this month several severe cases occurred among the out-patients of the Middlesex Hospital. In all there was more or less pain in the region of the uterus, increased by pressure, pyrexia, and diminished lochial discharge.

83	Case in a Mews near Portman Square. Natural labour. January, 1830.	Sixth day.—Continued well for six days after delivery, when fever of a typhoid character came on, with slight abdominal pain; puffy swelling over the left wrist, and on one of the thighs; slight tympanites.	Sulphate of quinine and stimulants.	Died. Uterus large; the left spermatic vein through its whole course lined with false membranes, its coats thickened, the lower part filled with pus and lymph; the upper part distended with coagula of blood; the veins at left superior angle of uterus lined with lymph, and filled with a bloody, purulent fluid; the veins on the right side of uterus gorged with pus; the right spermatic vein was healthy, also both hypogastrics.
84	Sophia Humphries. 30th January, 1830.	Third day.—Acute pain of uterus, increased by pressure; headache; tongue white; pulse 100; lochia scanty; bowels confined; blood cupped and buffed.	V.S. ℥ij, calomel, cathartics.	Recovered.
85	Jones; 48, Marshall Street. Natural labour. 11th February, 1830.	Third day.—Pyrexia; acute uterine pain; lochia suppressed; rigors; pain and swelling of left iliac region; cough; suppuration at the brim of the pelvis; the pus escaped under Poupart's ligament. Recovered after five months.	Leeches often repeated, cataplasms, bark, wine, stimulants; abscess opened artificially.	Recovered
86	Honeyman; Angel Street, City. Natural labour. 12th February, 1830.	Fourth day.—Acute uterine pain; violent rigor; headache; lochia suppressed; pulse 115, strong; respiration hurried.	V.S. ℥xxx, leeches xxiv., calomel, antimony, cathartics, diaphoretics.	Recovered.
87	Case in the Edgeware Road. 20th February, 1830.	Second day.—Pain in the region of the uterus; rigors; lochia and milk diminished; slight delirium; pulse 115; tongue white; great tenderness in the situation of right uterine appendages.	V.S. ℥j, leeches, calomel, antimony.	—— In the month of April, 1830, three cases occurred, which all yielded speedily to venesection, leeches, calomel, antim., Dover's powders, &c. The details of these cases are not preserved.

88	Mrs. Hadden; æt. 30; 3, Castle Street, Bloomsbury. Arm presentation. —	Fourth day.—Uterine pain; lochia suppressed; rigors; pain in right groin; pulse 100; tongue white. The pain was not effectually relieved till cathartics were freely administered.	V.S. ℥xij., leeches xvj., calomel, antimony, cataplasms, cathartics.	Recovered.
89	Mrs. Sears; æt. 26; 23, Church Lane. Natural labour. 20th June, 1830.	Fourth day.—Great uterine pain; pulse 100, full; lochia suppressed; rigors; blood cupped and buffed.	V.S. ℥xvj., leeches xxiv., calomel, antimony.	Recovered.
90	Mrs. Allen; æt. 26; 12, Phœnix Street, St. Giles's. Natural labour. 10th June, 1830.	Fourth day.—Uterine pain; lochia suppressed; tongue brown; vomiting; pain in right groin; pulse 130; respiration hurried.	V.S. ℥xxvj., calomel, antimony, opium, cathartics, saline effervescing draughts.	Recovered.
91	Sankey; 35, Wardour Street. Protracted labour. June, 1830.	Soon after delivery, a sudden attack of fever, with severe pain in the right iliac region and left groin and thigh; rigors; tongue loaded. July 12: the left iliac region is hard, swollen, and painful on pressure,—the hardness extends half way down the thigh, in the course of the femoral vessels; great constitutional disturbance. Aug. 6: a great quantity of pus discharged above Poupart's ligament. A slow but complete recovery.	Leeches, poultices, anodyne.	Recovered.
92	Mrs. Gyde; æt. 22; Brewer Street, Golden Square. Natural labour. 26th June, 1830.	Second day.—Rigors, and pain of the lower part of the abdomen, with pyrexia and suppression of the lochia. 29th: pain but slightly relieved; fever continues. July 4th: intense pain of the whole abdomen, and distension; pulse rapid and feeble; constant sickness and vomiting; tongue brown. 6th: symptoms aggravated. Died on the tenth day from attack.	V.S. ℥xij., leeches xij., opium, leeches, a blister, cathartics.	Died. lb. ij. of dark-coloured sero-purulent fluid in peritoneal sac; the whole abdominal viscera inflamed; small intestine, omentum, and uterus, all glued together with lymph; an abscess under the peritoneum of the uterus, near its fundus, on the left side; a small abscess in the body of the uterus on the left side; uterine appendages on both sides vascular, and coated with lymph.

93	Phillips; æt. 32; 2, Sussex Street. 30th July, 1830.	Fifth day.—Great uterine pain; pulse 130; violent headache; exquisite tenderness, increased by pressure, in the left side of the uterus, which gradually diminished, and the pulse became less frequent. A slow recovery.	V.S. ℥x., leeches xij., calomel, antimony, opium, cathartics.	Recovered.
94	Mrs. Chapman; æt. 36; 9, Belton Street, Long Acre. Natural labour. 19th August, 1830.	Fifth day.—After drinking cold beer, seized with sudden uterine pain; rigors; headache; delirium; pulse 120, weak; tongue dry and brown; constant vomiting and diarrhœa; delirium; great debility; coma; hurried respiration. Duration of disease nine days.	Leeches xii. to the temples, calomel, opium, pulv. cretæ comp. c. opio, fomentations, &c.	Died. Ovaria red, soft, and enlarged; left tube filled with pus; muscular coat of the uterus at the fundus where the placenta had adhered so soft, that the fingers passed through it in removing the parts; no inflammation of peritoneum or effusion into the abdominal cavity.
95	Keene; æt. 34; 2, Little Earl Street. Tedious labour. 2d September, 1830.	Third day.—Uterus large, hard, and painful, especially on the left side; headache; slight rigor; pulse 132; lochia continue.	V.S. ℥rj., leeches xij., calomel, antimony, opium, cathartics, pulv. ipecac. co.	Recovered.
96	——; æt. 30; Stewart's Rents, Long Acre. 5th October, 1830.	Third day.—Great uterine pain, increased by pressure; dyspnœa, and pain in right side of thorax; distension of abdomen. Duration of disease, five days. Dying when first seen.	V.S. copious leeches, fomentations, &c.	Died. Pleura and substance of lungs on right side inflamed; the left inferior lobe coated with lymph; two quarts of serum in the peritoneal sac; small intestines covered with lymph; uterus imbedded in lymph; uterine appendages inflamed; veins of uterus healthy.
97	Mrs. Wall; æt. 32. Protracted labour from distortion of pelvis. 1st November, 1830.	Attacked the day after delivery.—Acute uterine pain; uterus large and hard; lochia suppressed; pulse 100, soft; pain in left groin; pulse rapid; countenance dejected; great debility.	V.S. ℔ ss., leeches xx., calomel, antimony, opium, cathartics.	Died. Two pints of a dark-coloured serum in the peritoneal sac; uterine peritoneum inflamed; both ovaria soft, red, and large, and when cut into seemed filled with a purulent gelatinous fluid; the absorbents of the uterus on the left side filled with pus; veins and muscular coat healthy.

98	Saxton; æt. 30; British Lying-in Hospital. Hæmorrhage. 19th December, 1830.	Third day.—Great uterine pain; lochia suppressed; headache; rigor; countenance dusky; pulse rapid and feeble; distressing flatulence; tympanites.	V.S. ℥xix., leeches xxxvj., calomel, antimony, opium, cathartics, &c.	Died.
99	Jones; æt. 24; British Lying-in Hospital. Natural labour. 20th December, 1830.	Second day.—Intense pain of uterus and both groins; lochia suppressed; rigors; headache; vomiting; features collapsed; abdomen swollen; hurried respiration; pulse 120. Duration of disease, three days.	V.S. ℥rij., leeches xxxvi., calomel, &c.	Died. The placenta had been attached to the left side of the fundus uteri; the veins here were lined with lymph and gorged with pus; the absorbents on the left side distended with pus; both ovaria large, and so soft that they were broken down by a small stream of water falling upon them; tubes inflamed; ℥iv. of serum in peritoneal sac, and patches of lymph over the small intestines.
100	Cecilia Boyd; æt. 31; 32, Peter Street. Natural labour. 28th December, 1830.	Fourth day.—A rigor; great pain in the region of the uterus; slight delirium; pulse 120, from the time of delivery; countenance pale; abdomen tumid; hypogastrium and iliac fossæ painful on pressure; constant dozing; tongue dry and brown; vomiting; flatulence; distension of abdomen; pulse rapid and feeble, and irregular.	V.S. ℥rij. (followed by syncope), leeches xxrj., calomel, opium, antimony, poultices, mercurial friction.	Died. Abdomen distended with gas; ℥vi. of red serous fluid in its cavity; peritoneum healthy throughout, except that portion covering the posterior surface of the uterus and its appendage; pus in cellular membrane under peritoneum of uterus behind; both spermatic veins contained pus in considerable quantities, as did also the venous branches at the angles and inferior portion of the uterus; the fallopian tubes vascular; the muscular coat of uterus healthy; no appearance of pus in the orifices of the veins at that part to which the placenta had been attached.

ON THE
PROPER METHOD OF STUDYING
CHEMISTRY

AS A BRANCH OF PROFESSIONAL AND GENERAL EDUCATION,

Forming part of a Lecture, concluding the Chemical Course in the University of Glasgow, April 25, 1843,

DELIVERED BY DR. ROBERT D. THOMSON.

BEFORE bringing the chemical winter session to a close, I trust I may be excused if I direct your attention very briefly to the importance of the study of chemistry, and to the proper mode of acquiring a knowledge of the science. And in order to place this in a practical point of view before you, I think I cannot avail myself of a better method than to detail to you shortly the results of some of the investigations which have been undertaken during the past winter in the laboratory. Chemistry being a truly practical science, it is only by *working* that one can become familiar with its details. Lectures on chemistry can only assist you in practically working out a knowledge of the science. They are powerful, nay necessary auxiliaries; but by attending lectures alone, no man ever became a chemist, while by working, even without lectures, many chemists have been produced. In these observations I refer to lectures in which the lecturer alone performs the experimental illustrations. But there is another kind of lectures which have been introduced latterly into many schools, erroneously known under the title of Practical Chemistry, in which a number of students are formed into a class, headed by their lecturer, and are made to perform, by dictation, as many experiments as they conveniently can execute during one hour per day, or in some cases three times per week. The second kind of lectures, when arranged so as to make each student personally perform the experiments, is a decidedly important addition to the first kind of lectures; but if they are allowed to degenerate into a mere *short course of lectures* of the first description, and dispense with practice in the laboratory, which is very liable to happen, it may with some truth be apprehended, that the shadow is substituted for the substance, and thus students are led to believe that they are practically acquainted with chemistry, while, in fact, they have not been taught to handle a crucible. Those who have passed through the ordeal of their studies, and have engaged in their practical application to the business of life, reflecting upon the disadvantages under which they have laboured in their subsequent career, from a misdirection of their minds in their own practical education, must ever sympathise with their juniors who may be liable to suffer from similar influences. It is therefore usual with lecturers to bewail their own inattention to study in their youth, and to ascribe their deficiency to idleness. There may be some truth in this conclusion, but much depends on the proper direction of the mind to study.

Having had peculiarly extensive opportunities of comparing the methods of teaching chemistry in various parts of this country, and likewise on the continent of Europe, I have no hesitation in affirming, that the only method of studying practical chemistry is that introduced first by Dr. Thomson into Edinburgh, in the beginning of the century, and afterwards by him, in 1817, into Glasgow, viz., by the students personally working in the laboratory.

By combining analytic operations in the laboratory with the practical lectures alluded to, I believe that much good may be effected, and during the winter the laboratory pupils have accordingly been formed into a class during one hour, in which they have been exercised in the preparation of substances, and in manipulations, arranged in a systematic order.

The student, on commencing practical chemistry, should occupy himself with a simple analysis. To take to pieces a body consisting of two or three ingredients will probably be enough for him to manage in the first instance. With a medical student, some medicinal salt,—with the manufacturer, some ingredient employed in the arts,—and with the farmer, some simple constituent of the soil, may properly form their respective introductions to the practice of chemistry. He may then proceed to the analysis of minerals, and to more complicated substances. I shall only, however, allude to two of these, as they are not destitute of interest. Dr. Black examined the water of hot springs from Iceland, and found it to contain, in solution with soda, silica, or sand, a substance which, under ordinary circumstances, is well known to be insoluble in water. This was a most important observation, because it afforded a key to the explanation of the various appearances which silica assumes, whether as chalcedony, opal, or agate, and indicated the existence, at some period, of hot springs in those localities where such minerals are met with. Deposits in the neighbourhood of hot springs, it might be presumed, would contain much silica, and this is proved to be the case by the following analysis of a deposit from a hot spring in New Zealand :—

Silica	77·35
Alumina	9·70
Peroxide of Iron	3·72
Lime	1·55
Water	7·66
	99·98

Another mineral analysed, from New Zealand, was the native Prussian Blue, or phosphate of the protoxide of iron. Its constituents were found to be—

Water	28·4
Organic Matter	2·8
Silica	5·2
Phosphate of Iron . . .	62·8
	99·2

Both of these analyses were made by Mr. Robert Pattison.

I notice this substance more readily because it was in directing the analysis of it that my attention was again recalled to a proper mode of separating phosphate of iron from other phosphates, or iron from earthy oxides; and I think that by the use of cyanide of potassium, as prepared by Professor Liebig's easy process, or also by the use of tartaric acid, this separation can be easily effected. The study of this mineral was therefore a good introduction to the numerous analyses of soils which have been conducted in the laboratory during the session, principally by agricultural students.

In the following Table the results of four analyses of the same soil, from Erskine, are given, as executed by Messrs. Michelmore and Watson :—

COMPOSITION OF THE SOIL			When fresh.		After being some days in the laboratory.	
			Watson.	Michelmore.	Watson.	Michelmore.
1. Silica			249·86	214·5	247·1	213·87
2. Water of decomposed Soil . .			111·17	110·60	90.5	53·95
3. Stony Matter			70·80	74·50	49·0	93·20
4. Organic Matter, containing of .	Carbon		20·82	9·25	20·50	8·15
	Azote			2·15		1·8
	Hydrogen, Oxygen .			...		...
	Water of undecom. Soil			7·55		...
5. Perox. Iron and Phosphates	Perox. Iron . .		...	55·74	41·29	53·93 / 1·9 / 2·9 / 1·2 } 59·93
	Phos. Iron . . .		...			
	Phos. Lime and Magnesia . . .		...			
	Phos. Alum . .		...			
6. Carbonate of Lime			5·97	9·1	18·24	24·79
7. Alumina			15·40	16·40	6·23	6·19
8. Magnesia			...	...	2·27	2·20
9. Sulphate of Lime			...	...	0·60	1·00
10. Chloride of Potassium . . .			...	...	0·06	0·06
11. Chloride of Sodium			...	...	...	0·14

In this table I may call your attention to what must be viewed as an improvement in the analysis of soils. I found that the results by the old plan, of determining the organic matter of soils, were erroneous, and I have accordingly been in the habit of late of ascertaining the quantity of carbon and azote (the important elements for the nutrition of plants) by organic analysis. The expensive nature of oxide of copper induced me to try black oxide of manganese and red oxide of iron as a substitute for the combustion of the organic matter, and in every instance the resulting carbon was so much in excess that I was obliged to abandon these bodies. Mr. Michelmore obtained the following results with the above soil :—

1.	10 grains of soil gave 5·4 per cent carbon, with red oxide of iron.				
2.	10 grains	"	6·8	"	"
3.	10 grains	"	7·05	"	with black oxide of manganese.
4.	10 grains	"	1·85	"	with black oxide of copper.
5.	10 grains	"	1·63	"	"

The soils were in each experiment from the same parcel, and all at the same temperature,

But the analysis of a soil is of little value without the analysis of the grain which grows upon it ; because it is by a comparison of the two results that we are enabled to determine whether a soil is calculated to produce a crop of a particular grain ; for as the grain derives its inorganic constituents from the soil, it is obvious that this affirmation must hold with truth in all cases. Analyses of grain grown with different manures have, therefore, engaged our attention, and some analyses of this kind I present to you, executed by Messrs. Michelmore and Watson, of oats, including the husks, grown at Erskine with—

	Foreign Guano.	Sulph. Soda.	Brit. Guano.
Organic Matter	967·25	970·58	972·24
Silica	11·37	15·28	13·37
Alkaline Phosphates	1·87	2·00	3·75
Phosphates of Lime and Magnesia . . .	8·76	11·63	10·64
Phosphate of Alumina	0·60	0·50	trace
Phosphate of Iron	trace	trace	trace

For the quantity of inorganic matter in other specimens of oats, I refer you to the "Proceedings of the Philosophical Society of Glasgow," No. 6, just published.

There is still a kind of inquiry relative to agriculture, which forms the connecting link between that art and the science of health, and is, therefore, of equal value to the student of medicine and agriculture—I refer to the determination of the amount of the nutritive part of grain. Bread, we found in a preceding part of the course, contains the elements of the blood, and in proportion as the amount of these principles calculated to produce this fluid are greater or less in the aliment consumed, so is the latter possessed of superior or inferior nutritive power. The table annexed gives the result of a series of experiments upon the bread and flour of different countries.

The foreign bread was brought by myself from the towns mentioned; the flour was supplied by Mr. Wilson, Baker, of Gordon Street. The analyses were made by myself, and some of them were repeated by Mr. Watson and Mr. Michelmore. The numbers in the table were obtained by determining the quantity of ammonia which can be formed from the azote contained in the flour. The process is exceedingly simple, and can soon be acquired. The second column is read thus : 100 parts of Naumburg bread are equal in nourishing power to 150 of States flour, &c.

Nutritious Principles.

	Per Cent.	Equiv.
Naumburg Bread (Prussia)	16·49	100·
Dresden Bread	14·30	115·31
Berlin Bread	14·21	116·04
Canada Flour	13·81	117·23
Essex Flour	13·59	121·33
Glasgow unfermented Bread	13·39	123·15
Lothian Flour	12·30	134·06
United States' Flour . .	11·37	145·03
Ditto Ditto . .	10·99	150·00

The process, exhibited to you in a former lecture, for the mechanical analysis of flour, is equally interesting to the farmer and surgeon, and should be mastered by both. The following was conducted by Mr. Michelmore, and was the specimen from the United States noticed in the table. The coincidence in respect to the nutritive principles between the results of the two analyses conducted in different ways, is highly striking :—

		Per Cent.	
Starch		902·	68.73
Gluten { Fibrin	116·8	130·4	9·93
Casein	5·27		
Glutin and Oil . .	3·04		
Loss—Water . . .	5·29		
Albumen		14·0	1·06
Gum		60·4	4·60
Sugar		16·3	1·24
Water		189·3	14·44

3 oz. = 1312·5 grs. 100·00

Your time will not permit me to enlarge further upon the subject of practical chemistry, that is, the dedication of as much time as possible in the laboratory to operations which require, on the part of the pupil, the exercise of the mind and hands ; but before concluding, I cannot too much insist upon the indispensable nature of this study to the manufacturer, farmer, and medical man ; for it is the essence of the arts of calico printing, dyeing, bleaching, &c. and we can in vain look for any permanent advance in agriculture until farmers are educated practically in the elements of chemistry, just as they learn to plough, sow, and reap, or to sum up accounts. Without such a knowledge they will either be compelled to be sceptical or apathetic, as the chemical language addressed to them must be that of an unknown tongue, or they must ever be subject to be misled by the popular fallacies of the chemical empiric. To the surgeon and physician, practical chemistry, such as I have defined it, is as requisite as practical anatomy, and soon we may expect to find a session in the laboratory a part of the medical curriculum. The school which shall first take this position will show itself most alive to the progress of science.

The expense has been much overrated; and I believe the arrangements now adopted in the Glasgow College Laboratory will bring practical chemistry within the reach of most young men who desire to improve their minds by the study of one of the most valuable and interesting sciences with which man can occupy himself. But, as a branch of general education, I know of no study equally calculated to develop the mind. To make an analysis, that is, to divide a body composed of many parts united together into its ultimate constituents, a student must remember and reason, if he is properly taught; and if he enters upon a research, that is, a combination of analyses, one experiment arising out of another, until the united results enable a conclusion to be drawn, he becomes a disciple of Lord Bacon—an inductive philosopher, the safest condition for all study and for every profession. Irrespective, then, of the important knowledge to be acquired in the laboratory, the training which the mind undergoes is of the highest value, and I may appeal with confidence to all those who have passed through the studies of the laboratory, whether, whatever their future occupation in life has been, they have not had their powers of observation sharpened, and their appreciation of evidence improved, by their chemical education.

OBSERVATIONS
ON THE
CLIMATE OF THE BRITISH COLONIES OF NEW ZEALAND, NEW SOUTH WALES, AND VAN DIEMAN'S LAND,

AS COMPARED WITH THAT OF THE BRAZILS, MADEIRA, AND THE CONTINENT OF EUROPE:

From personal remarks, and the most recent authentic statistical data.

WITH A

FEW REMARKS ON THE DISEASES OF THE "ABORIGINES," AND THOSE INTRODUCED BY EUROPEAN COLONIZATION.

BY JAMES B. THOMPSON, M.D.

(*For the London Medical Gazette.*)

HAVING, during my recent sojourn in the colonies, made some reports on the vegetable and mineral productions of New Zealand in particular, and which are published in the first number of the New South Wales Magazine for 1843, it may not be deemed uninteresting to offer a few remarks on the subjects with which this paper is headed.

I have selected the statistical facts from the most correct and authentic sources that were available during my brief sojourn in antipodean regions.

From the most recent and approved medical standard works on pulmonary complaints, (Sir James Clark, Williams, Stokes, and Louis), it would appear that the people of this country are subject, in a more than ordinary degree, to diseases of the chest and lungs; and that greater mortality arises from this than from any other class of disease. Now whatever difference of opinion may be entertained as to the extent to which this peculiar liability is attributable to the unequable character of the English climate, the influence of climate on pulmonary disease is universally admitted to be by no means inconsiderable. I arrived in Auckland, in New Zealand, on the 8th of October, 1842, and sailed for Sydney on the 3d of December, and during this stay of nearly two months I had an opportunity of visiting several of the native and European settlements, and had also an opportunity afforded me of observing the diseases prevalent amongst the natives—these being a form of scurvy called "fe fe," rheumatism, dysentery, diarrhœa, and ophthalmia. The venereal disease is now very prevalent at the Bay of Islands, which is the great whaling station, principally North American and French, and it is most painful to witness the awful and destructive ravages which this disease produces on the natives, male and female. They are naturally, from their mode of life and little regard to cleanliness or clothing, and exposure to night air, often lying in their damp coverlets after their fishing excursions during a hot day, predisposed to glandular affections: indeed, scrofulous affections seem to have been entailed on the present generation by this neglect, probably, on the part of their progenitors, and I would adduce this fact as a proof of the great fatality amongst the Aborigines generally when become diseased with venereal or any of our exanthematous complaints.

It is incredible in what a short time any of this latter class of diseases will run a destructive and fatal course—once the constitution of the native becomes tainted, nothing will effectually remove the germs of the virus:

they invariably become affected with pulmonary complaints, and no medical treatment seems capable of affording them permanent relief. If a case is seen at the very incipient stage, you may calculate upon being of some utility; but once beyond this, it is a hopeless case. Venereal, particularly, seems to run a quick and fatal course, producing the most extensive sloughing ulcers, and affecting the bones and cartilages in a more marked form than I have ever witnessed in any of our large British hospitals. The natives have a great objection to bleeding and vaccination, and in order to induce them to take any medicine, they will expect you to give them some present for so doing, as they imagine they are doing you a favour by acceding to your request on this point.

In the vicinity of the European settlements they are now beginning to appreciate the use of medicine, and the other many advantages likely to result from the attendance of a medical man, and have, in many instances, gone for advice and medicine to the colonial surgeon. The medical man must have recourse to more active and rigorous measures in all cases of fevers, inflammations, &c. than in England; he must, to make use of a homely phrase, be beforehand with the disease, and, as some of the old school would call it, be thereby enabled to "knock the disease under." This is the mode of practice requisite in all tropical climates, making it, of course, suitable to the previous history of the patient, and to meet the urgency of the individual case.

Having made a short visit to the Brazils on my return from the colonies, I had an opportunity of witnessing some diseases amongst the African slaves, both in the hospitals and amongst the out-door patients; and it would appear to me that they are predisposed to similar diseases with the Aborigines above alluded to, with the additional prevalence, probably, of dysentery, ophthalmia, and rheumatism. Those slaves who have been resident in Brazil for some years appear comparatively healthy, and whenever operated upon for any disease, the late much lamented Dr. Lowdon, surgeon for sixteen years to the British hospital at Pernambuco, informed me that they bore the operation well, and became convalescent in a much shorter period than some of the Europeans operated upon at the same time and for a similar affection.

The wounds heal and cicatrize very quickly, unless there be some previous delicacy: They also seem to be equally exposed to the fatal consequences of venereal and the exanthemata. As an instance in confirmation of this latter point, I will here mention a circumstance which occurred just previous to my arrival at Pernambuco in May last. A slave-ship had arrived, having sailed from the opposite coast of Africa, Angola, with 1000 slaves on board; during the voyage, which is, on an average, about five weeks, and, from the want of ventilation and other necessary requisites for the comforts of these poor creatures, they lost 100 before they landed at the coast of Brazil; and in about ten days after there were only 600 souls left, 300 having died of small-pox. This was told me by Mr. Cooper, the British Consul. In corroboration of the fact of these slaves soon getting well after being operated upon, I think it may be well to mention that I saw one man in hospital who had been operated upon for a malignant disease, it was stated, in which it was necessary to remove a portion of the lower jaw. The man was nearly well when I saw him, and he bore this painful operation with great patience and fortitude.

Though the month of May is about the commencement of their rainy season in the Brazils, still I found it rather disagreeably warm and oppressive. They have had very little rain for the last year. The country is generally very low and marshy, and would lead one to expect such a place as would be rife for those diseases arising from miasmata and the direct rays of a tropical sun: still, it is remarkable how free from all such complaints this country generally is; in fact, it would induce one to doubt the existence of malaria or contagion, at least from atmospheric influence, and still more lead one to question the mischief so much talked of as arising from swamps and vegetable decomposition. The summer comprises three-fourths of the year here, and is somewhat hotter generally throughout than in England. The spring and autumn have the temperature, and clear settled weather, of

78	Leaney; æt. 26; British Lying-in Hospital. Natural labour. 11th January, 1830.	Third day.—Headache; pyrexia; uterine pain; pulse 120; lochia suppressed; vomiting.	V.S. ʒxiv., leeches lx., calomel, opium, cathartics.	Recovered.
79	Mesalin; æt. 22; British Lying-in Hospital. Natural labour. 13th January, 1830.	Second day.—Uterus large, hard, and painful; rigors; headache; lochia nearly suppressed; pulse 100; dyspnœa; cough; skin hot; pulmonic attack; abdomen distended; uterus hard and painful on pressure; vomiting; exhaustion.	V.S. ʒxvi, V.S. ʒxiv, calomel, Dover's powder, &c.	Died. Caput coli and transverse arch of colon covered with patches of lymph; uterus uncontracted, its anterior surface of a uniform dusky red colour; the muscular tissue under this reduced to a soft reddish pulp; the veins of the fundus uteri on both sides inflamed, and filled with a quantity of pus; both ovaria enlarged, their structure destroyed; fallopian tubes soft and vascular; lungs gorged with blood, but not inflamed.
80	Meaden; æt. 20; British Lying-in Hospital. 15th January, 1830.	Second day.—Headache; rigors; uterus painful, large, and hard; anxiety; countenance pale; breathing hurried; pulse 110; lochia scanty. Convalescent in 24 hours.	V.S. ʒxx., leeches xxiv., pulv. ipecac. comp. gr. v. 3tia q. q. hora.	Recovered.
81	Case after natural labour; British Lying-in Hospital. 28th January, 1830.	Third day.—Pyrexia; severe pain of the uterus, increased by pressure. Depletion followed by immediate convalescence.	V.S. ʒxx., calomel, opium, fomentations and poultices to hypogastrium.	Recovered.
82	Williams; æt. 26; a patient of Dr. Hugh Ley's, Middlesex Hospital. Natural labour. 13th January, 1830.	Eighth day.—Vomiting; rigors; severe uterine pain; foul tongue; offensive lochia; pulse 120, soft.	V.S. ʒvj; leeches xij; calomel, antimony, and opium.	Recovered. During this month several severe cases occurred among the out-patients of the Middlesex Hospital. In all there was more or less pain in the region of the uterus, increased by pressure, pyrexia, and diminished lochial discharge.

No.	Case	Symptoms	Treatment	Result
83	Case in a Mews near Portman Square. Natural labour. January, 1830.	Sixth day.—Continued well for six days after delivery, when fever of a typhoid character came on, with slight abdominal pain; puffy swelling over the left wrist, and on one of the thighs; slight tympanitis.	Sulphate of quinine and stimulants.	Died. Uterus large; the left spermatic vein through its whole course lined with false membranes, its coats thickened, the lower part filled with pus and lymph; the upper part distended with coagula of blood; the veins at left superior angle of uterus lined with lymph, and filled with a bloody, purulent fluid; the veins on the right side of uterus gorged with pus; the right spermatic vein was healthy, also both hypogastrics.
84	Sophia Humphries. 30th January, 1830.	Third day.—Acute pain of uterus, increased by pressure; headache; tongue white; pulse 100; lochia scanty; bowels confined; blood cupped and buffed.	V.S. ℥ij., calomel, cathartics.	Recovered.
85	Jones; 48, Marshall Street. Natural labour. 11th February, 1830.	Third day.—Pyrexia; acute uterine pain; lochia suppressed; rigors; pain and swelling of left iliac region; cough; suppuration at the brim of the pelvis; the pus escaped under Poupart's ligament. Recovered after five months.	Leeches often repeated, cataplasms, bark, wine, stimulants; abscess opened artificially.	Recovered
86	Honeyman; Angel Street, City. Natural labour. 12th February, 1830.	Fourth day.—Acute uterine pain; violent rigor; headache; lochia suppressed; pulse 115, strong; respiration hurried.	V.S. ℥iv., leeches xxiv., calomel, antimony, cathartics, diaphoretics.	Recovered.
87	Case in the Edgeware Road. 20th February, 1830.	Second day.—Pain in the region of the uterus; rigors; lochia and milk diminished; slight delirium; pulse 115; tongue white; great tenderness in the situation of right uterine appendages.	V.S. ℥ij., leeches, calomel, antimony.	—— In the month of April, 1830, three cases occurred, which all yielded speedily to venæsection, leeches, calomel, antim., Dover's powders, &c. The details of these cases are not preserved.

88	Mrs. Hadden; æt. 30; 3, Castle Street, Bloomsbury. Arm presentation.	Fourth day.—Uterine pain; lochia suppressed; rigors; pain in right groin; pulse 100; tongue white. The pain was not effectually relieved till cathartics were freely administered.	V.S. ℥iij., leeches xvj., calomel, antimony, cataplasms, cathartics.	Recovered.
89	Mrs. Sears; æt. 26; 23, Church Lane. Natural labour. 20th June, 1830.	Fourth day.—Great uterine pain; pulse 100, full; lochia suppressed; rigors; blood cupped and buffed.	V.S. ℥xvj., leeches xxiv., calomel, antimony.	Recovered.
90	Mrs. Allen; æt. 26; 12, Phœnix Street, St. Giles's. Natural labour. 10th June, 1830.	Fourth day.—Uterine pain; pulse frequent and full; lochia suppressed; tongue brown; vomiting; pain in right groin; pulse 130; respiration hurried.	V.S. ℥xxvj., calomel, antimony, opium, cathartics, saline effervescing draughts.	Recovered.
91	Sankey; 35, Wardour Street. Protracted labour. June, 1830.	Soon after delivery, a sudden attack of fever, with severe pain in the right iliac region and left groin and thigh; rigors; tongue loaded. July 12: the left iliac region is hard, swollen, and painful on pressure,—the hardness extends half way down the thigh, in the course of the femoral vessels; great constitutional disturbance. Aug. 6: a great quantity of pus discharged above Poupart's ligament. A slow but complete recovery.	Leeches, poultices, anodynes.	Recovered.
92	Mrs. Gyde; æt. 22; Brewer Street, Golden Square. Natural labour. 26th June, 1830.	Second day.—Rigors, and pain of the lower part of the abdomen, with pyrexia and suppression of the lochia. 29th: pain but slightly relieved; fever continues. July 4th: intense pain of the whole abdomen, and distension; pulse rapid and feeble; constant sickness and vomiting; tongue brown. 6th: symptoms aggravated. Died on the tenth day from attack.	V.S. ℥iij., leeches xij., opium, leeches, a blister, cathartics.	Died. ℔. ij. of dark-coloured sero-purulent fluid in peritoneal sac; the whole abdominal viscera inflamed; small intestines, omentum, and uterus, all glued together with lymph; an abscess under the peritoneum of the uterus, near its fundus, on the left side; a small abscess in the body of the uterus on the left side; uterine appendages on both sides vascular, and coated with lymph.

No.	Name, age, address	Symptoms	Treatment	Result
93	Phillips; æt. 32; 2, Sussex Street. 30th July, 1830.	Fifth day.—Great uterine pain; pulse 130; violent headache; exquisite tenderness, increased by pressure, in the left side of the uterus, which gradually diminished, and the pulse became less frequent. A slow recovery.	V.S. ʒx., leeches xij., calomel, antimony, opium, cathartics.	Recovered.
94	Mrs. Chapman; æt. 36; 9, Belton Street, Long Acre. Natural labour. 19th August, 1830.	Fifth day.—After drinking cold beer, seized with sudden uterine pain; rigors; headache; delirium; pulse 120, weak; tongue dry and brown; constant vomiting and diarrhœa; delirium; great debility; coma; hurried respiration. Duration of disease nine days.	Leeches xii. to the temples, calomel, opium, pulv. cretæ comp. c. opio, fomentations, &c.	Died. Ovaria red, soft, and enlarged; left tube filled with pus; muscular coat of the uterus at the fundus where the placenta had adhered so soft, that the fingers passed through it in removing the parts; no inflammation of peritoneum or effusion into the abdominal cavity.
95	Keene; æt. 34; 2, Little Earl Street. Tedious labour. 2d September, 1830.	Third day.—Uterus large, hard, and painful, especially on the left side; headache; slight rigor; pulse 132; lochia continue.	V.S. ʒxvj., leeches xij., calomel, antimony, opium, cathartics, pulv. ipecac. co.	Recovered.
96	——; æt. 30; Stewart's Rents, Long Acre. 5th October, 1830.	Third day.—Great uterine pain, increased by pressure; dyspnœa, and pain in right side of thorax; distension of abdomen. Duration of disease, five days. Dying when first seen.	V.S. copious leeches, fomentations, &c.	Died. Pleura and substance of lungs on right side inflamed; the left inferior lobe coated with lymph; two quarts of serum in the peritoneal sac; small intestines covered with lymph; uterus imbedded in lymph; uterine appendages inflamed; veins of uterus healthy.
97	Mrs. Wall; æt. 32. Protracted labour from distortion of pelvis. 1st November, 1830.	Attacked the day after delivery.—Acute uterine pain; uterus large and hard; lochia suppressed; pulse 100, soft; pain in left groin; pulse rapid; countenance dejected; great debility.	V.S. lb. ss., leeches xx, calomel, antimony, opium, cathartics.	Died. Two pints of a dark-coloured serum in the peritoneal sac; uterine peritoneum inflamed; both ovaria soft, red, and large, and when cut into seemed filled with a purulent gelatinous fluid; the absorbents of the uterus on the left side filled with pus; veins and muscular coat healthy.

if attention be paid to the facts I have mentioned, there will be no need to part with a tried and established remedy for one whose mode of action is no doubt essentially similar.

I might also remark, that the nitrate of silver seems to possess an almost equally beneficial action when applied to the skin in the immediate vicinity of other inflamed or irritable mucous membranes. My opinion was requested by a medical gentleman some months back, on a patient of his who had been under his care for about four months. It was a case of gonorrhœa, which had been about eight months under treatment before it came under the care of the gentleman alluded to. The patient was a young man of full habit, and a wine merchant, who was tolerably fond of good living. Almost every plan of treatment that could be thought of had been carefully tried, and had failed, over and over again; and at the time of my seeing him there was still a considerable discharge of thick yellow matter from the urethra, much pain in making water, and occasional attacks of chordee. By my direction the nitrate was applied along the under surface of the penis, as far as the scrotum, and also slightly behind it. I again saw this gentleman about three days afterwards, when he informed me that he was better than he had been for months, that the discharge was nearly gone, and serous, and that he had no pain in making water.

Since that period I have not seen either the patient or his medical attendant, and am therefore unacquainted with the termination of the case; but I left him with an understanding that he was to paint over the course of the urethra with the tincture of iodine about twice a week, until all the symptoms were removed.

13, Bloomsbury Square.

PECULIAR SOUND OF THE HEART,

INDEPENDENT OF VALVULAR DISEASE.

———

To the Editor of the Medical Gazette.

Sir,

The following case has been thought so interesting, that I have been requested to publish it. It proves the possibility of the existence of certain sounds of the heart, frémissement cataire, and of a peculiar jerking pulse, supposed to be sure signs of valvular disease, when none existed.

Henry Hughes, æt. 31, admitted into the Brighton Hospital, March 15, 1843, died June 3, 1843; a tinman, of a full, bloated habit. He was in the hospital about a year before, and had a hard superficial tumor, the size of an egg, taken from the loins. His present symptoms are, pain in the back; acute pain in the loins, as if they were broken; urine scanty, turbid; violent cough; mucous expectoration, not copious; bronchial sibilant râle all over the chest; pulse from 120 to 160, small, jerking; sounds of the heart strong, as if the left ventricle were hypertrophied; frémissement cataire, as if from mitral regurgitation; biliary secretions healthy.

For these symptoms he was bled, cupped, took ipecacuan, colchicum, digitalis, diuretics.

Post-mortem Examination. — Hard encephaloid tumors all over the parietes of the chest, from the size of a pin's head to that of an egg, embedded more or less in the muscular substance; lungs full of the same; mesenteric glands all hard and enlarged; large mass of similar tumors beneath and about the base of the heart, pressing upon and binding the aorta and heart; similar tumors beneath the stomach. The gall-bladder unusually distended with healthy bile. Lumbar vertebræ carious, the interior absorbed, leaving only a shell, through which the knife passed with slight pressure. Bronchial glands enlarged and hardened. The heart and valves perfectly sound; the ventricles rather small; and the parietes rather thin.

The peculiar pulse and the sounds of the heart seem to have been caused by the number of hard tumors which pressed upon the aorta and heart, and in a degree strangulated and modified its action.—I am, sir,

Your obedient servant,

W. King,

Physician to the Brighton Hospital, Fellow
of the Royal College of Physicians.

Brighton, August 1843.

———

ANALYSES AND NOTICES OF BOOKS.

"L'Auteur se tue à allonger ce que le lecteur se tue à abréger."—D'ALEMBERT.

Lectures on the Comparative Anatomy and Physiology of the Invertebrate Animals, delivered at the Royal College of Surgeons in 1843. By RICHARD OWEN, F.R.S. Hunterian Professor to the College. From Notes taken by W. W. COOPER, M.R.C.S., and revised by Professor OWEN. Illustrated by numerous woodcuts. London, 1843. 8vo. pp. 392

IT is unnecessary to recommend a work on comparative anatomy by Mr. Owen; it is sufficient to announce its appearance.

The book consists of twenty-four lectures; and the Professor has added to Mr. Cooper's notes the details which, for want of time, Mr. Owen omitted in the theatre.

Spiders, it seems, generally have eight eyes, and never less than six:—
"The spiders which inhabit short tubes, terminated by a large web exposed to the open air, have the eyes separated, and more spread upon the front of the cephalothorax.

"Those spiders which rest in the centre of a free web, and along which they frequently traverse, have the eyes supported on slight prominences, which permit a greater divergence of their axes; this structure is well marked in the genus *Thomisa*, the species of which lie in ambuscade in flowers. Lastly, the spiders called *Errantes*, or wanderers, have their eyes still more scattered, the lateral ones being placed at the margins of the cephalothorax. The structure of these simple eyes resembles that which has been so well described by Müller in the scorpion; Lyonnet had recognised the crystalline lens. The iris, or process of pigment which advances in front of the lens, is green, red, or brown, in the diurnal spiders, and black at the back part of the eye. The nocturnal species, as *Mygale* and *Tarantula*, have a brilliant tapetum, but no dark pigment." (Page 256.)

Professor Owen's lectures will be eagerly perused by those who have leisure for the delightful science of which they treat.

Next year he will lecture on Vertebrated Animals.

On Feigned and Factitious Diseases, chiefly of Soldiers and Seamen, &c. By HECTOR GAVIN, M.D. &c. London, 1843. 12mo. pp. 436.

DR. GAVIN's Essay gained the prize proposed by the Professor of Military Surgery at Edinburgh, in 1835. It has been since altered and enlarged, and is a very creditable performance. We extract the following excellent observations with great pleasure. The author says that Scott, Forbes, and Marshall, "do not plead for the notorious malingerer; but when instances of deception become *frequent*, in any country, in any garrison or station, in any regiment, or in any ship of war, they presume that the question may be very reasonably asked—is there not something wrong in the arrangement of the place, in the government or administration of the particular portion of the community in which such frequent deceptions abound? something which, acting injuriously on the bodies or minds of the men, is therefore not beneath the consideration of the medical officers of the establishment, who alone can appreciate the mischief, and by whose mediation alone it is likely to be remedied? The privilege conferred by their profession, of being the *friend of mankind*, is one which ought not to be willingly resigned. A striking exemplification of the truth of the foregoing remarks was shown in Trinidad, on the completion of the emancipation of the slaves. *The hospitals were emptied;* the sick were cured, the lame healed, the blind were restored to sight, and the insane to their senses. The boy of the Monday before, belonging to the second or lower gang, was suddenly endowed with the strength and muscle of a man, and wanted a full task; whilst the feeble man, whose strength before would not allow him to go through the work of the first gang, found it instantly renovated to the necessary pitch: the whole being the miraculous result of the sanatory effects of freedom." (p. 45-6.)

If Dr. Gavin's book reaches a second edition, which it richly deserves, he should revise his Latin quotations, some of which are in a very perplexing state.

On the Curative Influence of the Climate of Pau, and the Mineral Waters of the Pyrenees, on Disease. With descriptive notices of the Geology, Botany, Natural History, Mountain Sports, Local Antiquities, and Topography of the Pyrenees, and their principal Watering-Places. By A. TAYLOR, M.D. London, 1842. 12mo. pp. 342.

THE work before us is divided into nineteen chapters discussing the various points relating to the Pyrenean watering-places which are likely to interest either the physician or the invalid. The places described are Pau, Bagnères de Bigorre, Capbern, Barèges, St. Sauveur, Cauterets, Eaux-Bonnes, and Eaux-Chaudes. If we might hint a fault, we would suggest that the author should completely translate a number of French sentences in the geological part, which have been left in a transition, or Anglo-Gallic state. For example : " The secondary formation is composed of grès rouge, grès blanc, grès schisteux, and poudingue. With the exception of some beds of limestone, these rocks do not contain any foreign strata. The minerals accidentally met with, disseminated in the grès rouge, are fer sulphuré, fer hydraté, and cuivre pyriteux. The baryte sulfatée laminaire, rarely accompanied with a small portion of cuivre carbonaté and ocre de fer, frequently forms veins in the red sandstone." (p. 129.) Dr. Taylor's book contains solid information, and will be consulted with advantage.

MEDICAL GAZETTE.

Friday, August 25, 1843.

"Licet omnibus, licet etiam mihi, dignitatem Artis Medicæ tueri; potestas modo veniendi in publicum ait, dicendi periculum non recuso."
                                             CICERO.

THE PLEA OF MONOMANIA IN CRIMINAL CASES.

ONLY two kinds of madness are recognized in popular language—the furious

and the melancholy. When these forms are strongly developed (as in the figures by Cibber, which adorned the front of the old Bethlem, in Moorfields,) the patients are unfit for any of the offices of life. Such patients can neither fill the higher stations of society, nor perform the humble duties of hewers of wood and drawers of water. But there is a third kind of insanity, which, though it must always have existed, has but lately obtained a fixed place in nosology. We mean *monomania*—a name first given by Esquirol some thirty years since.

If we were asked by a medical student where he could learn the nature of this mental disease, we should refer him to the wards of a lunatic asylum, where he would find plenty of examples; but if the question were proposed by a man of letters, disinclined to study insanity practically, we should say, " Read Don Quixote once more."

In the romance of Cervantes we find a gentleman of fine feelings and cultivated understanding, who has hung over the tomes of chivalry till the day-dreams which they suggest have swallowed up the dull realities of life. Yet, although actual existence must have appeared to him flat and unprofitable, he seems to have carried on his affairs, not well perhaps, but tolerably, until his monomania passed into the second stage, and he sallied forth in quest of adventures. And now Cervantes brings us to that delicate point, where monomania touches upon crime, and hallucinations lead to acts incompatible with the peace of society. The knight of La Mancha, taking Amadis of Gaul, or him of the Burning Sword, for his guide, resolves with his own right arm to redress the wrongs of the world :—

Parcere subjectis, et debellare superbos!

His delusions, meantime, are on the increase; his eyes, misguided by his brain, become very faithless interpreters of the external world, and turn a flock of sheep into an army, and a barber's basin into Mambrino's helmet. In short, his hallucinations lead him so widely astray, that without being a criminal in the vulgar sense of the word, Don Quixote is constantly on the verge of committing murder. To most readers his adventures seem ludicrous to the highest degree, and palpably impossible; yet we might say to the modern monomaniac,—

mutato nomine, de te
Fabula narratur !

Thus, some addle-headed mechanic imagines that the difficulties which perplex society can be solved by the simple expedient of destroying the head of the state, or the leading politician of the day; the knot of human affairs, too great for his capacity to unravel, can be severed, he thinks, by the knife or the bullet. What is to be done with the assassin? The old, and perhaps the best plan, was to hang him. Oh! no! cry many modern writers, you must not hang him; for the man is a lunatic, and lunatics, says the law, are not chargeable for their acts.

Here, then, is a forensic difficulty of no ordinary magnitude. On the one hand, no one would send a stark, staring madman to the gibbet.

On the other, while it is clear that these political or religious enthusiasts are not of perfectly sound mind, the same is true of all criminals whatsoever; and if we acquit every assassin whose crime appears to lack an adequate motive, and all who have appeared at any time whimsical or crotchety, additional Bethlems may entirely replace Australia and the gallows.

No human being can draw an unerring line between the madness which makes a man irresponsible for his crimes, and that which still leaves him answerable to the law. It is the effect of discussion, however, and the office of legislation, to clear up some of the extreme points; and it is plain that to treat the assassin as an innocent man, merely because he has added murder as a kind of climax to his previous deviations from right, is of the most dangerous consequence to society. If he had killed a hare, his eccentricity would not save him from jail : he has sacrificed a man, and his life should expiate the deed. "A rogue," said Coleridge, " is a round-about fool—a fool in circumbendibus;" but the knave cannot therefore claim the privileges of the untainted simpleton. Nor is it true that capital punishment would be useless as an example to other monomaniacs. The half-mad, who perfectly understand the meaning of the gallows, abound, and on them the execution of a murderer is by no means lost.

Hence the Frenchman who thought that homicidal insanity was best cured on the *Place de Grève*, was not far from the mark.

On a former occasion* we ventured to assert, that the jury did right to acquit Macnaughten, if they believed him to be destitute of the glimmering of reason which would enable him to see the link between murder and the gallows; but though most persons who have seen him agree that he is mad, it may be doubted if he could have been acquitted by our test.

Among the writers who have lately endeavoured to throw light on this intricate subject, is Dr. Stark, of Edinburgh, who has lately put forth a pamphlet on the responsibility of monomaniacs for murder.

Dr. Stark is not always consistent with himself. Thus, immediately after insisting on the capital punishment of murder, because it is enjoined in the Pentateuch, he asserts that murder is

---

* MEDICAL GAZETTE, March 24th, 1843.

the only crime for which life ought to be forfeited, forgetting how numerous were the offences punished capitally by the Mosaic law.

But passing over this, let us proceed to three important questions which he asks and endeavours to answer.

The first is, " *Are all monomaniacs necessarily led to acts of destruction ?*

" By no means," we should reply, and all the world with us. There are, however, two classes of destructive monomaniacs; those, namely, who have always been homicidal, and those who have become so, as a subsequent and accidental symptom in monomania of another form. Dr. Stark, however, will only allow of the latter kind, where the thirst for blood is engrafted upon the monomania of love, ambition, or fanaticism; and will not hear of it as a separate disease. Nevertheless, it exists ; yet, we should be loath to make its existence a shield for the murderer. Ought a Thug to escape the gibbet which he has earned so richly and so repeatedly, because he has been a murderer from his youth up, and wrong is to him right ?

The next question is, " *Does the existence of mental alienation on one point so confuse a man's intellects as to deprive him of the power of judging between right and wrong ?*"

Some will reply " Yes !" Dr. Stark answers " No !"

Instead of entering into all the intricacies of this difficult problem, we would again refer to the test we gave above, or to Lord Brougham's speech on the 14th of March last, as quoted by Dr. Stark. " Then what was the true distinction which the law drew between right and wrong ? Why lawyers told us that that which was according to law was right, and what was contrary to law was wrong. Then why not say so in so many words ? This was the test he suggested."

The third and last question is, " *Are monomaniacs impelled to commit murder or suicide by a power which they cannot resist, so that they do not act as free agents ?*"

Dr. Stark answers this question broadly in the negative. Whether this answer is universally true is of little importance. Let the legal test be applied to the assassin, and if he has enough reason to know that he is committing a capital crime, he has no cause to complain that the sentence of the law is executed in his person. It is quite certain, too, that the execution of a monomaniac checks the propensity to crime among other persons suffering under partial insanity. Dr. Stark observes, that the monomaniacs who committed murder in imitation of Henrietta Cornier amounted to a dozen at least, but not one of the imitative murders occurred till the result of the trial was known, that the prisoner, namely, had been acquitted on the plea of insanity.

Dr. Stark is astonished that judge and jury should be so much guided by the medical witnesses in trials where insanity is pleaded on behalf of the prisoner. " I say, I cannot understand how they allow this—how they allow themselves to be led by the *opinion* of a man who, however eminent his standing in his own profession may be, is far from being nearly so capable as the judge (aye, or even, perhaps, the jurymen themselves), of forming a sound opinion on the facts which he may have heard from the ordinary witnesses, or from his having seen the prisoner once or twice."

We suppose that judge and jury are guided by the old maxim, *cuique in suâ arte credendum est ;* and that they believe an old mad-doctor who has treated ten thousand lunatics to have more tact in discerning insanity than the most experienced draper in the jury-box. As to the quantum of insanity which makes a man irresponsible for his crimes, that is a different matter. It is a point of law rather than of physic, and can hardly be better explained than in Lord Brougham's speech.

In conclusion, we think that monomania can seldom be a valid defence to a charge of murder. The law has not lost its terrors for monomaniacs; a fact which might easily be deduced from their being amenable to discipline in a lunatic asylum.

REGULATIONS OF THE COLLEGE OF SURGEONS.

The Regulations of the College of Surgeons have just been altered in the following points :—

1. Students were formerly required to bring proof " of having studied anatomy and physiology, by attendance on lectures and demonstrations, and by dissections, *during three anatomical seasons or sessions, extending from October to April inclusive."*

The latter part of the rule now runs thus : " *during three winter sessions, of not less than six months each.*"

2. Each course of the practice of surgery, physic, chemistry, materia medica, and midwifery, was formerly of the obligatory length of seventy lectures : this is now left undefined.

Moreover, the following circular has been sent round to medical teachers :—

Royal College of Surgeons in London,
August 15, 1843.

Sir,—I am directed by the President of this College to transmit to you the inclosed copy of their Amended Regulations respecting the professional education of candidates for their diploma; and, at the same time, to express the opinion of the Council that it is highly inexpedient that the pursuits of the Students should be interrupted by a vacation at Christmas, or at any other period of the winter, and to state that they strongly recommend that the vacation hitherto allowed should be discontinued.

I am, sir,
Your most obedient servant,
EDM. BELFOUR, Sec.

These alterations are of different degrees of merit. The London College of Surgeons was the only educational body which required an anatomical session to continue seven long months, from October to April inclusive.] A change much desired by many teachers has now taken place. But the College might perhaps have done better had it required the anatomical session to continue from November to April, both inclusive; thus insuring its commencement on the 1st of November, and its continuance for six months only. It was scarcely advisable to abolish the present minimum of seventy lectures for a course, and substitute no other in its stead; and whatever may be thought of some subjects, seventy lectures are certainly not too many for a course on the practice of physic, surgery, or midwifery.

There is an obvious danger, that among so many schools under no observation or control, a very insufficient number of lectures may be given, even on the most important subjects.

We believe that the College thought the pupils over-lectured; while the Society of Apothecaries could not see this; and hence probably this imperfect attempt at legislation.

We do not like the scheme of abolishing all holidays at one fell swoop. Hard unvarying toil, unsweetened by the gaieties of festive seasons, and the charities of domestic intercourse, will not make better men, or better surgeons. The student should be allowed to leave his murky lodging for a while, and fly on railway wings to Devonshire or Cumberland. Give him extra examinations, if you please, but do not cut off his intervals of repose.

UNIVERSITY OF LONDON.

B.M.—EXAMINATION FOR HONOURS, 1843.

Thursday, Aug. 17.—Morning, 10 to 1.

Anatomy and Physiology.

Examiners, Mr. KIERNAN & Prof. SHARPEY.

State the dissection required to expose the glosso-pharyngeal nerve and its branches after its exit from the cranium; commencing at the integuments, and describing the several parts brought into view in the dissection. The tympanitic branch of the nerve not to be traced.

Afternoon, 3 to 6.

1. A line being drawn round the arm two inches above, and another two inches below the bend of the elbow, describe the soft parts seen in dissecting the included portion of the limb, both before and behind, in the order in which they appear. The joint not to be described.

2. Give an account of the structure and mode of distribution of the capillary vessels in general, with the differences they present in respect of size, number, and arrangement, in different textures, and in the same texture at different periods of life. What evidence can be produced for, and what against, the existence of colourless capillaries?

Friday, Aug. 18.—Morning, 10 to 1.

Chemistry.

Examiner, Professor DANIELL.

1. What are the analogies which subsist between light and heat? Why, in a bright winter's day, is the snow melted around a leafless shrub or a post, whilst it is little affected by the direct rays of the sun?

2. What do you mean by *specific electric induction?*

3. State Professor Ohm's theory of voltaic force and resistances; and apply his formulæ $\frac{E}{R+r}=A$ and $\frac{nE}{nR+r}=A$ to the explanation of quantity and intensity in the voltaic current.

4. To what is the (so-called) *polarization* of the plates and electrodes of a voltaic circuit to be ascribed; and how may it be prevented?

5. Describe the principal phænomena of magneto-electric induction.

6. Describe and exemplify the characters of *monobasic, bibasic,* and *tribasic* acids.

7. What is Professor Graham's view of the constitution of *double salts?*

8. Draw a parallel between the principal compounds of ethule and methule.

9. What would be the products, carefully *collected, of ten grains of* tartrate of silver

$(\overline{T} + 2 \text{ AgO})$ burned with oxide of copper; the silver to be determined by a separate experiment.

Afternoon, 3 to 6.

Materia Medica and Pharmaceutical Chemistry.

Examiner, DR. PEREIRA.

1. How is the presence or absence of copper in oil of cajuputi to be ascertained? If powdered rhubarb were adulterated with powdered turmeric, by what chemical test would you detect the fraud? By what chemical means would you determine the absence of poppy oil in a given sample of castor oil?

2. Describe the microscopic appearances of starch-grains, and point out by what characters you would detect the presence of potato starch in West India arrow root, illustrating your answer by a sketch of the shapes, &c. of these two kinds of amylaceous grains.

3. Describe the mode of preparing the *Antimonii Oxysulphuretum,* Ph. Lond.; explain the chemical changes which attend the process; and state the composition of this medicine.

4. Describe the effects and uses of arsenious acid; and especially point out those symptoms which are apt to follow the long-continued medicinal employment of this substance. State what remedies you would resort to in a case of acute arsenical poisoning.

5. Enumerate the principal purposes for which cold is employed as a therapeutical agent.

6. Describe the botanical characters and medicinal qualities of *Ranunculaceæ.*

7. Name the substances respectively numbered 1, 2, 3, 4, 5, and 6.

FIRST EXAMINATION.

The names are arranged in the order of proficiency.

Anatomy and Physiology.

Jackson, A. (*Exhibition and Gold Medal*) } University Coll.
Jemmett, B. L. (*Gold Medal*) King's College.
Hakes, J. .... University Coll.
Redfern, P. .... Queen's Coll., Ed.
Eyre, B. M. .... University Coll.
Littleton, N. H. .... University Coll.

Chemistry.

Hakes, J.(*Exhib. & Gold Med.*) Univerity Coll.
{ Jemmett, B. L. .... King's College.
{ Littleton, N. H. .... University Coll.

Materia Medica and Pharmaceutical Chemistry.

Hakes, J.(*Exhib. & Gold Med.*) University Coll.
Redfern, P. (*Gold Medal*) .. Queen's Coll., Ed.
Jemmett, B. L. .... King's College.
Jackson, A. .... University Coll.
Littleton, N. H. .... University Coll.

LUNATIC ASYLUM REPORTS.

BELFAST ASYLUM,

Health of inmates.—The general health which pervaded the whole establishment, throughout the past year, was extraordinarily good; even during the severest weather scarcely a cough was to be heard; and from the beginning of the month of November to the middle of the February following, a period of upwards of three months, not a death had to be recorded—a length of time unprecedentedly long, in the annals of the establishment, without a casualty of this kind. The total amount of deaths which occurred during the year was eighteen (an average of about 7¼ per cent.), being nine less than last year.

Restraint of lunatics.—The average daily number of patients, during the year, amounted to 249·44—last year's was 244·67. Amongst so large a number, the cases requiring recourse being had to temporary physical restraint did not amount to more than two per cent. throughout the whole year.

There was no greater day of excitement in the establishment, during the year, than on the 12th of July last, or one more loudly calling for the application of restraint; inasmuch as, on this remarkable anniversary, a regular pitched battle had well nigh taken place amongst some of the females, in support of their respective political opinions and predilections; and, to prevent which, the nurses had to use the utmost vigilance during the day, which, however, happily passed over without any thing very serious occurring.—*Thirteenth Annual Report, by Dr. Stewart.*

DUNDEE ROYAL ASYLUM.

THE treatment, medical and moral, is of course much the same as before—the former, varied according to the different kinds of disease; and the latter, though it may have presented new modes of enjoyment, or of relaxation, or exercise, has still been the same in principle as before.

It would be uninteresting both to the meeting and the public to detail the numerous opportunities of innocent enjoyment afforded to the inmates of the Institution, as they have been so often noticed in former reports. One occurrence of sufficient importance to have occupied your time, the visit to the Asylum of the celebrated Mr. Mainzer, has been already so fully described in the different newspapers, and by the Rev. Mr. Roxburgh in the Directors' Report, that it is unnecessary here to do more than allude to it. We may just remark, that the conduct of the patients on that occasion was becoming; several showing very striking proofs of self-control.

We have got an Accordion for the use of the patients, and hope soon to have an Organ. Rocking-horses are being made similar to those in other institutions.

On several occasions, George Duncan, Esq. Member of Parliament, the Sheriff, the Chairman, and other Directors and Office-bearers, dined at the Asylum with a select number of the patients.

Religious Services.—The benefits arising from the performance of Divine Service are still very apparent. The opportunity of attending the chapel is highly prized by very many of the patients. One of them, an epileptic, says, " Let me go, and should the fit come on I can just be carried out." The experiment of allowing some of them to take the Sacrament in Dundee, was again tried both in October and April last, and with the most beneficial results.

Restraint.—During the whole of last year there was not a single patient under personal restraint of any kind.

Many of the patients estimate highly the kindness and attention with which they have been treated. Two proofs of this, which occurred last year, may not be unworthy of notice. One of the pauper patients who was discharged cured, came on foot a distance of fifty miles to see his old acquaintances in the Asylum. Two persons who had formerly been patients, being seized with premonitory symptoms, presented themselves at the Asylum, and insisted on being admitted.

To the Directors we beg again to tender our respectful thanks, for the uniform kindness and attention which they have shown to us individually, and to the interest of the Institution generally.

To Mrs. Kilgour, the Matron, we beg also to express our thanks for the great zeal with which she has seconded all our efforts, and for many valuable suggestions.

PATRICK NIMMO, Physician.
A. MACKINTOSH, Surgeon,
Superintendent.

MONTROSE LUNATIC ASYLUM.

A TABLE which is given shows the admissions to have been 12 males and 18 females —making 30—equal to those of the preceding year. But, among the former, one individual is marked twice; as, though not having relapsed, he required treatment in the Infirmary for some weeks, after which he again occupied his old position.

In respect to age, the admitted may be ranked thus :—

Up to 20, two; thence to 30, six; to 40,

three; to 50, eleven; to 60, three ; to 70, two; and to 80, three. The average age is a fraction above 44.

In most of the cases, there was obviously bad health, or bodily disease in some form, at the time of entry—as paralysis, epilepsy, delirium tremens, among the males— hysteria, dyspepsia, scorbutic or rather scrofulous affections, with dropsy, in the other sex. On the whole, they required a greater amount and variety of purely medical treatment than any corresponding series during my charge. As, to a certain extent, confirming this remark, it may be mentioned that three, out of the six deaths occurring within the year, were of individuals received into the House since last Report. One of them was from dropsy—in a female ; the second occurred in a male, who, besides the direct consequence of intemperance, early assumed symptoms of typhus, which I have encountered only once before in the Asylum during five years; and the third, which took place suddenly, seemed to have arisen from epilepsy—the malady for which, a few months previously, he had been a patient in the Infirmary. To complete the list— though not exactly in due order—the remaining deaths, three, were all of persons advanced in life, and one of whom had been an inmate for more than 40 years—in fact the oldest and longest residenter in the House. His occupation in early life, I may add, connected him incidentally with a well-known disaster—the loss of the Royal George—on which he had worked as a carpenter. One of the three—a female— was admitted in 1831. She laboured long under epilepsy, but otherwise enjoyed tolerable health, though perpetually in bed ; and, in regard to moral qualities, was one of the most amiable and engaging creatures ever under my care. A man—deaf and blind— particularly noticed in a former Report, completed this trio. He sank gradually, without lucid intervals.

Sundry interesting features were presented in a few of the admitted ; but, saving one, I shall not advert to them on this occasion. It afforded an exemplification of derangement in the propensities, emotion,s or sentiments, without discoverable lesion of intellect ; and was the more remarkable, as well as more certainly receptive of sympathy, because unaccompanied by any spirit or disposition tending towards the injury of others. It might be characterized, in a single sentence, as a case in which terror predominated, totally in opposition both to reason and daily experience. For some time after admission, every new event, no matter how trivial, excited that demon, whom it was impossible to cast out, subdue, or even assuage. Under his dominion, the poor patient, an inoffensive and seemingly

well-principled female, proved at once a sore grievance and a laughing stock to her astonished sisters. On the one hand, her outcries and violent perturbation broke their usual quietude, On the other, such extraordinary disproportion—in fact, such entire contrariety—between her paroxysms of agitation, and the circumstances on which they depended, became, at times, the cause of merriment, if not a provocative to sarcasm. I found it practicable at times to work on her own sense of the ludicrous, to which some of her apprehensions, rightly interpreted, gave ample exercise. They latterly varied in kind or object, became gradually weaker, wore off, and then could be recollected as some thing like dreams. Now, strange as to some it may seem, this woman's perceptions of all objects, so far as I could judge, were quite correct ; while her judgement—I speak of the reasoning power—was perfectly adequate to her safe guidance under the usual occurrences of life. How, then, shall we explain her constant unmitigated wretchedness—for she really was altogether miserable—where every circumstance was regulated so as to secure her safety and promote her comfort ? I answer —simply by asking another question. How shall we explain the intense horror, or agonising distress—not to be escaped from—which there are few persons who have not experienced during some minutes— passing as long, long heavy hours—of sleep ? For theory and speculation on the topic, I have neither time nor liberty in discharging immediate duty. I cannot even advert to its intimate connection with a matter greatly debated of late, and, in sundry quarters, as I cannot help believing, most erroneously represented—that, namely, to which the doubly indefinite, and, consequently, very disputable, expression has been applied—the responsibility of monomaniacs. Somewhat prematurely, as I think, this patient was removed by her friends—greatly composed, but not entirely free from a tyranny that rendered her equally pitiable and troublesome.

Our state of health during last year continued generally good, and had only a few— and these trivial —interruptions. I think scarcely above six patients—and these at different periods — were bed-ridden, even throughout the rigour and storms of winter. There cannot be a doubt, that, under Divine goodness, exemption from serious or widespread disease was owing to the measures, in regard to diet, clothing, air, exercise, employment, and recreation, steadily pursued, and found to be efficacious. I can vouch also for the predominance in the House of order, peace, and contentment— for the reality as well as the display of which, Mrs Macfie (now, not a little unhappily, to be styled the late matron,) must receive a full meed of commendation. Her excellent endowments—for a short time put forth on the narrow field of action which Montrose presents—will be amply tested, as I hope earnestly they may be sustained, in the vastly wider dominion of Middlesex County Asylum.

The proportion of recoveries—or, at least, of restoration to ordinary life, during the year—say about 14 out of the total discharged—though not large, is as fair as, in my opinion, the state and circumstances of our inmates generally might lead the experienced to expect. Incurable cases are, so to say, the rule in all old Asylums, and certainly abound; while the promising and curable form exceptions to it—more to be wished for than calculated on.—*Report for the year ending June* 1, 1843, *by R. Poole, M.D.*

RETREAT NEAR YORK.

DURING the past year, extending from Midsummer 1842 to Midsummer 1843, there have been 21 patients admitted into the Retreat; being three more than during the preceding year. This is a rather greater number than has been admitted during any single year, for the last fifteen years; and at the present time there are 94 patients remaining in the house, or more than have been under care at one time, for three years. The average number, however, resident during the year has not exceeded the average for the three years now expired.

Of those admitted during the year, four were neither members of the Society of Friends, nor connected with it; and, at the date of this report, there remain twelve not so connected, under care.

There have been 10 patients discharged recovered during the year. This is a very satisfactory number; and, as was anticipated in last year's report, such as fully compensates for the smaller number reported for that year.

The general health of the inmates of the Institution has been good; and the deaths, which were 4 in number, have been rather below the average; giving 4.46 per cent. as the mean rate of mortality of the year. The mean annual mortality of the Institution, for the previous three years, 1839-42, was stated in last year's report at 4.53 per cent. and that for the entire period of its operation, of 47 years, from 1796 to 1843, is 4·77 per cent. Though, however, the mortality of the past year is somewhat below the average, it is obvious that, where the numbers under care are comparatively so small, little value can attach to the varying results of single years. The annual review

of these results may, however, become both interesting and useful, by suggesting the probable causes of the fluctuations which are observed in them; provided due caution be observed as to the inferences which are thus formed.

The diseases which proved fatal, during the year, were general paralysis with gangrene, in the male; and pulmonary consumption in one female, atrophy in a second, and disease of the heart in a third. The last of these patients was seventy-six years of age, and had been for forty years under the care of the Institution. The average age of those who died was sixty-three years and a quarter. * * *

The importance, however, of placing the patient under proper care at an early period of the disorder is not only apparent from a comparison of the results of treatment, but is equally inculcated by that aggravation of the disorder and increased difficulty of management, which are the nearly uniform results, when persons attacked by insanity are detained at home. The friends of the patient are not always aware of these facts; but when they are, are too often repugnant to stamp the case with the character, or, as some think, the stigma, of confirmed insanity. It is believed, however, that more correct views with respect to mental disorders, and such as cannot but prove more advantageous to the patient, are gradually diffusing themselves in the public mind. "Whoever," as Sir James Mackintosh wrote to the celebrated Robert Hall, "has brought himself to consider a disease of the brain as differing only in degree from a disease of the lungs, has robbed it of that mysterious horror, which forms its chief malignity." By these remarks, however, it is far from being intended to recommend the premature removal to hospitals for the insane, of persons attacked by mental derangement, or by delirious excitement. Such a course, in many cases, is altogether unnecessary, and, in some, would be positively injurious; and it should rarely, if ever, be resorted to except under the advice of a judicious medical practitioner.

Nothing material has to be reported this year with respect to the internal economy and management of the Institution. Were it indeed an object in these reports to record every modification of practice or addition to the plans of treatment, or to report the respective results of established means, such might in several respects be stated. As, however, it has become the annual practice to present a statement of the numbers more or less employed, as well as the modes of employment during the year, a Table has been prepared to exhibit these. From a comparison of this table with those of previous years, it will be seen that as large a proportion have been in different ways occupied during the past as during any former year. It is satisfactory to state that our conviction of the importance of agricultural pursuits, in the treatment of a large proportion of patients of the male sex, is confirmed by the experience of succeeding years.

It seems here due to the Committee and Directors of the Institution to mention the great addition to the cheerfulness and comfort of the establishment, during the winter months, which has resulted from the introduction of lighting by gas, as well as from the warming of the corridors by a hot-water apparatus.

In concluding this report, I can hardly avoid taking the opportunity of stating, as it is highly gratifying to me to be able to do, that during the past year the important duties of the attendants have been performed to general satisfaction; and that, to many of those filling the office, I feel much indebted for the efficient manner in which they have carried out my views and wishes, as well as those of the other officers of the establishment.

JOHN THURNAM.

METEOROLOGICAL JOURNAL.

Kept at EDMONTON, *Latitude* 51° 37' 32" N.
Longitude 0° 3' 51" W. *of Greenwich.*

August 1843.	THERMOMETER.	BAROMETER.
Wednesday 9	from 57 to 79	30·02 to 29·95
Thursday . 10	58 65	29·95 30·06
Friday . . 11	46 71	30·15 30·17
Saturday . 12	47 72	30·18 Stat.
Sunday . . 13	47 71	30·17 30·10
Monday . . 14	48 76	30 00 29·94
Tuesday . 15	60 77	29·89 29·87
Wednesday 16	from 70 to 60	29·94 to 29·96
Thursday . 17	54 75	30·02 30·05
Friday . . 18	57 81	30 04 29·96
Saturday . 19	59 81	29 83 29·70
Sunday . . 20	60 72	29·64 29·76
Monday . . 21	50 68	29·91 29·87
Tuesday . . 22	49 60	29·62 29·49

Prevailing wind, N. and N.E.

The 9th, morning clear; afternoon and evening cloudy; distant thunder, and vivid lightning continually in the W., S W., and N.W., from 10 P.M. till midnight. 10th, morning cloudy; afternoon and evening clear. 11th, 12th, 13th, and 14th, generally clear. 15th, cloudy; a little rain in the morning; thunder and lightning in the evening. 16th, morning cloudy; afternoon clear. 17th, 18th, and 19th, generally clear. 20th, cloudy, with a little rain. 21st, clear. 22d, cloudy, with frequent rain.

Rain fallen, ·365 of an inch.

CHARLES HENRY ADAMS.

RECEIVED FOR REVIEW.

Lectures on the Comparative Anatomy and Physiology of the Invertebrate Animals, delivered at the Royal College of Surgeons in 1843. By Richard Owen, F.R.S. With Notes taken by W. W. Cooper, M.R.C.S., and revised by Professor Owen.

On Ankylosis, or Stiff-Joint : a Practical Treatise on the Contractions and Deformities resulting from Diseases of Joints. By W. J. Little, M.D. &c.

The Vital Statistics of Sheffield. By G. Calvert Holland, M.D., Physician Extraordinary to the Sheffield General Infirmary, &c. &c.

ROYAL COLLEGE OF SURGEONS.

LIST OF GENTLEMEN ADMITTED MEMBERS.

Friday, August 4, 1843.

T. P. Pocock.—A. Poland.—E. J. Kennedy.—W. Pearson.—J. Reid.—G. S. Deane.—H. Mitchell. F. Cheesman.—T. Moore.—J. Stevehs.—E. J. L. Whitmore.

Friday, August 18, 1843.

H. S. Wharton.—E. H. Ambler, J. A. Poole.—J. T. S. Jolley.—W. F. Coles.—D. Davies.—J. Beddell.—P. Redfern.—B. S.—Tallan.—C. M. Wayte.

A TABLE OF MORTALITY FOR THE METROPOLIS,

Shewing the number of deaths from all causes registered in the week ending Saturday, August 12, 1843.

Small Pox	7
Measles	25
Scarlatina	48
Hooping Cough	26
Croup	2
Thrush	5
Diarrhœa	27
Dysentery	3
Cholera	5
Influenza	2
Ague	0
Remittent Fever	2
Typhus	24
Erysipelas	4
Syphilis	1
Hydrophobia	0
Diseases of the Brain, Nerves, and Senses . .	135
Diseases of the Lungs and other Organs of Respiration	204
Diseases of the Heart and Blood-vessels	20
Diseases of the Stomach, Liver, and other Organs of Digestion	81
Diseases of the Kidneys, &c.	8
Childbed	5
Paramenia	0
Ovarian Dropsy	0
Disease of Uterus, &c.	1
Arthritis	0
Rheumatism	0
Diseases of Joints, &c.	2
Carbuncle	0
Phlegmon	2
Ulcer	0
Fistula	2
Diseases of Skin, &c.	0
Dropsy, Cancer, and other Diseases of Uncertain Seat.	73
Old Age or Natural Decay	60
Deaths by Violence, Privation, or Intemperance	21
Causes not specified	2
Deaths from all Causes	801

THE

LONDON MEDICAL GAZETTE,

BEING A

WEEKLY JOURNAL

OF

𝔐𝔢𝔡𝔦𝔠𝔦𝔫𝔢 𝔞𝔫𝔡 𝔱𝔥𝔢 ℭ𝔬𝔩𝔩𝔞𝔱𝔢𝔯𝔞𝔩 𝔖𝔠𝔦𝔢𝔫𝔠𝔢𝔰.

FRIDAY, SEPTEMBER 1, 1843.

LECTURES
ON THE
THEORY AND PRACTICE OF MIDWIFERY,

Delivered in the Theatre of St. George's Hospital,

BY ROBERT LEE, M.D. F.R.S.

Historical account of uterine inflammation in puerperal women.

WE know from the ancient writers that puerperal women have been liable in all ages to attacks of inflammation of the uterine system. In the works, however, of the earlier authors, its history is short and imperfect; and it is probable that the disease did not attract the particular attention of physicians before the middle of the 17th century, when it occurred at Paris as a malignant epidemic in the lying-in wards of the Hôtel-Dieu, and the bodies of those who died of it were found to be full of abscesses. Since that period it has often been observed in the principal cities and lying-in hospitals of Europe, both in a sporadic and epidemic form, and has been denominated by medical authors puerperal fever, child-bed fever, puerperal peritonitis, peritoneal fever, puerperal typhus, the epidemic disease of lying-in women. Upwards of 200 cases of this disease have come under my observation since the spring of 1827, the histories of more than 160 of which have been reduced into a tabular form. I have watched the symptoms and progress of these cases with the closest attention; observed the effects of the different remedies employed, and where death took place I carefully examined the alterations of structure in the uterine and other organs. The bodies of a great number of women have been inspected by myself personally: this task was not delegated to others ignorant of the pathology of the uterine system; and in all, without one single exception, there was some morbid change, decidedly the effect of inflammation, either in the peritoneal coat of the uterus or of its appendages, in the muscular tissue, the

lining membrane, or in the veins or absorbents of the organ, which accounted in a most complete and satisfactory manner for all the constitutional disturbance which had taken place during life. The ganglia and nerves of the uterus were the only structures which were not examined. These observations entirely subvert the opinion that there is a specific, essential, or idiopathic fever, which attacks puerperal women, and which occurs independently of any local affection in the uterine organs, and may even prove fatal without leaving any perceptible change in the organization of any of their different textures. As the constitutional symptoms thus appear invariably to derive their origin from a local cause, as the local affection is always uniform, and nothing else is so in the history of the disease, I have thought that it would be more philosophical, and more consistent with the correct principles of nosological arrangement, to banish entirely from medical nomenclature the terms puerperal and child-bed fever, and to substitute in their place that of uterine inflammation, or inflammation of the uterus and its appendages in puerperal women. The confusion and error which have hitherto prevailed on this subject have recently been aggravated by a futile attempt to include under the term "puerperal fevers," not merely the disease usually known by the name puerperal fever, but puerperal intestinal irritation, which is a totally distinct affection; hysteralgia, or what has incorrectly been called false peritonitis, and milk fever. "If, under the head of *puerperal fevers*," says the author of this new and unscientific arrangement, "we are to include all the fevers to which lying-in women are liable, and that are peculiar to the puerperal state, we must not pass over what is commonly called *milk fever*."

Until a recent period, the pathological anatomy of the uterine organs in puerperal women had not received that attention which its importance demanded. In the histories of the different epidemic fevers which have prevailed amongst lying-in women since the middle of the 17th century,

3 E

the symptoms and the morbid appearances, though imperfectly described, nevertheless strongly confirm the conclusion that the whole phenomena, local and general, of these fevers, are to be referred to inflammation of the uterine organs, and that the symptoms vary according as the superficial or the deeper-seated structures are affected. The winter of 1746 at Paris was most destructive to puerperal women, and they died between the fifth and the seventeenth day after their confinement. The epidemic attacked the indigent, but much less frequently and severely those women who were delivered at their own habitations than in the Hôtel-Dieu. Of twenty women in child-bed affected with the disease in February of that year, in the Hôtel-Dieu, scarcely one recovered.

M. Malouin has giving this history of the epidemic:—"The disease usually commenced with a diarrhœa, the uterus became dry, hard, and painful; it was swollen, and the lochia had not their ordinary course; then the women experienced pain in the bowels, particularly in the situation of the broad ligaments; the abdomen was tense; and to all these symptoms were sometimes joined pain of the head, and sometimes cough. On the third and fourth day after delivery the mammæ became flaccid. On opening the bodies curdled milk was found on the surface of the intestines; a milky serous fluid in the hypogastrium; similar fluid was found in the thorax of certain women, and when the lungs were divided they discharged a milky or putrid lymph. The stomach, the intestines, the uterus, when carefully examined, appeared to have been inflamed. According to the report of the physicians, there escaped clots on opening the vessels of this organ." "This terrible disease," says M. Tenon, in the Mémoires sur les Hôpitaux de Paris, p. 243, "has shewn itself at different epochs, and its returns have been more frequent than ever; it reappeared every winter from 1774; it commenced usually about the middle of November, and continued till the end of January. It is met with at the other seasons of the year, even during spring, for it has come to prevail more and more, and to be as it were naturalized. Those who were attacked in the years 1774 and 1775 died between the fourth and seventh days after delivery, and seven out of every twelve women who were delivered were seized with the disease. Two distinct forms of it were successively observed, one a simple form, which was cured by ipecacuan; the other a complicated form, for which there was no remedy; so that there perished in 1816, one of every seven of those who were attacked with puerperal fever, and death took place from the sixth to the eighth day after delivery, and often much earlier. The first symptoms manifest themselves twenty-four, *thirty-six*, or forty-eight hours after de-

livery, and sometimes, but rarely, in the space of twelve hours. The symptoms of the simple puerperal fever are developed in the following order: rigor, slight pain in the region of the kidneys, intestinal colic, which in two hours affects the whole hypogastrium, and gradually becomes more acute. Pulse concentrated, fever moderate, lochia not suppressed; mammæ flaccid, tongue dry in the middle, covered with a yellow mucus on the edges; hiccup and vomiting of green-coloured matters. There was sometimes combined with these constant and characteristic symptoms of the disease which took place in the years 1774 and 1775, a diarrhœa of a bilious glairy matter, a considerable swelling of the hypogastrium, thirst, and remarkable retention of urine. In the complicated puerperal fever the pyrexia is stronger, with exacerbations, the tongue is black and dry, the belly is tense, distended, and tympanitic, and slightly painful. In some women the lochia have been either wholly suppressed or only diminished; others have experienced attacks of ophthalmia; in some the respiration was difficult; in general the blood shewed the buffy coat. On opening the abdomen, the stomach, the intestines, particularly the small intestines, were inflamed, adhering to one another, distended, filled with air and a yellow fluid matter. The uterus was contracted to its ordinary dimensions, and was seldom found inflamed. I had occasion to dissect two: in one the uterus contained a coagulum of blood; an infiltration of a milky appearance, or whey-like fluid existed in certain women in the cellular membrane which surrounds the kidneys. Sometimes, also, a thick white cheesy matter was met with when the lungs were gorged with blood, or inflamed, or emphysematous, an effusion of serum was found in each side of the chest. We did not observe the hæmorrhages which occurred in the epidemic of 1664, and the uterus was not found dry, hard, and tumefied, as in that of 1746. In the epidemic of 1774, the lochia flowed, but they did not flow in 1746. "Sauvages, chiefly on the authority of Sennert and Mauriceau," observes Dr. Craigie, in his Elements of the Practice of Physic, "referred the disease to the head of inflammation of the womb, of which he distinguished three forms; the puerperal, the typhoid, or that complicated with malignant fever, and the milky, or that from suppression of the mammary secretion; the first and third, however, equally inflammatory in nature and tendency. In 1770, there appeared in the Hospital of St. Mark, at Vienna, a puerperal epidemic, which Storck regarded as inflammatory; and the disease continued to prevail in the same city for the two ensuing years with great fatality; with considerable abdominal swelling and pain in the hypogastric region: on inspection after death the intestines were found covered by false membrane, and several viscera, and among others the womb, bore marks of inflammation and gangrene. About the same time, the disease, which had originally been noticed by Strother (1718), and Burton (1751), in England, began to attract particular attention. Dr. Denman, the first English author who gave an express account of it, does not appear to have formed any very decided opinion of its nature. He speaks, indeed, of the inflammation of the womb, of the tenderness and pain of the os internum, and of the signs of inflammation preceding those of putridity. But he admits that he never had an opportunity of examining the body of any one who died of this disease, and adopting the appearances mentioned by Lieutaud as accordant with the result of later dissections, is satisfied with saying that the milky matter (materia lactea), with which the intestines were said to be covered, is probably an inflammatory exudation (p. 39). Dr. Manning, who wrote shortly after (1771), like most authors of the day, confounded the pathological or proximate cause with the remote causes, and ascribes all its phenomena to the putrid tendency of the humors." Drs. Hulme and Leake considered inflammation of the omentum to be the proximate cause of the disease, and the latter suspected that the whole mass of circulating blood becomes contaminated by absorption of the fluids effused into the peritoneal sac. "Considering," observes Dr. Leake, "the suppuration of the omentum, and large quantity of purulent fluid found in the abdomen after death, it is easy to see how a secondary fever, which was truly inflammatory at the beginning, may soon become putrid, by absorption of that fluid, which like old leaven, will taint the blood, by exciting a putrid ferment in the whole mass, and change its whole qualities into that of its own morbid nature. Some of those who survived recovered very slowly, and were affected with wandering pains and paralytic numbness of the limbs, like that of chronic rheumatism. Some had critical abscesses in the muscular parts of the body, which were a long time in coming to suppuration, and when broke discharged a sanious ichor." Dr. William Hunter, on examining the bodies of those who died from puerperal fever, found the viscera and every other part of the abdomen inflamed. There was a quantity of purulent matter in the cavity of the abdomen, and the intestines were all glued together. Pain of the head and abdomen, with fever, were the symptoms which Dr. Lowder considered to be pathognomonic of the disease; and redness of the peritoneum, adhesion of the intestines, effusion of serum mingled with pus and lymph, the most frequent morbid appearances. The history of the symptoms and morbid changes of structure, by Drs. Joseph Clark, Gordon, Campbell, Mackintosh, and other writers, is nearly the same;

and the late Dr. Hamilton, who believed that puerperal fever was a fever sui generis, nevertheless admitted that the appearances on dissection were exactly similar to the descriptions generally given by these authors, and that acute pain of the abdomen was a primary and not a secondary symptom of the disease. In the epidemic puerperal fever, which prevailed at Aberdeen between the years 1789 and 1792, Dr. Gordon examined the bodies of three patients who died of the disease, and in each the peritoneum and uterine appendages were inflamed. "The omentum," he observes, "does not appear to be more especially affected than the other productions of the peritoneum; which are all equally and indiscriminately affected. The dissections which I have made prove that the puerperal fever is a disease which principally affects the peritoneum and its productions, and the ovaria. The peritoneum was inflamed, and the omentum, mesentery, and peritoneal coat of the intestines, were all promiscuously affected." He found blood-letting and cathartics to be the most important remedies. Dr. John Clarke admitted that in most cases of the true puerperal fever which he examined, there was some degree of inflammation in the cavity of the abdomen, and that the uterus and the ovaria sometimes partook of the inflammation. In the greater number there was a large quantity of fluid in the peritoneal sac, and all the surfaces of the viscera and of the peritoneum were covered with a crust formed of the solid part of this matter, resembling coagulable lymph. The parts, however, lying under this coat or crust, were not always inflamed. The attempt made by Dr. J. Clarke to distinguish uterine inflammation from the low child-bed fever sometimes epidemic, is now universally admitted to have been unsuccessful; there is no distinct limit which bounds them in nature; and all pathologists now admit that these copious effusions into the peritoneal sac are invariably the result of acute inflammation, and not of any peculiar disposition of the vessels of the part, as he supposed. The works of Dr. Armstrong and Mr. Hey contain the histories of two epidemics, in which the leading symptoms were those which are present in cases of abdominal inflammation, and the employment of copious blood-letting, cathartics, and other antiphlogistic remedies, was attended with decided benefit. The actual condition of the uterine and other organs, was not, however, ascertained by either of these writers, as they were not permitted to examine the bodies of any of those who were cut off with the disease. Pinel, Bichat, Laroche, and Gardien, found the peritoneum inflamed in so many fatal cases, that they have considered this disease, as Mr. John Hunter did, essentially to depend on inflammation of the peritoneum. A foreign author, who has subsequently observed the disease, and who entertains the same opinion of its nature, asserts that nothing can be more absurd, more chimerical, or more contrary to the spirit of analysis and observation, than the idea that there is a fever essential or peculiar to women recently delivered. The bodies of 56 women were examined who had died of puerperal fever in the General Hospital at Vienna, in the autumn of 1819, and in all of these, with the exception of two, where delivery had taken place a considerable time previous to death, effusions of sero-purulent fluid were found in the abdominal cavity, and traces of inflammation in one or more of the abdominal viscera. The ovaria and fallopian tubes were always more or less swollen, red, and tender, and the body of the uterus was in consequence of inflammation flabby, tender, and easily broken down with the finger. It is also stated in the report of this epidemic, that the accession of fever is always preceded by marked changes in the whole system, particularly in the uterus, clearly indicating an inflammatory state. The symptoms, indeed, were such that the inflammation combined with high fever could not be mistaken.

Still more recent, and far more extended and accurate researches, have been made on the morbid anatomy of the uterine system in those who have died of puerperal fever. Of 222 cases examined by M. Tonellé in 1829, at Paris, there were traces of peritoneal inflammation observed in 193. There was more or less redness, and increased vascularity, of the peritoneal coat of the intestines, or of the mesentery, omentum, or peritoneum covering the uterus, with more or less effusion of serum, pus, and lymph. Changes resulting from inflammation were observed in the uterus and its appendages in 197 cases; which proves that the uterine system was more frequently affected than the general peritoneal sac. Inflammation of the ovaria was observed in 58 cases, and suppuration of them in four, and it appears from another statement that inflammatory lesions of the ovaria were observed in 99 cases. Traces of inflammation of the peritoneum, and in the uterus or its appendages, were found variously associated in 165 cases, and they were found separated in 57. In the substance of the uterus and ovaria there was simple inflammation in 79; superficial softening in 29; deep-seated softening in 20; inflammation of the ovaria in 58; suppuration in 4. In 90 there was purulent matter in the veins; in 32 in the absorbents; in 3 in the thoracic duct; and 9 along with inflammation and suppuration in the lumbar, inguinal, and other glands: the total changes in the uterus thus amounting to 324. Suppuration within the veins was accompanied with suppuration *of the uterus* in 32 cases; with softening in 11; *with inflammation and softening combined in 5; with peritonitis without any other change, in 34;* or without any other

lesion in 8. Suppuration within the lymphatics was associated with phlebitis in 20 cases; with metritis in 13; with softening without suppuration of the uterus in 6; with simple peritonitis in 3; without other lesion in 2. Inflammation of the ovaria was distributed in the following manner: associated with simple peritonitis in 29 cases; various changes in the uterus in 27; simple inflammation in 8; softening in 7; suppuration of the vessels in 12; all the previous alterations united in 16.

From all these facts discovered by morbid anatomy, you can now be at no loss to comprehend why inflammation of the uterus in puerperal women is so frequently fatal, so little under the control of remedies, and why it has been so difficult to give a clear and correct delineation of its constitutional symptoms. The facts disclosed by morbid anatomy, observes the learned pathologist already quoted, show that all the original descriptions of puerperal fever, however elaborate, from Strother and Denman, to the present times, are more or less inaccurate, in so far as they confound together the symptoms belonging to lesions of different parts and tissues. "Much confusion, disorder, and discordance, indeed, have prevailed among practical writers on the number and nature of the distinctions which they admit of the several forms and varieties of puerperal fever. Nor in the recent descriptions by different obstetrical authors does it appear to have been made practicable to avoid ambiguity in distinguishing the symptoms into different forms. Most authors agree that there are varieties in the disorder; but on the number and characters of these great discordance prevails. The great difficulty consists in the circumstance that though very generally the disease begins with inflammatory symptoms more or less distinctly marked, yet in almost all cases these are quickly succeeded, and as it were masked or disguised, by symptoms, in which feebleness, languor, listlessness, and mortal oppression occupy a prominent part, and consequently present that general character to which many physicians have applied the name of putrid, typhoid, ataxic, and adynamic. We have seen that J. Clarke considered it as an epidemic low fever of specific character, yet was obliged to admit that it is attended with inflammation of various abdominal and pelvic organs. Peu, Tissot, White, Alphonse Le Roy, looked on it as a putrid, typhoid, or adynamic fever; Antony Petit and Selle thought it a nervous fever; Doulat ascribed it to a gastric disorder; and lastly Walter, Johnston, Forster, and Cruikshank, Baillie, Hull, and Hey, deemed it a local inflammation of the peritoneum. The systematic writers have not diminished this discordance, and by the multiplicity of division and refinement in distinction they have rather obscured than elucidated the subject. Boer, the most accurate observer of the nature, character, and tendency of this disorder, distinguished it in 1806 into four forms: the first, the benign puerperal fever not inflammatory; the second, inflammatory puerperal fever; the third, anomalous puerperal fever; and the fourth, the malignant puerperal fever not inflammatory. M. Vigarous distinguishes five species of puerperal fever—first, the gastro-bilious, marked by intense hypogastric pain; 2d, the putrid-bilious, distinguished by great debility, small intermitting pulse, hypogastric swelling, with frequent pain, and putrid symptoms; 3d, the pituitous or mucous; 4th, the phlogistic or uterine inflammation, denoted by sense of great weight in the pelvis, hypogastric swelling, pain and hardness, with acute fever; and 5th, sporadic puerperal fever, proceeding from mental emotion, distress, &c. Gardien recognises six varieties of the disorder—1st, the angiotenic or inflammatory; 2d, the adeno-meningeal or mucous; 3d, the gastric or bilious; 4th, the adynamic or putrid; 5th, the ataxic or nervous; and 6th, that complicated with affection of other organs. These varieties, M. Martin, of the Hôpital de la Charité, at Lyons, augments to seven in the following manner:—1st, the gastric, the most frequent, often complicated with worms, with epigastric pain, headache, and full pulse; 2d, the intestinal, also complicated with worms, with meteorismus, borborygmi, and diarrhœa; 3d, the epidemic puerperal, assuming the character of the prevailing epidemic constitution; 4th, puerperal fever from retention of the placenta, first inflammatory, then adynamic or typhoid, with hard painful hypogastrium, small pulse, and faintness; 5th, adynamic or putrid puerperal fever, succeeding the gastric variety; 6th, puerperal uterine inflammation, marked by fixed pain in the region of the womb, suppression of the lochia, hard pulse, redness of the margins of the tongue, dry skin, and porraceous vomiting; and 7th and lastly, puerperal fever consequent on mental emotions, profuse hæmorrhages, copious external suppurations, or purulent deposits in the substance of organs, always terminating in ataxic or nervous symptoms. Still more recently Dr. Samuel Cusack distinguished the disease into three forms — 1st, the genuine inflammatory, marked by acute abdominal pain and tenderness, quick hard pulse, and other symptoms of synocha; 2d, the low or typhoid, generally epidemic, and allied to erysipelas and typhus fever, and similar low disorders, without tenderness, but with dull weight in the hypogastrium, weak languid pulse, and a sense of great faintness; and 3d, a mixed form, partaking of the characters of both, with abdominal tenderness, yet with the pulse neither so hard and incompressible as in the first, nor so weak as in the second variety. M. Tonellé refers all the varieties of the distemper which he observed under

M. Desormeaux to three principal forms: an inflammatory form, a typhoid, and an anomalous or ataxic form; which, he thinks, correspond to the different lesions of the solids, of the fluids, and of innervation. The inflammatory form he further subdivides into two varieties: one in which the inflammatory symptoms were open, distinct, and permanent; the other in which they were transitory, and were speedily followed by typhoid symptoms. The second variety and the typhoid form were by far the most prevalent, and were generally, if not invariably, associated with softening of the womb, and purulent matter within the veins and lymphatics, whether that were the effect of venous inflammation, or received within their interior by absorption. This division has been modified by Mme. Boivin and M. Dugès, who admit only two forms, one the simple inflammatory, or metro-peritonitis angiotenica, with strong full hard pulse; the other the typhoid, in which, though the symptoms are at first inflammatory, a secondary adynamic state speedily ensues, with small, contracted, oppressed pulse, burning heat, intense thirst, and great oppression of all the vital and animal motions; and they refer to the latter both the typhoid and the ataxic form of MM. Desormeaux and Tonellé. Lastly, Dr. Lee, discarding the name and nosological characters of puerperal fever and puerperal peritonitis, as hitherto maintained by authors, considers the several febrile disorders ensuing on parturition as essentially dependent on inflammation of the womb and its appendages; and the different forms which they assume as referable to the circumstance of affection of the serous, muscular, or venous tissue of the organ. Little doubt can be entertained that, so far as our knowledge of the relations between the external symptoms and the affection of the internal organs goes, this view is the most rational. If it be still imperfect, that is rather to be attributed to the circumstance, that in very few cases, perhaps, is one tissue exclusively affected, and consequently it is difficult, if not impracticable, to connect in any given case the external signs with any single lesion. The symptoms of mere peritoneal inflammation are modified, or it may be obscured, by those arising from ovarian or tubal inflammation, inflammation of the substance or inner surface of the womb, or the symptoms of uterine venous inflammation. This circumstance shews at once that the terms of typhoid, or adynamic, or ataxic puerperal fever, whether applied to forms or stages of puerperal fever, must convey a most erroneous notion of the pathological nature of the disease, and are in every respect inadmissible. Puerperal and typhus fever agree in no circumstance, unless in their concluding stages, namely, the production of the fatal event."

TABULAR VIEW (No. 2) OF 62 ADDITIONAL CASES OF INFLAMMATION OF THE UTERUS AND ITS APPENDAGES,

Observed by me from January 1831 to the end of April 1835.

No.	Name, Residence, and Delivery.	Date of Attack and Symptoms.	Treatment.	Result and Morbid Appearances.
101	Holding; 4, Marshall Street, Golden Square. Natural labour. January 18, 1831.	Third day,—Severe uterine pain; rigors and headache; lochia suppressed; pulse 130; features pallid; enlarged painful veins at the top of left thigh; great debility; vomiting; pain ceased.	V.S. ʒxvj., leeches xlviij. thrice, calomel, cathartics, stimulants, &c.	Died. Intestines distended with air, their peritoneum healthy; peritoneal coat of the posterior part of the uterus coated with lymph; both ovaria large and soft, the right covered with lymph; the muscular coat of the uterus, at the superior and anterior part where the placenta had adhered, of a yellow colour, and easily torn; the veins at the neck of the uterus on the left side filled with pus; the absorbents at the left superior angle of the uterus, and between the broad ligaments, filled with pus.
102	——; æt. 22; Northumberland Street, New Road. Natural labour. February 7, 1831.	Third day.—Violent pain and enlargement of uterus; no rigor; pulse 140, feeble; incessant vomiting; tympanites; delirium; lochia not suppressed.	V.S. ʒxvj., leeches liv., blisters, mercurial friction, calomel, antimony, opiates.	Died.
103	——; Compton Place. Natural labour. February 22, 1831.	Fifth day.—Slight uterine pain; headache; pain and swelling of groin; lochia suppressed; delirium; tremors; pale and sunken countenance. March 2d: iliac fossæ painful and swollen; no pain in umbilical and epigastric regions; nervous tremors.	V.S. ʒxvj., leeches, cataplasms, stimulants, Dying when first seen.	Died.

No.	Patient	History and Symptoms	Treatment	Result
104	Mrs. Crampton; 75, Gray's Inn Lane. Natural labour. May 16, 1831.	Fifth day.—Acute uterine pain; severe pyrexia. On the 12th day hectic fever; a large abscess pointing at the groin, from which a quantity of pus was discharged.	Leeches xxiv, three or four times, poultices, cathartics, opiates.	Recovered.
105	Mrs. Baird; æt. 30; Meard Street. Natural labour. May 1831.	Third day.—Pain in the region of the uterus, increased by pressure; suppression of lochia.	V.S. ʒxviij, calomel, Dover's powder, &c.	Recovered.
106	A Lady; æt. 26; Great Prescott Street. Placenta retained six hours. June 19, 1831.	In a few days great tenderness of the uterus and fever, with great prostration of strength. At the end of three weeks pain and tension along the brim of the pelvis, and a colourless swelling of the whole left inferior extremity. July 21st: pulse 150; nausea, vomiting, diarrhœa; tongue brown; dusky hue of skin; cough, dyspnœa, and expectoration. Died 24th July.	Leeches, fomentations.	Died. Uterus greatly reduced in size; recent adhesions between the uterus and rectum, and a quantity of pus; peritoneal and muscular coats of fundus and body soft, and of an inky-black colour; branches and trunk of left hypogastric vein full of pus, and lined with dark-coloured false membranes; the coats of common external, iliac, and femoral veins thickened and filled with lymph and pus; the vena cava in the same state.
107	Mr. Morley's case; Queen Street, Seven Dials. July 24, 1831.	Second day.—Rigors; tenderness of the hypogastrium; suppression of the lochia; rapid feeble pulse. July 31st: slight distension of abdomen; delirium; sickness; vomiting.	V.S. ʒxij, leeches, calomel, antimony, cathartics.	Died. Double uterus; extensive peritonitis, with sero-purulent effusion; uterine appendages imbedded in thick masses of lymph; vein of cervix uteri on left side full of pus.
108	Williams; 1, Kennedy Court, Crown Street. Hemorrhage and retained placenta. July 29, 1831.	Second day.—Pain in the hypogastrium; rapid feeble pulse; suppressed lochia; no relief after the first leeches; great uterine tenderness; ptyalism, followed by a remission of all the symptoms.	Leeches xviij, twice, calomel and opium, and cathartics.	Recovered.

No.	Patient	Symptoms	Treatment	Result
109	Porter; 21, High Street, Long Acre. Instrumental labour. August 7, 1831.	First day.—Great tenderness of abdomen; pyrexia; lochia scanty; abdomen tympanitis. Continued conscious till death.	V.S. twice during labour and twice after delivery, leeches, &c.	Died. Extensive peritonitis; inflammation of the peritoneum, covering the uterus and intestines, and softening of posterior part of uterus; uterine appendages inflamed; great effusion into the abdominal cavity.
110	Case in St. Marylebone Infirmary. October 1831.	Acute pain in the region of the uterus; rapid feeble pulse; vomiting and tympanites.		Died. Inflammation of uterine peritoneum, ovaria and tubes; extensive effusion into the peritoneum.
111	Bentley; British Lying-in Hospital. Natural labour. December 1831.	Intense soreness in the region of the uterus, aggravated by pressure; lochia suppressed; pulse 120; rigors; severe headache; thirst; pain extending to umbilical region.	V.S. ℥x., leeches xxiv., calomel, opium, cathartic, Dover's powder.	Recovered.
112	Howard; Titchfield Street. December 1831.	Constant pain in uterus, increased by pressure; lochia suppressed; pulse natural; rigors; violent headache.	V.S. ℥viij., calomel, and opium.	Recovered.
113	Wood; St. James's Infirmary. December 19, 1831.	Second day.—Pain in right side of hypogastrium; chills, not rigors; lochia scanty; tenderness increased; pulse 135; vomiting.	V.S. ℥viij., leeches xij., calomel and opium, V.S. ℥vij., leeches xij., V.S. xviij.	Recovered.
114	A lady; æt. 26; Conduit Street. Natural labour. January 6, 1832.	Severe irritation of the bowels from a cathartic before labour; 16 hours after delivery diarrhœa, with severe pain, increased by pressure, over the whole of the hypogastrium; pulse 160; no rigor. This might have been considered a case of intestinal irritation, but the symptoms did not subside till leeches had been applied, and calomel and opium given.	Leeches, calomel, Dover's powder, a blister.	Recovered.
115	A lady; æt. 25; South Street, Manchester Square. Protracted labour. January 9, 1832.	Twenty-four hours after delivery had a severe rigor, followed by tenderness of the uterus, increased by pressure; uterus large and hard; lochia scanty; tongue furred, dry, brown; delirium; hurried respiration; pulse 160, soft and feeble; vomiting. Jan. 12th: great pain in the left side of the hypogastrium; tympanites; vomiting; delirium; diarrhœa. 18th: pulse 145; tympanites and other bad symptoms subsided, but she had nearly died afterwards from paralysis.	V.S. ℥xiv., a great number of leeches, and large quantities of calomel and opium, clysters, blisters, saline draughts.	Recovered.

No.	Case	Symptoms	Treatment	Result
116	Case; British Lying-in Hospital. January 9, 1832.	Second day.—Pain in the region of the uterus; pulse 130; seemed to recover after the bleeding, and subsequently died with symptoms of inflammation of the deep structures of the uterus.	V.S. ʒx. (blood not buffed), calomel, extr. of colocynth, mistura salina c. camph. et summonia, cmplant.	Died.
117	Case; British Lying-in Hospital. January 9, 1832.	Thirty hours.—Rigors; slight tenderness in the region of the uterus, increased by pressure; with quick pulse, loaded tongue, and suppressed lochia and milk.	V.S. not employed. Anodynes, stimulants.	Recovered.
118	——; æt. 26; 12, Chapel Place, Crown Street. Distorted pelvis. January 19, 1832.	First day.—Rigor of great severity, followed by pain in the region of the uterus; suppression of lochia; pulse 130; great heat of surface; tongue white; urgent thirst; no nausea. Jan. 22d: a large swelling in the situation of the right parotid, with erysipelas of the face, and suppuration.	V.S. (blood not buffed), leeches, calomel, opium, cathartics, ol. ricini.	Recovered.
119	Case; British Lying-in Hospital. Natural labour. January 30, 1832.	Feb. 1st.—After a rigor, seized in the night with constant severe pain in the hypogastrium; lochia and milk suppressed; pulse 120; exquisite tenderness; tongue white; urgent thirst; nausea; pain across the forehead; no pain in abdomen, except in the uterus. 4th: convalescent. After leaving the hospital had another severe attack, which yielded immediately to blood-letting.	V.S. ʒxvj. (blood buffed), leeches xxiv., calomel, opium, saline draughts, cathartics. Took 50 grains of calomel. Poultices, &c.	Recovered.
120	Tellbury; British Lying-in Hospital. Natural labour. February 4, 1832.	Second day.—Acute pain in uterus; lochia suppressed; rigors; headache; tongue white on the edges, dry in the middle; pulse 140; feeble; face flushed; respiration hurried; occasional cough; great diarrhœa followed the calomel.	V.S. ʒxviij. (followed by immediate relief), leeches twice, calomel, opium, saline effervescing draughts, cathartics.	Recovered.
121	Otley; æt. 32; British Lying-in Hospital. Natural labour. February 7, 1832.	Second day.—Rigor; pain in the hypogastrium; suppression of lochia; pulse 140; skin warm; headache. Feb. 10th: pain on pressure in the right side of uterus; pulse frequent; abdomen soft and puffy; tongue loaded.	V.S. ʒxiv. (blood buffed), leeches xxiv., calomel, opium, ol. ricini.	Recovered.

No.	Case	Symptoms	Treatment	Result
122	Wildman; æt.30; British Lying-in Hospital. Natural labour. January 27, 1832.	Obscure febrile symptoms a few days after delivery; no pain in region of uterus. Tenth day after delivery incoherent; a severe rigor; pulse 130; tongue dark glossy red; countenance yellow; left lower extremity swollen. Feb. 13th: conjunctiva of both eyes intensely red and swollen; right knee-joint painful; gangrene over the sacrum. 14th: eyes enormously swollen; pain in right knee, elbow-joints, and wrists. Died on the 18th; sight lost before death.	Leeches, calomel, opium, stimulants and anodynes, fomentations, &c.	Died. Uterus contracted; abscess in muscular coat of uterus; coats of the left common external iliac and femoral veins deep and superficial, thickened, and their cavities filled with coagula; lower part of vena cava coated with lymph; the uterine, vaginal, gluteal, and other branches of the internal iliac, gorged with pus, and lined with false membranes; uterine branches of right internal iliac also affected.
123	Norris; æt. 30; British Lying-in Hospital. Natural labour. February 18, 1832.	Second day.—Severe rigor; pain in the region of the uterus; pulse 120, full; skin hot; lochia suppressed; headache; tongue furred. 21st: tenderness in the region of the uterus; frequent cough.	V.S. ʒxx. (blood neither cupped nor buffed), 40 grains of calomel taken with opium, leeches xij.	Recovered.
124	Little; æt. 28; British Lying-in Hospital. Natural labour. February 23, 1832.	First day.—Rigor; pain of hypogastrium, increased by pressure; pulse 100; headache; tongue white. Twenty-fifth day: pain immediately relieved by the bleeding. Twenty-seventh day: slight return of pain.	V.S. ʒxx. (blood buffed), leeches xviij., calomel, opium, leeches.	Recovered.
125	Case at Teddington. After natural labour. End of February, 1832.	Second or third day.—Rigors; uterine pain; accelerated pulse; and other symptoms; which immediately yielded to copious bleeding, &c. A case occurred the following day, and with the same result.	Copious V.S., calomel, opium, and oil of turpentine.	Recovered.
126	A lady; æt. 26; Charlotte Street, Bloomsbury. Natural labour. February 24, 1832.	Third day.—Slight rigors; diffused pain, increased by pressure, over the abdomen, and especially on the sides of the hypogastrium; headache; pulse 100; lochia and milk diminished. One of the mildest cases contained in this table.	Leeches xviij., calomel, and opium.	Recovered.
127	Case; British Lying-in Hospital. After hæmorrhage and retained placenta. February 28, 1832.	First day.—Rigors; exquisite tenderness in the region of the uterus; headache; pulse 110, feeble; tongue white; nausea and thirst; March 1st: pulse 110; pain diminished. 2d: gone, and convalescent.	V.S. ʒviij. (blood not buffed), calomel, antimony, opium, leeches xxiv.	Recovered.

No.	Patient	Symptoms	Treatment	Result
128	Walter; æt. 29; British Lying-in Hospital. Twins. February 20, 1832.	Second day.—Low and depressed ever since delivery; pulse 120; irregular shiverings; countenance haggard. Has not complained of much pain in the abdomen; no vomiting. The symptoms were apparently produced by mere debility, without any local affection. Died fourteen days after delivery. The symptoms were very obscure.	Neither blood-letting, general or local, or any other remedies, were employed.	Died. The whole of the peritoneal coat of the intestines, liver, and uterus, thickly covered with lymph, and a considerable effusion of sero-purulent fluid; the uterine appendages much inflamed; muscular coat and veins healthy.
129	Gates; æt. 22; British Lying-in Hospital. Natural labour. March 2, 1832.	First day.—Rigors; quick pulse; tenderness, increased by pressure, in the region of the uterus. March 4th; incoherence; great pain of uterus continues; tongue brown; urgent thirst; no sickness; pulse 120; countenance sallow.	Leeches xviij.; calomel, opium, leeches, cathartics.	Recovered.
130	Case; British Lying-in Hospital. After natural labour. March 15, 1832.	Second day.—Rigors; pain in the region of the uterus; diminished lochia; quick pulse; loaded tongue. March 18th: relieved by the bleeding.	V.S. ℥xij. (blood buffed), large doses of calomel and opium.	Recovered.
131	A lady; æt. 28. Uterine hæmorrhage. March 27, 1832.	On the second day, great quickness of pulse; and on the third, pain, increased by pressure, in the region of the uterus, especially on the left side; lochia diminished; no milk; slight incoherence. In a few days there was great febrile excitement; pulse 130; delirium. Tenderness of the left groin followed, and crural phlebitis on the left side.	Leeches, calomel, opium, sedatives, quinine, wine.	Recovered.
132	Case; Lying-in Ward of St. Marylebone Infirmary. April 1, 1832.	Pain in the right side of the hypogastrium, increased by pressure; rapid pulse; suppression of lochia and milk; great delirium. Duration of disease nine days.	Leeches, &c.	Died.
134	Sweatman; æt. 30; British Lying-in Hospital. Natural labour. April 14, 1832.	Third day.—Pain in the back. Fourth day: rigor; great tenderness in the uterine region; pulse 120; tongue red and dry in the centre, white and moist on the edge; thirst; cough; lochia scanty; uterus felt large and hard. Nineteenth day: pain relieved; pulse 110; mouth sore from mercury. Twenty-second day: vomiting; delirium; rapid pulse; great swelling in the situation of the parotids; no swelling, pain, or tension of abdomen; conscious till she sank.	V.S. ℥xiv., calomel, opium, leeches xij.	Died. Omentum, liver, uterus, intestines, all matted together with lymph; a little serum in the peritoneal sac; right ovarium and tube inflamed severely; all the veins passing into the right spermatic vein filled with pus; a great part of the veins in the walls of the uterus filled with purulent fluid.

OBSERVATIONS ON
SOME OF THE
MORE IMPORTANT DISEASES OF
CHILDHOOD.

By CHARLES WEST, M.D.

Member of the Royal College of Physicians;
Physician to the Royal Infirmary for Children;
and Physician-Accoucheur to the Finsbury
Dispensary.

[Continued from p. 742.]

II. *On a peculiar form of croup which
occurs as a complication of measles.*

DURING the autumn of 1842 diarrhœa
prevailed to an unusual extent among
the patients at the Infirmary for Children. The period of its greatest prevalence was the month of August, when
71 out of 168 patients admitted under
my care, or 41 per cent., were suffering
from it. In September the cases of
diarrhœa sank to 24, in October to 14,
and in November to 8 per cent. of the
total monthly admissions. In proportion, however, as the diarrhœa declined,
catarrhal affections of the air-passages
became frequent. Bronchial catarrh,
which, in the month of August, existed
in only 11 per cent. of the cases, attacked
20 per cent. in September, and 28 per
cent. in October; and, though it became less frequent in November and
December, still 18 per cent. of all cases
admitted in December were affected by
it. In the month of July 1842, at
which time diarrhœa first assumed an
epidemic character, affecting 30 per
cent. of the patients, cases of measles
began to occur more frequently, and
the disease soon became epidemic,
though for many months it had occurred
only as a sporadic affection. Measles
continued to prevail epidemically
during the whole of the autumn, but
did not reach their maximum frequency
until the end of November and commencement of December, in which
latter month 20 per cent. of all patients
who came under my care were affected
with them. Measles became less frequent in the beginning of 1843, and
their place, as an epidemic, was taken
by hooping-cough, which has been the
sole epidemic of the present year.
The epidemic constitution of the
whole period from the autumn of 1842
until the following spring, which,
moreover, shewed its character by an
unusual prevalence of that form of
ulcerative inflammation of the mucous
membrane of the mouth known by the

name of stomatitis, appears to have
imparted something of its peculiarities
to the measles then epidemic, giving
rise to a very insidious and dangerous
complication, which consisted in an
affection of the mucous membrane of
mouth and air-passages more nearly
resembling diphtheritis than ordinary
croup.
In no English work have I found
any account of this complication of
measles, beyond the mention of the
occasional occurrence of croup during
the progress of the disease, or as one of
its sequelæ. The slight notice taken
of it by continental authors would likewise lead to the inference that it is not
often a grave complication of measles
in other parts of Europe. MM. Rilliet
and Barthez, the most recent and most
trustworthy writers on children's diseases, expressly state* that the inflammation of the pharynx and larynx
which supervenes in the course of
measles is generally of but slight importance, that its symptoms are seldom
grave, and the lesions which it produces
are seldom serious. To this general
rule, however, there are some notable
exceptions: thus, in the years 1837-38,
an epidemic of measles prevailed in the
district of Besigheim†, in the kingdom
of Wurtemberg, in which the period of
desquamation was often attended with
an extremely perilous secondary croup,
accompanied with very extensive formation of false membranes in the air-
passages. During the prevalence of an
epidemic of measles in the year 1835,
in Sigmaringen‡ and the adjacent
country, false membranes formed on
the tonsils and palate, accompanied
with other symptoms of croup; but
this diphtheritic affection existed only
in one parish, though a tendency to it
shewed itself in other parts by the formation of aphthous ulcers about the
tongue. A similar complication, too,
existed in some cases during the very
fatal epidemic of measles at Bonn, in
the years 1829 and 1830§. An examination of the periodical literature of
medicine would probably discover

* Traité des Maladies des Enfants, t. ii. p. 731.
† For an account of this epidemic, see Dr.
G. C. F. Hauff, Medicinische Abhandlungen, 8vo.
Stuttgart, 1839, S. 79.
‡ Described by Heyfelder, in his Studien im
Gebiete der Heilwissenschaft, Stuttgart, 1839,
8vo. ii. Band, S. 9.
§ Described by Wolff, De morbillorum epi-
demia annis 1829 et 1830. Bonnæ, etc. grassante.
Bonn, 1831.

many instances in which measles were complicated with croup or diphtheritis. My present object, however, is not to write a history of the epidemics of measles, but simply to describe what came under my own notice.

None of the six cases of which I have preserved a record presented, at the outset, any peculiarity. The preliminary catarrh was not more severe than usual, nor was the eruption of measles either more or less abundant than in cases where no such complication occurred. In one instance the throat affection came on on the second day of the eruption; but in the other cases not until its decline, or till the period of desquamation had commenced. In the first case that I met with, that of an infant at the breast, of the name of Newell, living at 19, Prince's Court, Commercial Road, Lambeth, the attack of measles had been comparatively mild; the child had reached the sixth day from the appearance of the eruption, and everything seemed to promise a favourable convalescence. On the seventh day there was slight drowsiness, with some increase of the morbillous catarrh, but there seemed to be so little to excite anxiety in the symptoms, that I did not visit the child till the ninth day. I found it then labouring for breath, with all the symptoms of croup in a far advanced stage, and with great prostration of strength. These symptoms had then existed for twenty-four hours, and in twelve hours more they terminated in death. The child had had considerable inflammation of the mucous membrane of the mouth, with small aphthous ulcers on it and on the tongue, from the third day of the eruption. I was not, however, at that time aware of their betokening the existence of more serious mischief.

Another case, in which the croupy symptoms were well marked, though not so rapidly fatal as in the preceding instance, was that of—

. John Mayhew, æt. 4½ years; residing at 2, James Place, Union Street, Southwark. This child had good health until January 20, 1843, when he was taken ill; and on the 22d the eruption of measles appeared on him abundanly: he seemed going on well until the night of the 25th, when he began to cough, and on the 26th his breathing became difficult, and from that time grew worse and worse.

His mother had applied four leeches to the throat, had given him medicine and fomented his chest without relief; and brought him to me on January 28.

The remains of the eruption of measles were still to be seen on his face and back, his countenance was heavy and oppressed, breathing difficult, rather hurried, loud wheezing attending the inspiration, occasional slight hoarse cough, without much clangor. Pulse full, bounding, but easily compressible. Tongue red and raw, with slight aphthous spots upon it, and one or two similar spots upon the tonsils, which, however, were not very red, nor covered with false membranes. He had had on that day, for the first time, some difficulty in swallowing, and also occasional attacks of dyspnœa, in which suffocation seemed impending.

No unnatural sound was detected in either lung, but the air entered very imperfectly.

The case did not appear to be one in which depletion was admissible. I therefore ordered a solution of half a grain of the sulphate of copper every ten minutes till free vomiting should be produced, and to be continued afterwards every hour, and a drachm of the strong mercurial ointment to be rubbed into the thighs every two hours.

At 7 P.M. I visited him again. He had taken nine doses of the medicine, after the second of which he vomited, but the vomiting had not recurred. There was rather less dyspnœa than in the morning, and the child was sleeping quietly when I came in, but was easily roused, and when awake his face presented much less of that expression of anxiety which it wore in the morning.

I now discontinued the sulphate of copper, but directed the mercurial ointment to be still rubbed in, and ordered gr. ij. of calomel with gr. ¼ of tartar emetic to be given every two hours.

January 29, 10 A.M.—Slept much through the night, but had had two or three accessions of very urgent dyspnœa, and his mother considered him worse. He had made one effort to vomit, but rejected only a little phlegm, and that without any relief; and his bowels had acted twice. He was sitting upright in the bed, with much anxiety expressed in his face; jugular veins much distended; inspiration hissing; cough painful; and more suppressed than on the previous day. He swallowed tolerably, but distressing cough sometimes followed deglutition. He complained of his chest, and said his throat hurt him when touched.

The skin of the body was hot, but the extremities were cold; the pulse was about the same in frequency as on the day before, but it had lost power. His tongue was still red and raw, but there was no great redness of the fauces, nor were there any specks of false membrane upon them; there was considerable ulceration of the gums, and some fœtor of the breath.

The calomel was now discontinued. The mercurial inunction was still employed : gr. ij. of ammonia with ℳx. of tincture of squills and half an ounce of the decoction of senega were given every two hours.

In the evening the child was much the same, but the pulse was 140, and interrupted by occasional paroxysms of dyspnœa. I found him at 10½ A.M. on January 30, sitting up in his mother's arms, being unable to lie down; his face flushed and extremely anxious, the perspiration standing in big drops on his forehead, looking round with an expression of unutterable distress, as if in quest of relief. Respiration hissing, voice quite reduced to a whisper, cough hoarse, and without any clangor; and air entering the lungs but scantily. Gums very sore, fauces red, a little false membrane on the tonsils.

A blister was now applied to the upper part of the chest, the inunction was continued every three, and the ammonia given every two hours.

In the course of the evening he became able to lie down, but sank into a comatose condition, in which he continued with occasional intervals during the 31st of January, and until 6 A.M. on February 3d, when he died.

On the day before his death he appeared to breathe with far greater facility than he had done for some days. His face lost much of its anxious expression; the respiration became noiseless and unattended with effort; the cough less smothered; the voice, though still a hoarse whisper, was more distinct, and when aroused he answered rationally, and his mind no longer

wandered. At midnight, on February 2d, however, these treacherous appearances vanished, and in six hours he died.

On examining the body after death, the lower third of the lower lobe of the right lung was found in a state of red hepatization ; the bronchial glands were red and swollen.

The soft palate was thickened and œdematous, and there was a small ulcer on the right side of the uvula.

The under surface of the epiglottis, and the mucous membrane of the larynx, were generally rough and granular, looking as if eroded by innumerable little ulcerations. Their surface presented a dirty ash grey colour, was not coated with false membrane, but only with a little dirty mucus.

The trachea was red in patches, intensely so for an inch above the division of the bronchi. The larger bronchi were intensely red, and those on the right side contained a frothy reddish fluid, but the smaller bronchi were not injected.

The brother of this child, a fine infant about a year old, was taken with measles at the same time. In him the measles were complicated, almost from the outset, with pneumonia, and the croupy symptoms which came on on the third day were less distinctly marked. His gums became sore; his tongue red, raw, and ulcerated ; he lost his voice, had a croupy cough, though unattended with clangor : his dyspnœa was less urgent than in his brother's case, but, like him, he sank into a state of coma, and died on the seventh day. I was unable to obtain a *post-mortem* examination.

In all of the three above-mentioned cases the nature of the affection was sufficiently obvious, and in two the croupy symptoms were well marked. Sometimes, however, much greater obscurity attends the diagnosis. The child is evidently more ill than the mere existence of measles will account for, but it makes no definite complaint, and it cannot be ascertained that any organ in particular is suffering. There is considerable drowsiness, disinclination to swallow, and reluctance to speak, but cough may be absent; no croupy sound accompanies the respiration, and the child speaks in so low a tone that it is hardly possible to appreciate any alteration in the tone of its voice. In such a case I overlooked the dangerous complication till too late. The patient was a little girl, five years of age, named Jenkins, living at 13, William Street, Waterloo Road. She was attacked with measles, and I watched her the more sedulously because she had had several attacks of croup. The eruption came out naturally, and there was nothing unusual in the case except a preternatural drowsiness, which existed almost from the outset of the disease. The respiration was rather hurried; the pulse frequent, and without power; but there was neither cough nor croupy sound in breathing, nor did auscultation detect any serious mischief in the lungs. Still the child grew more and more drowsy; she took hardly any drink, never spoke, her pulse grew more frequent, and she sank into a state approaching to coma. I now bethought me of what I had hitherto neglected, and examined the state of the mouth. The fauces were very red and much swollen, and shreds of false membrane covered the tonsils and palate. Twelve hours afterwards, on the fifth day of the disease, the child died.

Ellen Douglas, aged 21 months, living at 7, Prince's Court, Commercial Road, Lambeth, was taken with measles on Dec. 9, 1842. She had a cough from the first, and the measles were associated with double pneumonia, which was combated by local depletion, and the administration of calomel and antimony. For a few days the child seemed to improve, but on the 16th she became worse, dozing for a short time, then suddenly starting up in the bed, as if in alarm. She grew habitually restless, was much troubled by hacking cough, and often refused drink, though she did not appear to have any particular difficulty in swallowing. Her voice became hoarse, this hoarseness terminating, some days before her death, into almost total aphonia. Still there was at no time any stridor in the breathing, or marked croupy symptom; but the tongue was red and raw, and little aphthous ulcers appeared at its edges, and the gums were sore; a circumstance attributed, probably erroneously, to the mercury that had been administered. Her restlessness increased, her strength declined daily, but no new symptom showed itself

until the 24th, when, though her dyspnœa did not seem increased in urgency, she would not lie down in bed, but continued sitting upright in her mother's arms, or in bed; and if laid down for a moment, she would instantly start up into the sitting posture. She continued thus until 6 A.M. on Dec. 25th, when she died.

After death, lobular pneumonia in the first stage was found in the upper lobe of the left lung; vesicular pneumonia, and grey hepatization of the greater part of the lower lobe. There was general lobular pneumonia, in the first stage, in the right upper lobe, with one patch of red hepatization; grey hepatization of the middle and lower lobes, with some vesicular pneumonia, in the lower.

The root of the tongue, and posterior part of the pharynx, were covered with shreds of false membrane, and the surface of the epiglottis presented a similar appearance, little excavated ulcerations seeming to occupy the site of the epiglottidean glands. The whole of the œsophagus was much congested, and lined by a complete tube of false membranes, which reached to within about an inch of the cardiac orifice of the stomach, and terminated in an irregular edge.

The lower surface of the epiglottis was coated with false membrane, and presented ulcerated spots just like those on its upper surface.

The mucous membrane covering the arytenoid cartilages was puckered and swollen, and the aperture of the glottis was much narrowed, partly by swelling, partly by deposit of false membrane.

Dirty greyish false membrane lined the larynx, filled up the interval between the true and false chordæ vocales, and obliterated the entrance to the sacculus laryngis. On removing the false membrane, the surface of the larynx appeared uneven as though worm-eaten, but not at all red or congested.

The false membrane did not extend below the larynx; the trachea was not at all congested, and contained only a small quantity of mucus.

The last case that I have met with was that of Evelina Turner, aged eighteen months, living in Pearl Row, Blackfriars Road, who was suffering, when admitted under my care, from diarrhœa following measles. The eruption had disappeared four days; the diarrhœa was severe, attended with tenesmus and bloody stools; and there were small aphthous ulcers in the inside of the mouth. For four days she appeared improving: she then was not brought to me for three days; and at the end of that time she returned with difficulty in deglutition, almost complete aphonia, slight croupy sound in breathing, and false membranes coating the intensely congested soft palate. In twenty-four hours more the child died.

The lungs were inflamed, and in some parts the pneumonia had reached the third stage.

The soft palate, fauces, epiglottis, and upper part of the pharynx, were intensely congested, and covered with false membrane, which was closely adherent, and extended for about an inch and a half into the œsophagus.

The larynx was lined with pus, and covered with a false membrane similar to that on the pharynx; its mucous membrane was intensely congested, but not ulcerated. This congestion terminated abruptly at the lower margin of the thyroid cartilage, and the trachea was quite pale, though containing some puriform fluid.

The foregoing details render any lengthened observations unnecessary. They show that an affection of the air-passages, dangerous in its character, often obscure in its symptoms, does occasionally occur as a complication of measles. They display a two-fold mode of attack, according to which the disease is either clearly marked, and attended from the first with obvious croupy symptoms, or its character is masked and its cause insidious. Its tendency is seen to be to produce a fatal result, while the violence of the symptoms during life affords no index from which to infer the amount of mischief which a post-mortem examination may reveal. Its hazard is further increased by the frequent coexistence with it of inflammation of the lungs, which, moreover, serves to throw the symptoms of croup into the shade. The existence of this affection, however, may be suspected wherever there are universal drowsiness, disinclination to swallow or difficulty in the act of deglutition, reluctance to speak, or alteration in the tone of the voice, even though there may be no croupy cough nor stridulous breathing. This suspicion would be raised almost to certainty, if the gums have a spongy appearance or be actually ulcerated, if the tongue be preternaturally red and raw, and if small aphthous ulcers be visible on its edges and on the lining membrane of the mouth. In such a case, an examination of the fauces, which ought never to be omitted, will usually disclose redness and swelling of the soft palate, and usually, though not invariably, the presence of false membrane.

A depressed state of the system, such as wholly to contraindicate depletion, accompanies the local affection. The employment of calomel, and of those measures usually resorted to in the treatment of inflammatory croup, is wholly inefficient; while it seems probable that success would attend the early and efficient application of caustics, as in ordinary cases of diphtheritis. Still the case of J. Mayhew shows that the development of false membrane on the fauces is not an invariable occurrence, that fatal mischief in the larynx may exist without it, and consequently that a favourable issue could not be anticipated in every case, even from the most timely use of cauterization.

TREATMENT

OF

CALCULI IN THE BLADDER.

To the Editor of the Medical Gazette.

SIR,

I MAKE no apology for offering the following case to the notice of the profession: the risks and anxieties necessarily following upon the operation render every ray of light welcome to the lithotomist; on which account I wish to give force to a suggestion offered by Sir B. Brodie in his "Lectures on the Diseases of the Urinary Organs;" for to that suggestion I was indebted for the steps taken, which although differing a little in mode, were adopted on the same principle, and followed by the same successful result.—I am, sir,

Your obedient servant,
HENRY CHARLES SHERWIN.

Hull, August 23d, 1843.

— Hartley, æt. 9 years, was brought to me by his mother (a widow), on the 8th of June, 1842, to be sounded for stone in the bladder. I detected one, if not two small ones. He had arrived the day before from near Ferrybridge, Yorkshire, a distance of 70 miles, and had suffered great pain during the journey. I was strongly importuned to cut him on the morrow, to which I imprudently consented: the operation was satisfactorily performed in the presence of my friends, Drs. Sandwith and Cooper, and two small calculi were removed in a few minutes; they were thinly coated with the triple phosphate of lime. An opiate was given, and the boy, without any apparent exhaustion of his vital system, was put to bed. As he had a rather deep perinæum, I made a very free incision through the intervening parts leading to the bladder, which induced me not to leave a canula in the wound, which I regretted afterwards. I will now quote from my notes.

Vespere.—Has slept; though calm, has a slight pain in the left groin; skin hot and perspiring; pulse 96, and full, apparently the effect of opium and reaction; the urine has flowed from the wound, which is smeared with lime.

10th, 9 A.M.—Has passed a painful and restless night; belly slightly tympanitic; there is acute pain beginning above the left groin, and extending upwards to the scrobiculus cordis; skin hot and dry; pulse 135, and small; tongue dry, and brown in the middle; countenance anxious; the upper lip retracted, with an expression of anguish. Some urine has passed by the penis as well as by the wound.

To apply half a dozen leeches to the left hypochondrium, followed by bran bag fomentations; to take Ol. Ricini ʒij. in mint water; to have a small warm-water enema.

4 P.M.—Has passed some loose stool and flatus with slight but temporary relief: symptoms much the same as in the morning; pulse 140, and weaker; belly more tympanitic; urine has come away as before.

To have 2 grs. of Dover's powder statim, and repeated after 4 hours; continue fomentations.

10 P.M.—No relief, except by occasional discharges of flatus; the wound is closing, and but little urine has passed that way.

To continue the fomentation, with an enema now and then to facilitate the discharge of flatus.

Pulse is 145, very feeble, soft, and intermitting.

I now felt convinced that I should lose him; as from the very onset of the attack, the vital powers seemed unable to sustain any depleting measures, and though having most of the characters of peritonitis, the symptoms precluded the antiphlogistic treatment. On referring the same evening to Sir B. Brodie's published "Lectures," I felt impressed with the fidelity of his description of the untoward symptoms following lithotomy. I caught at a suggestion he offers in a similar case, which he rescued by laying open the rectum with the wound, so as to give exit to a quantity of sanies: and I will take upon me here to remark, that the work alluded to, though offered to the profession in the simplest and most unostentatious style, is replete with the soundest principles of practice, and is a most excellent guide. But to return to my narrative.

11th, 7 A.M.—Found matters looking still worse; the boy had passed a wretched night, rolling from side to side in great pain; the belly hard and tympanitic; pulse feeble and fluttering, and hardly to be felt or counted, with more frequent intermissions; countenance of dusky leaden hue: occasional sighs and hiccoughs; tongue quite brown and dry. I now determined to open the wound, which was externally united: this was done with the handle of a scalpel, and having pushed up my finger to explore the parts, I gave exit to about 2 or 3 oz. of a pink-coloured sanies, having a foetid and ammoniacal odour. I was glad to find the opening in the bladder small and neatly contracted, with a well-defined margin, and scarcely admitting the tip of a finger. I broke up the entire wound in the perineum, and had the patient raised out of the hollow of his bed into a more depending position; gave a little brandy and water with a teaspoonful of castor oil.

11 A.M.—Much improved in every respect; countenance calm; had slept a little, and parted with a good deal of flatus; the pulse settled to 100.

9 P.M.—Has slept well; looks happy; pulse slower; tongue is moist; has asked for tea, and bread and butter. From this time the boy did well, and he returned to his home quite free from ailment in about three weeks after.

3 F

REMARKS.—The urine was alkaline, with considerable deposit of lime and mucus ; this (which ought to have been done before) was afterwards corrected by mineral acids, with Decoct. Pareiræ Bravæ, and Quinine. If, instead of giving a free vent to the sanies, I had treated the case as one of pure peritonitis, there can be no doubt but that he would have sunk in a few hours. Yet I committed an error in the first instance by operating so soon after a long journey. I relied too confidently on the youthfulness of the patient : time ought to have been allowed for the bladder and constitution to become tranquil before he incurred the additional risk of a formidable operation. Again, his bed was an inconvenient one ; it allowed his pelvis to sink into a hollow, which, with my neglecting to leave a canula in the wound, allowed some of the urine to lodge between the rectum and bladder ; a circumstance that has proved, probably, a more frequent source of mischief after lithotomy than is generally suspected. As an additional proof of the comparative immunity from risk enjoyed by young subjects, I would observe, that out of upwards of a dozen operations, and all successful ones, nine of them have been under the age of twelve, and only one turned sixty years, and, what is perhaps more worthy of note, eight of the former are the children of sloop-men from the banks of the Trent, Ouse, and their tributary rivers from thirty to sixty miles inland. With the exception of one, Mulberry, all the calculi mainly consisted of the mixed phosphates upon uric acid nuclei. Three of the boys (children of different parents) came from a small village adjoining Ferrybridge, where a large quantity of lime is burnt.

The eastern coast of Yorkshire, though subject to the same severe vicissitudes of climate as that of Norfolk, and quite as populous, does not yield many cases of stone in the bladder, especially when compared with the latter district; so that I am apt to think it still remains a problem how one district should abound in calculi so much more than others of a similar temperature. I have never been able to fix upon any one circumstance as tending more than another to originate this disorder; and on this account the fact of so large a proportion *of my cases* occurring in one class of the labouring poor (sloop-men) is worthy of note. In operating, I am careful to limit the opening in the bladder within the boundary of the prostate—a principle first publicly enjoined by Sir B. Brodie, and since very strongly confirmed by Messrs, Liston, Ferguson, &c.; and I quite agree with Mr. F. that when the stone is previously ascertained to be a small one, it is worse than needless to divide more of the deeper parts of the perinæum, preliminary to the section of the prostate, than will suffice for the easy introduction of the forceps. I use the knife and staff sold by Weiss, as Liston's the latter having a better defined groove than others, on account of its lower margin projecting beyond the upper one, and thereby rendering the groove more distinguishable when inserted, especially in the penis of a boy, whose parts are not so fully developed about the neck of the bladder as in man. The sound which has enabled me to detect a stone with the greatest facility is a straight one, having at its extremity a short turn, not exceeding an inch in length, which enables it to be freely turned in every direction.

ON

IRRIGATION AND WATER-DRESSING IN THE TREATMENT OF STUMPS AFTER AMPUTATION.

To the Editor of the Medical Gazette.

SIR,

I HAVE ventured to submit to your notice the subjoined cases on the good effects of irrigation and water-dressings in the treatment of stumps after amputation, should they merit that importance, and, in doing so, venture to hope the subject may attract the attention of more competent persons, whose opportunities for its trial may better appreciate its efficacy than my limited practice can afford.

My attention was first directed to this course of treatment after seeing the use of water-dressings more serviceable in the treatment of ulcers than sticking-plaster, as prescribed by the late Dr. Macartney, and followed, with increased success, in the practice of our intelligent and practical contemporary, Professor Liston ; the only difference betwixt their practice and mine being in the use of irrigation by stream upon the amputated limb at the first succeeding dressing subsequent to that of the operation, which, in my opinion, possesses advantages in contracting the capacity of the vessels, promoting the effusion of coagulable lymph, and retarding profuse suppuration to a greater extent than is to be derived from the use of water-dressings alone. However, should I not be able to establish this to your satisfaction, every unprejudiced surgeon must acknowledge the use of irrigation ensures cleanliness of the stump, comfort to the feelings, and has a decided preference over what may be justly deemed the opprobrium of surgery, viz., loading the amputated limb with adhesive stimulating plasters, bandages, &c.; thus exciting undue temperature of the stump, profuse discharges, and severe fever.

The use of strips of adhesive plaster to approximate the edges of the incision has no preference to isinglass spread upon gold-beaters' leaf; the difficulty of obtaining the latter, and its expense, alone precludes its use in provincial practice.

The manner in which irrigation was used was by a stream more or less elevated above the limb, or locally by saturating folds of lint with water, and applying them over the incision, and retaining the same with a bandage kept wet with water: the temperature of the water should vary from 60° to 80° Fah., according to the effect wished to be produced. If the object be to contract the capacity of the vessels, as after amputation, the temperature should be 60° Fah.; if, on the contrary, the desire be to promote gentle secretion with diminished capillary action, the temperature should be 80° Fah.—I am, sir,

Your obedient servant,

JESSE LEACH, M.R.C.S.L.
Fellow of the Royal Medical and Chirurgical Society of London, &c. &c.

Heywood, Lancashire, May 23, 1843.

CASE I.—A young man, of spare habit and healthy aspect, was caught by machinery, and had his wrist torn from his forearm, with fracture of the humerus. I performed the circular operation three inches below the elbow, and adjusted the fractured humerus in the usual way. The vessels being secured, the limb was sponged well with water of 60° Fah. until the bleeding from the small vessels had entirely ceased. I then drew the edges of the incision together by a strip of adhesive plaster, one inch broad and six long, using two such strips for the incision: a fold of lint was then applied around the limb, enclosing the end within its fold, to be kept constantly wet with water of 60° Fah. for six hours, when a wet circular bandage was applied, and kept as cool as agreeable to the feelings of the patient. On the fourth day the dressings were removed, and the limb, held by an assistant with a gentle declivity over a receiving mug, and five gallons of spring water, heated to 80° Fah., was poured from a jug in a stream held a foot above the limb, allowing the stream to come in contact with the limb four inches above the incision, and suffered to run over the wound.

For the space of two inches the wound is healed by the first intention, and the remaining portion is healthy: the temperature of the limb is natural: there is little fever or irritation. On every second day the irrigation and water-dressings were repeated, and in fourteen days from the accident the wound was healed.

The secretion of matter was small throughout, and destitute of fœtor; the granulations were clean and healthy, with little pain.

CASE II.—A collier, with scrofulous disease of the knee joint: the limb was very œdematous, the patient of very dissipated habits, but free from visceral organic disease: amputation was performed with the circular incision at the upper third of the thigh. The same dressings and after treatment were followed as in the preceding case, and the stump was healed in four weeks. A practical surgeon who assisted me in the operation, remarked that the case was likely to have a protracted healing, with a prospect of sloughing; the granulations at first were shining and flaccid; the cellular tissue discharged large quantities of serum: nevertheless, a perseverance in the water dressings, with irrigation, caused firm granulation, with a moderately healthy suppuration. The fever and debility in this case were counteracted by bark, ammonia, and wine. Although the patient recovered, and enjoyed good health for twelve months after, a reassumption of his old associates and intemperate habits brought on spontaneous mortification of the other leg, and the man sank under an accumulation of disease, until death put an end to his sufferings.

CASE III.—A young man was caught by machinery, and had his arm torn off above the elbow-joint: amputation was performed with the circular incision, four inches below the shoulder joint; the stump was dressed in the same manner as Case I., and the wound was healed in three weeks with little pain, moderate suppuration, healthy granulations, and a firm stump, although the family are of the scrofulous diathesis.

CASE IV.—A boy, 14 years old, was caught by machinery, and had his foot snapped off three inches above the ankle-joint; amputation was performed four inches below the knee. The wound was healed in three weeks. The same dressings and treatment were used as in the former case.

CASE V.—A man, 50 years old, of intemperate habits, and subject to epilepsy, with a bloated, doughy, and unhealthy aspect, had his right hand torn by machinery. The tendons, muscles, and bones, of the two first fingers and their metacarpal bones, were torn so as to coil like a cord in any direction; the bones of the thumb, ring and little fingers, were more or less injured. On a consultation with two other surgeons, Messrs. Pickford and Taylor, it was agreed that I should dissect off the two first fingers with their metacarpal bones, thus leaving a thumb, ring and little fingers, which were placed upon a flat board and dressed in the usual way: irrigation and water dressings were employed as in the preceding cases, and the wound was healed in five weeks from the receipt of the injury. A little stiffness remained for some time in the remaining fingers; but on the whole the man has a useful hand.

The intemperate habits, unhealthiness of the constitution, and extent of laceration, in this case, constituted important chances for sloughing and unfavourable termination.

CASE VI.—A young man, of healthy aspect, had his right arm caught in machinery, which laid bare the extensor tendons of the fingers by stripping the integuments and fascia off the *back of the hand* as high as the wrist,

fracturing in three situations the metacarpal bones of the index and second fingers, and severely crushing the fingers throughout their course. I dissected off the index and second fingers, with their metacarpal bones, secured the bleeding vessels, placed the remaining portion of the hand upon a flat board, and dressed with water, after binding the thumb and two fingers together with two strips of adhesive plaster.

The hand was very easy for the first two days, when he complained of pain and irritation. On removing the dressings on the fourth day, three live maggots were crawling in the metacarpal spaces in a mass of pus and coagulable blood, and on attempting to displace them they receded out of sight. I used the irrigation, but could not obtain a clean wound, the edges of the incision being of a dusky purple colour. I dressed the wound with pledgets of lint saturated with liquid chloride of lime, with a view of stimulating dormant vascular action, and destroying the live maggots which were still imbedded in the wound. In two days the dressings were removed; the wound was looking healthy, no maggots visible, and the mass of matter in the spaces becoming separable. I continued my chloride of lime dressings once more, which were succeeded, the next day with water dressings; and had the satisfaction to see the wound healed in four weeks from the accident.

Such, sir, are the results of six cases of amputated stumps, treated with irrigation by stream and water dressings. From their description, it will be manifest some were very unfavourable cases to make trial of its use and efficacy; yet there was neither a slough, tetanus, nor death, in any of the cases. Five out of six had little fever or constitutional derangement; and I am convinced a more speedy cure was accomplished in all than would have occurred under any other treatment.

In conclusion, it will be highly gratifying for me to hear that this treatment, when adopted, is as successful in the practice of other gentlemen of the profession as it has been in mine, and if, on trial, it be found so, it will confer comparative ease and comfort under affliction caused by loss of limb.

SOME OBSERVATIONS
ON THE
STATISTICS OF THE VIBRIO HUMANA.
(*Trichina Spiralis.*)

By Dr. Knox.

(For the London Medical Gazette.)

In the spring of 1836 a case occurred in the Practical Rooms, Old Surgeons' Hall, of the occurrence of this very curious entozoon infesting the human muscles. Numerous specimens of the worm and its sac were examined with great care by my brother and by myself, and the attention of the profession here was very generally directed to the case. The memoir was published in the July number of the Edinburgh Medical and Surgical Journal of the same year, viz. 1836. Since then, *one case only* has occurred in my Practical Rooms, viz. in October 1839, in almost every respect so much resembling the first, that it would be a waste of time to give any details respecting it. Now in the interval more than a hundred persons had been examined anatomically, and with such care as to render it nearly impossible that the presence of the worm could have escaped observation had it really occurred. Again, the comparative rarity of its occurrence in Scotland with what has been stated to be the case in England or in Ireland, induced me to address a note to my anatomical colleagues here, and from them I have very politely received the following answers to my queries.

Dear Sir,—I have not met with an instance of the very curious entozoon (the vibrio humana, or trichina spiralis of Farre) discovered by Messrs. Hilton and Paget, of London, although I have turned my attention to it. The number of bodies which have been dissected in my Rooms, and under my superintendence, amounts to one hundred and forty-three.—I am, dear sir,
Yours faithfully,
P. D. HANDYSIDES.
Feb. 6, 1840.

My Dear Sir,—In answer to your inquiry, I beg to state that I have seen but one subject in the muscles of which the trichina spiralis was developed. The subject was a female, about 50 years of age, and of rather spare habit; the muscles were pale and soft. The trichinæ were very numerous, at once detected with the naked eye, and contained, as usual, in a minute white cyst. I regret now that I did not take notes of all the muscles in which they were contained. I have superintended the dissection of between two and three hundred subjects, and this is the only case in which they were found.
I remain, my dear sir,
Yours sincerely,
ALEXANDER S. LIZARS.
1, Surgeons' Square, Edinburgh,
Feb. 13, 1840.

In addition to these notes from Drs. Handysides and Lizars, Mr. Mackenzie, who superintends Dr. Monro's Practical Rooms, has had the kindness to make me a lengthened verbal communication on the subject. He assures me that since the publication of my memoir the matter had received from him every attention, and he feels assured, that if any case had occurred in his Practical Rooms it could hardly have escaped observation; yet no case up to this date (February 1840), had ever occurred to him. Mackenzie comes therefore to the same conclusion as I and my other anatomical friends in town here have arrived at, viz. that the occurrence of the vibrio humana is very rare in Scotland, since of about 500 persons examined anatomically there had occurred but *three cases.* This of course refers more especially to the poorest class of society. What the average may be in the wealthier classes may, perhaps, be never ascertained.

REMOVAL OF DROPSICAL OVARIA.

To the Editor of the Medical Gazette.

Sir,

Having been so intimately connected with Mr. Walne's second case of ovarian operation performed on the 30th of May, 1843, it was with deep interest that I perused the details of Dr. Bird's case of the 26th of June, recorded in a recent number of your journal—a case so highly creditable to his management and tact.
It is not my intention to enter into the comparative merits of the major

and minor operations, and it is probable that I should not have addressed you on the subject at all, but for a remark in Dr. B.'s case as to his having "profited so little by Dr. Clay and Mr. Walne's recorded cases." Now, sir, in my perusal of Dr. Bird's case, what struck me most forcibly was the care with which he had pursued Mr. Walne's plan of treatment both before and after the operation (upon which, in my opinion, so much of its success depends), and I could not but feel how wisely he had acted in availing himself to the utmost of Mr. W.'s experience. Knowing, moreover, that the minute details of this *(then unrecorded)* operation, and its before and after management, were communicated to Dr. B. almost day by day during its progress, I regret exceedingly that he should have inserted such a paragraph in the report of his case.

It will, in my opinion, not lessen, but increase, the fair fame of every professional man to avail himself to the utmost of the experience of those who have gone before him; nay, it is a solemn responsibility which he is under to do so; but when communicating the results of successful experience let us do it in the spirit of the injunction of "in honour preferring one another."

I am, sir,
Your obedient servant,
JOHN M. CAMPLIN.

11, Finsbury Square, Aug. 29, 1843.

THE LATE SIR C. NIGHTINGALE.

To the Editor of the Medical Gazette.

SIR,

ON reading Mr. Lambert's account of the illness of Sir Charles Nightingale, and the post-mortem examination of the body, I was so surprised at the conclusion at which that gentleman seemed to have arrived, that I felt convinced there must be some circumstances omitted in the published account, which had materially influenced his judgment; his second communication, however, in no way removes the difficulty I felt in reconciling the inference drawn, with the symptoms from which it was deduced. Mr. Lambert's account of the case is very incomplete (for instance, there is no history given

of the symptoms previous to his first visit); but as he comes forward as the advocate of truth and justice, I will, with your permission, and with a view to elicit truth and to do justice, place the case in a different (and, as it appears to me, more natural) point of view to that taken by Mr. Lambert. The age of the deceased is not mentioned; but when a man at any age has emphysema of the lungs, dilatation of the left ventricle of the heart, chronic disease of the liver, and Bright's disease of the kidneys in an advanced stage, his constitution must have been a tolerably good one, if it has not given strong indications of what is commonly termed "breaking up." It would hardly surprise a medical man, who had arrived at a correct diagnosis in such a case, to find, in the latter stages of the combined diseases, effusion taking place into the cavities of the pleura and peritoneum; and if, urged by a desire to relieve his patient from some of his more urgent symptoms, he had recourse to the operation of tapping, it would scarcely be with a very sanguine hope that peritonitis would fail to swell the list of the allies of death. So far as we can judge from Mr. Lambert's account, this appears to have been the progress of the case; but we are not informed whether the tapping was done previous to his first visit, or subsequently; we are therefore left in uncertainty as to the operation being the cause of the peritonitis, the symptoms of which existed on the 4th.

Mr. Lambert, considering the combination of the diseases I have enumerated insufficient to cause death, seems to have cast about for some agent, the operation of which should satisfactorily account for the symptoms observed; and in "some irritant poison" he finds the solution to the difficulty. It is true, that in opposition to this idea stands the fact, that not only were there no symptoms during life indicating the action of poison, but that "there was not the slightest appearance in the mucous membrane (of the stomach) of inflammation or ulceration; it was more than usually pale." But Mr. Lambert gets over this difficulty very easily: he says, "but what *would* have been the appearances in the stomach *if* the vessels had not emptied themselves by secretion during the last stages of life?"! Panting is one of the symptoms on which much stress is laid by Mr. Lambert. One cannot help suspecting that the mode of breathing observed is inaccurately described by the term "panting," for, with emphysema of one part of the lungs, congestion of another part, and effusion of fluid into both pleural cavities, it is difficult to conceive how the deep, hurried respiration, properly called panting, could be performed. That the breathing should be disordered, even had the lungs been healthy, would excite no surprise, for it is commonly observed to be so in peritonitis. Another symptom of peritonitis, the continual drawing up of the legs, is ascribed to "spasmodic action of the flexor muscles," depending on spinal irritation. The mucous secretion, the vomiting, panting, icy coldness of the hands, are ascribed to irritation communicated to the solar plexus of nerves and spinal marrow; and the cause of this irritation is assumed to be poison!

It appears to me that Mr. Lambert, in his earnestness to advance the cause of truth and justice, has necessarily, either by publishing unfounded suspicions, and giving to them the weight of his character as a medical man, seriously compromised the character of innocent persons; or he has subjected himself to the imputation of doing so by omitting to state some of the grounds on which he comes to the conclusion he has drawn. If poison was the cause of death the symptoms must have corresponded with those usually produced by some known poison, which, in my opinion, they do not; and the circumstances under which the illness commenced would have been such as to indicate the mode of its administration. We do not learn from Mr. Lambert that such was the case. Disliking as much as Mr. Lambert controversial discussion, I think it hardly consistent with justice to insinuate criminality and deprecate inquiry.—I am, sir,

Your obedient servant,
G. D. HEDLEY, M.R.C.S.

Bedford, Aug. 28, 1843.

MEDICAL GAZETTE.

Friday, September 1, 1843.

"Licet omnibus, licet etiam mihi, dignitatem Artis Medicæ tueri; potestas modo veniendi in publicum sit, dicendi periculum non recuso."
CICERO.

VITAL STATISTICS OF SHEFFIELD.

MUCH has been done of late years to describe to Englishmen the state of England; to show one half of society how the other half lives; and thus to lighten the task of the legislator and the philanthropist, by pointing out what evils are the most pressing, and the most capable of being alleviated. Reports and books of this kind continue to appear in swarms. But as they commonly assume the shape of statistical works, a middleman, (or commentator) is required between the author desirous of being read, and the reader affrighted by long rows of figures; and we have, therefore, often thought it our duty to give the pith of a folio in an article, and lend the wings of the MEDICAL GAZETTE to facts which would otherwise have slumbered for ever on the shelves consecrated to Parliamentary literature. A work on the Vital Statistics of Sheffield, lately published by Dr. Holland, of that town, belongs partly, though not altogether, to this species. It will be consulted rather by members of parliament, and political economists, than by our professional brethren; and we shall therefore be doing some service to the latter, if we eliminate a few facts from the statistical volume of Dr. Holland.

The geological position of Sheffield is the foundation of its prosperity. Iron ore, and excellent coal, are plentiful; carboniferous limestone (used as a flux in smelting) is within the distance of a few miles; magnesian limestone for building costs only a few shillings a ton; while quarries of freestone exist in every direction round the town.

With these advantages, Sheffield has long been the head-quarters for the manufacture of hardware; in addition to which it is also a great, or perhaps the chief source of plate and plated goods. The hardware is exported to the whole world; the plated goods are chiefly for home consumption.

The working men of Sheffield are higher in morals, intelligence, and physical condition, than in towns, such as Leeds and Manchester, where machinery is extensively used, and where the steam-engine has too often brought down its human fellow-labourer to the starving point. Yet distress, severe distress, has now been the lot of the population of Sheffield for several years. The proofs of this are but too manifest. Nevertheless, so delusive are figures, unless we know all the elements on which they depend, that in one instance an important fact which seems to prove the increase of distress among the poor, is annulled by comparing it with another fact. The number of uninhabited houses at Sheffield in 1831 was 914; in 1841 it was 3,260. The second or corrective fact, however, is, that while the population of Sheffield and the neighbouring townships had only increased from 91,692, in 1831, to 112,492 in 1841, the number of inhabited houses had increased from 18,331 to 22,753; so that the population had rather more room to live in than before. In a word, the prodigious number of uninhabited houses arose not from a greater crowding of the poorer classes, but from the mania of speculators in building

On the other hand, an equally false conclusion might be drawn, and often has been drawn, from the prosperity of Savings' Banks. At Sheffield, for instance, in the years from 1838 to 1842 (both inclusive), the number of depositors increased from 5046 to 3257, and the sum total deposited from £152,560 to £162,170.

In spite of this, however, distress has been constantly on the increase. How can this be? The answer is a simple one. A part of the depositors consist of persons not dependent on trade, and a part of persons but little affected by its fluctuations. Thus among the depositors we find 221 cutlers. It is not difficult to imagine that of the 5000 cutlers of Sheffield, 221 may get constant employment in the worst times, while a great part of the remainder, men of average skill and conduct, may suffer the pangs of extreme want.

The four hundred and fifty or five hundred workmen employed in the silver plated manufacture, furnish 89 depositors; yet even this prosperous division of Sheffield workmen has, no doubt, its share of hunger and nakedness; so that while the poorest classes of workmen furnish some depositors, the richest must send out many claimants of charity. The greatest proportion of depositors, says Dr. Holland, "is found amongst the best paid artisans, as forgemen, edge tool makers, steel melters, scythe and saw makers." This is natural enough; yet Dr. Holland thinks, in the same chapter, that it is questionable whether prosperity be as conducive to the augmentation of the deposits, as adversity! He means, we believe, that times of general distress increase the predisposition to save among those who are unscathed by the calamities around them.

So that, on the whole, while a host of contributors to a given savings' bank show that the distress in that town is far from universal, they are far from proving the absence of a large mass of misery.

In his comparison between past and present periods of manufacturing distress, Dr. Holland triumphs in the economy with which relief is now doled out to the distressed poor. We cannot share in his exultation, especially when we read what he says in another place, that " the deaths of hundreds in this town are to be traced to a deficiency of the necessaries of life. They may die of disease, but this is induced by poor living, conjoined with laborious exertion. We speak from a personal and extensive knowledge of the condition of the working classes."

According to the scale of relief to the casual poor, a single man receives for six days' work, eighteen pence in money, with nine pounds of bread and three pints of soup.

Supposing the soup to be a *potage à la poor-law*, or *Decoct. Avenæ dil.*, we may set down its value at a penny a pint; and if the bread is worth twopence a pound, the wages of the man's labour will be 3s. 3d. a week—a reward which certainly does not err on the side of extravagance.

As an additional illustration of the doctrine that while the poor are sinking into misery, the upper and middle classes may be rising into luxury, we may quote the instance of Sheffield. " The immediate neighbourhood gives evidence of new life, activity, and happiness; and the changes in the picture have been effected chiefly within the last ten years. All classes, save the artisan and the needy shopkeeper, are attracted by country comfort and retirement. The attorney, the manufacturer, the grocer, the draper, the shoemaker, and the tailor, fix their commanding residences on some beautiful site, and adorn them with the cultivated taste of the artist." The Sheffield attornies, in particular, flourish exceedingly. Out of sixty-six, " fortyone live in the country, and generally in the most costly mansions; and of

the twenty-five remaining in the town, ten have been in practice only about five years."

Many points concerning the good town of Sheffield we must pass over with the briefest notice. The public roads in the township are good; the sewers very tolerable. The new houses or cottages are built with the slightest possible outlay of materials. Dr. Holland's account reminds one of the old pleasantry about houses in the outskirts of London, where dancing is forbidden in the leases, lest it should bring the walls down. " In ordinary buildings, the bond timber which is inserted into the walls is generally three inches thick; but in these modern structures it is usually an inch, and occasionally not more than threequarters of an inch."

The deaths from typhus fever at Sheffield are few to an inexplicable degree. Out of 100,000 deaths in Leeds, 4,688 are from this disease; 5,338 in Birmingham; 7,855 in London; and 6,390 in England and Wales; but only 1,551 in Sheffield. Whether this is an accident arising from the mean of only three years having been taken, or whether there is something febrifuge in the air of Sheffield, remains for time to show.

Among the causes which tend to lower the tone of morals in a manufacturing population, Dr. Holland enumerates—1. The crowding together of the working classes into filthy lanes and alleys. 2. The fluctuation of manufactures: prosperity produces dissipation, and penury breaks down the self-respect of the starving artisan. 3. The early employment of children. 4. The employment of women and girls. No school can be worse for a future wife than the workshop.

Dr. Holland truly says, that " the progress of civilization must not be measured by the creation of wealth, nor does the latter afford a just indication of the amount of happiness pervading society. * * * The imposing expression of independence and affluence in the few must not mislead us in our estimate of the condition of the many. To appreciate this, we must take into consideration the urgent difficulties experienced by the masses to procure the common necessaries of life; the melancholy failure of the attempt, as shown by the appalling fact, that in many manufacturing districts from one-seventh to one-tenth of the population is altogether dependent on parochial relief."

Dr. Holland, who is unfortunately a Malthusian, approves of the New Poor Law, which, he says, was passed to prevent the upper and middle classes being swallowed up in the growing degradation and necessities of the masses. He observes that we have enlarged our prisons, and made the paying of debts very easy, "yet when it is proposed to educate the poor, we are at once in arms, afraid that they will be enlightened and made good according to an established system, when the great truths of this system are the common truths on which all believers rest."

We must postpone to another occasion the account of the principal trades carried on at Sheffield, with the resources and relative position of the workmen.

COLLEGE OF SURGEONS — NEW CHARTER.

WE understand that the College of Surgeons have not actually obtained a new charter, but have every prospect of speedily doing so. The chief changes contemplated are:—The establishment of a body of "Fellows," amounting to 300, to be composed of members of a certain standing, not practising pharmacy. The Council to be periodically elected by the Fellows. The Court of Examiners to be appointed by the Council, but not necessarily to be members of that body.

CIRCULAR TO LECTURERS.

Royal College of Surgeons in London,
August 15, 1843.

Sir,—I am directed by the President of this College to transmit to you the inclosed copy of their Amended Regulations respecting the professional education of candidates for their diploma; and, at the same time, to express the opinion of the Council that it is highly inexpedient that the pursuits of the students should be interrupted by a vacation at Christmas, or at any other period of the winter, and to state that they strongly recommend that the vacation hitherto allowed should be discontinued.—I am, sir,
Your most obedient servant,
EDM. BELFOUR, Sec.

REGULATIONS OF THE COUNCIL.
Respecting the professional education of candidates for the diploma, August 15, 1843.

I. Candidates will be required, in addition to a Certificate of being not less than twenty-one years of age, to bring proof

1. Of having been engaged in the acquirement of professional knowledge for not less than four years; during which period they must have studied practical pharmacy for six months, and have attended one year on the practice of physic, and three years on the practice of surgery, at a recognised hospital or hospitals in the United Kingdom* ;—three months being allowed for a vacation in each year.

2. Of having studied anatomy and physiology, by attendance on lectures and demonstrations and by dissections, during three winter sessions, of not less than six months each.

3. Of having attended at least two courses of lectures on the principles and practice of surgery, delivered in two distinct periods or seasons, and one course, on each of the following subjects, viz. the practice of physic—chemistry—materia medica—and midwifery with practical instruction.

II. Members and licentiates in surgery of any legally constituted College of Surgeons in the United Kingdom, and graduates in

---

* By a Resolution of the Council on the 7th of November, 1839, no provincial hospital will in future be recognised by this College which contains fewer than 100 patients, and no metropolitan hospital which contains fewer than 150 patients.

surgery of any university requiring residence to obtain degrees, will be admitted for examination on producing their diploma, license, or degree, together with proofs of being twenty-one years of age, and of having been occupied at least four years in the acquirement of professional knowledge.

III. Graduates in medicine of any legally constituted College or University requiring residence to obtain degrees, will be admitted for examination on adducing, together with their diploma or degree, proof of having completed the anatomical and surgical education required by the foregoing regulations, either at the school of the university where they shall have graduated, or at a recognised school or schools in the United Kingdom.

IV. Certificates will not be recognised from any hospital unless the surgeons thereto be members of one of the legally constituted Colleges of Surgeons in the United Kingdom ; nor from any school of anatomy, physiology, or midwifery, unless the respective teachers be members of some legally constituted College of Physicians or Surgeons in the United Kingdom ; nor from any school of surgery, unless the respective teachers be members of some legally constituted College of Surgeons in the United Kingdom.

V. Certificates will not be received on more than one branch of science from one and the same lecturer ; but anatomy and physiology—demonstrations and dissections —will be respectively considered as one branch of science.

VI. Certificates will not be received from candidates for the diploma who have studied in London, unless they shall have registered their tickets at the College, as required by the regulations, during the last ten days of January, April, and October, in each year ; nor from candidates who have studied elsewhere, unless their names regularly appear in the registers transmitted from their respective schools.

N.B. In the certificates of attendance on hospital practice and on lectures, it is required that the dates of commencement and termination be clearly expressed ; *and no interlineation, erasure, or alteration will be allowed.*

Blank forms of the required certificates may be obtained on application to the Secretary, to whom they must be delivered, properly filled up, ten days before the candidate can be admitted to examination ; and all such certificates are retained at the College.

By order of the Council,

EDM. BELFOUR, *Sec.*

———

FELLOWES' CLINICAL PRIZE REPORTS.

BY ALFRED J. TAPSON.

University College Hospital, 1842.

[Continued from p. 751.]

———

CASE XVI.—*Acute bronchitis, with vesicular emphysema and cretaceous concretions in the lungs; dilated hypertrophy of the heart, and disease of the aortic valves; also disease of the liver, kidneys, &c.; fatal termination; sectio cadaveris.*

MARY M——, ætat. 42, admitted May 9, 1842, under Dr. Taylor. She is a tall, slight, pale and nervous looking woman ; is married, and has had three children, besides miscarrying three times ; her father is living and healthy ; her mother died of consumption. Her habits of life have been regular, and she has never been in want ; is a native of Scotland, but has been living near Tottenham Court Road for three years, in a close damp house, and has never been well since she has been there. She is habitually delicate, subject to headache and indigestion, with rising of a bitter greenish fluid into her mouth whenever she drank any beer or spirits, or took more food than usual. Menstruation perfectly regular. She had the measles and hooping-cough when six years old, and has ever since had a hard cough, especially in the winter ; and for nearly twenty years she used to spit up blood occasionally ; but this last symptom ceased ten years ago, about the time she was married. Her breath is always short, particularly in the night, and in foggy weather ; and lately she has frequently had fits of asthma. She never had palpitation or pain in the region of the heart, and was never laid up with rheumatism, though she has had many slight attacks of it.

She attributes her present illness to a cold which she caught two months ago, from walking out in very thin shoes when the weather was very cold. She was attacked with pain in the left side, increased difficulty of breathing, and her cough was much worse. During the last fortnight the pain has increased, and the cough has been very severe, and attended with expectoration of mucus.

Present symptoms.—Her face is rather pallid, but there is notwithstanding a slight amount of lividity ; the lips are swollen, and of a very deep red colour ; the nose is also very red. She complains of a severe pain in the left side, rather low down, about the ends of the false ribs, and also in the pit of the stomach ; it is increased by pressure and by a deep inspiration. The breathing is very quick and laboured, and increased in regular paroxysms, during which the urine passes off involuntarily. She has a good deal of cough, attended with frothy mucous expectoration. The skin is cool and moist; the pulse quick, but small and soft. She lies habitually on her left side, but can lie on either side. She complains of numbness of the left hand and fore-arm.

Physical signs.—Anteriorly the right side of the chest seems rather fuller than the left; during inspiration the ribs rise in a perpendicular plane with the sternum, and very little expansion takes place. The sound on percussion is very clear under both clavicles; it is rather clearer on the left side than on the right, in the lower third of the chest: on the right side percussion is dull below a line drawn from the lower end of the sternum to the sixth ribs laterally, and the dulness extends two or three inches below the margin of the ribs. The respiration is very loud, but scarcely any vesicular murmur can be heard, and there is a good deal of sonorous rhonchus. Posteriorly there is dulness on percussion over the lower third of the right lung, and sonorous and a little mucous rhonchus in the lower part of the chest, loudest on the left side. There is a distinct double murmur with the heart's sound, heard most distinctly over the base and at the lower third of the sternum: it is heard also in the neck. The impulse of the heart is increased in extent.

Applic. Cucurb. Cruent. infra scap. sinist. ad f℥viij.

℞. Antim. Potassio-Tart. gr. ss.; Mist. Camph. f℥iss. ft. haust. 6tis horis sumend. Low diet.

May 10th.—Has had no sleep at all during the night, but her breathing has been easier ever since her admission into the hospital. She feels weak and faint, and sick; she vomited once after taking the medicine. The pain in the side is not much relieved, and the pain at the epigastrium is worse. She has not much cough, but spits up a good deal of mucous. The bowels have not been opened. The urine is scanty, and deposits a copious, light, flesh-coloured sediment, soluble in liquor potassæ; reaction acid, not albuminous.

In the evening the breathing was very distressing; the countenance livid; the abdomen swelled and tympanitic. She was ordered a purgative enema.

11th.—The bowels have been opened twice; the dyspnœa and cough are less troublesome, but she cannot lie on the left side, which is the side she usually does lie on. The skin is cool.

Sumat. Antim. Potassio-Tart. gr. ¼, tantum pro doti.

12th.—The pain in the side prevents her from sleeping, and she cannot lie down at all now from the dyspnœa; complains of palpitation; the abdomen tympanitic and swelled; the menses appeared last night, which is, she says, a week before the proper time.

Habeat haustus purgans.

About noon she had severe pain about the umbilicus, which was relieved by pressure and by hot drinks, which caused the evacuation of wind. After this she became very much excited and delirious; the countenance extremely pallid, pulse 116 and weak, and was obliged to be pillowed up in bed. The urine was scanty, sp. gr. 1030; it contained an abundant sediment, and also a considerable quantity of albumen, as shown by heat and nitric acid, the precipitate filling one-fifth of the test-tube after standing twenty-four hours.

13th.—Pain and dyspnœa diminished; cough easier; mucous expectoration abundant and tinged with blood; pulse 104, soft, and rather jerking; feet and ankles slightly œdematous; she states that they used to swell, but have not lately; the bowels have been freely opened, and the motions were of a deep yellow colour, whereas hitherto they have been pale; tongue flabby, and covered with a whitish fur; she is very thirsty, but says that when she attempts to drink it always chokes her; still feels sick after taking the medicine; physical signs much the same as on her admission.

Omittatur haustus Antimonialis.

℞. Pil. Assafœtid. Comp. gr. x. ft. pil. ij. ter die sumendæ. Low diet, and pint of milk.

14th.—Sleeps very little, and frequently screams in the night; the breathing and the palpitation are much relieved, and she can now lie down again; feels very weak, cries frequently, and is troubled with globus; complains of a burning pain in the epigastrium, and whatever she takes is immediately vomited; there is tenderness on pressure in the upper part of the dorsal spine on the left side; pulse 108, jerking; tongue dry and brownish; papillæ enlarged; thirst great; bowels very open; urine plentiful, acid reaction, sp. gr. 1022, tolerably clear, but still contains albumen. In the afternoon she was ordered—

Sp. Æth. Sulph. f℥ss.; Aq. Menth. Pip. f℥iss.

which gave her much relief.

15th.—Slept better last night, and feels more comfortable.

16th.—Has been very restless again, making a great noise, crying, &c.; the breathing is more free, but she still feels a catching if she lies down; has no palpitation;

pulse 104, tolerably full; tongue moist and brown; urine still decidedly albuminous.

17th.—Last evening she became very outrageous, crying and making much disturbance, and about 10 o'clock she was ordered a draught containing half a grain of morphia: she went to sleep after a time, and the nurse found her dead between 3 and 4 o'clock. She had died without any convulsion, &c.

Sectio cadaveris 60 *hours after death.*—We may mention that, in consequence of the examination being made at the house in which the deceased had lived, some points were not so fully examined as they otherwise would have been. The body generally was considerably emaciated. The head was not opened.

Thorax.—The lungs scarcely collapsed at all when the thorax was opened. The right pleura contained about two pints of serum, and the left about half a pint; there were some old firm adhesions at the upper and back part of the right lung, but none on the left side; both lungs were somewhat distended with air, and the air-cells were distinctly enlarged everywhere; when squeezed, the air readily passed under the pulmonary pleura. The apex of the left lung presented an irregular puckered appearance, and on cutting into the substance a little beneath this there were several small calcareous concretions found. On making a section of the lungs, a good deal of frothy reddish serum exuded, and the bronchial tubes projected from the cut surface, being much thickened and indurated; they contained the same kind of bloody mucus as had been expectorated during life: the mucous membrane was not redder than usual. The pericardium contained about two ounces of a reddish serum. The heart was considerably enlarged, weighing fourteen ounces. The left ventricle was dilated, and its walls as thick as natural. The aorta measured two inches and six lines in circumference; there were no spots on it: the aortic valves were much diseased; one of them had a large vegetation growing from it, and the other two were thickened and somewhat diminished in size. The mitral valve was of the natural size, and so was the left auricle. The right ventricle was enlarged, and its lining membrane rather opaque; the tricuspid valve of the natural size; the pulmonary artery measured the same in circumference as the aorta; the semilunar valves were healthy; the right auricle was somewhat dilated, and contained a large, thin, dark coagulum.

Abdomen.—The cavity of the peritoneum contained some serous effusion. The liver was enlarged, chiefly the right lobe, which was very thick, measuring quite three inches and a half at the thickest part; the cut surface had a mottled aspect, there being small isolated brown spots, surrounded by a light

yellow tissue, and on the upper surface, over a considerable part of the right lobe, there was nothing but this yellow tissue for the depth of half an inch, looking as if all the blood had been driven from this part. The stomach was very large, and was somewhat constricted in the middle, otherwise apparently healthy. The spleen was very much enlarged, being about twice the natural length, and having a large rounded projection on the upper and inner part, which received quite a distinct set of vessels. The substance of the spleen was very firm, and contained very little fluid matter. Both kidneys were enlarged, and a little uneven on the surface; the investing membrane was firm, and adherent to the subjacent substance, small portions of this coming away with it when it was removed; the substance was pale, and of about the usual consistence. The intestines were not opened. The uterus was apparently healthy; the right ovary was very hard, and contained several small hard bodies about the size of a pea, and a small cyst filled with a dark coagulum of blood; the left ovary also was hard, contained several small cysts on the surface and in the substance filled with blood and bloody serum, also some small bodies as hard as cartilage.

REMARKS.—It is evident, from the preceding account of the symptoms which existed during life, and of the appearances after death, that the patient had laboured under a complication of diseases, most of which were of long standing, but some more recent. We shall, for the sake of perspicuity, arrange the symptoms in groups according to the different diseases on which they may be supposed to have depended, and introduce with them as much of the previous history and post-mortem appearances as seems necessary for the elucidation of the different parts of the case. In this way we cannot avoid considerable repetition.

1st. *As to the diseases of the lungs.* (*a.*) *History.*—She was predisposed to phthisis, as her mother had died of that disease. She had hooping-cough when six years of age, and had ever since been troubled with a hard cough and shortness of breath; worse in the winter, and especially in foggy weather; also for nearly twenty years she used to spit up blood frequently. The cough and dyspnœa had been much worse for two months, and she had, during the same time, bad pain in the left side.

(*b.*) *General symptoms and physical signs on admission.*—Lividity of the features; great dyspnœa, increased in paroxysms; frequent cough, accompanied with copious frothy mucous expectoration, and pain in the left side. Peculiar costal respiration; very clear sound on percussion all over the front of the chest, except at the lower part of the right side, where, as well as posteriorly on the same side, percussion was dull (this was attributed to enlargement of the liver) ; very feeble vesicular murmur ; sonorous rhonchus, loudest on the left side, and a little mucous rhonchus posteriorly.

(c.) *Post-mortem appearances.*—Serous effusion in both pleuræ ; permanent distension of both lungs with air ; enlargement of the air-cells ; hypertrophy of the bronchial tubes ; bloody mucus in them ; puckering of the apex of the left lung, and calcareous concretions just beneath the puckered part.

Such were the most important points concerning the lungs as a whole, but as we believe that they indicate three distinct diseases, viz., emphysema, bronchitis, and tubercular remains, we must briefly rearrange them under these three heads. Thus, to the emphysema belong the longstanding dyspnœa, increased in paroxysms, the peculiar respiration, the cough, the morbidly clear sound on percussion, and feeble vesicular murmur, together with the distension of the lungs and dilatation of the air-cells observed after death, which are quite distinctive of emphysema: secondly, to the bronchitis (to the chronic form of which we presume she had been subject), belong probably part of the winter cough and dyspnœa, the great aggravation of these during the last two months, the frothy mucous expectoration, which became tinged with blood a few days before death, the pain in the left side of the chest, the sonorous and mucous rhonchi, together with hypertrophy of the bronchial tubes, and bloody mucus found in them after death : and thirdly, we believe that the frequent hæmoptyses during nearly twenty years, the puckering of the apex of the left lung, and the cutaneous matter found in the lung just beneath the puckered part, are sufficient, when taken in connection with the predisposition to phthisis and the winter cough, &c., to prove that tubercles had formed in the apex of the left lung, that they had undergone that series of changes which ends in the formation of cretaceous masses, and had produced the puckering of the surface by exciting pleuritis, with effusion of lymph, which subsequently contracted.

There is yet another point which requires notice before leaving the lungs, viz., the effusion that was found in the pleuræ after death, amounting to two pints in the right pleura, and half a pint in the left. Did this depend on pleuritis? We think not; because there were not any other marks of inflammation of the pleura, no redness, or recent lymph, or false membranes, &c. It was probably due to the same cause as had produced the œdema of the ankles during life, viz., the disease of the heart : this opinion is confirmed by the coexistence of effusion into the pericardium and peritoneum, and also by the strong probability that it only came on a day or two before her death, about the same time as the œdema came on. It is true that there was dulness on the right side even on her admission, and supposing this to have depended on fluid in the pleura it would also explain the fulness of the right side of the chest, and the great dyspnœa and inability to lie on the left side, and afterwards to lie down at all; yet we think that had so much fluid been present it would have been detected ; and even admitting that it might have escaped detection (for we should mention that it was very difficult to make a careful examination of the physical signs, owing to the very nervous and excited state of the patient), how are we to explain the disappearance of the orthopnœa, as is stated in the report of the 14th May, unless the fluid had been absorbed: besides there were other causes which would explain the dulness and the symptoms that were present.

2d. *Diseases of the heart. (a.)* The *previous history* did not throw much light on these. She had been subject to rheumatism, but had never had a severe attack, and never had any particular symptoms of disease of the heart, as pain, palpitation, &c., at least she said she had not ; but considering that she was always very nervous, any symptoms of the kind that might have existed would probably have been attributed to nervousness.

(b.) *The symptoms and signs* on her admission clearly indicated considerable disease of the heart ; probably the lividity of the face was partly due to this cause, and also the palpitation and œdema, which came on subsequently, and the jerking character of the pulse. The impulse was increased in extent, and there was a distinct double murmur, loudest over the base of the heart and lower half of the sternum, heard also in the neck. These would indicate hypertrophy of the heart, and probably such disease of the aortic valves as would cause obstruction and permit regurgitation.

(c.) *The post-mortem appearances* quite confirmed the diagnosis which was made during life. The heart was considerably enlarged, being nearly double the average weight of the heart in females ; both ventricles and the right auricle were enlarged, and the walls of the natural thickness : there was therefore " dilated hypertrophy." All the orifices were of the natural size, except the aortic, which was obstructed by the presence of a large vegetation on one of the valves, whilst the other two valves were thickened and rather diminished in size. The morbid growth was evidently such as would produce considerable obstruction to the flow of the blood into the aorta, and also, by preventing the perfect closure of the orifice, would permit of regurgitation into the ventricle, and was quite sufficient to explain the double murmur which had existed.

3d. *Disease of the liver.* (a.) *The previous history.*—States that she had always been subject to a rising of a bitter greenish fluid into her mouth on taking beer or spirits, or even a little more food than usual, but she had never had jaundice or any disease of the liver.

(b.) *Symptoms and signs on admission.*—The chief of these was the increased size of the liver, as indicated by the increased extent of dulness on percussion both upwards and downwards. We may notice in connection with the state of the liver that the bowels were costive and the evacuations pale in colour at first, though subsequently they became of a deep yellow colour, and there were several symptoms of indigestion, as pain in the epigastrium, tenderness on pressure, great flatulence, and afterwards vomiting, &c.

(c.) *Post - mortem appearances.* — The liver was considerably enlarged and presented the nutmeg appearance, isolated brown spots, surrounded by a continuous yellowish tissue, indicating therefore congestion of the hepatic veins in common with the rest of the venous system.

4th. *State of urine and kidneys.*—On every occasion on which we tested the urine, except the first, it contained albumen; the specific gravity varied at different times, but we never found it less than 1020; it also contained a sediment of the lithates.

After death the kidneys were found to be enlarged and pale; the surface rather uneven, and the capsule adhered so firmly to the subjacent substance as to tear away small portions of it when it was stripped off; the substance appeared healthy, except being pale.

With these facts before us, what is the conclusion we come to as to whether the albumen in the urine depended on disease of the kidneys, or on some other cause? We know that various causes will temporarily produce albumen in the urine, but its habitual presence there must indicate some deranged state of the kidneys. In this case it was not detected when the urine was first examined, but it was on every subsequent occasion. Other causes existed here which would account for the albumen: thus the disease of the heart and venous obstruction were sufficient causes, and the fact of the specific gravity not being below the healthy standard would rather favour the idea that it did not depend on granular degeneration of the kidneys; but on the other hand the post-mortem appearances were those which are said to indicate the early stage of this dis-

ease; this, therefore, may have been the cause, and the specific gravity, (though always low in the advanced stages of this disease, is not always so in the early stages. We cannot, however, decide with certainty whether the albuminous urine depended on the state of the kidneys, or on the obstruction in the circulation.

5th. *Menstruation and the state of the ovaries.*—The patient died five days after menstruating, and we mention this in order to place it in connection with the condition in which the ovaries were found: whether any of the appearances were due to the menstruation we cannot tell, but certainly the ovaries were affected with a chronic disease, which, if the patient had lived, might perhaps have gone on to ovarian dropsy.

It is scarcely worth while to say anything respecting the condition of the spleen; it was enlarged and indurated, and of a curious shape; the enlargement was probably due to the same cause as the enlargement of the liver, *i. e.* most likely to the state of the heart.

We have now to say a few words on the treatment, causes, prognosis, and cause of death. The disease for which she was admitted, and the only one of the many under which she laboured that was likely to receive much relief from *treatment*, was the bronchitis. We may remark here that notwithstanding the extent and severity of this disease, the skin was cool and moist, contrasting strongly with the great heat and dryness of the skin in the cases of pneumonia which we have reported, and which confirms the usual statement of the much greater heat of skin in the latter disease. The treatment adopted here was local bloodletting by cupping, and the administration of tartar emetic. The last remedy produced much greater inconvenience than it usually does; and this was probably due to the extremely nervous state she was in, and perhaps also to the condition of the digestive organs: it was continued for four days, in which time many of the symptoms of bronchitis were much relieved, but she became so hysterical that there was no possibility of ascertaining the state of the disease. She was then ordered some antispasmodic pills, which did her good, and she seemed much better on the whole, but was very weak and nervous, and she expired rather unexpectedly.

The *causes* of the emphysema must be dated back to the attack of the hooping-cough which she had when six years old; her breathing had been short ever since then, and this disease is well known to be a cause of vesicular emphysema. The same cause may have excited the development of the tubercles on which, we presume, the hæmoptysis depended. The bronchitis, that is, the last attack of it, was caused by walking out in very cold weather with very thin shoes on. The cause of the diseases of the heart is not very apparent; the hypertrophy may perhaps be attributed to the long-continued increased action consequent on the state of the lungs, and to the hypertrophy we must ascribe the disease of the liver and spleen.

The *prognosis* in a case so evidently complicated could not be otherwise than unfavourable ultimately, but there was no great reason why she should not get the better of this attack; at all events, there seemed to be no cause for immediate apprehension. On the 12th of May she appeared to be almost dying, but recovered again, and then seemed better, and after being exceedingly outrageous she had a very moderate anodyne draught, and went to sleep, and was found dead some hours after. The cause of death was very obscure; it may perhaps have been due to the diseased condition of the heart.

TREATMENT OF GONORRHŒA.

To the Editor of the Medical Gazette.

Sir,

In Mr. Child's paper relating to the "Treatment of Gonorrhœa by Superficial Cauterization of the Urethra," he wishes to know if any other practitioner than himself had adopted the same mode of treatment.

I had the pleasure of attending Dr. Pereira's lectures with Mr. C., who must well remember Dr. P. relating the cases of two students trying this mode, in one satisfactorily, in the other it produced testitis and a long train of evils. Whilst gonorrhœa can be so easily managed with *weak* injections of the nitrate of silver (gr. ij. ad. Aq. Distillat. ʒviij.), and sulphate of zinc (gr. ij. ad Aq. ʒj.) with or without Bals. Copaib. &c. I cannot think we ought to try this "bold" practice, especially as even in this treatment Bals. Copaib. c. Cubeb. combined must be given.

If Mr. C. will even adopt the injection of cold water frequently repeated, say every half hour or so, he will find the discharge sooner cured, and his patients better pleased, than with his or Dr. P.'s "superficial cauterization of the urethra."

I have the honour to be, sir,

Yours very obediently,

M.D.

Islington, Aug. 21, 1843.

ROYAL COLLEGE OF SURGEONS.

LIST OF GENTLEMEN ADMITTED MEMBERS.

Monday, August 21, 1843.

J. T. Roberts.—R. T. Wylde.—J. T. Winnard. —T. J. Heaton.—N. Chadwick.—C. A. Mercer.— M. Healy.—T. R. Drinkwater.—F. D. Mudd.— W. Hunter.—G. W. T. Jarvis.—T. Clark.

Friday, August 25, 1843.

W. F. T. Ivey.—J. Burgess.—R. Cottingham. —E. L. Ogle.—E. Kittson.—W. Poole.—C. A. Wakefield.—F. Field.—B. H. Jagoe.—W. Pollock.—T. Spain.—G. Pedley.—T. B. Keetley.— W. Watson.

A TABLE OF MORTALITY FOR THE METROPOLIS,

Shewing the number of deaths from all causes registered in the week ending Saturday, August 12, 1843.

Small Pox	8
Measles	25
Scarlatina	42
Hooping Cough	19
Croup	6
Thrush	14
Diarrhœa	34
Dysentery	10
Cholera	1
Influenza	1
Ague	2
Remittent Fever	1
Typhus	33
Erysipelas	3
Syphilis	1
Hydrophobia	0
Diseases of the Brain, Nerves, and Senses	120
Diseases of the Lungs and other Organs of Respiration	185
Diseases of the Heart and Blood-vessels	27
Diseases of the Stomach, Liver, and other Organs of Digestion	75
Diseases of the Kidneys, &c.	7
Childbed	4
Paramenia	1
Ovarian Dropsy	0
Disease of Uterus, &c.	0
Arthritis	0
Rheumatism	0
Diseases of Joints, &c.	1
Carbuncle	0
Phlegmon	0
Ulcer	0
Fistula	0
Diseases of Skin, &c.	1
Dropsy, Cancer, and other Diseases of Uncertain Seat	95
Old Age or Natural Decay	51
Deaths by Violence, Privation, or Intemperance	22
Causes not specified	2
Deaths from all Causes	**795**

METEOROLOGICAL JOURNAL.

Kept at EDMONTON, *Latitude* 51° 37′ 32″N. *Longitude* 0° 3′ 51″ W. *of Greenwich.*

August 1843.	THERMOMETER.		BAROMETER.	
Wednesday 23	from 47 to 65		29·56 to 29·61	
Thursday . 24	53	66	29·54	29·80
Friday . . . 25	48	67	29·80	29·63
Saturday . 26	57	68	29·63	29·73
Sunday . . 27	48	68	29·83	29·79
Monday . . 28	48	64	29·74	29·65
Tuesday . 29	48	68	29·66	29·72

Wind variable, S.W. prevailing.

23d, morning clear; afternoon and evening raining generally. 24th, morning cloudy; afternoon clear. 25th, morning and evening clear, otherwise cloudy. 25th, generally clear. 27th, morning foggy, otherwise clear. 28th, cloudy, with rain. 29th, generally cloudy.

Rain fallen, ·94 of an inch.

CHARLES HENRY ADAMS.

WILSON & OGILVY, 57, Skinner Street, London.

THE

LONDON MEDICAL GAZETTE,

BEING A

WEEKLY JOURNAL

OF

Medicine and the Collateral Sciences.

FRIDAY, SEPTEMBER 8, 1843.

LECTURES

ON THE

THEORY AND PRACTICE OF
MIDWIFERY,

*Delivered in the Theatre of St. George's
Hospital,*

BY ROBERT LEE, M.D. F.R.S.

LECTURE XLII.

*On the Treatment of Uterine Inflammation
in Puerperal Women.*

LIKE inflammation of other organs, that of
the uterine system varies greatly in severity
in different cases and at particular periods,
and in some individuals at all periods there
is a disposition to the disease manifested
after delivery, by tenderness of the hypogastrium on pressure, and by acceleration of
the pulse, where inflammation has not been
actually developed, or where it has taken
place in so slight a degree as to yield
readily to the exhibition of opiates, and the
application of warm fomentations and poultices over the region of the uterus. Some
practitioners have been so convinced of the
advantages and necessity of employing these
remedies with the view of preventing attacks
of the disease, that they caused all their
patients recently delivered to take, from
time to time, and at intervals more or less
distant, small doses of Dover's powder, and
have applied emollient poultices to the
hypogastrium. In cases of intestinal irritation, after-pains, and various spasmodic
affections of the uterus and abdominal
viscera, this plan of treatment will prove
successful. In slight inflammatory affections of other organs it is not unusual for
the symptoms to subside without the employment of more active remedies, and it
scarcely admits of a doubt that in some of
the milder varieties of inflammation of the

uterus a spontaneous solution of the disease
not unfrequently takes place. But where
inflammation of the peritoneal coat of the
uterus is fully developed, and where the
affection occurs in a severe sporadic or epidemic form, the soothing plan of treatment,
by opiates and warm poultices over the
hypogastrium, will prove wholly insufficient
to arrest its course, and unless blood-letting,
general and local, and other antiphlogistic
remedies, be early and vigorously employed,
it will, in most cases, proceed to a fatal
termination. In no inflammatory affection
of the internal organs are the good effects of
blood-letting, general and local, more strikingly displayed than in puerperal peritonitis;
but the results of my experience do not confirm the accuracy of the opinion, that in all
cases, by the employment of these means, we
can succeed in arresting the progress of the
disease, which is always attended with the
greatest danger, and not unfrequently rapidly
runs its course to a fatal termination in spite
of the most prompt and copious depletion,
and the application of all other remedies.
When the symptoms of puerperal peritonitis
manifest themselves as before described, and
especially when there is intense pain of
the uterus, increased by pressure, twenty or
even more ounces of blood should be immediately abstracted from the arm by a large
orifice, and while the patient has the shoulders and trunk considerably elevated in bed.
We should not be deterred from employing
the lancet freely, because the pulse is small
and contracted, provided it does not exceed
120 or 130 in the minute, for in some cases
the pulse has become fuller and stronger
during the time the blood has been flowing,
or soon after. Even where the pulse is still
more rapid and feeble, if the local pain be
very great—this is here a far safer guide
than the pulse—we must not be deterred from
employing venesection to the requisite extent, and in all cases, if possible, a decided impression should be made upon the system, and

where syncope or faintness follows the blood-letting, it increases the salutary effect. In no case of inflammation of the peritoneal surface of the uterus and peritoneal sac have I seen any bad consequence to result from depletion carried to this extent. and in many, from its early use, the force of the disease has at once been completely broken, which could not have been the case had the inflammation been erysipelatous or of a specific nature. In reflecting upon the cases contained in the accompanying tables, and observing the number which terminated fatally, it is impossible to avoid the conclusion, that some patients were lost from the want of active depletion at the commencement of the attack. In many, the disease had been fully formed twenty-four hours or longer before the patients were seen, and then blood-letting was employed so sparingly as to exert no influence on the progress of the disease. When the attack of peritoneal inflammation is violent, and when the pain is but slightly relieved, the venesection should be followed without loss of time by the application of one, two, or three dozen of leeches to the hypo-gastrium, proportioning their number to the urgency of the symptoms. When the leeches have fallen off, the bleeding from their bites should be encouraged by warm fomentations, or by a thin warm linseed meal poultice, which should be frequently renewed while the bleeding continues. At the same time five grains of calomel should be administered in combination with five grains of James's powder. and gr. iss. or gr. ii. of opium, or with six or eight of Dover's powder, and this should be repeated every three or four hours until the symptoms begin to subside. The exhibition of purgatives along with the calomel till the bowels are freely evacuated, is always of the utmost consequence. There are comparatively few cases in which it is necessary to have recourse to a second bleeding from the arm, and where the propriety of this is indicated by an imperfect relief, or renewal of pain, the quantity of blood taken away seldom ought to exceed fifteen ounces. The quantity which requires to be withdrawn in the first bleeding seldom exceeds ℥xxx. and in the second ℥xv.; but there are exceptions to this, and cases of puerperal perito-nitis undoubtedly have occurred in which more copious depletion was had recourse to with decided advantage. Where the pulse has become much more rapid and feeble after the first bleeding, and the strength has appeared to be much impaired, even if the uterine pain continues, blood should not be drawn a second time from the arm. Six or eight hours after the first bleeding, should the pain continue undiminished in violence, and the pulse be full and not very rapid, and *the strength* of the patient but little im-

paired, a second venesection to the extent above stated may be ordered, not only with safety but with decided advantage. The great mortality which has taken place in this and in the other varieties of uterine inflammation certainly cannot be attributed to the abuse of blood-letting, for you will observe in the tables that the greater number of those patients who were bled early and copiously recovered, and that most of those who died were either not bled at all or very late and sparingly, or took stimulants. After the violence of the attack has been subdued, it is proper to continue the use of the mercury, but in diminished doses. two grains instead of five every four or six hours, combined with opium or Dover's powder, will be sufficient, and this should be continued until the mouth becomes affected, or until the uterine tenderness be greatly relieved. The object in administering mercury in uterine inflammation is the same as in iritis; to remove the congested and inflamed state of the vessels of the peritoneum. and to prevent the disease from terminating by effusion, when all remedies are generally unavailing. Blood-letting, general and local. the exhibition of mercury with opiates and purgatives, are the principal means which we possess in the treatment of cases of puer-peral peritonitis, and they often check the progress of the disease. But they have little influence over inflammation of the veins, absorbents, and muscular coat of the uterus. and I am not aware of the existence of any means by which it is possible for us to stop the progress, or counteract the effects, of such destructive morbid actions as those which produce suppurative inflammation of the uterine veins, and of the ovaria and fallopian tubes, and gangrenous softening of the walls of the uterus. The greater number of these cases will, I fear, always terminate fatally whatever plan of treatment be adopted : the lesions discovered by morbid anatomy have rendered this too obvious. The symptoms in these cases from the commencement have generally been such as to contraindicate the use of general blood-letting. Where the re-action at the invasion of the inflammation has been violent, and venesection has been employed, the relief obtained has only been temporary, if at all experienced; in some. blood would not flow when a vein was opened in the arm; and in a few others, the abstraction of only a few ounces has produced alarming faintness. When the local pain is severe, which it seldom is, leeches and warm fomentations seem to be the appropriate remedies; but as I have already stated, we possess none which effectually control the progress of deep-seated inflammation of the uterus. Some foreign phy-sicians are, however, of a contrary opinion,

and are satisfied that we possess a powerful remedy, even in the worst cases, in mercury employed so as to excite salivation. In several cases of uterine phlebitis I have pushed this remedy, by inunction, to a great extent, and brought the system under the influence of mercury in less than 24 hours; yet the progress of the symptoms was not arrested, and the patients died as others had done where the remedy had not been administered. In other cases I have employed mercury to a great extent internally, without the slightest benefit; and it may justly be doubted, from the results of M. Desormeaux's practice, whether or not it possesses the influence M. Tonellé supposes; for of forty-three cases where mercury was used as the chief remedy, only fourteen recovered. In the latter stages of inflammation of the deep-seated structures of the uterus, the great depression of the powers of the system renders the liberal administration of stimulants necessary; and in a few cases of uterine phlebitis the lives of the patients appeared to be preserved by them.

In the Elements of the Practice of Physic, by Dr. Craigie, there is contained the following excellent account of blood-letting in uterine inflammation. You will see that he has recommended a much more vigorous application of it than I have done; and probably he is right in this, and that I would have been more successful if I had been more energetic in the use of the remedy.

"That blood-letting is a powerful and effectual remedy is shown, not only by the experience of Hulme, Leake, and Gordon, but more recently by that of Hey and Armstrong. But, in order that it be effectual, two things are requisite: first, that it be carried to sufficient length; and secondly, that it be practised as early as possible, at the commencement, or at least within the first twenty, in many within the first twelve, hours of the disease. On the quantity of blood to be taken a great revolution has taken place in this and other inflammatory disorders. Thus, Hulme and Leake talk of eight or ten ounces as a great bleeding, which will do much good; whereas Gordon carried it to twenty or twenty-four: and as all his patients who were blooded to that extent in the beginning had speedy and perfect recoveries he did not think it expedient to carry it further. It is different with Armstrong and Hey, the former of whom occasionally carried it to thirty ounces at the first, and the latter in one case to fifty-two ounces (24th); and I found it necessary to detract forty ounces from a plethoric young woman at once, with the best effect, in puerperal fever. But though I mention these facts to give some idea of the quantity requisite to

to produce some check on the disease, it must not be imagined that it is possible to fix it in precise terms. In one subject, sixteen or twenty ounces may produce as great an effect as thirty or forty in another; and the best rule is to bleed until we have proof that the effect is produced. The most decisive and least equivocal proofs are, either fainting, either approaching or actually come on, and abatement or entire cessation of pain in the belly. If one blood-letting be not succeeded by one or other of these effects, a second, third, or even a fourth, at the interval of even a few hours, ought to be practised. This is the manner in which Hey and Armstrong appear to have practised blood-letting, rather than by one copious evacuation; and in some instances fifty, sixty, or even eighty, ounces of blood were lost before the disease began to yield. In one of Armstrong's cases, fifty ounces were drawn in three operations; and in another, by four copious bleedings and two small ones, eighty ounces were lost before the abdominal inflammation was subdued. In like manner, in one of Hey's cases, thirty ounces within the first four hours were taken at one blood-letting; at a second, ten; and at a third, eleven — fifty-one before the symptoms of abdominal soreness had abated; yet, as pain returned, fifteen more ounces were taken from the arm, and a few from the belly, by cupping and leeches. In another case twenty-five ounces were drawn at the first; after the interval of a few moments nine ounces more; and before the arm was finally tied up six ounces more; —making in all forty ounces, after which the patient became faint, and the pulse fell from 112 to 88; yet pain recurred, and was relieved permanently only by taking eight ounces more about six hours after. In another (22d) twenty-four ounces were taken at the first, with the effect of causing faintness and reduction of the pulse from 100 to 72, and about twelve hours after, in consequence of the pain returning, twelve ounces more, in all thirty-six. In a fourth case, (25th,) five hours after the first sensations of pain, thirty-three ounces were taken from a large orifice, and quickly, with the effect of removing soreness and pain, but without causing fainting, and about twelve hours after twenty ounces ere the symptoms of the disease were sensibly abated. In short, the simplest rule is to detract blood quickly and from a large opening, till the pulse becomes softer, or less frequent, or the pain is relieved, or the patient begins to faint. In some cases the pulse remains unchanged, or, instead of becoming slower, becomes quicker; and then it is best to be guided by the approach or occurrence of allevia   ain · and in the

where syncope or faintness follows the blood-letting, it increases the salutary effect. In no case of inflammation of the peritoneal surface of the uterus and peritoneal sac have I seen any bad consequence to result from depletion carried to this extent, and in many, from its early use, the force of the disease has at once been completely broken, which could not have been the case had the inflammation been erysipelatous or of a specific nature. In reflecting upon the cases contained in the accompanying tables, and observing the number which terminated fatally, it is impossible to avoid the conclusion, that some patients were lost from the want of active depletion at the commencement of the attack. In many, the disease had been fully formed twenty-four hours or longer before the patients were seen, and then blood-letting was employed so sparingly as to exert no influence on the progress of the disease. When the attack of peritoneal inflammation is violent, and when the pain is but slightly relieved, the venesection should be followed without loss of time by the application of one, two, or three dozen of leeches to the hypogastrium, proportioning their number to the urgency of the symptoms. When the leeches have fallen off, the bleeding from their bites should be encouraged by warm fomentations, or by a thin warm linseed meal poultice, which should be frequently renewed while the bleeding continues. At the same time five grains of calomel should be administered in combination with five grains of James's powder, and gr. iss. or gr. ii. of opium, or with six or eight of Dover's powder, and this should be repeated every three or four hours until the symptoms begin to subside. The exhibition of purgatives along with the calomel till the bowels are freely evacuated, is always of the utmost consequence. There are comparatively few cases in which it is necessary to have recourse to a second bleeding from the arm, and where the propriety of this is indicated by an imperfect relief, or renewal of pain, the quantity of blood taken away seldom ought to exceed fifteen ounces. The quantity which requires to be withdrawn in the first bleeding seldom exceeds ℥xxx. and in the second ℥xv.; but there are exceptions to this, and cases of puerperal peritonitis undoubtedly have occurred in which more copious depletion was had recourse to with decided advantage. Where the pulse has become much more rapid and feeble after the first bleeding, and the strength has appeared to be much impaired, even if the uterine pain continues, blood should not be drawn a second time from the arm. Six or eight hours after the first bleeding, should the pain continue undiminished in violence, and the pulse be full and not very rapid, and the strength of the patient but little im-

paired, a second venesection to the extent above stated may be ordered, not only with safety but with decided advantage. The great mortality which has taken place in this and in the other varieties of uterine inflammation certainly cannot be attributed to the abuse of blood-letting, for you will observe in the tables that the great number of those patients who were bled early and copiously recovered, and that most of those who died were either not bled at all, or very late and sparingly, or took stimulants. After the violence of the attack has been subdued, it is proper to continue the use of the mercury, but in diminished does two grains instead of five every four or six hours, combined with opium or Dover's powder, will be sufficient, and this should be continued until the mouth becomes affected, or until the uterine tenderness is greatly relieved. The object in administering mercury in uterine inflammation is the same as in iritis; to remove the congested and inflamed state of the vessels of the peritoneum, and to prevent the disease from terminating by effusion, when all remedies are generally unavailing. Blood-letting, general and local, the exhibition of mercury with opiates and purgatives, are the principal means which we possess in the treatment of cases of puerperal peritonitis, and they often check the progress of the disease. But they have little influence over inflammation of the veins, absorbents, and muscular coat of the uterus, and I am not aware of the existence of any means by which it is possible for us to stop the progress, or counteract the effects, of such destructive morbid actions as those which produce suppurative inflammation of the uterine veins, and of the ovaria and fallopian tubes, and gangrenous softening of the wall of the uterus. The greater number of these cases will, I fear, always terminate fatally whatever plan of treatment be adopted: the lesions discovered by morbid anatomy have rendered this too obvious. The symptoms in these cases from the commencement have generally been such as to contraindicate the use of general blood-letting. Where the reaction at the invasion of the inflammation has been violent, and venesection has been employed, the relief obtained has only been temporary, if at all experienced; in some, blood would not flow when a vein was opened in the arm; and in a few others, the abstraction of only a few ounces has produced alarming faintness. When the local pain is severe, which it seldom is, leeches and warm fomentations seem to be the appropriate remedies; but as I have already stated, we possess none which effectually control the progress of deep-seated inflammation of the uterus. Some foreign physicians are, however, of a contrary opinion.

and are satisfied that we possess a powerful remedy, even in the worst cases, in mercury employed so as to excite salivation. In several cases of uterine phlebitis I have pushed this remedy, by inunction, to a great extent, and brought the system under the influence of mercury in less than 24 hours; yet the progress of the symptoms was not arrested, and the patients died as others had done where the remedy had not been administered. In other cases I have employed mercury to a great extent internally, without the slightest benefit; and it may justly be doubted, from the results of M. Desormeaux's practice, whether or not it possesses the influence M. Tonellé supposes; for of forty-three cases where mercury was used as the chief remedy, only fourteen recovered. In the latter stages of inflammation of the deep-seated structures of the uterus, the great depression of the powers of the system renders the liberal administration of stimulants necessary; and in a few cases of uterine phlebitis the lives of the patients appeared to be preserved by them.

In the Elements of the Practice of Physic, by Dr. Craigie, there is contained the following excellent account of blood-letting in uterine inflammation. You will see that he has recommended a much more vigorous application of it than I have done; and probably he is right in this, and that I would have been more successful if I had been more energetic in the use of the remedy.

"That blood-letting is a powerful and effectual remedy is shown, not only by the experience of Hulme, Leake, and Gordon, but more recently by that of Hey and Armstrong. But, in order that it be effectual, two things are requisite: first, that it be carried to sufficient length; and secondly, that it be practised as early as possible, at the commencement, or at least within the first twenty, in many within the first twelve, hours of the disease. On the quantity of blood to be taken a great revolution has taken place in this and other inflammatory disorders. Thus, Hulme and Leake talk of eight or ten ounces as a great bleeding, which will do much good; whereas Gordon carried it to twenty or twenty-four: and as all his patients who were blooded to that extent in the beginning had speedy and perfect recoveries he did not think it expedient to carry it further. It is different with Armstrong and Hey, the former of whom occasionally carried it to thirty ounces at the first, and the latter in one case to fifty-two ounces (24th); and I found it necessary to detract forty ounces from a plethoric young woman at once, with the best effect, in puerperal fever. But though I mention these facts to give some idea of the quantity requisite to be taken in order to produce some check on the disease, it must not be imagined that it is possible to fix it in precise terms. In one subject, sixteen or twenty ounces may produce as great an effect as thirty or forty in another; and the best rule is to bleed until we have proof that the effect is produced. The most decisive and least equivocal proofs are, fainting, either approaching or actually come on, and abatement or entire cessation of pain in the belly. If one blood-letting be not succeeded by one or other of these effects, a second, third, or even a fourth, at the interval of even a few hours, ought to be practised. This is the manner in which Hey and Armstrong appear to have practised blood-letting, rather than by one copious evacuation; and in some instances fifty, sixty, or even eighty, ounces of blood were lost before the disease began to yield. In one of Armstrong's cases, fifty ounces were drawn in three operations; and in another, by four copious bleedings and two small ones, eighty ounces were lost before the abdominal inflammation was subdued. In like manner, in one of Hey's cases, thirty ounces within the first four hours were taken at one blood-letting; at a second, ten; and at a third, eleven — fifty-one before the symptoms of abdominal soreness had abated; yet, as pain returned, fifteen more ounces were taken from the arm, and a few from the belly, by cupping and leeches. In another case twenty-five ounces were drawn at the first; after the interval of a few moments nine ounces more; and before the arm was finally tied up six ounces more; —making in all forty ounces, after which the patient became faint, and the pulse fell from 112 to 88; yet pain recurred, and was relieved permanently only by taking eight ounces more about six hours after. In another (22d) twenty-four ounces were taken at the first, with the effect of causing faintness and reduction of the pulse from 100 to 72, and about twelve hours after, in consequence of the pain returning, twelve ounces more, in all thirty-six. In a fourth case, (25th,) five hours after the first sensations of pain, thirty-three ounces were taken from a large orifice, and quickly, with the effect of removing soreness and pain, but without causing fainting, and about twelve hours after twenty ounces ere the symptoms of the disease were sensibly abated. In short, the simplest rule is to detract blood quickly and from a large opening, till the pulse becomes softer, or less frequent, or the pain is relieved, or the patient begins to faint. In some cases the pulse remains unchanged, or, instead of becoming slower, becomes quicker; and then it is best to be guided by the approach or occurrence of fainting, and alleviation of pain; and in the

where syncope or faintness follows the blood-letting, it increases the salutary effect. In no case of inflammation of the peritoneal surface of the uterus and peritoneal sac have I seen any bad consequence to result from depletion carried to this extent, and in many, from its early use, the force of the disease has at once been completely broken, which could not have been the case had the inflammation been erysipelatous or of a specific nature. In reflecting upon the cases contained in the accompanying tables, and observing the number which terminated fatally, it is impossible to avoid the conclusion, that some patients were lost from the want of active depletion at the commencement of the attack. In many, the disease had been fully formed twenty-four hours or longer before the patients were seen, and then blood-letting was employed so sparingly as to exert no influence on the progress of the disease. When the attack of peritoneal inflammation is violent, and when the pain is but slightly relieved, the venesection should be followed without loss of time by the application of one, two, or three dozen of leeches to the hypogastrium, proportioning their number to the urgency of the symptoms. When the leeches have fallen off, the bleeding from their bites should be encouraged by warm fomentations, or by a thin warm linseed meal poultice, which should be frequently renewed while the bleeding continues. At the same time five grains of calomel should be administered in combination with five grains of James's powder, and gr. iss. or gr. ii. of opium, or with six or eight of Dover's powder, and this should be repeated every three or four hours until the symptoms begin to subside. The exhibition of purgatives along with the calomel till the bowels are freely evacuated, is always of the utmost consequence. There are comparatively few cases in which it is necessary to have recourse to a second bleeding from the arm, and where the propriety of this is indicated by an imperfect relief, or renewal of pain, the quantity of blood taken away seldom ought to exceed fifteen ounces. The quantity which requires to be withdrawn in the first bleeding seldom exceeds ʒxxv. and in the second ʒxv.; but there are exceptions to this, and cases of puerperal peritonitis undoubtedly have occurred in which more copious depletion was had recourse to with decided advantage. Where the pulse has become much more rapid and feeble after the first bleeding, and the strength has appeared to be much impaired, even if the uterine pain continues, blood should not be drawn a second time from the arm. Six or eight hours after the first bleeding, should the pain continue undiminished in violence, and the pulse be full and not very rapid, and the strength of the patient but little im-

paired, a second venesection to the extent above stated may be ordered, not only with safety but with decided advantage. The great mortality which has taken place in this and in the other varieties of uterine inflammation certainly cannot be attributed to the abuse of blood-letting, for you will observe in the tables that the greater number of those patients who were bled early and copiously recovered, and that most of those who died were either not bled at all, or very late and sparingly, or took stimulants. After the violence of the attack has been subdued, it is proper to continue the use of the mercury, but in diminished doses; two grains instead of five every four or six hours, combined with opium or Dover's powder, will be sufficient, and this should be continued until the mouth becomes affected, or until the uterine tenderness be greatly relieved. The object in administering mercury in uterine inflammation is the same as in iritis; to remove the congested and inflamed state of the vessels of the peritoneum, and to prevent the disease from terminating by effusion, when all remedies are generally unavailing. Blood-letting, general and local, the exhibition of mercury with opiates and purgatives, are the principal means which we possess in the treatment of cases of puerperal peritonitis, and they often check the progress of the disease. But they have little influence over inflammation of the veins, absorbents, and muscular coat of the uterus, and I am not aware of the existence of any means by which it is possible for us to stop the progress, or counteract the effects, of such destructive morbid actions as those which produce suppurative inflammation of the uterine veins, and of the ovaria and fallopian tubes, and gangrenous softening of the walls of the uterus. The greater number of these cases will, I fear, always terminate fatally whatever plan of treatment be adopted: the lesions discovered by morbid anatomy have rendered this too obvious. The symptoms in these cases from the commencement have generally been such as to contraindicate the use of general blood-letting. Where the reaction at the invasion of the inflammation has been violent, and venesection has been employed, the relief obtained has only been temporary, if at all experienced; in some, blood would not flow when a vein was opened in the arm; and in a few others, the abstraction of only a few ounces has produced alarming faintness. When the local pain is severe, which it seldom is, leeches and warm fomentations seem to be the appropriate remedies; but as I have already stated, we possess none which effectually control the progress of deep-seated inflammation of the uterus. Some foreign physicians are, however, of a contrary opinion,

and are satisfied that we possess a powerful remedy, even in the worst cases, in mercury employed so as to excite salivation. In several cases of uterine phlebitis I have pushed this remedy, by inunction, to a great extent, and brought the system under the influence of mercury in less than 24 hours; yet the progress of the symptoms was not arrested, and the patients died as others had done where the remedy had not been administered. In other cases I have employed mercury to a great extent internally, without the slightest benefit; and it may justly be doubted, from the results of M. Desormeaux's practice, whether or not it possesses the influence M. Tonellé supposes; for of forty-three cases where mercury was used as the chief remedy, only fourteen recovered. In the latter stages of inflammation of the deep-seated structures of the uterus, the great depression of the powers of the system renders the liberal administration of stimulants necessary; and in a few cases of uterine phlebitis the lives of the patients appeared to be preserved by them.

In the Elements of the Practice of Physic, by Dr. Craigie, there is contained the following excellent account of blood-letting in uterine inflammation. You will see that he has recommended a much more vigorous application of it than I have done; and probably he is right in this, and that I would have been more successful if I had been more energetic in the use of the remedy.

"That blood-letting is a powerful and effectual remedy is shown, not only by the experience of Hulme, Leake, and Gordon, but more recently by that of Hey and Armstrong. But, in order that it be effectual, two things are requisite: first, that it be carried to sufficient length; and secondly, that it be practised as early as possible, at the commencement, or at least within the first twenty, in many within the first twelve, hours of the disease. On the quantity of blood to be taken a great revolution has taken place in this and other inflammatory disorders. Thus, Hulme and Leake talk of eight or ten ounces as a great bleeding, which will do much good; whereas Gordon carried it to twenty or twenty-four: and as all his patients who were blooded to that extent in the beginning had speedy and perfect recoveries he did not think it expedient to carry it further. It is different with Armstrong and Hey, the former of whom occasionally carried it to thirty ounces at the first, and the latter in one case to fifty-two ounces (24th); and I found it necessary to detract forty ounces from a plethoric young woman at once, with the best effect, in puerperal fever. But though I mention these facts to give some idea of the quantity requisite to be taken in order to produce some check on the disease, it must not be imagined that it is possible to fix it in precise terms. In one subject, sixteen or twenty ounces may produce as great an effect as thirty or forty in another; and the best rule is to bleed until we have proof that the effect is produced. The most decisive and least equivocal proofs are, fainting, either approaching or actually come on, and abatement or entire cessation of pain in the belly. If one blood-letting be not succeeded by one or other of these effects, a second, third, or even a fourth, at the interval of even a few hours, ought to be practised. This is the manner in which Hey and Armstrong appear to have practised blood-letting, rather than by one copious evacuation; and in some instances fifty, sixty, or even eighty, ounces of blood were lost before the disease began to yield. In one of Armstrong's cases, fifty ounces were drawn in three operations; and in another, by four copious bleedings and two small ones, eighty ounces were lost before the abdominal inflammation was subdued. In like manner, in one of Hey's cases, thirty ounces within the first four hours were taken at one blood-letting; at a second, ten; and at a third, eleven — fifty-one before the symptoms of abdominal soreness had abated; yet, as pain returned, fifteen more ounces were taken from the arm, and a few from the belly, by cupping and leeches. In another case twenty-five ounces were drawn at the first; after the interval of a few moments nine ounces more; and before the arm was finally tied up six ounces more; —making in all forty ounces, after which the patient became faint, and the pulse fell from 112 to 88; yet pain recurred, and was relieved permanently only by taking eight ounces more about six hours after. In another (22d) twenty-four ounces were taken at the first, with the effect of causing faintness and reduction of the pulse from 100 to 72, and about twelve hours after, in consequence of the pain returning, twelve ounces more, in all thirty-six. In a fourth case, (25th,) five hours after the first sensations of pain, thirty-three ounces were taken from a large orifice, and quickly, with the effect of removing soreness and pain, but without causing fainting, and about twelve hours after twenty ounces ere the symptoms of the disease were sensibly abated. In short, the simplest rule is to detract blood quickly and from a large opening, till the pulse becomes softer, or less frequent, or the pain is relieved, or the patient begins to faint. In some cases the pulse remains unchanged, or, instead of becoming slower, becomes quicker; and then it is best to be guided by the approach or occurrence of fainting, and alleviation of pain; and in the event of this last symptom, with or without quick pulse recurring, it is always wisest to repeat the evacuation. If the pain and soreness of the belly be not removed or very materially alleviated in six hours, the blood-letting ought to be repeated; nor should a considerable degree of faintness, or even absolute *deliquium animi*, warrant the opinion that further blood-letting is either unsafe or unnecessary, so long as pain of the belly continues.

" The rapid course of this disease renders early blood-letting of the utmost importance. It is not well ascertained at what precise period of the disorder the inflammation may be incapable of being rendered amenable to suitable evacuation. Hey remarks, on this subject, that the disease may terminate fatally in forty-eight, or even in twenty-four hours, and he records one in which this took place in less than eighteen hours. But though these facts be of some consequence in showing with what promptitude remedial measures ought to be administered, they do not inform us how far blood-letting may be expected to be beneficial at any given period of the disease. The great point is to institute this remedy before effusion of sero-purulent fluid has taken place, or at least before it has gone to much extent; but as nothing very certain is known regarding this, further than that it will take place at different periods in different cases, it is manifest that no general rule can be established, and that the practitioner must draw his conclusions as to the propriety of using it, from the history of the case and the existing symptoms. Hey states that he knew blood-letting successful in a few cases in which a delay of more than twenty-four hours had been incurred, and he instances several of his own cases in which blood-letting was practised with success, thirty, and even forty hours after the commencement. This delay, however, ought never, if possible, to be permitted to take place, and it is always desirable to institute the evacuation at least within twelve hours from the first sensations of pain in the belly. In cases where earlier notice is given, this evacuation will be more effectual the nearer it is performed to the commencement of the disease. The most difficult and delicate point is to determine when it is too late to practise blood-letting. It is evident that the longer it is deferred, the more violent will the disease become; and as its effects very early begin to take place in lymphy exudation, and sero-purulent effusion within the peritoneum into the substance of the ovaries and the fallopian tubes, the great object is either to prevent or to arrest this process by timely suspension of inflammatory action. For the purpose of establishing

a rule as to the time and period of blood-letting, Armstrong has divided the disease into the two stages of excitement and collapse, in the first of which only this remedy is admissible. But as it may terminate in twenty hours, or extend to seventy in the acute forms of the disease, and is even more protracted in that which is termed subacute, it is obvious that no very precise rules can be derived from this principle. It is also to be remembered that, in not a few cases of puerperal fever, especially if attended with symptoms of uterine *phlebitis*, even the first or inflammatory stage presents so many marks of languor, oppression, and weakness, that an experienced observer might imagine the termination of the disease to be at hand, when blood-letting, if not injurious, must at least be useless. It is therefore indispensable not only to attend to the existing symptoms, but to inquire into their previous course and duration. When this has been determined, blood-letting should be performed, only if pain of the belly be still felt, if the skin and extremities are not cold and moistened with sweat, and if there be reason to believe that effusion has not taken place or is inconsiderable. If, on the contrary, there is no pain but weight of the belly, if, with an extremely quick thready pulse, the extremities are cold, and the person covered partially with chill damp sweats, and if the belly be distinctly distended with much sero-purulent fluid, no benefit can be expected from blood-letting."

Other means, besides those now described, have been recommended by different authors in the treatment of uterine inflammation; such as oleum terebinthinæ, ipecacuan, digitalis, colchicum, and camphor.

Since the oil of turpentine was introduced into practice by Dr. Brenan, the most contradictory statements have been published respecting its effects. In a paper published in the Dublin Hospital Reports, Dr. Douglas observes that in the epidemical and contagious puerperal fever, ʒiii. of the ol. terebinth., with an equal quantity of syrup and ʒvi. of water, should be given three or four hours after the exhibition of the first dose of the calomel; and that after the lapse of another hour this should be followed by an ounce of castor oil, or some other briskly purgative medicine. In some instances the oil of turpentine and castor oil may be combined in one draught. The internal use of turpentine is not to be repeated more than twice in any case whatever. " In several cases," Dr. Douglas adds, " where the debility is very considerable, the local bleeding may also be omitted; and in this case a flannel cloth, steeped in oil of turpentine, should be applied to the abdomen, and allowed to remain on for the space of fifteen minutes. This external application of turpentine, without either its internal use or the aid of bloodletting, I have frequently experienced to be entirely efficacious in curing puerperal attacks; and although I have hitherto omitted to speak of turpentine for the cure of the other varieties of this disease, yet I would not feel as if I were doing justice to the community if I did not distinctly state that I consider it, when judiciously administered, more generally suitable and more effectually remedial than any other medicine yet proposed. I can safely aver I have seen women recover apparently by its influence from an almost hopeless condition; certainly after every hope of recovery under ordinary treatment had been relinquished."

I have not ventured to prescribe in many instances the internal use of ol. terebinth. either in the superficial or deep-seated inflammatory affections of the uterus; but whenever this has been done, it has not only produced a renewal of the pain, but has excited the most distressing nausea and sickness. The results of my own observations, and those of the most accurate observers in this country, coincide very nearly with those which are described as having taken place in the practice of Dr. Joseph Clarke. " In addition to the usual routine of practice," he observes, in his letter to Dr. Armstrong, " numerous trials were made of the rectified oil of turpentine, in doses of from six to eight drachms, sometimes in plain water, sometimes combined with an equal quantity of castor oil. The first few doses were generally agreeable to the patient, and seemed to alleviate pain. By a few repetitions it became extremely nauseous, and several patients delared ' they would rather die than repeat the dose.' In more than twenty trials of this kind not a single patient recovered." In favour of the use of digitalis and colchicum in puerperal fever, little evidence that is satisfactory has hitherto been adduced.

Willis, White, and other physicians, employed *emetics*, and more particularly ipecacuan, in the treatment of puerperal fever, before the year 1782, when Doulcet recommended the exclusive use of these remedies at the Hôtel Dieu. Most exaggerated reports of the success of his method of treatment were speedily propagated throughout Europe, and many were disposed to consider the results at the Hôtel Dieu as affording unequivocal proofs of the power of emetics to arrest the progress of the disease when occurring in the most malignant forms. Two hundred women were represented as having been saved to society in the course of one epidemic in Paris, by the administration of ipecacuan at the onset of the attack. It

appears, however, from the statement of Alphonse le Roi, that the recovery of so many individuals was attributed, without any just ground, to the peculiar treatment adopted; for the employment of ipecacuan and Kermes mineral, according to him, was commenced by Doulcet in the lying-in wards of the Hôtel Dieu when the epidemic was ceasing, but these means were wholly inefficacious in the months of November and December, and at the beginning of the following year, when the mortality was greater than in 1780, before the remedy of Doulcet was known. M. Tenon affirms that in 1786 the complicated puerperal fever was curable by no means then discovered. From the intense pain of the abdomen, aggravated by the slightest pressure of the hand or by compression of the abdominal muscles, and from the early occurrence of nausea and vomiting in the worst cases of the disease, emetics obviously appear to be little calculated for the relief of the symptoms, and few enlightened practitioners have employed them in this country for the last forty years. Some have gone so far, indeed, as to declare that they are sufficient to produce inflammation where it does not already exist, and that their employment is not only useless, but dangerous and absurd.

Several distinguished continental physicians, as Hufeland, Osiander, and Desormeaux, have, however, continued to employ emetics in the treatment of puerperal fever, and have supposed that they have derived benefit from their use. M. Tonellé states that M. Desormeaux first made trial of them about the end of 1828, and that great advantage resulted from it. During the greater part of the following year they were again employed, but they succeeded in only a few isolated cases, and most frequently they entirely failed; they never, however, appeared to produce any aggravation of the pain or other symptoms. A new trial was made of them after this, and they were again followed by the most happy results. At the commencement of September, 1829, in the course of a fatal epidemic, and during a cold and moist season, emetics were again had recourse to; and for the two months during which this treatment was pursued, all the sick were not relieved, but a great number were delivered from their sufferings as if by enchantment, and for an instant there seemed to be a renewal of that brilliant success which had followed the adoption of this method by Doulcet and the physicians of the Hôtel Dieu. But at the end of October emetics gradually lost their influence; and towards the middle of November no advantage whatever was derived from them. In some of the successful cases related by M. Tonellé it ought to be observed, that forty leeches, and warm cataplasms, had been applied to the hypogastrium before the emetic was given, and in those where the relief was most decided the ipecacuan either produced a profuse perspiration, or acted freely upon the bowels, causing numerous, copious, and bilious alvine evacuations. It is highly probable, from the histories of the successful cases, that the effects of the treatment were referrible rather to the action of the ipecacuan on the skin and intestines than on the stomach, for the relief experienced did not immediately follow the vomiting. M. Tonellé admits that where effusion or suppuration had taken place, emetics were of no avail; and he also relates a number of cases in which the application of leeches to the hypogastrium, and the employment of other antiphlogistic remedies, were followed by speedy and complete relief where emetics had entirely failed to procure this. In the milder forms of uterine inflammation (and many of the cases related by Tonellé were of this description), it is highly probable that an emetic, which would produce a sudden determination to the skin and a free action of the intestinal canal, would relieve the congested and inflamed state of the uterus, and thus cut short the disease. I have met with no case, however, in which I have considered it safe to administer emetics in any stage of the complaint, and I cannot conceive it possible for a case to occur in which the treatment should chiefly or exclusively be conducted upon the plan of Doulcet.

The application of blisters to the hypogastrium and inside of the thighs and legs, has often been found advantageous where the pain of the hypogastrium has continued severe after the general and local bleeding. The external use of the oleum terebinthinæ has also in some cases unquestionably been followed by considerable relief of the pain; and its effect is more sudden than that of a blister.

Both general and local warm baths have been highly recommended by foreign practitioners. Where the skin was hot, the pain moderate, the strength of the patient not much depressed, the immersion of the whole body in warm water was often followed by a general perspiration and relief of all the symptoms. On the other hand, they state, that when the pains were excessive, when there was great anxiety, a profuse general or partial perspiration, the strength much reduced, the respiration hurried and anxious, and the face red with intense headache, the patient could not support the warm bath, and derived no benefit whatever from it. The hip-bath was found more generally useful, and was employed almost indiscriminately by M. Desormeaux in all the different varieties of the disease I have now

repeatedly tried the warm bath, but without benefit.

Recolin, Dance, and Tonellé, highly recommend the injection of warm water into the vagina and cavity of the uterus, by means of an elastic gum canula. These injections were repeated three or four times in the course of the day, and they not only washed away the putrid matters adhering to the internal surface of the organ, but they appeared to relieve the irritation and inflammation of the organ itself. This practice I have seen followed by good effects, and now generally recommend it. In many cases of puerperal fever severe irritation of the stomach supervenes in the progress of the disease, and this symptom seems occasionally to be aggravated by anodynes and saline effervescing draughts. A drachm of subcarbonate of potash should be added to ʒv. of aquæ menth. virid., and an ounce of this mixture given every two or three hours. The effect of this medicine in allaying the irritability of the stomach has been very remarkable indeed in some cases related to me, but I have often tried it without deriving any advantage from it. Should diarrhœa take place spontaneously, or result from the use of the mercury, it must be moderated by opium. The starch and laudanum clyster is by far the best mode of administering the anodyne.

During the first stage of uterine inflammation, cinchona, camphor, and stimulants, are wholly inapplicable; but when the acute symptoms have been subdued, and the patient is left in a state of great exhaustion, quinine, ammonia, wine, and other stimulants, sometimes produce the happiest effects in rousing the powers of the system. I cannot too strongly urge the necessity of continuing to employ these remedies, and whatever else is judged useful, whilst the slightest hope of recovery can be entertained.

The importance of the prophylactic treatment must be obvious from all that has now been stated. A puerperal woman ought to be as careful of exposing herself to cold and fatigue for a week after delivery, and committing any imprudence in diet, as an individual who is recovering from an attack of continued fever, or inflammation of some important organ. The administration of acrid cathartics should always be avoided for some days subsequent to delivery. After-pains, if severe, should be relieved by anodynes; and the lochial discharge, when scanty, promoted by warm fomentations and poultices over the hypogastrium, and other suitable means. The greatest care should always be taken during the labour, if an operation is required, to avoid inflicting any injury on the uterus.

TABULAR VIEW (No. 2) OF 62 ADDITIONAL CASES OF INFLAMMATION OF THE UTERUS AND ITS APPENDAGES,

Observed by me from January 1831 to the end of April 1835.

[Continued from p. 795.]

No.	Name, Residence, and Delivery.	Date of Attack and Symptoms.	Treatment.	Result and Morbid Appearances.
135	Case; St. Marylebone Infirmary. April 16, 1832.	Second day.—Rigors; acute pain in the region of the uterus; quick pulse and other characteristics; immediate relief followed the bleeding.	V.S. ʒxiv. (blood not buffed), leeches, calomel, opium, poultices.	Recovered.
136	Mrs. Gray; æt. 30; British Lying-in Hospital. Natural labour. April 18, 1832.	Slight rigor; tenderness on pressure in the region of the uterus; tongue white; thirst; bowels open. Twenty-first day: pain gone; pulse rapid; milk secreted. Twenty-seventh day: has continued entirely free from pain; great debility; pulse 120; delirious; tympanites.	Leeches xij., calomel, and opium.	Died.
137	Case with Mr. Prout; Titchfield Street. Natural labour. April 17, 1832.	Second day.—Rigors; pain in the back and left side of the uterus; intense headache; retching; diarrhœa; a tedious recovery after several weeks.	Opium and cathartics.	Recovered.
138	Three cases; British Lying-in Hospital. Between May 12 and 28, 1832.	They all had the characteristic symptoms of peritonitis within three days after delivery; rigors; uterine pain; quick pulse.—In the early part of June a fatal case occurred in the St. James's Infirmary, another in the St. Marylebone Infirmary, and a third in the British Lying-in Hospital.	Copious bleedings, calomel, opium, and cathartics, the only remedies.	Recovered.
139	Mrs. Foster; æt. 30; British Lying-in Hospital. June 25, 1832.	Second day.—Pain in the region of the uterus; no rigor; lochia not suppressed; uterus large and hard; pulse 110; tongue white and dry; pain relieved by the leeches, but returned and extended; nausea; vomiting; swelling of abdomen; delirium.	Leeches xviij. twice, calomel, opium, saline effervescing draughts.	Died.

No.	Case	Symptoms	Treatment	Result
140	A lady in New Bond Street. Natural labour. July 12, 1832.	Seen in consultation.—The day after slight pain in the region of the uterus; rigors; quick pulse. Sixteenth day: pain in the left groin, and swelling of the left leg and thigh. Eighteenth day: dyspnœa; cough; rapid feeble pulse. Twenty-first day: stupor; face flushed; pupils dilated: pulse 120; tongue covered with aphthæ; left shoulder painful, and a large red patch over it; diarrhœa.	Digitalis, diuretics.	Died.
141	Case; Kilburn. Natural labour. July 1832.	Third day.—Rigor; slight pain in the left side of the uterus; rapid pulse; furred tongue; great cerebral excitement. July 23d: pulse 120, not feeble; milk and lochia both continue; face flushed; slight delirium; diarrhœa; no sickness or vomiting.	Leeches xxij., starch and laudanum clysters, head shaved, cold lotions, blister to the hypogastrium.	Recovered.
142	Case in a public institution. Distorted pelvis, forceps, and perforation. September 1832.	Did not see the patient for several days after delivery; then vomiting; slight uterine tenderness and great debility; rapid pulse; died on the sixth day.	No treatment adopted at the onset of the disease.	Died. The mucous and muscular coat of the orifice, cervix, and lower part of body of uterus, softened and of a dark colour, broken down, and disorganised; the orifice lacerated in two parts.
143	Case; Leicester Square. Natural labour. June 24, 1832.	Third day.—Slight tenderness along the brim of the pelvis, on the left side; great depression of spirits; pulse little affected. July 1st: pain in the calf of the left leg, followed by swelling, and tenderness along the course of the iliac and femoral vessels of the same side.		
144	Case at Paddington. After natural labour. September 24, 1832.	Third day.—Acute pain on each side of the uterus, with rapid and feeble pulse; loaded tongue; dusky countenance; lochia not suppressed. Twenty-eighth day: pain relieved by bleeding, but the pulse became more rapid, and she gradually sank; tympanites before death.	V.S. twice, calomel, opium, and saline medicines.	Died. Both ovaria greatly enlarged, softened, and their structure completely disorganised; the fallopian tubes red and inflamed; peritoneal sac healthy; ℥v. of red serum effused.
145	Case; British Lying-in Hospital. November 3, 1842.	Did not see the onset of the disease.—Sickness and acute pain in the region of the uterus; rapid feeble pulse; vomiting; soon sank.	V.S. not employed. Leeches, calomel, and opium.	Died. Uterus large, soft, and thickened; uterine appendages on both sides of a dark livid colour; ovaria pulpy; coats of the upper part of the uterus in a soft shreddy state, torn by the slightest touch; a portion of the uterus behind retained the healthy structure.

No.	Case	Symptoms	Treatment	Appearances
146	Case; St. James's Infirmary, Retained placenta. November 6, 1832.	Eighth day.—Pulse rapid and feeble; dyspnœa; slight pain in the left side of the chest; no pain in the uterine region; sank soon, with diarrhœa and urgent dyspnœa; died 15th of November.	Leeches to the hypogastrium, a large blister to the chest, &c.	Died. No effusion into the peritoneal sac; uterus had contracted and sunk down into the pelvis; near the right round ligament there was an adhesion between the uterus and bladder; an abscess here under the peritoneum of the uterus; ovaria enlarged, red, and soft; at the neck of the uterus the veins full of pus, and the cellular membrane around inflamed; extensive pneumonia on the left side.
147	Mary Gane; near St. Thomas's Hospital. Natural labour. October 21, 1832.	Third day.—Pain and stiffness about the hypogastrium and inguinal regions, extending down the thighs, with pyrexia and headache; rigors; pulse frequent; offensive lochia. Thirtieth day: severe rigors; pain in the symphysis pubis and right groin; thigh swollen, and femoral vein painful; the left limb became affected; diarrhœa; gangrene over the sacrum, and over the right ankle.	V.S. at the commencement, leeches and cupping-glasses, fomentations, calomel, and Dover's powder.	Died. Symphysis pubis separated to the distance of an inch and a half, and its cartilages gone; pus had escaped from it into the pelvis; right femoral vein plugged up with fibrine, and the saphena major filled with pus; vena cava inflamed to a great extent; peritoneum of uterus inflamed.
148	Case; Paddington. Twins; retained placenta; flooding. October 1833.	Six weeks after delivery.—Complained of dyspnœa and pain in the right side of the chest; no rigor. Four days before death, extreme prostration of strength; irregular hectic fever; fœtid expectoration; lungs previously healthy.		Died. Pleuritis and hepatization of the lung on both sides; uterus greatly reduced in size; the ovaria and tubes healthy; left spermatic vein healthy, but the spermatic vein to its right, from the uterus to its termination in the vena cava, was greatly enlarged, and the coats thickened, and the cavity filled with a layer of lymph and clot of blood of a vermilion tint.

149	Case seen with Mr. Gosna; St. Martin's Parochial Infirmary. After natural labour. November 1833.	Cough; dyspnœa and pain in the chest a week or ten days after delivery; and also tenderness in the region of the uterus; the symptoms of pulmonary disease gradually became worse, and she died five or six weeks after her confinement.	Blisters to the chest, and other remedies to relieve the disease of the lungs.	Died. Extensive inflammation and hepatization of the lungs on both sides; the uterus within the pelvis and reduced to the usual size a month after delivery; the left fallopian tube adhering to the uterus low down behind; the veins of the cervix and body of the uterus filled with pus on the left side; all the branches of the internal iliac and common iliac inflamed, and lower part of vena cava; pus in pulmonary veins.
150	Case seen with Dr. Fergus; St. George's Parochial Infirmary. After tedious labour. July 2, 1834.	Did not see the patient during life; was informed that she had no pain in the region of the uterus; no rigor nor quickness of pulse; but that there was great debility, low muttering delirium; that the skin had a peculiar dark hue; and that the lochia were offensive.		Died. Brain perfectly healthy; red serum effused into the sacs of the pleura; one of the lobes of the lungs hepatized; veins of the fundus uteri on the left side filled with pus; veins of the cervix in the same condition; many absorbents on this side full of pus.
151	Case; St. James's Infirmary. After twins, and hæmorrhage. July 23, 1834.	Fifth day.—Intense headache; countenance pallid; slight convulsive twitches of the head and extremities; pulse 140, small; acute pain of uterus for a short time. July 29th: sinking; tremors; mucous rale; abdomen swollen; hypogastrium painful.	V.S. copious, and leeching, stimulants, and cordials.	Died. Peritoneum of posterior part of uterus, broad ligaments, and peritoneum of intestines and liver, coated with lymph; lb.iij. of sero-purulent fluid effused; ovaria large and soft, and tubes filled with pus; absorbents on left side of uterus full of pus.
152	Case of an idiot; St. George's Infirmary. July 24, 1834.	Dr. Fergus stated that the symptoms were: rapid feeble pulse; vomiting and diarrhœa: no uterine pain; purulent discharge from the vagina; the perinæum and also os uteri torn during the labour; death took place about a week after delivery. Present at the inspection of the body.	Anodynes, wine, and other stimulants,	Died. Examined the body with Dr. Fergus—slight peritonitis; veins of the cervix and fundus uteri gorged with pus; inflammation of veins appeared to have commenced near the part where os uteri was lacerated.

No.	Case	Symptoms	Treatment	Result
153	Case; St. Marylebone Infirmary. January 16, 1834.	Tenth day.—Great tenderness confined to the region of the [?]terus; pulse feeble; lochia scanty and very offensive.	Leeches, calomel, antimony, opium, cathartica.	Recovered.
154	Case of twins; British Lying-in Hospital. November 21, 1834.	Fever f[?]m the time of delivery. Fifteen days after: conjunctiva of right eye became red and swollen, and the eye-ball enlarged. Twenty-first day: eye destroyed; left eye similarly affected; excruciating pain in the left elbow and shoulder-joint; tongue brown; no delirium; [?]se 150; no tenderness in the region of the uterus; slight fulness along the brim of the pelvis, left side; cough, with dyspnœa, [?]sion; [?].		Died. The v[?]lle d[?]t spermatic vein inflamed, and filled with pus; pus [?]d copiously from the orifice of the veins in the lining [?]ne of the [?]us, [?]ld ([?]d; when cut open, this part of the uterus was like a sponge [?]d in pus.
155	A young man; 71, Clarendon Street, Portland Town. N[?]al labour. December 3, 1834.	Saw this patient first two days l[?]fce [?]h.—Pulse rapid; rigors; cold extremities; left lower extremities swollen, not discoloured; foot and leg pit on pressure; [?]ins around the knee swollen; great [?]n[?]ms in the course of c[?]ral vin; delirium; offensive odhia; [?]neral abdominal tenderness; delirium; diarrhœa; [?]ghs over m.	[?]p, stimulants, wine.	Died.
156	Case with the late Mr. Powell, 66, Grove St[?]ret, Camden Town. December 8, 1834.	The [?]nl symptoms of [?]me inflammation a few days [?]r delivery; in two months, when I [?]st saw the patient, crural phlebitis in the left [?]wer extremity, and the [?]tal symptoms declining. The right inferior [?]mity had previously been scarcely affected.	Leeches, fomentations, calomel, and opium.	Recovered.
157	Case; Saffron Hill. After natural labour. January 1835.	A female attended in labour by a surgeon [?]ho was at the time obliged, twice or thrice a day, to dress the leg of a gentleman [?]icted with phlegmenoid ery[?] [?]las; soon after delivery [?]he [?]man [?]aked.	V.S. 3xx.	Died. Extensive peritonitis, and inflammation of the veins of the uterus.
158	Mrs. ——; Poland Street. January 19, 1835.	In 30 hours after the birth of a putrid child, attacked [?]th the most violent [?]ym[?]m; [?]lle; [?]tupor; [?]ms of [?]mth; [?]vere pain in the [?]wer part of the [?]pe, comparatively [?]ttle on the [?]halen; eyes became enormously swollen and inflamed before death; pulse 120; nervous symptoms severe; great agitation; evidently fatal from the onset; countenance changed, overwhelmed with the disease at first; rapid pulse; hurried breathing.	V.S. 3xij, calomel, opium, leeches, cathartica. Every thing escaped by vomiting.	Died. The child died of erysipelas of the nates and abdomen; violent inflammation of the eyes.

159	A lady in Westminster. Protracted labour. June 17, 1835.	Acute pain, increased by pressure in the hypogastrium; sickness and vomiting; extreme restlessness; breathing hurried; pulse rapid; lochia not suppressed; pulse rapid and feeble; symptoms relieved for a short time by the bleeding and leeches, but they returned; the abdomen became tympanitic; there was incessant vomiting, and she died in 30 hours. Died 18th of January. Dr. Merriman saw this case in consultation.	V.S. ʒxxiv., leeches xxv., calomel gr. x., opium gr. iss., 2da q. q. hora.	Died. Her infant died soon after from erysipelas.
160	Case; British Lying-in Hospital. Twins. April 25, 1835.	Did not see this patient during life, but was informed that the pain in the region of the uterus had never been intense, that the abdomen became swollen and tympanitic, the tongue dry and brown, with great debility towards the termination. No sickness nor delirium before death.	Depletion not employed. Anodynes and saline diaphoretics I believe were the remedies, and afterwards wine and stimulants.	Died. Uterus and intestines coated with lymph; left appendages destroyed by inflammation; the placenta had adhered to this side of the uterus; veins of this contained a thin purulent fluid; pus between the muscular fibres of the part, not contained in veins, was a thick yellow lymph; a small quantity of pus in the vein of the cervix.
161	Case; Bruton Street. A young unmarried woman. May 9, 1835.	A young woman who had for some time been chlorotic, and had menstruated sparingly. Suffered for some time from pain in the back and left hip, and fever. Two days ago a swelling took place in the upper part of the foot, then in the calf of the leg and thighs. The whole left inferior extremity smooth, swollen, hot, colourless, looking like alabaster. Superficial veins of the limb distended with blood. The femoral vein in the upper part of the thigh hard and painful along its whole course. Vomiting, and symptoms of low typhoid fever, took place, and she died on the 21st May. Exposed to cold.	Leeches repeatedly, calomel, opium, &c.	Died. Vena cava, left common and internal iliac veins, and femoral, thickened, lined with false membrane, and plugged up with coagula and blood; the internal iliac was most severely inflamed, and its branches contained lymph and pus; the disease of the femoral vein originated in the vein of the cervix uteri.
162	Case; British Lying-in Hospital. Natural labour. May 11, 1835.	A woman died on the eleventh day after delivery. On the second day after delivery, slight uterine tenderness, which yielded readily to leeching. Diarrhœa took place, with fever, and the conjunctive of both eyes became red and swollen. I saw this patient only once or twice, but was not present when the body was examined.	Leeches, fomentations, calomel, opium, saline medicines.	Died. Examination made by Dr. H. Davies and Mr. Moss; no peritonitis; pus in considerable quantity in the veins of the fundus uteri, near the superficial angles; the veins gorged where the placenta had adhered.

| 163 | A lady at Kennington. Natural labour. April 30, 1835. | Third day.—Unusual tenderness of the uterus, rapid pulse, and shivering. The symptoms were relieved, and she seemed to be recovering for some days. May 11th: rapid feeble pulse, 120; tongue foul; sickness; severe nervous symptoms; no tenderness in the region of the uterus; drowsy stupor; profuse perspirations; occasional rigors. May 12th: conjunctive of both eyes red and swollen; vision nearly lost. 13th: symptoms aggravated. 14th: tongue dry and brown; teeth covered with sordes; right eye and eyelids greatly swollen; pulse very feeble. Died on the 12th day after delivery. Nervous tremors. I thought suppuration was going on about the uterus. | V.S. ℨxij., leeches, calomel, Dover's powder. Wine and stimulants in the latter stage. | Died. Examined the body with Dr. John Webster, May 17, 1838; the muscular coat of the uterus of a dull yellow colour; the fingers penetrate its substance like a rotten apple; no pus in the veins or absorbents the greater portion of the uterus affected in this way; whole inner surface of uterus coated with a yellow lucid layer. |

OBSERVATIONS ON

SOME OF THE

MORE IMPORTANT DISEASES OF CHILDHOOD.

By CHARLES WEST, M.D.

Member of the Royal College of Physicians; Physician to the Royal Infirmary for Children; and Physician-Accoucheur to the Finsbury Dispensary.

[Continued from p. 742.]

III.—On some forms of Paralysis incidental to Infancy and Childhood.

IN his work on the " Nature and Treatment of the Distortions to which the Spine and the Bones of the Chest are subject," Mr. Shaw devotes a chapter to an " Enquiry into the causes of the partial paralysis and wasting of one of the limbs during infancy, which frequently produce distortion of the spine." He describes some cases in which there was simple atrophy of one limb, unattended with much defect either in the power of motion or of sensation; though a measure of impairment in the motive power came on almost imperceptibly as the wasting of the limb grew by degrees more and more obvious. In other cases to which he alludes, the affection comes on suddenly, almost instantaneously; and the loss of voluntary power over the affected muscles is immediate. Mr. Shaw regards cases of the former kind as being induced by a deranged state of the bowels; "the affection of the brain being, as it were, intermediate between the disturbance of the bowels and the paralytic muscles." Those of the latter kind he conceives to depend on a sudden change in the brain or spinal cord, or in the nerves which supply the affected parts; though they, too, will often be found to be more remotely connected with disordered digestion. These cases occur especially about the period of weaning, and are commonly ascribed to the irritation of teething; sometimes they come on at a late period of childhood, and are consequent on some severe attack of illness, especially of fever, or of the exanthemata. He enters, however, into comparatively few details on the subject, his object being rather to excite general attention to it.

To the best of my knowledge, Dr. Underwood was the first writer on the diseases of children who noticed this affection; but he does not attempt to discriminate between those cases in which palsy is the result of organic disease of the brain, and those which depend on less grave causes. He was aware, however, that serious disease of the brain was not invariably present, and mentions that such curable cases usually recover very rapidly under the employment of brisk purgatives.

Feiler,* relates, under the title of "Aridura Crurum," a case of atrophy of one lower extremity in a girl between twelve and thirteen years of age. The patient was greatly benefited by friction and various stimulant applications to the wasted limb, and to the loins; but the observation is related as an isolated instance of an affection to which nothing analogous had since come under his notice.

In Dr. Marshall Hall's work, " On the Diseases and Derangement of the Nervous System," are some brief remarks on paralysis from dentition,† together with the particulars of a very interesting case of the disease. His observations, however, are rather suggestive, and he enters into no details on the subject.

Dr. Henry Kennedy,‡ has written a valuble paper on the subject of Infantile Paralysis. He seems to be most familiar with the affection as it occurs in the infant at the breast; in whom the upper extremity is in his opinion most frequently attacked. He notices the suddenness of the seizure, and its occurrence during apparently perfect health. He further remarks, that the lower extremity is sometimes affected in a similar manner; that sometimes instead of being paralysed he has seen it contracted and drawn up close to the body; and that in some instances not only is the power of motion gone, but the sensibility of the affected limb is greatly increased, the child crying on the slightest touch. Derangement of the bowels, and the irritation of teething, are the two causes to which he thinks the disorder may usually be referred; but he has also seen it occur after remittent fever. Lancing the gums, purging, and alterative remedies, are the chief means which he recommends for the cure of this affection.

The greater part of the essay, however, is occupied, not with details concerning the disorder itself, but with remarks on other affections with which it may be confounded. These are, either disease of a joint; injury to a limb, as, for instance, fracture; injury to a nerve, as when the arm is allowed to hang over the back of a chair; paralysis dependent on disease of the brain or spinal cord, and lastly, arthritis with suppuration.

A brief notice of paralysis in teething children is contained in a recent number of the American Journal of the Medical Sciences, by Mr. G. Colmer. The writer, whose communication does not exceed a few lines, mentions having seen a child so affected in a village through which he passed, and states that the inhabitants informed him that several infants in the neighbourhood had suffered in a similar manner.

Dr. M'Cormack, of Belfast, has published in the Lancet for May 27, 1843, some remarks on Infantile Paraplegia. He relates two cases of the disease affecting both lower extremities in children; but the history of each is very deficient in detail. He inclines to the opinion that this impaired power over the lower extremities arises from concussion of the spinal cord, or from injury to the sciatic nerve, and does not appear to have met with any case in which either upper extremity suffered a similar loss of motor power.

It will be my aim in this paper to supply in some slight degree the absence of detail with reference to this, and other similar paralytic affections, by relating the particulars of some of the cases which have come under my own notice.

In doing this it is my intention to leave out of consideration those cases in which certain limbs or certain muscles become palsied during the progress of organic diseases of the brain or spinal cord. Palsy from such a cause is less common during childhood than in the adult, though instances of it are by no means unusual. Thus, during the past summer, a girl, aged about three years, was brought to me suffering from hemiplegia, with very marked reflex movements of the palsied limbs, induced by the spinal marrow having become affected in the progress of scrofulous disease of the vertebræ. A boy, too, eight years old,

* Pädiatrik, etc. 8vo. Sulzbach 1814, p. 350.
† Ib. p. 198.
‡ Dublin Medical Press, Sept. 29, 1841.

is at the present moment under my care, in whom all the indications of cerebral tubercle exist, and in whom the motor power of one side of the body is very considerably impaired. In both of these instances, as well as in many others which might be adduced, the paralysis is only a secondary incident, merely a symptom betokening the advances of a grave and incurable malady; and to enter upon their examination would be foreign to the present purpose.

It may perhaps be convenient to arrange these cases in three classes; of which—

The first will include those instances in which the paralysis was congenital.

The second, those in which it accompanied or followed convulsions, or other symptoms of cerebral disorder.

The third, those in which the paralysis occurred without any indication of cerebral disease.

1st. Cases of congenital paralysis.

Rebecca Swan, aged eight years, 19, Regent Street, Poplar, one of ten children, of whom nine are still living. One died at the age of two months, but all the others are said to be strong and healthy. Her father is healthy, but not robust. Her mother is in the last stage of consumption; and this disease is hereditary on her mother's side.

Rebecca was a delicate child from birth, and her relatives assert that from her very earliest infancy she has had imperfect use of her right side.

She is of a spare habit, and rather sickly appearance; but her manner is cheerful, and her intellect does not seem at all defective.

The palsied condition of her right side is very obvious: she limps in her walk, treads always on her toes, with her heel raised very considerably above the ground, and turns her foot inwards at every step she takes.

She can use her right arm, though but imperfectly; the fingers of the right hand are constantly flexed and drawn into the palm; and though by a great effort she can extend them, yet the moment her attention is withdrawn they return to their former flexed position.

Sensation is as perfect in the right limbs as in the left; but their wasted condition and smaller size, as compared with the left extremities, show that nutrition has been but very imperfectly carried on.

The left arm measures, from the acromion to the end of the radius, 14¼ inches; right, 13 inches.

The girth of the left arm at the middle of the humerus, 5¾ inches; right, 5 inches.

From the left trochanter to the heel, 24 inches; right, 22½ inches.

The right leg and thigh measured considerably less in circumference than the left; but I have not preserved an account of their exact dimensions.

A similar case, but one in which the deformity was still more marked, came under my notice some months since at the Finsbury Dispensary. The patient in this instance was a girl aged eighteen years, in whom not only were the left extremities much shorter and smaller than the right, but the left half of the face also was very much smaller than the right. The parent of the girl stated that the inequality in size of the two halves of the body had existed from earliest infancy, and had not succeeded to a fit or any other indication of acute cerebral disease. The left side was weak, and motion imperfect, but sensation seemed to be unimpaired. The patient in this case was rather deficient in intellectual endowments.

2d. Cases in which the paralysis accompanies or follows convulsions or other symptoms of cerebral disorder.

The cases included in this class are of more frequent occurrence, and of greater practical importance, than the former, since they often excite great solicitude; though they for the most part eventually do well. The morbid phenomena are very frequently connected with disturbance in the process of dentition; and it will be seen that, in the former of the two following cases, they occurred during the period of teething. In this instance, however, there were but few indications of disorder of that process; nor did the fluctuations in the child's condition, nor its ultimate recovery, appear to be in any way influenced by the eruption of teeth.

Walter Scott Taylor, aged fourteen months, living at 39, Great Hunter Street, Old Kent Road, was the delicate child of parents who had lost two children in what they called a decline. In the first week of January 1840 he had a mild attack of measles, from which he recovered without any unfavourable symptom; but his parents placed him under medical care on

January 28th, on account of rickety swellings of his joints, which however were very slight.

On January 30, at 4 P.M. he was suddenly seized with convulsive movements of the left arm; his mouth was stated to have been drawn to the left side, and his left eyelid drooped. This condition lasted for about an hour, and when it went off he seemed as well as before, and slept moderately in the night. At 8 A.M. however, on the 31st, a fit came on similar to that of the preceding night, and lasted for nearly an hour. It returned at 11 A.M. and was then accompanied with rotatory motion of the head. Before the fit came on he cried much, as if in pain, and afterwards frequently threw back his head. In the course of the day it was observed that he did not use his left arm; and on the following morning, after having passed a good night, the arm hung powerless by his side, and the hand was useless. As day advanced, he gradually regained the use of his arm; and in the afternoon, when I visited him for the first time, he could move his fingers, though the hand was weak, and he employed the right arm in preference to the left. No remains then existed of the paralysis of the face or eyelid; both pupils acted equally under the stimulus of light. The child seemed quite cheerful; the bowels acted regularly, and the tongue was clean.

I ordered no medicine for the child; but visited him again on the 7th, when I found him in much the same state as before. He could move the left arm, but not the hand; and his mother thought that he limped somewhat with the left leg, dragging it behind the other. His head was rather hot; but he seemed quite cheerful, rested well at night, and all his functions were performed naturally.

I ordered small doses of mercury and chalk every evening.

On Feb. 17, there was no increase of power in the hand; he still dragged the left leg in walking; did not close the left eye so completely as the right. He was still cheerful, but the tongue was white, and his bowels were constipated.

On the 22d, at 4 P.M. his mother noticed that he could not use his left leg. He continued unwell and fretful until he was freely purged by castor-oil, after which he recovered his usual health. I saw him on the 25th, when he had acquired more power over the left hand, but the left leg was quite powerless, and he dragged it behind him as though it did not belong to him. He was still quite lively and cheerful; his tongue was moist and clean, but his gums were slightly swollen. I lanced the gums, continued the use of the Hydr. c. Cretâ, and ordered a liniment to the leg.

On the 28th the state of the leg was much the same, but the child had acquired more power over the hand. The Hydr. c. Cretâ was now discontinued, and a liniment was ordered for the leg.

March 3d.—Has recovered some use of the left leg, but it still does not serve him in walking. His bowels are disposed to be costive, unless castor-oil is given daily.

From this time he continued to improve, under the use of purgatives and stimulant liniments to the leg. His recovery, however, was very gradual, and could not be considered complete until the end of April.

William Cheshire, aged 3½ years: was never a strong boy, being always what his mother calls nervous, though he had not suffered from any particular illness until Dec. 30, 1840, when he had a fit, which lasted for five minutes; during it he struggled much, and his mouth was drawn to the left side.

On Dec. 31, some one opening his bed-room door suddenly, another fit came on, which lasted for ten minutes; during the fit he struggled, squinted, and his mouth was drawn to the left side; and the squint and distortion of the face continued for some time after the fit was over.

He was brought to me on Jan. 1, 1841. He was a fair, delicate boy, with blue eyes and a strumous aspect; his manner was quite natural, and there was no heat of head. His mouth was drawn slightly to the left side; he could not close his right eye; and in frowning or crying the muscles of the left side of his face only were brought into action, the right side remaining quite motionless. Sensation was perfect on both sides of the face. His bowels were open; tongue moist, but coated with brown fur; pulse 105, with power.

I ordered him two grains of calomel every night, and a senna draught every morning.

On the 5th he had no return of the fits, but the paralysis of the face continued, and the child complained of pain behind the right ear.

Four leeches were applied behind the right ear, and gave immediate relief to the pain; the same medicines as had before been given to him were persevered in, and the child regained the use of the right side of his face so rapidly, that by the 9th of January the signs of paralysis had almost entirely disappeared. The purgative treatment was continued for a few days longer, and a stimulant embrocation was ordered for the face, and by the end of the month the child was discharged cured.

3d. Cases in which the paralysis occurred without any indication of cerebral disease.

These cases are of the most frequent occurrence; they often run a very chronic course, and sometimes appear to be incurable, though for the most part gradual recovery takes place.

In some instances, children, apparently in perfect health, are suddenly attacked by this form of paralysis, but more frequently it follows an attack of measles or scarlatina, or comes on in strumous and debilitated children, in whom it is usually associated with obstinate constipation of the bowels. Of the sudden supervention of paralysis in a perfectly healthy child the following may serve as an instance.

Isabella Smith, aged 2 years and 9 months: was always a healthy child, and had had none of the diseases of infancy, with the exception of hooping-cough.

In the middle of June, 1841, she went to bed in perfect health, but when she arose in the morning she was quite unable to move her right leg, or to stand.

Her mother took her to a surgeon, who ordered something to rub the leg, and the child had since so far recovered as to be able, when brought to me in February 1842, to stand, and to walk, though with difficulty. In walking she turned the right foot quite out at right angles with the body, and did not raise the foot above the ground.

The right leg was half an inch smaller in girth round the calf than the left, and it felt considerably colder to the touch. The child was fat, looked healthy, her bowels were open, and all her functions were performed naturally.

I never saw this patient again.

Henry Barrett, aged 16 months, 4, Cottage Place, Granby Street, Lambeth: the healthy child of healthy parents: went to bed quite well on the evening of July 20, 1841. In the course of the night he became restless and very feverish, and in the morning his mother found that he had completely lost all power over his right leg. In other respects he continued well, except that his bowels were constipated.

He was brought to me on July 23, 1841. I found him to be a well-grown, fair child, pale, and of a weakly appearance, but presenting no marks of scrofula, nor of any serious derangement in his system.

He moved his limbs perfectly, with the exception of the right leg. On that limb being pinched, he cried, and moved his toes slightly, but was quite unable to draw back his foot or leg, or to move the thigh. I ordered him a small dose of jalap immediately, and directed it to be repeated every other morning.

July 27th.—Child's bowels were still confined, not having acted more than two or three times since last note. His health was still good, and he had gained a little more power over the limb: he could not move the leg at all, but moved the thigh slightly.

Aug. 6th.—The child had taken the powders daily since July 27th. His bowels were now regularly open, his health good, and he had acquired more power over the palsied limb. He could stand, but was unable to put the foot flat to the ground; he could move the leg a little, but did so chiefly by means of the muscles of the thigh.

He was still improving, when he was attacked by pneumonia, of which he died at the beginning of September. I could not obtain permission to examine the body.

Alfred Appleby, aged 7½ years, living at 2, Clifford Street, Walworth, the child of healthy parents, had had good health since he was four years old; before which time he had frequent attacks of croup.

He seemed in his usual health, when, on February 6, 1841, his mother noticed that he used his left limbs much less than his right.

He was brought to me on Feb. 27: he was a pale delicate boy, whose pulse was extremely feeble, bowels rather constipated, and tongue slightly furred. In walking he dragged his left leg, and turned the foot inwards; and though he could use the left hand, yet he was unable to grasp any object as firmly, or to hold any thing as tight, as with the right hand. Sometimes, when walking or standing, his left leg gave way under him, and he fell to the ground, though not in a fit, nor with any impairment of his senses.

I ordered him purges of calomel and senna daily, which acted violently, but did not at all improve his condition. I therefore began on the 2d of March to give the vinum ferri, and discontinued the employment of purgatives. Within a week he had acquired considerably more power over the leg, but the condition of the arm was much as before. I now ordered a stimulating liniment for the arm, directed the application of a flannel roller to the limb, and continued the use of the iron. The child now improved considerably; and after persevering in this plan of treatment was discharged on April 20th, in much more robust health than before, and having perfect use of both sides of the body.

Somewhat similar to the preceding is the case of Sarah Macartney, aged 4 years, who was brought to me on July 2, 1841. She had always been a delicate child, and about eighteen months before had had a very serious attack of measles, attended with inflammation of the lungs. She was in her usual health, however, last February, when, after having been for some days very heavy in her head, her mother noticed that she had lost the use of her left leg and arm. After taking medicine, the power over the left leg returned in the course of a few weeks, but she had not regained the complete use of her left arm.

The child's appearance was extremely unhealthy, and she was suffering from strumous ophthalmia. Her pulse was frequent and feeble, her bowels are confined, and the evacuations dark; tongue pale and moist; appetite bad; thirst considerable.

She had perfect use of all her limbs, with the exception of the left arm, which she could move slightly, but could not raise it to her mouth or head, nor grasp any thing with that hand. The fingers of the left hand were flexed, and the thumb was drawn into the palm.

She was unable to extend her fingers by any effort of the will, but could straighten them with the other hand without pain or difficulty. Sensation was perfect in the affected limb.

I ordered a small dose of the iodide of iron, three times a day, with a powder composed of rhubarb and the Hydr. c. Cret. to be taken every night, and a liniment for the arm.

In a fortnight she had acquired more power over the fingers, could grasp a little with the hand, but the state of the arm was unchanged.

She was now sent into the country: at the end of a week her general health was much improved; she could straighten her fingers, and had acquired much more power over the left arm, though she was still unable to raise it to her mouth or head.

On August 13, the same plan having been persevered in, her recovery was almost complete; she was now able to use the left arm freely, and could put the left hand on the top of her head, or bring it to her mouth.

At the end of the month she was discharged quite well.

Permanent palsy of the limb appears to be the result in some cases. This seems to have occurred to William Hinton, aged 3½ years, who, though of a strumous and unhealthy appearance, was reported by his mother to have always had good health. About ten months before he came under my notice it was observed that his left leg and arm seemed weak. As his general health continued good, no remedial measures were employed, although the impairment of power over his left extremities continued. He never completely lost the use of his left leg, but after some weeks began to regain power over it, and when brought to me could use it as well as the other. The left arm, however, grew worse, until it became completely useless, the boy having no power to move it, nor could he bend his wrist, though he could move his fingers.

The deltoid and other muscles of the left arm were so much wasted that its circumference was not much more than half that of the right. The left humerus, too, hung out of the socket, so that a finger could be placed between the head of the bone and the acromion, and a piece of tape extended from the top of the acromion to the tip of the index finger of the hand, measured—

On the left side 12¼ inches.

„ right „ 12 „

Sensation was perfect in the paralysed limb.

Of the subsequent history of the boy I am ignorant, since he was not brought to me again.

The cases now related may serve as specimens of the usual characters of this affection. In the majority of instances it is important rather from the anxiety it occasions the relatives than from any thing really grave in its nature.

It will be perceived, that, though perhaps most frequent in teething children, it is by no means confined to the period of dentition. It often involves both the upper and lower extremity, in which case, as in adults affected with hemiplegia, the lower always recovers much the more rapidly. The paralysis is usually incomplete, some power of moving the fingers or toes remaining, while neither the arm nor leg can be moved. Sensation, as far as one can judge, is unimpaired, and I have not in any instance observed reflex movements. Occasionally sensation is exalted; a circumstance which, when the lower limb is the seat of the affection, and the paralysis is incomplete, may lead to the apprehension of hip-joint disease. In such a case the child bears all its weight on the healthy limb, turns the foot of the affected side inwards when walking, and stands with the toes of that foot resting on the dorsum of the foot of the healthy side. Still it will usually be found that the exaggerated sensibility of the paralysed limb varies greatly at different times, while that extreme increase of suffering produced in cases of hip-joint disease by striking the head of the femur against the acetabulum by a blow upon the heel, and the fixed pain in the knee of the affected side, so characteristic of disease of the hip-joint, are absent; and these points of difference will, I should imagine, usually suffice to distinguish between the two affections.

With reference to another important point—how we may discriminate between paralysis from structural changes in the brain, and those less grave forms of which this paper treats—I would observe, that the paralysis which occurs in cases of tubercle of the brain does not usually supervene suddenly, nor

does it for the most part at *first* involve both the upper and lower extremity, but the upper is generally the first affected. In cases of tubercle of the brain, headache, and other vague indications of cerebral disease, have usually existed for a longer or shorter time, when the power over one limb is observed to be impaired. The patient at first uses that limb less willingly than the opposite one, but still moves it, though in a tremulous manner, nor is it till after some time that any thing approaching to complete paralysis comes on; and when it does it is usually associated with an involuntary tremor or twitching of the limb.

The cases with reference to which most doubt will exist are those in which the paralysis has succeeded to an attack of convulsions. Even here, however, there are circumstances which will often help us to discriminate between the graver and the less formidable malady. In tubercle of the brain it is but very seldom that any thing approaching to complete paralysis follows the first attack of convulsions, but usually, firm contraction of the fingers of one hand, or of some joint of one or other extremity, succeeds to the convulsion, and continues for some hours, or even longer, and it is only gradually, and after the recurrence of several fits, that the paralysis of the limb becomes very obvious. Cerebral tubercle, too, is almost always attended with headache, and a peculiar stupor, which usually precede, and almost invariably follow, any convulsive seizure.

The prognosis may usually be favourable, but the probably tedious convalescence should be borne in mind. The case of Hinton, however, shows the possibility of the paralysis being permanent; and Dr. Abercrombie relates an instance in which paralysis of the right leg, coming on in an infant of 18 months, continued during the subsequent life of the patient, who, when a tall and strong young woman of 20 years, still remained entirely paralytic of her right lower extremity.

It has been seen by the details of the cases how largely purgatives entered into the plan of treatment. That state of habitual constipation, however, which is often met with in weakly children, as in some of the subjects of the foregoing observations, is not best overcome by the employment of drastic purgatives, but rather by the persevering use of gentle aperients. The cases of Appleby and Macartney both illustrate the benefits of a tonic plan: in Appleby's case very free purging had been previously used without the slightest good effect. Stimulant liniments have often appeared to be of great service; but I have had no experience of the effects of electricity, though I had purposed trying it in Hinton's case if he had continued under my care.

ABSCESS IN THE INGUINAL CANAL.

To the Editor of the Medical Gazette.

Sir,

I shall feel obliged by the insertion of the following case in your very useful journal.—I am, sir,

Your obedient servant,
HENRY EWEN,
Member of the Royal College of Surgeons.
Long Sutton, Aug. 17, 1843.

Aug. 11, 1842.—I was requested by a professional neighbour to visit Robert Fendrick, a gardener, æt. 67, who was supposed to be suffering from strangulated hernia, and to require an operation for his relief. He complained that his bowels were constipated, and that his illness commenced five days ago with sickness, but he has not vomited since the day of attack. Four days since he observed a tumor in the situation of an inguinal hernia on the left side: there is now a tumor in that situation: the integuments covering it are red, tender, and like a phlegmon: the induration of the integuments extends as far as the linea alba on the inner side, upwards, not quite half way from the spinous process of the pubes to the umbilicus; outwards and above Poupart's ligament, nearly as far as the anterior and superior spinous process of the ilium. The spermatic cord is swollen to the size of my thumb, tense and tender, and nearly blocking up the external abdominal ring. He is pale and thin, and of lax fibre; tongue white; pulse 72, soft. The symptoms could hardly be considered as those of strangulated hernia, and I stated to my friend that I thought the case merely inflammation of the contents of the inguinal canal. Twelve leeches were

ordered, to be followed by fomentations and poultices: calomel and compound rhubarb pill, with salts and magnesia in peppermint water, were prescribed to unload the bowels.

12th.—He is much relieved; the cord is less tense and tender; the bowels have been well opened. He continues the fomentations and poultices.

20th.—The tumor is moderately easy; bowels open; urine loaded with purulent deposit. He continues the fomentations and poultices, and takes an aperient occasionally. Ordered the following:—

℞. Decoct. Uvæ Ursi, ʒxvss.; Liquoris Potassæ, Tinct. Hyoscyami, aa ʒij. M. sumat cochl. iij. ampl. ter quotidie.

28th.—A considerable quantity of pus has been discharged from an opening near the abdominal external ring: the urine is pale and limpid, and free from deposit.

30th.—The induration of the integuments has increased considerably; tongue clean; bowels open; urine natural; pulse 60.

September 5th.—Convalescent.

From Mr. Lawrence's remarks on the diagnosis of inguinal hernia (page 248, 5th edition), I should infer such cases as the one I have related are not of very common occurrence.

FERRI CITRAS.

To the Editor of the Medical Gazette.

Sir,

Should the accompanying memoranda suit your pages, their insertion will oblige   Your obedient servant,

G. M. MOWBRAY.

36, Paternoster Row,
Aug. 1843.

If we add citric acid in solution to iron filings, and invert the vessel so as to exclude atmospheric air, the solution will be colourless, depositing, at the same time, flakes of proto-citrate of iron. Light does not affect either the solution or the deposited flakes. By adding to 1 iron filings 7 citric acid, and 12 gallons of water, heating to the boiling point, and leaving to digest for 24 hours, a greenish-yellow solution may be obtained, sp. gr. at 55° F. 1025, which reddens litmus. The addition of 12 gallons more water to the sediment (after removing the previous solution) and boiling, leaving to digest for 24 hours, affords also a somewhat lighter coloured greenish yellow solution, which reddens litmus, and has a sp. gr. at 56° F. of 1008·6. A further addition of 12 gallons of water to the sediment, and boiling, affords a solution which *bleaches* litmus paper (owing to absorption of oxygen by the iron), and has a sp. gr. of 1002·5 at 60° F.

If to each or all of the above solutions, when mixed, liq. ammonia be added, a blackish precipitate is thrown down (the magnetic oxide of iron), and if the ammonia be added to such excess as to smell distinctly, and the liquor is evaporated over a water-bath, the solution gradually reddens at the edges, until, at the termination of the process, it assumes a most brilliant garnet hue, giving out, at the same time, a peculiar and somewhat acetous odour.

Collected on plates, this ferro-citrate of ammonia, or ammonio-citrate of iron, resembles an article now sold as the citrate iron (June 1842.) The first, or acid solution, sp. gr. 1025·, gives a product possessing the richest tint: the after solutions require the addition of more acid, in order to increase the solubility of the subsalt in the first instance, and afterwards to take up the peroxide which forms during evaporation.

If a quantity of the nearly insoluble proto-citrate of iron be diffused in water, and exposed to the atmosphere for a considerable length of time, say from eight to twelve months, according to the temperature of the season, the solution gradually darkens; more and more of the once colourless and almost insoluble salt dissolves, until it is entirely taken up, whilst during the same period a corresponding deposit of hydrated peroxide of iron ensues, and finally we obtain a most brilliant, deep ruby tinted solution of a persalt, possessing a peculiar odour and somewhat sweetish taste. If now we pour off this solution, and permit it to remain exposed, the whole of the iron is precipitated in the form of red (somewhat orange red), flocculi of hydrated peroxide of iron: the supernatant fluid, which is colourless, no longer contains citric acid, but retains the sweetish taste and acetous odour, reminding the operator of that peculiar smell which pervades a chamber wherein the ammonio-citrate, or ammonio-tartrate, of iron is being evaporated to dryness; and which, indeed, characterizes these remedies when they have been recently prepared. The addition of a small quantity of ammonia hastens these changes, whilst a large excess of citric acid modifies them, since the change first observed in the latter case is a film of mildew, forming in the solution and floating thereon: this, however, disappears during the progress of the changes narrated above.

The facility with which one atom of citric acid is converted by heat into either one atom of malic acid or three atoms of aconitic acid, the change being as under—

$$C_{12} \quad H_{10} \quad O_{11} = \bar{C}i \qquad \text{1 atom citric acid.}$$
$$H_2 \quad O_1 = aq \qquad \text{1 atom water}$$
$$\text{1 atom malic acid } \overline{C_{12} \quad H_{12} \quad O_{12}} = 3\,\overline{At.} = 3 \text{ atoms aconitic acid.}$$

together with the fact of the similarity of the phenomena before described—in the one case occurring by evaporation in a water bath, and in the other by the action of the atmosphere at ordinary temperatures—suggests this question: Is the salt which has been sold as the citrate of iron, or ammonio-citrate, by whichever term convenience may have designated it, to be ranged among the salts termed citrates? Is not the citric acid of the normal solution, or a portion of it, decomposed? The analysis of such decomposition I must defer until a future occasion. Meanwhile its investigation will amply repay such of your readers as take an interest in tracing the conversion of the carbonic acid of the atmosphere by the living plant, into tartaric, citric, malic, and other acids; being precisely the reverse of such process.

RUPTURE OF THE VAGINA.

To the Editor of the Medical Gazette.

Sir,

I send you a case of rupture of the vagina from sphacelation, terminating fatally. Should you be of opinion that it possesses sufficient interest, you would oblige me by its insertion.

Your obedient servant,
W. H. O. Sankey.

Margate, Aug. 28, 1843.

Mrs. M——, æt. 47, of a very relaxed and debilitated habit of body, exposed continually to malaria, having also undergone during her pregnancy, which is the 18th, much mental anxiety, bodily fatigue, and deprivation of food, was taken in labour on 8th of August, at 10 o'clock. Her previous labours had been severe; she had suffered at various times from hæmorrhage, adherent placenta, and convulsions.

For six weeks she had been unable to rise from her bed on account of the weight of the pregnant womb. The womb was pendulous, the abdominal parietes extremely flaccid and attenuated : when she sat up in bed, which she did constantly, though unable to get off it, the womb was observed to sink deeply into the pelvis : the pains about 11 o'clock came on regularly and tolerably strong. On the first examination I found the waters had broken, and the os uteri of the size of a crown-piece; vagina hot ; the labia œdematous, with slight œdema about the os uteri. I introduced repeatedly pieces of unmelted lard to cool the parts, and placed a broad bandage round the abdomen, and waited patiently. The pains continued till about 12 or 1, strong and good; they then began gradually to flag, and became weaker, till about 5 o'clock : the head of the child was partially protruded through the os uteri. Hoping from the cessation of pains she might obtain some sleep, I left her. About 7 o'clock I was again summoned. She had had no pains since I had left, but was taken sick ; she vomited slightly, and as she attempted to sit up in bed she experienced a burning heat in the lower part of her body, and found she had no power over one of her limbs, and the same time a bloody, grumous discharge escaped to the amount of 7 or 8 ounces, from the vagina.

I found her breathing rapidly and laboriously, with a very anxious expression of countenance; pulse very rapid and weak. I repeated small doses of cold brandy and water, and ordered the preparation of Mist. Vin. Gallici to be got ready; and sent for my friend, Mr. G. Hoffman, of this place.

The head was found in the same position as at 5 o'clock, half protruding through the os uteri.

The possibility of the rupture of the uterus presented itself both to Mr. Hoffman and myself, yet the non-receding of the head, and the absence of all uterine pain at the moment of the seizure, militated against it. We examined carefully for rupture of the os uteri, but could find none : that partial separation of the placenta caused the discharge seemed unlikely, on account of its black grumous nature, and the extreme depression of the patient; and the great anxiety, too, remained by that diagnosis unexplained : the impossibility of uterine pains being re-established plainly indicated the necessity of delivery by artificial means. We called in the aid of a third practitioner, Mr. Price, who concurring in the opinion, and the Mist. Vin. Gall. having been exhibited, and the usual precautions as to the contents of the bladder and rectum, &c. being taken, I proceeded to deliver.

The instruments which were the readiest at hand were a pair of short and straight forceps : the head not being out of the womb, an imperfect hold only was obtained, but the head advanced easily, assisted by some uterine pains. After the head was in the vagina, it, however, receded gradually from the grasp of the instruments. In attempting to re-apply them the head glided before my hand into the womb, and even receded within the os uterus. A delay of 20 minutes occurred before the long forceps were procured : the head was then so moveable, and the womb so flaccid, notwithstanding attempts to fix it externally by pressure, that it was found that turning would be much easier to accomplish : this was accordingly done, and a blackened dead child extracted.

A rather copious discharge of dark blood followed ; the placenta was in the vagina, and easily removed. Endeavouring to pass my hand into the womb to ascertain if it was duly contracted, it passed into what at first appeared to be the uncontracted womb, filled with large coagula, the parietes being so thin as to give my hand the sensation to Mr. Hoffman, who was making gentle pressure externally, as being merely covered with a glove. I felt also a large tumor, which, for a second, appeared like the head of a second child, but passing my hand down I found it to be fixed, and in fact to be the external or peritoneal surface of the contracted womb: my hand was therefore, for a few seconds, in the peritoneal cavity: what appeared at first coagula, were the intestines. On withdrawing the hand I found the os uteri entire, the rupture having taken place on the posterior wall of the vagina.

We placed a greased plug in the vagina, secured with a T bandage, and administered cordials; but the patient sank about 2½ hours afterwards, remaining perfectly sensible to the last.

Examination, 24 hours after death.— Great emaciation; copious frothy discharge from mouth.

Abdominal parietes in the mesial line not more than a quarter of an inch in thickness. Abdominal muscles pale, and extremely emaciated, scarcely to be detected. Peritoneum highly injected*. Uterus contracted and empty: natural, except in its peritoneal coat. Vagina blackened, its walls three quarters of an inch in thickness, ruptured longitudinally to the extent of four or five inches; the whole of posterior wall sphacelated; the bladder blackened and engorged. Rectum sound.

REMARKS.—It is evident that the state of the vagina was produced previous to commencement of the labour, and as the os uteri was sound, I imagine it took place by a kind of intussusception, especially as the rectum did not participate in the sphacelation; as it would have done had it been from pressure of the head or womb. That it did not take place during the labour is evident from the same cause, and from the short duration of the labour, lasting barely seven hours. That the rupture did not take place by the instruments, which are acknowledged to have slipped, is evident to my own mind from the gradual manner in which the head escaped from their grasp; and moreover, the rupture, which was extensive, must have been detected by the other practitioners, as well as myself, who made an examination previous to sending for the long forceps; and the rupture, if made by forceps, would have been most probably in a transverse direction. The morbid state of the vagina rendered it undilatable, crisp, and easily liable to tear, and the passage of the child, which was large, caused the rending of its walls.

* The peritoneum passed over full five inches of the vagina before it was reflected on to the rectum.

The hurried and laborious breathing took place immediately after the first symptom of the rupture: was this occasioned by the shut sac of the peritoneum having burst, and therefore no longer moving as one body upwards against the diaphragm by the action of the abdominal muscles? It is evident that, where an aperture existed in the peritoneum, the contraction and expansion of the abdominal parietes would merely act in a manner to force air in and out of its cavity, and the sac would cease to act as a body on the diaphragm.

MEDICAL GAZETTE.

Friday, September 8, 1843.

"Licet omnibus, licet etiam mihi, dignitatem *Artis Medicæ* tueri; potestas modo veniendi in publicum sit, dicendi periculum non recuso."
CICERO.

VITAL STATISTICS OF SHEFFIELD.

ONE of the most prosperous trades in Sheffield is the silver and plated manufacture. Until the last two years it has not shared the distress experienced by all engaged in making cutlery. The workmen belonging to this branch amount to 400, and form several unions, the restrictive laws of which are effective even in times of bad trade. The earnings of men vary from 18 to 42 shillings, and of women from 8 to 15 shillings a week.

The workmen in this manufacture are sober, intelligent, steady, and are, or were, in tolerable circumstances. This is attributable to various causes. First, the rule of the trades' union, which prohibits the masters from taking apprentices, has reduced the number of workmen, formerly superabundant. Secondly, the expensive materials and tools used in this trade prevent that sudden conversion of men into masters which is so common in so many other occupations. Thirdly, children are rarely employed in this trade much under fourteen years of age. Fourthly, the workmen are not liable to be thrown out of employment by machinery. This occupation is neither particularly detrimental to health, nor conducive to longevity. In the Silversmiths' Benefit Society, the mean age attained by those who die above the age of 40 is 59.12; while among the working classes generally, of Manchester, Leeds, and Liverpool, it is 58.97; so that the advantage in favour of the silversmiths is slight indeed. In rural districts the mean age attained by persons above 40 is 68.76. What a difference!

Next come the *saw manufacturers.*

"The workmen in this branch of trade are, perhaps, in no degree inferior in intelligence, sobriety, and general good conduct, to those in the manufacture of which we have just treated. They have both equally their respective unions, which regulate wages, the introduction of apprentices, and which, in time of sickness, afford a weekly allowance."

In the branch called *par excellence* saw making, there are 208 journeymen, of whom about 20 are not in union; 130 boys—being, indeed, more than the rules of the union allow; and about one woman or girl to every eight men.

Nine-tenths of the men are in sick clubs; nineteen out of twenty can read and write; and their average wages are 28 shillings a week, the extremes being 24 shillings and 45 shillings.

The *saw grinders* are fine healthy men, who generally live in the country, and often add the cultivation of a plot of ground, or even a small farm, to their mechanical occupation. They are peculiarly liable to accidents, and of 42 saw grinders who have died since 1821, 5 were killed by the breaking of stones. Dr. Holland gives a list of 13 accidents, being a part of those which have happened to 78 living members in union. Most of them are very serious, *e. g.* "3. Drawn over the stone; severely hurt; in bed nine months."

"9. Arm severely lacerated; lame three months."

The *edge-tool makers* are well paid, but are a less intelligent class than those previously mentioned. The number of *foremen* and *strikers* is equal in this trade; the former are said to earn, on the average, £1. 14s., and the latter £1. 2s. a week.

The account is furnished by a manufacturer, and, thought no doubt accurate as far as it goes, is defective in an important point. We do not learn from it how many months in the year the men are in work. The prices have been strictly enforced, even during the last three years, but for what portion of that time have the men obtained them?

Three-fourths of the workmen in this branch are in sick clubs; but only one among five adults can read and write. Trades that require strong arms rather than acute heads will be favourable rather to sensuality than intelligence; a blacksmith drinks more than he reasons; and Dr. Holland finds that the forgers of Sheffield have big occiputs, but low, retreating foreheads.

The spring knife makers are badly paid, and badly educated. "A few superior workmen may earn from 30s. to 40s. per week. In the first manufactories of the town the average is from 16s. to 25s. But in many of the inferior manufactories, the workmen are receiving no more than 12s. or 16s."

Moreover, when Dr. Holland was writing, in June 1843, this scale of wages was very greatly reduced.

This branch is not in union; not above half of the adults can read, and not one-fourth moderately well; about two-thirds only of the adults are in sick clubs.

Two circumstances combine to depress wages in this department. The most important is the smallness of the capital required to set up as a cutler. A few pounds are sufficient. The other one is the facility which this branch offers for the employment of children at an early age.

The *file trade*, as regards the circumstances of those employed in it, holds a middle place between the silversmiths and saw-makers, who are above, and the spring knife cutlers, who are below them.

The branch of the file trade called *forgers* consists, like the edge-tool makers, of foremen and strikers; but the profits are more equally divided between the two classes of workmen in the present instance; a foreman averaging £1. 12s. 10d. a week, and a striker £1. 6s. 9d.

As to *file-cutters*, by reference to thirty books of file-cutters, men of *steady* habits, each having the assistance of a boy, the average per week was found to be £1. 18s. 6d. Eighty per cent. of the adults can read, and seventy can write. The proportion among the boys is rather greater; which may either show that education is making way, or that a certain number of adults forget their little scholastic learning.

The *fork-grinders* carry on the most unwholesome trade in the kingdom. Fork grinding is always performed on a dry stone, and the clouds of stony and metallic dust produced in the process clog up the respiratory organs, and cause grinders' asthma, a disease which carries off its victims in a majority of cases before the age of thirty!

The better the state of a given trade in Sheffield, says Dr. Holland, the smaller is the proportion of minors employed in it. Thus in the silver-plated branch, the minors are to the adults as 16 to 100; and among the edge-tool makers, as 12¼ to 100. In the spring-knife branch the percentage is about 25; but among the fork-grinders the minors actually outnumber the adults, as there are 100 boys and only 97 men! Of the ninety-seven, about thirty are

at this moment suffering from grinders' asthma. It is remarkable that in this destructive trade the men are ill paid, but Dr. Holland does not say what their wages are. Nor is their education superior to their condition; for of the 197 men and boys, 109 can only read, and 69 can write.

Can nothing be done for the fork-grinders? The substitution of wet for dry stones, if this is practicable, would save numerous lives, and if the task is too difficult for unaided philanthropy, legislation might lend its assistance. We should not consider the difference of a farthing in the price of a fork a fatal objection. The Sick Clubs and Friendly Societies are very numerous, and their accumulated capital amounts, in Dr. Holland's opinion, to at least £70,000. The most ancient of them, the "Old Union," has been established for more than a century.

The error has sometimes been committed at Sheffield, as elsewhere, of making the terms of a benefit society too advantageous, so that it is ruined in twenty or thirty years by the increase of sickness and deaths among its members.

Dr. Holland has a chapter on "the amount of religious instruction and education in the several townships of the Sheffield Union."

The schools, though numerous, are insufficient. The pupils amount to 22,000; but one half of these attend only the Sunday schools, and thus receive a very trifling amount of instruction. Dr. Holland says of the Sunday schools that the knowledge imparted by them is extremely superficial; and a little further on, "for the little good which they effect we are grateful, and they richly deserve encouragement;" but two pages further on, he asserts that "not one-third of the youth of Sheffield can be regarded as receiving any education at all."

More day schools are evidently wanted, and Sheffield, like the rest of the kingdom, has reason to regret the loss of the late ministerial measure on education. Dr. Holland wishes that fewer churches and more schools had been built in Sheffield, forgetting that churches are schools, and that if the old catechetical discipline were restored, they might be made very effective Sunday schools. However, we do not differ from Dr. Holland when he asks for more schools; the National Society has set on foot a fresh subscription for this purpose, and we would suggest that he might contribute the profits of his book. We will touch but on one point more—the saddest and dreariest in his book—we mean his talk about medical charitable institutions. Four years ago Dr. Holland published a pamphlet, recommending the world not to be so charitable to the sick, on which we commented with some severity.* Time, we are sorry to see, has not mellowed the Doctor's feelings on this point. He still thinks that the Sheffield Hospital was intended for a few choice cases of unutterable distress, and gives a long extract from his former Malthusian essay. He "will not insult the memories of the good" by supposing that they intended the hospital for the working classes in general; and he thinks it "not difficult to define some of the conditions which ought to exclude from a participation in the charity."

Neither single men if employed, nor married men in work with small families, nor married men with several children and high wages, nor operatives with several sons or apprentices working for them, nor servants in place, are proper objects for the Sheffield hospital.

But what is to be done with a poor single man, without friends or money,

* MEDICAL GAZETTE, May 11th & 18th, 1839.

attacked with fever or pneumonia? We know what the founders of hospitals would answer; let us hear the reply of an economist: — " If they are not too ill to be incapacitated from pursuing their vocations, it is a gross imposition to extend to them the charity, and if otherwise, they have always homes. It may perhaps be urged in objection, that they will necessarily incur debts in providing at this time medical assistance. This, so far from being an objection, is an exceedingly powerful argument for throwing them on their own resources. They will thus be taught practically the injurious effects of misconduct: the struggle to overcome the subsequent difficulties is indeed [more] calculated to awaken reflection, and suggest rules for future guidance, than any discourse, however beautiful and just its views."

But what if the needy fork-grinder is not "taught practically," but only dies? Slips through your fingers for want of charitable aid, while you are intent on giving him a splendid Malthusian lesson?

COLLEGE OF SURGEONS — NEW CHARTER.

WE made an important mistake in our notice of this last week. It appears that there is to be no exclusion of those who practise pharmacy or midwifery from the body of Fellows, the admission to which is not to be according to standing, but by examination. Those who practise pharmacy or midwifery, however, are excluded from the council.

ASSOCIATION OF MEDICAL OFFICERS OF HOSPITALS FOR THE INSANE.

AT the Second Annual Meeting of this Society, held in Lancaster, June 1, 1842, and subsequent days—

It was resolved—" That the Governors of all Public Lunatic Asylums in the United Kingdom be solicited to further the objects of this Association, and that the Honorary

Secretary be deputed to explain by letter to such parties its nature and views."

This having been done to the Governors or Visitors of those Asylums *only* which the Associated wished *immediately* to visit—at the Third Annual Meeting of the Society, held in London, June 1, 1843, and subsequent days—

It was resolved—" That it is the wish of the Association that the Governors, Visitors, and Officers, of each Hospital for the Insane, be forthwith made acquainted, by Circular, with the existence of the Association, and with the objects it seeks to accomplish."

Gloucester, Aug. 25, 1843.

Sir,—In obedience to the above Resolutions I beg to inform you that " The Association of Medical Officers of Hospitals for the Insane" was formed in the summer of 1841, by medical gentlemen, officers of public lunatic asylums—that it was then proposed to consist of all the medical officers of such institutions in Great Britain as *ordinary* members—and of such medical gentlemen having the private care of the insane—of such persons not medical, known to take an interest in those afflicted with insanity—and of such distinguished foreigners, as the Society shall at any time think proper to elect, as *honorary* members.

The intentions and objects with which the Association set out, were—

1. " To improve the management of lunatic asylums."

2. " To improve the management of the insane."

3. " To acquire a more extensive and a more correct knowledge of insanity."

To effect these objects the members of the Association meet, annually, at some town or place in which there is a public lunatic asylum. They solicit the permission of the Governors or Visitors to visit the asylum, and to *inspect* it thoroughly, and afterwards to assemble in the committee-room of the asylum to speak freely, openly, and in good faith, upon the merits or defects they may have observed in the management of the asylum or in the treatment of the patients. On the same occasions such members as think proper read essays or papers on subjects connected with insanity ; and all communicate and compare their respective experience. At these meetings the governors or visitors are respectfully requested to attend.

The more effectually to compare their respective experience, the Association has adopted a register for the use of its members, whereby the leading features in the history and character of every case, placed under the care of each member, may be *uniformly* recorded. By this a great mass of similar facts will be simultaneously collected in all parts of the kingdom, and at the same time so arranged as to shew a record of insanity,

not as presented to one lunatic asylum, but as occurring throughout the kingdom. To this the Association begs respectfully to draw the attention of the governors and visitors of lunatic asylums.

The Association is collecting plans of all the asylums at present erected, and copies of such designs as from time to time may be projected. It collects also the printed reports and other published documents of different asylums.

The Association has already been permitted to prosecute its objects at the Gloucester, Nottingham, Lancaster, Middlesex, and the Surrey County Asylums, and at the Hospital of St Luke's, in London ; and it has been most kindly invited to the Kent, the Wakefield, the Northampton, Belfast, and Glasgow Asylums.

As the objects of the Association are solely directed to a public good—as they are in no degree, however remote, connected with a private end—and as the Society sustains itself by the exertions and resources of the members themselves—it feels assured that it is only necessary to make these facts known to secure the countenance and encouragement of the governors or visitors of the different establishments for the reception of the insane.—I have the honour to be,

Your most obedient servant,

SAMUEL HITCH, M.D.

Hon. Sec.

ACADEMY OF SCIENCES.

The Tartar on the Teeth. By M. MANDL.

A SOFT substance, of a whitish or yellowish colour, is habitually deposited upon the teeth, and sometimes becomes firmly fixed to them. This substance may accumulate in greater quantities, and growing firmer by degrees may form the hard and dry concretion known under the name of tartar. It increases in bulk by the fresh layers deposited on its surface. According to an analysis made by Vauquelin and Laugier, tartar consists of 66 parts of phosphate of lime, 9 of carbonate of lime, 14 of animal matter (of a yellowish white, different from the gelatine of bones,) and 3 parts of oxide of iron and phosphate of magnesia. Other chemists have found the proportions different ; sometimes the phosphate of lime was more abundant, and sometimes the animal matter (or mucus.)

Authors have been much occupied with the manner in which this substance is produced. Is it a secretion, as some have written ? Is it a deposit of the earthy salts contained in the saliva, and precipitated by a chemical agent, as medical books have repeated for ages ? Is it an earthy exhalation from the capillaries of the blood, to which the mucous membrane of diseased gums is prone?

Not one of these hypotheses has been proved; not one has the sanction of direct experience. Moreover, they are all sufficiently refuted by the following investigations into the composition of tartar.

It results from the experiments of M. Mandl that tartar is nothing but a deposit of the skeletons of dead infusoria, agglutinated by dried mucus; nearly as certain earths, according to the researches of M. Ehrenberg, are composed almost entirely of fossil infusoria.

In fact, if we take some of the mucous matter which is accumulated upon and between the teeth, and dilute it with a little distilled water previously warmed, we shall immediately perceive a host of infusoria, which move about with great liveliness. Their size varies from $\frac{1}{100}$ to several hundredths of a millimetre; and their shape is the same as that of the infusoria described by authors under the name of *vibriones*.

The presence of infusoria in mucus was pointed out by Leuwenhoek; but M. Mandl sets forth in all their details, the shape, liveliness, and other qualities of these infusoria.

These animals also exist in great quantity in patients who have been several days on low diet. They also constitute the greatest part of the mucous coating of the tongue in persons whose digestion is disordered. (According to an analysis by M. Denys, the chemical characters of this coating agree with those of tartar.)

After having ascertained the presence of infusoria in the mucus of the mouth, M. Mandl tried to find out whether these animals assist in forming the tartar also. For this purpose, he softened a particle of tartar in a drop of water for twenty or thirty minutes, and after compressing it between the two pieces of glass, he distinctly saw that the tartar was composed of dead vibriones, of different sizes, but generally measuring several hundredths of a millimetre, united by an organic substance (dried mucus,) the quantity of which is variable. The tartar is often almost entirely composed of these vibriones.

Hence it follows that these vibriones are provided with a shell, or inorganic skeleton [*squelette inorganique*], since tartar is found consisting entirely of these vibriones.

This shows, too, why cleanliness, and the use of tonic or alcoholic fluids, prevent the formation of tartar by preventing the production of the infusoria.

To recapitulate, it appears:

1. That there is a great number of vibriones in the mucus which accumulates around and between the teeth.

2. That tartar arises from an accumulation of dead vibriones, and consequently cannot be considered either as a calcareous substance deposited by the saliva, or as a peculiar secretion.

This discovery of the composition of tartar is as new, with reference to Leuwenhoek's observation, as the researches of Ehrenberg touching the composition of diluvial soils were new in reference to the well-known fact of the existence of infusoria in water.—*Gazette Médicale.*

A SIMPLE MEANS TO PREVENT OR STOP NERVOUS COUGHING.

THERE is a curious and rather interesting paper with the above title in a number of the French Gazette for February, and from it we have extracted the following passages. M. Diday, the author, makes a few prefatory remarks on the power which a mere strong effort of the will often gives to resist the impulse of a strong sensation (*besoin*, the French would say), like that of sneezing or coughing; and he goes so far as to assert that "it is always possible to prevent a fit of either by an energetic and sustained effort of the will, *if this be done from the very commencement.*" In old established coughs, as a matter of course, such an attempt is quite inadmissible, at least with any reasonable hopes of success. Whenever, indeed, the cough depends upon the presence of any matter to be expectorated, it is obvious that the effect cannot be checked as long as the cause remains. It is therefore almost exclusively to coughs depending upon nervous irritation that the following remarks are intended to apply.

The attempt also must be made before the annoyance has got, as it were, root in, or hold of, the system. At first, it is especially necessary that the patient acquire the habit of drawing in his breath slowly and not too deeply, and that he should avoid all hurried and irregular inspirations.

That most people have it in their power to arrest, at least to a certain extent, the frequent recurrence of fits of coughing and sneezing, is obvious from the very circumstance that these acts are not unfrequently the effect of mere—we might almost say *wilful*—imitation; as in churches, lecture-rooms, &c.; and we know that, whatever may be acquired by the will, may be as readily checked by it. Dr. Diday tells us that one of the most eminent physicians of La Pitié hospital is in the habit of bawling out, on entering any of the wards, "I will have no coughing during my visit; whoever cannot stop himself, shall be put on low diet;" and true it is that all the patients are wonderfully still as long as his visit lasts. It is an old saying, that very few people know what they can do until they try; and every one can testify from his own experience, that when the attention is suddenly engaged elsewhere, he ceases to feel a desire to some natural act, as to sneeze, to pass urine, &c., although this desire or *besoin* had been urgent just before.

M. Diday gives the following account of his observations.

"The first idea that occurred to me on this subject was suggested by what I observed to take place during sneezing. It is well known to many people that this act may be very often prevented by rubbing the edge of the eyelids or of the lips, or the tip of the nose, with your finger, when the disposition to sneeze is felt. I have repeatedly advised this expedient to my friends and patients, and it has invariably succeeded. In one case in particular, that of a young priest, who had been for some time much annoyed by the almost invariable recurrence of fits of sneezing that were apt to come on during his performance of mass, this simple means afforded a speedy and complete relief. In the performance of certain delicate surgical operations about the face and throat, such as that for hare-lip, fissure of the palate, &c., it is a matter of the greatest consequence that the patient should avoid all movement of the parts in the neighbourhood, and nothing disarranges everything so much as a fit of coughing or sneezing.

Now as the latter of these acts—which, by the by, is nothing else but a cough of the nasal passages, and of the back of the throat—may be so easily and effectually controlled in the manner we have just mentioned, we are naturally led to expect the same in the former; and so I have found it to be the case not only in myself, but in several other persons who have tried the experiment under my direction.

By merely rubbing pretty smartly with the point of a finger the edge of the lips or of the eyelids, or of the tip of the nose, when the first intimation of the 'besoin' to cough is felt, the act may often be entirely prevented. When this feeling returns very frequently, it will be found useful to employ the revulsive friction first on one of the parts, and then on the others in quick succession."

M. Diday says that the object in the rubbing is not to supersede the exercise of an effort of the will, but only to aid and augment its efficacy. He accounts for its effects on the principles of the excito-motory doctrines of Marshall Hall and Müller respecting the nervous system.

The impression made on the extremities of certain branches of the trifacial nerve acts as a sort of derivative, or counter-irri-

tant, to the morbid sensibility of the extremities of the glosso-pharyngeal and pneumogastric nerves. We often observe the effects of this revulsive action in a somewhat analogous case, that of nausea; for we know that the disposition of the stomach to take on an inverted action may often be checked by rinsing the throat with a mouthful of spirits. If the stomach be not too much overloaded, this simple means will not unfrequently prevent vomiting. Here, then, is an instance where, by making a peculiar lively impression on certain sensory nerves, a tendency to muscular contraction—or, to use the language of a modern school, an excito-motory action—in another part, more or less removed from it, is prevented and controlled; and yet every one knows that a different kind of impression, that of titillation, made on the same organs, is one of the surest methods of exciting this very sympathetic action. Much, therefore, evidently depends upon the kind or degree of the irritation produced. While gentle tickling promotes, firm rubbing will often serve to check, a sympathetic movement in a distant part.—*Gazette Médicale*; and *Dublin Journal of Medical Science.*

LUXATION OF THE PATELLA ON ITS AXIS,

By Dr. P. Gazzan, of Pittsburg.

JAMES, aged twenty-one years, son of Judge Porter, of Pittsburg, was thrown while wrestling, and immediately found himself unable to rise.

On seeing him about an hour after the accident, I found the patella of the right leg dislocated on its axis, *i. e.* it was lying on its edge, presenting the posterior face outward, and the anterior face inward, the inner edge resting in the groove between the condyles of the femur.

Flexing the thigh on the pelvis, and straightening the leg, I endeavoured to replace the bone by pressing its edges in opposite directions, but failing (after repeated trials), I requested that the patient should be brought to town (the accident happened three miles out of the city), and additional advice procured.

At about twelve o'clock the patient was brought to his father's house, where I met Dr. Addison. After repeated unsuccessful attempts at reduction it was thought well to lessen the tension of the joint by dividing the ligament of the patella. This I did, by introducing beneath the skin a narrow-bladed knife, and cutting the ligament close to the tubercle of the tibia. Again we attempted the reduction, but failed. The patella could be moved on its edge more freely than before the cutting, but resisted all our efforts to replace it.

Dr. Speer was now joined to the consultation, and, in accordance with his suggestion, the patient was placed erect, a vein opened, and the blood allowed to flow until the approach of syncope, when the efforts at reduction were renewed; but although the patella could be moved on its edge, it could not be lifted out of the groove in which it rested. It was now agreed to let the patient rest for a few hours.

The thigh was now strongly flexed on the pelvis, and the heel elevated. Then the leg was flexed steadily and forcibly on the thigh, and suddenly straightened. At the moment of straightening the leg I pressed very strongly against the lower edge of the patella from without, with the head of a door-key well wrapped, while Dr. Addison pressed with both thumbs against the upper edge of the bone towards the external condyle. On the fourth trial this manœuvre succeeded, the bone springing into its place with a snap. A cushioned splint was placed behind the knee and secured by a bandage; an evaporating lotion was used, and the patient kept at rest. Recovery was uninterrupted, and the young man has now perfect command of the limb.—*American Journ. of Med Sciences.*

OVARIAN DISEASE.

To the Editor of the Medical Gazette.

SIR,

I MAY perhaps not be singular when I confess myself at a loss to understand the motive that has induced your correspondent, Mr. Camplin, to put himself to the trouble of addressing you on the subject of my recent case of ovarian disease. The charge which he appears desirous of preferring against me needs no other refutation than that afforded by the narration of the case; and if Mr. C. had but read with as much care as " interest," he would, I think, scarcely have attempted to play the critic on grounds alike frivolous as untenable.

It is urged that I have adopted similar treatment to that employed by Mr. Walne, and that I have made use of the expression of " apparently having profited so little by the recorded cases of Dr. Clay and Mr. Walne." It is with true regret that I find Mr. Camplin descending to that lowest grade of criticism, which seeks its support in the selection of half sentences quoted without the accompanying context. In the few remarks appended to my case, I referred the chief causes of its successful issue to three heads, under the last of which I alluded solely to the manner of operating: in that paragraph the half sentence so inge-

niously isolated by your correspondent occurs, and has reference to no feature in the case other than that of the operation itself. I would beg to remind him, that the operations practised by Mr. Walne and myself are essentially different. Two methods of operating were many years ago introduced: one in which the abdominal incision was of very considerable length; the other having the opening into the abdomen not more than " an inch and a half or two inches long,"—the former being a severe, the latter probably a more dangerous one. Desirous of combining the advantages of both, I employed an incision sufficiently large to admit of the removal of the emptied cyst, and the application of the necessary ligatures, without the employment of any force, and at same time avoiding the increased pain consequent upon a very extensive wound of the integuments. In the first-named operation the sac is removed entire; in my own case its fluid contents were previously evacuated. It must be sufficiently obvious that I have not adopted the method of operating practised by Dr. Clay and Mr. Walne; and it was only in connection with this subject that I made use of the expression which has induced your correspondent to honour me with his remarks: whilst in the following sentence I have distinctly stated that I had carefully perused Dr. Clay's and Mr. Walne's cases, and had drawn somewhat different deductions from those arrived at by their authors.

But I will even concede to your correspondent that which he has gratuitously assumed, namely, that I denied having profited by the results of Mr. Walne's late case in the treatment of my own, and he is then placed in a more untenable position than before, for Mr. Walne's patient suffered from phlegmasia dolens, and mine did not. Surely Mr. Camplin will not assert that I adopted Mr. Walne's treatment by prescribing for a disease which did not exist. But the evidence is before him; let him compare the medical treatment of both cases, and then, as one of those trifling circumstances worthy of his criticism, he may probably discover that I have carefully abstained from administering a remedy to which much importance is attached, both by Dr. Clay and Mr. Walne,—the ox-gall, which, used by those gentlemen on several occasions, was not once employed by myself.

Your correspondent has not been less unfortunate in selecting the second case of Mr. Walne, as that from which I culled my ideas of treatment. Mr. Walne's first case was already published, and in its subsequent history corresponded much more closely to my own. Could not that fact content Mr. Camplin? He has thought otherwise, and has therefore indulged in the construction of an obscure little paragraph, by which I am informed that I received so large a number of bulletins of the condition of Mr. Walne's patient. I have no right to allude to any attendant circumstances of a case, however trivial and unimportant they may be, if not previously published; I may, however, briefly state that all that Mr. Camplin can mean is, that at about the time of Mr. Walne's operation I happened to be in attendance upon a lady, one of whose medical attendants had frequent opportunities of watching Mr. Walne's patient, and that I thus occasionally heard of the progress of the case.

It has not been without hesitation that I have replied to the letter of Mr. Camplin, and I cannot but feel that something like an apology should be offered to Mr. Walne for the very frequent reference made to his cases. Such apology is due from your correspondent; and in conclusion I would beg him (and the caution seems necessary) not to again misunderstand me. I trust I shall not fall into the equal absurdity of refusing to learn from recorded experience, or accusing others of having done so. I have derived both pleasure and instruction from the perusal of the writings of Mr. Walne, and shall be always glad to profit by the experience of one who so advantageously employs it; and let me add, if Mr. Camplin will kindly inform me where I can meet with any addition he has ever made to medical science, I shall be happy to profit by that also.

Allow me to remain, sir,
Your obedient servant,
FREDERICK BIRD, M.D.
38, Craven Street, Sept. 2, 1843.

MEDICAL ATTENDANTS ON UNIONS AND PARISHES.

To the Editor of the Medical Gazette.

SIR,
As it is of great importance that medical men should be aware of the nature of the qualifications required to enable them to hold situations in Unions, Parishes, &c., under the English Poor Law Act, it would, I feel assured, be conferring a favour on the profession your giving publicity to the following statement:—

By the General Medical Order of the Poor Law Commissioners, of date March 12, 1842, the guardians were instructed that no medical person, not possessing purely English qualifications in medicine and surgery, was legally qualified for holding offices in the Unions, &c. In consequence of remonstrances made against this order to the Secretary of State for the Home Department, by various Scotch and Irish medical bodies, the commissioners were instructed

by him to take a law opinion from Her Majesty's Attorney-General as to the state of the law on the matter. The Attorney General, and Mr. Martin, (another Counsel who was consulted,) have stated it to be their opinion "that as far as surgery is concerned, those persons who have a *surgical* diploma, or degree, from a Royal College or University in Scotland or Ireland are (in point of law) as competent to be appointed and to act as medical officers, under the statute referred to, as the persons who have the diploma of the Royal College of Surgeons in London.

It is important to medical men to be informed, that, in consequence of this opinion, the Poor Law Commissioners have intimated their intention "to admit persons having a surgical diploma or degree from a Royal College or University in Scotland or Ireland, to the same rights under the Poor Law Amendment Act, as members of the Royal College of Surgeons of London, and to make such modifications in their general medical order of the 12th April [March?] 1842, as may be necessary for giving effect to the above recited opinion of the Attorney-General."

If not too long for insertion, it would be highly satisfactory to medical men to find published in full in your widely circulated Journal the letter of the Poor Law Commissioners of date 21 August, 1843, and the opinion of the Attorney General, dated August, 8th, 1843, which was circulated along with it.—I am, sir,

Your obedient servant,
MEDICUS.
Edinburgh, August 2, 1843.

STRICTURE OF THE RECTUM.

To the Editor of the Medical Gazette.

SIR,
A VERY melancholy case occurred at this place about ten days ago. A lady of rank was supposed to have stricture in the rectum. Her surgeon, after several attempts at different times, at length succeeded, as he thought, in passing the bougie through the obstruction, but instead of this he fairly ran the instrument through the gut, and death followed in about 24 hours!!!

The body was opened, and, as some predicted, no stricture (or any trace of disease) was discovered. This sad event has, as you may imagine, led to much discussion among medical men. Some maintain that there is no such thing as *simple stricture* of the rectum—that it is never seen amongst the the poor (only among the rich, who can afford to pay for it), that it is never found on dissection, and that they doubt the accuracy of the statements they find in books, without impugning the veracity of the writers.

On the other hand, a few maintain that they have met with the disease, and cured it too. Now it would be a great satisfaction to know the opinion of your great London surgeons on this point. If there is such a disease, some of them must have met with it in their extensive practice, and it must have been often seen in the dead-rooms of the different hospitals.

The rectum was greatly *patronised* in this city some years ago, and it is still a favourite with one or two surgeons, who doubtless find it a fruitful source of income.

I am, sir,
Your obedient servant,
A SUBSCRIBER.

Bath, Aug. 25, 1843.

[The above is authenticated.]

SYDENHAM'S WORKS.

To the Editor of the Medical Gazette.

SIR,

I BEG to call your attention to an advertisement on the sheet of your excellent journal, by the honorary secretary of the Sydenham Society, of the 25th of August, announcing editions of works shortly to appear, the first of which seems to be in Latin.

" 1st. A complete edition of Sydenham's Works in Latin, by Dr. Greenhill, of Oxford."

With all due deference and respect to the proceedings of the Council of the Sydenham Society, I beg to remind them that, should this edition be published in Latin, as announced, without an English translation, it will not be read or appreciated by far the greater portion of the more practical members of the profession, from want of time and classical knowledge. An English translation would be far preferable to a Latin edition, and would better answer the good intentions of the society. With every desire for its substitution myself, I am, sir,

Your obedient servant,
A MEMBER OF THE SYDENHAM
SOCIETY.

Heywood, Lancashire,
Sept. 2, 1842.

RECEIVED FOR REVIEW.

Some Account of the Epidemic of Scarlatina, which prevailed in Dublin from 1834 to 1842 inclusive; with Observations. By Henry Kennedy, A.B., M.B., T.C.D., L.R.C.S.I., &c.

The Retrospect of Practical Medicine and Surgery: being a half-yearly Journal containing a Retrospective View of every Discovery and practical Improvement in the Medical Sciences. Edited by W. Braithwaite, Surgeon to the Leeds General Eye and Ear Infirmary, &c. Vol. vii. Jan.—June, 1843.

Appendix to the Reports regarding the Royal Infirmary of Edinburgh, 1843.

ROYAL COLLEGE OF SURGEONS.

LIST OF GENTLEMEN ADMITTED MEMBERS.

Monday, August 28, 1843.

E. T. Rendall.—B. Barrett.—F. Wildbore.— T. Orton.—C. R. Morgan.—T. H. Baker.—T. Engall.—C. Cooper.—T. C. Lewis.

A TABLE OF MORTALITY FOR THE METROPOLIS,

Shewing the number of deaths from all causes registered in the week ending Saturday, August 26, 1843.

Small Pox	4
Measles	25
Scarlatina	34
Hooping Cough	15
Croup	8
Thrush	6
Diarrhœa	23
Dysentery	11
Cholera	6
Influenza	0
Ague	1
Remittent Fever	0
Typhus	33
Erysipelas	1
Syphilis	1
Hydrophobia	0
Diseases of the Brain, Nerves, and Senses	149
Diseases of the Lungs and other Organs of Respiration	215
Diseases of the Heart and Blood-vessels	16
Diseases of the Stomach, Liver, and other Organs of Digestion	87
Diseases of the Kidneys, &c.	3
Childbed	8
Paramenia	0
Ovarian Dropsy	1
Disease of Uterus, &c.	2
Arthritis	0
Rheumatism	3
Diseases of Joints, &c.	3
Carbuncle	0
Phlegmon	0
Ulcer	0
Fistula	0
Diseases of Skin, &c.	1
Dropsy, Cancer, and other Diseases of Uncertain Seat	94
Old Age or Natural Decay	45
Deaths by Violence, Privation, or Intemperance	25
Causes not specified	2
Deaths from all Causes	842

METEOROLOGICAL JOURNAL.

Kept at EDMONTON, *Latitude* 51° 37′ 32″N. *Longitude* 0° 3′ 51″ *W. of Greenwich.*

August 1843.	THERMOMETER.		BAROMETER.	
Wednesday 30	from 61 to 71		29·80 to 29·94	
Thursday . 31	60	72	29·89	Stat.
September.				
Friday . . . 1	55	77	29·94	29·96
Saturday . 2	57	77	30·00	29·22
Sunday . . 3	54	78	29·96	29·93
Monday . . 4	68	55	29·93	29·99
Tuesday . 5	43	68	30·02	Stat

Wind variable.

30th cloudy, except the evening. 31st, morning cloudy; afternoon and evening clear. September 1st, morning foggy, otherwise generally clear. 2d, 3d, 4th, and 5th, clear.

CHARLES HENRY ADAMS.

WILSON & OGILVY, 57, Skinner Street, London.

THE

LONDON MEDICAL GAZETTE,

BEING A

WEEKLY JOURNAL

OF

Medicine and the Collateral Sciences.

FRIDAY, SEPTEMBER 15, 1843.

LECTURES

ON THE

THEORY AND PRACTICE OF MIDWIFERY,

Delivered in the Theatre of St. George's Hospital,

BY ROBERT LEE, M.D. F.R.S.

LECTURE XLIII.

On Crural Phlebitis.

WHEN inflammation commences in the uterine branches of the internal iliac or hypogastric veins, it sometimes extends into the common, external iliac, and femoral veins, and thus gives rise to the swelling of the lower extremities, and to all the other local and constitutional symptoms of phlegmasia dolens, œdema lacteum, œdeme des nouvelles accouchées, depôts laiteux, les infiltrations laiteuses des extremités inferieures, hysteralgia lactea, or metastasis lactis. In the works of Hippocrates, Rodericus a Castro, and Wiseman, there are obscure notices of this disease. Mauriceau was the first author who pointed out distinctly its most characteristic symptoms. I have seen, he says, several women after being safely delivered, who have had their whole legs and thighs, from the groin to the side of the foot, sometimes on one side, at other times on both, remarkably swollen and œdematous. This accident, he says, often occurs after a sciatic pain caused by a reflux upon the parts of certain humours which ought to be evacuated by the lochia. "Cet accident survient souvent ensuite d'une douleur sciatique causée par un reflux, qui se fait sur ces parties, des humeurs qui devroit être evacuées par les vuidanges, dont le gros nerf de la cuisse s'abreuve quelquefois tellement, qu'il en peut rester à la femme une claudication dans la suite, comme il est arrivée à une de mes tantes, qui quoiqu'elle fut très bien faite, et fort droite auparavant, est restée tout-a-

fait boiteuse d'une jambe depuis trente-huit ans par un semblable accident, ensuit d'une de ses couches." Mauriceau does not state that he ever saw the disease prove fatal, but he knew that it was dangerous when the pain and swelling of the limbs were great, accompanied with fever, difficulty of respiration, and much tension and soreness of the hypogastrium. When the swelling was slight and unaccompanied by fever, he knew that the affection was without danger, and would soon disappear by the use of diuretics. A far more full and exact description was given of the symptoms of crural phlebitis by Puzos, in two Memoirs, entitled Sur les Depôts Laiteux, appellés communement Lait Repandu, in 1759. He states that it is a painful and protracted, and sometimes a fatal disease, and that it occurs most frequently about the twelfth day after delivery, though sometimes as late as the sixth week. He also observed that one limb only is at first affected, and that the pain and swelling commence in the groin and superior part of the thigh, and descend along the course of the crural vessels to the ham, and thence along the calf of the leg to the foot. He observed likewise that the disease sometimes attacked the other limb, and that it presented the same appearances as the first affected. The extent of the evil, he remarks, is readily recognised by a painful cord formed by the infiltration of the cellular tissue which accompanies the crural vessels. "Quand le depôt laiteux se fait sur les extremités inferieures (p. 345), il n'en attaque qu'une à la fois. Souvent le mal guerit d'un coté, pour passer ensuite à l'autre. La douleur et l'enflure commencent toujours dans l'aine, and par le haut de la cuisse : le mal descend ensuite tout le long du cordon des vaisseaux ; c'est à dire, qu'il s'etend de haut en bas ; il gagne le jarret, le gras de la jambe, and vient se terminer au pied." At page 350 he says, again, "C'est dans l'aine, et dans la parte superieure de la cuisse, que le depôt commence à donner des signes de sa presence par la douleur que l'accouchée y ressent, et la douleur suit ordinairement le trajet des gros vaisseaux qui descendent le long de la cuisse ; elle est même plus vive dans tout ce trajet. On reconnoit l'etendue du mal par une espèce de corde douloureuse que forme l'infiltration du tissue cellulaire qui accompagne ces vaisseaux ; et l'enflure se joint presque toujours à la douleur " In the treatment of the disease, which Puzos considered to depend on metastasis of milk, he recommends repeated venesection, cathartics, and sudorifics, and various local applications, as fomentations and embrocations. The daughter in law of M. Clement, one of the most distinguished accoucheurs at the time, but an enemy to blood-letting in this disease, was attacked with pain in the thigh on the fifteenth day after a natural labour; violent fever and great swelling of the thigh speedily followed, and she died from the depôt laiteux, as it was called, on the twentieth day after her confinement, and the fifth day of the disease. Puzos admits that this was not the only case he had seen which had terminated fatally, and that copious blood-letting was not an infallible remedy. " J'ai eu le malheur de perdre plus d'une malade, malgre toutes les saignées que j'avois pu faire : non que les saignées eussent été contraires ; mais elles avoient été insuffisantes pour ces cas las, parceque le mal étoit plus puissant que le remede, and qu'il n'y en avoit pas d'autre."

Levret's description of crural phlebitis (1761), coincides in every respect with that of Puzos, and he refers the disease to the crural vessels, in so direct a manner, that it is wonderful some opportunity did not occur to enable him to discover its precise nature. When the disease attacks one side, a swelling more or less considerable, he observes, is felt in the iliac fossa.   The cord of crural vessels is also painful through a great part of its course.

In a manuscript copy of Dr. William Hunter's Lectures, taken in 1775, no account is given of the disease; but from the following note written by Mr. Cruickshanks to Mr. Trye, at the time he was engaged in the publication of his work on the subject, it is evident that Dr. Hunter had seen cases of crural phlebitis, and was convinced that the opinions of Puzos and Levret respecting the nature of the disease had no solid foundation. " They have imputed the swelled leg, which happens after lying-in, to a depôt de lait, but it is not; to something wrong in the constitution. The patient is first seized with pain in the groin ; the pulse becomes smart, and the part becomes tender ; the pain and tenderness get gradually lower down, and the muscles are stiffened into hard bumps, and an oedema frequently succeeds the inflammatory swelling. It is ge-

nerally called a cold, but it is not. In some it is over in a short time, in others it will last some months ; it generally does well." In 1784, Mr. White, of Manchester, published an " Inquiry into the nature and cause of the swelling in one or both of the lower extremities, which sometimes happens to lying-in women ;" and he suggested or adopted the opinion, that the disease depends on obstruction, detention, and accumulation of lymph in the limb, or on some other morbid condition of the lymphatic vessels and glands of the affected parts. He considered it to arise from some local accident during labour, and to be a purely local disease. Mr. White saw fourteen cases either during or subsequent to the attack ; but as none of them proved fatal, an opportunity was not afforded him to determine the truth of his hypothesis by an examination of the actual condition of the different textures of the affected extremities An Essay on the swelling of the lower extremities incident to lying-in women, was published in 1792, by Mr. Trye, of Gloucester, in which he referred the symptoms to rupture of the lymphatics as they cross the brim of the pelvis under Poupart's ligament. Six cases came under the observation of Mr. Trye, and in all recovery likewise took place. He clearly perceived, although he was unable to explain the fact, that an intimate relation subsists between uterine inflammation or puerperal fever, and the swelled leg of lying-in women. Dr. Ferriar soon after maintained, without furnishing the slightest evidence in support of his opinion, that there is a general inflammatory state of the absorbents in this disease. Dr. Hull, of Manchester, published, in 1800, an essay on crural phlebitis, which he called phlegmasia dolens, in which he showed that it was impossible to account for the phenomena on the supposition that the lymphatics were affected independently of a considerable primary affection of the sanguiferous system of the limb. He considered the proximate cause to consist in an inflammatory affection, producing suddenly a considerable effusion of serum and coagulating lymph, from the exhalants into the cellular membrane of the limb. All the textures, muscles, cellular membrane, lymphatics, nerves, glands, and blood-vessels, he supposed to become affected. The primary seat of the inflammation he believed to be in the muscles, cellular membrane, and inferior surface of the cutis ; but it was a mere supposition. Dr. Hull thus describes the symptoms of the disease :—" It has in many instances attacked women who were recovering from puerperal fever, and in some cases has supervened or succeeded to thoracic inflammation. It not uncommonly begins with coldness and rigors. These are succeeded by heat, thirst, and other symptoms of pyrexia; and then pain, stiffness, and other symptoms of topical inflammation supervene. Sometimes the local affection is from the first accompanied with, but is not preceded by, febrile symptoms. Upon other occasions the topical affection is neither preceded by puerperal fever nor rigors, &c.; but soon after it has taken place, the pulse becomes more frequent, the heat of the body is increased, and the patient is affected with thirst and headache, &c. The pyrexia is very various in degree in different patients, and sometimes assumes an irregular remittent or intermittent type. "The complaint generally takes place on one side only at first, and the part where it commences is various; but it most commonly begins in the lumbar, hypogastric, or inguinal region, on one side; or in the hip or top of the thigh, and corresponding labium pudendi. In this case the patient first perceives a sense of pain, weight, and stiffness, in some of the above-mentioned parts, which are increased by every attempt to move the pelvis or lower limb. If the part be carefully examined, it generally is found rather fuller or hotter than natural, and tender to the touch, but not discoloured. The pain increases, always becomes very severe, and in some cases is of the most excruciating kind. It extends along the thigh; and when it has subsisted for some time, longer or shorter in different patients, the top of the thigh and the labium pudendi become greatly swelled, and the pain is then sometimes alleviated, and unaccompanied with a greater sense of distension. The pain next extends down to the knee, and is generally the most severe on the inside and back of the thigh, in the direction of the internal, cutaneous, and crural nerves. When it has continued for some time the whole of the thigh becomes swelled, and the pain is somewhat relieved. The pain then extends down the leg to the foot, and is commonly most severe in the direction of the posterior tibial nerve. After some time the parts last attacked begin to swell, and the pain abates in violence, but is still very considerable, especially on any attempt to move the limb. The extremity being now swelled throughout its whole extent, appears perfectly or nearly uniform; and it is not perceptibly lessened by an horizontal position, like an oedematous limb. It is of the natural colour, or even whiter; is hotter than natural, excessively tense, and exquisitely tender when touched. When pressed by the finger in different parts, it is found to be elastic, little if any impression remaining, and that only for a very short time." After describing the manner in which the constitutional and local symptoms subside, Dr. Hull further observes, that "hitherto the disease has been described as

affecting only one of the inferior extremities, and as terminating by resolution, or the effusion of a fluid that is removed by the absorbents; but, unfortunately, it sometimes happens that, after it abates in one limb, the other is attacked in a similar way. It also happens, in some cases, that the swelling is not terminated by resolution; for sometimes a suppuration takes place in one or both legs, and ulcers are formed, which are difficult to heal. In a few cases gangrene has supervened. In some instances the patient has been destroyed by the violence of the disease, before either suppuration or gangrene has happened."

It is a very remarkable circumstance in the history of crural phlebitis, that above a century and a half should have elapsed from the time when it was first clearly pointed out by Mauriceau, and the seat of the disease distinctly referred, at a later period, to the crural vessels by Puzos and Levret, before an opportunity was presented or embraced of ascertaining by dissection the precise nature of the disease. There had indeed been opportunities to determine the accuracy of the different hypotheses which had been advanced, but these had been neglected; and the seat of the disease in the crural veins, and its commencement in the uterus, were imperfectly understood before the year 1829.

In January 1823, M. Bouillaud related in the 2d vol. of the Archives Générales de Médecine, p. 188, several cases and dissections, in which the crural veins were obliterated in women who had suffered from a swelling of the lower extremities after delivery; and he distinctly stated that he considered obstruction of the veins to be the cause, not only of the oedema of the lower extremities in lying-in women, but of many partial dropsies. He has adduced various facts and observations in support of the opinion, that in many cases venous obstruction, and not general debility, is a common cause of dropsy. A woman, æt. 20, was admitted into the hospital Cochin, on the 19th July, 1822, affected with tubercles of the lungs, and oedema of both lower extremities. She died in 45 days, and on opening the body a cancerous tumor was found in the pelvis, which involved the uterus, rectum, and the cellular tissue, and glands around. The hypogastric and iliac veins, which traversed this enormous mass, were obliterated by an old red fibrinous coagulum; the obliteration extended downward along the whole course of the crural veins, and upward into the vena cava, to the level of the right kidney.

Anne Vilard, æt. 55, entered the same hospital on the 19th of November, 1822. She died 59 days after, from chronic peritonitis, cancer of the ovaria, and an encysted abscess in the left hemisphere of the brain.

The two inferior extremities were infiltrated. On examination after death, the crural, external, and common iliac veins, were obliterated, and rendered impervious by the presence of solid fibrinous coagula.

A man, æt. 60, was admitted on the 16th of April, 1822, with pleurisy and chronic peritonitis. The lower extremities were swollen, and the scrotum and trunk of the body soon also became infiltrated. The dropsy of the trunk disappeared, and the abdomen was seen covered with large veins. The patient died in 75 days, and on opening the body, the right kidney was found greatly enlarged, and affected with encephaloid cancer. The tumor lay over the vena cava, was filled up with a fibrous, friable, pultaceous matter ; the emulgent veins, the veins of the pelvis, and those of the inferior extremities, were equally obliterated by old coagula.

Virginie Aubert, æt. 21, much affected with ataxic, adynamic fever, of three weeks duration, entered on the 8th of November, 1822. The left lower extremity was at this time infiltrated and painful. She died in nine days, and on examining the body, the veins of the swollen limb were found obliterated by a long, solid, red fibrinous coagulum, which extended into the vena cava. The veins on the opposite side contained fluid blood.—The two following cases are examples of genuine crural phlebitis, or phlegmasia dolens, in puerperal women, and they are the first cases, I believe, that were ever published, in which the crural veins were examined after death. Elizabeth Perfu, æt. 38, was received into the Cochin Hospital on the 27th of April, 1822, two months after her delivery. She had tubercles of the lungs, and infiltration of the left inferior extremity. The body was in a state of great marasmus. The veins of the affected extremity were found after death plugged up with a very old, red-coloured, easily broken down, fibrinous coagulum, which extended into the common iliac vein, where its consistence diminished. The vena cava, and veins of the other extremities, contained more or less fluid blood.

Marguerite Colliere, æt. 30, was delivered by the forceps in the Maternité, about the end of January, 1822. She entered the same hospital on the 20th of March following, having the left lower extremity greatly swollen. She died on the seventh day after. On opening the body, an enormous abscess was found in the pelvis, which appeared to have commenced on the left side of the cavity, before and within the psoas muscle. All the surrounding parts were extensively disorganised, and softened like lard. The veins of the swollen extremity, without excepting the great saphena, were obliterated by a solid, fibrinous, friable coagulum.

" It is known," adds M. Bouillaud, " that infiltration of one or both of the lower extremities is not unfrequently observed in women recently delivered, and that in the bodies of those who die, the crural veins are obliterated ; compression and inflammation are the causes to which he attributes this. On sait qu'il n'est pas rare de voir l'infiltration s'emparer de l'un ou des deux membres abdominaux chez les nouvelles accouchées. Eh bien ! on trouve sur les cadavres de celles qui succombent, des oblitérations des veines crurales. Les 5e et 6e observations que j'ai rapportées en fournissent des examples. MM. Chaussier, Meckel, Travers, en ont recueilli de semblables."

An Essay on the proximate cause of the disease called Phlegmasia Dolens, by Dr. David D. Davis, was read to the Medical and Chirurgical Society, May 6th, 1823, and subsequently published in the 12th vol. of the Med. Chir. Transactions. The following is the first case related.

" Caroline Dunn, æt. 21, of a weak constitution, was delivered of a male child on the 7th of February, 1817, after a severe labour of 27 hours' duration. Some loss of blood was sustained both before and after the birth of the child. On account of the latter hæmorrhage, the placenta was removed artificially by the introduction of the hand into the uterus. On the following day the pulse was full, and regular at 90 ; the tongue was white, but moist, and there was a slight thirst. Pressure upon the abdomen occasioned no pain, but a soreness was felt in the vagina. During the days immediately succeeding, the symptoms were moderate." On the 13th, the case was reported as follows. Slight fever; pulse quick and full; bowels costive ; tongue white and dry ; labia pudendi inflamed, swelled, and œdematous ; some headache ; respiration difficult ; appetite bad; a copious yellow discharge from the vagina, having the consistence of cream, but without fœtor.

17th.—The report was, better generally; discharge much decreased ; inflammation subsided ; bowels well relieved ; pulse regular at 86; tongue natural in its appearance; thirst still great.

21st.—Much better ; sleep good ; sat up out of bed for four hours.

22d.—Better still ; complained of slight pain, like cramp, as the patient herself expressed it, in the left leg.

26th.—Worse ; left leg and thigh much swollen ; pain in the inguinal region ; skin hot ; no signs externally of inflammation ; no pitting on pressure ; bowels costive; slight cough; respiration difficult ; pulse very quick and small ; headache.

Feb. 28th to March 2d.—No better ; leg pitted on pressure ; countenance depressed ; languor ; giddiness at intervals ; pulse 80 ;

freedom from pain; no appetite; bowels twice relieved.

3d.—Total insensibility; limb equally swollen; countenance sunk; pale, and emaciated.

4th.—Died at noon this day. Mr. Lawrence examined the body on the 6th of March, 1817, and gave the following description of the morbid appearances. "The left lower extremity presented an uniform œdematous enlargement without any external discolouration, from the hip to the foot. This was found on further examination to proceed from the ordinary anasarcous effusion into the cellular substance. The inguinal glands were a little enlarged, as they usually are in a dropsical limb, but pale coloured, and free from the slightest sign of inflammation. The femoral vein from the ham upwards, the external iliac, and the common iliac veins, as far as the junction of the latter with the corresponding trunk of the right side, were distended and firmly plugged with what appeared externally a coagulum of blood. The femoral portion of the vein, slightly thickened in its coats, and of a deep red colour, was filled with a firm bloody coagulum closely adhering to the sides of the tube, so that it could not be drawn out. As the red colour of the vein might have been caused by the red clot every where in close contact with it, it cannot be deemed a proof of inflammation. The trunk of the profunda was distended in the same way as that of the femoral vein; but the saphena and its branches were empty and healthy. The substance filling the external iliac, and common iliac portions of the vein, was like the laminated coagulum of an aneurismal sac, at least with a very slight mixture of red particles. The tube was completely obstructed by this matter, more intimately connected to its surface than in the femoral vein; adhering, indeed, as firmly as the coagulum does to any part of an old aneurismal sac. But in its centre there was a cavity containing about a tea-spoonful of a thick fluid of the consistence of pus, of a light brownish red tint, and pultaceous appearance. The uterus, which had contracted to the usual degree at such a distance of time from delivery, its appendages and blood-vessels, and the vagina, were in a perfectly natural state. There was not the least appearance of vascular congestion about the organ, nor the slightest distension of any of its vessels. Its whole substance was on the contrary pale, and the vessels every where contracted and empty. The state of the abdominal cavity and its contents was perfectly natural. That the substance occupying the upper part of the venous trunk, and the fluid in its central cavity, had been deposited there during life from inflammation of the vessel, does not admit of doubt." "I am

also," observes Mr. Lawrence, "decidedly of opinion, in consequence of its firmness, and close adhesion to the vein, that the red coagulum in the femoral vein was the result of a similar affection extending along the tube; and that the passage of blood through it in the whole tract submitted to examination must have been completely obstructed before death."

I have examined the preparation of the diseased veins, and there can be no doubt that the appearances here described were produced by inflammation of their lining membrane. If you look at the coloured engraving which accompanies the paper, and observe the thickened state of their coats, and the coagulum adhering to their inner surface, you will entertain no doubt of this. The greater part of the coagulum in the femoral vein is blood; it does not adhere to the lining membrane, but a coagulum similar to that in the common and external iliac is never seen but as the consequence of inflammation. No light is thrown by this dissection on the origin of the disease, and you might be led to infer from the observation of Mr. Lawrence, that the uterus and its appendages, and blood-vessels, were healthy; that the inflammation did not commence in the uterine branches of the hypogastric vein, or internal iliac; but it does not appear that the course of this vein was traced to its ramifications in the uterus, and unless the attention had been directed in a particular manner to the internal iliac vein, its morbid state might easily have escaped detection. Dr. Davis has also related the following case.

A lady died suddenly in the midst of apparent health on the 20th of September, 1819, in the sixth week after her second labour. The day after her delivery she was seized with violent peritoneal inflammation, the acute symptoms of which were subdued by antiphlogistic treatment. The febrile excitement was nevertheless not completely subdued, and ten days after she complained of a deep-seated pain in the groin, and along the tract of the great vessels of the thigh. The limb was observed to be swelled and exquisitely painful. By leeching and blistering, the new inflammation was speedily reduced, and in about a week from its commencement the swelling had entirely subsided, and the patient had recovered the full power of contracting and extending the extremity without suffering pain. From this period she recovered rapidly and satisfactorily. Her death took place instantaneously, whilst in the act of changing the recumbent for the sitting position, soon after dinner, and in a moment of slight excitement. The left external iliac vein, including about half an inch of the upper portion of its corresponding femoral vein, were found strongly attached by adhesions of its cellular coat to the parts around. Its parietes still retained a morbid thickness, and its internal tunic was studded in several places with deposits of adherent lymph. The portion most remarkable for this incrustation, and otherwise most diseased, was the part of the vein immediately under Poupart's ligament. The tube of the vessel was still manifestly pervious, though it had suffered a diminution of capacity amounting to perhaps one half of its natural diameter. The inguinal glands were also diseased. The right iliac vein was also in a perfectly healthy state. These appearances have also been represented in this coloured engraving, and there can be no doubt that they are the result of inflammation.

A case of fatal phlegmasia dolens, which occurred to Mr. Oldknow, has also been recorded by Mr. Davis as follows. "Jane Elliott was delivered in September, 1820, having an easy and natural labour. Until the 20th day after the delivery she was doing well; on that day she was seized with a violent purging, for which astringents were given with success; but the pulse continued quick, and she had considerable fever; on the 30th day the purging returned, and the left lower extremity became swollen and painful, with considerable increase of fever. She died on the 34th day." On examining the swollen limb the day after her death, "I found the femoral vein," says Mr. Oldknow, "one-third down the thigh, and all the iliac veins much enlarged, and containing adherent layers of coagulated blood, similar to that found in aneurismal sacs, together with a sort of grumous fluid of a brown colour, more or less mixed with air, and almost obliterating the venous canals. The same appearances, but in a much less degree, extended along the vena cava as far as the entrance of the renal veins. The coats of the veins were highly inflamed, and intimately attached to the surrounding parts. The absorbent vessels and glands were slightly enlarged as high as the lumbar regions, but no otherwise affected. The uterus had regained nearly its natural size." The appearances here described have also been represented in this coloured engraving, and there can be no doubt that the veins were inflamed. A fourth case has been related by Dr. Davis. "Mrs. L——, a lady of a delicate constitution, and of a very irritable habit, was delivered of her fifth child on the 2d day of July, 1821. She had been subject to feverish affections in several of her former confinements. On this occasion she was doing well until the 7th day after her delivery, when she was taken out of bed and placed upon a sofa, between the fire and a large loosely hung window. In this situation she was seized with a violent rigor. During the gradual

development of the succeeding hot fit she experienced a pain of the left side of the chest, which increased rapidly in intensity. She was freely bled before I saw her, without experiencing adequate relief. She was afterwards bled, leeched, and blistered. The pain of the chest was then in a great measure subdued; but this flattering advantage was not accompanied by any material reduction of the attendant fever. The pulse, on the contrary, continued quick, and the general distress and restlessness were so little mitigated as to call for much sympathy, and to excite serious alarm. In the evening of the same day, unequivocal symptoms of phlegmasia dolens declared themselves. The patient died on the 23d of the month. The pleura costalis on the left side was found inflamed. All the surfaces and viscera of the abdomen were apparently in a perfectly sound state. The left lower extremity, from the hip to the toe, was considerably but not greatly enlarged, and there was an evident fulness of the labium pudendi of the same side. The iliac veins of both sides were unusually turgid with blood; but presenting no other external manifestation of disease. They were entirely free from attachments to the contiguous parts. The inguinal glands were certainly not diseased, nor even visibly enlarged. On making a careful incision into the left internal iliac, it was first found to contain a coagulum of blood of firm consistence; but not at that part adherent to the internal surface of the vein. Upon opening, however, the common iliac portion of the vessel, adhesion of the same column of coagulum had obviously taken place; an appearance which is now distinctly to be seen in the preparation. The left internal iliac was greatly inflamed, and its diameter was so much contracted by the morbid thickening of its parietes, that it was rendered almost impervious. The right iliac vein, including both its common and external portions, was distended with a similar coagulum; or rather the same coagulum was prolonged over the angle of their common junction with the vena cava, from one iliac to the other." These appearances have also been represented in this coloured engraving. From these cases Dr. Davis inferred that the proximate cause of phlegmasia dolens is a violent destructive inflammation of the iliac veins and their contributory branches, including in some cases the inferior portion of the vena cava. "The principal veins of the pelvis are necessarily exposed to great pressure," he says, "from the uterus during the latter months of gestation. A well-known effect of this pressure is a varicose dilatation of the superficial veins, together with œdema of the lower extremities: a state of the limbs indicative, in the opinion of practical writers, of a predisposition to phlegmasia dolens."

"Phlegmasia dolens," he adds, "is a disease which almost always occurs in an excited state of the organs of circulation, and when that is not the case it is known to take place during a period of predisponency to inflammatory action of the great blood-vessels within the pelvis, and their immediate ramifications. Hence its occurrence after labours and miscarriages, before the perfect re-establishment of the balance of the circulation; and at those time more particularly after profuse hæmorrhages, or during phlegmasia of other parts; or from the application of occasional causes of whatever kind which may have the effect of exciting a febrile disturbance in the system. All the veins liable to much pressure, or to enlargement of diameter during pregnancy, appear to be more or less predisposed to inflammation upon the sudden removal of those agencies by the consummation of the act of parturition. Hence the predisposition to hysteritis and peritonitis during the first week after labour, and to the swelled leg, and to mammary abscesses, at a more advanced period."

For six years after the publication of these cases by M. Bouillaud and Dr. Davis, there was perhaps no subject on which a greater difference of opinion prevailed than on the pathology of phlegmasia dolens; and many remained in doubt whether these cases should be considered as examples of genuine phlegmasia dolens, or be viewed as essentially different diseases, and analogous in their nature to those formidable attacks of phlebitis which sometimes succeed to venesection and wounds. In opposition to their views, it was forcibly urged, that if phlegmasia dolens depended on inflammation of the iliac and femoral veins, the majority of those affected with the disease would die; whereas death does not take place in one case in a hundred where that disease is distinctly marked. Even that distinguished anatomist and pathologist, Mr. Lawrence, who had examined the first fatal case which occurred to Dr. Davis, and whose history of the morbid appearances threw more light on the nature of the affection than all the hypotheses that had previously been advanced —which were mere speculations, unsupported by facts—declared in the Medical and Chirurgical Society, as late as 1828, that he was fully convinced, from what had subsequently fallen under his observation, that Dr. Davis's views were incorrect, and that phlegmasia dolens did not arise from inflammation of the iliac and femoral veins.

In the next lecture I shall relate to you the cases, and exhibit the various preparations and drawings, which appear to me to demonstrate, not only that inflammation of the iliac and femoral veins gives rise to all the phenomena of phlegmasia, but that, in puerperal women, it originates in the uterine branches of the hypogastric veins, and subsequently extends from them into the iliac and femoral trunks of the affected side.

SPIDERS DISCHARGED FROM THE EYE*.

HYSTERIC MONOMANIA.

By A. Lopez, M.D. Mobile, Ala.

I was requested, on the 5th of February, 1840, to visit a young lady, from whose mother I received the following statement:— The patient had left the city of Charleston, S. C. (at which place I then was), to visit a friend who resided in the country. On the night of the 29th of January, while conversing in bed, she was sensible that some object had fallen from the ceiling of the apartment, upon her cheek, just below the inferior lid. This caused her to apply the hand briskly and forcibly in order to brush off what she supposed to be some one of the many insects so common in country houses, upon which the friend with whom she slept observed, that, as the room was much infested with spiders, it was probable that the object which had fallen was one of them. In the course of the night she was awakened by a feeling of intense pain in her left eye, which continued at intervals until morning, when, upon examination, the eye was discovered to be highly inflamed and lachrymose. Ordinary domestic means were applied, and during the morning, feeling an intense degree of itching and irritation, she rubbed the lids together upon the ball and removed two fragments which were readily recognised as the dismembered parts of a spider. Her alarm in consequence became very great, and was much heightened when the same thing was repeated in the afternoon. She left for home and arrived in Charleston on the 2d of February. During the voyage her mind was much perturbed and under considerable excitement from the event, and when I paid my first visit on the 5th, the date mentioned in the early part of my statement, the following was her condition: the right eye unaffected; the left turgid, inflamed, and weeping; and there had been removed from it, that morning, a spider, imbedded in a mucous covering. It was entire with the exception of two legs. The two preceding days before I had seen her, three others had been removed; and were now exhibited to me. I immediately submitted the eye to as close an examination as the irritable condition of

* From the American Journal of the Medical Sciences—July 1843.

the parts permitted, without being enabled to discover the minutest portion of any foreign substance. In order, however, to combat the pain and inflammation, I ordered leeches, saline-antimonial medicines, and evaporating lotions. I thenceforward visited her daily until the 19th, and at every visit I removed either an entire or dismembered spider from the same eye. Before proceeding it will be well to mention that during the interval between the 5th and 19th, I invited, to an examination of the case, Professors Geddings and Dickson, and Doctors Bellinger and Wurdeman. Dr. Dickson on one or two occasions also removed these objects from the patient's eye. I made, assisted by Professor Geddings, the most minute scrutiny with a view of discovering—first, whether there could possibly exist a nidus within the orbit for these animals; secondly, whether a sac containing their ova was there concealed; and, thirdly, if any communication between the eye and nose could account for their appearance. For these purposes, the superior and inferior palpebræ were everted with great care, traversed thoroughly with a blunt probe, and afterwards I threw injections around the internal lining, but all to no avail. The anterior and posterior nares were closely examined by strong light, both of the sun and candle, yet we could not perceive the slightest trace of any means by which either ova, insect, or nidus, could be retained.

The sensations always precursory to their removal were : a sense of burning in the ball, a pricking of the superior lid, proceeding more or less severely around the orbit, until it assumed a fixed pain within the lower lid, upon the eversion of which, by myself, if present, or her mother, in my absence, the spider, always dead, would be discovered enshrouded in its mucous bed, and removed by means of the finger or probe. I now resume the order of their discharge. From the 19th they were removed from both eyes, and so continued until the 23d, when again they became confined to the left, and afterwards from each eye alternately until the 5th of March, when a truce was had until the 10th. During this interval, the eyes resumed their normal condition, but again on the 10th the inflammation was renewed and the discharge of spiders recommenced, the right eye being now chiefly the depository. Up to the date, during which time my visits were unremittingly made, none other than general observations were kept, but, the spider-making power appearing so inexhaustible, a more circumstantial diary was thought necessary.

March 10th.—Two spiders.

11th.—Two. Pain over right orbitar region, passing gradually over the frontal

sinus to the left. Sharp pricking pains upon pressure.

12th.—Previous to my visit, one from the left eye, which was much less inflamed than the right.

13th.—Eyes much improved in appearance. One discharged since my last visit, and another just previous to my departure this morning. As this discharge served greatly to perplex the views at which I shall arrive before I conclude this paper, it may not be irrelevant to notice it. I have mentioned the scrupulousness with which the eye and its appendages were examined, in order to elicit, if possible, any clue by which to unravel this enigma, and the fruitlessness of those exertions. It appears, then, that on the day of this visit (the 13th) a spider was removed before my arrival. A servant was despatched for it to a neighbour's whither it had been sent for examination. Some time elapsed before her return, during which time I sat in such a relative position to the patient as to preclude all possibility of deception, and I had this day, as was my wont at every visit, made a careful examination of the eye without discovering a vestige of any kind of substance. Upon the return of the servant I arose to depart, at which moment the patient complained of pain, and, in a few seconds, by turning down the lid, I removed another spider.

15th.—Eyes extremely healthy and clear. On the 13th, just after my visit, the mother removed three spiders, two entire and one broken ; also a putrid substance, the precise nature of which I could not define. No others discharged to date.

17th.—None since the 15th. Right eye more affected ; upper lid much irritated and swollen. Left eye healthy.

18th.—Right eye still inflamed—discharged a portion of web from the inner canthus.

19th.—Eyes the same ; another piece of web.

20th.—Eyes perfectly natural. After my departure on the 19th, there was removed a sacculum containing ova.

27th.—None since the 20th until to-day. The left eye being inflamed and painful she was advised by a friend to insert an eyestone, which, at its exit, protruded one spider of the long-legged kind, entire.

April 6th.—None since the 27th ultimo. Eyes healthy, and generally improved in their appearance.

13th.—None since the 6th. Eyes healthy ; has used them since my last visit, in sewing and reading without inconvenience.

May 14th.—None since the 13th of April. Eyes healthy until a few days past ; to-day they are weak, lachrymose, and slightly injected. They however improved under remedial measures, and the case terminated.

The total number of spiders removed from the commencement were between forty and fifty. During the progress of this very singular case, the treatment was regulated according to the greater or less degree of local or general disturbance. The patient was restored to good health, and continued so uninterruptedly to the date of my leaving Carolina, in November 1840.

I have presented the facts as succinctly as possible, and here, perhaps, in the opinion of many, it should rest; but other considerations may offer themselves to warrant a further notice. They are these: 1st, a case so anomalous and of so unusual occurrence, could not well exist, without necessarily exciting an intense degree of public curiosity, and, in fact, becoming, as it did, a subject of general notoriety and discussion in the various public presses of the union, all of which, however, were strictly unprofessional, as this is the first entire and correct statement yet made on the subject by myself. 2dly, the character and respectability of the patient as well as her mother, being familiarly known to me for many years, preclude the remotest suspicion of any desire to impose, or to acquire a spurious notoriety on the part of the daughter, or of the countenance of fraud by the mother. 3dly, the pathological history of the patient, which I will proceed to give, and which has induced me to distinguish this case as one unequivocally of Hysteric Monomania.

In adopting this rationale I am of opinion that I conform more strictly to the category within whose scope are embraced so many equally singular and otherwise inexplicable perversions of the nervous system, and under the influence of which the most remarkable anomalies have been produced. I, moreover, am disposed to regard it rather as a melancholy, though interesting feature of disease, than a subject of levity to be classed among the nine-day wonders of every day report. The patient from her childhood exhibited a due inheritance of that temperament, which became more strongly developed at that age, which, in females so strikingly calls into action the consentaneous play of every nervous affinity. The establishment of the catamenial period corresponded with this complication. Her natural disposition was variable, at times cheerful, sometimes gloomy, but more commonly timid and reserved.

In 1839 I attended her for an attack of chorea, during which many peculiarities were observable, and a few months preceding the invasion of the case now under consideration she was under my case for a neuralgic affection, terminating in a tremulousness of her upper extremities corresponding with what Good in his Neurotica recognises as

"synclonus tremor," except that here the morbid action is exhibited on attempt at voluntary motion, whereas in this case it was indepedent of such causes. In the presence of these facts, to wit, the entire confidence entertained not only by myself but all others, in the strict veracity and irreproachable integrity of the parties; the predisposing and salient qualities in the idiosyncrasy of the patient, and the indisputable, though too frequently unexplained effects resulting from a morbid condition of the nervous system,—effects impressing their astounding influences not only upon the physical but also upon the psychological nature of man,—can we, without becoming amenable to the charge of an indifference incompatible with the proper spirit of inquiry which is so peculiarly the province of medical philosophy, refrain from devoting a little time to the investigation of this case.

Previously to any considerations touching the mental agency involved in this history, I will refer in abstract to a few instances, which, if not even in strict analogy, are nevertheless not devoid of interest, either as objects of science or curiosity.

1. In the "Mémoires de la Société Médicale," (Année 5me, p. 181,) M. Silvy relates a case in which an immense number of pins and needles were swallowed, and their exit from parts remarkably singular. These were doubtless swallowed under an erratic condition of the mind.

2. In the Med.-Chir. Rev. vol. ii. No. 22, Oct. 1825, p. 559, will be found the extraordinary "Copenhagen Needle Case," in which it is stated that a young woman from Aug. 1807 to Dec. 1823, discharged from nearly every part of her body 400 needles. This case is reported conjointly by Professor Heckoldt and Dr. Otto. In 1825 she was living and in good health in Frederick's Hospital, at Copenhagen. No account is given by which we are to infer that so immense an amount of needles were accidentally introduced, and the presumption is legitimate that they were either swallowed or thrust in under a state of mind beyond the patient's control. These are instances which would seem to owe their existence to influences such as constitute the pathological features of the case under review. They are only a few from the many with which medical history abounds. Nor are these records silent with regard to insects and larvæ being discharged from the human body, and from places so unusual as to excite surprise; and while I refer to a few of the most prominent, I do not conceive their characters parallel with my case, because in the former there are palpable grounds for explanation, whereas, in the latter, there is one of two modes alone, by which to obtain a solution,—either gross

fraud and premeditated concert, or a morbific condition dependent upon extreme exaltation of the nervous system. I will, nevertheless, briefly condense a few of the cases referred to.

In 1828, M. Cloquet reported to the Philomathic Society of Paris, the case of a rag-gatherer who in a state of intoxication laid himself down to sleep near some dead horses. He slept for twenty-four hours. On awakening he felt as if he were swelled out with much unusual pain. On his return home, a number of blisters arose about his head, and worms crawled out of his nose and ears, and other natural openings of his body. He went to the Hospital St. Louis. More came from his head when the swellings were lanced. His skin produced them every instant. The nurse collected three plates full. The conjecture was that the flies from the dead horses laid their eggs in the pores of the man's skin during sleep, as well as in the natural openings of his body, and that warmth hatched the eggs which produced the worms."—American Journal of Medical Science, No. 3, May 1828, p. 228.

Animals are frequently found in situations of the human body, for whose location it would be difficult to account. The doctrines of equivocal and spontaneous generation have been taxed through all the bearings, and still leave us as much benighted as ever. I will merely refer to the several authorities, and give their cases in brief. Worms in active motion under the conjunctiva. Blot, of Martinique, removed by incision two from a similar position in the eye of a negress. They were thread shaped, 38 milimetres long, with a black protuberance adapted for suction. The worm lay on the outside of the eye, and sometimes turned around a portion of the cornea, causing stinging pains and nervous symptoms from fear. The patient, an African, was unable to give any account of herself, or the liability of her country people to this disease.

Bajou, of Cayenne, in 1768, observed a worm in serpentine motion in the eye of a negress; upon incision being made it removed, but was secured by forceps and dislodged. He saw another case in 1771. (Am. Journ. Med. Sci., May 1840, p. 194.) The LOND. MED. GAZ. Aug. 1833, records a case of a little girl, ætat. 6, under whose conjunctiva, and resting upon the sclerotica, there was found a *cysticercus cellulosa* perfect in all its parts.

Some years since the Baltimore Sun related the case of an insect resembling a snake in the eye of a horse. It grew in two months from a half inch to three and a half or four inches in length. It moved with great rapidity, and incessantly.

Dr. Yule, in the Edinburgh Philosophical Journal, July 1825, p. 72, records cases of insects in the human stomach :—One, of a countryman, from whose stomach, after several weeks of intense suffering, there was ejected a large hairy caterpillar, supposed to be of the common dragon fly. The opinion is, that it must have lived several weeks in the stomach, and grown to its full size.

Dr. Reeve mentions the fact of larvæ inhabiting the human stomach. He cites a case, where the larvæ of the *musca domestica*, or common house fly, were voided by a girl. —New England Med. and Surg. Journal, Jan. 1821.

Kirby and Spence relate a case where several beetles were vomited by a boy.

In the Amer. Journ. Med. Sci., No. xlii. Feb. 1838, p. 473, will be found a case of a beetle discharged from the urinary bladder.

It now remains to attempt some explanation as to the means by which the spiders obtained their "local habitation" in the eyes of my patient. As might be supposed, conjectures were not idle, and the reasons assigned assumed their complexion in proportion as the credulity or scepticism of individuals prevailed. Those who yielded to the first, of course resorted to the intervention of miraculous agency, while the latter class believed it to be an artful endeavour to impose upon the community. I need not reiterate how unjust and unphilosophical such suspicions must appear under the historical features of this case. The only attempt to explain it by a natural and direct probable cause, was published by a Mr. Meddler, of Erie, Pennsylvania. In a letter addressed to the postmaster of Charleston, he gives the natural history and habits of the wood spider, which, he says, unlike the rest of that class of insects who propagate their young from eggs, " bring them forth in perfect form," and the female carries them about, attached to the extremity of the tail. Mr. Meddler thinks, therefore, that it was one of this class which fell upon the young lady's cheek, and that the effort to brush it off separated the young from the point of attachment, upon which they took different directions, some into the eyes and others into the nostrils, whence they "could easily pass" to the eyes, and become killed there by the touch. He also thinks that the spiders discharged from the eyes " were at different stages of maturity, and not of different species."

Now, Mr. Meddler errs in every particular. The wood spiders " bring forth their young in perfect form." We have shown that one of the articles removed on the 20th March, was a sacculum containing ova. Again, his idea of their passage into the eye at the moment of accident is disproved, because I have stated the extreme care with which I repeatedly examined that organ and all its appendages; and surely if the extraordinary number discharged from first to last had been lodged therein, they could not have escaped observation. They were not in the nostril, for I have also said that due exploration was there made: moreover, the communication between the nose and eyes, even in a healthy condition, could not possibly have admitted the passage of bodies as large as many of these spiders were, much less under the high state of inflammation and swelling in which they were almost constantly found. Lastly, Mr. Meddler, deriving his history of the case solely from newspaper reports, originating with persons unacquainted with its character and progress, errs in thinking that the spiders were only " at different stages of maturity," and not of different species. The spiders removed from the eye were subjected to close microscopic examination by myself, assisted by several professional gentlemen accustomed to scientific investigations, among whom was the Rev. Dr. Bachman, whose reputation precludes all doubt, and we discovered at least three different species, distinguished by the anatomical classification of Latreille, Walkenar, and Hentz. But even supposing them to have been lodged " in perfect form," the fact that they were subjected to a residence in depraved secretions unfit to preserve the lives of insects, forbids the belief that they could have reached the different stages of size and maturity which they presented; much less so, then, could we suppose them to have been hatched by incubation either in the eyes or nostrils. I am, then, constrained to discard from my mind the presumption that they were lodged and perfected previously to their discharge, or that they were placed there by the patient in a healthy condition of feeling and with a desire to impose.

The only suggestion left for my adoption is this,—that from all the preceding history of my patient, there existed a want of nervous integrity, so operating upon the mind as to produce the form of disease which I have distinguished in my text as hysteric monomania; and I am induced to think that the various types of mental irregularities, which an unbalanced nervous system is so familiarly known to produce, sustain the belief. It is needless on this occasion to investigate the diversified operations of the human mind in its physical and pathological relations, or to refer to the multiform phases it is capable of assuming under the excitement to which it is subjected by the agents which are perpetually at work upon its impressionable nature; suffice it to say, that the history of the different forms of insanity, from the highest degree of concentrated fury

to the most subtile shade of the mind's day-dream, present arguments and examples sufficiently numerous to render my view of this case at least plausible.

At the incipiency of the case, I do not for an instant doubt the presence of those fragments of spiders, and perhaps one or two entire; but my opinion is, that subsequently, terror, superinduced upon the idiosyncrasy described, dethroned the judgment; hallucination usurped its seat; a morbid concatenation was excited, and the patient under the control of this influence was urged irresistibly to introduce them from day to day, until the morbid series was exhausted. I cannot express myself more forcibly than by adopting the language of M. Ollivier, addressed to the court at Paris, in behalf of a young girl arraigned for the murder of an infant. She confessed to have given it ten pins to swallow from time to time. M. Ollivier said, " he was inclined to attribute the present act to one of those unaccountable perverse impulses which are not unfrequent in certain females, more especially about their menstrual periods." (Lancette Française, 1839.) M. Dupuytren says, " I have seen at the Hôtel-Dieu a great number of women and children, who had been affected with the strange mania of swallowing pins and needles." He then gives the case in detail, and concludes by saying, " on examining the body after death, several hundred pins and needles were found scattered through the viscera, muscles, cellular substance, &c."

I will, lastly, merely refer to that extraordinary form of insanity described in the Journal de Progrès, for 1828, under the title of Periodical Vino-Mania. It is reported by M. Pierquin who says, " The disorder commenced fifteen years ago in the shape of an irresistible impulse to swallow wine day and night without the possibility of satiety. The paroxysm lasts from two to three months, with an interval of equal duration, when it returns again without any prodrome that might indicate its approach."

I here close this case, extraordinary in its character under any aspect, and if my view of it be a correct one, it will afford another to the many which are to be found in nearly every work professing to analyze the yet inscrutable character of the human mind.

Mobile, Ala., April 26, 1843.

N.B.—The spiders are in my possession, and were exhibited with a statement to the Medical Society of this city.

CONTRIBUTIONS
TO
ANATOMY AND PHYSIOLOGY.

By Robert Knox, M.D. F.R.S.E.

Lecturer on Anatomy and Physiology, and Corresponding Member of the French Academy of Medicine.

(For the London Medical Gazette.)

I.—*Obliteration of the cavity of the Tunica Vaginalis Testis in middle and aged persons.*

During the last eight or ten years, I have remarked, in the dissecting-rooms I conduct, four or five cases of obliteration of the cavity of the tunica vaginalis testis, unconnected, so far as we could ascertain, with any operation or accident. In these persons the cavity was generally entirely obliterated; but without any other morbid appearance either in the testicle or in the cord. The tunica vaginalis itself could be forced from off the testicle by dissection ; and near the parietal portion it resembled common cellular tissue, but shewed no traces whatever of its having ever been inflamed.

In mentioning these cases during my lectures on the anatomy of textures, I have generally taken occasion to say, that I agreed with Baron Portal, and some others, in the theory, that adhesions of serous membranes, so extensive as entirely to obliterate their cavities, may take place altogether independent of inflammation ; and that I felt assured that I had seen this twice happen to the serous cavity of the pericardium. In quoting Portal's opinion as coinciding with my own as to the real nature of such adhesions, I do so from memory, having failed in recollecting the particular part in the Baron's voluminous works in which he mentions this doctrine.

II.—*On a Congenital Deformity of the Head and Neck of the Femur.*

In 1827, I published in the Transactions of the Medico-Chirurgical Society of Edinburgh, the brief history of a case in which, as it appeared to me, there had existed from infancy, perhaps even congenitally, a shortening of the neck of the thigh bone, with *sessile* head, and a general shortening of the whole extremity : as a consequence of this change upon the femur, the head of the bone was depressed as low at least as the level of the trochanter major. The particulars of the case, in so far as they require to be detailed here, were simply these. A child about two years of age, and of a suspected scrofulous constitution, died in consequence of an extensive inflammation of the right pleuræ, producing empyema. But although the child was suspected to be of a scrofulous habit, we found nothing in any of the textures confirming this opinion, excepting a slight tubercular appearance in the left lung.

Whilst examining the body of this child in order to ascertain the cause of death (which we have seen to depend on the state of the left pleura), I observed that one of the limbs was obviously shorter than the other, and suspecting that there existed some disease in the hip-joint, leave was got from the parents to examine the joint ; they assuring me, however, at the same time, that the child had never walked lame. On cutting into the joint every texture was found to be healthy, shewing no appearance whatever of diseased structure; but the neck of the femur had almost entirely disappeared, and the head of the bone, *sessile*, was on a level with the trochanter major. The specimen bore a very great resemblance to those described by Mr. Benjamin Bell, Sir A. Cooper, and others, under the name of interstitial absorption of the neck of the femur, and which had been so often mistaken for fracture of the *cervix femoris*, followed by osseous union.

Of the nature of this change upon the neck and head of the femur there have been held several opinions : some, as Beclard, considering the change to be the effects of age ; others ascribing it to chronic rheumatism ; and some, as Mr. Gulliver (in an excellent memoir published in the Edinburgh Medical and Surgical Journal, for July 1836), viewing it as a change in the structure of the bone, to be traced, in some instances at least, to a direct injury inflicted on the joint by a fall. The object of the present brief notice is not, however, to discuss the causes which may give rise to a shortening of the neck of the thigh-bone with occasional alteration of its cartilages, which causes may even be more various and obscure than is at present supposed, but to submit to the medical world a second case, in which, as it seems to me, the shortening of the neck of the femur, and greatly altered form of the head of the bone, was a *congenital malformation* altogether independent of any accident, or of any diseased condition of the bone, or its investing cartilage.

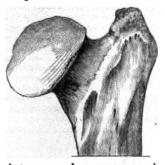

A strong muscular young person, who had died of acute pericarditis, was brought into the dissecting-room. The body, remarkably well formed in other respects, shewed this peculiarity, that the left lower extremity was obviously about half an inch shorter than the right. The limb could be moved freely in most directions, and had evidently been used equally with the other during life; but it could not be abducted so freely as the right leg, and when flexed, so as to allow the dissector to dissect and examine the perineum, the heel interfered considerably with the view of the left side of the perineum; the foot, in fact, projecting in front of this region in such a way as to conceal it to a great extent.*

On observing these facts, I drew the inference, that the hip-joint could not be altogether sound, and that the neck of the femur, more especially, could not possibly be so long as that of the opposite side. A careful dissection of the joint shewed that every structure was healthy, but that the head and neck of the femur presented the appearance delineated in the figure: the

* In other words, when placed in the usual position for performing the operation for lithotomy, the left foot lay in front of the perineum in such a way as to conceal the left side of the region from the dissector.

head was sessile, and had descended to a level with the trochanter; the cervix femoris was greatly shortened, but in all other respects the bone and joint generally were perfectly healthy: the opposite femur had the usual form in persons of this age.

Some may be disposed to think that there are no proofs adduced here of this being a congenital malformation, and I admit that after perusing Mr. Gulliver's accurately detailed cases of a similar change in the form of the femur seemingly produced by violence, the proofs I have to offer in favour of my own opinion are far from being convincing; but still, on reviewing the whole case, and the appearances on dissection, comparing it with that of the child of two years old, and of Sandifort (referred to by Mr. Gulliver), I feel much inclined to adhere to my first opinion, viz. that occasionally there is met with a congenital malformation of the femur in one or other limb, such as I have described.

It ought to have been added, that the left os innominatum partook of the change, being obviously weaker in its pubic portion than the corresponding bone of the opposite side.

I find that I ought to have added to the above brief notice, the condition of the skeleton of this person generally, and the texture of the left femur. Now in regard to the first, it appeared healthy throughout; and in respect to the second, it was found that all trace of epiphysis in the femur had disappeared: the intimate texture was white, firm, and, as appeared to me, remarkably dense and solid.

Observations on the muscle of the lachrymal sac, or tensor tarsi.

My attention to this muscle, as a part distinct from the orbicularis palpebrarum, was, with most anatomists I presume, first directed by Dr. Horner, of Philadelphia, about the year 1821. On re-examining the muscle at that time, it appeared to me—1st, that many would be disposed to view the tensor tarsi merely as a more or less detached portion of the sphincter. 2dly, What was most evident to myself, its anatomy had not been given correctly by Dr. Horner. From that time to the present I have often had occasion to repeat these remarks, but did not deem the matter worthy further notice. Lately, however, I observe that a very distinguished oculist and surgeon, Dr. W. Mackenzie, of Glasgow, has reviewed the matter in an historical point of view, contesting the discovery of the muscle with Dr. Horner, and restoring it to Du Verney, to whom the merit of having first described it evidently belongs. This called my attention again to the muscle; and as both the descriptions of Du Verney and of Dr. Horner are inaccurate, conveying to the student of anatomy and physiology a false notion of the shape, extent, uses, and connection of the muscle with the orbicularis, I have thought it worth while to submit the following brief observations.

In 1805, Rosenmüller gave a drawing of the muscle, and a method of dissecting it. There can be no objection made to his method of display, but the drawing is very imperfect. He recommends the eyelids to be cut from the edge of the orbits, and laid down over the nose, and of course towards the opposite side : the membrana nictitans comes in view, which is then to be dissected off; below it will be found a quantity of fat, cellular substance, and nervous filaments, with a firm though delicate fascia of cellular membrane covering the surface of the muscle. On removing this with the scalpel, a muscle of the size stated by Rosenmüller comes into view; it arises as if fleshy, and at once from the back of the os unguis, or where that bone meets the orbitar plate of the ethmoid, and proceeding forward and outward (but forward and inward as looked at during the dissection), soon divides into two portions, proceeding to the inner surface of the tarsal cartilages. Now instead of stopping at the puncta lachrymalia, as described by Rosenmüller, and as is represented in his drawings, and as is described, I presume, by most anatomists of the day, the bifurcated muscle runs on quite to the opposite extremity of the eyelids, thus doubling that part of the sphincter coming from the upper and lower part of the tendo oculi, and forming in itself the more immediate and most powerful part of the sphincter of the eyelids. This at least is what I have often seen.

By this arrangement the sphere of action of the muscle, when fully developed, is much more extended than is generally supposed. It supports the eyelids, draws them forcibly towards the inner canthus, and in the most efficient way, being bound down by cellular substance to the lachrymal sac, retains the eyelids in apposition to the eyeball, which no part of the orbicularis, as it is now arranged, could have done. Relaxation of the eyelids may depend, I imagine, on a relaxed condition of this muscle; and that peculiar and contracted condition of the eyelids, which every surgeon must have observed in some persons subject to ophthalmia with inversion of the eyelids, in all probability may depend occasionally on a spasmodic state of this muscle.

I ought to have added, that there is a very good description of the tensor tarsi in the French translation of Meckel's Anatomy.

ON VIVISECTION.

By ROBERT HULL, M.D.

(For the London Medical Gazette.)

I FIND a recent author, who is in every respect to be treated with attention—from his honourable personal character and his didactic position—making the following excuse for the infernal practice of vivisection ; *videlicet*—

"The surgeon's hand becomes tutored to act with steadiness, while he is under the influence of the natural abhorrence of giving pain to the subject of experiment, and he himself is thus schooled for the severer ordeal of operating on the human frame."

Now against such a reason for vivisection, I deem it a duty to enter a most solemn protest.

If young men are to learn steadiness of hand, whilst torturing animals, that they may be "schooled" to steadiness when they have to inflict pain on human patients, they become not chirurgeons but carnifices.

Is it meant that the tyro should vanquish his natural terror at pain-giving ? or that, the terror remaining, the hand should get steady in spite of it ? In either sense, *this* advocacy of vivisection is as unreasonable as it is unfeeling.

As to a victory over the natural abhorrence, the surgeon ought never to lose his sympathies; it is the feeling horror at the infliction of pain that induces him to master the science of anatomy, that he may cut his living subject as precisely and as quickly as he can. No superfluous incision; no protracted agony! His very sympathy with the *pained* victim tends to give him steadiness and dispatch. The softer his heart, the rapider his hand.

The most slow, nay bungling operators, that I have ever witnessed, have been cold-hearted, unfeeling men. They have carved and sliced the living organs, as they would the nonsentient corpse. Is not our natural abhorrence from giving pain implanted for reasonable purposes? Intended to make us treat others as ourselves would like to be treated? The more the operator *feels*, the more science, dexterity, dispatch, he will bring to the case of his fellow man.

"Natural," indeed, is our abhorrence, and this very circumstance might induce a tormentor to desist, and examine the propriety of his conduct. Considering this instinctive horror at mutilation as implanted by the great spirit of the universe for wise purposes, he might ask himself, when meditating torture, whether, in the particular instance, sobriety of views, a judicious selection of his miserable victim, an *imperative* demand on science, justify his process? No torture, save what is *needful*, can be approved by the great *Father* of his sensitive creatures. Is this or that particular experiment *needful?* If not, the manipulator is guilty of barbarity, of murder-like conduct. If needful, who is he that says so? The apprentice? The student? The young chirurgeon? The *unread* man? Prove, sirs, the *necessity*, before you dare to torture a being quite as deserving protection and happiness as yourselves!

If it be meant to say that no attempt should be made to eradicate our native tenderness; but that the sentiments subsisting, the mere hand should be made steady on the brute sufferer; such a disciple had better not aim at surgery; having commenced, he had best leave the profession. Nature has never intended him for it! Nature intends that steadiness of hand should result from clearness of head and benevolence of heart; that we might master the studies, before we commenced the practice. His heart informs the surgeon of the great misery he *must* inflict; his head instructs him not to make it greater than needful; and in exact proportion as he is fitted by his anatomical skill, will he approach his patient with steadiness of hand. Conscious skill is the true source of steadiness; not the mere acquirement of a *habit* of hearing with callosity the cries of the wounded. If he cannot boast *this* steadiness, and still must cut, let him take to sculpture! In this art his slowest incisions will bring him nearest to humanity. The marble will do him credit; and he *may* come to be classed with Pygmalion, Canova, and Chantrey. To me it is not unquestionably established that any of the great discoveries in surgery have been *essentially* connected with vivisection: that the results could not have been worked out by other and innocent processes. But, admitting that the grand discoveries by unquestionable philosophers could never have been effected without animal agony, I protest most vehemently against the mutilation of God's *feeling* creatures by boys, by students, by unphilosophical hands.

The Earl of Carnarvon, in a speech at the last general meeting of the Royal Society for the Prevention of Cruelty to Animals, gave utterance to sentiments which do him infinite honour—which add immense splendour and richness to his coronet and ermine. Let the chirurgic operator peruse this speech, and subscribe to that society! Let him see how the world at large is opening its eyes to the practices of the cruel experimenters; nor fancy any longer that the frightful howlings of their pitiful victims are muffled within the walls of the anatomical slaughterhouse! "I have," says this noble nobleman, "high professional authority for believing, that in an immense majority of instances those inhuman operations are performed for the sole purpose of illustrating what has already been established, or in an idle attempt to obtain results, which the extreme anguish and disturbances of system created in the unhappy victim by these operations, prevent men from attaining.

I do not wish to harrow up your feelings, or to work on them more than is necessary to impress you with the necessity of ultimately looking to legislative remedies for the correction of these monstrous abuses. Nor is it only for the sake of the victims that the legislature should interfere; they are bound to rescue the youth of England, who are intended for the profession of surgery, from such contaminating scenes; so horrible, that no religious parent could bear to see his child exposed to them.

I will read you a letter which comes from a distinguished gentleman of Germany. It refers to a work published a few months ago, alluding to a case of the kind I have just recorded, and which was justly stigmatised in one of our reviews as hellish."

[Here the letter was read, expressing abhorrence of vivisection, as pursued in England, and of the facts detailed respecting Sir Astley Cooper, in the Life recently published; concluding with Abernethy's opinion, that no medical man, who could be guilty of such practices to animals, was fit to attend a family.]

" Most fully do I coincide," said the feeling nobleman; most deeply do I coincide with him: and in language stronger than any which has been used, I fain would clothe my expressions. But what language can find a stronger term than "hellish;" and this is the language of the Quarterly Review; that glorious publication, which has always advocated the proprieties and virtues; which has thus openly declared itself against vivisection; and which cannot fail, supported as it is by writers of manly hearts and clear heads, to exhibit the zoicides to British scorn and horror.

The horrid practice of vivisection, according to one philosopher, is more important than common mortals can imagine.

" Shall it be said that the objects of physiological science are not worth the sacrifice of a few animals? Men are constantly forming the most erroneous estimates. Of what importance is it now whether Antony or Augustus filled the imperial chair? What will it matter, a few centuries hence, whether England or France swept the ocean with her fleets? But mankind will always be interested in the great truths deducible from physiologic experiments." Oh yes! The names of fiendish

vivisectors will be applauded when those of Antony and Augustus, Nelson and Wellington, are pronounced no more:—*but not till then.*

The vivisectors have never made out an undeniable justification of their revolting practices. Until they do, and on them lies the burthen, they have, whether or not they feel it, the settled dislike of mankind; nobody permitting to them the unreproved boast—

ἐκ τῶν γὰρ αἰσχρῶν ἐσθλὰ μηχανώμεθα.

Norwich, Sept. 1843.

DR. WIGAN ON TINEA CAPITIS.

To the Editor of the Medical Gazette.

Sir,

Having recently been in correspondence with Dr. Wigan on the subject of that obnoxious and very intractable disease, tinea capitis, he has favoured me with the following statement of the method he pursues.

Desirous that a mode of treatment professing to be uniformly successful, should be extensively tested, I have obtained his sanction to publishing his letter. Should it attract attention, he will, I have no doubt, furnish a fuller detail; but his present impression seems to be, that no one can obtain notice unless he possess a public appointment.—I am, sir,

Your obedient servant,
Thomas Willis, M.D.

20, Old Steine, Brighton.
August 30, 1843.

Dear Sir,—To give a full answer to your queries as to my treatment of tinea capitis, would require a pamphlet instead of a letter—at least, if I were to enter into all the minute characteristics by which the disease is distinguished, the degree and mode of its propagation, and the combinations by which it is often mystified.

I waive, therefore, all these considerations for the present, and suppose the disease to be clearly recognised. When this is the case, I do not hesitate to say that there is no other mode of treatment which can be compared with mine for certainty, rapidity, and absence of collateral or consequent inconveniences, and I have seen, I believe, all modes, as well of the Continent, as of Great Britain and Ireland. If any faith is to be placed in firm convictions, I am exempt from prejudice, but as this is every man's opinion of himself, I only put it forth *(quantum valeat)* as presumptive evidence that my mind was not lightly made up.

My plan, although never published (in the usual sense of the term), was made known by me many years ago to some hundreds of medical men in London and its environs; but I really believe that the absolute terms in which I spoke of instantly curing a disease which has for ages been the *opprobrium medicorum*, indisposed the great majority to put faith in my statements, and to give the plan a trial; because it sounded so like quackery.

My mode is this—

Unless the quantity of hair on the head is exceedingly small and offers no obstacle to the complete examination of the skin, I insist on the head being shaved very carefully, twice.

The reason is obvious: with a moderate quantity of hair you may be curing the parts which first attract notice, while others which have been infected are gradually progressing to a visible disease, and the cure is thus indefinitely prolonged. I do not, however, object to a little circlet of hair round the face, if there be no sign of disease apparent in it, and if it be carefully washed with hot common vinegar. This is a concession to parental vanity which may be safely made, and without which sometimes it would be impossible to obtain confidence.

My remedy is Beaufoy's *concentrated* acetic acid—pyroligneous acid, as it is still called—though no longer made from wood.

As a preliminary, however, I use the acid diluted with three times its weight of water. I call this the detector acid. On its application a number of spots which looked perfectly healthy become red patches. They are indications that infection had been taken, but had not gone through its stages, which period I believe (after great experience), to be eight days. This assertion is not lightly hazarded.

Having by this reconnaissance ascertained the numbers and position of your enemy, your course is clear. One vigorous assault, and there is an end of the matter. With a piece of fine sponge either tied to the end of a stick or held in a pair of silver sugar-tongs, I imbue each spot thoroughly with the concentrated acid for the space of three or four minutes, and the business is finished.

The only reason why it is necessary to see the patient again, is, that as a crust is generally formed, and an appearance of "worsening" takes place, the friends require to have their confidence renewed from time to time by explanation and encouragement. I have often applied the acid more than once, but it was always (I firmly believe) unnecessary, when the preliminaries above stated had been gone through properly upon the *shaved* and *tested* head.

The crust gradually grows up with the hair, which soon sprouts again if the eruption be recent, and as soon as a pair of fine scissors can be inserted underneath, it should be removed; but this should not be done prematurely, lest a sore place be produced.

When first proposed, a good deal of correspondence took place respecting the plan with those who had tried it without success. I found, however, that in *every case* they had either used a much weaker acid (it is sold of all strengths), or that they had continued the use of it long after the disease was cured, and thus produced that not very rare result, "*disease of the Doctor.*" In the latter cases it was only necessary to discontinue the acid, and wash the head with warm water.

It is so difficult in the present day to attract notice to any plan of treatment, the result of common sense and experience, unless accompanied by a plausible theory, that I quite despair of obtaining attention, were I to publish my sentiments on this subject. I introduced nearly twenty years ago a German invention (if so simple a contrivance deserves the name), by which a man with broken leg is enabled the same day that it has been put into order to move in and out of bed without any assistance, and without the slightest risk of displacement. It is not adopted by any but those who have seen it in use; and to this day patients are allowed to linger weeks or months in the rheumatic gout, with frequent metastasis to heart, loss of its elasticity, hypertrophy, water in the chest or pericardium, to terminate in a painful death, who might not have been cured in twenty-four hours by a remedy simple, safe, and *certain*, which I published ten years ago, and from the use of which no ill consequences have ever resulted.

Had I done nothing more for my fellow-creatures than this, I have not lived in vain. I consider that my mode of treating rheumatic gout, introduced after a long, careful, and discriminating attention, much thought, and cautious experiment, is as great a benefaction to society (compared with the smaller numbers of the sufferers) as vaccination itself.

This boast, which would have been indecorous and ridiculous while I was in practice, may be pardoned now.

No man can obtain attention in the present day unless he possess a public appointment, or be connected with a Medical School.—I am, my dear sir,

Yours very truly,

A. L. WIGAN.

The complications of tinea capitis with other diseases of the scalp produce a few and slight modifications of the treatment, especially the common eruption, porrigo favosa; but even this is often a very simple eruption, and will get well without aid.

ON

BRONCHIAL BLENORRHŒA, &c.

CONSIDERED IN CONNECTION WITH RHEUMATISM.

By R. R. CHEYNE, SURGEON.

(*For the London Medical Gazette.*)

THE metastasis of diseased actions is one of the most curious and interesting subjects that can occupy the attention of the practitioner of medicine, whether we class it in reference either to the treatment or to the pathology of disease. The phenomena of this phenomenon may be, in general terms, attributed to the operation of the functions of the nerves and to the sympathy, supposed to exist, between similar and different organs and the same, but yet it must be admitted that the cause which regulates such hints

tions from one mere usual course of disease are ill-defined and obscure.

Gout and rheumatism seem to be remarkably prone to transfer the morbid action in which they consist to the fibrous and mucous tissues, and the diagnostic powers we possess are often called forth to enable us to discover the real disease under the strange mask it assumes. Rheumatic affections of the fibrous tissues, such as those of the periosteum, pericardium, pleura, diaphragm, dura mater, and sclerotic coat of the eye, are, it is well known, exceedingly common, both as primary affections and as the result of metastasis: and it is a well-recognized principle in practice that they require a mixed treatment, viz. that of rheumatism, combined with the antiphlogistic, when inflammation exists, which, it must be borne in mind, is here much altered in character by the rheumatic diathesis. My own opinion is, that the term inflammatory is often very vaguely applied to many of these affections, and that infinite mischief may be done in omitting to follow the indications afforded by their specific nature.

The latter remark will bear still more forcibly upon that peculiar irritation of one or more of the several tracts of mucous membrane which from time to time is set up, whilst the system is struggling (if I may use the expression) to throw off an attack of rheumatism or gout. The result of this struggle may be, in one case, the development of bronchitis; in another, of dyspepsia or diarrhœa; and in a third, of irritation of the genito-urinary mucous membrane. But, whatever the form of the secondary disorder, it must, if possible, be traced to its cause, otherwise the treatment we adopt cannot fail to be empirical and inefficient. It is not, however, always easy to unravel the intricacies of these perplexing cases, and it is fortunate that nature now and then gives us a broad hint, which serves to guide us out of the path of error, and directs us how to prescribe for our patient with the greatest precision and success.

The above remarks may properly introduce the subject of this paper.

My observation has been for some time past turned upon a well-marked form of what may be called bronchial blenorrhœa, which is clearly dependent upon the metastasis of rheumatism, or, at least, upon the rheumatic diathesis, and which is as clearly unconnected with bronchitis. As this affection, as far as I know, has not been described, I will sketch a case which, in most respects, may be considered a type of the whole class; and, at the same time, I will point out the remedies which, in my hands, have been strikingly and uniformly beneficial.

CASE.—Mr. B., æt. about 60, a strong healthy man, whose occupation exposed him, for many hours daily, to a very high temperature, and subjected him constantly to profuse perspirations, became in June last affected with troublesome cough, without expectoration or dyspnœa. His pulse was natural, and skin cool; his appetite was deficient; he became weak and out of spirits, perspired profusely at night, and passed little urine, which was loaded with the lithates. At the end of a week he began to expectorate large quantities of muco-purulent fluid, without relief to his cough; he got weaker, and lost flesh; so much so, that his friends feared consumption, to which view of the case, however, auscultation gave the negative, inasmuch as, at first, no morbid condition whatever could be detected, and it was only when free secretion was taking place that rhonchi could be heard shifting about in every ramification of the air-tubes. Besides, percussion elicited a clear sound over the whole of the chest. Now, the treatment of this patient, during a fortnight, consisted in the application of a blister, the use of mild doses of mercury and ipecacuanha until the gums were slightly touched, and of occasional opiates at night to relieve the cough; at the same time the diet was strictly regulated. This plan, which was steadily pursued, failed in controlling the symptoms. My patient was then sent a few miles into the country, where I continued to visit him daily; and (as the enormous expectoration was producing great debility, and there was a total freedom from fever), I changed the treatment, and prescribed quinine with iron, and a liberal diet. Nevertheless, the disease still defied the remedies, after three weeks' duration. I must confess I was now puzzled, until *one morning I found my patient complaining of an attack of severe* pain in

the ankle-joint, which was not accompanied by either swelling or redness; and, in addition, I then learnt that he had been for a year or two occasionally subject to pain and slight puffy swelling of the right knee-joint, though never to the degree of confining him to his house. He now, also, recalled to mind, that he had felt great weakness in the knee, but not in the ankle, just before his present illness. These invaluable hints of the true origin of the complaint I was not slow to act upon. I at once ordered for him a pill composed of two grains of the acetous extract of colchicum, and three grains of the compound extract of colocynth, to be taken at night, as an aperient; and, in the course of twenty-four hours, a mixture containing of Iodide of Potassium ℈j., of liquor Potassæ, and Tincture of Henbane aa. ʒj. in Mist. Camph. ʒvj. He was also directed to place his feet every night and morning in a hot mustard and water bath.

In so short a period as three days, under these remedies, the bronchial blenorrhœa was reduced to half its former quantity, and at the end of a week it had ceased altogether. Soon afterwards his cough left him; and his health and strength were rapidly restored.

Two facts may, I think, be fairly deduced from the history of this case; viz. first, that a peculiar irritation of the bronchial mucous membrane, with profuse secretion, constituting a distinct kind of bronchial blenorrhœa, may be induced by the rheumatic diathesis; and secondly, that iodide of potassium (as in the above formula) is, undoubtedly, a medicine of astonishing power over this state of the mucous membrane. I may add, that colchicum, in my hands, has frequently proved to be of greatly inferior efficacy.

I can, certainly, come to no other conclusion but that the description I have given of the above disease cannot, with any regard to accuracy, be identified with that of any form of bronchitis, unless the latter term be used, without the least reference to the actual symptoms.

Having thus endeavoured to shew, by analysis, the existence of a rheumatic form of bronchial blenorrhœa, I will now, in order to make the evidence as conclusive as I can, examine the subject, by a method

like that of syuthesis, in briefly alluding to a class of morbid phenomena,
often excited in another tract of mucous
membrane; viz. the genito-urinary,
which phenomena clearly evince the
close connection that obtains between
either irritation, or simple discharge
from that membrane, and the development of rheumatism, in individuals who
possess the rheumatic diathesis. For
example, gonorrhœa, urethral blenorrhœa, and even the irritation and discharge sometimes brought on by the
passage of a bougie (as I have again,
and again witnessed), may be excitants
of rheumatism. Leucorrhœa, also, is
often attended by the same complication, especially in the form of neuralgia,
to which young women are extremely
predisposed. Lastly, I may observe,
that, for the supervention of rheumatism, it is by no means necessary that
this irritation, and increased secretion,
be of a specific nature, as in gonorrhœa. It was with reference to what
has been named gonorrhœal rheumatism, that Swediaur*, who first noticed
it, asks the question, whether in such
cases, gonorrhœa is not rather arthritic
than syphilitic; and I am, myself,
almost disposed to agree with Richter†,
and others, who attribute some forms
of these discharges to transferred rheumatic action.

43, Berners Street.
Sept. 7, 1843.

TUMOR OF THE PHARYNX,

To the Editor of the Medical Gazette.
  SIR,

SHOULD you consider the brief outlines
of the following case sufficiently interesting, their insertion in your valuable journal will much oblige
      Your obedient servant,
          CHARLES DEAZELEY.
Late Demonstrator of Anatomy,
   Westminster Hospital.

Mrs. H——, the wife of a military
officer, having suffered for a long
period from a dull aching pain in the
head, extending down the neck to the
chest, and often producing fainting
and insensibility, requested me to examine her throat, as she said it was

* Traité des Mal. Syphilitiques, tom. ii. ch. vii.
† Chir. Bibl. b. iv. p. 506.

becoming so narrow that she could
neither breathe nor swallow without
extreme pain and difficulty.

On examination, I found a tumor
about the size of a small strawberry,
which it somewhat resembled in appearance, growing from the back of the
pharynx, about opposite the third cervical vertebra, and to a great extent
diminishing the passage for the food
to the stomach. When seized by the
forceps, it felt firmly attached and
unyielding, leading me to suppose that
it originated from, or adhered to, the
body of one of the vertebræ; it was
evidently not a polypus, from the hardness of its structure, and the force
required to move it with the forceps.
I applied the lunar caustic to its surface for a few days, under the use of
which it appeared rather to increase,
and certainly to become much more
painful. I then resolved to remove it
cum ferro. Having the head made
steady by the aid of an assistant, and
depressing the tongue by means of a
broad spatula, I was enabled to see the
tumor distinctly, and with one sweep
of a long bistoury to remove it completely from its attachment, which was
done as nearly as possible to its connexion with the vertebra. It required
considerable force to cut through the
base, which communicated to the
touch a sensation similar to that experienced when cutting through bone
in a state of caries. The tumor, however, was not of the latter description,
but rather of a fibro-cartilaginous
nature, with gritty particles of ossific
matter developed in its interior. The
operation caused but little hæmorrhage,
and the application of the argenti
nitras occasionally for a few days subdued the irritation and produced complete cicatrization. More than six
months have now elapsed since the
operation, and there is not the slightest
appearance of the tumor returning. It
is worthy of remark that prior to the
removal of the tumor the lady suffered
very often from fainting fits, for which
every medicine prescribed was only
of temporary benefit; but since, the
fits or headache have not returned, and
she enjoys excellent health, often
facetiously amusing her friends by
relating the anecdote of a doctor having
cut her throat to save her life.

I think it very probable that the
swooning and headache, which were

always worse after eating, may have arisen from the pressure of the tumor, in the efforts to swallow, on the numerous filaments of the sympathetic nerve with which it must have come in contact. It is true, the difficult respiration might account for the other symptoms, and *vice versâ*. Certain it is, however, that since the tumor has been removed the paroxysms have ceased.

MEDICAL GAZETTE.

Friday, September 15, 1843.

" Licet omnibus, licet etiam mihi, dignitatem *Artis Medicæ* tueri; potestas modo veniendi in publicum sit, dicendi periculum non recuso."

CICERO.

A LATE INQUEST IN THE NORTH.

WE have been favoured with copies of the Carlisle Patriot and the Carlisle Journal of the 2d instant, both giving an account of an inquest held just before their publication, at Beaumont, near Carlisle. So great an interest has been excited by this inquiry that the Patriot devotes eight columns to its report, and the Journal five. This interest is of a medico-political stamp. It appears that a feud has long raged among the practitioners of Carlisle, and the grave of James Clark is the battle-field of the contending factions.

The mere dry facts, or skeleton of the case, are as follows.

James Clark, a countryman, æt. 50, was admitted an out-patient of the Carlisle Infirmary in October 1842. On the 14th of December, he was made an in-patient, and was discharged January 11th, 1843. He then returned to Beaumont, his usual residence, where he remained without advice till the month of April. He was then attended by some practitioners from Carlisle (not those of the Infirmary) grew worse and worse, and died August 25th. He was buried on the 27th; on the 28th his grave was just opened, so that the jury might take a

glance at his body, for form's sake; and the inquest was held on the 28th and 31st. The jury found that the deceased had laboured under rheumatism and disease of the hip-joint; that he had died of the latter; and that he had been properly treated.

So much for the broad features of the history, which we give to serve as a general guide to what follows; the interest of the case depends, of course, on the minuter and more controverted facts.

James Clark, when admitted as an out-patient, was labouring under rheumatism and disease of the hip-joint. But though *morbus coxarius* was set down by Dr. Barnes, his physician, as one of his diseases, its symptoms do not appear to have been very prominent; had they been so, indeed, it is reasonable to suppose that the patient would have been placed under the care of the surgeon of the hospital, rather than the physician. During Clark's attendance as an out-patient, he was bled, cupped, blistered, and rubbed with tartar emetic ointment, and took a dose of Epsom salts and one of Dover's powder. A mixture of spirits of turpentine was also given internally. During this period of eight weeks the patient used to go from Beaumont to Carlisle once a week in a cart, and return the same day. Had his disease been in an advanced stage this would have been impossible.

He was now admitted into the Infirmary, where he remained four weeks.

The ticket placed at the patient's bed-head, on which the prescriptions were entered, has not been preserved; but the Physician's Register, kept by the House-Surgeon, contains the following abstract of it.

" 1843, No. 8. James Clark, aged 50, married; residence, Beaumont; occupation, labourer; date of admission, Dec. 14, 1842; date of discharge, Jan. 11, 1843; disease, rheumatism,

&c.; relieved; treatment, quinine, cupping; subscriber's name, Mr. Thurnam."

Besides the treatment mentioned in this abstract, Clark took calomel and Dover's powder, and the house-surgeon thinks he also had blisters.

While Clark was in the Infirmary, repose was not insisted upon. Dr. Barnes desired him to keep his bed a good deal; but as he said that the heat of the bed increased his pain, he was allowed to sit up. As Dr. Barnes found neither enlargement of the hip-joint, nor matter in its cavity, nor ulceration of the cartilages, he allowed the patient to walk about. Clark liked to walk about, though it gave him pain to do so. Was this permission to walk warrantable ? *Judicent peritiores.* The witnesses against the Infirmary doctors lay much stress on perfect rest as the most essential part of the treatment of *morbus coxarius.* The authorities are, no doubt, with them; yet there are exceptions to this great rule. Thus, when delivering the treatment of inflammation of the synovial membranes of joints, Sir Benjamin Brodie says, "The chronic inflammation is relieved more slowly. In the first instance the joint should be kept in a state of perfect quietude."

But soon after we read, that "when the inflammation is in great measure relieved, a moderate degree of exercise of the joint is beneficial rather than otherwise*."

Whether the disease, in Clark, had reached this favourable turning-point, may, of course, be a matter of doubt. Another question which, if solved, would throw light on this difficulty, is the one, was Clark relieved when discharged from the Infirmary on the 11th of January? Had the four weeks' walking in the wards of the Carlisle Infirmary made him better or worse?

* *Pathological and Surgical Observations on the Diseases of the Joints,* 3d edit. pp. 35 and 37.

There is plenty of evidence to show that he was better, some to show that he was just the same, none to say that he was worse.

All the formal or official evidence goes to prove that he was better. The Physician's Register, as we have seen, says "relieved." Mr. Page, surgeon to the Infirmary, deposes that Clark, on his discharge, said to the Committee that he was much better. Mrs. Masterman, matron of the Infirmary, says, "he thanked me for my attention, and very grateful he was. He expressed himself as better. I think he was better. When he first came, he required help to get up the steps; when he went out, he had only the aid of his sticks. He was less lame than when he entered. I used to say to him he altered as the weather altered."

Grace Reay, who was a nurse in the Infirmary when Clark was an in-patient, deposes, that when he left he told her he was much better than when he came.

John Davidson, a pensioner, and an intimate acquaintance of Clark, used to conduct him to the infirmary as an out-patient, helped him up the stairs when he was taken into the house, and received him when he came out. Clark told Davidson that he was much better when he left the infirmary than when he went in. "He was not so much better as he would like.."

John Graham deposes, that when Clark came out of the Infirmary he said he was easier.

The Rev. Robert Robinson, the clergyman of the parish, deposes that thanks were returned in the church for the relief obtained by James Clark in the Cumberland Infirmary. Moreover, Clark attended church once or twice after being at the Infirmary, and told Mr. Robinson that he thought himself a little better.

The parish clerk deposes that he got the paper (of thanks) which he gave to

Mr. Robinson, either from Clark or his wife.

Per contra there are four witnesses. The first is the widow of the deceased, who deposes that when he left the Infirmary he did not feel himself any better; and that he informed her that he had told Dr. Barnes that he did not think he had got any benefit, and might as well go home as not.

Secondly, James Sewell, of Beaumont, farmer, deposes that he saw Clark shortly after his return from the infirmary, and he was much the same as when he went. "Some of our folk told me (I was not there myself) that James Clark had returned thanks in the church to Almighty God for being relieved at the infirmary; and I was uncommonly hurt at this, because he was not a bit better."

When this honest husbandman was told that returning thanks was only a form, he replied: "let us be duin with forms and ceremonies, and give us the reality o't thing." He adds, in his evidence, that Clark "was not a stroke better when he returned from the infirmary."

. It is impossible not to sympathize with this sturdy Cumbrian farmer in his contempt for shams and flams; let us hope that the coming age may be blessed with many such reformers!

Thirdly, Thomas Todhunter, who lives in the village of Beaumont, and was a near neighbour of Clark's, saw him on the night of his return from the infirmary, and he was no better than when he went.

Lastly, John Hodgson, surgeon, of Carlisle, was told by the deceased that the doctors of the infirmary had done him no good.

How shall we balance this conflicting evidence? Probably, James Clark, when he left the infirmary, was substantially in the same condition as when he entered it; yet for a day or two he might enjoy sufficient ease to

give him the hope of recovery. In a genial or polite moment he might return thanks to his doctors; in his candid hours (no longer a hero to his *valet de chambre*) he might confess that he had not improved, and might exclaim, as he did, while an out-patient, to frank farmer Sewell, that "there was no betterness for him in this world."

The remainder of the history we must dispatch briefly.

We do not hear anything farther of the progress of the case until Easter Sunday, when he was seen by Mr. Hodgson.

On that day Clark hobbled after him on two sticks, said he was rapidly getting worse, and that he would be glad if Mr. Hodgson or any of his medical friends could do anything for him.

On the 27th of April, Clark was visited by Dr. Jackson and Mr. Elliott, of Carlisle, and he was seen again by Mr. Hodgson in the beginning of May. "He was in bed: there was a large abscess discharging from the front of the thigh—the limb was shortened an inch and a half. There was great pain on the slightest motion. Matter was spreading among the muscles of the thigh, so that when the lower part of the thigh was pressed, matter came out at the anterior and upper part of the thigh."

About this time a seton was put in his groin, and pus was freely evacuated. "Many gallons of matter ran from the wound," says his wife; meaning, of course, during the seventeen weeks that the patient was confined to his bed. After his discharge from the infirmary, he was not seen by any of the medical officers of the institution, excepting on the day of his death, by the house-surgeon.

It would be difficult to affirm that the treatment of Clark in the infirmary was the most vigorous that the case admitted, *especially now that we know its subsequent progress.* It would be still more difficult to conclude that the treatment was very bad, considering the age of the patient, and want of prominence in the symptoms ; and also recollecting that he went out at least as well as he came in; but it would be most difficult, and almost impossible, to believe that this inquest could have taken place, had it not been for the internecine war waged by the medical men of Carlisle. Whether it befits practitioner to pick holes so eagerly in the coat of his brother practitioner, we leave to the good sense and good feeling of our readers.

THE CARLISLE CONTROVERSY.

SINCE writing the above, we have received the Carlisle papers of Saturday, the 9th inst. We subjoin a couple of extracts; and, to make the matter clearer to our readers, we add the following elucidations.

The Infirmary at Carlisle was founded about two years ago, and at the present moment contains twenty patients. Dr. Barnes is the physician, Mr. Page the surgeon, and Mr. Burch the house-surgeon. In the present controversy, and, we believe, in the feuds which preceded it, the Carlisle Patriot has taken the side of the medical officers of the Infirmary, while the Carlisle Journal has espoused the cause of the critical lookers-on.

Mr. Steel, editor of the Carlisle Journal, is a governor of the Infirmary, and a chief promoter of the attack on the present officers.

The Patriot, on the other hand, calls the discontented practitioners " Medical Trades Unionists," and can see errors in them alone. The supposed facts, therefore, of the two journals, and the arguments built upon them, must be taken with some grains of allowance.

The first two extracts are from a letter by Mr. Steel to the Bishop of Carlisle.

From the Carlisle Journal of Sept. 9th.

" And first as to the inquest. It has been said that it was " an investigation without a parallel in this or any other country." If this had been an assertion founded in ignorance, the writer might have some claim upon our pity; but when put forth as a wilful perversion of well-known facts, loathing and contempt are the only feelings excited by it. Inquests on persons suspected to have " died of the doctor" are of common, almost every-day occurrence, as must be well known to every reader of the daily journals or works of medical jurisprudence. Then Mr. Nanson, who appeared before the coroner as the advocate of the governors—though what advocacy *they* required I am at a loss to conceive—appeared to think he had made a great point when Dr. Jackson and Mr. Elliott candidly admitted that *they* had called upon the coroner to hold the inquest; and I am aware that attempts have been made to treat this act of theirs as little less than a crime. My Lord, they who thus speak have surely forgotten all that has passed, or are wilfully blind to what has been passing under their noses. If Dr. Jackson and Mr. Elliot had not taken steps to call for an inquest, they must have been content to sit down under the stigma of having been accessory to the death of James Clark. At the public meeting of the governors of the Infirmary, held on the 1st of August, at which your Lordship so ably presided, Dr. Barnes made this statement:—

" ' It might well be said he (Clark) was relieved. When he came to the Infirmary he could not walk, but when he left it he could walk well. *He had since that been operated upon by other medical gentlemen :* when he left the Infirmary he was rapidly recovering, and walking about; but SINCE OTHER MEDICAL GENTLEMEN ATTENDED HIM, *he was now in bed and in great danger.*' "

From the Carlisle Journal of Sept. 9th.

" Three medical men connected with the infirmary were examined. Dr. Barnes, the physician, says Clark was labouring under rheumatism and disease of the hip-joint. Mr. Page, the surgeon, swears it was debility, rheumatism, and disease of the hip-joint. Mr. Burch, the house surgeon, looked upon it as rheumatism alone—he so records it on the only records kept, and it appears never to have struck him that Dr. Barnes was treating the patient for anything else.—This is confirmed by the nurse, who says she applied blisters to the man's *knee* by Mr. Burch's direction. Mr. Page's evidence, to be sure, can go for very little, for he seems to be wonderfully oblivious of everything connected with the case. He might have seen him, or he might not have seen him—it is probable he saw him—it is probable he treated him —*but he has no entry of him in his book.* My Lord, is this the practice of the Infirmary, which gives the Committee "full confidence" in the "ability and attention" of their medical officers? A patient enters labouring under the most dangerous of all surgical diseases—and his case is never entered in the surgeon's book!

The patient says he was first seen by Mr. Page, who ordered him a blister on the *knee*, thus showing that he entirely mistook the nature of his complaint— and then turned him over to Dr. Barnes, the physician—thus affording another proof that he had either not examined the man as he ought, or that he was unable to distinguish between the cause of disease and its symptoms. Your Lordship will doubtless think this still more strange, after hearing Mr. Page declare that he (a young gentleman with a year and a half's practice) had seen "hundreds of cases of hip-joint disease"—a degree of good fortune to a practitioner which, I shall venture to say, was never enjoyed by Sir Benjamin Brodie himself, in all his long experience*. But the truth is, my Lord, Mr. Page's evidence proves nothing— except that he turned his patient over to his colleague as a *medical* case, and that his colleague immediately entered the man as labouring under a *surgical disease!*" "When I left I said to Dr. Barnes I think I'll go out, for I am getting no better, and if I was at home I could toddle about there. He said, well, if you think you are no better you may go. My leg was then as bad as ever. I thanked the gentlemen (committee) for their kindness. I got a paper from the committee to return thanks in church for being cured."

Mr. Gilkerson. — "I was in the

* Why should Mr. Steel limit Mr. Page's experience to the year and a half that he has been surgeon to the Infirmary? He must allow him the cases which occurred at the hospitals where he learned surgery.—*Ed. Med. Gazette.*

church, and heard the words 'than—— either for being cured or relieved, I am not sure which."

Patient.—"Miss Margaret Blamire called to see me after church-time, and remarked that it was odd I should return thanks for being cured, when I was no better."

Mr. Gilkerson.—"He was worse, and everybody remarked it."

From the Carlisle Patriot of Sept. 9th.

"We do not consider a general newspaper the proper medium for discussing a medical question, or we could multiply our quotations from authors of great authority to show, that, at the very least, 'doctors differ,'—but, in point of fact, we believe it will be generally understood from the evidence, that Clarke had for many years been labouring under chronic inflammation of the fibrous structures around the joint; for that there was no disease in the joint itself while the patient was in the Infirmary, is proved by Dr. Barnes and Mr. Burch, who rotated or moved the limb in every direction; and a part so labouring under chronic disease was more liable to active inflammation, which a fall or other accidental cause might set up, and which might, if unattended to, go on to the destruction of the joint. But be this as it may, we wish to press upon the attention of our readers a fact which we consider decisive as to whether Clarke's case was best understood by the officers of the Infirmary, or by Dr. Jackson and Mr. Elliott—and it is this, that the treatment adopted by Dr. Barnes aimed at *relieving* the patient, and it succeeded in accomplishing that result; but the treatment adopted by Dr. Jackson and Mr. Elliott, which also aimed at relieving the patient, did not succeed in affording him any relief, as it is distinctly stated in evidence that poor Clarke said that he never knew what pain was until subjected to the treatment they adopted.

But there remains another interpolation in the *Journal's* report, of still greater importance. With a desperate determination to save the 'Medical Trades' Unionists from the odium to which they had subjected themselves, the reporter for the *Journal* has appended to the verdict of the jury a statement that "the jury were unanimously of opinion, that the treatment of Dr. Jackson and Mr. Elliott was correct, and all that could be done for him under the circumstances." This admits of but one sort of contradiction. It is a deliberate and desperate falsehood. No such statement was made in the court; and we have ascertained, on inquiry, that no such opinion was ever expressed, or meant, or intended to be expressed by the jury."

INFLUENCE OF THE SEASONS.

THE results to which the foregoing facts and reasonings lead may be briefly stated as follows :—

1. The amount of sickness in the central districts of London during the year 1842 varied directly as the temperature, being a maximum in August, the hottest month of the year, and a minimum in January, the coldest month.

2. The diseases which determined the order of sickness were febrile and catarrhal affections, the contagious exanthemata, and the disorders of the digestive organs; to which may be added, the mixed group, consisting of gout, scrofula, &c.

3. The diseases of the organs of respiration followed the inverse order of those already mentioned, and were inversely as the temperature, being most numerous in the colder, and fewest in the hotter months.

4. The temperature did not appear to exercise a marked influence on the other classes of disease : with the exception, perhaps, of those which form a measure of the activity of the sexual passion, which were in excess during the hottest months of the year—a fact which corresponds with, and corroborates, our experience of the influence of the seasons on crimes against the person, &c.

5. The hygrometric state of the air appeared to have little effect on disease, and if it produced any effect it was on the diseases of the organs of respiration, which were in excess during the months in which the quantity of moisture in the air was the greatest; but these were also the coldest months.

6. The mortality for the metropolis during the year 1842 was greatest in the first quarter, and least in the second, and was inversely as the sickness, except that the mortality of the third quarter exceeded that of the fourth.

7. The diseases which chiefly influenced the order of the quarters in respect of mortality, were those of the chest; to which may be added, as following the same order, the decay of nature in the aged. It is well known that the most common cause of death in the aged is an affection of the lungs, called "bronchitis senilis."

8. The order of the seasons in respect of sickness and mortality differs year by year, and does not admit of being reduced to any precise rule.

9. As a general rule, but one admitting of many exceptions, it may be stated, that the amount of sickness tends to vary directly, and the amount of mortality inversely as the temperature.

These results must be received with some reserve, as they are founded on a comparatively small number of facts; but they are probably not very far from the truth. At any rate they may prove suggestive of future inquiries, founded upon a broader basis. At present the materials for a comprehensive theory of the influence of the seasons and weather upon sickness and mortality are wanting, and are not likely to be supplied till the example set by one or two public hospitals and dispensaries shall have provoked imitation. In the meantime the present attempt, if it accomplish no other purpose, may serve as an example of the mode by which such inquiries must be conducted.

In the course of this inquiry it is scarcely possible that some hypothesis should not have suggested itself as the most likely to prove true; and it may not be amiss to bring this attempt to a conclusion, by stating in few words that which I have been led to form.

The causes of sickness are twofold, consisting of atmospheric changes which may be submitted to measurement, and of certain more subtle changes in the composition of the air, which at present can neither be analysed nor estimated. To the former class belong the temperature, moisture, and pressure of the air; to the latter those emanations from the earth, or from human beings themselves, which give rise to the majority of epidemic, endemic, and contagious diseases. As the number of cases of sickness produced by these latter causes is generally considerable, the influence of the pressure, temperature, and hygrometric state of the air, will not be observed in those years in which these causes are in operation; but in the absence of epidemics, the temperature will be found to be the most influential cause of sickness. When the temperature of the summer is high, there will be such an amount of sickness in the summer months as to cause a large return of sickness for the entire year; so, on the other hand, a severe winter will swell the total sickness of the year, by producing a great excess of affections of the organs of respiration. A summer or winter of unusual length, beginning early and ending late, will also cause an increase of sickness on the entire year; but the nature of the sickness will be different as the temperature is higher or lower than usual. The order of the seasons in respect of sickness will also be mainly determined by the degree in which the temperature of these seasons exceeds, or falls short of, the average temperature.

The mortality, in like manner, in non-epidemic years will be chiefly dependent upon the temperature, varying in the several seasons inversely as the temperature, except in those years in which the summer is unusually warm, when the mortality of the summer may even exceed that of the winter season. In other instances, the mortality of the summer months will rank next to that of the winter or autumn.—*Dr. Guy, in Quarterly Journal of the Statistical Society.*

ON THE PREPARATION OF HYDRIODIC ACID.

In consequence of a remark made at a recent meeting of the Pharmaceutical Society, recommending the use of hydriodic acid in the manufacture of iodide of potassium, we have been applied to by two or three correspondents for a description of the best and easiest method by which this acid can be obtained. A correspondent, who writes from Birmingham, seems to consider the process an intricate and difficult one ; but in this opinion we do not coincide, at least with reference to the liquid acid, which of course would be used in the case alluded to. The process recommended in most chemical books consists in mixing iodine with water, placed in any suitable vessel, and passing a stream of sulphuretted hydrogen through the liquid, until the whole of the iodine has disappeared. The sulphuretted hydrogen (H S) on coming in contact with the iodine, is decomposed, the hydrogen quitting the sulphur, which is precipitated, and combining with the iodine to form hydriodic acid (H I), which is held in solution. On heating the liquid to expel free sulphuretted hydrogen, and separating the sulphur by filtration, a colourless solution of pure hydriodic acid is obtained. There is, surely, nothing complicated in this process ; it is a case of simple substitution.

In conducting the operation, there are two or three practical points to be attended to, on which the success and facility with which it is conducted will greatly depend. The iodine should be reduced to fine powder, by rubbing it down in a mortar, and in doing this it will be well to add a small quantity of the water with which it is to be mixed. The iodine (half an ounce) and water (eight ounces) are now to be placed in an open vessel, such as a beaker glass, or a cylindrical pint-measure glass, and a glass rod of suitable size provided, for the

purpose of agitating the mixture during the transmission of the gas through it.

It is necessary to have an abundant supply of the sulphuretted hydrogen gas, and the following is the best means of obtaining it :— In the first place, provide a gas generating bottle ; a six or eight ounce wide-mouthed bottle, to which is fitted a cork with a bent tube of sufficient length to reach the bottom of the vessel containing the iodine, will answer the purpose. Into this bottle put an ounce or two of sulphuret of iron, in pieces about the size of a pea. The best sulphuret of iron is made by heating a bar of iron at a blacksmith's forge, to a white or welding heat, and while the iron is at this temperature, holding a stick of roll sulphur against the end of it, over a pail of cold water. The sulphuret and warm water enter into combination, and the resulting sulphuret flows in a state of fusion into the water. This sulphuret is an indispensable item in every practical laboratory, and some of it, as above directed, should be kept in a gas-generating bottle, ready for use. On pouring a few ounces of diluted sulphuric acid into the bottle, a copious evolution of sulphuretted hydrogen takes place, which is to be conducted to the bottom of the vessel containing the iodine and water, by means of the bent tube. As the gas is thus made to pass through the mixture, the iodine should be stirred up with the glass rod from the bottom. Notwithstanding this precaution, however, it will be found difficult to keep the iodine diffused through the liquor, for the sulphur, as it separates, forms a spongy mass, in which the iodine becomes enveloped, and shielded from the action of the gas. This constitutes a practical difficulty, and indeed the only one which occurs in the operation, as it becomes necessary to continue the transmission of the gas for a much longer time than would otherwise be the case.

It is very easy to obviate this difficulty, in making the hydriodic acid for the purpose we are contemplating, namely, the employment of it in the manufacture of iodide of potassium. Instead of mixing the iodine with the water, in which case the greater part of it remains undissolved, the four drachms of iodine should be mixed with six drachms of iodide of potassium, or a sufficient quantity of the solution of iodide of potassium under operation, so as to form a clear solution. On sending the sulphuretted hydrogen gas through this solution, the decomposition is effected in a very short time, and without the slightest difficulty, the acidification of the iodine being completed in about two minutes.

The completion of the process is ascertained by the entire discolouration of the liquid; and this being effected, the gas-delivering tube is to be removed, and the acid being poured away from the remaining sulphuret of iron contained in the bottle, the latter will be for use on a subsequent occasion. We now have a solution of hydriodic acid mixed with iodide of potassium; and this may be used for neutralizing the alkalinity of the iodide of of potassium liquor; while any remaining portion, not required for this purpose, should be saturated with potash, and then added to the other liquor.—*Pharmaceutical Journal.*

OPERATIONS FOR FISSURE OF THE SOFT AND HARD PALATE.

By J. Mason Warren, M.D.

The form of operation which I have practised will be best illustrated by the relation of the first case in which it was put into execution.

The patient was a young man, 25 years old, with a congenital fissure of the soft and hard palate, the bones being separated quite up to the alveolar processes, with a deviation to the left side. On looking into the mouth, the whole posterior fauces were exposed, with the openings of the eustachian tubes and the bottom of the nasal cavity of the left side distinctly visible. The speech of the patient was rendered so indistinct by this misfortune, that it was with the greatest difficulty that he could make himself understood. Deglutition had always been imperfectly performed, liquids, particularly, being swallowed with much difficulty, and often regurgitated through the nose. At the first glance the soft parts were scarcely perceptible, being almost concealed in the sides of the throat from the action of the muscles. On being seized by a forceps they could be partially drawn out, though with great resistance. So far as any of the old methods were applicable to the relief of this extensive fissure, the patient was beyond surgical aid. I determined, however, to put in practice the operation which had before appeared to me practicable.

The patient was placed in a strong light, his mouth widely opened, and the head well supported by an assistant: with a long double-edged knife, curved on its flat side, I now carefully dissected up the membrane covering the hard palate, pursuing the dissection quite back to the root of the alveolar processes. By this process, which was not effected without considerable difficulty, the membrane seemed gradually to unfold itself, and could be easily drawn across the very wide fissure. A narrow slip was now removed from the edges of the soft palate, and with it the two halves of the uvula. By this means a continuous flap was obtained, beginning at the roots of the teeth and extending backwards to the edges of the velum palati. Finally, six sutures were introduced, on tying of which the whole fissure was obliterated. The patient was directed to maintain the most perfect quiet, and to abstain from making the slightest efforts to swallow even the mucus which collected in the throat, which was to be carefully sponged out as occasion required.

The following day he was doing well. He complained of some pain or rather sensation of excessive emptiness of the bowels, which was relieved by the use of a hot spirituous fomentation. On the third day, a slight hacking cough commenced, owing to the collection of thick ropy mucus in the throat and air-passages. The cough was temporarily relieved by an injection of a pint of oatmeal gruel into the rectum; during the night, however, it again increased so much as to tear away the upper and lower ligatures. I now allowed him to take liquid nourishment, which at once quieted the irritation in the throat. The other four ligatures were removed on the following days; the last being left until the sixth after the operation. This patient returned home into the country at the end of three weeks, a firm fleshy palate being formed behind, and half the fissure in the bony palate obliterated.

In the following spring I again operated on the remaining fissure in the hard palate, and succeeded in closing about half the extent of it; the tissues yielding with some difficulty, owing to the inflammation caused by the former operation. The small aperture which remained I directed to be closed by a gold plate. His speech was very much improved at once, as well as the powers of deglutition, and he will no doubt, ultimately, as the soft parts become more flexible, to a great degree recover the natural intonations of the voice.

Since performing this operation, I have had occasion to repeat it in thirteen different cases, which with one exception have terminated successfully, either in the closure of the whole fissure, or of both hard and soft palate, or so far that the aperture which remained in the bones could be easily closed by an obturator fitted to the adjoining teeth. Some of these cases have been exceedingly interesting.—*New England Quarterly Journal of Medicine and Surgery;* and *Dublin Journal.*

A CAUTION RESPECTING NITRIC ACID.

WE not unfrequently see prescriptions in which five or six minims of nitric acid are ordered for a dose, diffused in an ounce or an ounce and a half of fluid. This is a strong dose when the acid is of sp. gr. 1.4, as was the case with the acid generally used until lately. But since the publication of the remarks of Mr. Phillips on the subject, which drew attention to the fact that the acid ordered in the Pharmacopœia is of sp. gr. 1.504, the manufacturers have supplied the article according to the correct standard ; and the circumstance not having been sufficiently made known in the medical profession, patients have sometimes suffered from the inconvenience of taking a dose considerably stronger than was intended. In such cases we conceive it to be the duty of the pharmaceutical chemist to impart that information to the prescriber which shall enable him to regulate the dose accordingly.

The maximum dose of acidum nitricum dilutum is stated in the Pharmacopœia to be minims (equal to four minims of the forty acid) ; and we have no hesitation in stating that this quantity is quite sufficient, *unless largely diluted*, to act injuriously on the enamel of the teeth. On reference to some other authorities, we see the dose of strong nitric acid stated as " from five to ten minims ;" and on this account might have felt a delicacy in animadverting on the subject, if we had not repeatedly heard serious complaints from patients. An instance lately occurred in which six minims were taken in an ounce of fluid, three times a day. In the course of two or three days the teeth were found to be seriously injured, to the great annoyance of the medical attendant, who was not aware that he had ordered more than might be taken with perfect safety. In all cases in which it is desirable to administer large doses of this powerful acid, care should be taken to dilute it sufficiently, and the patient should be directed to rinse the mouth with water, or a solution of carbonate of potash, immediately after having taken each dose. These precautions should never be neglected, by those who consider the preservation of a good set of teeth of any importance.

We may also observe, that the strong nitric acid should never be used in dispensing in small quantities, as it is impossible to measure a few minims with so much accuracy as a proportionate quantity of the diluted acid.

Nitric acid of sp. gr. 1.504, always contains a considerable portion of nitrous acid, which gives it a pale yellow colour. The action of light and air occasions the liberation of oxygen, and the consequent conversion of a further portion of nitric into nitrous acid. According to M. Millon this is the case, more or less, with commercial nitric acid of all densities, but more particularly when highly concentrated ; consequently, the Acidum Nitricum P.L. is not a convenient preparation for general use, and should be kept in the dark, and not unnecessarily exposed to the action of the air by the frequent removal of the stopper.—*Pharmaceutical Journal.*

FLUID EXTRACT OF SENNA.
By PROFESSOR CHRISTISON.

TAKE fifteen pounds avoirdupois of Tinnevelly senna, and exhaust it with boiling water by displacement : about four times its weight of water is sufficient. Concentrate the infusion in vacuo to ten pounds ; dissolve in the product six pounds of treacle previously concentrated over the vapour-bath, till a little of it becomes nearly dry on cooling ; add twenty-four fluid ounces of rectified spirit (dens. .835) ; and, if necessary, add water to make fifteen (16 oz.) pints—the object being that the preparation shall be of such strength that every fluid ounce shall correspond to one avoirdupois ounce of senna. Mr. Duncan, of Edinburgh, generally makes eighty pounds of senna into this extract in one operation. The numbers given are those by which he worked in the first instance. The dose is two drachms for an adult; it very rarely causes griping. It tastes precisely like treacle, and the absence of disagreeable taste is owing to the fact that pure senna has but a feeble mawkish taste, which treacle easily covers.—*Pharmaceutical Journal.*

ON ROARING IN THE HORSE.

I FIND in my own practice, says Mr. Webb, and in that of others, so few cases of roaring successfully treated that, perhaps, it will not be deemed presumption on my part if I send the account of one in which I have been fortunate.

The patient, a thorough-bred chestnut stallion, was considered to be entirely useless, on account of his being a confirmed roarer. The sound was occasionally so loud that his master was ashamed to be seen driving him, and requested me to do what I could with him.

Upon careful examination of him, the seat of disease seemed to be confined to the larynx. The treatment which I adopted was to have the compound iodine ointment well rubbed into the throttle during three months.

I am glad to say that the roaring has entirely ceased. He is used in harness, and to ride ; and not the least noise can be heard.—*Veterinarian.*

NEW HERNIA KNIFE.

DR. T. CAMBELL STEWART has described in a late number of the "American Journal," a new form of knife for the purpose of dividing the stricture in cases of strangulated hernia, and said not to be open to the sources of danger attending upon the employment of the instruments commonly in use; he particularly advocates its use in cases of inguinal and crural hernia. The knife consists of a small convex blade concealed in a hollow canula, presenting at half an inch from its extremity a notch of about two lines in length, and one line deep, for receiving the membranes which constitute the structure ; the opening is closed at the top by a steel blade, presenting at one end a small shoulder, and at the other a wire spring concealed in the handle. The knife, small and convex, is strengthened by a shoulder on either side, projecting a little higher than itself, and protecting its edge from contact with the canula.

The instrument is directed to be used in the following manner :—

So soon as the sac constituting the hernia shall have been laid bare and opened, the canula containing the knife is to be introduced flat, between the intestine and the stricture ; so soon as it has entered, the instrument is turned, so as to bring its upper surface in contact with the part to be divided, and then pushing gently and cautiously onwards : after penetrating a short distance, its further progress is arrested by a small shoulder, the blade of which, however, being terminated by the spring. yields to continued pressure so far, and so far only, as may be necessary to admit the constricting membranes. These being now engaged in the excavation, the knife is made to move forwards and backwards by pushing and withdrawing a button placed beneath the handle, with the index finger of the right hand, so as to incise as much of the membranes as may be thought necessary to permit the reduction of the hernia. The structure may be thus divided, above, below, or on either side of the intestine.

SCENES ON THE NIGER.

WE were soon at Bullock's island, and about nine we reached its upper extremity. The island seemed to be swamped throughout. An egret and a few other birds were the only living things appearing on it. A short way above this a human body was seen floating downwards with the stream ; on coming near to it, we found the face downward, the nates and abdomen distended, the viscera of the latter protruding ; the hands and feet seemed blanched ; the back appeared as if it had been scorched. A band ornamented with beads crossed the loins, and a cincture round the head was similarly adorned. At twelve, the Albert entered a passage between the left bank and a group of islands in the middle of the river. This delightful passage was about four or five miles long, and varied in breadth from fifty to sixty yards, and its banks were richly clothed. The stately bombax from its enormous trunk reared its wide-spreading branches in the midst of cassiæ, and other shrubs and trees of endless variety of tint and shade. The amount of cultivation of yams, bananas, and plantains, indicated more extensive habitation than we had yet seen, with the exception of Aboh.—*Dr. Macwilliam's Medical History of the Expedition to the Niger.*

TREATMENT OF
HEMICRANIA & TIC DOULOUREUX
BY CAUTERIZING THE PALATE.
By M. DUCROS, of Marseilles.

IN the most intense hemicrania, and in the most obstinate *tic douloureux*, whether fronto-facial or temporo-facial, the pain disappears instantaneously on the application of ammonia at 25°*, to the palatine arch, by means of a [camel's-hair] brush ; the brush being allowed to remain on the part, till a copious flow of tears has been excited. I have tried this for the last three months in a very great number of cases, and the pain has always ceased. If the pain returns, a fresh application again produces a cessation of the neuralgia.—*Gazette Médicale.*

ANALYTICAL TABLES
OF THE CASES OF DISEASES TREATED AT THE INFIRMARY OF THE PARISH OF ST. MARYLEBONE FOR THE YEAR 1841.

THE chief object held in view in the arrangement of the following tables has been to show the influence of age, of sex, and of season, upon disease, as occurring amongst the pauper population of this section of the metropolis, during one year.

The first table includes the total number of the cases treated, with the exception of

---

* *i. e.* A solution of ammonia, showing 25° on Baume's hydrometer, — a specific gravity of ·906. The Liquor Ammoniæ fort. of the London College is of the sp. gr. ·882.—*Translator's Note.*

about 900, of such a nature as would only be admitted to the infirmary of a workhouse, or establishment similarly constituted. This table contains also the age, the sex, and the results of disease, at the four periods of life.

The second table shows in a more condensed form, the prevalence, and the mortality, of each class of disease, according to sex, and the period of life.

The third table comprises the whole of the cases contained in the preceding, and the rate of morta'ity, at the different quarters of the year.

The fourth table contains the gross number of patients admitted into the lying-in ward and into the infirmary in each quarter; the average number under treatment and average duration of their residence in the house; distinguishing them into medical and surgical.

An abstract of the expenditure of the establishment has been added, with the average number of patients of all classes indoor and out.

In the first table it may be observed, that the females far outnumber the male. This fact has been remarked in former years; as also that the mortality among the females is inferior to that of the former, being 1 in 6, the latter 1 in 5.3.

When we look at the different classes of disease, singular facts are presented; in those of the digestive organs, there is a preponderance of one-third on the part of females. This disproportion depended mainly on the more frequent occurrence of inflammatory affections of those organs in the female than the male, the number and the mortality of those affections being more than twice greater in the former than the latter. The tendency to diarrhœa was nearly equal in both classes, but the mortality was greatest in the males.

In the diseases of the respiratory organs the numbers were nearly alike in both sexes, but the mortality was greatest among males, being about 43½ per cent., and in females 37 per cent. The present tables confirm the incorrectness of that opinion which assigns a greater mortality from pulmonary consumption to women than to men.

Dropsy was most frequent amongst females.

The diseases of the vascular system fell more heavily on the females than the males. To some extent this is owing to derangement in menstruation; and so far as concerns the heart, the preponderance is owing to affections of that organ being less frequently complicated with disease of the respiratory organs in woman than in man.

Nothing particular is to be remarked of diseases of the genito-urinary organs. Venereal cases, however, have been much more numerous among females than males.

Diseases of the nervous system have fallen most heavily on females, which may be accounted for, from hysteria having been exclusively confined to them, and also the greater frequency of insanity among them in this house. The rate of mortality, however, is nearly equal in both sexes, from the more frequent occurrence of apoplexy and *delirium tremens* in males.

Diseases of the locomotive organs and cellular tissue, are, as might have been expected, more frequent in males than females.

Fever seems to affect both sexes almost indifferently; but in those of an eruptive kind, the mortality has been greatest in the female, and chiefly confined to the first period of life. So much for the comparative frequency of different diseases, and the mortality in both sexes.

An analysis of the second table shows us that diseases of the digestive organs chiefly prevail between twenty and forty-five years of age, the mortality being greater as life advances.

In the diseases of the respiratory organs the prevalence was greatest after 45, but the mortality was enormous in infancy. This fact is so striking, that, if returns from other institutions correspond with the present, it will call loudly for the necessity of excluding young children from crowded establishments in large towns.

Diseases of the vascular system prevailed most in adult and advanced life, and were most fatal at the latter period.

Diseases of the nervous system were most numerous between twenty and forty-five, but the greatest mortality occurred after that period.

There were but few cases of disease in the locomotive organs and cellular tissue, until after the first period of life, when they became pretty equally distributed over the three last periods.

The peculiarities respecting fevers have already been pointed out.

The effects of season upon particular diseases, as is shown in the third table, are very remarkable. Those of the digestive organs are most numerous, but least fatal, during the summer months. Those of the respiratory organs most frequent in winter.

Diseases of the vascular system were most numerous in the first quarter; the mortality was greatest in the first and last quarters; syphilitic cases were most numerous in the last quarter. This may partly be owing to the inclemency of the weather forcing a greater number to seek an asylum at that season.

Common fever was most frequent and fatal during the first quarter, and least so in the last quarter.—*Edin. Med. and Surgical Journal.*

STRICTURE OF THE RECTUM.

To the Editor of the Medical Gazette.

SIR,

YOUR last number contains a letter from a correspondent in relation to stricture of the rectum, which letter you, judiciously consulting the reputation of its author, have imparted to your readers anonymously.

I do not address you for the purpose of supporting or protecting the professional character of the individual who is stated to have committed the unfortunately fatal error, although I take pleasure in asserting, that having known him almost from his infancy, I may, without fear of contradiction, affirm that the profession does not contain a man of better education, more sterling integrity, or general practical information.

Your correspondent writes, in allusion to the existence of stricture of the rectum, " Now, it would be a great satisfaction to know the opinion of your great London surgeons on this point. If there is such a disease, some of them must have met with it in their extensive practice, and it must have been often seen in the dead-rooms of the different hospitals. The rectum was greatly patronised in this city some years ago, and it is still a favourite with one or two surgeons, who doubtless find it a fruitful source of income." Being a London surgeon, but without the wish or intention of assuming to myself the term "great," I would answer his inquiries so far only as may be requisite for the furtherance of science, and the amelioration of human suffering, by assuring the profession that simple stricture of the rectum does exist, and is commonly met with among the poor,—a fact of which your correspondent may be convinced by investigating the practice of this charity, which is open gratuitously to the medical public, while in the museum thereto attached are many preparations of the disease, varying in its position from the sigmoid flexure of the colon to the anal extremity of the rectum.

I am, sir,

Your obedient servant,

FREDERICK SALMON.

12, Old Broad Street, Sept. 13, 1843.

MEDICAL ATTENDANCE ON THE POOR.

THE Poor-Law Commissioners have signified their intention of hereafter admitting those gentlemen who hold a Scotch or Irish diploma in surgery, to the same rights under the Poor-Law Amendment Act, as members of the College of Surgeons in London. For this purpose they are to make the necessary alterations in their order of the 12th of March, 1842.

WOUND OF THE AORTA AND PERICARDIUM.

THE following case is interesting in a medico-legal point of view :—A Spanish refugee was struck by one of his companions with a knife in the back. The blade broke at a little distance from the skin. The patient walked to the hospital, where he died two hours after. At the *post-mortem* examination, it was found that the knife had penetrated between the seventh and eighth dorsal spines, that it had cut or broken a portion of one of these processes, crossed obliquely the vertebral canal, traversed the body of the vertebra from below, and a little to the right side of thecentre, and then wounded the aorta below its arch. The pericardium was divided to the extent of five millimetres; it contained three grammes of blood. The pleuræ, but more especially the left, were filled with a considerable quantity. The spinal cord was not affectd.—*Bull. de Ther.*, June 1842 ; and *Dublin Journal of Medical Science.*

A TABLE OF MORTALITY FOR THE METROPOLIS,

Shewing the number of deaths from all causes registered in the week ending Saturday, Sept. 2, 1843.

Small Pox	4
Measles	29
Scarlatina	38
Hooping Cough	24
Croup	3
Thrush	9
Diarrhœa	53
Dysentery	16
Cholera	6
Influenza	1
Ague	0
Remittent Fever	0
Typhus	33
Erysipelas	3
Syphilis	1
Hydrophobia	0
Diseases of the Brain, Nerves, and Senses	147
Diseases of the Lungs and other Organs of Respiration	219
Diseases of the Heart and Blood-vessels	35
Diseases of the Stomach, Liver, and other Organs of Digestion	98
Diseases of the Kidneys, &c.	5
Childbed	40
Paramenia	1
Ovarian Dropsy	1
Disease of Uterus, &c.	2
Arthritis	0
Rheumatism	3
Diseases of Joints, &c.	5
Carbuncle	0
Phlegmon	0
Ulcer	1
Fistula	0
Dropsy, Cancer, and other Diseases of Uncertain Seat	105
Old Age or Natural Decay	44
Deaths by Violence, Privation, or Intemperance	20
Causes not specified	5
Deaths from all Causes	909

WILSON & OGILVY, 57, Skinner Street, London

THE

LONDON MEDICAL GAZETTE,

BEING A

WEEKLY JOURNAL

OF

Medicine and the Collateral Sciences.

FRIDAY, SEPTEMBER 22, 1843.

LECTURES

ON THE

THEORY AND PRACTICE OF MIDWIFERY,

Delivered in the Theatre of St. George's Hospital,

BY ROBERT LEE, M.D. F.R.S.

LECTURE XLIV.

On the Origin, Symptoms, and Treatment of Crural Phlebitis.

No unequivocal example of phlegmasia dolens was recorded in the medical literature of this country, where the actual condition of the affected parts was ascertained by dissection, from the year 1823 to 1829, when the history of the following case was published in the fifteenth volume of the Medico-Chirurgical Transactions. Several eminent physicians and surgeons examined the patient during the progress of the affection, who was under the care of Dr. Nathaniel Grant, Thayer Street, and none of them expressed a doubt as to the disease being genuine phlegmasia dolens. The hard painful femoral vein in the groin was supposed by some to be an inflamed absorbent vessel, but the dissection proved this opinion to be incorrect.

I. Mrs. Jones, æt. 31; delivered on March 10, 1827. On the 14th she began to experience a sense of pain in the left groin and calf of the leg, with numbness in the whole left inferior extremity, but nothing unusual was perceived in the appearance of the limb, except a slight tumefaction of the inguinal glands, where pressure occasioned great uneasiness. She had rigors; the tongue was furred, and there was much thirst; bowels open; pulse 80; the flow of milk and lochia natural. 16th (the sixth day after parturition), the pain of the left thigh and leg continued with increased severity, particularly from the groin to the knee, along the inner surface of the limb, where a swelling of a glistening white appearance was observed;

the pulse still 80; and the general functions but little deranged. 19th. The pain had diminished, but the swelling had greatly increased, and extended to the leg and foot, which were both very tense, and did not pit upon pressure; there was no discolouration of the skin; the pain of the limb was relieved by placing it in a state of moderate flexion. 21st. The pain in the groin had abated, and the swelling appeared to decrease. 24th. Pain of the limb aggravated particularly on moving it; pulse more accelerated; skin hot and moist; she was extremely irritable and desponding. 25th (the fifteenth day after delivery), when I first saw her, the whole extremity was much swollen, the intumescence being greatest in the ham and calf of the leg. The integuments wore a uniform smooth shining appearance, having a cream-like colour, and every where pitting on pressure, but more readily in some situations than in others; the temperature to the touch did not differ from that of the other limb, though she complained of a disagreeable sensation of heat throughout its whole extent, and much pain was experienced in the upper and inner part of the thigh on moving it. Immediately below Poupart's ligament, in the situation of the femoral vein, a thick hard cord, about the size of the little finger, was distinctly felt. This cord, which rolled under the fingers, and was exquisitely sensible when pressed, could be distinctly traced three or four inches down the thigh in the course of the femoral vessels, and great pain was experienced on pressure as low down as the middle of the thigh, in the same direction. The pulsations of the femoral artery were felt in the usual situation below Poupart's ligament: pressure over this vessel excited little or no uneasiness. Pulse 90, and sharp; tongue much furred; thirst urgent; bowels confined; the lochia had nearly disappeared; leeches were applied to the left groin and upper and inner part of the thigh; these were followed by cold evaporating lotions to the affected parts, and

3 L

mild cathartics and anodynes were administered internally. 30th. The acute pain on pressure and motion of the limb had subsided, and the extremity was universally œdematous. For two months after this period the limb remained so feeble as to disable her from walking, and continued larger than the other. Eleven months after the attack the general health of the patient was completely restored, and she again became pregnant. Because she recovered perfectly from the attack of phlegmasia dolens, I was not unfrequently afterwards reminded by one of the physicians who had seen her of the mistake he believed I had committed in supposing that the hard painful cord in the groin was the inflamed femoral vein, and not an inflamed absorbent. On the 5th of November, 1828, she was delivered of a still-born child, and died soon after from uterine hæmorrhage. On dissection the whole of the left inferior extremity was considerably larger than the right, but no serous fluid escaped from the incisions made through the integuments, beneath which a thick layer of peculiarly dense granular adipose matter was observed. The common and internal iliac and femoral veins and arteries, inclosed in their sheath, were removed from the body for examination. The common iliac, with its subdivisions, and the upper part of the femoral veins, so resembled a ligamentous cord, that on opening the sheath, the vessel was not, until dissected out, distinguishable from the cellular substance surrounding it. On laying open the middle portion of the vein, a firm thin layer of ash-coloured lymph was found in some places adhering close to and uniting its sides, and in others clogging it up, but not distending it. On tracing upwards the obliterated vein, that portion which lies above Poupart's ligament was observed to become gradually smaller, so that, in the situation of the common iliac, it was lost in the surrounding cellular membrane, and no traces of its entrance into the vena cava were discernible. The vena cava itself was in its natural state. The entrance of the internal iliac was completely closed, and in the small portion of it which I had the opportunity of examining the inner surface was coated with an adventitious membrane. The lower end of the removed vein was permeable, but its coats were much more dense than natural, and the inner surface was lined with a strong membrane, which diminished considerably its calibre, and here and there fine bands of the same membrane ran from one side of the vessel to the other. The outer coat had formed strong adhesions with the artery and the common sheath ; the inguinal glands adhered firmly to the veins, but were otherwise in a healthy condition. No appearance of recent disease existed, and the density and firmness of the morbid tex-

tures evidently showed that the whole was the result of inflammation, which had occurred at a remote period. An accurate coloured drawing of the appearances was made immediately after the removal of the vessels from the body, which I shall now hand round, with the preparation of the morbid parts, and which I entreat you to examine rigorously At the period when this occurred I was wholly unacquainted with the important pathological fact, that the inflammation of the iliac and femoral veins in plegmasia dolens commences in the uterus, and I could obtain no satisfactory explanation of the cause why the disease did not occur during pregnancy, which it must have done had it been owing to pressure of the gravid uterus on the vessels : and why a certain period should always elapse after delivery before the disease commences. Neither in this nor in the following case, which has also been recorded in the fifteenth volume of the Medico-Chirurgical Transactions, were the internal iliac veins examined with a view to discover the commencement of the disease in the uterus, because at this time no suspicion existed that it originated in the uterine veins, and that crural was the result of uterine phlebitis.

II. Mrs. Edwards, æt. 35, No. 54, King Street. 16th of April, 1829, was delivered of her second child, three weeks ago, after a natural labour, and on the 9th inst. was attacked suddenly with a pain in the calf of the right leg, and loss of power in the whole right inferior extremity. On the 13th, a considerable swelling, without discolouration, had taken place from the ham to the foot, and great tenderness was experienced along the inner surface of the thigh to the groin. The extremity is now universally swollen, painful, and deprived of all power of motion. The temperature along the inner surface of the limb is increased ; the integuments are pale and glistening, and do not pit upon pressure. There is no pain in the hypogastrium, but pressure along the course of the crural vessels excites great suffering, and the vein from the groin to the middle of the thigh is indurated, enlarged, and exquisitely sensible. There is also great sensibility in the ham, and along the inner surface of the leg to the ankle, where some branches of the superficial veins are hard and painful on pressure. Pulse 80 ; tongue much loaded ; thirst ; bowels open. There was no rigor, or symptom of pyrexia, at the invasion of the disease. She states, that the veins of the right extremity were more distended during pregnancy than those of the left. Twelve years ago, after the birth of her first child, the patient and her relatives report, that she experienced an attack similar to the present, in the same limb, and that it remained in a weak condition for several months afterwards, but ultimately recovered its natural size and power. April 18th.— The tension and increased heat along the inner surface of the limb are somewhat diminished, but the pain continues in the course of the vessels. May 1st.—Affection declining. The femoral vein cannot now be felt, but there is still a sense of tenderness in its course down the thigh. No pitting on pressure. She has suffered, during three or four days, considerable uneasiness between the umbilicus and pubes, as well as in the loins, and has had rigors, with quick pulse, loaded tongue, and thirst. The abdomen is soft, but tender on pressure around the umbilicus. 9th.—The swelling of the limb is nearly gone, as is the tenderness in the course of the femoral vessels. For several days past, she has experienced attacks of acute pain in the umbilical region, loins, and back, which have assumed a regular intermittent form. Every afternoon there has been a violent rigor, of an hour's duration, followed by increased heat and profuse perspiration. In the course of the last and preceding nights, there was slight delirium. The skin is now hot and dry; the pulse 125; the tongue brown and parched; bowels open. The abdomen is neither tense nor swollen. On pressing around the umbilicus, she complains of a deep-seated feeling of soreness. A strong vibratory motion, corresponding with the pulsations of the heart, is perceived in the epigastrium. 21st.—The febrile attacks gradually declined in severity, and she appeared to recover, until yesterday, when she had a long and violent fit of cold shivering. The countenance is now expressive of great anxiety, and the pulse extremely quick and feeble. There remains no visible trace of the affection of the lower extremity. 23d.—Has been vomiting ever since yesterday, at intervals of half an hour. Complains of great pain in the left side, increased upon taking a deep inspiration. The pulsation in the epigastrium diminished, although it is still clearly perceived: pulse 120, and soft.

24th.—Symptoms continue without alleviation. Has had a severe shivering fit of long duration. Skin hot and dry; pulse 140; tongue brown and parched; diarrhœa. The pulsation in the epigastrium has entirely disappeared; the pain in the left side of the thorax is diminished; but the respiration is hurried, and there is frequent cough. Great prostration of strength. Surface of the body has assumed a peculiar sallow tinge. She has been delirious in the night, but is now perfectly conscious when roused. The conjunctiva of the right eye has suddenly become of a deep red colour, and so much swollen, that the eyelids cannot be closed. The cornea is dull, and she makes little complaint of pain in the eye, and there is no intolerance of light. The vomiting has ceased. 25th,—

Has again had repeated attacks of vomiting. Debility rapidly increasing; respiration hurried; incessant hacking cough; pulse 140, extremely feeble; surface of the body cold and clammy; the tongue and teeth covered with dark sordes; diarrhœa. The left eye has also become red and swollen, without much increased sensibility. 26th.— Great debility; when undisturbed she is delirious, but is conscious when roused, and complains of pain in the left side of the chest. Pulse above 140. Tongue black and dry. Conjunctiva of the left eye also affected with swelling and intense redness. The cornea is dull, and shreds of lymph appear to have been effused over the left iris. 28th.—Had so violent a rigor in the afternoon that the bed shook under her. She is now completely insensible. The eyes are red and swollen, and there is a copious secretion of an opaque fluid from their surface and from the eye-lids, which cannot be closed. The respiration hurried. Pulse 140. 31st.—Has recovered her consciousness, and drank cider and porter with great eagerness. Pulse rapid and feeble. Eyes so much swollen that they seem pushed forward from their orbits. Vision entirely lost; but hearing and the other senses remain. 2d June.—Great debility. A red puffy swelling has suddenly appeared over the right elbow-joint. Tongue dry and black; diarrhœa; frequent, or rather constant wandering, except when spoken to, when she answers questions distinctly, and complains only of pain in the chest, with difficult respiration and cough. 10th.—Little change has taken place in the symptoms; but she has become much weaker. The vision is lost, but the hearing is perfect, and she makes no complaint of pain in any part of the body, 15th June.—Died this morning.

Morbid appearances on examining the body of Sarah Edwards on the 16th of June.— Present, Drs. Sims and Locock.

Thorax.—In its left cavity were contained upwards of two pints of a thin purulent fluid, and extensive recent adhesions existed between the pleura covering the lower margin of the superior lobe, and the pleura costalis. The surface of the inferior lobe was coated with a thick layer of flocculent coagulated lymph, as was a corresponding part of the pleura costalis. The substance of this lobe was of a dark colour, approaching to black, and soft in texture, so as to be readily broken down with the fingers. In its centre about an ounce of thick cream-coloured pus was found deposited in the dark-coloured and softened lung. This was not contained in any cyst or membrane, but infiltrated into the pulmonary tissue.

In the right cavity of the chest recent adhesions also existed at the inferior part. A considerable portion of the right inferior lobe was entirely changed from the healthy structure, being converted into a dense, solid, dark red coloured mass.   On the anterior surface of this lobe the pleura was elevated as if by a hard irregular tumor ; but when cut into, no pus escaped from this part, and it presented only the appearance of the surrounding portions of lung with a greater degree of condensation. *Vena cava inferior:* Coats of the vessel considerably thickened, and the internal were visible, of a scarlet colour; its whole cavity occupied by a coagulum, distending it to its utmost extent, and terminating in a loose pointed extremity about an inch below the entrance of the vena cava hepatica. The coagulum, covered with a membranous-like investiture of a bright red colour, throughout firmly, and in many places inseparably, adherent to the inner lining of the vein. The substance within it varied in consistence and colour : in some parts it presented the appearance of coagulable lymph ; in others it was a pultaceous, dull yellow mass, made up apparently of pus and lymph blended together. The exterior of the firmer portions were separated into layers, which gradually disappeared as they approached the centre. The mouths of all the veins emptying themselves into the cava were sealed up, the emulgents excepted, the coagulum near the entrance of these vessels hanging loosely within the cava. *Left common iliac and its branches:* Its interior plugged up with a continuation of the coagulum from the cava, and differing in no respect from it either as to consistence, colour, or the firmness of its adhesions to the inner tunic of the vein; it was continued beyond the entrance of the internal iliac (which it completely closed), and terminated in a pointed extremity about the middle of the external iliac ; neither the remainder of this vessel nor the femoral vein exhibited any morbid changes. The internal iliac was much contracted, and lined with a thick adventitious membrane. *Right common iliac and its branches:* This vessel was contracted to more than one-half its natural size ; it was firm to the touch, and of a greyish blue colour; to its internal coat adhered an adventitious membrane of the same colour, containing within it a firm coagulum, made up of thin layers of dense lymph.   The internal iliac was rendered quite impervious by dense dark-coloured bluish membranes, and, at its entrance into the common iliac, was converted into a solid cord. The contracted external iliac contained within it a soft yellowish coagulum, similar to the one in the cava ; its coats were three or four times their natural thickness, and lined with dark-coloured membranous layers. The *femoral vein*, from Poupart's ligament to the middle of the thigh, was diminished

in size, and almost inseparable from th artery. Its tunics were thickened, and its interior coated with a dense membrane surrounding a solid purple coagulum strongly adherent to it. The superficial and deep femoral veins were in a similar condition, and the saphena major and minor differed from the femoral veins only in the size of the coagulum they contained, which was slender, and had formed no adhesions with the layers of lymph lining their cavity. The cellular membrane and other textures of the limb were in a perfectly healthy condition, and in size and appearance there was externally no visible difference between the two extremities. The morbid alterations of structure now described can still be distinctly seen in the preparation of the diseased veins, and have been represented with great accuracy in this beautiful drawing, made by Mr. Perry, from the parts immediately after their removal from the body. These I shall likewise hand round, that you may have an opportunity of comparing them with this description, and verifying its accuracy.

In this case, the connection between inflammation of the vena cava and of the iliac and femoral veins, and the destructive inflammation of the eyes in puerperal women, was so obvious, that it could not be overlooked, and I supposed had long been admitted as an undoubted fact. In the article Puerperal Fevers, by Dr. Locock, published in the first volume of Dr. Tweedie's System of Practical Medicine (1840), p. 361, there is the following statement :—" The remarkable destructive inflammation of the eye, which has been already mentioned, rare as it is, can hardly, perhaps, be placed as a symptom peculiar to this form of puerperal fever, but we have witnessed four instances of it, and in each there were purulent deposits in various parts of the body. In the five cases related by Dr. Marshall Hall, which also occurred after delivery, the same fact is noticed ; there is the same rapid pulse, with constitutional disturbance, lasting for many days before the inflammation of the eye was discovered. In Dr. Hall's cases the left eye was uniformly the one inflamed, and it is curious that such was the fact in the four which have come under our own knowledge. In only one of Dr. Hall's cases was any decided abdominal pain and tenderness noticed, whereas three out of the four of our cases had such symptoms. In none could any post-mortem inspection be obtained. Dr. Robert Lee (Cyc. Pract. Med. art. Puerperal Fever) has alluded to two cases under his care where this destructive inflammation of the eye occurred in both eyes. He is inclined to believe that this remarkable affection is the attendant upon ' the morbid condition of the veins of the uterus,' the purulent or other depraved secretions entering the system, and acting as a poison on the whole mass of blood. In Dr. Hall's cases and our own no examination took place to elucidate this theory, and *Dr. Lee does not quote any dissections to confirm it.''*

The following statement, contained in the same article, is so completely at variance with all my experience respecting uterine inflammation in puerperal women, that it would have been much more satisfactory had the author mentioned where and when the cases occurred, and by whom the most careful but unsuccessful search was made for morbid alterations of structure in the veins, the absorbents, the muscular structure, and the lining membrane of the uterus, and of the adjacent parts. " In Gooch's Treatise on Peritoneal Fevers, already quoted, several cases are recorded in which death ensued after certain symptoms, and in which no morbid appearances were discovered on dissection. Dr. Lee would reply to this that the examination was not pushed far enough, and that a more close inspection must have discovered some of the changes he has described. But after Dr. Lee's researches into these subjects were known, several cases similar to those related by Gooch occurring in our own practice, and in that of others, convinced us that in these something might therefore be found. The most careful search was made for morbid alterations of structure in the veins, the absorbents, the muscular structure, and the lining membrane of the uterus and of the adjacent parts, and nothing could be found to explain the cause of death.''

III. Mrs. Foster, æt. 25, No. 27, Little Windmill Street, out-patient of the British Lying-in Hospital. May 8, 1829. Previous to her confinement, six weeks ago, she had been affected for several months with pain in the chest, difficulty of respiration, cough, with copious expectoration of a matter tinged with blood, profuse perspirations in the night, and had become greatly emaciated. During the last fourteen days she has been suffering from attacks of pain in the bowels, and diarrhœa. On the 4th instant she experienced a sense of soreness in the left groin, which gradually extended along the inner surface of the thigh to the ham, and from thence along the posterior surface of the leg to the foot. She stated, that for two or three days before the occurrence of pain in the groin she had felt great uneasiness in the region of the uterus, that this suddenly quitted the hypogastrium and passed into the groin, and that from thence it extended downward along the inner surface of the thigh and leg. The limb became swollen twenty-four hours after the invasion of the pain. The whole left inferior extremity is now affected with a hot, painful, colourless swelling, no where pitting on pressure except over the foot. The thigh is double the size

of the other, and any attempt to move the limb produces excruciating pain along the inner surface of the thigh; and the pain excited by pressure along the tract of the femoral vein is so acute that the condition of this vessel cannot be ascertained. Several branches of the saphena major above the knee are distended and hard; pulse 120; respiration quick and laborious; tongue peculiarly red and glossy; diarrhœa continues. 10th. Pulmonary affection aggravated. The limb continues extremely painful, and is still more swollen. The groin is so tender that she cannot endure the slightest pressure over it. The same is the case with the inner surface of the thigh. The branches of the saphena vein are still hard and painful. 11th. The femoral vein, under Poupart's ligament, can now be felt indurated and enlarged, and it is exquisitely painful when pressed, as is the inner surface of the thigh, the ham, and the calf of the leg. There is comparatively little tenderness along the outer surface of the limb; pulse 120; skin hot. 17th. Diarrhœa, emaciation, colliquative sweats, and difficulty of respiration, increasing. The left inferior extremity is still much swollen, but there is less pain at the groin and in the course of the femoral vessels. The foot and ankle pit on pressure. 26th. Calf of the leg still swollen and painful. June 19th. The pulmonary affection aggravated, and she is now reduced to a state of extreme debility. The limb is still considerably swollen, and is universally œdematous. 24th. Died this morning from the disease of the chest. *Dissection*—present Dr. Sims and Mr. Prout. *Thorax:* Extensive adhesions between the pleuræ on both sides. Scarcely a portion of lung could be observed which did not contain tubercles in various stages of their growth. The right and left superior lobes contained several large tuberculous excavations. The vena cava and right common external iliac veins were in a sound state. The left common external and internal iliac veins were all impervious, and had undergone various alterations of structure. The common iliac, at its termination, was reduced to a slender tube, about a line in diameter, which was lined with a bluish slate-coloured adventitious membrane. The remainder of the common and the external iliac veins were coated also with a dark-coloured membrane, and their centre filled with a brownish ochrey-coloured tenacious substance, rather more consistent than the crassamentum of the blood. The left hypogastric or internal iliac vein was in the same condition, but in some places reduced to a cord-like substance, and its cavity throughout completely obliterated. The branches of this vein taking their origin in the uterus, and usually termed the uterine plexus, were found completely plugged up with firm reddish coagula of lymph. From the commencement of the branches of this plexus of the hypogastric vein to the termination of this vein in the iliac, the whole had become thickened, contracted, and plugged up with coagula and adventitious membranes of a dark blue colour. The same changes had taken place in the uterine plexus and trunk of the right hypogastric vein, from the uterus to its unusual termination in the left common iliac vein. The coats of the left femoral vein were thickened, and closely adherent to the artery and surrounding cellular substance; its whole interior lined with an adventitious membrane, and distended with a reddish-coloured coagulum. The same morbid changes presented themselves in the deep and superficial branches as far as they were examined down the thigh. If you examine this drawing made of the

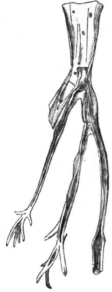

parts by Mr. Perry, immediately after their removal from the body, and this preparation of them, you will require no further evidence to convince you that the inflammation of the left iliac and femoral veins which produced phlegmasia dolens in the left lower extremity, commenced in the uterine branches of the hypogastric vein. The following case, which has likewise been published in Vol. XV. of the Medico-Chirurgical Transactions, with a coloured engraving, demonstrates this fact in the most conclusive manner.

IV. Mrs. Mason, æt. 42, No. 3, Little *Vine Street*, August 29th, 1829, four weeks ago, *was delivered of twins*, and before the expulsion of the placenta had nearly perished from uterine hæmorrhage. Considerable tenderness of the uterus succeeded and remained until the 27th instant, when, without any apparent cause, she had a violent fit of cold shivering, followed by febrile symptoms, and pain in the right iliac region and groin. Yesterday morning the pain increased in severity, and extended down the inner surface of the thigh towards the ham, and in the evening the whole thigh and leg was perceived to be considerably swollen. At present the whole right interior extremity is affected with a general intumescence, and is completely deprived of all power of motion. The temperature of the limb, particularly along the inner surface, is much higher than that of the other, but the integuments retain their natural colour, and do not pit on pressure. The femoral vein, for several inches under Poupart's ligament, is very distinctly felt enlarged, and is very painful when pressed. Out of the course of the crural vessels little uneasiness is produced by pressure. In the right side of the hypogastrium there is also great tenderness; pulse 120; tongue furred. She appears pale and depressed, and complains of deep-seated acute pain in the lower part of the spine when she attempts to move. August 31st.— The pain continues in the groin, and along the inner surface of the thigh. The glands in the groin are painful and tumid. The limb is considerably swollen, and the temperature is increased. Febrile symptoms continue. Sept. 8th.—There is less pain in the limb, but the femoral vein can still be felt large and hard, and is painful on pressure. The foot and leg pit. She has suffered much from rigors, and has had repeated attacks of diarrhœa; pulse quick, with great prostration of strength. 14th.—The limb is now œdematous, and nearly free from pain. She has complained of tenderness in the left groin and thigh, but nothing unusual can be perceived in the seat of the pain. During the last four days she has had repeated attacks of cold shivering, and has suffered severely from diarrhœa, and deep-seated pain in the lower part of the back; pulse 130, and feeble; tongue white. From the 13th to the 22d, when she died, she was occasionally delirious, and made no complaint of pain except in the back; pulse 140; tongue dry and furred. Frequent attacks of diarrhœa and severe rigors. Both inferior extremities were œdematous. *Dissection:* present Mr. Prout. The veins presented nearly similar appearances to those observed in the preceding cases, and the drawing and preparation will convey a more correct idea of the changes they had undergone, than any verbal description. The divisions of the vena cava were in this instance both affected. On the left side, the cavities of the iliac and femoral veins were filled with a dark purple coagulum, their coats being not much thicker than natural; whilst, on the right side, the coats of these veins were dense and ligamentous, and the cavities blocked up by adventitious membranes, or lymph of a dull yellow colour. The lower part of the vena cava, for the space of two inches, as well as the right common iliac, was obstructed by a tough membrane of lymph surrounding a soft semifluid yellowish matter. The right, common, external, and internal veins were imbedded in a mass of suppurating glands, the purulent fluid of which had escaped into the adjacent cellular membrane, and forced its way downwards in the course of the psoas muscle, as low as Poupart's ligament. The right hypogastric vein was reduced to a small impervious cord, and its membranes distended with coagula of lymph of a bright red colour. The right femoral and its branches were in like manner impervious, their coats being greatly thickened, and their interior occupied by coagula. The cavities of the left common external iliac and hypogastric veins contained soft coagula, disposed in layers, which adhered to the inner tunic of the vessel. The trunk of the left hypogastric vein was contracted, its coats somewhat thickened, as well as its branches filled with red-coloured, worm-like, coagula. The spermatic veins were healthy. The lower extremities were both infiltrated with serum.

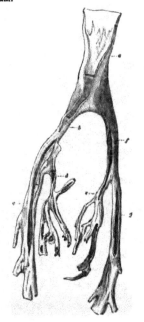

V. A lady, 26 years of age, was delivered on the 19th of June, 1831. The labour was protracted, and the placenta, after having been retained in the uterus six hours, was removed artificially by the practitioner with some difficulty. In the course of a few days after, great tenderness of the uterus, with pyrexia, followed. The pain subsided after the application of leeches to the hypogastrium, but the fever, with remarkable prostration of strength, continued till the end of the third week. A painful sense of tension then came to be experienced in the brim of the pelvis, on the left side, and in a few days the whole left inferior extremity became affected with a hot, tense, painful, and colourless swelling. On the 21st of July (four weeks after delivery) I was requested by Mr. Cleland, her medical attendant, to see this lady in consultation with him. The pulse was 150, and feeble; there was constant nausea, vomiting, and diarrhœa; tongue of a dark brown hue; great debility; the countenance and whole surface of the body of a dusky colour; respiration hurried, with frequent cough and expectoration; occasional delirium; the whole left inferior extremity was swollen to more than double the size of the other; the femoral vein, exquisitely painful on pressure, was felt indurated and enlarged in the upper part of the thigh, and there was fulness and tension above Poupart's ligament, in the situation of the iliac veins; the foot and ankle pitted upon pressure, but the integuments of the thigh were hot and tense, and did not retain the impression of the finger. 22d. Great prostration of strength; pulse 160; respiration laborious; tongue dry and brown; diarrhœa and vomiting continue; is conscious at intervals, and then complains of great pain along the inner part of the left thigh and in the ham; there is also tenderness of the hypogastrium, and sense of throbbing in the direction of the abdominal aorta; abdomen tympanitic. 23d. Sinking; cold extremities; pulse feeble and intermittent; singultus. 24th. Died. Inspection: present Dr. Sims and Mr. Cleland:—The uterus had sunk down into the pelvis, and was as much reduced in size as it usually is four weeks after delivery. The peritoneum at first sight appeared every where healthy, but, on closer inspection, an adhesion, by means of false membrane, was found to exist between the posterior part of the uterus and rectum. More than a pint of purulent fluid was contained between the uterus and rectum. The peritoneal and muscular coats of the fundus and body of the uterus were so soft as to be readily torn with the fingers, and of an inky black colour. The coats of the common external iliac and femoral veins, to the middle of the thigh, were all thickened, and their cavity filled with soft coagula of lymph and pus. The vena cava, to about two inches below the entrance of the hepatic veins, was completely blocked up with a coagulum of lymph, which partially adhered to the inner surface of the vessel. Several glands in the vicinity of the vena cava and iliac veins were in a state of suppuration. The coats of the left internal iliac vein, at its termination in the oncomm iliac, were in a soft shreddy state. The right common, internal and external iliac and femoral veins, were all in a healthy state. You may hand round the preparation of the parts, in which all these appearances are still seen.

VI. Mrs. Wildman, 30 years of age, was delivered after a natural labour, in the British Lying-in Hospital, on the 27th of January, 1832. Obscure febrile symptoms took place a few days after delivery; but as there was no pain in the region of the uterus, and the patient would not admit that she was indisposed, I was not called to see her till the tenth day after her confinement; I was then informed that she had been incoherent in the night, and that she had suffered from a long and severe fit of cold shivering. The pulse was 130 and feeble; tongue of a dark glossy red colour; lips parched; tremors of the muscles of the face and extremities; the countenance of a dusky yellow colour. There was no tension, pain, or swelling of the hypogastrium; but there was exquisite pain on pressure along the course of the iliac vessels, on the left side, and down the inner part of the thigh. I now, for the first time, discovered that the whole left lower extremity was much swollen, hot, tense, and shining. 18th. The swelling of the left lower extremity, and pain in the course of the iliac and femoral veins, relieved by leeches and warm fomentations. Pulse 140, and extremely feeble; tongue dry and brown; but there is no vomiting, diarrhœa, or distension of abdomen. The conjunctiva of both eyes have suddenly become intensely red and swollen, and the vision is much impaired, if not lost; consciousness remains. The right knee-joint is now exquisitely painful when moved, but it is neither red nor swollen. A dark-coloured gangrenous spot has appeared over the sacrum. 14th. Eyes red, and enormously swollen; eyelids cannot be closed; pulse rapid and feeble; tongue, lips, and teeth, covered with sordes; severe pain in the right knee and elbow joints, and right wrist; left lower extremity less swollen. Died on the 18th. The body was inspected, at my desire, by the late Dr. John Prout, who had been present with me at the examination of all the preceding cases. The uterus had subsided into the pelvis, and no trace of disease was perceptible in the sac of the peritoneum. Both spermatic veins were healthy. The coats of the left common, external iliac, and femoral veins, deep and

superficial, were all thickened, and their cavities plugged up with firm coagula; the same was the case with the epigastric veins and circumflexa ilii. The glands in the vicinity of these veins were enlarged, red, and vascular, and closely adherent to the cellular membrane and outer surface of the vessels. The vena cava, to a short distance above the entrance of the left common iliac vein, had its coats thickened, and a soft coagulum of lymph adhering to its inner surface. The uterine, vaginal, gluteal, and most of the other veins which form the left internal iliac, were gorged with pus, and lined with false membranes of a dark colour approaching to black. The uterine branches of the right internal iliac vein were also filled with pus and lymph; but the inflammation had not extended beyond the entrance of the trunk of the vessel into the common iliac, and the right common, external, iliac, and femoral veins, were all in a healthy condition. In the muscular tissue of the cervix uteri, on the left side, was a cavity which contained ℥ij. of purulent fluid. The veins proceeding from this part of the cervix were filled with pus, and a large portion of the inner and muscular coats of the uterus was as soft as lard. The conjunctivæ, which before death had been red and swollen, were now almost colourless, scarcely a vessel containing red blood being discernible.

VII. Mary Gane, æt. 20, was delivered on the 21st October, 1832, of her first child, at her residence near St. Thomas's Hospital. The labour was natural, and she went on favourably till the third day, when she complained of pain and stiffness about the hypogastric and inguinal regions, extending down the thighs, with pyrexia and headache. 25th. Increased pain on pressure over the region of the uterus, extending down the right thigh; pulse frequent; rigors; offensive lochia. 30th. Rigors have been more frequent and severe, with great febrile disturbance. The pain of the uterus has never entirely gone off, and she now suffers severely from pain in the symphysis pubis. 31st. Pain of uterus diminished, but increased tenderness in the right groin, extending in the course of the femoral vessels, which are felt hard and cord-like, beneath Poupart's ligament, for a space of three inches down the thigh. The limb greatly swollen, and œdematous, and free from discolouration, except below the ham, where it is of a dark hue from distension of the saphena veins. November 1st. The limb is immensely swollen, but the femoral vein can no longer be felt in the upper part of the thigh; pitting upon pressure in different parts of the extremity; pulse rapid and feeble; tongue foul; diarrhœa; surface covered with perspiration; countenance pale and depressed. 4th. Pulse 130 and feeble; tongue loaded; diarrhœa continues; pain in the uterine region gone. 13th. Pain and swelling have taken place in the course of the left saphena vein; swelling of right lower extremity diminished; pulse 130, and feeble; distressing diarrhœa. The soft parts covering the sacrum have become affected with gangrenous inflammation, and also the right outer ankle and foot, from which there is a dark ichorous discharge. Several large dark-coloured vesicles have also appeared over the limb. Delirium and pain of the chest ensued, and she speedily sunk. On examination of the pelvis it was found filled with purulent fluid, which had escaped through the symphysis pubis, which was separated to the distance of an inch and a half, and its cartilages gone. The right femoral vein was plugged up with fibrine, and the saphena major filled with pus. Permission could not be obtained to examine the left lower extremity, to ascertain the condition of the internal iliac vein, though there could be little doubt that the inflammation commenced in the uterine branches of this vessel.

VIII. The preparation which I shall next shew you exhibits in a very striking manner the effects produced by inflammation on the lower part of the vena cava, and the left common, external, and internal iliac, and femoral veins. A woman became pregnant who had distortion of the pelvis, and this large fibrous tumor imbedded in the walls of the uterus which you now see. Premature labour came on, and the child was expelled without artificial assistance, but in a short time uterine and crural phlebitis took place in the left side, and she ultimately died. The fibrous tumor was partially in a softened state, and all the branches of the left hypogastric vein were filled with pus and coagula of blood. It is impossible to examine this beautiful specimen of crural phlebitis without being convinced that the inflammation did not commence in the common or external iliac, but in the branches of the left hypogastric vein.

IX. In the third lecture, the uterus, with all the veins connected with it, were exhibited in the recent state, which had been removed from the body of a woman who died on the 9th of October, 1842, four weeks after delivery, and who had phlegmasia dolens in both lower extremities, the left having been first and most severely affected. The symptoms were those which characterise uterine and crural phlebitis, and you saw all the veins of the cervix uteri in the left side filled with lymph and pus, and coated with false membranes. The left internal, common external iliac, and femoral veins, were all in the same condition. The vena cava was thickened as high as the diaphragm, and a rough false membrane adhered to the whole of its inner surface. The right common, ex-

ternal, and internal iliac, femoral, and saphena veins were all inflamed, though in a slighter degree than on the left side. There was a quantity of serous fluid in the cellular membrane of the limb, but no disease of the absorbents that could be discovered. This dissection demonstrates in the most conclusive manner that in this case of phlegmasia dolens, as in all the preceding cases, the inflammation commenced in the uterine branches of the hypogastric veins, and subsequently extended from them into the iliac and femoral trunks of the affected side.

Many authors have confounded diffuse cellular inflammation with crural phlebitis, and have in consequence been led to deny that inflammation and obstruction of the crural veins is invariably the cause of phlegmasia dolens. "Drs. Otto, Duncan, and Craigie," observes Dr. Copland, "refer phlegmasia dolens to diffuse inflammation of the cellular substance, but I think on insufficient evidence. If this tissue be really inflamed in that disease, other structures participate, and it certainly is not the part first affected. In the cases which I have seen examined after death, only three in all, the nerves and veins were the parts to which the symptoms of disorder were first referred, the veins being obstructed in all the cases." Cases of diffuse cellular inflammation of the thigh in puerperal woman, which had extended from the peritoneum of the uterus, have most erroneously been represented by some as genuine cases of phlegmasia dolens, though none of the pathognomonic symptoms of the disease were present; where the pain and swelling were in fact on the outside of the thigh, and not in the course of the femoral vessels. It has also been asserted "that phlegmasia dolens has manifested itself to a very considerable extent in some cases without any inflammation of the veins whatever;" but when and where such cases happened no information is given, and in opposition to this I will affirm that no such cases have been recorded during the last sixteen years in the medical writings of this country. I believe no example of genuine phlegmasia dolens has occurred in England during this period, in which the iliac and femoral veins were not affected before the cellular membrane, lymphatics, and nerves, and other textures of the limb.

In a Work on the Pathology and Treatment of some of the most Important Diseases of Women (1833), cases and dissections are related by me, which prove that crural phlebitis is not peculiar to women who have been recently delivered, but that it may also arise from suppressed menstruation, malignant ulceration of the os and cervix uteri, polypus of the uterus, and other organic diseases of the uterine organs. Cases are also related in which crural phlebitis occurred in the male sex, and where the disease commenced either in the hæmorrhoidal, vesical, or in some of the other branches of the internal iliac veins, in consequence of inflammation or organic changes of structure in one or more of the pelvic viscera,—or in the superficial veins of the legs, which extended upwards and involved the great venous trunks of the thigh and pelvis. The following is the description of puerperal crural phlebitis, which was then given, and the accuracy of which subsequent observation has confirmed. In seven of the twenty-two cases which I have observed, the disease has commenced between the fourth and twelfth days after delivery, and in the remaining fifteen it appeared subsequent to the end of the second week after parturition. In most of the patients there was either an attack of uterine inflammation in the interval between delivery and the commencement of the swelling in the lower extremity, or there were certain symptoms present which I have before described as characteristic of venous inflammation, viz.: rigors, headache, prostration of strength, a small rapid pulse, nausea, loaded tongue, and thirst. The sense of pain at first experienced in the uterine region has afterwards been chiefly felt along the brim of the pelvis, in the direction of the iliac veins, and has been succeeded by tension and swelling of the part. After an interval of one or more days the painful tumefaction at the iliac and inguinal regions has extended along the course of the crural vessels, under Poupart's ligament, to the upper part of the thigh, and has descended from thence in the direction of the great blood-vessels to the ham. Pressure along the course of the iliac and femoral vessels has never failed to aggravate the pain, and in no other part of the limb has pressure produced much uneasiness. There has generally been a sensible fulness perceptible above Poupart's ligament, before any tenderness has been experienced along the course of the femoral vessels; and in every case at the commencement of the attack I have been able to trace the femoral vein proceeding down the thigh like a hard cord, which rolled under the fingers. A considerable swelling of the limb, commencing in the thigh and gradually descending to the ham, has generally taken place in the course of two or three days, and in some cases immediately after the pain has been experienced in the groin. In other cases the swelling has been first observed in the ham or calf of the leg, and has spread from these parts upward and downward, until the whole extremity has become greatly enlarged. The integuments have then become tense, elastic, hot, and shining, and, in most cases, where the swelling has taken place rapidly, there has been no pitting upon pressure, or

discolouration of the skin. In several well-marked cases, however, of crural phlebitis, at the invasion of the disease, the impression of the finger has remained in different parts of the limb, more particularly along the tibia; but, as the intumescence has increased, the pitting upon pressure has disappeared, until the acute stage of the complaint has passed away. At the onset of the disease I have also observed, in several cases, a diffuse erythematous redness of the integuments along the inner part of the thigh and leg. In one individual only has suppuration of the glands taken place in the vicinity of the femoral vein; but in several, by an extension of the inflammation, the inguinal glands have become indurated and enlarged. In some women the inflammation of the femoral vein has appeared to be suddenly arrested at the part where the trunk of the saphena enters it, and the inflammation has extended along the superficial veins to the leg and foot. The swelling and pain in these instances have been greatest along the inner surface of the thigh in the course of the saphena veins. In most cases of crural phlebitis, not only the whole lower extremity, but the nates and vulva, have been affected with a hot, colourless, and painful swelling, which has not retained the impression of the finger. The power of moving or extending the leg has been lost after the disease has been completely formed, and the greatest degree of freedom from pain has been experienced by the patients, in the horizontal posture, with the limb slightly flexed at the knee and hip-joints. The severity of the pain and the febrile symptoms has usually diminished in a few days after the occurrence of the swelling; but this has not invariably happened, and I have seen some individuals suffer from excruciating pain, and violent febrile disturbance, for many weeks, or through the whole period of the acute stage of the disease. The duration of the acute local symptoms has been very various in different cases. In the greater number they have subsided in two or three weeks, and sometimes earlier, and the limb has then been left in a powerless and œdematous state. The swelling of the thigh has first disappeared, and the leg and foot have more slowly resumed their natural form. In one case, after the swelling had subsided several months, large clusters of dilated superficial veins were seen proceeding from the foot, along the leg and thigh, to the trunk, and numerous veins as large as a finger were observed over the lower part of the abdominal parietes. In some women the extremity does not return to its natural state for many months or years, or even during life. In the summer of 1831, a lady was placed under my care, for an affection of the left lower extremity, who, forty years before, had suffered from an attack of puerperal crural phlebitis in the same side. The left thigh and leg had remained larger and weaker than the other during the whole of this long period, and was liable to suffer severely from fatigue and slight changes in the atmosphere. In four cases of this affection, after the symptoms had begun to subside, the same appearances were observed in the iliac and femoral veins of the opposite extremity, and the other thigh, the leg, and the foot, became similarly affected. In two individuals only has the disease attacked the same extremities twice.

Puzos, as has already been stated, recommended repeated and copious venesection in cases of crural phlebitis; but, in all the cases which I have seen, there has been so much feebleness of pulse, and prostration of strength, that I have not ventured to draw blood from the arm. Many individuals attacked with crural phlebitis have already suffered from hæmorrhage and uterine inflammation, and are not in a condition to lose much blood. But there are cases occasionally met with where the symptoms require, and are immediately relieved by, a general bleeding. An example of severe crural phlebitis after delivery occurred some years ago, in the practice of a medical friend, where the abstraction of twenty ounces of blood seemed at once to break the force of the attack. In a great proportion of cases venesection is not required, and the inflammation will be subdued by the repeated application of leeches above and below Poupart's ligament in the course of the crural veins. From two to three dozen of leeches should be applied immediately after the commencement of the disease, and the bleeding should be encouraged by warm fomentations and poultices. Should the relief of the local pain not be complete, it is requisite soon to re-apply the leeches, in numbers proportioned to the severity of the attack, and to repeat them a third or even fourth time, at no very distant intervals, should the disease not yield. It is requisite, in the progress of the disease, not only to apply leeches along the course of the iliac and femoral, but of the saphena veins, or to any parts of the limb where the swelling is great and the pain very acute. Some patients experience greatest relief from the use of warm cataplasms to the limb, others derive most advantage from the application of cold, or a tepid evaporating lotion. The bowels are often much disordered in this disease, but the employment of strong cathartics is always injurious. Repeated small doses of calomel and antimonial powder, and Dover's powder, should be given, with some mild purgative, not only with the view of correcting the disordered state of the bowels, but to subdue the local inflammation and the

great constitutional disturbance usually present. I believe no good is derived from mercury to salivation in this disease. It is of importance also to administer saline and diaphoretic medicines, and to procure rest and relief from pain, by anodynes, until the acute symptoms pass away. The diet should be the same as that usually allowed to patients who are labouring under inflammatory and febrile diseases. I have seen no advantage derived from the employment of digitalis in any stage either of uterine or crural phlebitis. Dr. Sims informed me that the swelling, pain, and tension of the limb, in a case of phlegmasia dolens, were strikingly relieved by puncturing the skin in different parts with a fine needle. In other cases this has done little or no good.

When the inflammatory symptoms have passed away, the limb remains in a weak œdematous state, and great uneasiness is often experienced from congestion of blood in the veins. Until the collateral branches which are to carry back the blood to the heart become enlarged, it is impossible by any means we possess to afford complete relief: the obstructed vein can never again be rendered pervious. Much benefit may, however, be derived, in this stage of the complaint, from the occasional application of leeches to different parts of the limb, and by preserving it in the horizontal position. I have seen much mischief produced by having recourse too early to remedies intended to promote the absorption of the fluid into the cellular membrane. Blisters, frictions, stimulant embrocations, and bandages to the limb, are only useful when the inflammation of the veins has wholly subsided, and other vessels have become so much enlarged as to carry on the circulation of the blood in the extremity without interruption. In the acute stage of the disease our main object is to moderate the inflammation of the iliac and femoral veins; and in the chronic form, to promote the circulation in the collateral veins by all the means in our power, and to further the absorption of the fluid effused. I have not perceived any sensible benefit accrue from the use of mercurial ointment and iodine in crural phlebitis. The repeated application of blisters is a much more powerful means of exciting the absorbents. The local abstraction of blood at the commencement of the disease is you will perceive by far the most important remedy.

ON THE

TREATMENT OF PUERPERAL CONVULSIONS

BEFORE THE FULL TERM OF UTERO-GESTATION*.

By S. HARRIS, M.D. of Clarkesville, Va.

OF the many accidents incident to pregnancy, that of puerperal convulsions is among the most alarming, the most sudden, and the most unmanageable. Intimately connected with and dependent on the gravid uterus, there is no period of pregnancy exempt from its attacks. It is admitted by all, that cerebral congestion is the most common cause of these convulsions; but it is contended by some that they occur under an opposite state of the brain, and it cannot be denied that there are some facts to sustain this opinion. Be this, however, as it may, they are generally preceded by undoubted evidences of a fulness of the vessels of the head, such as a flushed face, headache, giddiness, drowsiness, tinnitus aurium, &c. They are most common in the latter stages of pregnancy, and in labour during the violence of the parturient pains; and it is said that they sometimes come on after labour has terminated. It is no part of my present purpose to describe this disease, as the symptoms are familiar to almost every practitioner. My design is simply to call the attention of the profession to a material point in its treatment, when the usual remedies fail, and we are compelled to resort to delivery, but the os uteri is found undilated, and undilatable by gentle means. We are advised, and on this point I believe all agree, to bleed the patient as long as the pulse will bear it, to give cathartics, and apply cold applications to the head. But in the event of these remedies failing, we must endeavour to evacuate the uterus with as little delay as possible. Different means of effecting this object are accurately and minutely pointed out, to be used according to the circumstances of the case. We are told to deliver with the forceps, if the head of the child be engaged in the pelvis and the os uteri dilated; or if not engaged in the pelvis, but above the

brim, and the membranes have not been ruptured, the hand must be introduced, and the child turned and delivered by the feet; or if this be impossible, the perforator must be used. Now all these operations are made to depend upon the condition of the os tincæ. If not dilated or dilatable by gentle means, we are advised not to attempt any thing. All the authorities that I have consulted disapprove of a forcible entry into the uterus under any circumstances. Now I am not disposed to question the correctness of this established principle, as a general rule of practice; but in the disease which we are now considering, it frequently happens that delivery or death are the only alternatives presented. And must we, then, quietly seat ourselves, and witness a certain triumph of this terrible disorder? Do not the tears and entreaties of husband and friends justify, and even demand, a last and desperate effort to ward off the fatal result?

We will suppose that a woman enjoying apparent good health is taken suddenly with these convulsions in the fifth or sixth month of pregnancy; she is bled as far as her pulse or strength will allow, cold is applied to the head, cathartics administered either by the mouth or per anum, without any or but slight abatement of the fits. On examination per vaginam, the os uteri is found nearly closed, hard, and callous, and no manifestations of uterine contractions. The patient, during the intervals of the fits, lies in a profound stupor, unconscious and helpless, with a stertorous breathing, the eyes fixed, with dilated or contracted pupils; the heart, though still true to its office, propels the blood with a weak and vacillating action; a cold clamminess spreads over the upper portion of the body, with other equally distinctive signs of approaching dissolution. What, I ask, is to be done under such trying circumstances? Must the case be given up to nature, or are we not justified in making a forcible entry into the uterus, and extracting its contents? I am decidedly in favour of this last painful resource. And hopeless as such an undertaking may seem to be, it is nevertheless practicable in most cases, unless, perhaps, in the very early stages of pregnancy. But, it may be asked, will this forced delivery, even if it can be accomplished without a laceration

* From the American Journal of the Medical Sciences—July 1843.

of the os and cervix uteri, save the life of the woman? I answer, that to judge from the few cases of the kind which I have seen, it probably will, unless pretty extensive effusion has taken place in the brain. In support of this opinion, I will relate a case that fell under my observation in the spring of 1838.

I was called in consultation to Mrs. ——, a strong, healthy, plethoric woman, about sixteen years of age, pregnant with her first child. She was in the fifth month, and up to the time of the attack of puerperal convulsions under which she was then labouring, had enjoyed robust health, with, perhaps, occasional transient pain and giddiness of the head, flushed face, and ringing in the ears. The convulsions came on suddenly, and recurred at intervals of twenty or thirty minutes. Up to the time I first saw her, which was probably ten hours from the commencement of the attack, she had had twenty-two or three distinct fits. A neighbouring physician, of some distinction, reached her in the morning, soon after the onset of the disease, and bled her freely, indeed I may say largely, and repeated the operation several times during the day. The bowels were likewise emptied, and irritants applied to the extremities. I found her, on my arrival, totally insensible to surrounding objects. The most glaring light produced no change whatever in the pupils of the eyes, which were fixed and distorted. The loudest noise excited no manifestations of consciousness. Deglutition, if performed at all, was involuntary, and the power of articulation was completely suspended. Her breathing was laboured and stertorous, and the pulse weak and fluttering, and sometimes not even perceptible at the wrist. There was no evidence of uterine action, and on examination the os tincæ was found almost entirely closed, hard, and unyielding. Viewing the case as nearly desperate, but still desirous of doing something, we determined to administer ergot, regardless of the rigidity of the os uteri. Several twenty-grain doses were accordingly put into the mouth, but from the inability to swallow, very little if any was conveyed to the stomach. No uterine contractions resulted from this experiment. The paroxysms continuing to recur with

unabated fury, I proposed as the only resource left to make an effort to deliver her. This my colleague in the case assented to, though reluctantly, as he considered it, if not impossible without certain death, to say the least of it rash and useless. I determined, however, to make an effort. Not having with me my obstetrical instruments, I was under the necessity of making a small crotchet for the purpose, out of the spindle of a cotton spinning wheel, such as is used in many families in the southern and western parts of the United States. As some of the readers of the American Journal of Medical Sciences may not be familiar with this domestic machine, I will describe that part of it which I used on this occasion, as well as on others of a like emergency, when time was not allowed to procure more suitable instruments. It is a small round iron spike, from twelve to fourteen inches long gradually tapering off from about the middle to a point at one end, while the other half remains of an uniform size, say one-fourth of an inch in diameter. The hook was readily made by heating the sharp point to a red heat, and bending it exactly as I wished. For the purpose of perforating the head of the fœtus, I wrapped with tape the blade of a common dirk-knife to within half an inch of the point. With these rude instruments I prepared for the operation, by placing the nates of the woman on the edge of the bed, with a chair and an assistant on each side to support the legs (the usual position in this country for turning). With the index finger of the left hand I soon found the os tincæ, and cautiously but firmly thrust it into the uterus. The second finger, by dint of perseverance, was likewise forced in by the side of the first. This effected a slight dilatation of the passage. and after ascertaining pretty satisfactorily that the fœtal head presented, I withdrew my fingers and carried up the point of the knife, carefully guarded with my finger until it reached the head, which I pierced readily by acting on the handle of the knife with my right hand exterior to the vulva. After perforating the head, I introduced the hook, and with some difficulty fixed the point in the bones of the cranium. These were, however, so soft as to yield under the slightest force. I succeeded ultimately in fixing the point among the bones at the base of the skull. The last situation enabled me to use as much force as I pleased; but bearing in mind the delicacy of the parts thus rudely assailed, I did not exert it beyond what I supposed would have been the natural expulsive power of the uterus, under ordinary circumstances in abortion, at the fifth or sixth month of pregnancy. Though occasionally interrupted by the recurrence of the fits, the efforts at delivery were kept up at short intervals for several hours, when finally the os uteri yielded, and I succeeded in extracting the fœtus and secundines. Little or no hæmorrhage ensued. The woman was then placed back on the bed in what appeared to be a truly forlorn and hopeless condition. Blisters and warm applications were immediately applied to the extremities, which were now cold and clammy. As is usually the case, she had two or three fits after delivery, but they were less severe, and occurred at longer intervals. She remained in a comatose state nearly twenty-four hours, frequently without any pulse at the wrist, or the ability to swallow either nutriment or medicine. Gradually, however, reaction came on, the breathing became less stertorous, the pulse slower and fuller, the surface warmer, the face less livid, and the eyes more natural in appearance. In this situation she remained for several hours, and finally waked up as if from a sound sleep, uttering moans and inarticulate cries of pain and anguish. Consciousness having returned, she was soon able to converse a little with her anxious friends, and take a little fluid nourishment; but the complete restoration of all her faculties was retarded for several days, in consequence of the severe shock which the brain had received. Mild laxatives, with an occasional mercurial purgative, a nutritious but not stimulating diet, frictions on the surface, with quiet but cheerful company, soon restored her to perfect health. As far as I was able to ascertain, neither the uterus nor its appendages sustained the slightest injury from the operation. She has since been pregnant three or four times, but has not as yet brought forth a living child. Generally she has an abortion about the fifth or sixth month, preceded by giddiness and pain in the

head; and on one occasion slight convulsions, which ceased after the expulsion of the fœtus, but a partial paralysis remained in one arm and hand for six or eight months afterwards.

The result of this case proves, I think, beyond all question, that we are not only justifiable, but in duty bound, when all else fails, to force our way into the uterus and remove the offending cause. The practicability of this too much dreaded operation, without serious or permanent injury to the organ, is likewise demonstrated in the following case.

I was called in the month of February 1839, with two other medical gentlemen, to see Mrs. ——, with puerperal convulsions, pregnant with her fifth child, and about thirty years of age. Naturally of a thin, nervous habit, she had never enjoyed robust health, and for several years previous to the attack, had been declining in strength and vigour. She was in the latter part of the fifth or first part of the sixth month of gestation. She had been labouring under the disease eight or ten hours when I first saw her, and had had probably a dozen severe paroxysms. The os uteri was undilated, and we were unable to discover any indications of labour. After bleeding freely and finding no relief, it was proposed to deliver her at once. This I accomplished in nearly the same manner as in the other case. She had only one fit after the extraction of the fœtus, but remained in a state of almost hopeless insensibility for many hours. The general aspect of the case was very similar to the one already detailed both before and after delivery; but it could not be viewed otherwise than as a more hopeless one, as this lady had neither the youth nor vigour of constitution of the other. The next day after the operation she became rational, but was unable to articulate distinctly. The following evening fever came on, attended with a low muttering delirium, and a slow but full pulse. There was no tenderness or swelling of the abdomen, nor were the vaginal discharges at all different from that which usually follows abortion. There was, however, a retention of urine for several days, which compelled us to use the catheter. In order to lessen the violence of the reaction, she was bled from the arm and cupped on the temples, cold applied to the head, and the bowels evacuated. Her case continued on for six days, with some slight remission of the symptoms in the forenoon, but a high fever with delirium in the evening. During all this time she enjoyed not one hour's refreshing sleep, nor did one-sixth of a grain of the sulph. morphia which we ventured to give her, produce more than an unquiet stupor. She would occasionally, in the morning, converse for a few moments on the subject of her children, or domestic concerns; at all other times she appeared unconscious of, or indifferent to what was passing around her. There was evidently in this case pressure on the brain, either from congestion or effusion, and the treatment pursued was strictly in accordance with this view of its pathological condition. She died on the seventh day. Had delivery been resorted to sooner, possibly the result might have been different.

We find that the os tincæ, though closed and rigid, will, by persevering efforts, generally admit one and sometimes two fingers, which will enable us to perforate the fœtal head, if presenting, without wounding the uterus. This being done, and a proper degree of tractive force applied, the passage will generally dilate and allow the fœtus to be extracted. It is admitted, I believe, by most of the standard authorities on the subject of parturition, that the child being forcibly impelled by the contractions of the uterus at the full period of utero-gestation towards the os uteri, contributes powerfully to dilate this opening, by overcoming the resistance of its circular fibres. Is it not probable, therefore, that if an equal degree of force be applied directly to the head of the child, and kept up at proper intervals for a reasonable length of time, that the same effect will be produced? Unaided by the concurrent action of the uterus itself, I grant that we might not so readily succeed; but it rarely happens that this sensitive organ fails to second our designs. Roused up by the rupture of the membranes, and the tractive efforts of the operator, the contractions of the body and fundus contribute more or less to the dilatation of the os uteri, and the ultimate delivery of the fœtus.

Not having seen a case of convulsions of the epileptic or apoplectic form, earlier than the fifth month, I am not prepared to give any positive opinion as to the practicability or utility of extracting the ovum in the first period of pregnancy. But so firmly convinced am I of the importance of the operation in such cases, that I should not hesitate one moment, other things having failed, to make the attempt. I have frequently seen this disease in the latter stages of pregnancy, and during labour at the full term of gestation, and I have not yet succeeded in checking it even until after delivery, either by the natural powers of the uterus, or by an operation.

In thus presenting to the public my views, in reference to this formidable malady, based on an experience so limited, I can only hope to direct the attention of others to the subject, rather than expect an imitation of my rashness. If I have subjected myself to the imputation of having violated an established rule of practice, in the two cases reported, I have at least the consolation of knowing that the bold innovation of forcibly entering the uterus and delivering the fœtus saved the life of one patient, and did not injure the person of the other. It is only as a *pis-aller* that I can recommend this course, and I venture to affirm, that if timely resorted to, it will, under guidance of reason and the promptings of ingenuity, result very often in the preservation of human life.

[Every proposition for the relief of so terrible a disease as puerperal convulsions is deserving of a respectful consideration, and therefore we have given place to the preceding well drawn up paper. The cautious practitioner will, however, doubtless require evidence of greater success from the practice advocated by our respectable correspondent, than has been adduced, and will duly weigh the consideration whether the forcible dilatation of the os uteri is not likely to be productive of more injury than the delivery will be of benefit.

Dr. Churchill, the author of one of the best works on diseases of women, and an experienced practitioner, remarks on this subject, " I believe there is no dispute that, until labour sets in naturally, interference would be injurious; so that in convulsions during gestation, we have nothing to do with the uterus, but must confine ourselves to the treatment of the convulsive disease." — *Diseases of Females*, Am. Ed. p. 403.

Dr. Rigby, equally high authority, states: "The practice in former times of dilating the os uteri, introducing the hand, and turning the child, has been long since justly discarded, for the irritation produced by such improper violence would run great risk of aggravating the convulsions to a fatal degree."—*System of Midwifery*, Am. Ed. p. 385.

Mr. J. T. Ingleby entertains similar views. "From the seventh to the ninth month," he observes, "delivery, when it is expedient, may certainly be accomplished, but every objection which attaches to artificial delivery at the full term of utero-gestation, applies with peculiar force to the performance of it if undertaken before the term is completed, since the cervix uteri will not have undergone its full development. In numerous instances death has speedily followed after artificial delivery; in others, the event has not been so immediately fatal. In an instance of very recent occurrence, the comatose state in which the patient died did not take place for many hours after delivery; she was in the eighth month of pregnancy, and labour succeeded the artificial evacuation of the liquor amnii. Even admitting that the convulsions which arise previous to labour depend *primarily* upon the condition of the uterus, it is important to recollect that labour is not always necessary for their removal, and that whether delivery be effected artificially, or by the violence of the paroxysms, the convulsions may continue in full force, notwithstanding the evacuation of the uterus; possibly indeed, the impression previously made upon the brain may be increased by the efforts which attend delivery." — *Facts and Cases in Obstetric Medicine*, p. 31.

Again, he says, "It has been already stated that convulsions sometimes cease under *natural* and *spontaneous* labour-pains, nevertheless it is equally true that manual interference is, at the moment, calculated both to renew the paroxysm and render it more violent:

thus Denman found the mechanical dilatation of the os uteri productive of these effects, and the best informed writers, including Chaussier, fully confirm his statement. The principle of forwarding the dilatation of the os internum by means of the fingers, can only be commended when the orifice is in a soft and yielding condition; under contrary circumstances, the practice cannot fail to be injurious."—*Op. cit.* p. 33.

Mr. Symonds, in a paper on puerperal convulsions (*Lancet*, 8th Feb. 1834), after detailing the particulars of four cases successfully treated—first, by depletion, cold to the head, blistering, the warm bath, and camphor and opium—concludes in the following words: "Instructed by my own experience, and fortified by the authority of such writers as Denman, Blundell, and Gooch, I would say with the latter, take care of the convulsions, and let the uterus take care of itself." In this as a general principle Mr. Ingleby says that he quite concurs, and adds, "but exceptions to it may arise." When the attack appears during actual labour, our line of practice is clearly defined; we must moderate excessive action, and deliver on the first favourable moment. But should the convulsions *precede* labour, the practice pursued by Dr. Joseph Clarke (very similar to that recommended by La Motte) is the most rational that can be followed, viz. to trust to nature's efforts, aided by medical treatment, until the patient's life appears to be *immediately* endangered by the continuance of the disease, and then to interfere in the speediest and safest manner to promote delivery. The circumstances which justify interference demand an impartial and dispassionate consideration, and should embrace the state of the uterus, the presentation of the fœtus, the period of gestation, and the violence of the symptoms. An apprehension lest the patient may die undelivered has often proved an incentive for undertaking delivery at any risk, and, doubtless, the interests of the mother alone ought to decide so momentous a question; indeed, under severe and frequent paroxysms, especially of the tetanic kind, the child is frequently still-born. In Collins's cases, 14 of 32 children, including two twin births, were born alive. Of 43 cases, including a twin birth, which occurred under Dr. F. H. Ramsbotham's observation, 21 of the infants survived. The death of the child is considered, by this gentleman, to depend rather upon a defective utero-placental circulation, than upon direct pressure; but the result may be occasioned by either cause.

"The want of success in delivering generally arises from one of two causes; the first—delivering too early, before the uterine orifice has undergone sufficient relaxation; the second—postponing the delivery until effusion has taken place, or a fatal impression been made upon the brain. Previous to delivery being attempted, sufficient relaxation of the uterus must therefore be obtained by bleeding or emetic medicines in nauseating doses, purgative enemata, and perhaps the application of belladonna to its orifice, otherwise we incur the risk either of an apoplectic seizure, or a laceration of the uterus or vagina.* This precaution has less regard to the degree of dilatation of the os uteri, (for the orifice is not unfrequently more or less open for many days before labour), than to its state of softness; and if a decided impression be made upon it during the paroxysm, the sooner delivery is accomplished the better. Although the uterine orifice often becomes relaxed earlier than we might à priori infer, a moderate degree of resistance is, in every delivery, both to be expected and desired: but a forcible entry into the uterus must be discountenanced by every rational practitioner. Ashwell considers that we may always dilate the uterus with the fingers: a statement which I cannot assent to, and it is with marked propriety that Collins strongly cautions the practitioner to 'avoid hasty measures for the delivery of the child.' " — Op. cit. p. 35, 36, 37.

All these considerations should be duly weighed, and we would particularly recommend to the junior practitioner a careful perusal of the admirable remarks of Mr. Ingleby on puerperal convulsions, in the work from which we have just quoted.—EDITOR.]

* Of five fatal cases recorded by Collins, three were complicated with laceration of the vagina.

ON VIVISECTION.

To the Editor of the Medical Gazette.

SIR,

HAVING derived great pleasure from a letter in your last number from Dr. Hull, on the subject of vivisection, and having for some years past devoted at intervals some time to the consideration of that subject, I venture to offer a few remarks in corroboration of the sentiments of your enlightened correspondent. In my endeavours to promote methods of pathological investigation more strictly instructive than those commonly employed, I have been necessarily led to the examination of the general bearings of experiments on animals on the progress of physiological and especially on pathological science, and the result of such examination is the conviction, that so far as regards experiments involving the suffering of the animal, that they waste time which I am prepared to show might be better employed; that, philosophically, they are to the last degree inconclusive, and that they are morally indefensible. Either or all of these positions I am quite prepared to defend. But let me be understood: I object to no experiment which does not involve cruelty, nor do I include in the catalogue of cruel experiments those which imply the killing the animal with the ordinary expedition. Not the least interesting fact of the many which investigation of this subject discloses is, that the moment experiments cease to be cruel, they begin to be instructive; or if they are not, it is owing to some want of circumspection in the conduct of the experiment. I shall be quite ready to illustrate all that I say, on conditions presently to be mentioned; but I will now observe that it is about five years since that I offered to the Society for the Prevention of Cruelty to Animals, to make a digest of the principal experiments on living animals within the last 100 years (involving cruelty), in order to show that they had either not in the least degree assisted us in relieving disease, (because it must be remembered that is our object) or that if they had shown any thing in relation thereto, it was only that which might be much more satisfactorily demonstrated by other and unobjectionable phenomena. The only condition was, that the Society should pay the expence of the publication; but although the offer was courteously received, either for want of funds, or some other reason with which I am unacquainted, I heard nothing more of the matter. Since that time two rather sharp illnesses have thrown some other matters in which I am engaged so much in arrear, that I cannot venture to repeat the offer; but if your or any other journal will open its columns for short demonstrations on the subject, and Dr. Hull and other gentlemen will lend their assistance, I promise to be a cheerful contributor. At pages 48, 52, and 54 to 56, of my last work, "Medicine and Surgery one Inductive Science," some remarks will be found on this matter, with a suggestion as to the mode of bringing the subject to the required test; but it is too long, I suppose, to quote. Suffice it to say, that I have plenty of material, and nothing would give me more pleasure than to see physiological science well rid of that which now misrepresents and disgraces it. One word as to coolness in operations. I agree with Dr. Hull, and having operated not a little, I know of no better rule than that of my old master Abernethy—"Never do an operation that you would not have performed on yourself, were you in similar circumstances." If, however, the leading motive should be lucre, display, or some others that I could mention, a surgeon may find himself obliged to dismiss his feelings, or lose his self-possession, and if any thing unexpectedly untoward happen, he may (as I have witnessed) be deprived of both.

I have the honour to be, sir,
Your obedient servant,
GEORGE MACILWAIN.

9, Argyle Place,
Sept. 16, 1843.

MR. LEE ON BELGIAN MEDICAL INSTITUTIONS.

To the Editor of the Medical Gazette.

SIR,

THE present brief notice of some of the Belgian medical institutions and practice may interest several of the readers of the MEDICAL GAZETTE, and may serve as a *pendant* to that which I sent last year of those in Holland.

I am, sir,
Your obedient servant,
EDWIN LEE.

September, 1843.

Liege.—Although containing a population of 60,000 inhabitants, chiefly manufacturing and commercial, Liege possesses no good hospital; the one termed de la Bavière was formerly an ancient convent, the church now forming the principal ward. The surgical wards are low and indifferently ventilated; the medical wards on the first floor are loftier and more airy. On the walls are images of Saints, &c.; the sick are superintended by sisters of charity. The number of beds does not exceed 120, including those for the medical and surgical cliniques. Two physicians and two surgeons perform the medical duties. The administration of this and the other charitable institutions (the Hospices, Bureau de bienfaisance, and Mont de Piété), is vested in a commission nominated by the regency. Among the most prevalent diseases at Liege, are phthisis, bronchial inflammation, scrofula, and rheumatic affections, which last are mostly treated by antiphlogistic measures, colchicum being very seldom employed. In scrofula, and incipient phthisis, the cod-liver oil is a common remedy. Inflammatory attacks, and fevers, are not usually treated by energetic depletory measures; contra-stimulants and cooling diuretic remedies, as the nitrate of potass, with an occasional laxative, being chiefly trusted to. Auscultation and percussion are not very generally employed, except by Dr. Lombard, who enjoys a high reputation in Liege. Stone cases are very uncommon.

The Hôpital de Santé is for chronic and syphilitic diseases. In order to be admitted, patients must obtain a certificate from the physician or surgeon, and from the Commissaire de Police. There are also at Liege a hospice for old men, one for old women, a lying-in and a foundling hospital, and out of the town a hospice for patients of either sex labouring under mental alienation, which, however, are little else than places of detention.

Many of the sick poor are visited at their own habitations. The University is a large detached building, containing a handsome library, cabinets of instruments, anatomical and pathological preparations. Lectures are delivered within the building, but the examinations of candidates take place at Brussels. The number of the students is 450, of which scarcely 100 attend the medical classes.

The following are professors in the faculty of medicine:—

Dean, and Professor of Obstetrics, Simon. Descriptive anatomy, and general therapeutics, J. B. Royer. (Physiology, and general anatomy—Spring.) Dissections and materia medica, Vaust. Pathological anatomy, and hygiene, Raikein. Internal pathology and therapeutics, Sauveur. Surgical pathology and ophthalmology, Asiaux. Medical cliniques, Lombard, and Frankinel. Surgical clinique, Delavacherie.

Brussels.—The old and ruinous hospital existing within the town was at the time of my visit about to be pulled down, and the patients transferred to the handsome new hospital St. John, in a more airy situation, on the Boulevard du Jardin Botanique, of which its extensive stone facade forms a chief ornament. It is built around a spacious court yard, at the extremity of which is a chapel, and contains 500 beds, including those for the cliniques. The interior organization, and the disposition of the wards, will apparently leave nothing further to be desired in this respect. The chief physician is M. Van Cutsem; the surgeon, M. Uytterhoeven. The hospital St. Pierre, founded as far back as 1179, stands in an elevated position at the opposite end of the town. It contains 350 beds. The wards are clean and well ventilated, those for surgical diseases being on the ground, the medical on the first floor. There are besides, wards containing about 100 beds for syphilitic patients, and sick children, as also several rooms for patients who pay from two to six francs a day. The medical service is performed by a chief physician (M. Graux), a chief surgeon (M. Sentin), and assistants. Clinical instruction is given at the bed-side of those patients whose cases present the greatest interest. There are no separate clinical wards. Typhoid fevers, pulmonary complaints, chronic gastro-enteritis, scrofula, and diseases of the kidneys, are inferior orders at Brussels. The treatment of typhoid fever is mostly by a moderate bleeding at the commencement, and subsequently a tonic or stimulating medication. When not counterindicated, the use of stimulants externally, as camphorated liniment, is likewise frequently combined with the internal measures. Aperients, and diaphoretics, are not much employed. Here, as in Paris, in almost all the patients who die from this disease, enlargement or ulceration of the follicular intestinal glands is met with. In inflammation of organs, energetic vascular depletion is not usually adopted; moderate general or local abstraction of blood, and blisters or other contrastimulants, with appropriate internal medicines, being the means mostly adopted; more attention being paid to the patient's general condition, &c. than to the local disease, as regards the exhibition of remedies. Tabes mesenterica is very common among children and young persons; occasional leeching, and the exhibition of ioduret of potass, with the application of the ointment to the abdomen, a bland diet, and tepid baths, being the measures from which the greatest amount of advantage has been derived.

M. Sentin has the most private practice among the Brussels practitioners, and is known in other parts of the continent as well as in England, more especially from his method of treating fractures by starched bandages, which he applies, in all cases, from the first. Even when there is considerable swelling, and in compound cases pasteboard splints moistened so as to adapt themselves to the form of the parts being laid laterally beneath the turns of the bandage, and the interstices formed by the varying thickness of the limb being filled up by cotton wool, which is also placed along the edge of the pasteboard splints, to protect the soft parts from pressure. The application is never removed till the cure, but when matter is formed, or the swelling of the limb has subsided so as to produce slackening of the bandage, it is cut open with scissors, the superabundant edges of the pasteboard are broken off, and another bandage, pasted with the starch solution by an assistant with a painter's brush at the time of its application, is bound over the previous one, remaining until consolidation of the bone is effected.

This practice, which, with some modifications, is now adopted in many European hospitals, and in private, is more particularly advantageous in fractures of the inferior extremity, from the circumstance of patients being thereby enabled to get about on crutches, or with a stick a few days after the accident, instead of remaining in bed for several weeks frequently, to the great detriment of the general health. In some cases which I treated at St. George's Hospital by Amesbury's apparatus—which, however, is too expensive and complicated, and requires more attention than the starched *appareil*—consolidation was procured within a much shorter period than by the old method, and in two or three instances the point where the tibia had been fractured could not afterwards be detected on feeling. In fractures of the upper extremity, however, this method presents little advantage over the ordinary one, nor is its application generally advisable in compound cases, for though the exclusion of the air from the wound, and immobility of the limb, are circumstances of the highest importance, still, where much injury of the parts has been inflicted, and suppuration is inevitable, serious consequences would often ensue, as was sometimes the case in the practice of Baron Larrey, who also had recourse to an analogous method of treatment in all cases in the hospital to which he was attached.

M. Sentin likewise employs the starched bandages in chronic diseases of the joints, and in some cases of tumor. Stone cases rarely occur in the hospitals at Brussels. Disease of the eyes, especially the ophthalmia formerly so prevalent in the army, now afflicts a large proportion of the inferior classes. Syphilitic cases, especially ulcerations of the face, are treated with great success by the ioduret of potass, to the extent in many instances of thirty grains daily.

Considerable sensation was excited in Brussels some time ago on account of a cataleptic patient who was magnetised at this hospital by M. Montère, in the presence of numerous physicians, students, and other persons, and who exhibited in a high degree the phenomena of clairvoyance, to the satisfaction of those present, including some members of the administration of hospitals. It is not my intention to enter into the details of this interesting case, but will

mention two or three of the circumstances.

While in somnambulism, she indicated the treatment to be pursued, and stated that she would be cured in six weeks if this treatment were followed; which in the successive *seances* was consequent, and never of a contradictory nature. After her eyes had been covered with a bandage she was able to indicate the persons behind her, their attitudes, the colour of their clothes, as well as some objects placed behind her head, notwithstanding one of the gentlemen present, as a further precaution, pressed his fingers upon the eyes over the bandage. Among others, the surgeon of the hospital of the Maternité held up behind her head several coins, which she immediately recognised; stating without any mistake which side of the coin was turned towards herself. M. Malvin, the director of the hospital, likewise addressed several questions to the somnambulist, to which she replied with the greatest exactness. Several experiments were tried to verify the abolition of sensibility, M. Sentin being present: among others, the flame of a candle was applied to her arm, without any sensation being evinced, notwithstanding she was seriously burnt. On awaking she experienced a slight degree of pain, at which she was surprised, not knowing the cause. M. Sentin having asked her whether he had any pain, she replied that he felt a pain in his left foot, which was the case, owing to a tight boot. The clairvoyance was not always present while she was in somnambulism, as she was sometimes lucid, at others not. The Hospice de l'Infirmerie is chiefly an asylum for 500 old people of both sexes. The Hospice de la Maternité contains about 50 beds: women are received in the last month of their pregnancy till after accouchement. There are also rooms for those persons who pay. A school of instruction in midwifery is attached. At the Enfans *trouvés* 500 infants is the average number of those annually received. They are for the most part sent into the country, and kept by the establishment till the age of 12 years. The *bureau de bienfaisance* supplies provisions and medical assistance at the houses of the sick poor, in different quarters of the city.

In my next I will give an account of the medical institutions of Ghent.

REPLY TO
A MEMOIR, BY M. MALGAIGNE,
ENTITLED,
RECHERCHES SUR LA FREQUENCE
DES HERNIES SELON LES SEXES,
LES AGES, ET RELATIVEMENT
A LA POPULATION.

BY ROBERT KNOX, M.D. F.R.S.E.
Lecturer on Anatomy in Queen's College, Edin-
burgh, and Corresponding Member of the
French Academy of Medicine.

DURING the winter session of 1836-37,
I read to the Medico - Chirurgical
Society in Edinburgh, a Memoir on
" The Statistics of Hernia in Man, with
some Observations on the Anatomical
causes which determine its Production," which memoir was soon after
published in the 128th No. of the
Edinburgh Medical and Surgical Journal, and shortly afterwards republished
by myself, with several other memoirs,
in a small fasciculus of Anatomical and
Physiological Memoirs.

These researches were originally
undertaken, on my own part, with a
view chiefly to shew that accurate data
were altogether wanting to determine
the ratio of hernia to the population,
viewing the question almost in every
way, and that consequently the statements of several estimable practical
surgeons and others, respecting the
great frequency of hernia, must, if extended to the population generally, be
extremely erroneous, or, at the very
least, entirely conjectural. Another
object kept in view in the composition
of my memoir was the ascertaining in
how far a peculiar conformation of the
pelvis contributed to produce hernia in
either sex.

Now, sensible that my objects were
these, I felt disposed at first to blame
myself for a certain want of perspicuity in the composition of my memoir,
inasmuch as one of the most candid
critics of the day (I had almost said
the most candid medical critic, the
writer of at least a portion of the
Medical and Surgical Journal, edited
by Dr. Johnston) has said, in the notice
he favoured my memoir with, that
" after having objected to the conclusions of all others, Dr. Knox has
arrived at none himself." But, reflecting again on the very object of my
memoir, I saw that no blame could
attach to me for not having put before
the public data which do not exist. I
repeat, my memoir was written to shew
that by far the greater number of
opinions then held by medical men
respecting the frequency of hernia,
were mere opinions, and not derived
from any proper statistics. Indeed, I
might have gone a little farther, and
said justly, though somewhat harshly,
that the greater number of the authors
whose opinions I quoted did not know
the right meaning of the word " statistics." So far, then, I think the criticism alluded to has no force in its application to me, since it merely blamed
me for not having obtained a ratio
where no data existed. Let it also,
however, be observed, that I certainly
did arrive at the conclusion, that whilst
hernia was " rather frequent," nay,
perhaps, might ultimately be found to
offer a comparatively high ratio in the
hard-working labouring and mechanical
class of the population, male and
female, but more especially the former,
there were classes remarkably free
from this disease ; amongst whom I
included the very idle, the very rich,
and, in this country, the aspirant for
military honours, who would rather
serve for sixpence a day, and do no
work, than live *independent* by the
sweat of his brow.

My next critic was a less candid one :
I allude to Mr. Marshall, whose notions
of statistics seem to me by no means
very good. He says, that the "data
drawn from dissecting rooms furnish
no sure information, and especially no
statistics to be depended on." Now,
on the part of Mr. Marshall, this is
speaking in great ignorance, and purely
at random about what he does not
understand ; and it were easy to show,
were it worth while, that the statistics
of the practical-rooms, at least in this
part of the kingdom, are much superior
to most of his army reports in every
sense. But it is not worth while to
do so: Mr. Marshall can have no experience on these points.

My third critic is M. Malgaigne,
who seems to me to be deficient in
candour in speaking of his contemporaries. What he has said in the way
of objection to my memoir may be
reduced simply to two heads. 1st. He
accuses me of having fallen into the
strange error of " taking the ratio of
hernia in a population of a certain age,
and applying this ratio to the general
population." I have looked over my

memoir with the greatest care and attention, and I cannot find a single passage warranting such an accusation. 2d. M. Malgaigne has pointed out a circumstance leading to error in my mode of estimating the ratio of hernia cases occurring amongst the conscripts of the French Army. The Athenæum, from which I took my information, simply stated that, of the 286,420 conscripts for 1833, there were 4,222 exempted from service as being affected with hernia. Unacquainted as I am with the routine of the French conscript laws, for the non-existence of which we Britons have every reason to be thankful to Providence, I could not possibly know that, of these 286,420 who appeared as conscripts, there were only 124,603 examined, of whom 4,222 were rejected for hernia. Thus, my average should have been rather more than three per cent. instead of one and a fraction. Now, after all, this correction makes the ratio approximate more nearly to my own conjecture. But admitting this correction to be right, as I presume it to be, does it really give us the ratio of hernia to the male population of the conscript age? I say it does no such thing; and this is precisely the conclusion I arrived at in my original memoir. The statistics of hernia (an extremely difficult question) is quite open for further inquiry, notwithstanding the laborious "Researches" of M. Malgaigne. In my observations on the Statistics of Hernia, I took occasion to point out several circumstances for which neither M. Malgaigne nor my other critics have given me credit.

1st. I believe I was the first to shew that the estimated valuations of the frequency of hernia to the general population, by Messrs. Turnbull, Munro, Sir A. Cooper, and others, were entirely worthless as statistical inquiries: this, at least, was coming to some conclusion, and not leaving the matter where I found it. 2d. The curious fact that, since the Anatomy Act came into force, hernia cases are very rarely met with in the Practical Rooms in Scotland. This I believe to be another *fact*, of which I am quite certain, in so far as regards my own Practical Rooms. 3d. I took the liberty of pointing out what I thought to be an extraordinary use or abuse of technical language on the part of Mr. Marshall, who, in the drawing up some official reports, made the following statement. "Of 82 recruits rejected for hernia, there were, inguinal 32, ventral 44, umbilical 6." I called the attention of the readers of my memoir to the extraordinary fact of an army surgeon meeting with 44 cases of ventral, and 6 cases of umbilical hernia, in a short space of time; being a greater number of such cases than had been seen by half the surgeons of the empire. I suggested the following queries:—Were these cases of hernia? were they not rather laxity of the abdominal parietes? Mr. Marshall's statistics depend on his diagnosis, which I hope he does not consider infallible; mine are the result of anatomical investigation, made in presence of large bodies of medical students. 3d. Again, I suggested that I had seen many hundreds of the dark races (Caffres), and I had not noticed umbilical hernia to be at all frequent in the adult, from which I presume that the laxity of the abdominal walls around the umbilical orifice, if it exist in the children of the Caffre, as it is said by Mr. Marshall to do in the negro, must after a time cease. 4th. In attempting a comparison between the two great races which inhabit France, the Celt and the Kymri (which races, with M. Tiers and Edwards, he seems to consider distinct), M. Malgaigne ought, in fairness, to have stated that I was the first to attempt this new line of inquiry; instancing the Saxon Dutch at the Cape of Good Hope as being much afflicted with hernia, or at least presumed to be so on good authority, but without venturing to give to such observations the name of "statistics."

MEDICAL GAZETTE.

Friday, September 22, 1843.

"Licet omnibus, licet etiam mihi, dignitatem *Artis Medicæ* tueri; potestas modo veniendi in publicum sit, dicendi periculum non recuso."
                                        CICERO.

WHAT IS QUACKERY?

WHAT is quackery? A question more easily asked than answered, though few perhaps really are, and fewer still suppose themselves to be, ignorant of its meaning. Dr. Johnson, while following the simple alphabetical order in his definitions, has thus suggested a remarkable development of the subject, a consideration of which may not only be interesting, but have great practical utility.

He begins with " To quack, *v. n.* (from the Dutch *quacken*, to cry as a goose) 1. to cry like a duck ; often written *quaake*, to represent the sound the better." Nothing can be more simple, more unsatirical, or inoffensive, than this primitive meaning. The word, or one like it, however, must surely have been used before Dutch was a language. It is impossible to believe that frogs were admitted to have cried out βρεκ-εκ-εξ, as Aristophanes writes their croaking choruses, earlier than ducks and geese were admitted to cry quack ; and the difficulty of writing the latter word in the Greek character without the digamma, would only prove to an ingenious controversialist the necessity for that obsolete and once disputed letter. Hear Johnson again : " 2. To chatter boastingly, to brag loudly, to talk ostentatiously.

> Believe mechanick virtuosi
> Can raise them mountains in Potosi,
> Seek out for plants with signatures
> To quack of universal cures.
> HUDIBRAS."

It may here be noted, that a neuter verb is the only one mentioned ; the active verb " to quack," in the sense of to coddle, to physic, or advise one's self or others, seems to be a very modern invention. Perhaps no one used the verb till after modern dilettanti had thoroughly established the practice. That it is not a mere omission of the Doctor's, which he would honestly have attributed to forgetfulness, or " sheer ignorance, madam," as he did another mistake, is probable from this, that in the same page of our edition, the last

that has his own corrections, " Quadrille" means only " a game at cards;" the dance and the doctoring were not yet subjects for the full flow of London talk. Next comes " Quack, *n. s.* from the verb, a boastful pretender to arts which he does not understand. ' The 'change, schools, and pulpits, are full of quacks, jugglers, and plagiaries.'— *L'Estrange.''*

The 'change did not, in the time referred to, as it does now, suggest only the notion of Spanish actives and the like, but was frequented by physicians as well as merchants, so that the art of physic, though not expressly mentioned, was not perhaps meant to be excluded from those touched by the writer. To resume. 2. " A vain boastful pretender to physic ; one who proclaims his own medical abilities in public places. ' At the first appearance that a French quack made in Paris, a boy walked before him publishing with a shrill voice, My father cures all sorts of distempers, to which the doctor added in a grave manner, the child says true.'— *Addison.* 3. An artful tricking practitioner in physic. " Despairing quacks with curses fled the place."— *Pope.* The natural sound of the well-known bird, the simple etymon, gradually made to include the idea of boastful yet hardly dishonest assumption, now conveys that of deceit and knavery. The awful brows of the literary giant must have been more closely knitted when he wrote as follows. " Quackery, mean or bad acts in physic;" *in physic! intra* muros peccatur. No example is given—could none be found? and did the doctor with a seer's eye merely imagine in that century a word, for a thing to be invented in a future one. Surely the man who read a dictionary, and complained that though the author seemed very clever, his style was rather unconnected, did not read attentively enough, or did not read Johnson. His dictionary, treated in the synthetical way, seems sometimes like a series of Essays—quite an anthology, from the abundance and beauty of its quotations; nay almost a poem, with the cantos shuffled.

To examine the subject more seriously. The regular practitioner is not more exempt from temptations to quackery, than the professor of religion is from temptations to hypocrisy, and a little attention will enable us to trace the progress of the former evil, the pathology of quackery from its first attack in the healthy subject, by following the alphabetical order of words in the dictionary.

The first symptom is a temptation merely to talk loud, to make himself heard—simply to quack (the verb neuter), natural to all, especially to youth, and harmless enough if it goes no further; but it is very apt to lead to *v. n.* 2—boasting, or making an undue parade of acquirements, real or [fancied; and as great modesty usually attends great knowledge, a want of it is generally found amongst the ignorant and superficial. Forwardness, then, shallowness, and ignorance, lead to boasting. A shallow man thinks much of his own powers, and has not yet discovered his deficiencies; he assumes a character that does not belong to him, but he does it in ignorance, and without intentional dishonesty; he speaks only what he thinks when he boasts of his knowledge; he is merely mistaken. Many remain in this happy state of ignorance, quacking away, *tout bonnement*, without meaning or knowing it, in the daily use of the neuter verb, 2.

But worse threatens. He who has for some time sustained a character for knowledge which he does not possess, however honestly he may have believed that he did, is liable one day to be undeceived on this point; and then, if he

have a conscience, he feels called upon to be modest — to leave off boasting. If he do this, all may be well—another stage of the disorder has been gone through safely; if not, and this abstinence is difficult to such persons, he is in danger of becoming what is accurately defined " quack, noun substantive;" from the verb 1, a boastful pretender to an art which he finds he does not understand as well as he once said he did; and when his medical abilities are proclaimed in public places —when his own peculiar proselytes cry out in their various shrill tones that he cures all or any manner of distempers, he admits with much gravity of countenance that they say very true, and thus he furnishes as good an example as that in the dictionary of *n. s.* 2.

From the passively appropriating unmerited applause to the actively becoming an artful tricking practitioner in physic, *n. s.* 3, is a very easy transition; it follows naturally on more boasting, more case-hardening by time and competition, and to one strongly predisposed is quite 'unavoidable. It is obvious that each of these stages had its premonitory symptoms, and that previously to each, conscience might have suggested salutary treatment, and saved the patient. Those in whom the malady has fairly run its course to this melancholy point, have by that time generally given proof of their state, by publishing either in bold whitewash, or by hand-bills, or by advertisement in that particular column which every newspaper dedicates to their especial use.

Is thy servant a dog, that he should do this thing? is the natural exclamation on witnessing these gross offences against professional and general morality; but there are certain of our authors, who, although they seem to be restrained by timidity, or, one would fain hope, some better motive, and who never get farther than a discreditable monograph on a popular malady advertised among the light reading of the day, yet differ, in reality, rather in degree than in kind from the most unblushing.

Against the boastful pretender to an art which he does not understand, the legislature confesses its inability or unwillingness to protect either the public or the profession. It must be evident, as we have elsewhere observed, that although acts of parliament may compass the punishment of particular quacks, yet they are powerless to prevent quackery. That portion of the public who have liberty to choose for themselves, who have intelligence enough to understand plausible arguments, but not knowledge enough to detect fallacies, must be, and always will be, the subjects to keep up the demand for quacks. Pretenders clever enough to get on without the realities of regular education, and powerful enough to despise its forms, will always be found to supply the demand. But even practitioners regularly educated will always be found in greater or less number to make up by quackery for those qualities which should have enabled them to compete with their professional brethren, and thus mislead many who would shrink from employing a professed and unlicensed quack.

The quackery of the dictionary — mean or bad acts in physic—can be prevented only by the prevention of meanness and badness in those who practise physic. A sound healthy training of the moral and intellectual faculties, diligence in the pursuit of science and cultivation of art, modesty in the self-estimation of attainments, moderation in desires for mere applause or emolument, whatever in fact strengthens the intellect or revives honesty, will conduce to this end.

A profession, every member of which had these qualities in abundance, might indeed have quacks for its rivals, but would triumph without a combat.

____

THE CARLISLE CONTROVERSY.

THIS unseemly feud still continues. The Carlisle Journal of Saturday, the 16th inst. contains a second letter from Mr. Steel, the editor, to the Bishop of Carlisle. He defends himself for having drawn the public attention to Clark's case, and says, " I undertook the unpleasant task, not in concert with the medical men — the 'Medical Trades Union,' as they have been called with as much vulgarity as indecency—but as a duty, which my position as a journalist, and a governor of the Institution, fairly imposed upon me."

He is highly indignant with the Committee of the Infirmary for having unanimously declared that the accusations of neglect and improper treatment against their medical officers were totally unfounded, as proved on the inquest. Mr. Steel, also, stoutly defends the calling of an inquest; and thinks it not only justifiable, but quite the usual sort of thing in such a case— an opinion in which few reasonable persons will agree with him. The instances which he cites to strengthen his argument are not in point. On the 17th of August, it seems, an inquest was held in Lancashire on an unfortunate pauper, who died of disease of the lungs, which had been overlooked by the parish surgeon, who pronounced his sickness all a sham. Or, as another example, an inquest was lately held on the body of a woman who died after delivery. In both these instances the supposed error of the practitioner was immediately followed by the death of the patient; in the Carlisle case more than seven months intervened, as well as a long treatment by other practitioners. Mr. Steel answers the charge of falsifying the verdict of the jury in Clark's case, by giving a letter from Mr. Carrick, the Coroner, who furnished the verdict published in the

Journal of the 2d inst. and affirms it to be correct.

The following extracts will interest our readers, as it is obvious that the controversy, though nominally carried on by the editors of the Journal and the Patriot, is really sustained by professional combatants. Each faction in Carlisle might say to the mouth-piece of its rivals—

Non me tua fervida terrent
Dicta, ferox; Dii me terrent, et Jupiter hostis.

From the Carlisle Journal of Sept. 16th.[*]

This, my Lord, settles the question of the coroner's duties and responsibilities, and I venture to prophecy that we shall not again hear a repetition of the threats which have been so abundantly thrown out within the last ten days, of instituting legal proceedings against him for doing that which, had he failed to do, would have subjected him to fine and imprisonment. Of Mr. Carrick's mode of conducting the inquest it is unnecessary to say much. The Coroner's Court is a Court of *inquiry*,—and, if it be not intended to frustrate the very object of its institution, a much wider latitude must be given to the examination of witnesses than is either necessary or required in our courts of record. In the one case, the coroner has often to grope his way in the dark, amidst unwilling or hostile witnesses, whilst in the other every thing is prepared, and it is known exactly what each individual can say, and the precise bearing of his evidence upon the case. Here strict rules may be observed; but were they to be applied by the coroner, in nine cases out of ten his inquiry would prove a total failure. The medical journals remark upon Dr. Jackson and Mr. Elliot being allowed to put questions to the witnesses. In making such remark, they were not aware that these gentlemen were present as accused parties—as men who, though courting the investigation, had been pointed to by Dr. Barnes as the men by whose treatment the death of Clark had been accelerated; and standing in that position, they were fully entitled, in that or any other court, to put such ques-

tions as were relevant to the object of the investigation.

With respect to Dr. Lonsdale's connection with this case, your Lordship, at all events, will not fail to appreciate the dishonesty of the attempt to detract from the weight of his evidence by insinuating the imputation of malevolence; as you will have no difficulty in estimating the amount of truth in the assertion that he was "an unsuccessful competitor with Dr. Barnes for practice in the district," whilst residing some years ago as a general practitioner in your Lordship's own neighbourhood. The very grossness of the assertion defeats its object.

From the Carlisle Patriot of Sept. 16th.

Mr. Steel then enlarges upon the treatment of the patient Clarke in the Infirmary, but it is clear that all his showy information upon this part of the subject is derived exclusively from the doctors who attended Clarke for four months previous to his death, and under, or in spite of, whose treatment he sunk. Dr. Jackson and Mr. Elliot agreed to consider Clarke's case one of that particular kind of scrofulous affection of the hip-joint commonly known as *morbus coxarius*, which is a surgical case, usually occurring in young children, and never within the reading or experience of even the Medical Trades Unionists, in adults of fifty years of age, as Clarke was. All their charge, all their treatment, and the *hope* of their conspiracy, rested upon the correctness of this view of his case. But in point of fact it has been proved, we may say to demonstration, that this patient's affection was one of "*rheumatism*," to which he had been constantly subject for eight years, and more, previous to his death, and with which several members of his family were affected; but it was accompanied by chronic inflammation of the ligaments and tendons surrounding the joint, and this constituted the kind of *morbus coxarius* for which Dr. Barnes treated the deceased. The erudition of Mr. Steel, therefore, however laboriously got up for the nonce, the reading and experience, such as it was, of the doctors who operated upon Clarke, and the testimony of those who subsequently saw him, and even of that "eminent" personage who pretended

---

[*] In our last number, the extract beginning, "When I left" (page 873, col. 1), and ending, "remarked it" (col. 2), should have been separated from the previous passage, as it is taken from a different part of the Carlisle Journal.

to give an opinion without having seen the case at all, were utterly inapplicable to the particular affection under which Clarke laboured when a patient of the infirmary, and in this opinion we are borne out to a considerable extent by the opinions of the medical journals, which we publish in full in our last page. * * * They gave him professional attendance for 17 weeks, and then the man died; upon which they requested the coroner to hold an inquest upon the body of one who had virtually become their own patient—because, forsooth, they did not feel easy at the imputations likely to attach to their treatment. They have attempted, therefore, to remove the blame from their own shoulders to the medical officers of the infirmary, who, it must be remembered, had not seen the man for nearly eight months, and who, therefore, could know nothing about the cause of his death, much less be held responsible for it.

REGULATIONS TO BE OBSERVED
BY STUDENTS
INTENDING TO QUALIFY THEMSELVES
TO PRACTISE AS
APOTHECARIES IN ENGLAND AND WALES, 1843.

[We have just received the new edition of the Regulations of the Society of Apothecaries, which we subjoin in full, believing it may be convenient for medical students to have them before they commence their winter courses.—ED. GAZ.]

EVERY Candidate for a Certificate of Qualification to practise as an Apothecary, will be required to produce Testimonials,

1. Of having served an Apprenticeship, of not less than five years, to an Apothecary:
No gentleman practising as an apothecary in England or Wales can give his apprentice a legal title to examination, unless he is himself legally qualified to practise as an Apothecary, either by having been in practice prior to or on the 1st of August, 1815, or by having received a certificate of qualification from the Court of Examiners. An apprenticeship for not less than five years to Surgeons practising as Apothecaries in Ireland and Scotland, gives to the apprentice a title to be admitted to examination.

2. Of having attained the full age of 21 years:
As evidence of age, a copy of the baptismal register will be required in every case where it can possibly be procured.

3. Of good Moral Conduct:
A testimonial of moral character from the gentleman to whom the Candidate has been an apprentice, will always be more satisfactory than from any other person.

4. And of having pursued a Course of Medical Study in conformity with the Regulations of the Court.

Course of Study.

Every Candidate whose attendance on Lectures commenced on or after the 1st of October, 1835, must have attended the following Lectures and Medical Practice during not less than three winter and two summer sessions: each winter session to consist of not less than six months, and to commence not sooner than the 1st nor later than the 15th October; and each summer session to extend from the 1st of May to the 31st of July.

First Winter Session.—Chemistry. Anatomy and Physiology. Anatomical Demonstrations. Materia Medica and Therapeutics; this course may be divided into two parts of fifty Lectures each, one of which may be attended in the Summer.

First Summer Session. — Botany and Vegetable Physiology; either before or after the first winter Session.

Second Winter Session.—Anatomy and Physiology. Anatomical Demonstrations. Dissections. Principles and Practice of Medicine.

Second Summer Session.—Forensic Medicine.

Third Winter Session. — Dissections. Principles and Practice of Medicine.

Midwifery, and the Diseases of Women and Children, two courses, in separate sessions, and subsequent to the termination of the first winter session.

Practical Midwifery, at any time after the conclusion of the first course of Midwifery Lectures.

Medical Practice during the full term of eighteen months, from or after the commencement of the second winter session; twelve months at a recognised hospital, and six months at a recognised hospital, or a recognised dispensary; in connection with the hospital attendance, a course of clinical lectures, and instruction in morbid anatomy, will be required.

The sessional course of instruction in each subject of study is to consist of not less than the following number of lectures:
One hundred on chemistry. One hundred

on Materia Medica and Therapeutics. One hundred on the Principles and Practice of Medicine. Sixty on Midwifery, and the Diseases of Women and Children. Fifty on Botany and Vegetable Physiology.

Every *examination* of an hour's duration will be deemed equivalent to a lecture*.

The lectures required in each course must be given on separate days.

The lectures on Anatomy and Physiology, and the Anatomical Demonstrations, must be in conformity with the regulations of the Royal College of Surgeons of London in every respect.

Candidates must also bring testimonials of instruction in Practical Chemistry, and of having dissected the whole of the human body once at least.

The above course of study may be extended over a longer period than three winter and two summer sessions, provided the lectures and medical practice are attended in the prescribed order, and in the required sessions.

Those gentlemen whose attendance on lectures commenced before the 1st of Oct. 1835, will be allowed to complete their studies in conformity with the previous Regulations of the Court.

Recognition of Lecturers and Schools.

No Member of the Court of Examiners will be recognised as a lecturer on any branch of medical science.

The Court will not recognise any lecturer unless he lectures in connection with a recognised medical school; nor will they recognise a lecturer on more than *two* branches of medical science; nor will they recognise a lecturer until he has produced very satisfactory testimonials of his attainments in the science he purposes to teach, and of his ability as a teacher thereof, from at least two persons of acknowledged talents and distinguished acquirements in the particular branch of science in question; nor will they recognise a lecturer until he has given a public course of lectures on the subject he purposes to teach; but if, after such preliminary course, the lecturer shall be recognised, certificates of attendance on that course will be received.

Satisfactory assurance must also be given that the teacher is in possession of the means requisite for the full illustration of his lectures, viz. that he has, if lecturing—

On Chemistry, a laboratory and competent apparatus:

On Materia Medica, a museum sufficiently extensive:

On Botany, a hortus siccus, plates or drawings, and recent plants:

* The Court particularly request attention to this clause.

On Midwifery, a museum, and such appointment in a public institution as may afford the means of practical instruction to the pupils.

The lecturer on the Principles and Practice of Medicine, if he lectures in London, must be a member of the Royal College of Physicians of London; and if in a provincial town, either a member of the Royal College of Surgeons of London, or a graduated Doctor of Medicine of a British University of four years' standing, unless prior to his graduation he had been for four years a licentiate of this Court.

The lecturer on Materia Medica and Therapeutics must be a member of the Royal College of Physicians, or a graduated Doctor of Medicine of a British University of four years' standing; or he must have been a licentiate of this Court for the same period.

The lecturer on Midwifery must be a member of one of the legally constituted Colleges of Physicians or Surgeons in the United Kingdom, of four years' standing, or he must have been a licentiate of this Court for the same period.

The names of the lecturers recognised by the Court may be known on application to the Secretary at the Hall of the Society.

The certificates of teachers recognised by the constituted medical authorities in Dublin, Edinburgh, Glasgow, and Aberdeen, as also those of the medical professors in Foreign Universities, are received by the Court.

Much inconvenience having arisen from the presentation of schedules signed by *lecturers unknown to the Court*, it is particularly requested that the Registrars of the medical schools will furnish a correct list of their recognised teachers to the Secretary of this Court, at the commencement of every winter session.

No Hospital will be recognised by the Court, unless

1. It contain at least one hundred beds:

2. It be under the care of two or more physicians, members of the Royal College of Physicians of London, or graduated Doctors of Medicine of a British University:

3. The physicians give a regular course of clinical lectures and instruction in morbid anatomy:

4. The apothecary be legally qualified, either by having been in practice prior to the 1st of August, 1815, or by having received a certificate from this Court.

No Dispensary will be recognised by the Court, unless it be situated in some town where there is a recognised medical school, and be under the care of at least two physicians and an apothecary legally qualified.

No Medical Practice will be available, unless it be attended in conformity with the course of study prescribed for pupils.

Registration of Testimonials.

All testimonials must be given on a printed schedule*, with which students will be supplied at the time of their first registration :
In London, at this Hall.
In Edinburgh, at Messrs. Mac Lachlan and Stewart's, booksellers.
In Dublin, at Messrs. Hodges and Smith's, booksellers.
In the Provincial Towns, from the gentlemen who keep the registers of the medical schools.
All students, in London, are required, *personally*, to register the several classes for which they have taken tickets ; and those only will be considered as complying with the regulations of the Court, whose names and classes in the register correspond with their schedules.
Tickets of admission to lectures and medical practice must be registered in the months of October and May ; but no ticket will be registered unless it be dated within *seven* days of the commencement of the course ; and certificates of attendance must be registered in the months of April and August. Due notice of the days and hours of such registrations will be given from time to time.
The Court also require students at the provincial medical schools to register their names in their own hand-writing, with the registrar of each respective school, within the first twenty-one days of October, and first fourteen days of May ; and to register their certificates of having duly attended lectures or medical practice within fourteen days of the completion of such attendance.
The registrars are requested to furnish the Court of Examiners with a copy of each registration *immediately* after its close, as those students only will be admitted to examination whose registrations have been *duly* communicated to the Court.

Names of Gentlemen having the care of the Registers.

Bath.—R. T. Gore, Esq. Lecturer on Anatomy.
Birmingham. — W. Sands Cox, Esq. Lecturer on Anatomy.
Bristol.—Dr. Wallis, Henry Clark, Esq. Lecturers on Anatomy.
Hull.—Edward Wallis, Esq. Lecturer on Anatomy.
Leeds.—Thomas Nunneley, Esq. Lecturer on Anatomy.
Liverpool. — Dr. Malins, Lecturer on Medical Jurisprudence.
Manchester. — Thomas Turner, Esq. ;

* It is particularly requested that the lecturer himself will fill up the blanks in the schedule, specifying the mode of attendance.

Thomas Fawdington, Esq. Lecturers on Anatomy.
Newcastle.—William Dawson, Esq. Lecturer on Midwifery.
Sheffield. — W. Jackson, Esq. Lecturer on Anatomy.
York.—John Hopps, Esq. Lecturer on Anatomy.

Preliminary Examination.

Students may undergo their Latin examination at any time after their first registration, except during the months of August and September. A book is opened at the Beadle's office at the Hall, for the signatures of those gentlemen who are desirous of undergoing this examination, to which twenty will be admitted on each successive Saturday ; but unless twenty names are entered on the list, no examination will take place. Candidates are required to attend at half-past three o'clock, and those who fail to pass this examination satisfactorily, will not be readmitted until they appear for their general examination.

Examination.

Every person intending to offer himself for examination must give notice in writing to the Clerk of the Society on or before the Monday previously to the day of Examination, and must at the same time deposit all the required testimonials at the office of the Beadle, where attendance is given every day, except Sunday, from *Ten* until *Four* o'clock.
The examination of the candidate for a certificate of qualification to practise as an Apothecary, will be as follows :—
In translating portions of the first four books of Celsus de Medicinâ, and of the first twenty-three chapters of Gregory's Conspectus Medicinæ Theoreticæ.
In Physicians' Prescriptions, and the Pharmacopœia Londinensis.
In Chemistry.
In Materia Medica and Therapeutics.
In Botany.
In Anatomy and Physiology.
In the Principles and Practice of Medicine. This branch of the examination embraces an inquiry into the pregnant and puerperal states ; and also into the diseases of children.
The examination of the candidate for a certificate of qualification to act as assistant to an apothecary, in compounding and dispensing medicines, will be as follows :—
In translating Physicians' Prescriptions, and the Pharmacopœia Londinensis.
In Pharmacy and Materia Medica.
By the 22d section of the Act of Parliament, no rejected candidate for a certificate to practise as an apothecary can be re-examined until the expiration of six months from his former examination ; and no rejected candi-

date as an assistant until the expiration of three months.

The Court meet in the Hall *every Thursday*, where candidates are required to attend at a quarter before four o'clock.

The Act directs the following sums to be paid for certificates.

For London, and within ten miles thereof, ten guineas.

For all other parts of England and Wales, six guineas.

Persons having paid the latter sum become entitled to practise in London, and within ten miles thereof, by paying four guineas in addition.

For an Assistant's certificate two guineas.

By order of the Court,

HENRY BLATCH, *Sec.*

Apothecaries' Hall,
   Aug. 1843.

For information relative to these Regulations, students are referred to the Beadle, at Apothecaries' Hall, every day (Sunday excepted), between the hours of ten and four o'clock.

It is expressly ordered by the Court of Examiners, that no gratuity be received by any officer or servant of the Court.

Information on all subjects connected with the "Act for better regulating the Practice of Apothecaries," may be obtained on application to Mr. R. B. Upton, Clerk of the Society, at the Hall every day (Sunday excepted) between the hours of one and three o'clock.

QUALIFICATIONS OF MEDICAL OFFICERS OF POOR LAW UNIONS.

(*From the Western Luminary.*)

WE have been favoured with the following letter and opinion relating to a matter of great importance to members of the medical profession, by Mr. J. G. Bidwill, clerk to the St. Thomas Union.

"Poor Law Commission Office, Somerset House,
               August 31, 1843.

" Sir,—In consequence of a communication made to them by Her Majesty's Principal Secretary of State for the Home Department, the Poor Law Commissioners have consulted the Attorney-General and another counsel on the competency of medical practitioners possessing Scotch and Irish qualifications to act as officers in a union or parish under the Poor Law Amendment Act.

"The effect of this opinion (a copy of which is annexed for your information) is as follows :—

" 1. That persons having a surgical diploma or degree from a Royal college or university in Scotland or Ireland, are legally

as competent to be medical officers under the Poor Law Amendment Act as persons having the diploma of the Royal College of Surgeons in London.

" 2. That persons having only Scotch and Irish medical qualifications are not, as such, competent to practise pharmacy in England and Wales.

"The commissioners think they are, by this opinion, justified in admitting persons having a surgical diploma or degree from a Royal college or university in Scotland or Ireland to the same rights under the Poor Law Amendment Act as members of the Royal College of Surgeons of London.

" The commissioners will, therefore, be prepared to consent to such arrangements, and to make such modifications in their general order of the 12th of March, 1842, as may be necessary to give effect to the above recited opinion of the Attorney-General.—I am, sir,

Your very obedient servant,

" E. CHADWICK, *Sec.*"

Question arising out of the Case. — "Whether persons on whom medical degrees, diploma, or licenses have been conferred by the universities or other medical authorities in Scotland or Ireland, are competent to be appointed and to act as medical officers under the 4th and 5th William IV., c. 76 ?"

Opinion.—" We are of opinion, that as far as the question of surgery is concerned, those persons who have a surgical diploma, or degree, from a Royal college or university in Scotland or Ireland, are (in point of law) as competent to be appointed and to act as medical officers under the statute referred to as the persons who have the diploma of the Royal College of Surgeons in London.

" With respect to pharmacy, the right to practise in England and Wales is confined to those who have the license or certificate of the Apothecaries' Company, and other persons whose rights are saved by the Apothecaries' Acts ; and in our opinion persons having Scotch and Irish medical degrees are not among such last named persons.

" F. POLLOCK.
" S. MARTIN."

NEWS FROM ANTIGUA.

WE are indebted to a correspondent for three numbers of the Antigua Weekly Register, being those for the 4th, 11th, and 18th of July. The most interesting article contained in them is the report of a trial for poisoning, which took place on the 14th of June. The prisoner, a woman named Patience, was indicted for having poisoned four of her half-brothers with arsenic. She had already been indicted for the same offence last December; but the jury were unable to agree upon their verdict; and the Commission having expired, the trial was necessarily cut short. This year the March sessions were postponed, on account of the earthquake in February.

The facts of the case are simple enough. The children died after eating porridge prepared by the mother; and arsenic was found not only in the porridge, but in the stomachs of two of the victims. Moreover, one Robert Brown, shopman to Dr. Fergusson, declared at the inquest that he had not sold any arsenic to Patience, but declared afterwards that he *had*. As this second declaration, however, did not take place till Brown's memory had been refreshed by a proclamation offering a reward for the discovery of the murderer, the jury do not appear to have believed it. We suppose that Brown was a witness at the trial, but in the report before us his evidence is merely given at second-hand by Dr. Fergusson.

When the earthquake occurred in February, " Patience was locked up in the room allotted to her on the upper floor of the jail, and as the walls fell she made her way through the crumbling masses, and leaping from the gallery into the yard, escaped without a contusion. Although it is unquestionable that she was frequently absent from the prison at night, owing to the insecure state of the ruins, she invariably returned, and remained in custody until the morning of her trial." This circumstance, no doubt, had its weight with the jury, who, after an absence of a quarter of an hour, returned into court with a verdict of acquittal.

" The prisoner was immediately discharged amidst the noisy and indecorous expressions of applause indulged in by the crowd which thronged the court and its approaches. Only one man was seized, who was joining in the uproar; and he was forthwith committed by the Bench to the Common Jail for thirty days."

This trial leaves an unsatisfactory impression on the mind : one is scarcely convinced of the innocence of Patience; and if she *is* innocent, what must Robert Brown be? The earth, vast as it is, is scarcely wide enough for both !

We will extract another paragraph from these Registers, of a more agreeable cast.

" We are informed that fifteen fugitive slaves, from Guadeloupe, arrived in a small boat at the Island of Montserrat last week."

Our colonies now enjoy, like their mother country, the privilege of giving freedom to the slave; to *him* every rock over which the British flag floats is a sanctuary, where " the wicked cease from troubling, and the weary are at rest."

VARUS MENTAGRA AND GUTTA ROSEA, THE SYCOSIS MENTI AND ACNE OF WILLAN,

TREATED WITH SULPHATE OF IRON EXTERNALLY.

By W. DAUVERGER.

OF all the modes of treatment recommended for these obstinate affections, the following appears to have been the most useful in the author's hands.

The sulphate of iron in different forms is the most efficacious local remedy for the pustular inflammation of gutta rosea, and mentagra.

It is used in solution, either by bathing the part affected, or by applying linen dipped in it, or by sprinkling the ulcerated parts of the mentagra with a mixture of charcoal and sulphate of iron. This mixture need not be finely levigated, for it then forms a crust too easily, becomes lumpy, and is not easily removed by washing the beard. In spite of his previous opinions, M. Dauverger also tried a pommade of sulphate of iron, but was obliged to give it up. The following are the formulæ employed by him.

No. 1. — Sulphate of iron twenty-five grammes. Distilled water two hundred grammes. Dissolve.

No. 2.—Sulphate of iron fifty grammes. Distilled water two hundred grammes. Dissolve.

No. 3.—*Ferro-carbonic powder*. Sulphate of iron ten grammes. Charcoal thirty-five grammes. Powder and mix.

The author first treats the inflammatory symptoms with emollients; when he thinks them sufficiently reduced, he orders the patient to bathe the part twice a day with two glasses of warm water containing one or two spoonfuls of the solution No. 1. A quarter of an hour afterwards, he prescribes a local bath of an emollient decoction; and afterwards, if possible, the application of a poultice of the same kind. When no further improvement takes place under this treatment, he has recourse to No. 2, which is twice the strength of the former, and proceeds in the same way. The author employs general means of treatment at the same time.—*Gazette Médicale*, Sept. 9, 1843.

CONVENIENT MODE OF ADMINISTERING OIL OF TURPENTINE.

By M. BOUCHARDAT.

THE oil of turpentine is very often used internally, and might be employed still more frequently, were it not that the usual formulæ for its administration, such as the terebinthinous ether, or Durand's remedy, turpentine emulsion, and the different terebinthinous mixtures, all fail in masking the disagreeable taste of this medicine. The following, however, is the form of an electuary which M. Bouchardat assures us may be administered with the greatest ease.

Take of gum acacia, ten grammes; mix it with ten grammes of water; add of white honey, fifty grammes; oil of turpentine, fifty grammes; carbonate of magnesia, q. s. Make a soft electuary.

The dose is from 2 to 10 grammes (36 to 180 grains) a day, in unleavened bread.

In some cases a little opium, or from 10 to 20 drops of Rousseau's laudanum, may be added to the mucilage in the above mixture.—*Bulletin Général de Thérapeutique,* and *Gaz. Médicale.*

ADULTERATION OF COMMON SALT AT PARIS.

THREE years ago, it was found that of three thousand samples of common salt taken from the druggists of Paris, more than a tenth part was adulterated. The same fraud has just been discovered among a number of grocers. On making the visits enjoined by the law (which ought to take place in the other towns of France likewise), it was found that some samples showed traces of copper, and were adulterated with a large proportion of impure carbonate of soda *(sel de varech),* containing iodine. Three specimens contained small crystals of a salt of copper.—*Gazette Médicale,* August 26th.

NARROW ESCAPE OF A DRUGGIST.

A DRUGGIST was lately summoned before the police tribunal of the Seine, for having infringed the 34th article of the law of the 21st Germinal of the year XI, which enacts that poisons are to be kept in a separate place, and to be locked up, under a penalty of 3000 francs. The court was of opinion, however, that the sale of the poison was necessary to bring the offence within the meaning of the enactment; and as this had not occurred in the case before them, they merely put into execution the 471st article of the penal code, and adjudged the druggist to pay a fine of five francs, and the expenses.—*Gazette Médicale.*

APOTHECARIES' HALL.

LIST OF GENTLEMEN WHO HAVE RECEIVED CERTIFICATES.

Thursday, September 14, 1843.

H. Morley, London.—E. Thomas, Pullheli, North Wales.—J. Robinson, Bahamas.—T. Tar-drew, Carmarthen.—J. Yate, Madeley, Salop.—J. C. Wickham, Didmarton, Gloucestershire.—G. J. Gunthorpe.—N. C. Latham, Wigan.—H. R. Norris, South Petherston.

A TABLE OF MORTALITY FOR THE METROPOLIS,

Shewing the number of deaths from all causes registered in the week ending Saturday, Sept. 9, 1843.

Small Pox	9
Measles	17
Scarlatina	41
Hooping Cough	26
Croup	5
Thrush	13
Diarrhœa	51
Dysentery	12
Cholera	6
Influenza	1
Ague	0
Remittent Fever	0
Typhus	45
Erysipelas	4
Syphilis	1
Hydrophobia	0
Diseases of the Brain, Nerves, and Senses	130
Diseases of the Lungs and other Organs of Respiration	307
Diseases of the Heart and Blood-vessels	16
Diseases of the Stomach, Liver, and other Organs of Digestion	36
Diseases of the Kidneys, &c.	7
Childbed	7
Paramenia	0
Ovarian Dropsy	1
Disease of Uterus, &c.	3
Arthritis	0
Rheumatism	1
Diseases of Joints, &c.	4
Carbuncle	0
Phlegmon	0
Ulcer	0
Fistula	1
Diseases of Skin, &c.	1
Dropsy, Cancer, and other Diseases of Uncertain Seat	81
Old Age or Natural Decay	71
Deaths by Violence, Privation, or Intempe-rance	31
Causes not specified	0
Deaths from all Causes	880

METEOROLOGICAL JOURNAL.

Kept at EDMONTON, *Latitude* 51° 37' 32" N. *Longitude* 0° 3' 51" W. *of Greenwich.*

Sept. 1843.	THERMOMETER.		BAROMETER.	
Wednesday 13	from 52 to 68		29·85 to 29·75	
Thursday . 14	50	70	29·60	Stat.
Friday . . 15	59	72	29·56	29·64
Saturday . 16	54	74	29·72	29·76
Sunday . . 17	53	79	29·81	29·83
Monday . . 18	54	72	29·84	Stat.
Tuesday . 19	59	76	29·85	29·85

Wind on the 13th, N.E.; 14th, E. by N. and N.E.; 15th, 16th, and 17th, S.E.; 18th, S. by E. and N.W.; 19th, N. by E.

Clear, except the afternoon of the 14th, when a little rain fell.

Rain, fallen, ·145 of an inch.

CHARLES HENRY ADAMS.

WILSON & OGILVY, 57, Skinner Street, London.

THE

LONDON MEDICAL GAZETTE,

BEING A

WEEKLY JOURNAL

OF

Medicine and the Collateral Sciences.

FRIDAY, SEPTEMBER 29, 1843.

LECTURES

ON THE

THEORY AND PRACTICE OF MIDWIFERY,

Delivered in the Theatre of St. George's Hospital,

BY ROBERT LEE, M.D. F.R.S.

—

LECTURE XLV.

On Diseases of the Brain and Mammæ in Puerperal Women.

MILIARY fever, intestinal and remittent fever, ephemeral fever or weed, pneumonia, bronchocele, stranguary, paralysis, diarrhœa, tympanites, and various spasmodic and nervous disorders, have all been enumerated by systematic writers as peculiar to puerperal women, but as I have no observations of the slightest importance to make respecting these, I shall conclude this department of the course—the pathology of the puerperal state—with a few very general remarks on diseases of the brain and nervous system, and of the nipples and mammæ. From sympathy with the great uterine system of nerves after delivery, there is often a predisposition manifested to disease in the brain, and violent cerebral derangement is produced by causes which, at other times, would have had no effect. In the fifth vol. of the Transactions of the London College of Physicians there is a Paper, by Dr. J. Clarke, on the Effects of Certain Articles of Food, especially of Oysters, after Child-birth, in which are related fatal cases which followed the use of oysters in the puerperal state ; and the same effect has been produced by other articles of diet. Fourteen days after delivery a lady was attacked with giddiness, then with violent pain of the head, neither of which yielded to the common remedies. The symptoms increased rapidly ; she became senseless and delirious, and convulsions and death followed. Towards the close of the disease

it was ascertained that she had eaten oysters on the day preceding the attack. A young, healthy, plethoric woman, three weeks after a natural labour, was attacked with pain of the head. A day before she had eaten five or ten oysters, which had been dressed by boiling them in the liquor contained in the shells. Venesection, emetics, and purgatives, were employed, and the symptoms were mitigated for a time ; but convulsions came on, and compression of the brain, and she died in no long time. Dr. J. Clarke has also related the case of another young healthy woman, who began a few days after delivery to complain of headache, and a sense of internal fulness in the head. These symptoms not having yielded to bleeding, purging, and low diet, a state of coma came on, and she died in sixteen hours. On the day preceding the attack she had eaten twelve raw oysters. On the third day after a natural labour, a woman, who was recovering in the most favourable manner, was suddenly attacked with a severe fit of cold shivering, followed by violent headache, throbbing of the temporal arteries, intolerance of light and sound, and other symptoms which indicated the existence of a dangerous affection of the brain. The pulse was 130, skin hot, tongue loaded. The abdomen was soft and puffy, and not affected by pressure. I ascertained that the attack was produced by the patient having eaten a quantity of ham twelve hours before. The symptoms were relieved by calomel and purgatives. Another woman, on the eighth day after a natural labour, was suddenly attacked with insensibility and convulsions. Twenty ounces of blood were taken away by cupping from the temples, and repeated doses of active cathartics were administered, and she recovered. A few hours before the attack she partook rather heartily of roasted chicken and salted tongue, with a friend who had come to visit her.

Inflammation of the brain and its membranes, in puerperal women, is not a disease of frequent occurrence. The symptoms are those of common phrenitis, not of insanity. There is headache, flushing of the face, throbbing of the arteries, intolerance of light and sound, and delirium. General and local blood-letting, and active purgatives, should be had recourse to as soon as possible, and all the other remedies usually employed in inflammation of the brain: the patient should be kept in a dark room, and ice in a bladder applied over the shaven scalp. Puerperal mania is a much more common disease than inflammation of the brain, and the symptoms and treatment do not essentially differ from mania as it occurs in women who have not been pregnant, or even in the male sex. Without knowing the history of the patient, it would be impossible in any case to ascertain, from the phenomena alone, whether the disease had followed delivery. In puerperal women it assumes all the varied forms of ordinary insanity, occurring sometimes with symptoms of deep depression or melancholy, and at other times with symptoms of great excitement—talking incessantly and vehemently, pouring forth a torrent of words, and running from one subject to another without the least order in their ideas. In some cases the disease first manifests itself by want of sleep and restless nights, and a peculiar irritability of temper, the temper being ruffled at the merest trifles. Often it is first marked by some unreasonable dislike to the nurse, and she is accused unjustly of carelessness and inattention, or the husband is charged with infidelity, or some other crime. In some cases the aberration of mind is preceded by headache and other symptoms of cerebral irritation, quick pulse, and hot skin; while in others there is little derangement of the bodily functions, the circulation being almost natural, the skin cool, and the digestive organs very slightly disordered. Sometimes puerperal insanity is preceded by an attack of violent uterine irritation; there is pain of the hypogastrium, increased by pressure, and some other symptoms of uterine inflammation, which have speedily disappeared on the supervention of the mental disorder. In the greater number of cases puerperal mania occurs after natural labours, and has not been preceded by any peculiar derangement of the digestive organs during pregnancy, or uterine hæmorrhage during labour.

There is an hereditary predisposition to the disease in a considerable number of those who become affected, and some have suffered from it repeatedly in the puerperal state. The disease is attended with much greater danger when it occurs soon after delivery, with symptoms of violent excitement of the brain, than when it commences several months after, during suckling, in the form of melancholy madness. Dr. Burrows published a table of fifty-seven cases, of which ten died. Of *ninety-two patients* at the Salpetrière, six

died, or one in fifteen. Of these ninety-two cases recorded by M. Esquirol, sixteen occurred from the first to the fourth day after delivery; twenty-one from the fifth to the fifteenth day; seventeen from the sixteenth to the sixtieth day; nineteen from the sixtieth day to the twelfth month of suckling; and in nineteen cases it appeared after voluntary or forced weaning. M. Esquirol infers that puerperal mania occurs more frequently as the consequence of delivery than of nursing, and that the more distant the time at which it occurs from the period of delivery, the less it is to be feared. Of these ninety-two cases, eight were idiotical; thirty-five melancholic; and forty-nine maniacal. The ages of these numbers were as follows :—twenty-two from 20 to 35 years of age; forty-one from 25 to 30; and twelve were upwards of 40 : therefore, neither delivery nor suckling, according to this statement, modify derangement as far as age is concerned, for in this disease, produced by other circumstances, it most frequently occurs between the ages of 30 and 35. Sixty-three of the cases related by M. Esquirol were married women; twenty-nine single. Fifty-six out of the ninety-two were entirely restored to health; thirty-eight of these recovered in the first six months. The appearances on dissection, it is stated, threw no light on the nature of the disease. These ninety-two cases of puerperal mania were treated by mild purgatives frequently repeated, by blisters to the nape of the neck and limbs, enemata, and baths; bleeding was seldom indicated. In the treatment of puerperal mania the greatest attention should be paid to the state of the brain and of the digestive organs. If the countenance is flushed, the carotid and temporal arteries throbbing violently, the head should be shaved, and blood drawn by leeches from the temples. When there is strong general excitement of the circulation, combined with these symptoms of local determination to the brain, blood should be drawn from the arm in quantity proportioned to the severity of the symptoms. In ordinary mania, decided benefit is sometimes produced by moderate general depletion, and after this great advantage follows the application of ice, in a bladder, to the scalp, or a cold evaporating lotion. Light and noise should be carefully excluded, and a nurse accustomed to the charge of insane persons should have the care of the person. It must be a mild, but vigilant and firm control, which is exercised, and especial care taken that patients who are sometimes violent and vindictive inflict no injury upon themselves or those around them. The windows should be secured, and all sharp and cutting instruments should be put out of their way. Women are not unfrequently, at the commencement of the disease at least, fully aware of the disordered state of their minds; they feel that they have not their wonted power over trains of thought passing through their minds, and their ideas succeed one another with extraordinary rapidity, and in a manner different from what they did in a state of health. The condition of the mind during sleep or dreaming is also peculiar. Often when the disease is forming, the ideas have all a relation to the process of delivery. A lady now afflicted with puerperal mania was delivered unexpectedly at the end of the sixth month of pregnancy when sitting up—the child literally dropped from her, and had nearly fallen upon the floor ; she cannot now, though several months have elapsed, be persuaded that the same accident is not about to take place, and keeps her hands nearly all day long in a position to prevent it. The mother of this lady had one or more attacks of puerperal mania, and the disease was obviously hereditary. A disordered state of the digestive organs is not unfrequently a concomitant of puerperal insanity, and in a few cases this has appeared to be the exciting cause of the complaint, for relief has almost immediately followed the action of brisk cathartics. Whether we view deranged states of the digestive organs as causes or consequences of puerperal mania, these should be effectually removed by repeated doses of calomel and purgatives, and the condition of the alvine evacuations frequently ascertained. Bleeding, general or local, is not required in the greater number of cases of puerperal mania, and the frequent and long-continued use of active cathartics is injurious, especially when the disease is accompanied with symptoms of general debility and exhaustion. More benefit is then derived from narcotics, especially acetate of morphia, nourishing diet, and gentle exercise in the open air. Benefit has also been obtained, in some cases, after the acute stage of the disease has passed away, and convalescence has commenced, by allowing the patient occasionally to communicate with her relatives, from whom she had been separated.

The affections of the nipples and mammæ during suckling, though attended with little danger, often produce the greatest suffering. When the breasts have become suddenly distended after first labours, and where the child has not been applied sufficiently early, constitutional disturbance of great severity sometimes takes place. There is a rigor, succeeded by intense heat of skin, quick pulse, oppression of breathing, headache, flushed face, and sometimes slight incoherence or delirium. The tongue becomes dry, and there is urgent thirst. However violent the symptoms of milk fever may be, little danger is to be apprehended ; none, in comparison with uterine inflammation or puerperal fever, which ought not to be confounded in any way with milk fever. If the breasts are hard and distended on the third or fourth days after delivery, and there is no pain increased by pressure in any part of the hypogastrium, however severe the febrile disturbance may be, there is comparatively little risk, and the symptoms will gradually subside if the proper treatment is adopted. Active saline cathartics ought to be liberally administered, and diaphoretics at short intervals, and the over distension of the breasts should be relieved by warm fomentations, or frictions, and having the milk drawn off. The exhausting syringe, or glass tube and ball, are often employed for this purpose, but the safest and most efficacious method is to procure a child a few months old, and apply it to the breasts. Blood-letting is rarely necessary in milk fever, and it is better to relieve the determination of blood to the head, where it is great, by leeches to the temples, and a cold evaporating lotion. The early application of the child to the breasts, warm fomentations, and poultices, or occasional friction with oil or camphorated liniment, and the exhibition of cathartics and diaphoretics, and low diet, are the best means of preventing attacks of milk fever : where women are not to suckle their children, the secretion of milk should be lessened by the exhibition of saline purgatives soon after delivery, and the sparing use of liquids. The breasts may be covered with fine linen rag, moistened with the following, or some similar, tepid lotion. Camphor. ʒj. ; Spirit. Vin. Rectif. ʒjss. ; Aquæ ʒviii. Nurses sometimes cover the breasts with diachylon plaisters, and the pressure probably acts by arresting the secretion. Sometimes, however, this is done very imperfectly, and the breasts are very large and distended, and painful for two or three days, and then the secretion begins to diminish. The application of warm fomentations and emollient poultices are upon the whole better applications ; they are more soothing. They allow a small portion of milk to flow from the nipples, and the milk soon recedes, with low diet and cathartics. If the distension is very great and painful, and there is much constitutional disturbance in spite of all this, it is best to relieve the breasts by drawing off a portion of the milk.

Ulceration of the nipples occurs either as a simple superficial excoriation or as a deep crack. Some women suffer so severely after every confinement from excoriation and ulceration of the nipples, that they are altogether unable to suckle their children, however anxious to do so. No sooner does the child begin to suck, than the skin covering the nipple gives way, and if the suckling is continued, large foul painful superficial ulcers or deep cracks, take place, which bleed every time the child is applied. The pressure of the child's gums prevents the ulcers from healing, the edges of the sores are drawn asunder every time the child is applied, and they are thus prevented from healing. To obviate the effect of this mechanical irritation, shields and prepared teats are employed, but children often refuse to suck with these, and they are obliged to be put aside. If one nipple is excoriated, and the other is not, the child should be more frequently applied to the sound than the sore nipple. These excoriations and ulcerations of the nipples would all cicatrize, if it were possible to leave them sufficiently long in a state of rest. A great number of different applications have been recommended in these cases; but I am unable to explain to you precisely the principle upon which they act. The good they do is probably chiefly effected by allaying the excitement of the parts, or by acting as gentle stimulants and astringents, as similar applications act upon common ulcers in other parts of the body. The following are some of the applications in common use. ℞. Sodæ Sub. Borat. ʒj. Aquæ distill. ʒiijss. Spirit. Vin. rectif. ʒss. M. Or alum. sulph. gr. iij. Aquæ ʒj. M. or Zinc. Sulph. gr. xv. Aquæ Rosas. ʒiv. An ointment now extensively used, and with great advantage, consists of ʒj. of the Balsam of Peru to ʒvj. of Unguent. Cetacei. Sometimes the Unguent. Hydr. Nitr. Oxid. mixed with a small proportion of opium, answers very well, or ointment of bismuth, or zinc ointment, or simple cerate. Some sprinkle a little gum arabic over the nipple. Where there is a granulating surface, looking like a raspberry, a solution of lunar caustic, two grains to the ounce of water, applied with a camel's hair brush, answers very well. Another method of applying the lunar caustic is to touch the nipple, after carefully drying it, with a sharp pencil of nitrate of silver, and afterwards covering it with a little simple ointment. I have seen all these applications, and many others, tried without success, and the ulcerations have at last healed up under the use of a bread-and-water or linseed-meal poultice, spermaceti ointment, or the most simple unctuous application. Not unfrequently ulceration of the nipples gets well, where the applications have not produced the effect,—the last, however employed, generally receives all the credit for the salutary change.

Inflammation of the mammæ often occurs spontaneously, and cannot be referred to an ulcerated condition of the nipples, exposure to cold, external injury, improper diet, mental excitement, or any other adequate reason. It may take place during the whole period of suckling—three, six, or even twelve months, after delivery, and it has sometimes occurred after weaning. Most frequently, however, inflammation of the mammæ takes place within a month after delivery; sometimes it occurs before the end of the second week. A hard lump is often at first felt in the breast, which is painful on pressure, without any redness of the integuments covering it; but as the inflammation extends, the integuments assume an uniform redness, and this is more or less diffused according to the extent of the part affected. Rigors, quick pulse, headache, thirst, and other symptoms of constitutional disturbance, usually accompany the affection; but these vary very much in severity in different cases. Where the inflammation is in the cellular substance under the skin, or in a superficial portion of the gland, suppuration soon takes place, and the pus is often discharged through an opening in the skin near the root of the nipple. In other cases a large portion of the gland is inflamed, and the matter makes its way very slowly to the surface. Different modes of practice have been adopted in this disease. I believe it to be unnecessary here to abstract blood from the arm; and in a large proportion of cases warm applications are more useful than cold evaporating lotions. When there is much pain, tension, and hardness of the breast, apply twelve or eighteen leeches to the affected part, and foment the bites till a sufficient quantity of blood has been procured. Then a warm linseed-meal poultice should be laid over the part, which should be renewed every four or six hours. The bowels should be very freely opened by calomel, antimony, and some saline cathartic, as senna and salts, and afterwards the febrile symptoms allayed by saline diaphoretics, and rest procured by anodynes. If the inflammation is severe, it is often necessary to reapply the leeches a second or third time, and the poultices and fomentations should be continued, or warmth applied by means of these wooden bowls, till resolution or suppuration takes place; and when pus is formed, it is in general the best practice to allow the matter to make its way to the surface, and be discharged by ulcerative absorption of the parts intervening between the surface and the cavity of the abscess. The circumstances which ought to guide us in opening mammary abscesses have thus been clearly stated by Sir A. Cooper:—" If the abscess be quick in its progress, if it be placed on the anterior surface of the breast, and if the sufferings which it occasions are not excessively severe, it is best to leave them to their natural course, rather than to employ the lancet for the discharge of the matter. But if, on the contrary, the abscess in its commencement be very deeply placed; if its progress be tedious; if the local sufferings be excessively severe; if there be a high degree of irritative fever, and the patient suffer from profuse perspiration and want of rest, much time is saved, and a great diminution of suffering produced, by discharging the matter with a lancet." "Still, it is wrong to penetrate with the lancet through a thick covering of the abscess, as the opening does not succeed in establishing a free discharge of matter, for the aperture closes by adhesion, the accumulation of matter proceeds, and ulceration will still continue. On this account the opening should be made where the matter is most superficial, and the fluctuation is distinct; and it should be in size proportioned to its depth." "Several abscesses," adds Sir Astley, "sometimes form in the same breast, quickly succeeding each other, and lead to very protracted sufferings. In these cases opium and quinine will be required to lessen irritability, and support the strength of the system. Sometimes an abscess is produced at a great depth in the breast, and discharges itself by several different apertures, forming sinuses of various extent. The best mode of treatment in these cases, as far as I have had an opportunity of observing, is to inject them with a solution of two or three drops of the strong sulphuric acid to an ounce of rose water, and to apply the same solution by folds of linen cloth over the bosom, by which the secretion of milk is checked, and adhesion is produced."

ON THE MINERAL WATERS OF GREECE.

By Dr. John Bouros,

Professor of Special Medical Pathology, and of the Internal *Clinique*, at the University of Athens.

Greece possesses mineral waters varying extremely in natural and chemical composition. The greater number, however, are saline and sulphureous, and are consequently connected with volcanic phenomena of the soil. On the other hand, chalybeates, properly so called, are much less numerous, and I do not know of a single acidulous spring.

All our springs, therefore, may be divided into four classes: the first comprehending thermal sulphureous waters, the second thermal saline waters, the third cold saline waters, and the fourth thermal chalybeates.

Hot sulphureous springs.—Of the sulphureous springs, the most important in Greece, and perhaps one of the most important in the world, is one which rises in the northern part of Greece, in the ancient Phthiotis, about the distance of half an hour* from the city of Patraziki, towards the road that leads to Lamia. In a beautiful and

* If in Greece or Italy distances are calculated after the German fashion, this would be about one English mile.—*Translator's note.*

fertile plain surrounded on one side by lofty mountains, and on the other by the distant sea, the water smokes and boils, as it rises into a large and deep basin, in the middle of a kind of hill formed by the calcareous precipitate which it continually deposits. The temperature of the water in this basin varies in its different parts from 23° to 35° R. (83¾° to 110¾° of Fahr.); while in the centre it rises as high as 40° R. (122° Fahr.) and perhaps more. The water has a greenish tint, and is turbid; but as soon as it cools, it becomes limpid, and deposits a yellowish sediment. It sends forth a very penetrating odour of sulphuretted hydrogen, and has a saltish, acidulous, and not disagreeable smell.

Sixteen ounces of this water have been found, on analysis, to contain—

	Grains.
Muriate of Soda . . .	48.100
Muriate of Lime . . .	3.543
Sulphate of Magnesia .	1.800
Sulphate of Lime. . .	2.043
Carbonate of Lime . .	5.210
Carbonate of Soda . .	1.900
Silica	3.000
Extractive matter. . .	2.005

together with fifteen cubic inches of carbonic acid gas, and twelve cubic inches of sulphuretted hydrogen gas.

At the bottom of the basin is an abundant sediment, a kind of greasy and blackish mud, with a strong odour of sulphur. From the ingredients of this water one might infer its efficacy in some diseases, which has been fully confirmed by long experience. But as the springs have hitherto remained uncovered, and are at some distance from the town of Patraziki, they are but little frequented. At present, however, the royal medical council is occupied in building an establishment capable of containing a great number of patients.

Other springs of this kind, not less important to the physician, and far more interesting to the geologist, are contained in the island of Negropont, at its north-west extremity towards the harbour of Edipsus. In this place, with the sea on one side, and a mountain formed of transitional calcareous matter mixed with argillaceous schist and serpentine, on the other, at least twenty hot springs rise in the circumference of a square French league; and they deposit so much calcareous sediment, that they have formed entire mountains. In this space, which appears empty, and resembles the lid of a great cauldron, are plainly seen many spots which in other times gave exit to springs, but which are now closed; either through earthquakes, which, according to Strabo, once occurred, or from the great quantity of calcareous matter deposited by these springs.

The springs pour forth with vehemence and noise a great quantity of foaming and steaming water, which loses itself in the sea; but from one of them in particular the water issues in such abundance as to turn a mill, and with such force as easily to throw out large stones which may have fallen into the mouth of the spring.

Its temperature is very high, being 73° of Reaumur (196¼° Fahr.); so that it warms the sea, when calm, to the distance of fifty or sixty feet. The water is limpid, has a bitter taste, gives forth a penetrating smell of sulphur, and has a specific gravity of 1.016.

Sixteen ounces, when analysed by Signor Landerer, Professor of Chemistry in the University of Athens, were found to contain—

	Grains.
Muriate of Soda . . .	68.000
Muriate of Magnesia. .	3.500
Muriate of Lime . . .	2.084
Carbonate of Lime . .	2.043
Carbonate of Soda . .	.4.200
Sulphate of Magnesia .	11.240
Sulphate of Lime . . .	3.000
Silica	2.000
Iron	1.005

together with eight cubic inches of carbonic acid gas; thirty-two cubic inches of sulphuretted hydrogen; and a little extractive matter.

The abundant sediment of peroxide of iron which is seen all around might make one suppose that the quantity of iron contained in these waters is greater than Signor Landerer found in them. However this may be, the thermal waters of Edipsus are among the most efficacious, and their reputation as a remedy ascends to the remotest times. This is still shown by some remains of ancient baths and aqueducts, and is confirmed by a passage of Plutarch, where he says that Sylla frequented the thermal springs of Edipsus, in order to get rid of a species of gout by which he had been attacked at Athens.

In the great work of the French scientific expedition in the Morea, (t. ii. p. ii. p. 43 and 239) mention is made of another thermal water in the plain of Lelas, which enjoys a certain reputation among the natives; but as nothing more is said of it, it is impossible to know to what class it belongs.

Between the waters of Patraziki and Edipsus there is another spring of the same kind, on the mainland, which has given its name to that historic spot where Leonidas fell with the three hundred Spartans. I mean Thermopylæ (i. e. the warm gates.)

These ancient gates of Greece are composed on one side of Mount Œta, which is formed of transitional calcareous matter, mingled with argillaceous schist, and a little serpentine; and on the other of the Sinus Maliacus or Gulf of Zituni. At the foot of Mount Œta rises a hill entirely formed of a transitional calcareous stone, and giving free passage through various fissures to a copious thermal spring, which falls into the sea after passing through a plain about one French league long, and depositing calcareous sediment in various forms. The temperature of this limpid water is from 52° to 54° R. (149° to 153½° Fahr.); its taste is salt, its odour sulphureous and penetrating. Chemical analysis has shown that its constituents are the same as those of the spring at Edipsus.

In another part of Greece, which has undergone great volcanic revolutions, and at no very distant epochs, as Strabo reports, and as the very nature of the soil shows, namely, in that part of Peloponnesus which extends to the Saronic gulph, other sulphureous springs occur; particularly in the eastern part of the peninsula of Mettana, the greater portion of which is formed of trachite. Several springs of limpid water rise, within a circumference of 40 or 50 metres, above a small harbour surrounded on the west by rocks of porphyry, trachite, and calcareous matter; and they fall into a lake formed of sea water. Their temperature was 25° R. (88¼° Fahr.) while that of the atmosphere was 24° R. (86° Fahr.)

The constituents of these waters are not yet known, but we have placed them among sulphureous springs, on account of the great quantity of sulphuretted hydrogen gas which they emit, and which has given them the popular name of βρωμολίμνη, or stinking lake. This must be the fountain which, according to Pausanias, first appeared in the reign of Antigonus, King of Macedon, and whose appearance was preceded by a volcanic eruption on this spot.

On the north side of the peninsula, opposite the island of Ankistri, there is another spring of the same class. It is very near the sea, and mingles with it, so that its temperature cannot be exactly determined; but it must be high, as the water heats the sea for a circumference of about ten metres. However, a thermometer which M. Virlet immersed in the channel from which the water issues rose to 37° Centigr. (98¾° Fahr.) The inhabitants of Mettana give the name of βρῶμα (stink) to this fountain, from the odour of the sulphuretted hydrogen gas which it emits in abundance. It seems that this spring first rises, as M. Virlet asserts, from another level 50 or 60 feet higher, where some ruined baths, of mediæval construction, are still to be seen.

In the gulph of Patrias, on the mainland of Greece, to the west of Lepanto, and near the mountain of Kaki-Scala, there rises a thermal spring, which emits a strong smell of sulphuretted hydrogen, and is of the temperature of 32° R. (104° Fahr.) This fountain appears to have afforded considerable materials to the mythology of the ancients, who placed upon this smoking and stinking spot the tombs of the Centaurs who were buried under the mountain called *Taphius*, or the sepulchral; while they derived the old name of the inhabitants of these regions, the Ozoli (or, *strong-smelling*) from the stench of the spring.

The last spring of this class which we shall mention is one which rises in the island of Milos, on the south of mount Kalamo, from a grotto which the inhabitants call θειαφᾶιον *(sulphur mine)* because its walls are covered with crystallized sulphur, and the water emits a strong smell of the same mineral. Its temperature is 47° R. (137¼° Fahr.)

Hot saline waters.—The first place in this class is due to the one in the island of Thermia, which is at present so much used that it deserves especial mention. It is necessary to observe that near this spring there is another, called *Caccavo*, which from the quantity of iron that it contains, belongs to the class of chalybeates; but to avoid repetitions we will speak of both at the same time.

The island of Thermia appears a continuation of the promontory of Sunium (now Cape Colonna); and is formed of primitive mountains of micaceous and argillaceous schist, together with rocks of crystallized calcareous matter. This island offers a phenomenon hitherto unique in geology, I mean a spacious cavern in a schistous mountain, near the village of Sillaca; and in the whole island there is not a single fountain of water fit to drink, so that the inhabitants use wells.

There are three copious springs of thermal water, the first of which is called λουτρὸν *(the bath)*, and the remaining ones, which are very near each other, and hardly 50 metres from the *bath*, are known under the name of *Caccavo (cauldron)*.

Not the slightest mention of these waters occurs in ancient authors, although some small monuments and sepulchres found in these spots make us presume that the virtues of the springs were not unknown to our ancestors. The first historical indication of these waters that I know of is the name of the Island Thermia, which first occurs in Mela the geographer, instead of Ophiussa, Kythnos, or Dryopis, its ancient appellations; and there is no doubt that the name was conferred on the island, for the same reason that it was given to other places, and to Diana herself (θερμία) as the patroness of thermal waters. In the middle ages the

baths of Thermia were already in use, as may be seen from the remains of an aqueduct of that period.

The water of the *bath* is of the temperature of 32° R. (104° Fahr.) in the middle of the cistern; but at the mouth of the fountain I found it 33° R. (106½° Fahr.) when the atmosphere was 10° R. (54½° Fahr.) It has neither smell nor colour; its taste is saline and bitter; its specific gravity is 2·015*; it is limpid and deposits no sediment. Sixteen ounces of this water afforded by evaporation 117·333 grains of a white salt of a saline and bitter taste, the composition of which was as follows:—

	Grains.
Hydrochlorate of soda . .	42·096
,, lime . .	4·320
,, magnesia .	2·402
Carbonate of lime	3·614
,, soda	2·942
Sulphate of magnesia . . .	6·634
,, lime	2·004
Water	53·000

With traces of ioduret of soda, of bromide of soda, and of silica. It contained two cubic inches of carbonic acid gas.

According to the commission, the water of Caccavo is of the temperature of 45½° R. (134¾° Fahr.) I found it, however, to be only 42° R. (126½° Fahr.) while the atmosphere was at 10° R. (54½° Fahr.)

At its source it gives forth numerous bubbles, in the gases which it develops; it diffuses a weak sulphureous smell, has a light yellow colour, is limpid, has a specific gravity of 1·039, and deposits a copious sediment of peroxide of iron.

The chemical analysis of the commission afforded a great quantity of carbonic acid; and four ounces of the water gave by evaporation the following ingredients:—

	Grs.
Carbonate of iron	2
,, lime	8
,, soda	2
Muriate of soda	28
,, magnesia . . .	21
,, lime.	6
,, potash	9
Sulphate of lime	4
,, magnesia . . .	2
With traces of silica.	

The Commission could not discover any trace of hydrosulphuric acid.

According to Signor Landerer, sixteen ounces of this water afforded by evaporation 367 grains of salt, consisting of the following ingredients:—

---

* Probably a misprint for 1·205.—*Translator's Note.*

	Grains.
Carbonate of iron . . .	3·436
,, lime . . .	12·840
,, soda . . .	5·462
Hydrochlorate of soda . .	64·939
,, lime . .	12·402
,, magnesia	21·040
Water	206·000

Although the odour indicates the presence of hydrosulphuric acid, he could not find any; but he found both hydrobromate and hydriodate of soda.

These are the physical and chemical properties of the waters of Thermia, which have been shown by long experience to be very efficacious, particularly against chronic rheumatism and arthritis, paralysis, and some lymphatic swellings. His Majesty's government erected an establishment three years ago for those who frequent this bath.

At the western part of the island, near the ruins of the ancient city, in the centre of a small harbour called Apocriosis, and near a church dedicated to St. Nicholas, there is another spring, a very small one, which appears to have the same chemical qualities as the Caccavo water.

The island of Santorino contains several thermal waters of the same nature. In the western part of this singular island I met with a spring which rises near the sea from the trachite forming the base of an enormous rock. Its temperature was 28° R. (95° Fahr.), while that of the atmosphere was 14° R. (63½ Fahr.)

The water is limpid, without odour, and contains in sixteen ounces:—

	Grains.
Sulphate of magnesia . . .	12·500
Muriate of soda	8·740
,, magnesia	3·550
Carbonate of soda	2·143

with a small quantity of carbonic acid and extractive matter.

This fountain is called in the country Placa, and it seems to have been long used, as an artificial ditch is still to be seen there, covered with an arch, now ruined by the waves of the sea.

At a short distance south of the Placa, there is a place called Thermi, from another warm spring which rises very near the sea from trachitic rocks. Its temperature is 28° R. (95° Fahr.) The water is limpid, very salt, somewhat pungent, and diffuses an odour of sulphur.

The inhabitants of Santorino first used it against rheumatism in particular; but about the year 1816 they had given it up, from some untoward symptoms which it produced; in 1834 I found it again under a layer of sand above three metres thick.

By continuing to coast the island, towards the south, many springs of the same nature are found in different parts, which being on the shore of a very deep sea, are frequently covered by it.

The island of Milos certainly owes its existence (which is of no long date) to a volcano still burning, which penetrates it with its fire in such a manner that fissures and smoking caves are to be seen in many places; and if one digs anywhere a little below the surface, the temperature is high, and often insupportable.

This island naturally contains a great number of hot springs, but it would be superfluous to give a list of them all. It will be sufficient to mention one of them, which enjoys a certain reputation among the inhabitants of the island, and bears the name of "the salt-baths" (Λουτρὰ τῆς ἁλυκῆς).

To the south of the new city, at the distance of a quarter of an hour's walk from the harbour of Panagia towards the east, there is a low grotto of volcanic sandstone, 45 metres long. It seems to be artificial, from the seats cut in the sandstone, as well as from an aperture in the upper part to let in light. In this grotto there is water enough for a whole bath.; its temperature is 22½° R. (82½° Fahr.). When the thermometer, however, was plunged into the spot from which the water seemed to issue, I found the temperature to be 29° R. (97¼° Fah.); while the external air was hardly 16° R. (68° Fahr.) It was limpid, salt, and without smell; and on its surface were floating many pieces of a delicate crust composed of carbonate and sulphate of lime. Its ingredients are salts in the state of carbonates, sulphates, and hydrochlorates. According to some writers it also contains sulphate of alumina in small quantity. (Exped. Scient. en Morée, t. ii. p. ii. p. 289.)

The salt baths, not very long ago, were much more frequented for cutaneous diseases, rheumatism, and paralysis. In a barren plain, about 500 metres south-west of the grotto, a volcano phenomenon takes place which is worth mentioning; namely, that a kind of boiling mud is thrown up, from a subterraneous volcano, through numerous apertures; and when this is going on, it is observed that the quantity of the water mentioned above increases.

Mr. Ross, Professor of Archeology at Athens, has found a warm spring in the southern part of the island of Serfo, under a mountain containing much iron, and near the ruins of an ancient tower. Two leagues and a half from the city of Corinth, towards the north-east of the gulph bearing the same name, several warm springs rise from a compact calcareous rock, which have given the name of Lutraki (little bath) to a neighbouring village. One of these springs, spouting forth the greatest quantity of water, is called κεφαλόβρυσις (chief fountain).

About three leagues from this place, near the small harbour of Kenchriè, it seems that the thermal waters still exist which formed of old the "hot baths of Venus."

Lastly, the members of the scientific expedition to the Morea found another thermal water, copious and very salt, in the eastern part of the Peloponnesus, ten leagues from Patras, near the harbour called Kunupeli; its temperature was 28¼° R. (96¼° Fahr.)

Cold saline springs. — These are very common in Greece, and are much used as purgatives, whence the natives call them laxative waters, or, in some places, hard waters. They have not been accurately examined by any chemist. Among these are—

1. The mineral spring in the harbour of Munichia in Attica, which Professor Ross believes to be the Sirangium of the ancients. Remains of an artificial Roman basin are still to be seen there, showing that it was used in old times. This water in the dose of two pounds is slightly laxative; and I have myself observed good effects from its use in what are called obstructions of the abdominal viscera, particularly of the liver.

2. Upon the island of Ægina, not far from the city, there is a saline water, which seems to be of the same nature as the preceding one, and produces the same effect.

3. In the harbour of Naussa, in the island of Paros, hardly ten minutes' walk from the city of the same name, I found a saline spring which the inhabitants call *di Santi Anargiri,* and employ as a purgative in the spring. Its use seems to be at least as old as the middle ages, as I have already shown in the journal entitled *l'Esculapio.*

4. Dr. Röser, our illustrious and learned first physician, when accompanying his Majesty to continental Greece and the Peloponnesus, found other springs of this kind; but as they are not yet sufficiently known, we can merely indicate the places where they exist. At Malvasia, at St. Nicholas, at Marattonisi, (with an ancient inscription) at Levezora (with an ancient bas-relief), at Limeni, at Barboni, at Lutrò in the Gulph of Arta, at Vonixa, where the springs form marshes which infect the town, at Galaxidi, in the Gulph of Corinth, and at Aspra Spitia.

Chalybeate springs.—Besides the chalybeate water of Caccavo, which we mentioned in speaking of the island of Thermia, Greece possesses a spring of the same kind at Milos, but still richer in iron. Towards the south of the new city in this island, an hour's distance from Panagia, there arises on the beach, and in the very sea itself, from different springs, upon a soil formed of tertiary rocks, and covered by sand, a copious stream of the temperature of 45° to 48° R. (133¼°

to 140° Fahr.) It is saline, and rather astringent, with the odour of carbonic acid gas; and it deposits upon the sand a large quantity of a yellowish brown sediment, indicating the peroxide of iron. Sixteen ounces of it afforded :—

Carbonate of iron	16·000
,, lime	4·050
Muriate of lime	1·643
,, soda	75·000
Sulphate of lime	2·634
,, magnesia . . .	61·859

with carbonic acid in an undetermined quantity, and traces of bromate of soda.

The large quantity of iron shows that its medical virtues must be considerable, and the natives of the island use it with great success against paralysis, and some atonic diseases; but as the waters are still uncovered they cannot be easily frequented by foreigners[*].

CASES OF PHLEBITIS,

WITH SOME PRELIMINARY REMARKS ON ITS
PATHOLOGY AND TREATMENT[†].

By N. CHAPMAN, M.D.

Professor of the Theory and Practice of Medicine
in the University of Pennsylvania.

IT very rarely happens that phlebitis originates spontaneously. Never have I seen a case of it, or met with any on record which I would admit as indisputable. Cruveilhier, I am aware, it is said, has related one of the vena porta, which is often quoted. But so far from this being true, he expressly says, that the suppuration was of the cellular sheath,—the vein itself being perfectly sound. Generally it proceeds from some mechanical injury done to the vein by venesection, or other surgical operations, amputation, the extirpation of tumors, and such like deep and extensive incisions, involving large vessels. The tying of varicose veins, as was formerly practised so commonly, proved a very prolific source of it, and we are not without examples of its happening in the same way to the hemorrhoidal veins, of which, I once saw an instance, under the care of the late Professor Physick. Compression from adjacent tumors does also induce it, and much is imputed to the introduction of a virus into the circulation by

---

[*] From *Il Filocamo,* an Italian medical journal of considerable merit, published in Malta.
[†] From the American Journal of the Medical Sciences—July 1843.

inoculation, or otherwise. Breschet goes so far as to affirm, that it may be occasioned by bleeding with a lancet previously used in vaccination, not thoroughly cleaned, and he cites several cases, where it proceeded from the cuts of a scalpel charged with the matter of putrid bodies. Even the washing their excoriated hands, in water, employed in the protracted maceration of flesh, he saw do it in some of the attendants on a dissecting-room. Dance mentions an instance of a surgeon, who died of an attack of it, brought on by puncturing a small phlegmon with a carefully wiped bistoury, with which he had, a month before, laid open an anthrax. Numberless facts to the same purport might be adduced.

As a common cause, is also held to be the absorption of pus or acrid fluids from foul ulcers, or the secretion of various surfaces, as of the uterus and other organs, and parts, to which so much, we have seen, has been referred in the production of phlegmasia dolens, &c. But in respect to the latter, I have always been exceedingly distrustful, and cannot help believing, that under these circumstances, the inflamed veins, which may be detected, have become so by a derivation from the structure through which they pass being previously in that state. For example, in hepatitis, or pulmonitis, &c. discovering these vessels phlogosed, it is to be taken as the effect, and not the cause, the secondary and not the primary lesion. This proneness of the veins to be thus affected, was remarked by Hunter, especially in those who had died of amputation, compound fractures or gangrene, and the observation does not want confirmation. My impression on the whole, is, that phlebitis is owing almost exclusively to a wound of the vessel, and that it is perhaps never directly occasioned by a virus. Certainly, it may be excited independently of any. There are times and individuals, at all times, when the slightest incision or puncture, or even a scratch, will lead to the most disastrous results of this nature, from the cleanest instruments. Every practitioner is aware, that at particular seasons, phlebitis is very apt to follow venesection, and I have known a lady for thirty years who has never been bled during that period, however carefully the operation may have been performed, without suffering in some degree from it;—and on three occasions so severely, as to place her life in imminent danger. Even the pricking of a finger from a needle brought on immense tumefaction of the arm, up to the shoulder, with the other phenomena of well-marked phlebitis; — and the late Professor Physick, who saw the case with me, mentioned that he had met with two others precisely like it. The instances of tumefaction from the insertions of a virus, I presume to be affections of the lymphatics. Notwithstanding all which has been urged of late to the contrary, I cannot believe that veins in any mode are absorbents; —and it is truly said by an eminent authority, "that whatever may be found in those vessels, whether pus, or other unusual! matters, is generated within, and not introduced from without."

Except in traumatic phlebitis, and particularly from venesection, it is not uniformly easy to distinguish the disease, and when seated in the veins of the interior, never, perhaps, with any precision or certainty. The obscurity arises, under the most favourable circumstances, from the resemblance it bears to the inflammation of the lymphatics, and still more to that of the cellular tissue. Between these three affections, at their height, the difference is less appreciable, since the cellular membrane mostly becomes involved, in which event the peculiarities of the others are merged and concealed. Diffusive inflammation of this tissue fills up all interstices and inequalities, forming a perfect rotundity of surface, dense, smooth, and polished. But in the early or last stage, prior to excessive tumefaction, or in its subsidence, the phlogosed vein may be felt in a tortuous course, hard and knotty, and sometimes, also, the lymphatics enlarged and indurated.

That this is a dangerous disease sufficiently appears from the preceding history of it. Timely attended to, it is for the most part easily arrested. But permitted to proceed till the vein is intensely inflamed, and especially suppuration has freely taken place, with the establishment of the multiplied sympathetic affections incident to this stage of the case, our efforts are mostly impotent, and death is to be anticipated. Yet, in a state apparently so desperate, the natural resources are sometimes applied successfully.

By Hunter it was declared, that the veins in phlebitis reveal on dissection, inflammation, suppuration, and even ulceration. Experience has since fully confirmed the accuracy of his report, and to which, in relation to the appearance of the vein itself, little has been added. Beginning usually in the internal or lining tissue, the phlogosis, when intense and persistent, may pervade the whole of the vascular parietes. Extravasations of lymph are common, and distributed in a similar manner. Deposits of it are on either surface or both, and inter-tissual, or in other words between the membranes. The same may be said of pus, and of ulceration, existing in one or the entire coats. But of these several anatomical characters, something more must be said. The inflammation is faint, or of a rose, or of a deep scarlet, or brownish hue, in specks, or striated or arborescent, local or extending along to the heart, continuously or in detached patches, between which the intervening spaces are healthy. Collections of pus and of lymph are detected sometimes in the calibre of the vessel to an amount very seriously to embarrass, or even to obstruct the circulation, and coagula of blood have been seen, though seldom, separately or united to the other matters, having the same effect. There are instances, too, where, from adhesions of the sides of the vessel, a total obliteration is produced, and should recovery take place, it becomes ultimately a dense, impervious cord. The ulcers are few or many, superficial or deep. I once saw several that had gone entirely through the walls of the vessel. Lymph having been deposited on the exterior surface, it occasionally agglutinates the vein to the surrounding cellular surface, and abscesses are formed. Generally the texture of the vessel is softened, sometimes to pultaceousness, and in one instance, from the colour, the odour, and other circumstances, I had reason to suppose the existence of gangrene, as well of it as the adjacent cellular membrane.

These are the principal lesions, which may be restricted to a single vessel or extend to others more or less diffusely —or indeed, according to some writers, involve any one, or every organ of the body, at different times, in inflammation and its consequences. Excepting, however, the purulent depositions previously noticed, I am not sensible of any thing in the consequent derangements meriting further attention. Disseminated through the structure of the organ, they are detected from the size of a pea to a walnut, or sometimes double or treble, or quadruple the size; the number always larger as they are diminutive. They are infiltrations of pus collected at a point or points, and not properly abscesses, as they have seldom or never any regular cyst. The organ is usually found mostly inflamed immediately around the deposit. It is the fashion of the day to elevate in importance and frequency the diseases of the veins, and the accounts we receive respecting them are exaggerated, and must be received with qualifications. Even more than the heart and the arteries are they susceptible to *imbibition*; and mere redness, which I suspect has been too readily admitted as evidence of phlogosis, proves here equally delusive. Coloration, with injection of the vessels of the surface, warrants a suspicion of the existence of this state, though not conclusive. Demonstration of it is only afforded by the presence of lymph or pus, or thickening or softening of tissues, or other changes of structure.

Contemplating the pathology of this affection, we are at once struck with some circumstances in it exceedingly anomalous and heteroclite. The mode sometimes, of its origin, and that a trivial lesion of a vein, so often extensively injured with impunity, should lead to such wide constitutional disturbance, and this nearly always showing a tendency to typhoid debility and vitiation, are certainly very extraordinary. I have already alluded to the singular predisposition in these cases, without, however, assigning the nature of it, which I am unable to do. It occurs, perhaps, most frequently in various cachectic states, while on other occasions it is met with apparently in the soundest and most healthy conditions. Could it be demonstrated that the local inflammation was rapidly and widely diffused through the veins, so as to embrace any large portion of them, then an explanation would be afforded of the enormous mischief produced. Granting it sometimes happens, it cannot be averred that it generally does. The contrary, indeed, is nearer true, or that in a large number of instances of traumatic phlebitis, especially from venesection, the inflammation is restricted to a few inches from the wound, and though it may run up to the heart, it seldom involves other veins. The phenomenon is only explicable on the supposition of the sympathies of the rest of the veins with the affected one. Considering that these vessels form a natural and homogeneous system engaged in the same operations, it is presumable independently of other proof, that they have a very intimate consent of parts, by which there is a reciprocity of sufferings, oftener, however, of functional irritation than positive disease; or, in other words, that what was primarily a local phlegmasia is rendered a constitutional affection, without an extension of actual inflammation. Different, however, is it in a more advanced stage of the case, where the adynamic degeneration has supervened. Great reason is there to suppose that suppuration here exists, and that the immense change thus suddenly wrought in the character and physiognomy of the disease proceeds from the mingling of pus with the blood. Endo-carditis alone, to which it has been imputed, will not account for it. The phenomena of the two cases are dissimilar, and those of the veins are precisely such as are induced by injecting certain fluids, and above all, putrid fluids, into the circulation. Nor is the amount of matter secreted inadequate to the effect. In three extremely grave instances of phlebitis from bleeding, attended by me, at each visit I pressed out of the orifice of the vein half an ounce or more of an ill-conditioned or illaudable pus.

Not conversant with any other form of the disease than that of which I have just spoken, and entertaining the conviction it is the only one capable of recognition with any certainty, at all events in time to do any thing efficient, I shall confine my practical remarks to it. These, however, should a case of spontaneous origin be detected in season, will be equally applicable to it, so far, at least, as concerns the general treatment.

We are, in the first place, to support the limb, so as to secure an absolute state of rest, and which can only be attained by putting it into a nicely adjusted case. It is very much the custom here to have one carved, that it may be more exactly accommodated to the contours of the part, by which the main object is better secured, and the pain of motion prevented. The suspensory sling, made of a handkerchief, tied round the neck, commonly used elsewhere for the arm, is a miserable contrivance, having unquestionably often led to the most disastrous consequences. The antiphlogistic plan is now to be adopted, and, as part of it, venesection would seem to claim priority of attention. Experience, however, teaches, that the benefit resulting from it is never proportioned to what might be reasonably anticipated —that it is sometimes utterly unavailing—and that a very serious objection to it is, that it is very apt to be followed by a fresh attack of phlebitis, evidence of which has come under my own observation. It may therefore be best not to resort to it unless excitement is high and general—leeches, on the whole, being decidedly preferable. These are to be liberally applied along the course of the vein, and again and again repeated. Emollient cataplasms or fomentations may also be useful, and especially where the swelling is extensive. The case proving obstinate, menacing a serious career, of all remedies the one deserving of the greatest confidence is a blister. Numerous are the instances in which I have witnessed its superior efficacy; and I believe there is little division of sentiment as to its extraordinary value among the profession in this part of the country. From what I have seen and heard I cannot entertain a doubt that it will at once arrest a large majority of cases. But though coming from the late Professor Physick—published by him some forty years ago, and since frequently alluded to with the highest commendation in the writings of this country, it seems to have attracted scarcely any attention in Europe, or, at least, I do not find it noticed in the treatises on the subject I have consulted, with a solitary exception: Cooper, in his Surgical Dictionary, appropriates a paragraph to it, without praise or censure. The manner of application is, to place a narrow strip of epispastic plaster along the course of the vein, as far as it appears to be inflamed, cutting an opening in it at the orifice, over which a soft poultice is to be placed; and the blister having drawn, is to be so dressed as to be kept freely discharging. Little further of any peculiarity appertains to the management of this state of the affection. Evacuations of the bowels, and the ordinary antifebrile mixtures, are usually directed. But enormous doses of tartarised antimony are recently praised, and so is the profuse use of mercury. It is difficult to discern the motive for such practice; there is no evidence of its success, and much in it to condemn. Chiefly do I rely, at this juncture, on a combination of calomel, ipecacuanha, and opium, in moderate portions, and where pain and restlessness are prominent, increase considerably the latter article, or give at once the Dover's powder largely. The promotion of perspiration, I very strongly suspect, has not here been duly appreciated.

As the case advances, the indication arises to prevent the pus, the secretion of which may now be apprehended, from being transmitted to the heart; and with this view divers expedients have been suggested to interrupt the communication. Compression above the orifice was practised by Hunter, so as to obliterate the canal by adhesion of the sides of the vessel. But this having failed, after a fair trial, was abandoned, and a division of the vein substituted with probably no greater success. Discouraged from the further prosecution of it, a ligature was next advised, and which, though promising more fairly, I do not know has ever been attempted. The project, therefore, of arresting the pus, would seem to be deemed hopeless.

That the two first operations should not have answered is sufficiently intelligible. Compression adequate to the end could not be made, it is presumable, without at the same interrupting the arterial circulation; and independently of the pain induced by it, I doubt exceedingly its feasibility at all, in a limb so swollen as happens at the period when the experiment becomes justifiable. Cutting the vein in two does not intercept the progress of the blood effectually, while every objection to the ligature applies to this operation in an equal force. Determining, therefore, on any of these expedients,

the ligature should be preferred. Yet it must be confessed, that it would be a very serious affair to lay open and tie a vein in the state of parts so irritated as they are when the operation is most demanded, and whether it would be for good or for evil, is uncertain.

Caused as it may be, whether by the introduction of pus, as I think it is, or in any other mode, when the typhoid malignant stage sets in, whatever is calculated to uphold or renovate the vital forces is resorted to, with however seldom any advantage.

Designing to annex some cases, in which the treatment of this affection is more detailed, I have now, to avoid the prolixity of repetitions, presented only an outline of it. The first of these cases is probably the second on record of suppurative phlebitis, it having been preceded only by the one reported by Mr. Hunter, to which I have before alluded.

It is given as it was originally published, more than thirty years ago, in the Eclectic Repertory, one of our journals, which will account for some circumstances in the narrative not otherwise very intelligible.

CASE I.—In the month of March 1810, I was requested by the late Mr. Thomas W. Francis, of this city, to visit his coachman. On inquiring into the case, I learned that three days before, while on a journey, he had been attacked in the evening with slight symptoms of pleurisy, which very readily yielded to a moderate bleeding.

The next morning he felt for the first time some degree of pain and tension in the right arm, in which he had been bled. But the uneasiness was so trifling, and in other respects he was so well, that he continued on the journey. The exertion of driving, as might have been expected, aggravated exceedingly these affections. Yet such was his anxiety to reach home, that he studiously disguised his real situation, lest he might be left behind—and obstinately persevered, against every remonstrance, to perform his duties as coachman. But on the last day of the journey, overcome by the severity of his sufferings, he reluctantly consented to be placed in the carriage, and was in this way conveyed to the city.

My attendance on him commenced in the night, an hour or two after his arrival. Even at this early stage, the case presented a very serious aspect. The arm was swelled to perhaps twice its natural size, and the pain and inflammation were excessive. By pressure, a copious stream of purulent matter issued from the orifice, and I could distinctly trace the enlargement of the vein for several inches, imparting the sensation of a hard, inelastic tube, enclosed under the integuments.

Nor were these the only untoward circumstances of the case. There was also considerable pain in the left side, with a universal soreness pervading his body. Little or no fever was indicated by the pulse, which was weak, irregular, and quick;—of a contracted volume, and rather corded. It was more a disturbed than a febrile pulse—certainly evincing nothing of an inflammatory diathesis. But though apparently not much if at all feverish, he was greatly harassed by restlessness and inquietude. The temperature of his body was unequal and fluctuating. When his attention was fixed by conversation addressed directly to him, his mind seemed perfectly rational; but otherwise he quickly became flighty;—talking incoherently, and endeavouring to get out of bed. Whatever were my doubts as to the ultimate event, I entertained none respecting the nature of the complaint, or the cause which had produced it. I was at once satisfied that the whole of the existing mischief was attributable to inflammation of the vein, extending probably to the heart, and to the introduction of pus into the blood. To the latter cause I the more promptly imputed the train of nervous affections, as I had seen, in a series of experiments, phenomena of the same kind induced by the injection of pus, of milk, of oil, of mucilage, and other bland fluids, into the veins of different animals.

Nor could I hesitate long as to the practice to be pursued. To subdue the inflammation of the vein, and arrest the pus in its passage to the circulation, were obvious indications.

Notwithstanding the feebleness of arterial action, I bled him to the amount of twelve ounces. I suspected a state of depression, and thought it not unlikely that the pulse might rise by depletion. Where so large a vessel was inflamed, and seemingly too, the heart itself, it certainly was not unreasonable to conjecture that the want of diffused excitement was owing to this condition of the system. But my anticipations were not realized. The bleeding was indeed followed by' no sensible effect, and the blood was without any very peculiar appearances. It did not, it is true, separate as it ordinarily does. The serum and crassamentum were commixed, as if slightly stirred together. I could detect no pus in the blood.

I next enveloped completely the arm with a blister from the elbow to the shoulder, excepting at the puncture, which was covered with a small emollient poultice to facilitate the evacuation of the matter. During the night I ordered, moreover, that he should take at stated intervals a solution of salts till it purged him actively.

In the morning he appeared in some respects to be better. The blister had drawn well, and the pain and swelling were in consequence considerably reduced. Neither was he so restless or irritable, and his mind had ceased to wander.

When at night I again called, he was much as he had been at my preceding visit. The swelling of the arm was perhaps somewhat further abated. But in a few hours afterwards the pain in the side, which at no period had entirely subsided, reverted with violence. It did not, however, raise his pulse.

Convinced by a variety of considerations that the pain proceeded from inflammation of the heart, I placed a large blister over the region of that organ. Though relieved by this application of the pain, I had the mortification of seeing him the succeeding morning in a situation of increased danger. With a pulse weak, quick. and tremulous, he was wild and distracted. I directed that he should lose six or eight ounces of blood by cups, from the neck and temples, and to have a blister put on behind each ear.

It now appeared to me to be literally of vital importance to intercept the pus in its course to the circulation. I, therefore, resolved without delay to make use of compression, though it seemed still to be forbidden by the tumefaction of the limb. A bandage and compress were accordingly applied a short distance above the puncture. But nothing material was gained by these applications. The swelling of the arm however declined, and no inconvenience was experienced from the compression. The pus continued to flow profusely from the orifice : this was late in the evening.

My visit the next morning found him worse. To all the bad symptoms which previously prevailed, were now added some still more inauspicious. The morbid sensibility of his body had become so exquisite, that he could not bear the slightest touch, or scarcely the weight of the bedclothes without complaining. So sensibly alive was he to every sudden impression, that by opening or shutting the door, or walking across the room, or by a question put to him in a sharp tone of voice, or by a strong glare of light, he was startled and sometimes exceedingly agitated.

At this critical juncture I resorted to the advice of Dr. James, who very obligingly met me in consultation. We agreed to give the camphorated emulsion in large doses, and to have stimulating injections repeatedly administered. But this treatment was equally unavailing, and my patient progressively sunk. Low delirium, cold extremities, tremors of the nerves, and convulsive cough, soon supervened. His pulse became hardly perceptible. The pupils of the eyes were widely dilated, and his countenance assumed an expression uncommonly haggard, phrensied, and distressed. Desperate as I deemed the case, I did not permit my exertions to be relaxed. By the constant use of the most powerful stimulants, such as camphor and opium, the volatile alkali, the spirits of turpentine, ether, wine, and brandy, I protracted his existence for three days longer, without having however, during this interval, a single gleam of hope afforded me by any change of his recovery.

The morning after my patient expired, I made an examination, with a view of ascertaining the exact state of things. I exposed the vein from the wrist to the axilla. The external surface of the vessel was in many places inflamed, and especially above the puncture. Between this and the shoulder, matter had escaped from the vein by four distinct sinuses into the neighbouring cellular membrane, forming small abscesses. Two of these sinuses were high up the arm.

I dissected very carefully the parts adjacent to the wound. Directly around it there was an abscess containing, I presume, a large spoonful of pus, mixed with a dark fetid sanies. Sphacelus had already destroyed a portion of the cellular texture.

I next laid open the vein. There was inflammation more or less, from a little below the elbow to the final point of my dissection, without being anywhere very great. By the appearance of the coat of the vein there was, however, the amplest proof of its having existed in the highest grade, and which is abundantly shown by the formation of the sinuses, &c. Below and above the orifice for several inches, gangrene had taken place, bounded by an extensive erysipelatous blush, and the inner surface of the vessel within this space, had begun to slough.

The quantity of pus in the cavity of the vein was small. It ought, indeed, to have been stated that for two or three days prior to his death the discharge from the orifice had gradually diminished. No disposition whatever was evinced any where along the canal of the vein, to an adhesion of its sides. My wish to extend the dissection was frustrated. Enough however has been brought to light by this partial exposition, to confirm my original notions as to the nature and causes of this series of extraordinary affections.

In reflecting on the management of the case, I have only to regret having confided too much in compression as a means of promoting adhesion. But surely I shall escape censure, for having adopted a measure which had been approved by the very high and concurrent authority of Hunter, Cooper,

Abernethy, &c. &c. I had never before an opportunity of trying compression under such circumstances, or of seeing it employed. My conviction now is that it will rarely succeed. It is confessedly at all times difficult to produce a union in tubular or fistulous ulcers, even where pressure can be used. It is yet more so, to effect a coalescence between the opposite surfaces of blood-vessels, because, among other obstacles, the coagulable lymph which is the medium of attachment, must in a great measure be swept away by the circulation as fast as it is deposited. It is besides almost impracticable to make adequate compression on any of the veins of the arm, without interrupting the return of the blood. I confess, however, that these speculative objections to the practice, have less weight with me than the melancholy instance of its failure which I witnessed. In the case of my patient the experiment was fairly made,—for five days and nights successively, I continued the compression, and with the utmost vigilance to the due regulation of it. Distrusting, therefore, the efficacy of this expedient, if ever I should meet with a similar case I would apply a ligature to the vein. The operation, however, will not often be necessary. It can only be required where suppuration has taken place, and there are grounds for the apprehension that the matter is travelling into circulation. Cases of this sort are extremely rare. Few, at least, have been recorded. I have met in my researches with only one at all analogous. They have hitherto been contemplated by writers rather as a possible than an actual occurrence.

Injuries to the veins from bleeding are, for the most part, attended by only circumscribed inflammation. The suppurative process seldom ensues. Even when it happens it is generally limited to the vicinity of the wound, through which the pus is either freely evacuated, or is lodged in the surrounding cellular texture, and the abscess thus formed may be made by an opening to discharge externally, if, contrary to the ordinary course, it does not do it spontaneously.

CASE II.—It was in 1816, I think, for, owing to a casualty the date cannot be ascertained exactly, that I was requested by Dr. M. Phillips, a young physician of this city, to visit with him an elderly man, a native of Germany, whom he considered very strangely and alarmingly affected. Five days previously he had been bled for sciatica, and, according to the popular prejudice of his country, in the foot of the same side in which the pain was seated. Being relieved of the rheumatism by the loss of blood, he the next day resumed his occupation of driving a cart, and of course was much on his feet. Early in the evening he came home with severe pain shooting up the leg, ascribed to a return of rheumatism. This increasing during the night, with considerable swelling of the limb, Dr. Phillips was sent for, who, adopting a similar view of the nature of the case, treated it in the usual manner by general and local bleeding, purging, the mild diaphoretics, and divers local applications, fomentations, liniments, &c. Great as the pain and swelling were, his pulse had never been full or active, the temperature even of the part high, or, indeed, any very unequivocal evidence of fever, and though the orifice of the vein had not united, there was nothing very peculiar about it. The man becoming, however, restless and delirious, with chills, rigors, and other alarming symptoms, I was consulted. The preceding account I derived from the attending physician, and which was confirmed by the wife of the patient.

On entering the chamber I was struck with the wild and phrensied expression of countenance, and soon perceived that he was greatly agitated and distressed. Not content scarcely for a moment in any one position, he was alternately up and down, or tossing himself from side to side of the bed, and had evidently a sort of spasmodic jerking of the limbs. Examining the case, I found his intelligence very imperfect, the pulse feeble and tremulous, the skin cool, covered with a dewy sweat, especially about the forehead and neck, and there were nervous tremors, and difficulty both of articulation and deglutition. The whole of the leg, and part of the thigh, were prodigiously swollen, tense, and pale, and around the orifice, which was closed by some thick glutinous matter, was an abscess of nearly an inch in diameter that had not before been observed. By gently pressing it, a sanious fluid flowed out freely, and from stroking the vein above it, amounted altogether to an ounce and a half. The whole of the affected portion of the extremity was covered with a blister except at the orifice, over which a poultice was placed, and opium, the carbonate of ammonia, and brandy toddy liberally given. In the evening he appeared decidedly worse, having had several tetanoid spasms, and becoming so furiously deranged, that several men were required to restrain him from acts of violence. He died in the night in a convulsion, of which he had several previously. Every effort was resisted to get an autopsic inspection even of the vein.

CASE III.—Not long after the preceding, I saw, with Professor Physick, a third case of this affection. It was in a middle-aged lady, corpulent, plethoric, and of sedentary or even sluggish habits. Frightened by a recurrence of an apoplectic admonition, which she had experienced several times before, she determined at once to resort to venesection.

No longer, owing to extreme obesity, could blood be obtained from the arm, and on this occasion a vein in the hand was opened. Eleven days after this, and when the incision had completely healed, which indeed it did very promptly, she for the first time complained of sharp darting pains along the course of the vein up the limb. As Dr. Physick, her family physician, was confined at the period by sickness, the bleeder who had performed the operation was sent for, by whom she was told that a nerve or a tendon had been pricked, and that nothing was to be apprehended, as it was an injury temporary in its nature, and readily cured. Directing her to wear the hand in a sling, and to bathe it with an emollient liniment, he retired. But henceforward the pain and swelling of the forearm rapidly increased, and the same person was again consulted, who now advised the loss of blood by leeches, which were several times repeated, followed by poultices. No advantage, however, was gained by these applications, and she becoming a good deal weakened, and slightly wandering in her slumbers, Dr. Physick was urgently requested to see her. Discerning her perilous situation, and from the infirmities of his own health being incapable of paying her the attentions he thought she required, he waited in the house till I came to his assistance. The preceding history of the case was then related by him to me. This was late in the afternoon. Her general condition reminded us much of that of the incipiency of low typhoid fever. The eyes were injected, the pupils slightly dilated, with a swimming fatuous expression, and she felt some uneasiness of the head. Deep sighing was frequent, and though she had vomited once or twice she still complained of epigastric oppression and of nausea. There was some distension of the abdomen, probably owing to the loaded state of the bowels, as she was constipated; the temperature of the surface unequal; the extremities cool and pallid, while the head was preternaturally warm, and the face rather florid. Her pulse was quick, irritated, and corded, of very small volume, and so irregular as to be somewhat intermittent. Depression of spirits was very conspicuous, and she frequently declared that her sensations were such, that she was sure her death was inevitable.

To the elbow, the arm was much swollen and exquisitely tender, with little pain in it, either lancinating or pulsatory, and pretty nearly of the natural hue, except here and there some livid spots appeared. The orifice was inflamed, and its lips pouting, and slightly retorted. Discovering some sanguinolent matter on the poultice, the vein was delicately pressed, when there oozed out nearly a couple of drachms of pure pus.

We recommended that a stimulating enema should be immediately given to empty the bowels, and if not succeeding, an infusion of senna and salts, administered in repeated doses, till the effect was attained. The arm was also to be covered with a blister, except at the orifice, over which a poultice was to be placed, and then secured in a case. These instructions were faithfully executed, and on my return in a few hours, I learnt that she had been amply purged with the medicine. Yet her condition had deteriorated, by an aggravation of cerebral and nervous disorder, and of jactitation and wretchedness. An opiate was now ordered. The report of the morning was, that she had slept altogether some hours, with, however, much muttering delirium. No improvement could we discern in any respect; on the contrary, as related to the general condition, manifestly worse. The blister not having drawn, it was replaced by a fresh one very carefully prepared, and bound on the limb by strips of adhesive plaster. Dover's powder and wine whey were given during the day. Towards evening we saw her again, and thought her better. For several hours she had been comparatively tranquil, and took eagerly some nourishment, sago, with wine and nutmeg. The nervous system was more steady, the intelligence perfect, the swelling of the arm considerably reduced, of the purulent discharge scarcely any, and the aspect of the wound greatly improved. Having drawn well, the blister was removed, and dressed by a mixture of the basilicon and mercurial ointments. Her recovery henceforward advanced so rapidly that I ceased to take notes of the case.

This is one of the many instances, certainly, however, not of equal severity, which I could recite of the extraordinary control of vesication over phlebitis. Except it, nothing here was resorted to of any decided curative power, and the whole of the beneficial effects may be justly ascribed to it. With entire rest of the limb, I have much reason to suppose that it will arrest a very large proportion of these cases antecedently to the suppurative stage, and even then where the attack is mild. Endocarditis, however, taking place, or such a quantity of pus having entered the circulation as to induce a state of poisoning, with all those complications of typhoid affections consequent on it, then I believe that it, in common with every thing else hitherto devised, will prove nugatory. Fortunately, however, the most violent forms of the disease are not common. The inflammation in traumatic phlebitis is usually local, and when more extensive and suppurative, the quantity of pus secreted is small, or if copious, its introduction into the circulation is very often prevented by some of those provisions wisely instituted by nature, to which I have previously alluded.

ON SEMINAL DISCHARGES FROM THE URETHRA.

By James Douglas,

Lecturer on Anatomy at the School of Medicine, Portland Street, Glasgow, &c. &c.

(For the Medical Gazette.)

Since reading the papers in the Gazette, by Mr. Phillips, on involuntary discharges of spermatic fluid, I have always intended to send a note of my small experience on this subject, but have delayed rather too long for it to come into close enough relation with his. The readers of the Gazette will probably remember, however, that after describing the causes and the debilitating effects of these discharges, Mr. Phillips explained M. Lallemand's plan of treatment, by cauterising the prostatic portion of the urethra with the nitrate of silver, and gave an account of the cases in which he himself had put it in practice.

In October, 1837, I read a paper on spermatorrhœa before the Glasgow Medical Society, in which I gave an account of Professor Lallemand's opinions on this subject, and the history of a case which had occurred to myself. The patient was a medical man, and he was so impressed with the truth of M. Lallemand's doctrine, with which I had made him acquainted, that he formed the resolution of visiting Montpellier, and being operated on by the professor himself. This was accordingly done; but he did not remain sufficiently long under M. L.'s care to see that there should be no need for a repetition of the application. He was, however, greatly benefited, the discharges having become much more rare. Some months after he desired me to cauterise the prostatic urethra for him again, which I did very freely, and a renewed improvement was the result, although the discharges have never entirely ceased.

Last year a case occurred to me, which I treated with a different local application. As it appeared to me that the effect of the caustic on the urethra must be very much the same which its solution has on the conjunctiva, diminishing its sensibility or irritability, I thought that perhaps a solution of opium might serve the purpose as well, or perhaps better, attempting at the same time to give tone to the parts by the use of general means.

3 O

R. M'G., æt. 28. Nov. 20th, 1842. About six years ago fell into the practice of masturbation; at that time having never touched a woman. For about twelve months was much given to that bad practice, and ever since has continued it occasionally. About seven months after first commencing masturbation had sexual connection, and but seldom since.

Five or six months ago he complained to me of frequent slight headache, and giddiness in looking down, which he attributed to derangement of the stomach, and treated as such, with but partial success.

In August last he first noticed that he lost semen at night during sleep; not thrown out in the way of ejaculation, but running from him gradually, and without any pleasurable sensation; also without any lascivious dreams, and with scarcely any erection. About the same time he noticed the semen to be parted with when at stool, and frequently also when making water.

In the beginning of October he told me of this complaint. I inquired whether he had given up the bad practice which occasioned it, and he pled guilty to still polluting himself with it sometimes. I made him promise to give it up entirely, and this promise he has faithfully kept. I then put him on an ounce of steel (Tr. Mur. Ferri), and ordered the shower-bath, cold, every morning. By the end of October he said that he felt his general health improved, but that the emissions still continued. I then ordered a mixture of mucilage with watery solution of opium, 1 gr. of opium and 3 grains of acetate of lead to the ounce of the mixture, to be injected into the back part of the urethra, and even into the bladder. In ten days I doubled the strength of the opium. This was used three times a day. When the injection was first allowed to pass back, it produced a sensation of heat, and afterwards a pleasing soothing feeling. It has now been used for three weeks, and the improvement is very marked. He has now no nocturnal emissions, and very rarely when at stool, and these only to a very small extent.

I recommended him at this date to change the muriate of iron for the carbonate, and to continue the shower-bath and the injection.

Dec. 6th—Has improved very much *in his general* appearance. Uses the injection now only before going to bed. Has had no nocturnal emissions since former date (Nov. 20th), and very few when at stool, and none at all with his urine. I advised him to continue.

This summer I had occasion to see him on account of dysentery, and learned that he was almost entirely free of his annoyance, the only remedy which he still uses being the shower-bath.

Should this treatment, by injecting the solution of sugar of lead with opium, mixed with mucilage, be found generally serviceable, it will have the advantage of not requiring the confinement which is necessary for some days after the application of the nitrate of silver.

Glasgow, 35, North Frederick Street,
September 16, 1843.

EFFICACY OF WARM INJECTIONS IN STRICTURE.

To the Editor of the Medical Gazette.

SIR,

I READ some short time back, in one of the medical periodicals, an account of a case of stricture, in which the medical gentleman in attendance found use in applying a warm fluid to the strictured portion of the urethra, through the means of an ordinary catheter.

Now it struck me at once that an instrument much more fitted to the purpose, and much more likely to succeed, would be a catheter with its orifice at the extremity instead of at the side as is usual.

I had one made, therefore, and for greater convenience a stop-cocked syringe, holding about an ounce, fitted to its other end.

My mode of applying it is this: I fill the syringe with some warm bland fluid (oil, or barley-water, for instance), and I then connect it with the catheter, and gently pass the latter down to the stricture. The moment I feel the resistance, I turn the stop-cock with the index-finger of my right hand (steadying the penis with my left), and propel a jet of the warm liquid upon the strictured portion with moderate force, taking care, of course, not to press the apparatus forcibly against the urethra, but keeping all firm and ." well in hand."

I have tried this in four cases, and several times in each case, in which I had before failed entirely in passing the smallest catheter, and in all with decided and instant success, the instrument always passing freely, and without the slightest pain.

I do not know whether this is novel, but as I have not seen it before myself, and as we are all bound to do our best for suffering humanity, you may perhaps think· the observation worth a place in your widely circulating journal.—I am, sir,

Your obedient servant,
FRANK HUDSON.
2, Onslow Place, Brompton,
Sept. 18, 1843.

MR. LEE ON BELGIAN MEDICAL INSTITUTIONS.

To the Editor of the Medical Gazette.

SIR,

A VARIETY of interesting cases daily present themselves at the Eye Dispensary, which was established at Brussels some years ago by M. Cunier, who, in the treatment of ophthalmia and its consequences, seldom has recourse to vascular depletion, but trusts chiefly to derivatives, as laxatives, mercurials, and counter-irritants, with sedative or slightly stimulating lotions; the solution of nitrate of silver in variable proportions (from two grains to ten to the ounce of water), a few drops of which, instilled into the eyes at stated intervals, being one of the most frequent applications. Many patients, however, afflicted with the military ophthalmy (especially those from the country), frequently neglect to apply for relief until the disease has made such progress as to destroy the sight. M. Cunier has no exclusive method for the removal of cataract, sometimes performing extraction, at others depression. He has performed the operation for artificial pupil with great success in several bad cases. One of these patients, who had been blind for twenty-five years, in consequence of military ophthalmy, so far recovered his sight from the operation, as to conduct himself without any guide in the streets, and to read the larger letters on the printed bills. The case is recorded in the Annales d'Oculistique, a volume of which is published annually.

Prior to the revolution, medical practice and instruction was in a very backward state in Belgium; and during the existence of the provisional government, the medical professors of one of the universities created a *free* faculty of sciences, of which the diploma might be obtained by almost any applicant; and this had a most prejudicial effect. "All that there was in the country of barbers and ignorant men hastened to present themselves before this *soi-disant* faculty, to purchase the diploma of candidate of sciences, and thus prepare the way for the acquisition, with very little trouble, of that of doctor in the three departments of medicine. The persons cannot be sufficiently stigmatised who thus degraded the honourable profession of medicine, by inundating the country with those medicators who go about bleeding and purging the community without control*."

Shortly afterwards, however, a new organization of the profession was effected. A free university was inaugurated at Brussels in 1834, the *personel* of the secondary school, which had till then existed, forming the nucleus of the faculty of medicine; and a central jury of examination was instituted, before which candidates for the diploma from the other universities were bound to appear. A Catholic university was founded at Malines, and subsequently transferred to Louvain; the universities of Liege and Ghent remaining the national ones, and kept up by the state. An Academy of Medicine was likewise formed, which, with the medical societies of Ghent, Antwerp, and Bruges, greatly contributed to diffuse information by the publication of their memoirs, to raise the condition of the profession, and to form a closer union of its members. The community of language with France, and the reprints, in a cheap form, of most of the valuable works published in Paris, had likewise great influence in extending professional knowledge. There appear now in Brussels a Gazette Médicale, an Annales de Médecine, a Bulletin Médical Belge, and one or two other periodicals. The Encyclographie des Sciences Médicales, published monthly, gives the substance of whatever is valuable in the chief medical journals of France, England, and Germany.

"Clinical instruction," says an author,

* Coup-d'Œil sur les Institutions Médicales Belges, par C. Broex.

whose favourable account of medicine in Belgium, as compared with France, bears the impress of great partiality, "is acquired by each pupil having the charge of a certain number of patients, respecting whose cases he is interrogated at the bed-side, reporting upon their progress from day to day : the professor verifies the exactness of the report by comparing it with that of the *interne*, and by examining the case himself; a disputation being carried on respecting the progress of the disease, and the treatment to be adopted. On the admission of a patient, the pupil to whom he is confided is required to examine the peculiarities of the case, before the professor and the students. The most prominent symptoms are noted daily upon a paper, placed at the head of each bed, on which are likewise indicated the remedies prescribed. An autopsic examination is made of the patients who die; the pathological alterations, and their reference to the symptoms during the course of the disease, being remarked upon by the professor. In the surgical department operations are frequently performed by the *internes* and the more advanced pupils, in the presence of the professor, who superintends their performance. Professorships are not obtained by the method of *concours* in the Belgian universities. The free university of Brussels forms, however, an exception in this respect. The professors are appointed by the directors of the universities, who are guided in their choice by the previous reputation of the candidates, their scientific publications, or a personal appreciation of their merits[*]."

Another author, however, of the highest reputation in Belgium, (M. Guislain, Lettres Médicales sur l'Italie) on comparing the internal organization of the hospitals in his own country with that of others, acknowledges their superiority in some respects. "As regards their localities, several of our most important establishments are susceptible of great ameliorations: they are in many parts ancient buildings, with vast wards, most frequently without fire-places; the roofs displaying immense wooden rafters, supported by columns, whose antique capitals recal

[*] Parallele entre l'Enseignement Médical des Universités de Paris, Berlin et la Belgique, par le Doct. Van Meerbeck.

the epoch to which they belong. Almost always these buildings are faulty as regards the hygienic department, and also with respect to the patients being placed too closely together; for, except a few tolerable establishments, and two or three new institutions, all of them are in a state of degradation such as is unparalelled in other parts. There is much likewise to be desired as regards the furniture of our hospitals: the iron beds have no curtains, and where there are any they are not so appropriate to their purpose as in the establishments in the north of Italy. Our store-rooms, our kitchens, are far from presenting the abundance and comfort of those in the English hospitals; our baths and douches, where there are any, cannot be compared with those of Italy and France, which country might give us some excellent lessons in all that regards the internal administration of hospitals, which is generally neglected with us, and conducted in a mere routine manner.

"In Italy, there is an air of richness and profusion in the interior of charitable institutions, amidst the misery, often very great, which is met with in the streets. In Belgium, on the contrary, where there is a much greater amount of general comforts, our hospitals, and hospices, present an appearance, if not of indigence, at least of distress; a want of uniformity in the beds, in the colour and the material of the coverlets, which are for the most part coarse and old; a cloathing like the costume of Harlequin, patched all over; blackened walls, badly painted windows and doors, roofs which allow the rain to penetrate, and even snow to fall on the patients' beds; damp cells, in which the insane are crouched up in their dirt; doors which do not shut; 'windows broken and mended with paper.' Every where an inferiority is perceived in the administrative department, which, in many respects, is essentially egotistical, bureaucratical, wishing to economise in every thing, even in the common necessaries for patients; most frequently having recourse to that worst of all measures, that of contracting for the care and attention towards the unfortunate, and neglecting all direct control and superintendence. It is this deplorable system, which sends out, in many places, foundlings, orphans, the blind; the old; the insane to lodge with poor or avaricious peasants; it is this system which peoples our country places, as also our hospitals, with pallid, scorbutic, scrofulous individuals ; which causes a frightful mortality among the indigent, because the inadequate food which they receive is not sufficient to keep up their strength; because their clothing does not preserve them from the effects of atmospheric vicissitudes."

"There is, likewise, (continues M. Guislain), great room for improvement in the medical administration of our establishments, and particularly with reference to the appointment of the physicians and surgeons, who are generally nominated by the local authorities, upon the presentation of the administrative commissions of the civil hospitals. This method is essentially adverse to the interests of the science; we would wish to see the appointment of the medical attendants of these institutions determined by some learned body, capable of eliminating, in a proper manner, the merit of the candidates, either by a faculty of medicine, an academy, or a medical commission."

After citing the mode of election pursued at Lyons, as a model, M. Guislain further observes:—"Let us hope that our local administrations will follow the example, and abandon an old routine system directly opposed to all the principles of equity, and especially to the progress of the science. The position of a well-informed young physician is often very disheartening, amidst the obstacles by which he is surrounded, and which prevent the development of his capabilities. What a pinery for good subjects, what hopes, what a guarantee for the future, does not the method of the *concours* offer ! And compare this excellent institution to our nominations by favour, in which the number of friends, the always painful and humiliating supplications, intrigue, and low manœuvres, but too often gain the advantage over real and modest merit. The good of this method consists in its preparatory tendencies in the constitution of a school, for the development of talents formed for practice, and for the production of distinguished characters. Let it not be said that there exist insurmountable obstacles ; these can only come from men behind the spirit of the age; for experience has already decided as to the

value of the mode of competition, inasmuch as the trial has already been in operation for more than fifty years in the above-named city, as well as elsewhere. It is true we have already made a step forward in this direction, since the clinical professors of our state universities are now elected by *concours*." I have quoted thus largely the remarks of M. Guislain, as affording a more correct account of the administration of affairs in Belgium than could be given by a traveller through the country. His work, however, was published in 1840, and it appears to me that ameliorations have been effected in some respects since that period.

Belgium possesses some handsome and extensive military hospitals, and the government has lately established *hôpitaux des invalides,* where patients with incurable disease of the eyes are likewise received.

MEDICAL GAZETTE.

Friday, September 29, 1843.

" Licet omnibus, licet etiam mihi, dignitatem *Artis Medicæ* tueri; potestas modo veniendi in publicum sit, dicendi periculum non recuso."
CICERO.

THE CARLISLE CONTROVERSY.

"Adhuc sub judice lis est."—HOR.

IT was acutely observed by Cullen, that there are more false facts than false theories in the world. We might add, that most erroneous theories, when analysed, are found to consist of little more than imaginary facts in a state of temporary cohesion. But, alas ! facts are very difficult to ascertain ; the calm philosopher does not always succeed in his search; what chance has the sectarian, the party-man, the controversialist ? Our brethren at Carlisle continue their hopeless debates over the grave of James Clark, "and find no end, in wandering mazes lost."

A fresh series of facts has been published in the Carlisle Patriot of the 23d inst., which, if uncontradicted, would turn the scale greatly in favour of the medical officers of the Infirmary.

The committee of the Cumberland Infirmary, having considered the great difference between the evidence given at the inquest by their own medical officers, and that of the practitioners by whom Clark was attended during the last seventeen weeks of his life, resolved to investigate the matter farther. Accordingly, they requested Mr. W. N. Hodgson, Mr. Page, and Mr. Donald, to go down to Beaumont, and make farther inquiries respecting Clark's case. Mr. Page is, of course, the surgeon of the Infirmary; who the other two inquirers are, we know not. The first person whom they examined was Mr. John Hodgson, a farmer, who had been foreman of the coroner's jury. He told them that he had long known Clark, who had been lame for many years, and even eight years ago could hardly get home from his work, so severe were the pains in his limbs. "We used always to say James Clark was as good as a weather-glass. He could always tell the weather by the pains in his joints." Clark came out of the Infirmary about the same as he went in, and continued to go about until the doctors came, who cut him and put on a splint. After this he could no longer hobble about, and was in the most exquisite torture. Five days after the operation, "he shouted aloud with the pain."

We have already seen, that when Clark was an out-patient, he was able to go in a cart, to the Infirmary, once every week. We here find, from the evidence of William Irving, that Clark went in a cart on the Saturday before the operation to Thrustonfield Mill, three miles from Beaumont, each way; and even drove himself back. He repeated the journey in the following week, the morning before, or the very day, he was "cut." "He was not worse then, not any lamer, than he had been for a very long time before. I helped

to lift him out of the bed. He was then as bad as he could be. This was after he was cut."

Thomas Todhunter, one of the jurors, says that Clark "was completely done after they cut him," yet he was in great spirits, for the doctors said they would cure him with a stiff joint. Till the doctors cut him he was walking about, not more lame than usual. He often told Todhunter he wished the doctors had never come to him.

An important fact is mentioned by this witness, and confirmed by several of the others, which certainly lightens the complexion of the case for both sets of doctors, the Infirmary, and the anti-Infirmary ones. Some weeks before the operation, Clark had a severe fall; so serious, that one of the witnesses heard that "Jemmy Clark had got a fall out of his back door and knocked his haunch out. This was a common report in the village." In speaking of the fall, Clark said to Todhunter, "I thought I'd been killed altogether, I never suffered such pain in my life." It is obvious, on the one hand, that, after this accident, Clark's case may have been extremely different from the one treated at the Infirmary. On the other hand, it is possible that the inflammation produced by the fall may have rendered measures excusable, or necessary, which would have been inadmissible before; yet we see that in spite of the fall the patient was going about as usual up to the day of the operation.

James Pearson, who was also a juror, and knew Clark, says that when he came out of the Infirmary he could walk, and Pearson "saw no odds in his lameness between going in and coming out." After the operation, the scene was changed; he was then "bedfast."

John Graham, another juror, gives very similar evidence. Clark had been in the field where they were dressing sheep, a few days before he was cut. Graham gives the *before* and *after* as follows : —

Before. — " He said his pain had been removed in the Infirmary, but he was still weak, and he thought it would be a long time before he would be strong. He was in a kind of low-spirited way. He said doctors could'nt mend rheumatism."

After.—" I saw him a week or two after he was cut. Some methodists were praying with h m. He was then very bad. The doctors said at the inquest that they cut him and relieved him of pain, but they never said more wrong than that—it was an untruth altogether. Every one in Beaumont knows he was far worse of pain after he was cut." .

A strange illustration of Cullen's axiom remains still to be stated—it seems difficult, if not impossible, to ascertain what the verdict of the coroner's jury really was. In the Carlisle Journal of the 2d inst. it was made to include an approbation of the treatment pursued by Dr. Jackson and Mr. Elliot. In the Patriot of the 9th, this was characterized as a deliberate and desperate falsehood. In the Journal of the 16th appeared a letter from Mr. Carrick, the coroner, stating that he himself had furnished the Journal with the verdict characterized as false. On the 23d, the Patriot contains a statement signed by ten of the twelve jurymen, denying that the jury either expressed or entertained the opinion that the treatment of Dr. Jackson and Mr. Elliot was correct, and all that could be done for him under the circumstances. Of the remaining jurors, James Sewell cannot remember anything that was said or done on the day of the inquest ; while William Armstrong says " there has been a great deal too much fuss

about it already ; it is only a piece of spite of the doctors agaipt one another, and I shall say no more about it one way or another." But in answer to some questions by Mr. W. N. Hodgson, he denied that he had disapproved of the treatment of Dr. Barnes, or approved of that pursued by Dr. Jackson and Mr. Elliot.

In consequence of this evidence, and more of a similar kind, the Committee came to the conclusion that the evidence of all the persons examined at Beaumont was at variance with the statements made by the practitioners who last attended the deceased. " For instance," say the Committee in their minute. " they [namely, Messrs. W. N. Hodgson, &c.] learned that instead of Clarke being standing at his door and hobbling into the house when first seen by them, [*i. e.* Dr. Jackson and Mr. Elliot,] he was at the time sitting over the fire with his nephew—that instead of his being in the last stage of hip-disease, the slightest motion giving him the most excruciating pain, and his being just about dying, he had been, up to the time of his being operated on, in the habit of going about as usual, and on that very day had been a journey of six miles in his cart, before nine in the morning—that instead of his having no rheumatism, his rheumatism was considered as good as a weather glass in the village, and had been so for years—that instead of no hopes being held out when first seen by these medical men, he had told numerous persons that the doctors had promised to cure him, with a stiff joint —that instead of the palliative treatment having answered its end, it was well known in Beaumont that he was far worse of pain after he had been cut; that he had received a severe blow on the part where the abscess was found, three weeks before it was opened, and that the statement in the *Carlisle Journal*, that the jury were satisfied with the treatment of Dr. Jackson and Mr. Elliot, is altogether without foundation, they never having expressed, or even entertained, such an opinion."

Our readers will now be ready to exclaim—

Claudite jam rivos, pueri, sat prata biberunt;

but we must just touch on a point or two more.

In the first place, then, the Patriot of the 23d inst. contains a calm and judicious letter addressed by Sir John Fife, of Newcastle, to Dr. Barnes.

After observing that no man can judge of the treatment of a case which he does not see at the time, he adds, that "a medical coroner would have understood this, and if he committed himself by asking those who last treated the case what they thought of the former treatment, an impartial coroner would also have asked the first medical attendants what they thought of the treatment of those who saw the last of the case."

Secondly, supposing an inquest to have been held, which was certainly unnecessary, a post-mortem examination ought not to have been omitted.

Lastly, the machinery of the law is very defective in a case like this. The *venue*, we believe, cannot be changed in an inquest; yet a jury of Cumbrian villagers, and a group of medical practitioners eager to attack their rivals, do not seem very fit instruments for the investigation of hidden truth. The coroner, too, had been deeply tinged with the medical politics of Carlisle, and was evidently an Anti-Infirmary man to the backbone. Can any remedy be devised for these evils ? For justice, like Cæsar's wife, should not only be pure, but unsuspected.

A FREAK OF THE STARVATIONISTS.

"Vaulting ambition doth overleap itself," says Shakspeare; and it must be confessed that the " vaulting ambition" of our poor-law people sometimes overleaps itself most grotesquely. The subaltern imps, who endeavour to curry favour with the great Lords of Somerset House, overdo the thing in the excess of their zeal, forgetting that, in a country which possesses a free press, some measure of decency must be observed.

On the 8th of this month, three young men were brought up before Mr. Long, at the Marylebone Police Office, charged with refusing to work, and being otherwise disorderly, in the Strand Union Workhouse, Cleveland Street, Fitzroy Square.

It seems that the regular diet in this receptacle is as follows :—

" Six ounces of bread, with butter, and half a pint of gruel, in the morning. Three days a week they have five ounces of meat, and half a pound of potatoes for dinner; on three other days they have soup without meat, and on one day, making up the seven, suet-pudding weighing fourteen ounces. They have also six ounces of bread each day for supper, with some cheese if they like it*."

" Then they have no bread at dinner ?" asked Mr. Long.

" No, sir," replied the accusing Bunyard.

But the point of the epigram is yet to come. The men, having been idle and refractory, were condemned to pick an increased quantity of oakum, namely, six pounds a day, and with only six ounces of bread instead of twelve. They were willing to do three pounds of oakum daily; but no—halve the bread, double the oakum, is the rule in Cleveland Street Workhouse.

Mr. Long, however, thought that the usual diet could not be lessened with safety, and refused to interfere against the prisoners. This case, at any rate, requires no comment.

---

* From the evidence of Bunyard, porter of the Workhouse.—*Times*, Sept. 9, 1843.

PATHOLOGY.

Dr. Boyd has published a lengthened Report on Vital Statistics, to which Mr. Gulliver has added some interesting notes on the morbid parts, which last we subjoin.

Brain.

Yellow or rusty coloured matter in the site of old apoplectic affections was found to contain oily molecules and granular corpuscles, in a matrix of fine granular matter, and shapeless yellow fragments. Dr. Davy found the colouring matter to be peroxide of iron.

Yellow matter in the pia mater.—In two cases, in which old apoplectic cells existed in the brain, microscopic granular masses, of a deep yellow colour, were clearly seen in some parts of the *pia mater*, although the membrane had only a diffused yellowish appearance to the naked eye. The yellow matter seemed to be the peroxide of iron. In one of these cases, the *pia mater* was studded with microscopic crystals of an intense orange colour.

Old blood clots in the cerebrum.—Two were carefully examined. They had a dull red colour towards the centre, brownish nearer the surface, and yellow at the circumference. They contained a great quantity of minute molecules, larger oily globules, and granular corpuscles. Bits of the clots dried by heat on paper gave it a greasy stain. The yellow matter was peroxide of iron. Dr. Davy examined one of the clots, and found that it contained fatty matter, chiefly olein. The molecules and granular corpuscles, he concluded to be, at least in part, composed of olein; and in the lower portion of the clot he found yellow colouring matter consisting of peroxide of iron.

Lungs.

The inflamed lungs were not more commonly of a red or ruddy colour, than of a brown or leaden hue. The latter variety sometimes inclined to a slate tint. Whether the brown consolidation be or be not a chronic stage of the red,[*] the two kinds were found to differ in more respects than in colour. They were often more or less blended together; and occasionally existed distinctly in different parts of the same lung. The brown variety, though most commonly seen in old cases of phthisis, was repeatedly present in lungs quite free from tubercle.

Minute Molecules. — Smooth, circular, oil-like particles, varying in diameter from $\frac{1}{12000}$ to $\frac{1}{5000}$th of an English inch; pellucid and nearly colourless when examined singly, yet generally paler and brighter in red than in brown pulmonary consolidation. The molecules were especially abundant in the early stages of pneumonia, and usually rather plentiful at every period of the disease. The molecules seem to be analogous to the elementary granules of Henle.[*]

Pale Exudation Corpuscles,—commonly about $\frac{1}{3000}$ of an inch in diameter, but varying from $\frac{1}{5000}$th to $\frac{1}{700}$th, were the chief objects observed in red pneumonia. They generally resembled the corpuscles of fibrinous exudations; were more or less globular, not so frequently oval; pale or nearly colourless; semitransparent; and less distinctly granulated than the dark exudation corpuscles. A great many of the pale corpuscles often presented all the characters of pus globules, but this was seldom the case with the majority. Although the pale corpuscles usually contained merely minute molecules and very fine granular matter, the larger cells sometimes inclosed others which had still smaller nuclei. The pale exudation corpuscles appear to be allied to the elementary cells of Henle.[†]

Dark Exudation Corpuscles.—They appeared of a dull brown colour, nearly opaque, as frequently oval as globular, often shapeless, commonly $\frac{1}{1000}$th of an inch in diameter, but almost always varying from $\frac{1}{1500}$th to $\frac{1}{700}$th. Their dark appearance may arise from their opacity, as they may sometimes be seen to be whitish by reflected light. They were most distinctly granulated, being made up of molecules, sometimes with larger oil globules; had occasionally a nucleus, though generally not; were as frequently without as with an envelope; and when this existed, it generally formed a smaller proportion of the corpuscle than the cell-wall of the pale exudation globule. A quantity of very minutely granular matter was now and then seen in the dark exudation corpuscles. Sometimes the envelope was but partially full of the molecules, sometimes it was full to bursting. The dark exudation corpuscles are similar to the objects described by Gluge[‡] and Bennett[§] in softened brain, and by Dr. Henderson[||] in pneumonia; and to the aggregation or granular corpuscles of Gerber.[¶]

The dark exudation corpuscles were the chief and characteristic compound particles observed in brown consolidation of lung, just as the pale exudation corpuscles were the

---

[*] Dr. Williams observes that the colour of the inflamed part in chronic pneumonia, varies from a dary dingy red, to different lighter shades of reddish brown or buff.—On the Diseases of the Chest, 4th edition, London, 1840, p. 143.

[*] Anatomie Generale, par Jourdan, p. 161.
[†] Loc. cit. p. 150 et seq.
[‡] Prov. Med. Journ. No. 113, and Oestr. Med. Woch. January 22, 1842.
[§] Edin. Med. and Surg. Journ. Nos. 153 and 155.
[||] Lond. and Edin. Monthly Journ. October 1841.
[¶] General Anatomy, Atlas, p. 5.

principal objects in red consolidation. But the two kinds of corpuscles were frequently seen together, especially in those parts of the inflamed lung which were of a brownish hue; and in some old cases of phthisis, molecules and the dark corpuscles were found rather plentifully in portions of the lung not in the least consolidated, but rather emphysematous, yet of a dull-brown or lead colour.

Fatty Globules,—larger than the molecules, were very commonly noticed in every variety of pneumonia and pulmonary gangrene. The fatty matter was especially abundant in the brown consolidation occurring in phthisis. The fatty globules were usually isolated, often irregular in shape, or drawn out by adhesion to the object plate, as if semifluid, and quite destitute of any envelope. They were sometimes aggregated, with or without a matrix of minutely granular matter; occasionally they were attached to or contained in a flat membranous fragment like an epithelial cell; and it was not unusual to see them clustered within a dark exudation corpuscle.

Shining corpuscles, concentrically striated,—rounded, lenticular, or oval; margins smooth, sometimes undulating, the stripes running parallel to the circumference; generally single, but occasionally including one, two, or three bodies, more or less similar to the shell; diameter very variable, though commonly about $\frac{1}{1600}$th of an inch. These are probably identical with the lenticular spheres figured by Gruby[*] in the expectorated matter of phthisical patients. The striated corpuscles were occasionally observed in red pneumonia, unaccompanied by tubercular disease, and very commonly in brown pneumonia, especially in old cases of phthisis. The striated corpuscles sometimes occur in other diseases, and even where no disease is suspected. I have observed them in the thymus body.

Smooth pale Globules,—of different sizes, but usually about $\frac{1}{1600}$th of an inch in diameter, were frequently seen in red pneumonia. They were less commonly found in brown pneumonia. They are very delicate, soft, and fugitive; are destroyed by vegetable acids, and by water.

Colouring Matter.—Shapeless fragments of a bright-yellow, sometimes of a deep-orange colour, were often seen in red pneumonia. Their appearance was granular, obscurely crystalline, laminated, or rounded, and their colour was rendered more distinct by acetic acid. In the bronchial tubes of a still-born child, yellowish green matter was found in great abundance, which had exactly the same characters under the microscope as meconium from the same child. The pul-

monary parenchyma of this child had a healthy appearance, till examined microscopically, when the greenish matter was observed in considerable quantity. The black pigment of the lungs was, as usual, generally observed in irregular shapeless masses, composed merely of a congeries of extremely minute circular particles; but in many cases these particles were contained in distinct rounded cells about $\frac{1}{2000}$th of an inch in diameter, the intensely black contents contrasting strongly with the pale semitransparent cell-wall. In many cases, rounded masses of the black matter existed without any envelope; and occasionally a similar mass had about a third or fourth of its circumference occupied by a pale crescentic body, which sometimes appeared to be an imperfect cell-wall; and sometimes a smooth and rounded nucleus only partially covered by the pigmentary granules.

Tubercle.—The precise seat of pulmonary tubercle was often within the air cells;[*] and occasionally also in the filamentous tissue between them. In a child of eleven months the lungs were studded with small miliary tubercles, a careful examination of which showed the tubercular matter partly filling the interior of the air-cells, and partly the tissue situated exterior to them.

Chemical Observations.—Dr. Davy frequently examined the minute molecules, and found them to be chiefly composed of olein. In a recent examination of the pale exudation globules, he concluded that the cell-wall was in a great part formed by margarine, and the included molecules of olein. In the brown exudation corpuscles he found a considerable quantity of olein and some margarine.[†]

Although acetic acid, strong or dilute, often exerts no evident action on the juice of pneumonia, yet it is remarkable that this acid sometimes produces a tolerably copious precipitate or clot in the juice. Occasionally this clot is tenacious, and presents even a fibrous appearance when examined by the microscope. The same observations apply to the action of acetic acid on purulent matters.[‡]

A portion of lung (Dr. Boyd's case 490) in which the black pigment was remarkably abundant, was examined by Dr. Davy, who found that the colouring matter differed chiefly from soot in containing a little peroxide of iron, i. e. the black pulmonary matter yielded the oxide on incineration.

Liver.

Jaundiced Cells.—A woman, æt. 35, had

---

[*] See Dr. Goodfellows' Translation, Microscopic Journal, September 1842 to January 1843, plate 6, figs. 89-95.

[*] See Willis's Translation of Wagner's Physiology, part 2, p. 360, fig. 175.
[†] On this subject see Henle, l. c. p. 162 and 118; Acherson, Paget's Report, p. 7; Bennett, Edin. Med. and Surg. Journ. No. 155.
[‡] See Dr. Guterbock's account of Pyine, De pure et Granulatione, Berol. 1837; and Dr. Davy's Researches, Phys. and Anat. Vol. ii. p. 475.

many of the tissues jaundiced. The cells of the liver were surcharged with greenish yellow biliary matter, so as to contrast remarkably with the cells of the healthy liver. A like case occurred in a child, of which the notes made at the time will be subjoined, as the subject is interesting in relation to the question of the ultimate secreting structure.[*] October 14, 1842 : Dr. Boyd's case 515 ; a female fourteen days old ; received part of liver, aorta, and costal cartilages, all of which were of a deep yellow colour. Cells of the liver intensely yellow under the microscope, whether viewed by reflected or transmitted light ; the greater part of the colouring matter granular, or in minute shapeless fragments ; some of it apparently fluid, especially near the edges of the cells ; the granular part chiefly collected around the nucleus, though also irregularly scattered throughout the cell. Some of the cells, excepting a part near to the circumference, were rendered opaque by the accumulated colouring matter within them. Cells from the healthy liver of a child, aged three years, examined at the same time for comparison, afforded a striking contrast, as they were destitute of the colouring matter around the nucleus, were throughout of a light brownish colour, and nearly transparent. Some cells from the healthy liver of a woman, æt. 90, presented a similar contrast to the jaundiced cells.

Waxy-looking liver. — Some portions from two cases were nearly of the colour of crude bees'-wax, and stiff or tenacious in texture. These characters appeared to be owing to an unusual accumulation in the liver of viscid biliary matter. with a large proportion of mucus. In neither case did the organ contain more fatty matter than in the healthy state.

Kidneys.

Lithic acid in the tubules.—A female child, born prematurely, died nine days afterwards. The cut surface of the mammillæ of the kidneys presented a multitude of streaks, from distension of the tubules with a reddish-brown solid matter, which Dr. Davy ascertained to be either lithic acid or lithate of ammonia, most probably the former.

Yellow matter.—In the substance of the medullary and cortical part of the same kidneys there were numerous very distinct microscopic particles, of a very bright yellow colour. They had a granular appearance, were quite plain after several days' maceration in water, and not affected by acetic acid.

* See Goodsir on the Ultimate Secreting Structure, Trans. Royal Soc. Edin. Vol. xv. ; Carpenter on the Origin and Functions of Cells, p. 23, from Brit. and For. Med. Rev. No. 29 ; Henle, Anatomie Generale, par Jourdan, p. 211.

The quantity of the yellow matter was not sufficient to enable Dr. Davy to ascertain its nature ; but he agreed with me that it was different from the contents of the tubules.

Fatty matter.—The kidneys of a woman, aged 37, who died of chronic arachnitis, had a great number of white specks on the surface, and imbedded in the cortical part, very plain to the naked eye, though generally only from 1-100th to 1-50th of an inch in diameter. The specks were made up of a congeries of fatty globules, very characteristic under the microscope. In the kidneys, said to be affected with Bright's disease, from a woman, aged 58, there were in the juice a multitude of fatty globules, and a few small pearly crystalline plates. Dr. Davy extracted a little margarine, cholesterine, and a trace of olein, from a fragment of one of the kidneys.

Cysts containing margarine, olein, and yellow granular corpuscles.—In the cortical part of the kidneys of a man aged 55, who died of phthisis, there were several round or oval cysts, about a third of an inch in diameter, some of which contained a limpid yellow fluid, and others a pulpy matter, of the same colour. In some of the cysts this substance was tolerably stiff, resembling the meliceris and atheroma of authors. In the fluid were many round granular corpuscles, of an intense yellow colour, mostly with envelopes, and of very different sizes, but generally about 1-600th of an inch in diameter. There were also numerous pale fatty globules, often aggregated into clumps. In the pulpy and stiffer substance the fatty matter was so abundant as to render thick paper transparent when dried on it by heat.

Cysts containing cholesterine, and pale granular corpuscles.—In the preceding instances the fatty matter was chiefly margarine and olein ; in two other cases the fatty substance was nearly all cholesterine. There were cysts filled with a limpid fluid, and imbedded in the surface of the kidneys. Each cyst was about the size of a pea. A great quantity of plates of cholesterine were found, principally sticking to the walls of the cysts. The fluid also contained many pale, round, nearly transparent, and minutely granular corpuscles, generally about 1-1300th of an inch in diameter. The kidneys were otherwise healthy.

Testicles.

After middle life the seminal tubes were often more or less obstructed with molecules, generally aggregated into irregular masses, nearly opaque, either of a dull brown, yellowish, or lead colour. Occasionally they were aggregated into oval or round corpuscles, mostly destitute of an envelope ; and they were not unfrequently seen within bodies which were probably the seminal cells. This state of the tubes was almost always found in old subjects; it was by no means rare before 30 in persons who had died of lingering diseases; and was generally coincident with a fewness or total absence of the spermatozoa*. Larger oil globules were sometimes seen within the tubes. There is reason to believe that the molecules contain a large proportion of olein.

Black pigment in the intestinal mucous membrane.

Sometimes there were black specks, sometimes a diffused brown or black colour, of the mucous membrane of the large intestine†. The affection was most frequently observed in the rectum, especially in elderly people. The pigmentary granules were occasionally observed in rounded cells; but the black matter, like that of the lungs and bronchial glands, had generally no appearance of a special apparatus, but was scattered in shapeless masses, and had just the same chemical characters as the black pigment of the lungs.

Arteries.

Fatty degeneration. — This very commonly existed in the substance of the inner and middle membranes, often between them, and sometimes in the outer coat. Though most common in old age, it was twice seen in subjects not past 21, and once in a boy of 16. Even in the early stage of the disease, the fatty matter was easily recognizable in the well-known opaque whitish spots, or thickened parts of the inner tunic of the vessel. The disease was observed in the aorta and its valves, in the cerebral arteries, in the iliac and femoral arteries. In a man who died of apoplexy, the coats of the arteries of the brain, even of the smallest branches, were studded with, and made fragile by, fatty patches. I have elsewhere described the disease, and the nature of the fatty matter‡.

Black pigment. — Black and brown specks and patches were sometimes observed in the large arteries. This was caused by black pigmentary granules, in greater or less quantity, without any evident cells; generally confined to the inner membrane, but extending in one instance to the middle coat, and sometimes situated between these tunics. The pigment had the same chemical charac-

ters as that of the lungs. This discoloration of the arteries was observed where the inner tunic had become partially broken and detached near to old fatty and bony deposits.

Softened fibrine.

Several specimens from the veins were examined. The central pulpy part of the clot was found to consist chiefly of granular matter and minute molecules; larger fatty globules, and shrunken cells. Sometimes still larger compound granular corpuscles were also observed, either encysted and more or less opaque, or naked and appearing like a congeries of minute oil globules. Occasionally there were corpuscles resembling those of purulent matter; but the bulk of the softened fibrine was still granular matter, the corpuscles being much less abundant than in regular pus. The pus-like corpuscles of the fibrine were not enlarged by water; some of them were not much affected by acetic acid; others had the cell wall rendered fainter, or nearly invisible, by the acid, so as to expose nuclei resembling those of the pus globule*. Around the fluid or pulpy part, where the brine was tolerably firm, but had begun to soften, corpuscles of the character just mentioned were commonly abundant, often with an intervening tissue of very delicate fibrils, and the corpuscles were especially numerous in clots of a buff colour, opaque, with an appearance of commencing diffluence, although nowhere broken down or fluid. These clots were most commonly noticed in the heart; and they would sometimes form a viscid ropy compound, as is generally the case with fresh primary cells, when triturated with concentrated solutions of alkaline or earthy salts, or of pure alkalies.

PHYSIOLOGICAL NOTICES.

1. *The left ventricle* begs to announce to the Presidents, Vice Presidents, and Councils in Trafalgar Square and Lincolns' Inn Fields, that it cannot possibly continue to propel *venous blood through the liver* more than a quarter of a century longer. It will be happy to propel arterial blood through the hepatic artery until dooms-day, or any later period the authorities may be pleased to specify, but is fully determined to take the earliest opportunity of resigning the undignified office of propelling portal blood through the portal trunk, branches, plexuses, and hepatic veins.

2. *The spleen* humbly begs to inform the

---

* See a case of the seminal tubes of a bear obstructed by fatty matter, in my Observations on the Semen and Seminal Tubes. - Proc. Zool. Soc. of London, July 26th, 1842.

† See Dr Hodgkin's Observations on Colour. — Lectures on Morbid Anatomy, Vol. i. p. 297, et seq.

‡ In a paper read at the Royal Medico-Chirurgical Society, February 28, 1843. — Abstract in the Edinburgh Monthly Journal, No

* As to the action of this acid, see Dr Bennett's Observations, — Microscopic Journal, January, and Gerber's Anatomy, note, p. 95, fig.

same learned bodies that it (spleen) is the root of an unfortunate *vein* out of employment ; but which vein, *although* a vein, has certain remarkable peculiarities which render it perfectly competent to carry on the circulation through the liver, and serve in the triple capacity of recipient cavity, propulsive agent, and afferent vessel. An auricle, a ventricle, and an artery, do no more.—N.B. The duties of the office being slow and easy, a "nominal salary" only will be required.

3. *The thyroid gland* begs to express its conviction that the left ventricle cannot efficiently propel blood through the cerebrospinal capillaries by applying propulsive force to that blood only behind or on the arterial side of those capillaries. It has also to state, that if the honourable Presidents, Vice Presidents, and Councils Chirurgorum et Medicorum, will permit the left ventricle to send it (thyroid gland) plenty of blood laden with propulsive force, that it is ready to pledge its honour, as an organ, not to rob that blood of such propulsive force, but to see it duly conveyed to, and allow it to impinge on, the tardy currents in the internal jugulars and left vena innominata. By this *tour-de-maitre* the thyroid gland confidently believes it would be easy to increase the rapidity of the return of blood to the heart by the superior cava, and thereby to accelerate and strengthen the *cerebro-spinal circulation*, — the only function in which the thyroid gland can condescend to play a subordinate part.

4. *The thymus* is a remarkably sleepy organ, and therefore not a communicative one.

August 7, 1843.

DR. JOHNSON ON VIVISECTION.

[As the subject of vivisection has recently excited some discussion in our pages, we think it may not be uninteresting to give Dr. Samuel Johnson's remarks on the subject, as published in an early number of the *Idler*.]

THE idlers that sport only with inanimate nature may claim some indulgence ; if they are useless, they are still innocent ; but there are others, whom I not how to mention without more emotion than my love of quiet willingly admits. Among the inferior professors of medical knowledge, is a race of wretches, whose lives are only varied by varieties of cruelty ; whose favourite amusement is to nail dogs to tables, and to open them alive ; to try how long life may be continued in various degrees of mutilation, or with the excision or laceration of the vital parts ; to examine whether burning irons are felt more acutely by the bone or tendon ; and whether the more lasting agonies are produced by poison forced into the mouth, or injected into the veins. It is not without reluctance that I offend the sensibility of the tender mind with images like these. If such cruelties were not practised, it were to be desired that they should not be conceived ; but, since they are published every day with ostentation, let me be allowed once to mention them, since I mention them with abhorrence.

Mead has invidiously remarked of Woodward, that he gathered shells and stones, and would pass for a philosopher. With pretensions much less reasonable, the anatomical novice tears out the living bowels of an animal, and styles himself physician, prepares himself by familiar cruelty for that profession which he is to exercise upon the tender and the helpless, upon feeble bodies and broken minds, and by which he has opportunities to extend his art of torture, and continue those experiments upon infancy and age, which he has hitherto tried upon cats and dogs.

What is alleged in defence of these hateful practices, every one knows ; but the truth is, that by knives, fire, and poison, knowledge is not always sought, and is very seldom attained. The experiments that have been tried, are tried again ; he that burned an animal with irons yesterday, will be willing to amuse himself with burning another to-morrow. I know not, that by living dissections any discovery has been made by which a single malady is more easily cured. And if the knowledge of physiology has been somewhat increased, he surely buys knowledge dear, who learns the use of the lacteals at the expense of his humanity. It is time that universal resentment should arise against these horrid operations, which tend to harden the heart, extinguish those sensations which give man confidence in man, and make the physician more dreadful than gout or stone. —*The Idler*, No. 17.

CASE OF ARTIFICIAL ANUS.

By R. G. WHARTON, M.D.

Grand Gulf, Mississippi.

I WAS called in August, 1841, to see a negro child, five or six days old, belonging to Mr. D. G. Humphreys, whose umbilical cord had sloughed off close to the abdomen, leaving a circular opening at least one and a half inches in diameter, penetrating through the abdominal parietes and a corresponding portion of the intestinal canal. The gut adhered firmly to the circumference of the abdominal opening, and the bowels were evacuated exclusively through this channel. I could not ascertain what was the cause of the sloughing. Its general health was good, though it suffered a good deal from occasional paroxysm of pain proceeding apparently from irritation of the ulcerated opening. The inner surface of the exposed portion of the intestine was of a very deep red, owing probably to its exposure to the external air. I ordered simple poultices of powered slippery elm, made with the infusion of oak bark, to be constantly applied with a tolerably firm bandage, and emollient and oily enemata several times a day, to excite the action of the lower bowels. This last means afforded great relief to the pain, and after a few days fæcal matter was discharged in small quantities, per anum. The local applications were occasionally varied; and under this treatment the umbilical opening gradually contracted, so that in three or four months it had become quite small, only a small quantity of the fluid portion of the fæcal matter passing through it. I then touched it with argent. nit. which formed an eschar, and I suppose it had healed long ago, as I ordered it to be touched occasionally. At present (May 1843), however, there still remains a small circular ulcerated surface, very red, about two lines in diameter, from which there is a slight oozing of the watery part of the contents of the intestinal canal. This circular ulcer is surrounded by a large circular cicatrix, showing the original seat, though contracted about one third of the primary opening. I ordered the application of the nit. argent. and had the child watched so as to prevent his rubbing off the eschar, which seems to be the cause of its not having closed up before now. The child is large for its age, and perfectly healthy.—*American Journal of the Medical Sciences.*

CÆSAREAN SECTION ON A DWARF.

By Dr. CYRUS FALCONER.

THE patient was only three feet six inches in height, with ill-proportioned form. When seen by Dr. F. she had been in labour upwards of fourteen hours; the left foot of the fœtus was presenting at the os externum. On examination, Dr. F. found that "the sacrum projected towards the pubis so as to give the superior strait the character of a fissure; the antero-posterior diameter being certainly not over one inch and three-fourths. The leg of the presenting foot occupied the full breadth of the fissure, affording an evidence but too conclusive that nature was not competent to the delivery.

The os uteri was well dilated, and the pains incessant and severe."

The Cæsarean section was resolved upon, and executed in the following manner:—A somewhat oblique incision was made, "beginning at the upper part, near the margin of the linea alba, crossing towards its centre in the descent towards the pubis," this being necessary "in order to get an opening large enough to extract the fœtus." When the peritoneum was opened, much difficulty was experienced in preventing the escape of the intestines. The uterus being then divided, the fœtus was exposed, its back presenting to the incision, "Although," says Dr. F., "I began my incision considerably above the umbilicus, such was the relative size of the child that I found it impracticable to extract it, until I had extended the opening in each direction; approaching nearly to the cartilage of the lower true rib above, and the pubis below. During my efforts to accomplish the delivery, considerable extravasation took place. The relative size of the child and mother can only be conceived by the reader, when he remembers the height of the mother—three and a half feet—and learns that the child was about the ordinary size, weighing, by conjecture, from seven to eight pounds.

"I at length succeeded, by grasping the thighs, in elevating the breech, and delivered the child, as in a breech presentation; it soon cried lustily, and was separated from the cord. The uterus now contracted powerfully, the placenta was expelled, the extravasated blood removed as much as possible, and we then proceeded to dress the wound.

"Four or five points of the interrupted suture were employed—long adhesive strips were applied between the sutures, leaving a space at the lower portion, for the escape of any discharge that might accumulate. A broad compress was next applied, and the whole covered with a broad, firm bandage, tolerably tight.

"During the operation, the patient made very little complaint; she now said she felt very comfortable, and expressed much gratification at being relieved by an amount of suffering so much less than she had apprehended. An anodyne was administered, and finding her, at the end of a couple of hours, still comfortable, and inclined to rest, I left her."

Before morning, however, inflammation was developed, and the patient died on the eighth day.

"The child did well, and is now a vigorous, healthy, and well-formed little girl."—*Ibid.*

TREATMENT of VASCULAR NÆVUS.

Prof. N. R. Smith, of Baltimore, has devised the following method of treating vascular nævus. He saturates a thread with a saturated solution of caustic potash. This is dried by a fire, and a needle being armed with it, the base of the tumor is transfixed with the needle, and the thread quietly drawn through the part. This is repeated in different parts of the tumor. Dr. S. states that he has now under care a case treated by this plan, and the tumor is rapidly wasting, without any distressing symptoms having occurred. —*Maryland Med. and Surg. Journ.*

RESEARCHES
ON THE
DECOMPOSITION AND DISINTEGRATION OF PHOSPHATIC VESICAL CALCULI;

AND ON THE INTRODUCTION OF CHEMICAL DECOMPONENTS INTO THE LIVING BLADDER.

By S. ELLIOT HOSKINS.

The object of these researches was the discovery of some chemical agent, more energetic in its action on certain varieties of human calculi, and less irritating when injected into the bladder, than any of the fluids hitherto employed.

These indications not being fulfilled by dilute acids, or other solvents which act by the exertion of single elective affinity, the author investigated the effects of complex affinity in producing decomposition, and consequent disintegration of vesical calculi.

For this purpose an agent is required, the base of which should unite with the acid of the calculus, whilst the acid of the former should combine and form soluble salts with the base of the latter. The combined acids would thereby be set free in definite proportions, to be neutralized in their nascent state, and removed out of the sphere of action, before any stimulating effect could be executed on the animal tissue. These intentions the author considers as having been fulfilled by the employment of weak solutions of some of the vegetable super-salts of lead; such as the super-malate, saccharate, lactate, &c. The preparation, however, to which he gives the preference, is an acid-saccharate, or, as he calls it, a *nitro-saccharate of lead*.

This salt, whichsoever it may be, must be moistened with a few drops of acetic, or of its own proper acid, previous to solution in water, whereby alone perfect transparency and activity are secured. He further states, that the decomposing liquid should not exceed in strength one grain of the salt to each fluid ounce of water, as the decomposing effect is in an inverse ratio to its strength.

Having by experiments, which are fully detailed, ascertained the chemical effects of the above class of decomponents on calculous concretion *out* of the body, the author briefly alludes to the cases of three patients, in each of whom from four to eight ounces of these solutions had been repeatedly, for weeks together, introduced into the bladder, and retained in that organ, without inconvenience, for the space of from ten to fifty minutes.— *Proceedings of the Royal Society*, No. 56.

INSULT TO THE MEDICAL PROFESSION.

To the Editor of the Medical Gazette.

Sir,

Allow me to request your public reprobation of the accompanying "private and confidential" gross insult to the medical profession; and at the same time to suggest, that the shameful bargaining for attendance on Poor-Law Unions may possibly have appeared to promise it success.—I am, sir,

Your obedient servant,

C.

London, Sept. 1843.

PRIVATE AND CONFIDENTIAL.

23d June, 1843.

Sir,—As you must professionally know how very frequently funeral expenses press heavily on the funds of families, I beg leave to submit to you my plans, which combine economy with perfect decency at the smallest expense.

The highest prices combine funeral respectability, and even elegance, at very reduced charges; whilst the system tends to, and is, gradually abolishing walking funerals, by having a carriage to convey six mourners to and from any Cemetery at less cost; thereby giving to the poorest of the population the advantage of Cemetery interment, and mitigating the evil and disgust naturally attending many of the present grave-yards.

Should you be of opinion that by influencing families, in the hour of distress, to adopt my system, you are rendering them pecuniary service, and preserving public health, it will of course promote the interests of the "Cemetery and General Funeral Company," with which my patent carriages are united; and upon my being informed of such recommendations, I will pay into the Medical Benevolent Society, or to any hospital fund, 5 per cent. of the cost of such funerals.

Should it be preferred that such remuneration should be personal, the amount shall be privately and most confidentially paid on addressing a note that you have rendered this essential benefit to families, and to the public health of the metropolis.

I hope you will put the most favourable construction on the novelty of my plan, which is respectfully submitted to you; and apologizing for the intrusion,—I remain, sir,

Your most obedient servant,
GEORGE SHILLIBEER.

P.S. A visit to the principal establishments, at the City Road, adjoining Bunhill Fields Burial Ground, and at High Street, facing St. Marylebone Church, also one on a smaller scale, at 136, Union Street, Southwark, will no doubt convince you of the public usefulness of my project.

Should church-yards be preferred to cemeteries, the expense is the same, subject only, in many instances, to the higher church fees.

OVARIAN OPERATION.

(From a Correspondent.)

WE understand that Mr. Walne operated successfully, by the large abdominal section, in a third case of dropsical ovarium, on the 12th inst. The tumor, weighing twenty-eight pounds, was removed entire, and the patient, a lady under twenty years of age, is recovering rapidly and satisfactorily.

[We hope to be able to lay before our readers the full particulars of this case in our next number.—ED. GAZ.]

BOOKS RECEIVED FOR REVIEW.

Lectures on the Principles and Practice of Physic, delivered at King's College, London. By Thomas Watson, M.D. Fellow of the Royal College of Physicians, &c. &c. In two volumes.

Dr. Maclagan on the Bebeern Tree of British Guiana.

Pulmonary Consumption, successfully treated with Naphtha. By John Hastings, M.D. Senior Physician to the Blenheim Street Free Dispensary.

Lectures on Polarised Light, delivered before the Pharmaceutical Society of Great Britain, and in the Medical School of the London Hospital. Illustrated with Engravings.

APOTHECARIES' HALL.

LIST OF GENTLEMEN WHO HAVE RECEIVED CERTIFICATES.

Thursday, September 21, 1843.

J. L. Hanley, Westminster.—F. H. Secretan, Barnet, Herts.—T. Tarton, Denby.—J. Pickop, Blackburn.—J. H. Norton, Matlock.—J. Whitteron, Knaresbro', Yorkshire.

A TABLE OF MORTALITY FOR THE METROPOLIS,

Shewing the number of deaths from all causes registered in the week ending Saturday, Sept. 16, 1843.

Small Pox	5
Measles	22
Scarlatina	48
Hooping Cough	15
Croup	6
Thrush	11
Diarrhœa	69
Dysentery	7
Cholera	4
Influenza	0
Ague	0
Remittent Fever	1
Typhus	36
Erysipelas	6
Syphilis	1
Hydrophobia	0
Diseases of the Brain, Nerves, and Senses	177
Diseases of the Lungs and other Organs of Respiration	210
Diseases of the Heart and Blood-vessels	16
Diseases of the Stomach, Liver, and other Organs of Digestion	98
Diseases of the Kidneys, &c.	4
Childbed	2
Paramenia	2
Ovarian Dropsy	0
Disease of Uterus, &c.	2
Arthritis	0
Rheumatism	3
Diseases of Joints, &c.	5
Carbuncle	0
Phlegmon	0
Ulcer	2
Fistula	0
Diseases of Skin, &c.	0
Dropsy, Cancer, and other Diseases of Uncertain Seat	83
Old Age or Natural Decay	44
Deaths by Violence, Privation, or Intemperance	18
Causes not specified	8
Deaths from all Causes	915

METEOROLOGICAL JOURNAL.

Kept at EDMONTON, Latitude 51° 37' 32" N. Longitude 0° 3' 51" W. of Greenwich.

Sept. 1843.	THERMOMETER.		BAROMETER.	
Wednesday 20	from 53 to 72		29·84	Stat.
Thursday . 21	46	71	29·84 to	29·92
Friday . . . 22	48	68	30·03	30·06
Saturday . 23	48	69	30·14	Stat.
Sunday . . 24	50	64	30·12	30·05
Monday . . 25	46	67	29·95	29·86
Tuesday . 26	42	58	29·83	29·71

Wind on the 20th N. and S.E.; 21st S.E. and N. by W.; 22d, N. and N.E.; 23d, N. by E.; 24th, N.W. and N. by E.; 25th, N. and N.W.; 26th, N.W.

Generally clear, except the 24th and 25th, a little rain on the afternoon of the 25th.

CHARLES HENRY ADAMS.

INDEX TO VOL. XXXII.

(VOL. II. FOR THE SESSION 1842-43.)